INTERDISCIPLINARY PEDIATRIC PALLIATIVE CARE

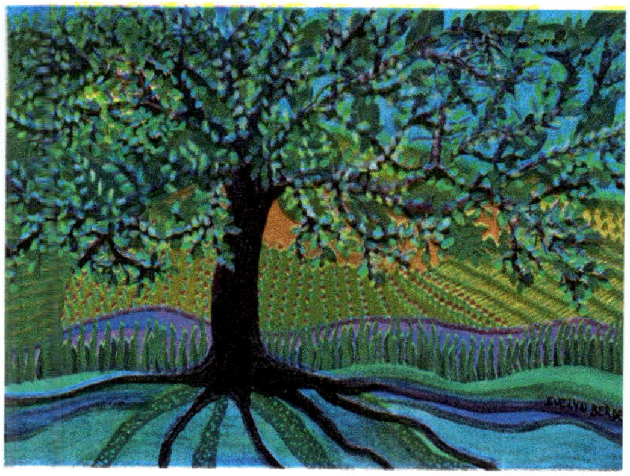

INTERDISCIPLINARY PEDIATRIC PALLIATIVE CARE

EDITED BY

Joanne Wolfe, Pamela S. Hinds, and Barbara M. Sourkes

OXFORD
UNIVERSITY PRESS

OXFORD
UNIVERSITY PRESS

Oxford University Press is a department of the University of Oxford. It furthers the University's objective of excellence in research, scholarship, and education by publishing worldwide. Oxford is a registered trade mark of Oxford University Press in the UK and certain other countries.

Published in the United States of America by Oxford University Press
198 Madison Avenue, New York, NY 10016, United States of America.

Library of Congress Cataloging-in-Publication Data
Names: Wolfe, Joanne, editor. | Hinds, Pamela S., editor. |
Sourkes, Barbara M., editor.
Title: Interdisciplinary pediatric palliative care / [edited by] Joanne
Wolfe, Pamela S. Hinds, Barbara M. Sourkes.
Other titles: Textbook of interdisciplinary pediatric palliative care
Description: 2. | New York, NY : Oxford University Press, [2022] |
Preceded by Textbook of interdisciplinary pediatric palliative care / [edited by]
Joanne Wolfe, Pamela S. Hinds, Barbara M. Sourkes. 2011. |
Includes bibliographical references and index.
Identifiers: LCCN 2021027440 (print) | LCCN 2021027441 (ebook) |
ISBN 9780190090012 (hardback) | ISBN 9780190090036 (epub) |
ISBN 9780190090043 (online)
Subjects: MESH: Palliative Care | Child | Patient Care Team |
Professional-Patient Relations | Professional-Family Relations |
Terminal Care | Infant | Adolescent
Classification: LCC RJ249 (print) | LCC RJ249 (ebook) | NLM WS 220 |
DDC 618.92/0029—dc23
LC record available at https://lccn.loc.gov/2021027440
LC ebook record available at https://lccn.loc.gov/2021027441

DOI: 10.1093/med/9780190090012.001.0001

9 8 7 6 5 4 3

Printed by Sheridan Books, Inc., United States of America

To Drs. David Nathan, Sam Lux, and Ed Benz, long-time sponsors and allies,
for supporting pediatric palliative care and innovation that has transformed from
afterthought to essential forethought in the care of seriously ill children and their families,
and
As always, to Sam, Hannah, Ben, and Michael with love.
Joanne Wolfe

To every child who has suffered and to every child's family that has observed that suffering,
and to my husband, children, and grandchildren who have shared my caring about ill children.
Pamela S. Hinds

In memory of my parents,
teachers of the heart,
and
for Talia Jade
my shining heart.
Barbara M. Sourkes

And to the colleagues from whom we have learned
and the children and families for whom we have had the privilege to care.

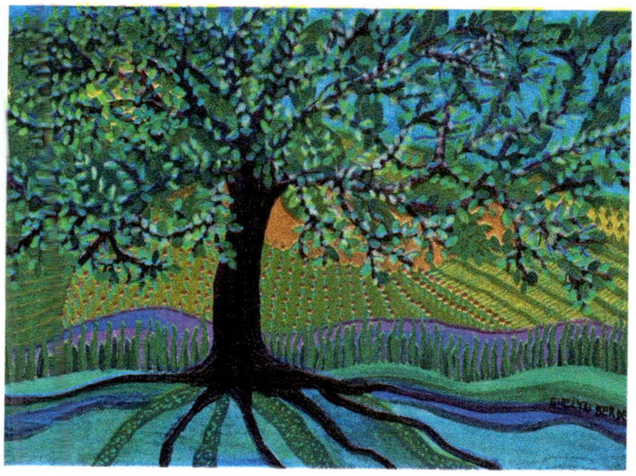

CONTENTS

SECTION IV ILLNESS AND TREATMENT EXPERIENCE

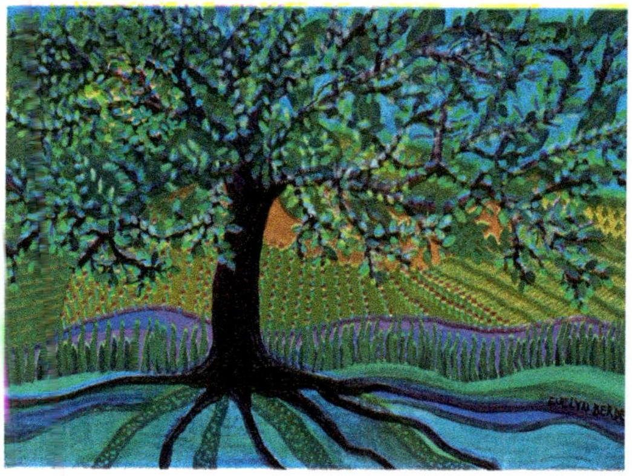

FOREWORD

"We have such a long way to go," said the boy. "Yes, but look how far we have come," sighed the horse.

Charlie Mackesy (The Boy, the Mole, the Fox, and the Horse)

Over the past 25 years the field of pediatric palliative care has grown exponentially from its early beginnings in the children's hospice movement to its current status as a pediatric specialty and the professionalization of team members' respective disciplines in palliative care. In 1998, the World Health Organization first published its guideline on "Cancer Pain Relief and Palliative Care in Children," setting a public health framework for a global call to action to provide palliative care to children with life-threatening illnesses and their families. In 2001, in the United States, the Institute of Medicine (now the National Academy of Medicine) published its seminal report entitled "When Children Die." This groundbreaking review of the care of dying children in the United States concluded that care was neither competent nor compassionate, identified a host of barriers, and offered a series of wide-ranging recommendations to address this serious public health need. In 2011, the first edition of this textbook was published, offering an interdisciplinary evidenced-based compilation of the growing knowledge base in this nascent field with an expansive perspective on what constitutes the field of pediatric palliative care. In the ensuing years, numerous national and international policies have supported the integration of pediatric palliative care into healthcare systems, with the World Health Organization's Resolution in 2014 calling it "an ethical responsibility of its member states."

Now, in 2021, this second edition demonstrates how the research expertise, clinical practice, educational efforts, and policy reform have evolved to assure that humane, competent, and compassionate care to children with serious illness and their families is possible. This publication comes at a time when the International Children's Palliative Care Network estimates that up to 21.5 million children worldwide are in need of a palliative care approach and up to 8 million require specialty palliative care, with the majority who require care living in low- and middle-income countries. The need for wide dissemination of this textbook as an educational resource is compelling.

For the reader, the text's format models the concept of interdisciplinary team care, with each of the editors being internationally recognized clinician educators, researchers, and champions in pediatrics, nursing, and psychology. All of the chapters are team-authored and showcase the growing range and depth of expertise and scholarship in the fields of pediatrics, psychology, social work, rehabilitation, chaplaincy, and child life. With a thoughtful and intentional approach to using poetry, art, clinical vignettes, and reflections, the authors demonstrate the art and science of providing physical, psychological, and spiritual care to the seriously ill child and family.

The book is divided into four sections that frame the critical thinking and domains of care in pediatric palliative care, setting the stage for individual chapters that discuss a range of essential topics including age-appropriate communication methods, shared decision-making, ethical challenges, family dynamics, experienced ways to navigate "a careful dance" with the other pediatric experts caring for the child and family, symptom control, the importance of healthcare provider's introspection and self-care, and much more. In multiple chapters, the authors identify the need for more research in, for example, symptom assessment and control, new technologies and better payment methods to further the evidence base for standardized protocols, treatment guidelines, and economic data that are essential aspects to assuring full integration into healthcare systems.

This unique format and scope allows learners to become educated in the basics of best practices in pediatric palliative care while serving as a compendium of referenced educational materials for those engaged in providing, teaching, or learning specialty palliative care. For each of the disciplines reading this book, the text is a combination of the basic skills that needs to be mastered and the advanced knowledge the specialist in pediatric palliative care needs to know.

This new comprehensive second edition is an up-to-date reference and guide capturing the complexity and challenges that healthcare providers face in caring for children with serious illness, some of whom will die. It shows a way forward while emphasizing an important principle: every encounter offers the clinician "the opportunity for a sense of connection and meaning."

Caring for these sick children and their families is a privilege and a responsibility. Access to pediatric palliative care is a human right imbedded in the right to health and in the right to freedom from cruel, inhumane, and degrading treatment. Fostering interdisciplinary care and arming new pediatric teams with the knowledge and experience presented in this textbook furthers the call to action to make palliative care a reality for all children in need.

Kathleen M. Foley, MD
Memorial Sloan Kettering Cancer Center
Member Emeritus
Weill Cornell Medical College Professor Emeritus,
Department of Neurology

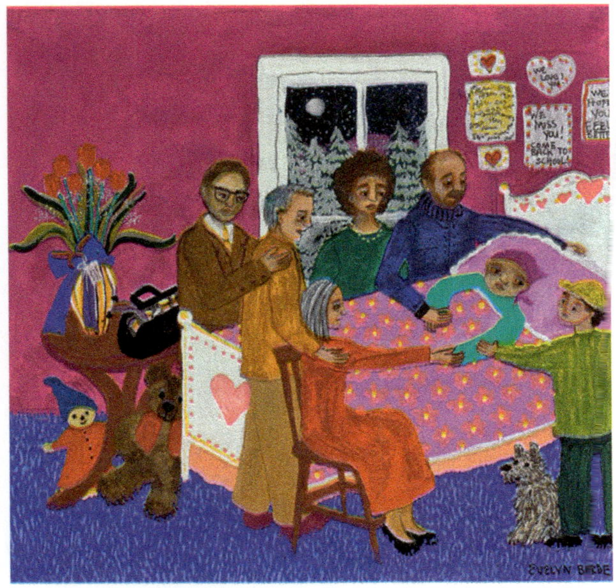

Holding the Moment by Evelyn Berde, (2007)

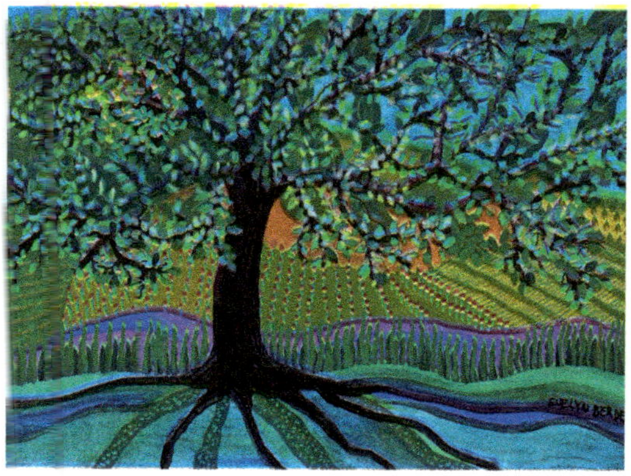

PREFACE

The field of palliative care is based on the fundamental principle that an interdisciplinary team is optimal in the care of seriously ill patients and their families throughout the illness trajectory. The *Textbook of Interdisciplinary Pediatric Palliative Care (TIPPC)* (2011) was the first of its kind to be written by and for interdisciplinary clinicians (rather than by or for a single target discipline) caring for children and adolescents with serious illness, their families, and their healthcare providers. The editors come from medicine (Wolfe), nursing (Hinds), and psychology (Sourkes).

Since *TIPPC* was first published in 2011, the field of pediatric palliative care has developed at an astonishing rate. No longer is there a need to focus on its basic foundation and assumptions; rather, innovative initiatives in clinical care, research, and education are emerging from a spectrum of disciplines. The editors have thus led the production of this tenth anniversary edition to reflect these developments—the progress, the obstacles, and the dilemmas.

Similar to the first edition, a crosscutting feature of this text is consistency of language. Most palliative care publications lack uniformity of language. The highest quality of communication is required for all interdisciplinary palliative care team members to deliver effective palliative care, yet communication expertise is often lacking. Basic words such as "palliative care," "end-of-life care," and "terminal care" are often used interchangeably, yet they convey very different meanings to clinicians, patients, and families and can lead to unintentional harmful consequences. As stated by Dr. Eric Cassell, "Similar to scalpels for surgeons, words are the palliative care clinician's greatest tools. Surgeons learn to use their tools with extreme precision, because any error can be devastating. So too should clinicians who rely on words." A primary focus of the textbook is to ensure consistent terminology throughout (as explicated in Chapter 1), as a means of exemplifying this critical tenet of palliative care.

All the chapters in this textbook are co-authored by an interdisciplinary group. The organization and content of the textbook purposefully encompass perspectives across and between disciplines. Although the chapters address the specific needs and responsibilities of individual professions, we feel that the interwoven perspectives from many disciplines best convey the dynamism and creativity of our field. Importantly, even in the most effective of integrative palliative care teams there are clinical situations of role or discipline tension. They most likely stem from diverse team members arriving at the same care conclusion but at different times or not agreeing with certain care considerations or priorities. This tension is of concern to all members of interdisciplinary teams and is often attributed to having different perspectives about the care situation. Part of the focus of our text is on acknowledging those periods of tension that are of concern to all members and using them ultimately to benefit patient and family care outcomes.

One final enhancement is based on the premise that pediatric palliative care is delivered in partnership with families, and each chapter includes a box highlighting a family perspective.

We will be honored and pleased if this second edition of *Interdisciplinary Pediatric Palliative Care* proves valuable to trainees and new and experienced clinicians who practice in multiple settings. Our overriding hope is that the volume adds meaning for all clinicians in their experience of providing pediatric palliative care. We thank all of our authors and our publishers, Marta Moldvai and Tiffany Lu, who have been great partners in developing this text. We are grateful to Evelyn Berde for allowing us to reprint three pieces of her vivid artwork on the cover and the frontispiece pages. Finally, we thank Dr. Kathleen Foley for her unwavering advocacy for pediatric palliative care and for her insightful foreword.

Joanne Wolfe, Pamela S. Hinds,
and Barbara M. Sourkes

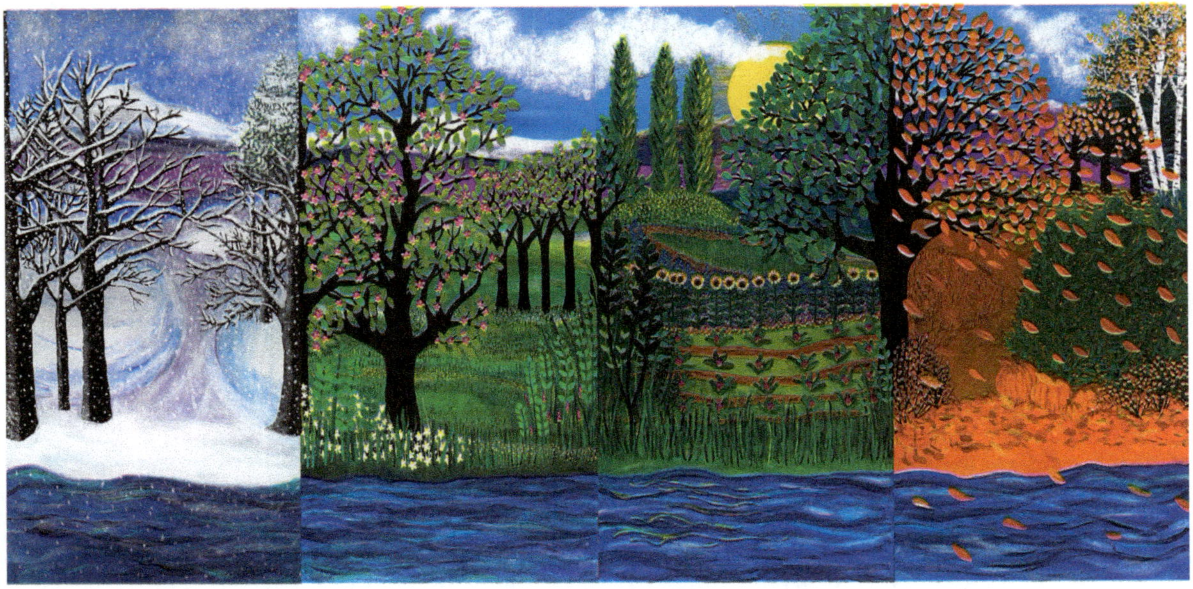

The Four Seasons by Evelyn Berde, (2008)

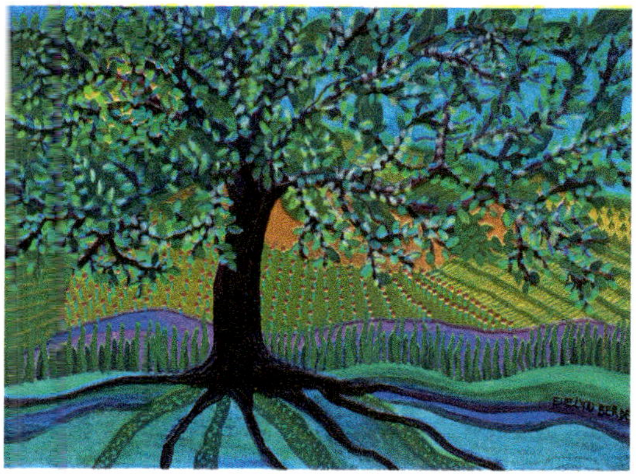

ABOUT THE ARTIST

Evelyn Berde grew up in the old "West End" of Boston, a neighborhood of European, African-American, and Latin immigrants. Today, many of her images and colors reflect her passion for Native American, Southeast Asian, Latin American, and African art, but also, her paintings still somehow recall for her the world she lived in as a child in the West End. Evelyn brings much of her life experiences to each painting. Her work resembles the patchwork of her childhood and adult life, as an artist, mother, wife, and teacher. Evelyn incorporates her connection to people and their "stories," her surroundings in everyday life, inspirations, and dreams. Evelyn's artwork has been commissioned by Children's Hospital Boston for the Anesthesia Department Library, the Children's Hospital Chapel, and the patient family house at 241 Kent Street. In creating these works, Evelyn notes, "I try to talk with many patients, parents, and staff members before I create a piece of art. The colors, lights, textures, and lines of each painting hopefully reflect the thoughts and feelings of each person I have met."

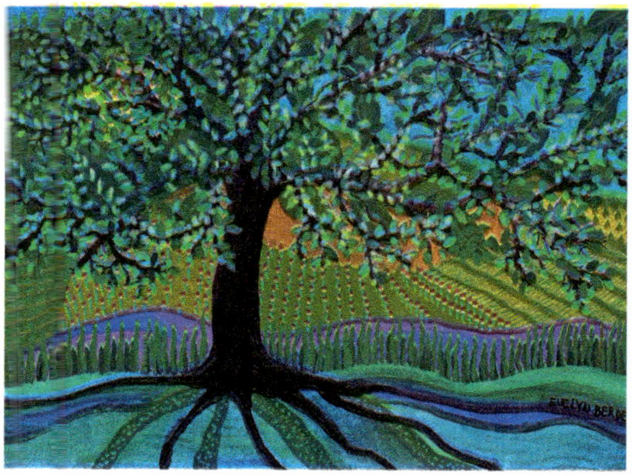

CONTRIBUTORS

Allistair Abraham, MD
Assistant Professor of Pediatrics
Division of Blood and Marrow Transplantation
George Washington University School of Medicine and Health Sciences, Children's National Hospital
Washington, DC, USA

Toluwalase A. Ajayi, MD
Medical Director of Palliative Medicine
Scripps Mercy Hospital San Diego
San Diego, CA, USA
Assistant Clinical Professor
Department of Pediatrics
University of California San Diego and Staff Researcher, Scripps Research Translational Institute
San Diego, CA, USA

Terrah Foster Akard, PhD, RN, CPNP, FAAN
Director, PhD Nursing Science Program
School of Nursing
Vanderbilt University
Nashville, TN, USA

Melissa A. Alderfer, PhD
Center Director (Delaware Valley) & Principal Research Scientist
Center for Healthcare Delivery Science
Nemours Children's Health System
Wilmington, DE, USA

Justin Baker, MD, FAAHPM
Chief
Division of Quality of Life and Palliative Care
Full Member
Department of Oncology
Memphis, TN, USA

Raymond Barfield, MD, PhD
Palliative Medicine Specialist
Director of Palliative CareMemorial Health University Hospital
Savannah, GA, USA

Mark Bartel, MDiv, BCC
Manager
Spiritual Care
Orlando Health Arnold Palmer Hospital for Children
Orlando Health Winnie Palmer Hospital for Women & Babies
Orlando, FL, USA

Renee Bartle, BS, RRT, RCP
Respiratory Therapist
Duke University Health System
Durham, NC, USA

Margarita Bidegain, MD, MHS-CL
Professor of Pediatrics
Division of Neonatology
Duke University Medical Center
Durham, NC, USA

Elizabeth D. Blume, MD
Associate Professor
Director
Advanced Cardiac Therapies
Boston Children's Hospital
Boston, MA, USA

Jori Bogetz, MD
Acting Assistant Professor of Pediatrics
Division of Bioethics and Palliative Care
Department of Pediatrics
University of Washington School of Medicine
Seattle Children's Hospital and Research Institute
Seattle, WA, USA

Amber Borucki, MD
Anesthesiologist
Center of Pain, Palliative and Integrative Medicine
Benioff Children's Hospitals
University of California at San Francisco (UCSF)
San Francisco, CA, USA

Renee Boss, MD, MHS
Rembrandt Foundation Professor of Pediatric Palliative Care
Director, Pediatric Palliative Care
Associate Professor, Division of Neonatology
Johns Hopkins Hospital
Baltimore, MD, USA

Kimberly A. Bower, MD, FAAHPM, HMDC
Attending Physician
Rady Children's Hospital San Diego
San Diego, CA, USA

Debra Boyer
Associate Professor of Pediatrics
Harvard Medical School
Associate Medical Director, Lung Transplant Program
Boston Children's Hospital
Boston, MA, USA

Amie Brandtjen, MSW, LICSW
Hospice Social Worker
Fairview Home Care and Hospice
Minneapolis, MN, USA

Katharine E. Brock, MD, MS
Assistant Professor
Department of Pediatrics
Director, Supportive Care Clinic at the Aflac Cancer and Blood Disorders Center
Emory University, Children's Healthcare of Atlanta
Atlanta, GA, USA

Michelle R. Brown, PhD
Clinical Professor of Psychiatry
Stanford University School of Medicine
Stanford, CA, USA

Michele R. Burdette-Taylor, PhD, MSN, RN, CWCN, CFCN, NPD-BC
Associate Professor
College of Health
University of Alaska Anchorage
Anchorage, AK, USA

Rachael Burgess, CPNP-AC
Pediatric Palliative Care Nurse Practitioner
Maine Medical Center
Portland, ME, USA

Jillian Campbell, MS, RN, CPNP-PC
Advanced Practice Nurse Practitioner
Sickle Cell Program, Center for Cancer and Blood Disorders
Division of Pediatric Hematology, Children's National Hospital
Washington, DC, USA

Kris Catrine, MD
Medical Director
Department of Pain Medicine, Palliative Care and Integrative Medicine
Children's Minnesota
Minneapolis, MN, USA

Jody Chrastek, RN, DNP
Pediatric Advanced Complex Care Team Coordinator
Fairview Home Care and Hospice
Minneapolis, MN, USA

Harvey Cohen, MD, PhD
Professor
Department of Pediatric
Stanford University
Stanford, CA, USA

Moshe Cohn, MD, HEC-C
Assistant Professor
Pediatric Critical Care, Pediatric Advanced Care Team (PACT)
Hassenfeld Children's Hospital at NYU Langone
New York, NY, USA

Erin Collins, MSW, LCSW
Administrative Social Work Supervisor and Bereavement Program Coordinator
Hassenfeld Children's Hospital at NYU Langone
New York, NY, USA

Christopher A. Collura, MD, MA
Assistant Professor of Pediatrics, Division of Neonatal Medicine
Department of Pediatric & Adolescent Medicine
Mayo Clinic College of Medicine, Mayo Clinic
Rochester, MN, USA

Melissa K. Cousino, PhD
Associate Professor
Department of Pediatrics
University of Michigan
Director of Psychosocial Services and Research
Congenital Heart Center, C. S. Mott Children's Hospital
Ann Arbor, MI, USA

Lauren Cramer, MSW, LICSW
Clinical Social Worker
Pediatric Advanced Care Team
Boston Children's Hospital
Boston, MA, USA

Christy Cummings, MD
Assistant Professor of Pediatrics
Division of Newborn Medicine
Boston Children's Hospital
Boston, MA, USA

Janet A. Deatrick, PhD, FAAN
Professor Emerita of Nursing
University of Pennsylvania
Philadelphia, PA, USA

Elisabeth Potts Dellon, MD, MPH
Professor of Pediatrics
Department of Pediatrics, Division of Pulmonology
University of North Carolina School of Medicine
Chapel Hill, NC, USA

Ami Doshi, MD
Director of Inpatient Palliative Care
Department of Pediatrics
Rady Children's Hospital-San Diego
San Diego, CA, USA

Janet Duncan, MSN, CPNP
Editor
Educational Content and Training
Courageous Parents Network
Boston, MA, USA

Donna Eull, RN, CNS, PhDc
Clinical Practice Specialist
Department of Pain Medicine, Palliative Care and Integrative Medicine
Children's Minnesota
Minneapolis, MN, USA

Angela M. Feraco, MD, MMSc
Attending Physician
Dana-Farber/Boston Children's Cancer and Blood Disorders Center
Associate Program Director
Pediatric Hematology/Oncology Fellowship Program
Instructor of Pediatrics
Harvard Medical School
Boston, MA, USA

Chris Feudtner, MD, PhD, MPH
Director of Research for the Justin Michael Ingerman Center for Palliative Care
Department of Medical Ethics
Children's Hospital of Philadelphia
Departments of Pediatrics and Medical Ethics and Health Policy, Perelman School of Medicine
University of Pennsylvania
Philadelphia, PA, USA

Dawn Freiberger, RN, MSN, CCTC
Lung Transplant Coordinator
Department of Pulmonary
Boston Children's Hospital
Boston, MA, USA

Jenna E. Freitas, MSN, RN, CPNP
Pediatric Nurse Practitioner
Director
Pediatric Advanced Care Team Nurse Practitioner Fellowship
Boston Children's Hospital
Boston, MA, USA

Stefan J. Friedrichsdorf, MD
Professor in Pediatrics
University of California at San Francisco (UCSF)
Medical Director
Center of Pain, Palliative and Integrative Medicine
Benioff Children's Hospitals
University of California at San Francisco (UCSF)
San Francisco, CA, USA

Sarah Gall, MD
Assistant Professor of Pediatrics
Duke University Health System
Durham, NC, USA

Jessica Goggin, PhD, RN
Director, Pulmonary Services
Division of Pulmonary, Critical Care and Sleep Medicine
UC San Diego Health
La Jolla, CA, USA

Michelle Goldsmith, MD
Clinical Associate Professor of Child and Adolescent Psychiatry
Stanford University School of Medicine
Stanford, CA, USA

Julie Good, MD
Clinical Associate Professor
Stanford University School of Medicine
Department of Anesthesiology, Perioperative and Pain Medicine and by Courtesy, Pediatrics
Stanford Children's Health
Stanford, CA, USA

Cristina Gordon, MD
Voluntary Clinical Instructor
University of California San Diego
San Diego, CA, USA

Julie Hauer, MD, FAAHPM
Medical Director
Seven Hills Pediatric Center
Groton, MA, USA

Lauren Heathcote, PhD
Postdoctoral Researcher
Department of Anesthesiology, Perioperative, and Pain Medicine
Stanford University School of Medicine
Palo Alto, CA, USA

Lynne Helfand, MSW, LICSW, MPH
Clinical Social Worker
Lung Transplant Program
Boston Children's Hospital
Boston, MA, USA

Chelsea Heneghan, MSN, CPNP-AC/PC, CPHON
Nurse Practitioner
Division of Pediatric Palliative Care
Boston Children's Hospital and Dana-Farber Cancer Institute
Boston, MA, USA

Pamela S. Hinds, PhD, RN, FAAN
The William and Joanne Conway Chair in Nursing Research
Executive Director, Department of Nursing Science, Professional Practice, and Quality Outcomes
Research Integrity Officer, Children's National Hospital
Professor
Department of Pediatrics
The George Washington University
Washington, DC, USA

Lisa Humphrey, MD
Director of Hospice and Palliative Medicine
Nationwide Children's Hospital
Columbus, OH, USA

Jennifer Hwang, MD, MHS, MSEd
Assistant Professor
Clinical Pediatrics
University of Pennsylvania
Director of Education, Pediatric Advanced Care Team
Children's Hospital of Philadelphia
Philadelphia, PA, USA

Shana Jacobs, MD
Associate Professor
Children's National Hospital
Department of Pediatrics
The George Washington University
Washington, DC, USA

Emily Johnston, MD, MS
Assistant Professor
Pediatric Hematology/Oncology
University of Alabama at Birmingham
Birmingham, AL, USA

Danielle Jonas, MSW, LCSW
PhD Student
New York University, Silver School of Social Work
New York, NY, USA

Megan Jordan, MD
Medical Director Pediatric Palliative Care
Assistant Professor of Medicine and Pediatrics
Duke University Health System
Durham, NC, USA

Marsha Joselow, LCSW
Clinical Social Worker
Pediatric Advanced Care Team
Dana-Farber Cancer Institute and Boston Children's Hospital
Boston, MA, USA

Tammy I. Kang, MD, MSCE
Texas Children's Hospital
Baylor College of Medicine
Houston, TX, USA

Timothy Klouda
Division of Pulmonary Medicine
Boston Children's Hospital
Boston, MA, USA

Blyth Lord, EdM
Executive Director
Courageous Parents Network
Newton, MA, USA

Wei Li Adeline Koay, MBBS, MSc
Infectious Diseases Attending
Department of Infectious Diseases
Children's National Hospital
Washington, DC, USA

Kathie Kobler, PhD, APRN, PCNS-BC, CHPPN, FPCN, FAAN
Coordinator
Center for Fetal Care
Advocate Children's Hospital
Park Ridge, IL, USA

Eunice Koh, MD
Clinical Assistant Professor of Pediatric Critical Care
Stanford University School of Medicine
Stanford, CA, USA

Deborah A. Lafond, DNP, PPCNP-BC, CPON, CHPPN, FPCN, FAAN
Clinical Director
PANDA Palliative Care Team
Children's National Hospital
Washington, DC, USA

Kristen Lakis, MSW, LCSW, MDiv
Pediatric Palliative Care Social Worker
Duke University Health System
Durham, NC, USA

Emily Layok, MS, CCLS
Child Life Specialist
Duke University Health System
Durham, NC, USA

Shih-Ning Liaw, MD, FAAP
Program Director
Harvard Interprofessional Pediatric Palliative Care Fellowship
Boston Children's Hospital/Dana-Farber Cancer Institute
Boston, MA, USA

Stephen Liben, MD
Director
Pediatric Palliative Care Program
Professor of Pediatrics
McGill University
Montreal Children's Hospital
Montreal, QC, Canada

Becky Lois, PhD
Clinical Associate Professor
NYU Grossman School of Medicine Department of Child and Adolescent Psychiatry
Pediatric Psychology Director
Integrated Behavioral Health Programs
Hassenfeld Children's Hospital at NYU Langone
New York, NY, USA

Debra Lotstein, MD, MPH
Chief, Division of Comfort and Palliative Care
Children's Hospital Los Angeles
Associate Professor of Clinical Pediatrics
Keck School of Medicine of the University of Southern California
Los Angeles, CA, USA

Robert Macauley, MD
Professor of Pediatrics
Cambia Health Foundation Endowed Chair in Pediatric Palliative Care
Oregon Health and Science University
Portland, OR, USA

Kevin Madden, MD
Assistant Professor
Department of Palliative Care and Rehabilitation Medicine
Division of Cancer Medicine
The University of Texas, MD Anderson Cancer Center
Houston, TX, USA

Margaret M. Mahon, PhD, CRNP, FAAN, FPCN
Pain and Palliative Care
Dermatologic Conditions and Symptom Control
National Institutes of Health
Bethesda, MD, USA

Daniel P. Mahoney, MD
Assistant Professor of Pediatrics
Texas Children's Hospital
Baylor College of Medicine
Houston, TX, USA

Meghan L. Marsac, PhD
Associate Professor
University of Kentucky College of Medicine
Lexington, KY, USA

Sarah Matthews, MD, AAHIVS
Fellow
Hospice and Palliative Medicine
University of California San Diego
San Diego, CA, USA

Julia McBee, RN, MSN, CPNP
Pediatric Advanced Care Team (PACT) Nurse Practitioner
Hassenfeld Children's Hospital at NYU Langone
New York, NY, USA

Sarah McCarthy, PhD, MPH, LP
Assistant Professor of Psychiatry and Psychology, Division of Child and Adolescent Psychology
Department of Psychiatry and Psychology
Mayo Clinic College of Medicine, Mayo Clinic
Rochester, MN, USA

Michael McCown, DO
Chief, Pediatric Pulmonology
Walter Reed National Military Medical Center
Bethesda, MD, USA

Elissa G. Miller, MD
Chief, Division of Palliative Medicine
Division of Palliative Medicine
Nemours/Alfred I. DuPont Hospital for Children
Wilmington, DE, USA

Kim Mooney-Doyle, PhD, RN, CPNP-AC
Assistant Professor
University of Maryland School of Nursing
Baltimore, MD, USA

Sue E. Morris, PsyD
Senior Psychologist
Director Bereavement Services
Department of Psychosocial Oncology and Palliative Care
Dana-Farber Cancer Institute
Assistant Professor
Harvard Medical School
Boston, MA, USA

Alexis Morvant, MA, MD, FAAP
Chief of Pediatric Palliative Care
Children's Hospital New Orleans
Assistant Professor
Louisiana State University Health Sciences Center
New Orleans, LA, USA

Jeffrey Moss, PharmD
Clinical Specialist Pharmacist
Pediatric Intensive Care Unit
Department of Pharmacy
Lucile Packard Children's Hospital Stanford
Palo Alto, CA, USA

Jonathan Mullin, MD
Assistant Professor of Pediatrics
Washington University School of Medicine
St. Louis, MO, USA

Sara Munoz-Blanco, MD
Assistant Professor
Neonatal-Perinatal Medicine/Pediatric Hospice and Palliative Medicine
Section of Palliative Care, Department of Internal Medicine
University of Texas Southwestern
Dallas, TX, USA

Anna C. Muriel, MD, MPH
Associate Professor of Psychiatry
Harvard Medical School
Division Chief
Pediatric Psychosocial Oncology
Department of Psychosocial Oncology and Palliative Care
Dana Farber Cancer Institute
Boston, MA, USA

Tessie October, MD, MPH
Associate Professor of Pediatrics
Department of Pediatrics, Division of Critical Care Medicine
Children's National Hospital
Washington, DC, USA

Katherine Ort, MD
Clinical Assistant Professor of Child and Adolescent Psychiatry and Pediatrics
NYU Grossman School of Medicine Department of Child and Adolescent Psychiatry and Department of Pediatrics
New York, NY, USA

Maryland Pao, MD
Clinical and Deputy Scientific Director
National Institute of Mental Health Intramural Research Program
Bethesda, MD, USA

Danai Papadatou, PhD
Professor of Clinical Psychology
Faculty of Nursing National and Kapodistrian University of Athens
Athens, Greece

Priyal Patel, DO
Assistant Professor
Hospice and Palliative Medicine
Pediatric Hematology/Oncology/Blood and Marrow Transplant
Nationwide Children's Hospital
Columbus, OH, USA

Kathleen Perko, MS, PPCNP-BC, CHPPN, CPON, CPLC, FPCN
Pediatric Palliative Care Certificate Track Director
Palliative Care Training Center
University of Washington
Seattle, WA, USA

Thaddeus M. Pope, JD, PhD
Professor of Law
Mitchell Hamline School of Law
St. Paul, MN, USA

Nicholas Purol, MSW
Social Worker
Psychosocial Oncology and Palliative Care
Dana-Farber Cancer Institute and Boston Children's Hospital
Boston, MA, USA

Kimberly A. Pyke-Grimm, PhD, RN, CNS, CPHON
Nurse Scientist
Department of Nursing Research and Evidence-Based Practice
Clinical Assistant Professor, Division of Hematology/Oncology
Department of Pediatrics
Lucile Packard Children's Hospital Stanford
Palo Alto, CA, USA

Elliot Rabinowitz, MD
Division of Pulmonary Medicine
Department of Psychosocial Oncology and Palliative Care
Boston Children's Hospital and Dana-Farber Cancer Institute
Instructor of Pediatrics
Harvard Medical School
Boston, MA, USA

Lindsay Ragsdale, MD, FAAP, FAAHPM
Chief, Division of Pediatric Palliative Care
Kentucky Children's Hospital
Associate Professor of Pediatrics
University of Kentucky
Lexington, KY, USA

Natella Rakhmanina, MD, PhD
Director of HIV Services and Special Immunology
Children's National Hospital
Washington, DC, USA

Anke Reineke, PhD, BCIAC
Pschologist
CSH Inpatient Pain Program
Rady Children's Hospital San Diego
San Diego, CA, USA

Stacy S. Remke, MSW, LICSW
Senior Teaching Specialist
Division of Pain and Palliative Care and Social Work
Minneapolis, MN, USA

Valerie E. Rogers, PhD, RN, CPNP
Retired
University of Maryland School of Nursing
Baltimore, MD, USA

Karen Ron-Li Liaw, MD
Clinical Associate Professor
NYU Grossman School of Medicine Department of Child and Adolescent Psychiatry
Service Chief
Hassenfeld Children's Hospital at NYU Langone
New York, NY, USA

Abby R. Rosenberg, MD, MS, MA
Associate Professor
Department of Pediatrics
University of Washington School of Medicine
Seattle, WA, USA

Rachel Rusch, LCSW, MSW, MA
Clinical Social Worker
Division of Comfort and Palliative Care
Children's Hospital Los Angeles
Los Angeles, CA, USA

Chase Samsel, MD
Assistant Professor of Psychiatry
Harvard Medical School
Medical Director
Psychiatry Consultation Service
Department of Psychiatry and Behavioral Sciences
Attending Psychiatrist
Pediatric Transplant Center
Boston Children's Hospital
Department of Psychiatry and Behavioral Sciences
Boston Children's Hospital
Boston, MA, USA

Michael Sangster, BScPT, MBA, DPT
Physiotherapist
Clinical Specialist (Pain Science)/Clinical Associate
IWK Health Centre/Dalhousie University
Halifax, NS, Canada

Caitlin Scanlon, MSW, LCSW
Clinical Social Worker
Pediatric Palliative Care Team
Riley Hospital for Children
Indiana University Health
Indianapolis, IN, USA

Rose Sharpe, MSN, CPNP
Nurse Practioner
Pediatric Palliative Care NP
Duke University Health System
Durham, NC, USA

Richard J. Shaw, MD
Professor of Child and Adolescent Psychiatry and Pediatrics
Stanford University School of Medicine
Stanford, CA, USA

Bryan Sisk, MD, MSCI
Assistant Professor
Department of Pediatrics, Division of Hematology and Oncology
Department of Medicine, Bioethics Research Center
Washington University School of Medicine in St. Louis
St. Louis, MO, USA

Jennifer M. Snaman, MD, MS
Assistant Professor
Dana-Farber Cancer Institute
Department of Psychosocial Oncology and Palliative Care
Dana-Farber Cancer Institute
Department of Pediatric Oncology
Boston, MA, USA

Barbara M. Sourkes, PhD
Professor
Department of Pediatrics
Stanford University School of Medicine
Stanford, CA, USA

Barbara Speller-Brown, DNP, CPNP, MSN
Assistant Professor of Pediatrics
Division of Pediatric Hematology
George Washington University School of Medicine and Health Sciences
Lead Sickle Cell Translational Research APN
Director SCD Transition Clinic
Children's National Hospital
Washington, DC, USA

Anne Sullivan, MD
Instructor in Pediatrics
Attending Neonatologist
Division of Newborn Medicine
Boston Children's Hospital
Boston, MA, USA

Amanda L. Thompson, PhD
Chief, Pediatric Psychology
Life with Cancer
INOVA Schar Cancer Institute
INOVA Health System
Fairfax, VA, USA

Christy Torkildson, PhD, RN, PHN, FPCN, PACT
Team Coordinator
Complex Pain and Palliative Care
UCSF Benioff Children's Hospital Oakland
Senior Clinical Practice Consultant
Hospice and Palliative Care, Banner Health
Gilbert, AZ, USA

Paula Tran, MD
Clinical Assistant Professor of Child and Adolescent Psychiatry
Stanford University School of Medicine
Stanford, CA, USA

Christina Ullrich, MD, MPH
Assistant Professor
Harvard Medical School
Clinical Director
Pediatric Advanced Care Team
Senior Physician
Psychosocial Oncology and Palliative Care
Pediatric Hematology/Oncology
Dana-Farber Cancer Institute and Boston Children's Hospital
Boston, MA, USA

Elisha Waldman, MD, FAAHPM
Chief, Division of Palliative Care
Ann & Robert H. Lurie Children's Hospital of Chicago
Associate Professor of Pediatrics
Northwestern University Feinberg School of Medicine
Chicago, IL, USA

Meaghann S. Weaver, MD, MPH, FAAP
Adjunct Associate Professor
Department of Palliative Care
University of Nebraska Medical Center
Omaha, NE, USA

Jennifer Webb, MD, MSCE
Assistant Professor of Pediatrics
Division of Pediatric Hematology
George Washington University
School of Medicine and Health Sciences
Children's National Hospital
Washington, DC, USA

Kimberley Widger, RN, PhD, CHPCN(C)
Associate Professor
Lawrence S. Bloomberg Faculty of Nursing
University of Toronto
Toronto, ON, Canada

Lori Wiener, PhD
Co-Director, Behavioral Health Core
Director, Psychosocial Support and Research Program
Pediatric Oncology Branch Center for Cancer Research, National Cancer Institute
National Institutes of Health
Bethesda, MD, USA

Megan Wilkins, PhD
Associate Member
Divisions of Infectious Diseases and Psychology
St. Jude Children's Research Hospital
Memphis, TN, USA

Conrad Williams IV, MD, FAAP, FAAHPM, HMDC
Assistant Professor of Pediatrics
Medical University of South Carolina
Medical Director
Palliative Care Program
MUSC Children's Health System
Charleston, SC, USA

Joanne Wolfe, MD, MPH
Attending Physician, Pediatric Advanced Care Team
Dana-Farber Cancer Institute and Boston Children's Hospital
Professor of Pediatrics
Harvard Medical School
Boston, MA, USA

Eric S. Zhou, PhD
Assistant Professor
Staff Psychologist
Dana-Farber/Boston Children's Cancer and Blood Disorders Center
Boston, MA, USA

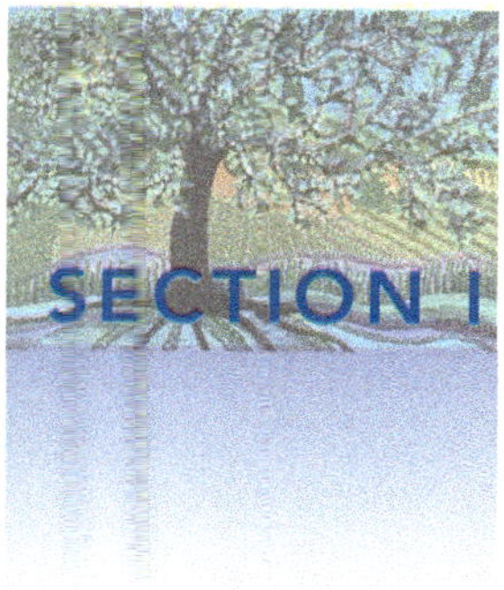

SECTION I | SETTING THE STAGE

Children are born with rainbows in their hearts and you'll never reach them unless you reckon with rainbows.

CARL SANDBURG

We hope that the lives of all children will be filled with possibility, with open horizons and rainbows into the future. Children with serious illnesses, their families, and those who care for them confront the realization that "not everything is possible," that, despite dramatic scientific and medical advances, the life spans of some children will be shortened. This threat of premature loss heightens the sense of time for children and families alike and challenges clinicians to create new pathways of hope for them.

The interdisciplinary field of pediatric palliative care has emerged over the past three decades, with rapid development in clinical care, education, research, and policy. In this section, "Setting the Stage," themes, constructs, and emerging evidence that are foundational to the spectrum of pediatric palliative care provide a conceptual framework for this book and this field.

Words define, clarify, and communicate experience; their potential impact is powerful in both positive and negative ways. The importance of a common language cannot be underestimated when clinicians from many disciplines care for children and families who face extraordinary challenges. The opening chapter, "The Language of Pediatric Palliative Care" sets this foundation.

Who are these children? Who are the parents and families who care for them? Chapter 2 on the epidemiology of pediatric palliative care portrays the distribution of conditions, their trajectories and symptoms, and trends in mortality. The chapter also contains a declaration that pediatric palliative care is a firmly established field. Families are discussed regarding their structure, the "work of care" for the child, coping, and financial issues. Overarching both the child and family variables are epidemiological factors in healthcare systems at regional, national, and international levels.

In Chapter 3, "Children's Voices," children and their siblings provide another type of portrait: through their own words and images they convey their experience of *living* with illness: their awareness of its life-threatening nature, the undercurrent of anticipatory grief, and their role in decision-making. These experiences are a perfect prelude to the very next chapter, Chapter 4, which is on settings of care. This is because the settings are now wherever a child needs palliative care. The nature of this care has broadened and so, too, have the number of settings.

Chapter 5, social considerations and disparities, directly addresses how the culture that creates disparities in healthcare in general can also create disparities in pediatric palliative care. Cultural humility is defined and described as a way of giving palliative care that welcomes how individuals (children, families, care providers) can discover how they are both different from each other and the same. These discoveries guide best-fit palliative care for the ill child, family, and care situation.

Pediatric palliative care programs have expanded, and this unfolding of programs is described in Chapter 6, which shows their growth and networking connections in a non-linear manner. Programs are now characterized by links beyond hospital settings to communities. Being informed by business plans has become a necessity. Relatedly, Chapter 7 frames education and training as benefitting from interdisciplinary approaches that span settings and consider the skills of each learner and the knowledge gaps of each as well. The knowledge and learning of an *individual* can translate through planned actions to interdisciplinary *team* knowing.

"Setting the Stage" closes with Chapter 8, on quality in pediatric palliative care and defines quality care as being based on knowing the goals of all involved—the child, family, and care professionals. Care based on goal awareness of all involved yields safe, effective, patient-centered, timely, efficient, and equitable care. Providing that kind of pediatric palliative care will help pediatric palliative care providers from diverse disciplines to "reckon with rainbows" of all ill children.

1 | THE LANGUAGE OF PEDIATRIC PALLIATIVE CARE

JOANNE WOLFE, PAMELA S. HINDS, AND BARBARA M. SOURKES

The Word
Oh, a word is a gem, or a stone, or a song,
Or a flame, or a two-edged sword;
Or a rose in bloom, or a sweet perfume,
Or a drop of gall is a word.

You may choose your word like a connoisseur,
And polish it up with art,
But the word that sways, and stirs, and stays,
Is the word that comes from the heart.

You may work on your word a thousand weeks,
But it will not glow like one
That all unsought, leaps forth white hot,
When the fountains of feeling run.

ELLA WHEELER WILCOX

Words are, in my not-so-humble opinion, our most inexhaustible source of magic. Capable of both inflicting injury, and remedying it.

J. K. ROWLING *(Harry Potter and the Deathly Hallows)*

INTRODUCTION

Basic words such as "palliative care," "end-of-life care," and "terminal care" are often used interchangeably yet they convey very different meanings to clinicians, patients, and families and can lead to unintentional and harmful consequences. As stated by Dr. Eric Cassell, "Similar to scalpels for surgeons, words are the palliative care clinician's greatest tools. Surgeons learn to use their tools with extreme precision, because any error can be devastating. So too should clinicians who rely on words" (personal communication). A primary focus of this second edition of *Interdisciplinary Pediatric Palliative Care* (IPPC) is to ensure that all contributors use consistent, predefined terminology as a means of exemplifying this critical tenet of palliative care.

Family Reflection

Several months into our son Steve's cancer treatment, we experienced one of many stressful situations.

Because Barb is a nurse, the doctors generally directed their technical medical explanations to her, even when we stood side by side. Barb quickly developed the habit of pointing at me and instructing them to make sure I understood the information they were trying to convey—translate it into civilian language—and let me ask questions.

In this particular incident, however, that was not the problem. Throughout his hospitalizations Steve frequently endured extremely high fevers and severe rashes. One of these incidents landed him in the ICU. After a very difficult night, the head of the ICU stopped in and casually said something along the lines of, "Your son is the sickest child in the unit." We were floored. Did we really need to know that? How did comparing him to other patients provide us with actionable information? Our worries skyrocketed. Since we were in the largest children's hospital in a major metropolitan area, we started to wonder if Steve was the sickest child in the city that day. Was his death imminent?

While we stood there trying to process that news, Steve's oncology fellow managed to track us down in the ICU. She approached us with a cheerful smile on her face. Unaware of the news we just received, she excitedly told us that his recent scan showed that his tumors were shrinking!

We were constantly searching for hope, but wondered how exactly should we process this news? How does it align with the words of the ICU head? Was our family having a good day or a bad day?

Seventeen years later, we still think about this.

Bob & Barb Calla
In memory of our son, Steven Calla

DEFINITION OF TERMS

The definitions of words in this chapter were derived through consensus. Specifically, for the first edition of this textbook, the list of terms and definitions were generated by the editors and distributed to all authors for review. Any suggested edits were then considered by the editors, and, if consensus agreement was reached, the edit was incorporated. Additional terms were also suggested by chapter authors, and the same process was used to determine whether such terms should be included in this overview. For the current edition, the editors re-examined all terms and suggested updated terminology when indicated.

Illness. The subjective experience of a patient with an underlying disease or medical condition.[1]

Life-threatening, life-limiting, or serious illness? The term "life-threatening" suggests a range of possible outcomes including living a long or shortened life, and that the outcome is uncertain. The term "life-limiting" may imply that there is no realistic hope for a long life or that the condition limits the fullness of the life experienced. "Serious illness" is a health condition that carries a high risk of mortality and either negatively impacts a person's daily function or quality of life or excessively strains the caregiver.[2] In this text we recommend using the broadest terms, either *life-threatening* or *serious illness*.

Children with complex chronic conditions. Formally defined by Feudtner et al., these are children with chronic conditions that involve different organ systems or one organ system severely enough to require specialty pediatric care and probably some period of hospitalization in a tertiary care center.[3] Many, though not all of these children have life-threatening illness.

Palliative care (from Latin *palliare*, to cloak). The World Health Organization (WHO) defines palliative care as an approach to care that improves the quality of life of patients and their families facing the problems associated with life-threatening illness through the prevention and relief of suffering by means of early identification and impeccable assessment and treatment of pain and other problems, physical, psychosocial, and spiritual.[4]

Palliative care

- considers the child/patient and family as the center of the unit of care;
- provides relief from pain and other distressing symptoms;
- affirms life and regards dying as a normal process;
- intends neither to hasten or postpone death;
- integrates the psychological and spiritual aspects of patient care;
- offers a support system to help patients live as actively as possible until death;
- offers a support system to help the family cope during the patient's illness and in their own bereavement;
- uses a team approach to address the needs of patients and their families, including bereavement counseling if indicated;
- aims to enhance quality of life and may also positively influence the course of illness;
- is applicable early in the course of illness, in conjunction with other therapies that are intended to prolong life, and includes those investigations needed to better understand and manage distressing clinical complications.

WHO definition of palliative care for children (adapted)[4]: Palliative care for children represents a special, albeit closely related field to adult palliative care. The WHO's definition of palliative care appropriate for children and their families is as follows:

- Palliative care for children is the active total care of the child's body, mind, and spirit and also involves giving support to the family.
- It begins when illness is diagnosed and continues regardless of whether or not a child receives treatment directed at the disease.
- Healthcare providers must evaluate and alleviate a child's physical, psychological, and social distress.
- Effective palliative care requires a broad interdisciplinary approach, one that includes the family and makes use of available community resources; it can be successfully implemented even if resources are limited.
- It can be provided in tertiary care facilities, in community health and hospice centers, and in children's homes.
- Care should be developmentally appropriate and in accordance with family values.

Primary palliative care and specialty palliative care.[5] As described, palliative care is an *approach* to caring for seriously ill people and their families. This approach can be delivered by a *primary* interdisciplinary team, such as a cardiology team caring for someone with advanced heart disease, or a *specialty* palliative care team. All clinicians caring for the seriously ill should have basic primary palliative care skills in communication, advance care planning, symptom management, and coordination of care. The role of the specialty palliative care team is severalfold: (1) to provide added expertise for more complex clinical circumstances; (2) to provide education and training to clinicians caring for the seriously ill; (3) to advance the field of palliative care through innovation, quality improvement, and research; and (4) to advocate across systems for improved care of the seriously ill.

End-of-life care or terminal care (from Latin *terminalis*). Unlike most of palliative care, which is often delivered in the context of prognostic uncertainty, the terms "end-of-life care" or "terminal care" refer to the care delivered when the prognosis of death is almost certain and close in time. Examples include a patient with advanced refractory metastatic cancer who is expected to die within days or weeks, or a patient with end-stage lung disease being maintained on high ventilator settings and this technological support is being discontinued. Needless to say, exceptions arise and patients may survive well beyond what was expected to be an earlier death. *Comfort care* is often used to describe the interdisciplinary care provided at end of life. However, there is little consensus on what comprises comfort care, and, as such, the term should be avoided.

Hospice. In the United States, *hospice* is a Medicare and Medicaid benefit and is defined as a special way of caring for people who are *terminally ill*. Hospice care involves a team-oriented approach that addresses the medical, physical, social, emotional, and spiritual needs of the patient. Hospice provides support to the patient's family or caregiver as well. Hospice care is given by a public agency or private company approved by Medicare. It is for all age groups, including children, adults, and the elderly during their final stages of life. The goal of hospice is to care for a terminally ill patient and family, not to treat the underlying illness.

Outside the United States, "hospice" is a term used to describe a philosophy of care which focuses on the palliation of terminally ill patients. The term is also often used in association with a building that may house patients receiving terminal care and/or a hospice program serving patients in the community.

Dying. "Dying" refers to the period when a patient is approaching death within days, hours, or moments. Although in conversations with patients clinicians may echo terms used by patients and/or family members such as "passing away" or "at life's end," these gentler terms are not used in this text unless being used as a communication example.

Hospice and palliative care. "Hospice and palliative care" is the term used to denote the interdisciplinary field as a whole.

Hospice and palliative medicine. "Hospice and palliative medicine" is the term used by the American Board of Medical Subspecialties to denote this physician subspecialty, established in 2006.

Multidisciplinary. A collection of disciplines in which each discipline retains its methodologies and assumptions without change or development from the others. It is a linear model—the disciplines run parallel to one other.

Interdisciplinary or interprofessional. An integrative model wherein people from multiple disciplines or professions work together in addressing a common challenge. This model can be seen as overlapping circles (as in a Venn diagram) where each specialty maintains its own identity while also sharing some common methodologies and assumptions with other disciplines in the web. This collaborative work is more typical of pediatric palliative care and is the underlying tenet of this book (as per the title!). Notably, there is some debate in the literature regarding which of these two terms is better. "Interdisciplinary" can refer to healthcare providers with the same foundational training but different specialties, such as physicians who are oncologists and surgeons. At the same time, the term can refer to those with different foundational training, such as nursing and child life. Some suggest that "professional" is a more empowering and inclusive term,[6] however, it is behavior rather than a term that leads to more inclusive outcomes. Of note, "interprofessional" is used at times in this textbook in the context of education and training.

Transdisciplinary. A term used with increasing frequency that does not yet have a stable, consensus meaning. Usage suggests that a transdisciplinary approach dissolves boundary between disciplines. In a still emerging field, porous boundaries may create confusion and undercut the richness and uniqueness of each discipline.

Medical provider, medical caregiver, or clinician? Psychosocial clinician? The most general term we would recommend using to refer to a practitioner of palliative care would be "clinician," no matter what the underlying discipline, including physician, nurse, pharmacist, etc. "Medical provider" may connote physician, and "caregiver" is often used in referring to a layperson such as a family member who cares for a patient. Other acceptable terms include healthcare provider and mental health provider for psychologists, social workers, etc. However, if referring to a skill set unique to one of these types of clinicians, then that discipline is explicitly named.

Child life specialist. Child life specialists provide both therapeutic play interventions and social recreation for children on an individual and group basis.

Chaplain. A chaplain is typically (although not always) a member of the clergy who serves in specific settings, including hospitals and hospices. Chaplains provide spiritual guidance and counseling for families as well as carry out religious rituals. In most instances, chaplains will meet with families of any faith, regardless of their own denomination, unless the family makes a specific request.

Opioid. An opioid is a chemical substance that has a morphine-like action in the body. These agents work by binding to opioid receptors, which are found principally in the central nervous system and gastrointestinal tract. The receptors in these two organ systems mediate both the beneficial effects and the undesirable side effects. Although the term "opiate" is often used as a synonym for opioid, it is more properly limited to the natural opium alkaloids and the semi-synthetics derived from them.

There are a number of broad classes of opioids:

- *Natural opiates*, alkaloids contained in the resin of the opium poppy including morphine and codeine.
- *Semi-synthetic opiates*, created from the natural opioids, such as hydromorphone, hydrocodone, oxycodone,

oxymorphone, desomorphine, diacetylmorphine (heroin), nicomorphine, dipropanoylmorphine, benzylmorphine, and ethylmorphine.

- *Fully synthetic opioids*, such as fentanyl, methadone, and tramadol.
- *Endogenous opioid peptides*, produced naturally in the body, such as endorphins, enkephalins, dynorphins, and endomorphins.

The term "narcotic" is believed to have been coined by the Greek physician Galen to refer to agents that benumb or deaden, causing loss of feeling or paralysis. It is based on the Greek word ναρκωσις (narcosis), the term used by Hippocrates for the process of benumbing or the benumbed state. Because the term is often used broadly, inaccurately, or pejoratively outside medical contexts and often instills fear in families, because of such associations, we prefer the more precise term "opioid."

Resuscitation status and do-not-resuscitate. Resuscitation status refers to the outcome of a discussion (or a series of discussions) between a patient and family and a clinician regarding the potential use of certain medical interventions in the care of a patient with life-threatening illness. Most healthcare facilities have a specific order form, entitled "do not resuscitate" (DNR), that is used to denote the patient's resuscitation status. The exact content of a DNR order varies widely depending on legal jurisdiction and individual facility interpretation. Terms such as "do not attempt resuscitation" (DNAR) and "allow natural death" (AND) have been proposed to replace DNR in order to emphasize differing qualities of such orders. For example, DNAR negates the underlying assumption that if an intervention is employed, the outcome will be successful. AND has been recommended as a more acceptable term from a patient perspective, although this has not been explicitly studied among families of children with serious illness. *To add and clarify*: the expression "the parents signed the DNR" is misleading since in most settings they are not required to do so. It is more accurate to state that the parents "agreed to the recommendations of the healthcare team regarding resuscitation status."

TERMS TO AVOID

Aggressive care. Aggressive is often used to describe an approach to treatment of serious illness which can have positive and negative connotations. Similar to "fighting" and other battle terminology, the implication is that, with an aggressive approach, the patient will win; that is, defeat the illness. However, these words imply that the patient has control over the outcome of their illness, whereas the reality is that outcomes are beyond their control (Box 1.1).

Aggressive care is also often used to describe a negative approach to care, such as "overly aggressive care at end of life." Labeling care in this manner undermines an approach that may be entirely goal concordant. We favor the term "intensive" to describe interventions or an approach that may involve more medical intervention.

BOX 1.1 NATE CAVALLO EULOGY: DECEMBER 14, 2015

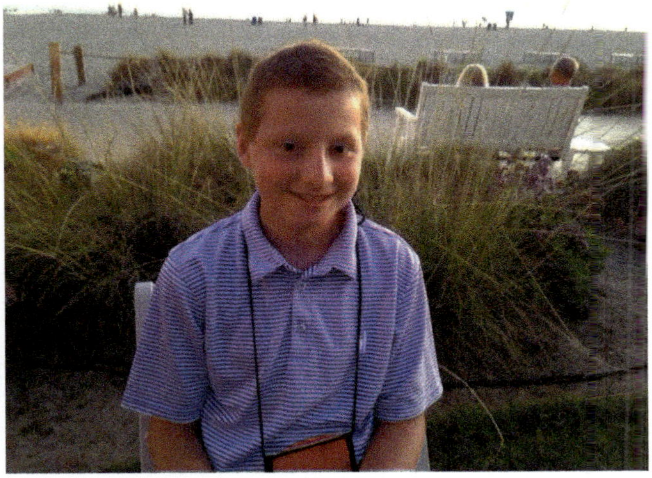

Nate
Funny, Active, Creative, Wise
Sibling of Lexi and Bennett
Lover of Halloween and Christmas
Who fears pitch dark
Who needs my Mom
Who gives a happy attitude
Who would like to see Disneyworld
Resident of Lexington
Cavallo

So insightful, even at a young age, this is how Nate described himself in a poem he wrote in Ms. Klein's third grade class at Fiske School.

Three and a half years ago, Nate was dealt an unimaginable curve ball when he was diagnosed with stage 4 cancer within days of graduating from Fiske Elementary School. While most people, myself included, may have been derailed by this, Nate rallied and somehow only got stronger and more courageous as time went on.

Often we hear about a child battling cancer as if he is at war with his own body, but this metaphor is unfair. It assumes that the child somehow has control over his disease and plays a role in his own success or failure to cure it. Nate understood the complexity of his situation and chose to focus on making every day count. A few months ago, Nate posted a picture of himself on Instagram and was angered by somebody's comment "keep fighting." To the rest of us, it seemed like a perfectly reasonable comment, but Nate said, "Why do people think I spend my time fighting everyday? I am just living like everyone else."

Curative versus palliative. To "cure" implies eradication of a disease. For example, some cancers can be cured. A person, however, cannot be "cured" because even if a serious disease is eliminated, the person does not revert to their prior self; rather they are forever transformed by the illness experience. Disease-directed treatment, especially in cancer care, is often referred to as "curative" or "palliative" in intent. This dichotomous labeling, however, suggests only two outcomes are possible. In reality outcomes are much more nuanced, complicated, and uncertain. Specifically, while a disease may be eradicated, the person may be left with current or future serious illnesses/conditions such as organ dysfunction or risks for secondary cancer and may be at risk for poor quality of life and social outcomes. "Palliative intent" connotes that the disease will not be cured. Here again, outcomes are more nuanced. For example, treatment of the underlying disease may lead to life prolongation and enhanced well-being. Furthermore, labeling treatment intent may simply be a back-hand way of communicating prognosis, which requires sophisticated communication skills. Finally, families often hold multiple "intents" or "hopes" for disease-directed therapy,[7] and labeling can undermine these aspirations.

Transition to palliative care/redirecting care/do nothing. *Transition* means the process of changing from one state or condition to another. In considering our seriously ill patients, clinicians often refer to a distinct "change in direction" of care and use phrases such as "transitioning to palliative care" or "redirecting care." As discussed earlier, palliative care is not a phase of care: it is an approach to care that is integrated throughout the serious illness trajectory. To transition suggest that something new is being offered, when a palliative approach should have been present throughout the illness. "Redirecting care" connotes an abrupt change and, similar to "comfort care only," is vague and can be differentially interpreted, leading to miscommunication and care that is not aligned with family goals. Finally, we should never suggest "doing nothing" as an alternative to disease-directed treatment. Indeed, no matter what the prognosis we will always provide care, often "concurrent care" or a "blended approach" including disease-directed treatment along with palliative care.

Withdrawal or withholding of support/care. The frequently used term "withdrawal" or "withholding of support" results in the unintended message that all care is ending, rather than just the particular intervention that is being stopped. We would greatly prefer to model language such as, "ventilator support will be discontinued or forgone because it is no longer clinically indicated, and maximal supportive care will be continued."

Closure. The word "closure" is used all too often, especially around bereavement, to denote some completion of a psychological process. This quote from a *Newsweek* article illustrates how "closure" can be misused.

> "Morrison's ambivalence spilled over recently when Oprah broached the death of Morrison's son. During her last month of TV shows last year, Oprah invited her "most memorable guests" back to share "life-changing lessons." Still in mourning, Morrison consented to be flown into Chicago on a private jet and put up at the Four Seasons. But she bristled when Oprah suggested the show would help her get "closure" on Slade's death. "Don't ever say that word," Morrison said. "There's never closure with the death of a child." She says now that she was happy to discuss her son, but not in detail. "There's no language for that"—especially not the language of closure[8] (visit https://nymag.com/news/features/toni-morrison-2012-5/index.html).

The child failed. The expression "the child failed treatment" or "the child failed extubation" implies that the child was at fault for the intervention not succeeding. Truly no one has failed anything or anyone (neither the child, nor the clinical team); rather, a treatment or procedure was not successful. As such, the word "failure" should be avoided. Similarly, we often hold the child responsible for the outcome through statements like, "your child is in charge" or "we will follow your child's lead." We recommend avoiding these terms.

Labeling the child with his or her disease. A frequently used shortcut is to label the child with the name of the underlying illness, for example, "The leukemic child" or "The hypoplast." A preferable approach, though slightly longer, is "the child with leukemia" or "the child with hypoplastic left heart syndrome."

"Mom" and "Dad." These terms are frequently used when talking about or with parents. The only time "mom" and "dad" should be used is when the child talks to them or about them with another family member or friend. In written vignettes, we use "the mother," "the father," "the parents," or an initial or pseudonym.

Noncompliance. Unintentionally or not, this term has come to suggest a *willful* ignoring of instructions, although many factors often contribute to an inability to follow through with medical recommendations. As such, healthcare professionals prefer to talk about "adherence" to a regimen rather than "compliance."

Dependence. Commonly, children are referred to as "wheelchair dependent," "trach dependent," and "g-tube dependent". The term "dependent" confers a reliance on and being lesser able. Alternate phrasing, while less succinct, confers less judgment, such as "uses a wheelchair," "uses a trach," or "uses a g-tube."

To complain of. When referring to a symptom reported by a patient, the clinician typically states, "The patient complains of pain." The implication of "complain" is that patient is annoyed or dissatisfied. "The patient *reports* pain" confers less judgment.

Moral distress. Commonly, when conflict between families and clinicians arises, clinician distress is often termed "moral" distress. The term "moral" implies that there is a clear right or wrong and that the clinician knows what is right and, by extension, what the parents are doing is not only wrong, but immoral. No question, staff distress is real and, as defined by Jonas and Bogetz, "is defined as the negative experience that occurs when a person cannot do what they feel is right."[9(p. 679)] The necessity of the word "moral" is highly questionable.

HELPFUL TERMINOLOGY

There are many words that should always be a part of our communication toolbox and can facilitate effective communication. The following are some notable ones.

Icebreakers. When patients and family members first meet clinicians, it is not uncommon to first ask about the patient's illness, which is what families are used to. We suggest beginning with, "Tell me about yourself/your child? What are they like as a person? What do they enjoy? Tell me about your family." In so doing, the family immediately understands that you are authentically interested in them. For infants, asking such questions may be awkward. As an alternative, it is often informative to ask a parent how they chose the child's name. There is almost always a story, including simply that they liked it, to something more in-depth about family history.

Responding to emotion. When a patient or family member expresses a strong emotion, it can be hard for clinicians to continue a discussion. We may instinctually want to ask the family if they need some time alone. However, sitting with family as they integrate the emotion can be comforting, so silence is often well received. Naming the emotion can also be helpful, "You seem very worried, is that right?" although it is almost never helpful to tell someone they seem angry. Rather, you may want to say, "You seem upset, can you tell me more about why you are feeling that way?" One of the most impactful statements can simply be, "I can't imagine what this must be like for you." Importantly, do not say you *can* imagine, because we simply cannot.

Loving parents. As eloquently described by Weaver et al.,[10] parents strive to be "good parents" for their child. Consistent with this desire, it is often helpful to name that "equally loving parents" may make different decisions.

I wish . . . I worry. As will be described in many chapters, it is critical to explore patient and family hopes. It is also important to recognize and accept that families hold multiple and, at times, conflicting, hopes. When a child is near end of life and we want to gently guide a family toward a comfort-focused approach, it may be helpful to use the phrase, "I also wish that [parent hope] were possible. At the same time, I worry that time is short. Would it be OK to consider how we should take care of your child should we not achieve [parent hope]?" Notably, asking permission to talk about a difficult topic is a gentle way to introduce the topic.

I wonder. . . . At times it is helpful to interject during team meetings or meetings with families when you have something to add or are trying to change the focus of the discussion. To gently interrupt, it is often helpful to start with the phrase, "I wonder" and follow that with, "if it may be helpful to take a step back," or "if perhaps we can look at this a different way."

Strategies to limit the duration of discussions. As clinicians caring for seriously ill patients and families, we are committed to spending the time needed for effective communication. At the same time, discussions with patients and families can go on for extended periods of time, sometimes longer than necessary. Thus, it is helpful to employ strategies that help guide the amount of time we can devote to a visit. To set the stage for a specific duration, you may want to tell a family, "I have about 30 minutes." Then when nearing the end of the time together, it is important to summarize by saying, "So what I am hearing is. . . ." And, finally, you can initiate the wrap by saying, "I am aware of the time." Notably, you can always set up a time for a follow-up discussion.

CONCLUSION

There are many other words used by clinicians in the care of children with life-threatening illness which can relay unintended and potentially harmful messages to children, families, and members of the interdisciplinary team. Even simple words can be harmful. For example, Macdonald and Murray describe in detail how the term "appropriate" has replaced "normal" to describe what is suitable for a particular person, situation, or place.[9] Its use is "appropriate" when being used as a descriptor for the physical condition of the patient, for example, "The child's growth was *appropriate* for his age." However, they argue that the term is increasingly used to pass moral judgment, for example, "The mother's tears were *appropriate* given the news she had just received" or "The father's series of questions were *inappropriate*." From this example they conclude that there are many hidden values behind one's choice of words and phrases and eloquently state, "It is essential that we bring an awareness to our language . . . and reflect on what we mean, what messages we are [trying] to convey"

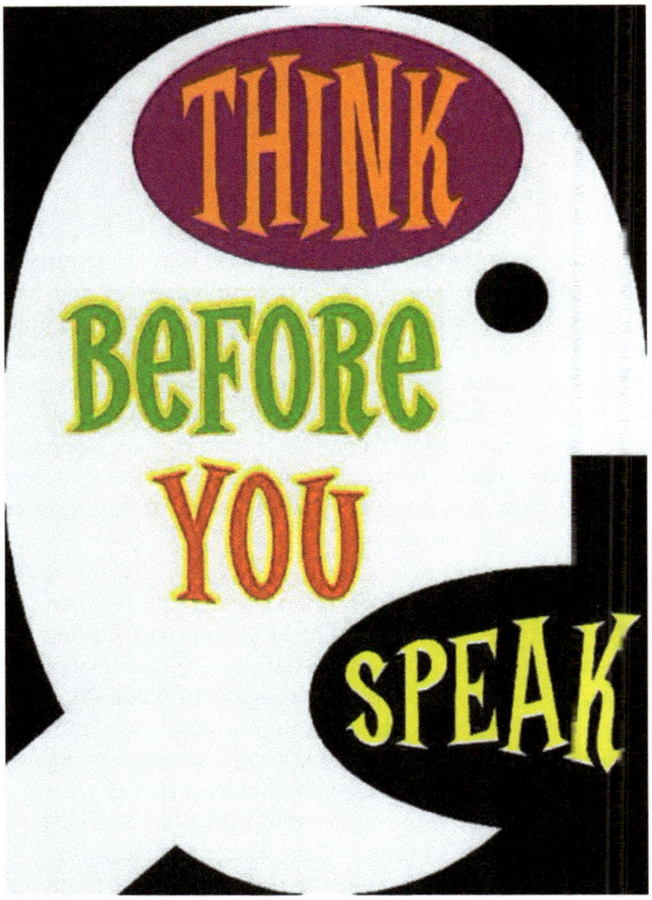

Figure 1.1 *"Thinking Before Speaking No. 2," a painting by John Osgood.* Reproduced with permission from John Osgood.

[1, p.71]. This emphasis on language is not intended to impart a heightened sense of anxiety around communication, rather to underscore the importance of "thinking before speaking" (see Figure 1.1). Furthermore, as eloquently articulated by Ella Wheeler Wilcox in her poem, speaking with authenticity and caring truly conveys meaning. And, if ever something comes out "wrong," it is always "appropriate" to apologize.

REFERENCES

1. Jennings D. The confusion between disease and illness in clinical medicine. *CMAJ*. Oct 15 1986;135(8):865–870.
2. Kelley AM, Bollens-Lund E. Identifying the population with serious illness: The "Denominator" challenge. *J Pall Med.* Mar 1 2018; 21(Suppl 2):S-7–S-16.
3. Feudtner C, Christakis DA, Connell FA. Pediatric deaths attributable to complex chronic conditions: A population-based study of Washington State, 1980–1997. *Pediatrics*. 2000;106(1, pt 2):205–209.
4. WHO Definition of Palliative Care. http://www.who.int/cancer/palliative/definition/en/. Accessed October 30, 2020.
5. Quill TE, Abernethy AP. Generalist plus specialist palliative care: Creating a more sustainable model. *N Engl J Med.* 2013;368:1173–1175.
6. Seaman JB, Lakin JR, Anderson E, Bernacki R, Candrian C, Cotter VT, DeSanto-Madeya S, Epstein AS, Kestenbaum A, Izumi S, Sumser B, Tjia J, Hurd CJ; Sojourns Scholar Interprofessional Working Group. Interprofessional or interdisciplinary: Why terminology in teamwork matters to hospice and palliative care. *J Pall Med.* 2020;23(9):1157–1158.
7. Bluebond-Langner M, Belasco JB, Goldman A, Belasco C. Understanding parents' approaches to care and treatment of children with cancer when standard therapy has failed. *J Clin Oncol.* 2007;25(17):2414–2419.
8. *Newsweek*, May 7, 2001. https://nymag.com/news/features/toni-morrison-2012-5/index.html
9. Jonas DF, Bogetz JF. Identifying the deliberate prevention and intervention strategies of pediatric palliative care teams supporting providers during times of staff distress. *J Pall Med.* 2016;19(6):679–683.
10. Weaver MS, October T, Feudtner C, Hinds PS. "Good-parent beliefs": Research, concept and clinical practice. *Pediatrics.* 2020:145e20194018.
11. Macdonald ME, Murray MA. The appropriateness of *appropriate*: Smuggling values into clinical practice. *Can J Nurs Res.* 2007;39(4):58–73.

2 | THE NEW AND CHANGING LANDSCAPE OF CHILDREN RECEIVING PEDIATRIC PALLIATIVE CARE IN THE US

An Evidence Base Emerges

BRYAN SISK, KIMBERLEY WIDGER, AND CHRIS FEUDTNER

I did then what I knew how to do. Now that I know better, I do better.

MAYA ANGELOU

Team Reflection

In the late 1970s, when a child was born with hypoplastic left heart syndrome, which is a fatal congenital cardiac condition, the babies would be born, they would be OK for a few hours, and then they'd start getting sick. There would be some kind of emergency workup. You would realize, "Oh my gosh, this baby has only one ventricle," and you would gather and say, "Oh, we're sorry there's nothing we can do," and the baby would live for a day or so. And that was hypoplastic left heart. Well, now in 2019, number one, those children are diagnosed at 20-weeks of gestation. They're diagnosed long before they're born, and then there's an opportunity to plan for their delivery. They're delivered in a high-risk center and then there are a series of three complicated surgeries available to the family, so the family can be counseled. "Yes your baby is going to have rough road ahead, but it's certainly not going to be fatal, and the likelihood is your child is going to live, and maybe live through these three surgeries and maybe on to have a heart transplant, and end up in college and beyond," so there are those kinds of developments that create an entire need for palliative care. I mean, if you define palliative care broadly, which includes multidisciplinary support for continuity of care throughout the trajectory of the illness and assisted decision-making, then pediatric palliative care for that child with hypoplastic left heart begins about 5 months before that baby is born and then continues on through all of those different phases of treatment. It's an entirely different ball game.

Now again, back in the '70s, if you were treated for acute lymphoblastic leukemia and then you relapsed, often you died. Now, if you're treated and you relapse, then you go on to a more intensive chemo therapy regimen, and then if you relapse again, you go on to bone marrow transplant, and then if that fails, you usually have a second bone marrow transplant, and if that fails, then you're referred on to CAR-T cell therapy. And so these diseases that were once quite short and fatal are now prolonged and variably successful and so they create and entire need for palliative care along the way.

Ross Hays, MD, Pediatric Palliative Care Physician, Seattle Children's Hospital, excerpted from *Pediatric Palliative Care Oral History Project,* Becker Medical Archives, Washington University School of Medicine.

INTRODUCTION

Pediatric palliative and hospice care (PPC) is now firmly established as a clinical discipline across multiple countries. The evidence base to support PPC practice has grown considerably over the past two decades, but many gaps in knowledge persist. In this chapter, we briefly review the history of foundational PPC research that began more than 50 years ago. We then discuss the current state of PPC research related to the patient experience, the family experience, communication studies, symptom-directed interventions, outcome measure development, and systems of care. We end by highlighting areas in need of further study.

HISTORY OF PEDIATRIC PALLIATIVE AND HOSPICE CARE RESEARCH

PPC did not become a widely recognized clinical specialty until the 21st century, but research into the experiences of children with serious illnesses dates back to the 1950s.[1] In the 1950s and 1960s, pediatricians and psychologists began publishing accounts of the psychological experiences of children with "terminal" illnesses (most commonly cancer) and their mothers. For example, Bozeman, Sutherland, and Orbach published one of the earliest studies of this kind in 1955, in which they described the blunted responses of children with cancer.

> The children were extraordinarily quiet, sometimes apathetic. . . . Their physical condition during hospitalization was largely responsible for limited activity, but the anxiety over separation from their mothers created additional limitations. Crying and moaning were common when mothers were present and increased shortly after they had left.[2]

Others similarly described the experiences of these children and their parents over the ensuing decade.[3–5]

By the 1970s, this psychological research shifted toward more rigorous studies, exemplified by the work of Spinetta and Bluebond-Langner. Spinetta, a psychologist, explored children's awareness of their impending death and their adaptation to this knowledge. He focused on children's anxiety, highlighting their perceptions that nurses and doctors distanced themselves as their disease progressed. Spinetta's work contributed to the development of psychosocial standards for the International Society for Pediatric Oncology (SIOP).[6–10] Bluebond-Langner, an anthropologist, performed ethnographic observations in a pediatric cancer ward, culminating in her landmark book, *The Private Worlds of Dying Children*.[11] Bluebond-Langner's work explored the role of relational and social networks in the way families processed and worked through their children's fatal cancer diagnoses. Notably, her work further explored the concept of mutual pretense that was originally proposed by Glaser and Strauss.[12]

Infants fared even worse than young children. In the mid-1980s, Anand and colleagues published a series of studies demonstrating that infants have robust hormonal and biochemical stress responses after surgery, thus indicating that infants could feel pain in a meaningful way.[16–18] Prior to this work, many physicians commonly believed that infants were unable to experience pain. Some thought that a high pain threshold was evolutionarily adaptive to protect infants from the pain of birth.[19] Additionally, pain prior to that time was viewed as "a subjective phenomenon."[19] Given that infants had limited cognitive capacity, many believed they were unable to experience pain in the same way as adults. Instead, most clinicians believed the infant's manifestations of "pain" to be merely physiological reflexes, similar to tapping the knee with a reflex hammer and watching the leg kick. Even if infants did experience painful stimuli, some argued they were probably unable to remember it after the event. (Surprisingly, this lack of a memory for painful events was reassuring to some clinicians.) As a result of these beliefs about pain, infants routinely underwent major surgeries, even thoracotomies, with paralytics and sedatives but no analgesia.[20]

By 2000, a growing body of literature had begun to explore the physical, psychological, and social experiences of children with life-threatening illnesses. Yet few studies explored actual clinical practices. Wolfe and colleagues published a pair of landmark studies in 2000 that highlighted inadequacies in communication and symptom management for children with cancer at the end of life.[21,22] Soon after, Hilden and colleagues found that pediatric oncologists endorsed "a strikingly high reliance on trial and error in learning to care for dying children."[23] In 2002, Contro and colleagues studied the experiences of bereaved parents, finding evidence of "confusing, inadequate, or uncaring communications regarding treatment or prognosis; preventable oversights in procedures or policies, failure to include or meet the needs of siblings . . . and inconsistent bereavement follow-up."[24] Concurrently, children began to be involved and included in their own care, leading to open communication and engagement in decision-making, especially advanced directives.

From this foundation in the early 2000s, PPC research has expanded rapidly into a growing evidence base. The initial focus on pediatric cancer in PPC research has broadened to include many complex diseases, thus contributing to a shift in PPC from a focus on end of life to a focus on quality of life (QOL), no matter how long or short it might be.

In the following sections, we summarize the current state of research in PPC, and we end by identifying future directions for investigation and development of interventions.

PATIENT EXPERIENCE

While each child receiving PPC services is unique, there are discernable patterns of conditions and diseases, mortality and prognosis, and concerns about symptoms and QOL.

CONDITIONS AND DISEASES

Not all children who die receive PPC services, but national profiles of children who die provide the strongest epidemiological evidence to characterize the conditions and diseases of children receiving PPC. Examining mortality data in the United States between 1999 and 2006, one notices immediately that infant deaths are due mostly to specific perinatal conditions, such as premature birth and congenital syndromes or chromosomal disorders, whereas older children are most likely to die from external causes, such as traumatic injury (Figure 2.1).

We can examine the number of children who die from complex chronic conditions (CCCs) as one statistic that can inform the field of PPC. CCCs are defined as

- Any medical condition that can reasonably be expected to last at least 12 months unless death intervenes,
- Any medical conditions that involves either several organ systems or one organ system severely enough to require specialty pediatric care, with a likelihood of some period in a tertiary care center.

For childhood deaths in the United States, congenital and chromosomal abnormalities were associated with 20.3% of infant and 4.4% of child deaths, while diseases of the nervous system were attributed to 1.3% of infant and 4.8% of child

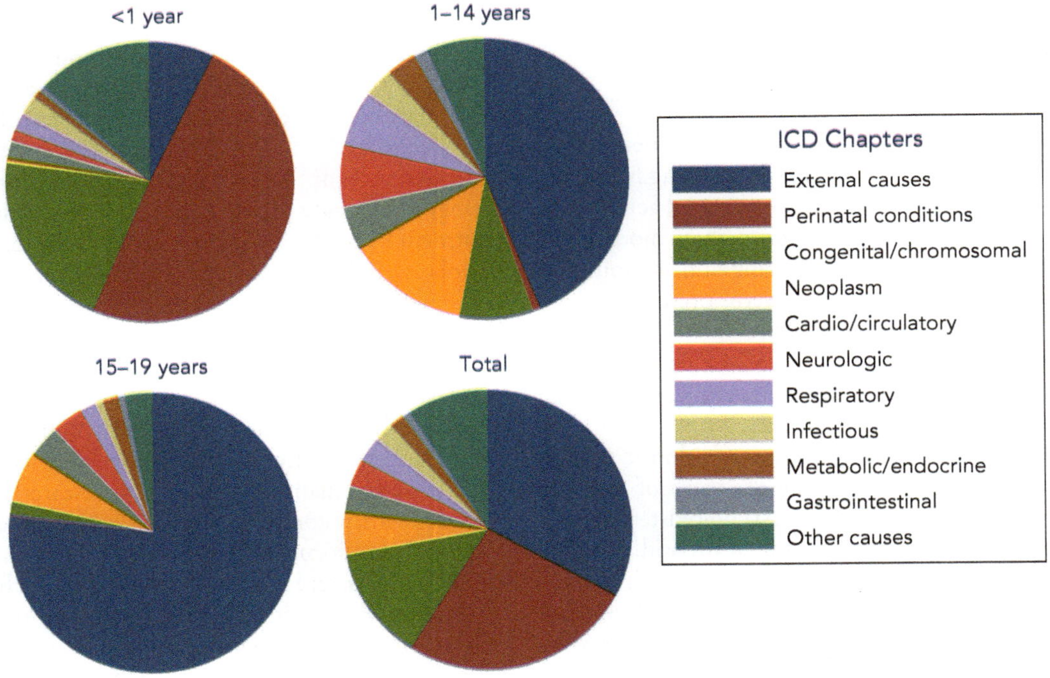

Figure 2.1 Causes of death by age

deaths. Deaths from cancer, which is perhaps the condition most strongly associated with the imagery of palliative care in the mind of the public and much of the healthcare professions, accounted for only 0.5% of infant deaths and 8.9% deaths past infancy.

A few studies of patients enrolled in PPC programs support the evidence of diverse conditions in this population. In a study of 13 PPC programs in Canada, patients had as their primary diagnosis nervous system disorders (26.8%), cancer (15.8%), or perinatal-onset conditions or congenital anomalies (36%).[25,26] At a large children's hospital in the United States, 41.8% of patients who were referred for specialist PPC services had a primary diagnosis of cancer and 38% had congenital or genetic disorders.[27] Moreover, another study evaluated the complexity of patients admitted to a large tertiary children's hospital, finding that nearly half of all children admitted to the hospital suffered from CCCs, and 82% of children were diagnosed with rare diseases.[28]

MORTALITY AND PROGNOSIS

Over the past century, child mortality has been declining for both children suffering from trauma and from CCCs. Examining US mortality data from 1979 to 2006, the rates of death attributed to CCCs as well as injury, sudden infant death syndrome, and other causes declined substantially, with the corresponding numbers of deaths also declining, but less so since 2000.

One published study focused on the interval between 1979 and 1997, when the annual death rate due to non-cancer and cancer-related CCCs declined for almost every age group (from a 7.1% decline for infants with cancer to a 49.9% decline for 1- to 4-year-olds dying from non-cancer CCCs). The one exception to this decline was the mortality attributed to non-cancer CCCs among 20- to 24-year-olds, for whom the rate of death actually increased by 11.6% over this 18-year interval, which may be due to the longer life spans of children with CCCs dying at later ages, such as those with cystic fibrosis and Duchesne's muscular dystrophy.[29] For this reason, studies of pediatric deaths and palliative care need to include the experiences of young adults, perhaps into their 20s or 30s, who are living with these congenital or childhood-onset conditions (Figures 2.2 and 2.3).

PATIENT SYMPTOMS AND QUALITY OF LIFE

The management of physical and psychological symptoms is of utmost importance in PPC. Most research in this area has been conducted with bereaved parents of children with cancer, beginning with Wolfe and colleagues who found a high degree of suffering and lack of treatments offered.[21] Subsequent studies have replicated these findings in multiple countries. In one such study, 96 bereaved Australian parents of children with cancer reported that, in the last month of life, 84% of children suffered from at least one physical symptom (pain, fatigue, poor appetite, constipation, dyspnea, nausea/vomiting, diarrhea, and seizures), with pain, fatigue, and poor appetite as the most frequent complaints.[30] Nearly half (43%) of children in this study suffered from three or more of these symptoms. Parents also reported that 42% of children had been "more than a little sad," 38% experienced "little or no fun," and 21% were "often afraid."

In a Swedish study of 449 bereaved parents of children with cancer, physical fatigue was the most frequently reported

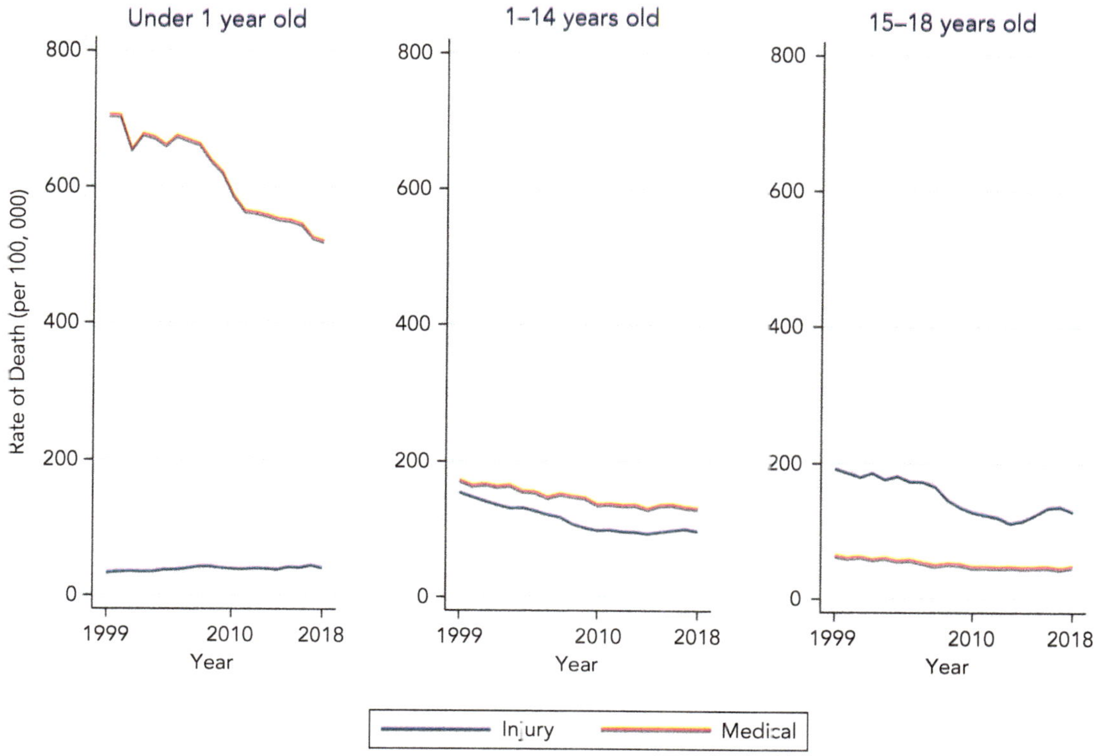

Figure 2.2 Rate of death by age injury vs medical

symptom (86%) that had a moderate or high impact on the child's well-being. Reduced mobility (76%), pain (73%), and decreased appetite (71%) were also major concerns.[31] Parents were also more likely to report anxiety in children older than 9 years of age than in younger children. Children also suffered from difficulties in swallowing, depression, reduced mobility, impaired speech, swelling, disturbed sleep due to anxiety, and urinary problems. Problems with breathing during the last day of life, and with loss of motor function in the last week of life, were also reported in a study of 28 bereaved parents

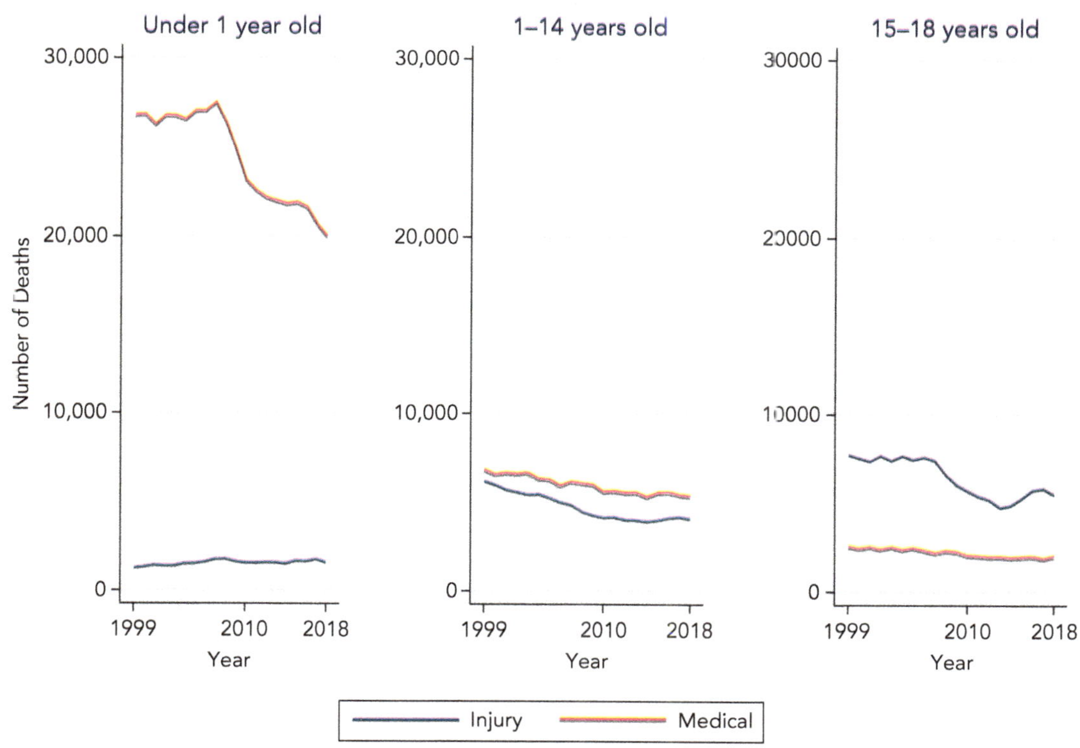

Figure 2.3 Number of deaths by age injury vs medical

whose children had been enrolled in a pediatric hospice program in St. Louis.[32] A study of 65 parents (of 52 children) reported similar symptoms, which did not differ according to patient gender, disease, or location of death.[33] Bereaved parents of 48 children who died of cancer in another study reported that their children suffered from anxiety, which was not treated effectively.[34]

More recently, additional studies of children with cancer have characterized symptoms during therapy and near the end of life. A study in 2010, for example, found that 96% of parents reported that their child with cancer reported fatigue in the last month of life, and 50% reported significant suffering from this fatigue. Of these children, only 13% received any fatigue-related therapy, and only 3% of children received effective treatment for fatigue.[35] Outcomes from the PediQUEST trial identified the following prevalence of symptoms reported primarily by children (or their parent when the child was too young or unable) being treated for advanced cancer: pain (48%), fatigue (46%), drowsiness (39%), and irritability (37%). Reports of pain within the final 12 weeks of life increased to 62%.[36] A subsequent analysis of data from the PediQUEST trial found that children from low-income families were also more likely to report pain (64% vs. 42%). Other measures of psychological distress and QOL did not reach statistical significance, but point estimates of all measures suggested worse outcomes for children from low-income families.[37-40] Much remains to be done in improving the treatment of symptoms in this population.

Researchers have focused less on QOL in the face of serious illness. The PediQUEST study demonstrated strong associations between distressing symptoms and QOL, [41] but few other studies have evaluated QOL in PPC. A key barrier is the lack of instruments specifically developed for use in this population and the evidence that existing generalized instruments may not be suitable for this population of children.[42,43] Currently available instruments tend to focus primarily on physical functioning as a key component of QOL, yet children with cancer have highlighted the importance of social functioning throughout the illness experience.[44] Health professionals have suggested additional domains of QOL, such as living in the present moment and experiencing pleasure, which may be important in the assessment of QOL particularly in advanced illness.[45]

FAMILY EXPERIENCE

When a child has a CCC, the entire family is affected. Furthermore, the ability of the family to adapt to their child's condition can affect (negatively or positively) the experience of the child. For example, the structure and membership of a family, as well as patterns of family organization and function, can influence the care of children with CCCs.[46] Family structure shapes how tasks are divided and roles are assigned in caring for the child. One parent might assume primary physical care for the patient, while the other parent or other family members manage care of the household and siblings. Structure also dictates how families respond to and regulate their intense emotional reactions to a child's illness, which influence daily symptom management, soothing the ill child, and making critical end-of-life decisions. Family structure critically affects how care is performed and is in turn affected by the family's finances, their social and cultural backgrounds or community, and their religious and spiritual beliefs and practices. Additionally, several aspects of care can affect how parents cope with their child's illness and/or death. To varying degrees, the healthcare literature provides useful data and knowledge about each of these topics.

FAMILY STRUCTURE

Parents of children with serious illness report negative effects in many aspects of their lives including family life, finances, social life, and physical health.[47,48] Social support may serve as a protective factor for some families.[49,50]

Families vary in how they function, and some families may be characterized by high conflict levels, poor cohesion, poor communication, and a tendency to reject healthcare.[51,52] Even within a family, parents may differ in how they experience and cope with a child's illness.[53,54] Such families may be considered "difficult" families by clinical staff, especially if there is a history of limited family support, inconsistent caregivers, and multiple living environments.[55]

Some research initially suggested that two-parent married households of children receiving palliative care who died were at higher risk for divorce[56], but later research found that these parents were not necessarily at greater risk for divorce.[57] In fact, some may experience positive benefits, such as feeling closer as a family and supporting each other, which offset the stresses.[58] One study of families of children diagnosed with cancer found that, while many families went through a period of difficulty and stress in terms of marital, parent–child, and sibling conflict, the majority of families were able to weather the storm and maintain good family relationships.[59] Caregiver- and family-focused interventions may help families cope with the stress of caring for a child with a life-threatening illness.[60–62]

When parents are divorced, remarried, or have never been married, complex relationships (spouses, ex-spouses, step-children, step-siblings, other extended family) and a history of conflict may undermine communication and support efforts by clinicians,[63] especially when the nonresidential parent has a different opinion about the child's care than that of the custodial parent.[64] Having multiple or discordant decision-makers within the family can contribute to conflicts both within the family and with clinical staff.[65]

Single-parent households have been less frequently studied,[66] but some evidence suggests that single mothers of children with serious illness may have higher stress-related symptoms, their children might have higher hospitalization rates, the parent may engage in fewer health-maintaining behaviors, and the parent may feel more isolated.[67,68] Other studies on children with disabilities and children being treated with cancer suggest that single parents had greater difficulty with finances[69] but also were more flexible in adapting to new family roles and arrangements.[70] Children in the foster care system with serious illness may have unique needs because of a history of prior trauma and abuse.[71] These prior traumas could impact the child's coping responses and exacerbate psychological and social insults from their disease process. In these scenarios, psychologists and social workers provide critical skills and guidance to PPC teams.

Social and cultural characteristics of families can also affect family functioning. Numerous studies indicate that racial and ethnic minorities may have difficulties with poverty, less trust and poorer communication with the medical profession, and different belief systems and family structures.[72–76] Religion and spirituality are very important to many families, but the impact of these beliefs is not uniform or prescriptive.[77–79] Some families appreciate spiritual and religious support from clinicians but prefer that such support be initiated by the family based on their needs.[80,81] Discussing religion and spirituality with families is considered an advanced communication skill that not all clinicians are comfortable with.[82,83]

THE WORK OF CARE

Although most children with serious illness die in the hospital, some children with serious illness are cared for and die at home.[84,85] Although this allows families to spend more time together at home, it also requires much work on their part.[86] This work of care consists of the effort, labor, and various tasks in which parents and other family members engage in to care for the child with a CCC and for the family system. Daily tasks include administering medications, feeding and bathing, providing emotional support, and monitoring any changes in the child's health.[87–91] Some parents are responsible for maintaining complex technology such as ventilators, which, in addition to the stress of keeping the ventilator going, may wake parents up in the middle of the night when alarms go off.[92,93] Parents also are responsible for managing their child's medical care by arranging and bringing their child to appointments and filling out copious amounts of paperwork[94] while creating an environment in which their child can have as normal a life as possible.[95] These efforts can occupy a great deal of time.[96] One study of parents whose children had gastrostomy tubes, compared to parents whose children did not, found parents in the first group devoted more than 7 hours a day to technical and nontechnical care of the child compared to 3 hours in the second group.[97] How this work is organized, distributed, and completed likely varies across family structures, and some evidence also exists that stronger family function is related to better execution of disease management activities.[98–100]

PSYCHOLOGICAL DISTRESS AND COPING

Parents of children with serious illness can experience acute emotional distress and high levels of uncertainty about their child's future.[101–105] Parents and siblings have been observed to suffer from an array of psychological and physical forms of distress: parents report depression, grief, guilt, and anxiety as well as problems such as insomnia, headaches, and musculoskeletal pain. One study of parents of children with severe cardiac disease, compared to parents of healthy children, found substantial decrements in the parents' QOL in general and specifically regarding emotions, physical health, and vitality.[98] Also, posttraumatic stress disorder (PTSD) was first described in survivors of childhood cancer in the late 1980s.[106,107] Subsequent research has documented the presence of PTSD in 10% of mothers of childhood cancer survivors but noted that 95% of mothers met the criteria for one component of PTSD, namely re-experiencing.[108] PTSD symptoms have been noted in other populations including parents of children who received care in critical care settings.[109] Bereaved parents also report symptoms of PTSD long after their child's death. One study surveyed parents 13 months after their child died in an intensive care unit (ICU), finding that many parents reported symptoms of PTSD (35% of mothers and 24% of fathers) and depression (35% of mothers and 30% of fathers).[110] Another study evaluated parents 5 years after their child was diagnosed with cancer, finding that 19% of mothers and 8% of fathers reported symptoms of PTSD. For bereaved parents, 20% of mothers and 35% of fathers reported PTSD symptoms.[111] In another study of parents 5 years after their child was diagnosed with cancer, 66% of parents reported low peace of mind, regardless of their child's relapse status. This low peace of mind was associated with persistent worries about relapse, new toxicities, and persistent limitations on their child's life as a result of the cancer and its treatment.[112]

For families of children with CCCs, engagement and effective communication with clinical teams might support coping and adaptations. In a qualitative analysis of focus groups, bereaved parents highlighted the importance of maintaining relationships with the clinical team, the benefits of high-quality communication, and the impact of negative interactions with clinicians on their grief.[113] Furthermore, a study of parents whose children received PPC found a positive association between higher ratings of communication and continuity of care with lower levels of long-term parental grief. Higher reports of the child's symptom burden, however, were associated with higher levels of long-term grief.[114] Some of this grief might be related to the challenges parents face in meeting the needs of everyone in their family. One mixed-methods study found that parents engage in "parenting triage," a process by which parents make difficult tradeoffs in their perceived responsibilities and obligations to all the children in the family. Parents described the "emotional and relational consequences of agonizing decisions made addressing needs of one family member over needs of another." These parents felt "torn, guilty, overwhelmed, frustrated, afraid, exhausted, and heartbroken."[115] Another study focused on population-based data on the psychological outcomes of mothers and siblings of children with cancer, finding that mothers and siblings were more likely to seek psychological care than the general population, with the risk being highest among mothers who were younger, of lower socioeconomic status, and of rural residence.[116]

The impact of a sibling's death can be long-lasting. Siblings may struggle with fears, traumatic reactions, isolation, difficulties in school and social settings, and the behavior problems that result.[117] Nearly all bereaved siblings in one survey-based study reported that their sibling's death still affected them 12 years later, and half of these respondents reported that this death affected their current educational and career goals.[118] When asked for advice in another study, one-third of bereaved siblings said they had needed better medical information when their sibling was alive. Also, these participants recommended that clinicians provide clear guidance to parents about how to engage their other children before and after their child's death.[119]

Beyond these findings, few methodologically rigorous studies have examined the impact of a child's death on family members or the family structure. Much of what is known about parental reactions to a child's death is based on samples of those who present for psychological treatment; presumably, a much larger percentage of bereaved families experience essentially normal patterns of grief and other mental health consequences from the death of a child without ever presenting for clinical care. Estimates of psychopathology in bereaved parents are therefore likely to be erroneously high.

FINANCIAL CONCERNS

A family's financial concerns are related to both the work of care and coping. Many parents of children with serious illness report struggling to figure out how to cover the expenses associated with medical care and lost income due to missing work to care for the child.[37,69,120,121] In particular, three areas of finances—insurance, paid work, and out-of-pocket expenses—are affected by caring for a child with a CCC. Due to the high costs of care, families may have difficulty finding or keeping insurance coverage and may find that certain services are not covered or that caps on spending prevent other services from being used.[122] Often in families caring for a child with a CCC, one family member, usually the mother, decides to stay at home, forsaking the income and benefits provided by paid work.[123,124] For example, 52% of parents in one study reported a change in their job status due to their child's illness, and only 52% of parents reported that their current job allowed them sufficient time to care for their child.[125] Out-of-pocket expenditures are also very high and might further impoverish families.[126] Although the Family and Medical Leave Act has provided some protections, parents report "difficulties in accessing and using benefits, including lack of knowledge by employers, complexity of rules and processes, and inadequacy of the benefits themselves."[127] Furthermore, only about half of Americans are eligible for these benefits, and the protected time off is unpaid, which can exacerbate financial distress.

COMMUNICATION STUDIES

Communication is an essential tool for palliative care clinicians, especially in pediatrics. Clinicians must navigate the communication preferences and needs of the child, the parents, and the siblings. In some situations, parents might also request support in communicating with their extended family or social support network.

Although communication is central to the role of palliative care clinicians, research on communication in pediatrics has largely focused on the pediatric oncology population. Additionally, most published studies are descriptive in nature, with limited (if any) studies of interventions to bolster communication outcomes. However, this body of literature continues to grow, and recent psychosocial palliative care standards reinforce the central role of communication in palliative care.[128,129] Here, we briefly highlight key findings and limitations in this communication literature, focusing on communication with parents and communication with children.

COMMUNICATION WITH PARENTS

Most parents of children with life-threatening illnesses report a desire for disclosure of difficult information, such as poor prognosis or future limitations for the child. For example, most parents of children with cancer indicate that they value and prefer transparent disclosure of this information, even if it is upsetting.[130,131] Despite clinicians' concerns about negative effects of this disclosure, many parents report that such information actually supports their hope despite its upsetting nature because it resolves uncertainty about the future.[132]

Yet many parents' communication needs are unmet. A national survey study from Denmark found that 42% of bereaved parents felt that information about their child's end of life was given too late, and 31% felt they were "deprived of the option to say goodbye to their child in their preferred manner."[133] Even when parents of children with cancer report "high-quality" communication, many still hold inaccurate estimates of prognosis and future limitations.[134,135] In part, these inaccuracies might result from the positive framing of this communication. For example, a study of neonatal ICU (NICU) family conferences found that discussions were optimistically framed and focused on the functional needs of the child rather than QOL for the infant or family. In this study, "most parents left the conference believing their infant's prognosis to be more optimistic than did clinicians." [136]

COMMUNICATION ACROSS CULTURES

Communication among individuals from different social or cultural backgrounds poses additional challenges. For example, parents of color report higher unmet information needs. One study in pediatric oncology found that 87% of parents wanted as much detail as possible about their child's prognosis, and this preference did not vary by race or ethnicity. However, significantly more physicians believed that black and Hispanic parents were less interested in this information.[137] Similarly, parents did not vary in their preferred role in decision-making by race or ethnicity. Yet physicians were significantly less likely to accurately predict the preferred role of parents of color (53% for white parents, 23% for black parents, 37% for Hispanic parents, and 43% for Asian/other race parents).[138] Additionally, parents of color held more active roles in decision-making than they preferred, which has been associated with increased decisional regret in other studies.[139] These challenges can be further exacerbated when parents speak different languages and clinicians must rely on interpreters.[140] However, most communication research samples have underrepresented people of color and non-English speakers. Moving forward, more research is needed to ensure communication practices are meeting the needs of all families, regardless of race, ethnicity, or culture.

COMMUNICATION WITH CHILDREN

Communicating with children who have CCCs can challenge clinical teams for many reasons. First, some children with CCCs have limited cognitive capacity, which can impede communication efforts. Additionally, children will undergo substantial physical, developmental, and social changes as they grow. In each stage of development, children have different concerns, capacities, and preferences for involvement in their care.[141] Parents and clinicians can also feel a sense of duty to protect the child from any harms of communication.[142] Given these complexities, it is unsurprising that most communication literature has focused on adolescents and young adults (AYA) rather than young children. As such, we will focus this section on AYA studies.

Similar to studies of parents, most AYA patients with life-threatening illnesses value information about their treatment prognosis, and future limitations. One oncology study, for example, found that 85–96% of AYA patients reported that prognostic information was very or extremely important throughout the first year after diagnosis of cancer. Additionally, 76–85% of patients reported that a numeric estimate of prognosis was very or extremely important.[143] Another study of 10- to 18-year-old patients with cancer found a widespread desire for more communication about QOL, pain and symptom management, and prognosis.[144] However, many of these communication needs are unmet. For example, one study found that AYA patients' involvement in communication about their relapsed cancer was limited to responding to questions and participating in the history and physical examination.[145] Recent research highlights the importance of communicating directly with the AYA patient as there is not always strong congruence between patients' reported needs and their families' understanding of these needs.[146] Despite this desire for information, AYA patients need the information tailored to their social and cognitive development. Otherwise, clinicians might be viewed as "aloof, patronizing or cold."[147]

Other studies have explored the preferred role of AYA patients in decision-making. Again, nearly all of these studies have focused on cancer populations. One study, for example, found that 53% of AYA patients with cancer wanted to share in decision-making with their physician, and 51% preferred their parents to have limited involvement.[148] Another study found that AYA patients with advanced cancer or HIV infection "want to be able to choose and record (1) the kind of medical treatment they want and do not want, (2) how they would like to be cared for, (3) information for their family and friends to know, and (4) how they would like to be remembered."[149] Such goals can be supported by advanced care planning guides,[150] and many AYA patients have the desire and capacity to engage in such meaningful deliberation.[151] However, only a minority of AYA patients with life-threatening illnesses utilize such advanced care planning tools.[152] Much work is needed to better understand how to communicate effectively with children of all ages who have life-threatening illnesses, especially illnesses beyond cancer.

LIMITATIONS IN THE COMMUNICATION LITERATURE

The literature on communication in PPC is growing, but still has several limitations. First, nearly all studies have been observational or descriptive, with limited development of communication interventions. In a 2019 review article of communication interventions in oncology, no studies specifically targeted communication in pediatric oncology.[153] Although a similar review article does not exist for communication interventions in PPC, we suspect similar limitations exist.

Some studies have attempted to determine the effect of specialist PPC consultation on improving communication with parents, but these studies tend to be methodologically flawed. For example, a systematic review from 2019 explored the impact of specialist PPC consultation on communication experiences for parents. The authors concluded that studies suggest some positive benefit, but they rated 58% of studies as poor quality. The poor quality of these studies limits the utility of these results.[154]

Another challenge in communication research is the dearth of reliable measures of communication effectiveness. For example, the previously mentioned oncology review article found that 88 communication intervention studies used 188 different outcome measures for communication, with 156 of these measures used only by single studies.[153] Without consistent and theory-driven outcome measures that are used across studies, comparison of results will remain a challenge.

INTERVENTIONS AND OUTCOMES

Most research in PPC to date has described patient characteristics, symptom burdens, and communication practices, among other topics. These descriptive studies have created the foundation for PPC research, but intervention studies are necessary to improve the care of children with CCCs. In recent years, the number of intervention studies in PPC has started to grow. Next, we describe the current state of studies on pharmacological and nonpharmacological symptom management. Similar to the need for interventions, this field also needs robust and reliable outcome measures to test and monitor the effectiveness of PPC interventions. Here, we also review the current literature on outcome measures in PPC.

PALLIATIVE CARE SERVICES

Several studies (including randomized control trials and observational designs) have examined the impact of receiving palliative care services, essentially as a bundle of different interventions, on patient and family outcomes. Patients receiving PPC experience reduced suffering, receive fewer medications and procedures, and are more likely to have medical orders setting limits on care received.[155,156] Early integration of PPC has been found to be both feasible and beneficial for families.[157–159] Other researchers have shown the benefits of providing PPC in outpatient and home settings.[160–162]

INTERDISCIPLINARY, TEAM-BASED CARE

Providing palliative care to children with CCCs requires collaborative, interdisciplinary care. No single clinician or profession can provide appropriate care and attention to the child's psychological, social, spiritual, emotional, and medical needs. Despite a growing body of evidence on team science,[163–166] little work in PPC has focused on the functioning of interdisciplinary teams. In one study of parents whose children had refractory cancer, only 47% of parents described their medical team's teamwork as excellent.[167] Other studies have explored the role of teamwork in communication, identifying several barriers to inclusion of nurses in difficult conversations.[168,169] Interdisciplinarity is the hallmark of effective PPC, and future studies must further explore the functioning of teams and develop data-driven best practices.

PHARMACOLOGIC TREATMENTS

Medications are one of the mainstays of modern medicine. Polypharmacy is usually considered a problematic phenomenon among geriatric patients, but children admitted to children's hospitals are typically exposed to five different medications (median count) during their hospitalization, with 10% of the patients exposed to 14 or more medications. By the time pediatric patients have been hospitalized for a month or more, the 10% receiving the most medication have been exposed to 40 or more medications.[170]

The drugs used to treat children who are receiving palliative or hospice care have not yet been well-described. In a cohort of 834 pediatric patients enrolled in hospices across the United States, the most commonly used class of drug was opioids (72% of all patients), followed by hypnotics (60%), laxatives and other medications for the bowels (50%), antacids and other medications for the stomach (41%), and anti-epileptic drugs (38%) (unpublished data). In the United Kingdom, a small study found that 21 children being treated by hospice services received a median of 10 medications, ranging from 3 to 23. The most commonly used drugs were anti-epileptics (27%), analgesics (16%), laxatives (8%), anti-reflux agents (6%), muscle relaxants (6%), and anti-cholinergic agents (5%).[171]

The use of specific medications appears to vary substantially across hospitals and hospices. For instance, in a study of 626 children's and general hospitals (which include many NICUs) in the United States, among terminal hospitalizations the exposure to opioids varied across hospitals from 0.7% to 99.1%, with the interquartile range extending from 35.3% to 59.5%.[172] Studies of more specific pharmacologic interventions in PPC have been rare. Most pertinent studies have focused on children with cancer. For example, some groups have studied topical and systemic treatments for peripheral neuropathy,[173] phantom limb pain,[174] pain with needle insertion,[175] and opioid-refractory cancer-related pain.[176]

NONPHARMACOLOGIC TREATMENTS

Medications are only one of many possible interventions used in PPC to ameliorate symptoms or improve QOL. Much less is known about the epidemiology of other interventions, such as a child's exposure to complementary and alternative medical (CAM) practices. In one study of 92 parents of children with cancer in the United States, 49% reported that their children used at least one type of CAM and 20% used herbal remedies, homeopathy, or vitamins in the 2 months preceding the survey,[177] which suggests that, if any of these children died, some may have continued to receive CAM treatments at the end of life.

A small number of clinical trials from other medical disciplines have evaluated nonpharmacological approaches to pain and symptom management. Some of these interventions have focused on psychological interventions to improve symptom management. For example, trials have tested cognitive-behavioral therapy[178] and yoga[179] as adjuvant treatments for pain for children with sickle cell disease. Others have studied the use of guided imagery to decrease pain and anxiety for children undergoing surgery[180] Additionally, the PRISM study evaluated the impact of a brief intervention targeting stress management, goal-setting, cognitive reframing, and meaning-making on supporting resilience for children with cancer or diabetes mellitus type 1.[181,182] Similar interventions should be developed and evaluated in PPC in the future.

OUTCOME MEASURES

To ensure that interventions and PPC services are benefiting patients, researchers and clinical teams need reliable and appropriate outcome measures. Currently, researchers and clinicians have not identified consensus definitions or measures of value or effectiveness. This deficiency presents a major barrier to ensuring the quality and efficacy of specialized PPC. For example, a 2019 scoping review of outcome measures in PPC identified 46 studies that compared specialized PPC with usual care. Of these studies, one was a randomized controlled trial. The most commonly used indicators were location of death, length of stay in hospital, and number of hospital admissions. Overall, these studies used 82 different indicators, and only 22 of these indicators were defined the same way in at least two studies.[183] Another group performed a systematic review of instruments to measure outcomes in PPC. They found 15 articles that utilized quantitative measures and 9 of these measures were estimated to have at least moderate quality. Only 5 of these measures included patient-reported outcomes. Also, the authors noted, "We had no access to the developmental process of the instruments used to present the underlying concepts that were underpinning the constructs."[184]

MULTILEVEL SYSTEM OF CARE

Children with CCCs receive care in a broad range of settings, spanning from the child's home to ICUs, with each level of this complex overall system of care playing important roles for these children and their families.

CARE IN THE HOME

PPC in the home is intended to increase the QOL of patients and families, and some, if not a majority, families prefer being at home to care for the child.[88] From 1989 to 1993, only 12.3% of children with CCCs died in the home; from 1999 to 2003, 17.7% of children with CCCs died in the home. In the same period, hospital deaths declined and deaths at all other sites and care institutions remained comparably stable.[185] This pattern of a rising proportion of pediatric deaths attributed to CCCs occurring at home is traceable to 1979, shortly after the first study demonstrated that families could support dying children in their homes.[186] Over the same time periods, stark differences in the proportion of deaths that occurred at home are evident and persistent among patients classified on their death certificates as white, Hispanic, or black.[185]

Home care usually involves the partnering of skilled nurses with the parents, who are able to share knowledge and divide tasks related to the work of care.[187] Issues to be considered in home care include the work of care, impact on the family, the likelihood of adverse events, and cost.[88,188–191] In a study of parents of 48 children who died from cancer, 88% of parents chose "at home" as the most appropriate location of death in hindsight, but only 41% of parents provided palliative care in the home and 48% of children died at home.[34]

HOSPICE CARE

The term "hospice" has different meanings in different contexts. In the United States, hospice care is defined operationally by insurance coverage benefits and is provided by dedicated hospice agencies and their staff; care is almost always in a patient' home or in a specific hospice facility or hospital. In Canada, hospice typically refers to a free-standing building. In the United Kingdom, hospice care can refer to either palliative care in general or to the buildings where respite care and end-of-life care are provided for children.

A study of Florida Medicaid pediatric patients who died revealed that only 11% received any hospice services, but those who did were more likely to be non-Hispanic whites than non-Hispanic black and have chronic conditions and longer Medicaid enrollment than non-hospice users.[192] In a study of pediatric oncologists, physicians with access to hospice that accepted patients receiving chemotherapy had more patients die outside the hospital, but not all hospices admit patients actively receiving chemotherapy.[193] A broader survey of pediatric medical providers experienced in end-of-life care reported that 86% of responders thought hospice was beneficial, especially in the provision of nonmedical services.[194]

HOSPITALS

While there is a trend of increasing hospice and home-based PPC, pediatric death still occurs mostly in the hospital setting. From 1989 to 2003, 80.1% of childhood deaths resulting from CCCs occurred in the hospital (down from 85.7% in 1989 to 2003), with considerable variation in the location of death by CCC category.[185] The same study also demonstrated that infants and children from racial and ethnic minorities were more likely to die in the hospital than were older children and nonminority children.

Hospitalizations of children with CCCs who subsequently died were characterized by long lengths of stay, mechanical ventilation during their terminal admissions, and death in the ICU. In a study that linked information from death certificates to hospital use records from 1990 to 1996 in Washington state, 458 infants with CCCs who died under a week of age spent 92% of their lives in the hospital, and 286 infants with CCCs who died during the second to twelfth months of life spent 41% of all their lives in the hospital.[195] For children and young adults with CCCs, the median time spent in the hospital in the year preceding death was 18 days, and a third of this group was hospitalized until the last week of life. Across all age groups, rates of hospital use increased closer to the child's death. Half of hospitalized infants and 19% of children and young adults with CCCs were mechanically ventilated during their terminal admission. Studies from hospitals in a range of countries (the United States, Australia, and the Netherlands) suggest that although a number of deaths take place in the operating room and emergency departments, most pediatric deaths occur in the ICU.[196–199] In a study of a UK children's hospital, infants with congenital malformations and perinatal conditions were most likely to die in the ICU (odds ratio [OR] 2.42; 95% confidence interval [CI]1.65, 1.35), and older children with cancer were the most likely to die outside the ICU (OR 6.5; 95% CI 4.4, 9.6).[200]

A more recent Canadian study of 1,620 children evaluated the costs associate with end-of-life care, finding that most children who died in Ontario received end-of-life care in acute care settings. The average cost of healthcare in a child's last year of life was $78,332 (Canadian), with a median cost of $18,450. Two-thirds of these costs were incurred in acute care settings. The vast majority of children with perinatal/congenital illness (88%) and chronic illness (80%)

died in acute care settings. Only 33% of children received any home care during their last year of life.[201]

Over the past decade, hospital-based palliative care services have begun in many pediatric hospitals across the country. An evaluation of the impact of one such interdisciplinary program in Boston documented, after the program's establishment, an increased frequency of hospice discussions (76% vs. 54%, for an adjusted risk difference of 22%), earlier documentation of do-not-resuscitate orders (18 vs. 12 days), and fewer deaths in the ICU or in other hospitals (decrease of 16%). Parents also reported that their child suffered less pain (adjusted risk difference of 19%) and that they felt more prepared during their child's last month of life and at the death.[202] In another study on the impact of a PPC program in Germany, 69% of families preferred to have their child at home for the death compared to 18% of families before the program was instituted.[203] Yet barriers to consultation persist. A systematic review of specialist PPC initiation in pediatric cancer, for example, found that 55% of pediatric oncology patients received any specialist PPC services prior to their death. The first discussion of PPC and initiation of PPC often occurred shortly before the child's death.[204]

RESPITE AND OTHER MODALITIES OF CARE

Beyond hospital and hospice care, other modalities of care might also be useful for seriously ill children. Broadening the definition of the population in need to encompass children with complex or special healthcare needs, respite care provides parents with time off from being in charge of this care. Respite care also has different meanings and purposes attributed to it by different families.[205] In a study among caregivers of children with cerebral palsy in Canada, 46% of caregivers reported using respite services in the past year, and 90% of caregivers indicated that respite was beneficial for both the child and family.[206] In another study of children with special healthcare needs, researchers demonstrated that a program in an emergency department setting to provide telephone advice and care coordination enhanced parental satisfaction with emergency care.[207] Furthermore, respite care through a pediatric hospice can serve as an entry point to palliative care services for families who initially have concerns about seeking these services.[208]

FUTURE DIRECTIONS

PPC is now firmly established as a professional medical discipline across multiple countries. The body of research to support this field is growing, but many unanswered questions remain. For guidance, we will refer to the results of a workshop of PPC leaders and researchers, in which they identified seven priorities for future research. These should be prioritized as PPC investigators develop research agendas in the future (Box 2.1).

BOX 2.1 SEVEN PRIORITIES FOR PEDIATRIC PALLIATIVE CARE RESEARCH

Bolster training and development of PPC investigators
Develop core resources
Advance symptom measurement (and measurements of other exposures and outcomes)
Improve symptom management and quality of life interventions
Improve communication, elicitation of goals of care, and decision-making
Understand family impact and facilitate or improve family adaptation and coping
Analyze and improve systems of care, policy, and education

Adapted from Feudtner C, Rosenberg AR, Boss RD, et al. Challenges and priorities for pediatric palliative care research in the U.S. and similar practice settings: Report from a pediatric palliative care research network workshop. *J Pain Symptom Manage.* 2019;58(5):909–917.e3.

REFERENCES

1. Sisk BA, Feudtner C, Bluebond-Langner M, Sourkes B, Hinds PS, Wolfe J. Response to suffering of the seriously ill child: A history of palliative care for children. *Pediatrics.* 2019:e20191741.
2. Bozeman MF, Orbach CE, Sutherland AM. Psychological impact of cancer and its treatment. III. The adaptation of mothers to the threatened loss of their children through leukemia. I. *Cancer.* 1955;8(1):1–19.
3. Orbach CE, Sutherland AM, Bozeman MF. Psychological impact of cancer and its treatment. III. The adaptation of mothers to the threatened loss of their children through leukemia. II *Cancer.* 1955;8(1):21–33.
4. Richmond JB, Waisman HA. Psychologic aspects of management of children with malignant diseases. *AMA Am J Dis Child.* 1955;89(1):42–47.
5. Morrissey J. Children's adaptation to fatal illness. *Social Work.* 1963;8(4):81–88.
6. Spinetta JJ, Maloney LJ. The child with cancer: Patterns of communication and denial. *J Consult Clin Psychol.* 1978;46(6):1540–1541.
7. Spinetta J. Adjustment in children with cancer. *J Pediatr Psychol.* 1977;2(2):49–51.
8. Spinetta J, Maloney J. Death anxiety in the outpatient leukemic child. *Pediatrics.* 1975;56(6):1035–1037.
9. Spinetta JJ, Rigler D, Karon M. Personal space as a measure of a dying child's sense of isolation. *J Consult Clin Psychol.* 1974;42(6):751–756.
10. Spinetta JJ, Rigler D, Karon M. Anxiety in the dying child. *Pediatrics.* 1973;52(6):841–845.
11. Bluebond-Langner M. *The Private Worlds of Dying Children.* Princeton, NJ: Princeton University Press; 1978.
12. Glaser BG, Strauss AL. *Awareness of Dying* (1st ed.). New Brunswick, NJ: Aldine Transaction; 1965.
13. Eland JM, Anderson JE. The experience of pain in children. In Jacox AK, ed. *Pain: A Source Book for Nurses and Other Health Professionals.* New York: Little, Brown; 1977:453–478.
14. Beyer JE, DeGood DE, Ashley LC, Russell GA. Patterns of postoperative analgesic use with adults and children following cardiac surgery. *Pain.* 1983;17(1):71–81.
15. Schechter NL, Allen DA, Hanson K. Status of pediatric pain control: A comparison of hospital analgesic usage in children and adults. *Pediatrics.* 1986;77(1):11–15.
16. Anand KJ. The stress response to surgical trauma: From physiological basis to therapeutic implications. *Prog Food Nutr Sci.* 1986;10(1–2):67–132.
17. Anand KJ, Brown MJ, Bloom SR, Aynsley-Green A. Studies on the hormonal regulation of fuel metabolism in the human

newborn infant undergoing anaesthesia and surgery. *Horm Res.* 1985;22(1-2):115–128.

18. Anand KJ, Brown MJ, Causon RC, Christofides ND, Bloom SR, Aynsley-Green A. Can the human neonate mount an endocrine and metabolic response to surgery? *J Pediatr Surg.* 1985;20(1):41–48.
19. Anand KJ, Hickey PR. Pain and its effects in the human neonate and fetus. *N Engl J Med.* 1987;317(21):1321–1329.
20. Harrison H. Why infant surgery without anesthesia went unchallenged. *New York Times.* 1987, December 17.
21. Wolfe J, Grier HE, Klar N, et al. Symptoms and suffering at the end of life in children with cancer. *N Engl J Med.* 2000;342(5):326–333.
22. Wolfe J. Suffering in children at the end of life: Recognizing an ethical duty to palliate. *J Clin Ethics.* 2000;11(2):157–163.
23. Hilden JM, Emanuel EJ, Fairclough DL, et al. Attitudes and practices among pediatric oncologists regarding end-of-life care: Results of the 1998 American Society of Clinical Oncology survey. *J Clin Oncol.* 2001;19(1):205–212.
24. Contro NA, Larson J, Scofield S, Sourkes B, Cohen HJ. Hospital staff and family perspectives regarding quality of pediatric palliative care. *Pediatrics.* 2004;114(5):1248–1252.
25. Widger K, Davies D, Rapoport A, et al. Pediatric palliative care in Canada in 2012: A cross-sectional descriptive study. *CMAJ Open.* 2016;4(4):E562–E568.
26. Widger K, Davies D, Drouin DJ, et al. Pediatric patients receiving palliative care in Canada: Results of a multicenter review. *Arch Pediatr Adolesc Med.* 2007;161(6):597–602.
27. Thrane SE, Maurer SH, Cohen SM, May C, Sereika SM. Pediatric palliative care: A five-year retrospective chart review study. *J Palliat Med.* 2017;20(10):1104–1111.
28. Bösch A, Wager J, Zernikow B, et al. Life-limiting conditions at a university pediatric tertiary care center: A cross-sectional study. *J Palliat Med.* 2018;21(2):169–176.
29. Feudtner C, Hays RM, Haynes G, Geyer JR, Neff JM, Koepsell TD. Deaths attributed to pediatric complex chronic conditions: National trends and implications for supportive care services. *Pediatrics* 2001;107(6):E99.
30. Heath JA, Clarke NE, Donath SM, McCarthy M, Anderson VA, Wolfe J. Symptoms and suffering at the end of life in children with cancer: An Australian perspective. *Med J Austral.* 2010;192(2):71–75.
31. Jalmsell L, Kreicbergs U, Onelov E, Steineck G, Henter JI. Symptoms affecting children with malignancies during the last month of life: A nationwide follow-up. *Pediatrics.* 2006;117(4):1314–1320.
32. Hendricks-Ferguson V. Physical symptoms of children receiving pediatric hospice care at home during the last week of life. *Oncol Nurs Forum.* 2008;35(6):E108–115.
33. Pritchard M, Burghen E, Srivastava DK, et al. Cancer-related symptoms most concerning to parents during the last week and last day of their child's life. *Pediatrics.* 2008;121(5):e1301–1309.
34. Hechler T, Blankenburg M, Friedrichsdorf SJ, et al. Parents' perspective on symptoms, quality of life, characteristics of death and end-of-life decisions for children dying from cancer. *Klin Padiatr.* 2008;220(3):166–174.
35. Ullrich CK, Dussel V, Hilden JM, et al. Fatigue in children with cancer at the end of life. *J Pain Symptom Manage.* 2010;40(4):483–494.
36. Wolfe J, Orellana L, Ullrich C, et al. Symptoms and Distress in Children With Advanced Cancer: Prospective Patient-Reported Outcomes From the PediQUEST Study. *J Clin Oncol.* 2015;33(17):1928–1935.
37. Bona MF, Al-Sayegh H, Ma C, et al. The relationship between household income and patient-reported symptom distress and quality of life in children with advanced cancer: A report from the PediQUEST study. *Cancer.* 2018;124(19):3934–3941.
38. Steele R, Siden H, Cadell S, et al. Charting the territory: Symptoms and functional assessment in children with progressive, non-curable conditions. *Arch Dis Child.* 2014;99(8):754–762.
39. Baume ED, Balkin EM, Aiyagari R, et al. Parental perspectives on suffering and quality of life at end-of-life in children with advanced heart disease: An exploratory study. *Pediatr Crit Care Med.* 2014;15(4):336–342.
40. Friedrichsdorf SJ, Postier AC, Andrews GS, Hamre KE, Steele R, Siden H. Pain reporting and analgesia management in 270 children with a progressive neurologic, metabolic or chromosomally based condition with impairment of the central nervous system: Cross-sectional, baseline results from an observational, longitudinal study. *J Pain Res.* 2017;10:1841–1852.
41. Rosenberg AR, Orellana L, Ullrich C, et al. Quality of life in children with advanced cancer: A report from the PediQUEST Study. *J Pain Symptom Manage.* 2016;52(2):243–253.
42. Huang IC, Shenkman EA, Madden VL, Vadaparampil S, Quinn G, Knapp CA. Measuring quality of life in pediatric palliative care: Challenges and potential solutions. *Palliat Med.* 2010;24(2):175–182.
43. Coombes LH, Wiseman T, Lucas G, Sangha A, Murtagh FE. Health-related quality-of-life outcome measures in paediatric palliative care: A systematic review of psychometric properties and feasibility of use. *Palliat Med.* 2016;30(10):935–949.
44. Anthony SJ, Selkirk E, Sung L, Klaassen RJ, Dix D, Klassen AF. Quality of life of pediatric oncology patients: Do patient-reported outcome instruments measure what matters to patients? *Quality of Life Res.* 2017;26(2):273–281.
45. Avoine-Blondin J, Parent V, Lahaye M, Humbert N, Duval M, Sultan S. Identifying domains of quality of life in children with cancer undergoing palliative care: A qualitative study with professionals. *Palliat Support Care.* 2017;15(5):565–574.
46. Patterson JM. Integrating family resilience and family stress theory. *J Marriage Fam.* 2002;64(2):349–360.
47. Zimmermann K, Bergstraesser E, Engberg S, et al. When parents face the death of their child: A nationwide cross-sectional survey of parental perspectives on their child's end-of life care. *BMC Palliative Care.* 2016;15(30).
48. Silva-Rodrigues FM, Pan R, Pacciulio Sposito AM, de Andrade Alvarenga W, Nascimento LC. Childhood cancer: Impact on parents' marital dynamics. *Eur J Oncol Nurs.* 2016;23:34–42.
49. Stremler R, Haddad S, Pullenayegum E, Parshuram C. Psychological outcomes in parents of critically ill hospitalized children. *J Pediatr Nurs.* 2017;34:36–43.
50. Boyden JY, Hill DL, Carroll KW, Morrison WE, Miller VA, Feudtner C. The association of perceived social support with anxiety over time in parents of children with serious illnesses. *J Palliat Med.* 2020 Apr;23(4):527–534.
51. Schuler TA, Zaider TI, Li Y, et al. Perceived family functioning predicts baseline psychosocial characteristics in US participants of a family focused grief therapy trial. *J Pain Symptom Manage.* 2017;54(1):126–131.
52. Schuler TA, Zaider TI, Li Y, Hichenberg S, Masterson M, Kissane DW. Typology of perceived family functioning in an American sample of patients with advanced cancer. *J Pain Symptom Manage.* 2014;48(2):281–288.
53. Sood E, Karpyn A, Demianczyk AC, et al. Mothers and fathers experience stress of congenital heart disease differently. *Pediatr Crit Care Med.* 2018;19(7):626–634.
54. Bailey-Pearce O, Stedmon J, Dallos R, Davis G. Fathers' experiences of their child's life-limiting condition: An attachment narrative perspective. *Clin Child Psychol Psychiatry.* 2018 Jul;23(3):381–397. doi:10.1177/1359104517730115.
55. Meltzer LJ, Steinmiller E, Simms S, Grossman M; Complex Care Consultation Team, Li Y. Staff engagement during complex pediatric medical care: the role of patient, family, and treatment variables. *Patient Educ Couns.* 2009 Jan;74(1):77–83. doi:10.1016/j.pec.2008.07.051.
56. Martin P. Marital breakdown in families of patients with spina bifida cystica. *Develop Med Child* Neurol. 1975;17(6):757–764.
57. Cappelli M, McGarth PJ, Daniels T, Manion I, Schillinger J. Marital quality of parents of children with spina bifida: A case-comparison study. *J Dev Behav Pediatr.* 1994;15(5):320–326.

58. Barbarin OA, Hughes D, Chesler MA. Stress, coping, and marital functioning among parents of children with cancer. *J Marriage Family.* 1985;47(2):473–480.
59. Katz LF, Fladeboe K, Lavi I, et al. Trajectories of marital, parent-child, and sibling conflict during pediatric cancer treatment. *Health Psychol.* 2018;37(8):736–745.
60. Sheng N, Ma J, Ding W, Zhang Y. Effects of caregiver-involved interventions on the quality of life of children and adolescents with chronic conditions and their caregivers: A systematic review and meta-analysis. *Quality of Life Res.* 2018;28(1):13–33.
61. Rosenberg AR, Bradford MC, Junkins CC, et al. Effect of the Promoting Resilience in Stress Management Intervention for Parents of Children With Cancer (PRISM-P): A randomized clinical trial. *JAMA Network Open.* 2019;2(9):e1911578.
62. Barrera M, Alexander S, Atenafu EG, Chung J, Hancock K, Solomon A, Desjardins L, Shama W, Mills D. Psychosocial screening and mental health in pediatric cancer: A randomized controlled trial. *Health Psychol.* 2020 May;39(5):381–390.
63. Lichtenthal WG, Kissane DW. The management of family conflict in palliative care. *Prog Palliat Care.* 2008;16(1):39–45.
64. Ganong L, Doty ME, Gayer D. Mothers in postdivorce families caring for a child with cystic fibrosis. *J Pediatr Nurs.* 2003;18(5):332–343.
65. Forbat L, Sayer C, McNamee P, Menson E, Barclay S. Conflict in a paediatric hospital: A prospective mixed-method study. *Arch Dis Child.* 2016;101(1):23–27.
66. Brown RT, Wiener L, Kupst MJ, et al. Single parents of children with chronic illness: An understudied phenomenon. *J Pediatr Psychol.* 2008;33(4):408–421.
67. Macpherson C, Redmond AO, Leavy A, McMullan M. A review of cystic fibrosis children born to single mothers. *Acta Paediatr.* 1998;87(4):397–400.
68. Wiener L, Viola A, Kearney J, et al. Impact of caregiving for a child with cancer on parental health behaviors, relationship quality, and spiritual faith: Do lone parents fare worse? *J Pediatr Oncol Nurs.* 2016;33(5):378–386.
69. Bona K, London WB, Guo D, Frank DA, Wolfe J. Trajectory of material hardship and income poverty in families of children undergoing chemotherapy: A prospective cohort study. *Pediatr Blood Cancer.* 2016;63(1):105–111.
70. McCubbin MA. Family stress and family strengths: A comparison of single- and two-parent families with handicapped children. *Res Nurs Health.* 1989;12(2):101–110.
71. Lindley LC, Slayter EM. Prior trauma exposure and serious illness at end of life: A national study of children in the U.S. foster care system from 2005 to 2015. *J Pain Symptom Manage.* 2018;56(3):309–317.
72. Rehm RS. Cultural intersections in the care of Mexican American children with chronic conditions. *Pediatr Nurs.* 2003;29(6):434–439.
73. Elfert H, Anderson JM, Lai M. Parents' perceptions of children with chronic illness: A study of immigrant Chinese families. *J Pediatr Nurs.* 1991;6(2):114–120.
74. Williams HA. A comparison of social support and social networks of black parents and white parents with chronically ill children. *Soc Sci Med.* 1993;37(12):1509–1520.
75. McCubbin HI, Thompson EA, Thompson AI, McCubbin MA, Kaston AJ. Culture, ethnicity, and the family: Critical factors in childhood chronic illnesses and disabilities. *Pediatrics.* 1993;91(5 Pt 2):1063–1070.
76. Watts KJ, Meiser B, Zilliacus E, et al. Communicating with patients from minority backgrounds: Individual challenges experienced by oncology health professionals. *Eur J Oncol Nurs.* 2017;26:83–90.
77. Feudtner C, Haney J, Dimmers MA. Spiritual care needs of hospitalized children and their families: A national survey of pastoral care providers' perceptions. *Pediatrics.* 2003;111(1):e67–e72.
78. Robinson MR, Thiel MM, Backus MM, Meyer EC. Matters of spirituality at the end of life in the pediatric intensive care unit. *Pediatrics.* 2006;118(3):e719–729.
79. Superdock AK, Barfield RC, Brandon DH, Docherty SL. Exploring the vagueness of Religion & Spirituality in complex pediatric decision-making: A qualitative study. *BMC Palliat Care.* 2018;17(1):107.
80. McNamara LC, Okoniewski W, Maurer SH, Moehling K, Hall DE, Schenker Y. "Give them the door but don't push them through it": Family Attitudes Toward Physician-Led Spiritual Care in Pediatric Palliative Medicine. *J Relig Health.* 2020 Dec;59(6):2899–2917
81. Uveges MK, Hamilton JB, DePriest K, Boss R, Hinds PS, Nolan MT. The influence of parents' religiosity or spirituality on decision making for their critically ill child: An integrative review. *J Palliat Med.* 2019;22(11):1455–1467.
82. Ford DW, Downey L, Engelberg R, Back AL, Curtis JR. Discussing religion and spirituality is an advanced communication skill: An exploratory structural equation model of physician trainee self-ratings. *J Palliat Med.* 2012;15(1):63–70.
83. Kaye EC. Finding faith. *JAMA.* 2020;323(7):609–610.
84. Hoell JI, Weber HL, Balzer S, et al. Advance care planning and outcome in pediatric palliative home care. *Oncotarget.* 2018;9(25):17867–17875.
85. de Banate MA, Maypole J, Sadof M. Care coordination for children with medical complexity. *Curr Opin Pediatr.* 2019;31(4):575–582.
86. Kuo DZ, Cohen E, Agrawal R, Berry JG, Casey PH. A national profile of caregiver challenges among more medically complex children with special health care needs. *Arch Pediatr Adolesc Med.* 2011;165(11):1020–1026.
87. Monaghan MC, Hilliard ME, Cogen FR, Streisand R. Nighttime caregiving behaviors among parents of young children with Type 1 diabetes: Associations with illness characteristics and parent functioning. *Fam Syst Health.* 2009;27(1):28–38.
88. Wang KW, Barnard A. Caregivers' experiences at home with a ventilator-dependent child. *Qual Health Res.* 2008;18(4):501–508.
89. Kirk S, Glendinning C, Callery P. Parent or nurse? The experience of being the parent of a technology-dependent child. *J Adv Nurs.* 2005;51(5):456–464.
90. Sullivan-Bolyai S, Deatrick J, Gruppuso P, Tamborlane W, Grey M. Constant vigilance: Mothers' work parenting young children with type 1 diabetes. *J Pediatr Nurs.* 2003;18(1):21–29.
91. Koch KD, Jones BL. Supporting parent caregivers of children with life-limiting illness. *Children (Basel).* 2018;5(7).
92. Kuster PA, Badr LK. Mental health of mothers caring for ventilator-assisted children at home. *Issues Ment Health Nurs.* 2006;27(8):817–835.
93. Meltzer LJ, Mindell JA. Impact of a child's chronic illness on maternal sleep and daytime functioning. *Arch Intern Med.* 2006;166(16):1749–1755.
94. Osterlund CS, Dosa NP, Arnott Smith C. Mother knows best: Medical record management for patients with spina bifida during the transition from pediatric to adult care. *AMIA Annu Symp Proc.* 2005:580–584.
95. Williams C. Alert assistants in managing chronic illness: The case of mothers and teenage sons. *Sociol Health Illness.* 2000;22(2):254–272.
96. Curran AL, Sharples PM, White C, Knapp M. Time costs of caring for children with severe disabilities compared with caring for children without disabilities. *Develop Med Child Neurol.* 2001;43(8):529–533.
97. Heyman MB, Harmatz P, Acree M, et al. Economic and psychologic costs for maternal caregivers of gastrostomy-dependent children. *J Pediatr.* 2004;145(4):511–516.
98. Arafa MA, Zaher SR, El-Dowaty AA, Moneeb DE. Quality of life among parents of children with heart disease. *Health Quality of Life Outc.* 2008;6:91.
99. Fiese BH, Wamboldt FS, Anbar RD. Family asthma management routines: Connections to medical adherence and quality of life. *J Pediatr.* 2005;146(2):171–176.
100. Lewin AB, Heidgerken AD, Geffken GR, et al. The relation between family factors and metabolic control: The role of diabetes adherence. *J Pediatr Psychol.* 2006;31(2):174–183.

101 Oxley R. Parents' experiences of their child's admission to paediatric intensive care. *Nursing Children and Young People.* 2015;27(4):16–21.
102. Kearney JA, Salley CG, Muriel AC. Standards of psychosocial care for parents of children with cancer. *Pediatr Blood Cancer.* 2015;62 Suppl 5:S632–683.
103. Diaz-Caneja A, Gledhill J, Weaver T, Nadel S, Garralda E. A child's admission to hospital: A qualitative study examining the experiences of parents. *Intens Care Med.* 2005;31(9):1248–1254.
104. Bally JMG, Smith NR, Holtslander L, et al. A metasynthesis: Uncovering what is known about the experiences of families with children who have life-limiting and life-threatening illnesses. *J Pediatr Nurs.* 2018;38:88–98.
105. Katz LF, Fladeboe K, King K, et al. Trajectories of child and caregiver psychological adjustment in families of children with cancer. *Health Psychol.* 2018;37(8):725–735.
106. Y.N. Posttraumatic stress disorder in children with cancer. In Pyncos ESaR, ed. *Posttraumatic Stress Disorder in Children.* Washington, D.C.: American Psychiatric Press; 1985:121–132.
107. Pot-Mees, C.C. *The Psychological Effect of Bone Marrow Transplantation in Children.* Delft: Eburon; 1989.
108. Kazak AE, Alderfer M, Rourke MT, Simms S, Streisand R, Grossman JR. Posttraumatic stress disorder (PTSD) and posttraumatic stress symptoms (PTSS) in families of adolescent childhood cancer survivors. *J Pediatr Psychol.* 2004;29(3):211–219.
109. Shaw RJ, Bernard RS, Deblois T, Ikuta LM, Ginzburg K, Koopman C. The relationship between acute stress disorder and posttraumatic stress disorder in the neonatal intensive care unit. *Psychosomatics.* 2009;50(2):131–137.
110. Youngblut JM, Brooten D, Cantwell GP, del Moral T, Totapally B. Parent health and functioning 13 months after infant or child NICU/PICU death. *Pediatrics.* 2013;132(5):e1295–1301.
111. Ljungman L, Hoven E, Ljungman G, Cernvall M, von Essen L. Does time heal all wounds? A longitudinal study of the development of posttraumatic stress symptoms in parents of survivors of childhood cancer and bereaved parents. *Psychooncology.* 2015;24(12):1792–1798.
112. Sisk BA, Weng S, Mack JW. Persistently low peace of mind in parents of cancer patients: A five-year follow-up study. *Pediatr Blood Cancer.* 2019;0(0):e27609.
113. Snaman JM, Kaye EC, Torres C, Gibson DV, Baker JN. Helping parents live with the hole in their heart: The role of health care providers and institutions in the bereaved parents' grief journeys. *Cancer.* 2016;122(17):2757–2765.
114. van der Geest IM, Darlington AS, Streng IC, Michiels EM, Pieters R, van den Heuvel-Eibrink MM. Parents' experiences of pediatric palliative care and the impact on long-term parental grief. *J Pain Symptom Manage.* 2014;47(6):1043–1053.
115. Mooney-Doyle K, Deatrick JA, Ulrich CM, Meghani SH, Feudtner C. Parenting in childhood life-threatening illness: A mixed-methods study. *J Palliat Med.* 2018;21(2):208–215.
116. van Warmerdam J, Sutradhar R, Kurdyak P, et al. Long-term mental health outcomes in mothers and siblings of children with cancer: A population-based, matched cohort study. *J Clin Oncol.* 2020;38(1):51–62.
117. Alderfer MA, Labay LE, Kazak AE. Brief report: Does posttraumatic stress apply to siblings of childhood cancer survivors? *J Pediatr Psychol.* 2003;28(4):281–286.
118. Rosenberg AR, Postier A, Osenga K, et al. Long-term psychosocial outcomes among bereaved siblings of children with cancer. *J Pain Symptom Manage.* 2015;49(1):55–65.
119. Lovgren M, Bylund-Grenklo T, Jalmsell L, Wallin AE, Kreicbergs U. Bereaved siblings' advice to health care professionals working with children with cancer and their families. *J Pediatr Oncol Nurs.* 2016;33(4):297–305.
120. Bilodeau M, Ma C, Al-Sayegh H, Wolfe J, Bona K. Household material hardship in families of children post-chemotherapy. *Pediatr Blood Cancer.* 2018;65(1).
121. Thomson J, Shah SS, Simmons JM, et al. Financial and social hardships in families of children with medical complexity. *J Pediatr.* 2016;172:187–193.e181.
122. Satchell M, Pati S. Insurance gaps among vulnerable children in the United States, 1999–2001. *Pediatrics.* 2005;116(5):1155–1161.
123. Thyen U, Kuhlthau K, Perrin JM. Employment, child care, and mental health of mothers caring for children assisted by technology. *Pediatrics.* 1999;103(6 Pt 1):1235–1242.
124. Porterfield SL. Work choices of mothers in families with children with disabilities *J Marriage Fam.* 2002;64(4):972–981.
125. Siden H, Steele R. Charting the territory: Children and families living with progressive life-threatening conditions. *Paediatr Child Health.* 2015;20(3):139–144.
126. Lukemeyer A, Meyers MK, Smeeding T. Expensive children in poor families: Out-of-pocket expenditures for the care of disabled and chronically ill children in welfare families. *J Marriage Family.* 2000;62(2):399–415.
127. Chung PJ, Garfield CF, Elliott MN, Carey C, Eriksson C, Schuster MA. Need for and use of family leave among parents of children with special health care needs. *Pediatrics.* 2007;119(5):e1047–1055.
128. Wiener L, Kazak AE, Noll RB, Patenaude AF, Kupst MJ. Standards for the psychosocial care of children with cancer and their families: An introduction to the special issue. *Pediatr Blood Cancer.* 2015;62(S5):S419–S424.
129. Weaver MS, Heinze KE, Kelly KP, et al. Palliative care as a standard of care in pediatric oncology. *Pediatr Blood Cancer.* 2015;62 Suppl 5(Suppl 5):S829–833.
130. Sisk BA, Greenzang KA, Kang TI, Mack JW. Longitudinal parental preferences for late effects communication during cancer treatment. *Pediatr Blood Cancer.* 2018 Jan;65(1).
131. Sisk BA, Kang TI, Mack JW. Prognostic disclosures over time: Parental preferences and physician practices. *Cancer.* 2017;123(20):4031–4038.
132. Nyborn JA, Olcese M, Nickerson T, Mack JW. "Don't try to cover the sky with your hands": Parents' experiences with prognosis communication about their children with advanced cancer. *J Palliat Med.* 2016;19(6):626–631.
133. Lykke C, Ekholm O, Schmiegelow K, Olsen M, Sjøgren P. End-of-life communication: A nationwide study of bereaved parents' perceptions. *BMJ Support Palliat Care.* 2019 Jul 11:bmjspcare-2018-001709.
134. Kaye E, Mack JW. Parent perceptions of the quality of information received about a child's cancer. *Pediatr Blood Cancer.* 2013;60(11):1896–1901.
135. Mack JW, Cronin AM, Uno H, Shusterman S, Twist CJ, Bagatell R, Rosenberg A, Marachelian A, Granger MM, Glade Bender J, Baker JN, Park J, Cohn SL, Levine A, Taddei S, Diller LR. Unrealistic parental expectations for cure in poor-prognosis childhood cancer. *Cancer.* 2020 Jan 15;126(2):416–424.
136. Boss RD, Lemmon ME, Arnold RM, Donohue PK. Communicating prognosis with parents of critically ill infants: Direct observation of clinician behaviors. *J Perinatol.* 2017;37(11):1224–1229.
137. Ilowite MF, Cronin AM, Kang TI, Mack JW. Disparities in prognosis communication among parents of children with cancer: The impact of race and ethnicity. *Cancer.* 2017;123(20):3995–4003.
138. Sisk BA, Kang TI, Mack JW. Racial and Ethnic Differences in Parental Decision-Making Roles in Pediatric Oncology. *J Palliat Med.* 2020 Feb;23(2):192–197.
139. Sisk BA, Kang TI, Mack JW. The evolution of regret: decision-making for parents of children with cancer. *Support Care Cancer.* 2020 Mar;28(3):1215–1222.
140. Davies B, Contro N, Larson J, Widger K. Culturally-sensitive information-sharing in pediatric palliative care. *Pediatrics.* 2010;125(4):e859–865.
141. Stein A, Dalton L, Rapa E, et al. Communication with children and adolescents about the diagnosis of their own life-threatening condition. *Lancet.* 2019;393(10176):1150–1163.

142. Sisk BA, Bluebond-Langner M, Wiener L, Mack J, Wolfe J. Prognostic disclosures to children: A historical perspective. *Pediatrics.* 2016;138(3):pii: e20161278.
143. Sisk BA, Fasciano K, Block SD, Mack JW. Longitudinal prognostic communication needs of adolescents and young adults with cancer. *Cancer.* 2020 Jan 15;126(2):400–407.
144. Levine DR, Liederbach E, Johnson LM, Kaye EC, Spraker-Perlman H, Mandrell B, Pritchard M, Sykes A, Lu Z, Wendler D, Baker JN. Are we meeting the informational needs of cancer patients and families? Perception of physician communication in pediatric oncology. *Cancer.* 2019 May 1;125(9):1518–1526.
145. Frederick NN, Mack JW. Adolescent patient involvement in discussions about relapsed or refractory cancer with oncology clinicians. *Pediatr Blood Cancer.* 2018 Apr;65(4).
146. Friebert S, Grossoehme DH, Baker JN, et al. Congruence gaps between adolescents with cancer and their families regarding values, goals, and beliefs about end-of-life care. *JAMA Network Open.* 2020;3(5):e205424–e205424.
147. Zebrack B, Chesler MA, Kaplan S. To foster healing among adolescents and young adults with cancer: What helps? What hurts? *Support Care Cancer.* 2010;18(1):131–135.
148. Mack JW, Fasciano KM, Block SD. Adolescent and young adult cancer patients' experiences with treatment decision-making. *Pediatrics.* 2019:e20182800.
149. Wiener L, Zadeh S, Battles H, et al. Allowing adolescents and young adults to plan their end-of-life care. *Pediatrics.* 2012;130(5):897–905.
150. Zadeh S, Pao M, Wiener L. Opening end-of-life discussions: How to introduce Voicing My CHOiCES, an advance care planning guide for adolescents and young adults. *Palliat Support Care.* 2015;13(3):591–599.
151. Needle JS, Peden-McAlpine C, Liaschenko J, et al. "Can you tell me why you made that choice?": A qualitative study of the influences on treatment decisions in advance care planning among adolescents and young adults undergoing bone marrow transplant. *Palliat Med.* 2019:269216319883977.
152. Needle J, Smith AR. The impact of advance directives on end-of-life care for adolescents and young adults undergoing hematopoietic stem cell transplant. *J Palliat Med.* 2016;19(3):300–305.
153. Sisk BA, Schulz GL, Mack JW, Yaeger L, DuBois J. Communication interventions in adult and pediatric oncology: A scoping review and analysis of behavioral targets. *PLoS One.* 2019;14(8):e0221536.
154. Streuli JC, Widger K, Medeiros C, Zuniga-Villanueva G, Trenholm M. Impact of specialized pediatric palliative care programs on communication and decision-making. *Patient Educ Couns.* 2019;102(8):1404–1412.
155. Seddighzadeh RP, Lawrence K, Hamby T, Hoeft A. Influence of palliative care on medical treatment of pediatric patients with complex chronic diseases at cook children's medical center. *J Palliat Med.* 2018;21(11):1617–1620.
156. Gans D, Kominski GF, Roby DH, et al. Better outcomes, lower costs: Palliative care program reduces stress, costs of care for children with life-threatening conditions. *Policy Brief UCLA Cent Health Policy Res.* 2012(PB2012-3):1–8.
157. Callahan K, Steinwurtzel R, Brumarie L, Schechter S, Parravicini E. Early palliative care reduces stress in parents of neonates with congenital heart disease: Validation of the "Baby, Attachment, Comfort Interventions." *J Perinatol.* 2019;39(12):1640–1647.
158. Hendricks-Ferguson VL, Haase JE. Parent perspectives of receiving early information about palliative and end-of-life care options from their child's pediatric providers. *Cancer Nurs.* 2019;42(4):E22–e30.
159. Liberman DB, Song E, Radbill LM, Pham PK, Derrington SF. Early introduction of palliative care and advanced care planning for children with complex chronic medical conditions: A pilot study. *Child Care Health Dev.* 2016;42(3):439–449.
160. Brock KE, Snaman JM, Kaye EC, et al. Models of pediatric palliative oncology outpatient care-benefits, challenges, and opportunities. *J Oncol Pract.* 2019;15(9):476–487.
161. Kaye EC, Rubenstein J, Levine D, Baker JN, Dabbs D, Friebert SE. Pediatric palliative care in the community. *CA: Cancer Journal for Clinicians.* 2015;65(4):316–333.
162. Friedrichsdorf SJ, Postier A, Dreyfus J, Osenga K, Sencer S, Wolfe J. Improved quality of life at end of life related to home-based palliative care in children with cancer. *J Palliat Med.* 2015;18(2):143–150.
163. Cannon-Bowers J, Salas E, Converse S. Shared mental models in expert team decision-making. In: Castellan J, NJ, ed. *Individual and Group Decision Making: Current Issues.* Hillsdale, NJ: Erlbaum; 2001:221–246.
164. DeChurch LA, Mesmer-Magnus JR. Measuring shared team mental models: A meta-analysis. *Group Dynamics: Theory, Research, and Practice.* 2010;14(1):1–14.
165. Kosty MP, Hanley A, Chollette V, Bruinooge SS, Taplin SH. National Cancer Institute-American Society of Clinical Oncology Teams in Cancer Care Project. *J Oncol Pract.* 2016;12(11):955–958.
166. Weaver AC, Callaghan M, Cooper AL, Brandman J, O'Leary EJ. Assessing interprofessional teamwork in inpatient medical oncology units. *J Oncol Pract.* 2015;11(1):19–22.
167. Feraco AM, Ananth P, Dussel V, Al-Sayegh H, Ma C, Rosenberg AR, Feudtner C, Wolfe J. Parent Perceptions of Team-Delivered Care for Children With Advanced Cancer: A Report From the PediQUEST Study. *J Pain Symptom Manage.* 2020 Oct;60(4):811–817.
168. Anderson WG, Puntillo K, Boyle D, et al. ICU bedside nurses' involvement in palliative care communication: A multicenter survey. *J Pain Symptom Manage.* 2016;51(3):589–596.e582.
169. Newman AR, Haglund K, Rodgers CC. Pediatric oncology nurses' perceptions of prognosis-related communication. *Nurs Outlook.* 2019;67(1):101–114.
170. Feudtner C, Dai D, Hexem KR, Luan X, Metjian TA. Prevalence of polypharmacy exposure among hospitalized children in the United States. *Arch Pediatr Adolesc Med.* 2012;166(1):9–16.
171. Mtunzi NM, Baba M. Polypharmacy in paediatric palliative care. *Arch Dis Child.* 2019;104:A187–A188.
172. Womer J, Zhong W, Kraemer FW, et al. Variation of opioid use in pediatric inpatients across hospitals in the U.S. *J Pain Symptom Manage.* 2014;48(5):903–914.
173. Rossignol J, Cozzi B, Liebaert F, et al. High concentration of topical amitriptyline for treating chemotherapy-induced neuropathies. *Support Care Cancer.* 2019;27(8):3053–3059.
174. Wang X, Yi Y, Tang D, et al. Gabapentin as an adjuvant therapy for prevention of acute phantom-limb pain in pediatric patients undergoing amputation for malignant bone tumors: A prospective double-blind randomized controlled trial. *J Pain Symptom Manage.* 2018;55(3):721–727.
175. Cozzi G, Borrometi F, Benini F, et al. First-time success with needle procedures was higher with a warm lidocaine and tetracaine patch than an eutectic mixture of lidocaine and prilocaine cream. *Acta paediatrica (Oslo, Norway: 1992).* 2017;106(5):773–778.
176. Gibbons K, DeMonbrun A, Beckman EJ, et al. Continuous lidocaine infusions to manage opioid-refractory pain in a series of cancer patients in a pediatric hospital. *Pediatr Blood Cancer.* 2016;63(7):1168–1174.
177. Martel D, Bussieres JF, Theoret Y, et al. Use of alternative and complementary therapies in children with cancer. *Pediatr Blood Cancer.* 2005;44(7):660–668.
178. Schatz J, Schlenz AM, McClellan CB, et al. Changes in coping, pain, and activity after cognitive-behavioral training: A randomized clinical trial for pediatric sickle cell disease using smartphones. *Clin J Pain.* 2015;31(6):536–547.
179. Moody K, Abrahams B, Baker R, et al. A randomized trial of yoga for children hospitalized with sickle cell vaso-occlusive crisis. *J Pain Symptom Manage.* 2017;53(6):1026–1034.
180. Vagnoli L, Bettini A, Amore E, De Masi S, Messeri A. Relaxation-guided imagery reduces perioperative anxiety and pain in children: A randomized study. *Eur J Pediatr.* 2019 Jun;178(6):913–921.
181. Rosenberg AR, Bradford MC, McCauley E, Curtis JR, Wolfe J, Baker KS, Yi-Frazier JP. Promoting resilience in adolescents and young adults with cancer: Results from the PRISM randomized controlled trial. *Cancer.* 2018 Oct 1;124(19):3909–3917

182. Rosenberg AR, Bradford MC, Junkins CC, Taylor M, Zhou C, Sherr N, Kross E, Curtis JR, Yi-Frazier JP. Effect of the Promoting Resilience in Stress Management Intervention for Parents of Children With Cancer (PRISM-P): A randomized clinical trial. *JAMA Netw Open*. 2019 Sep 4;2(9):e1911578.
183. Widger K, Medeiros C, Trenholm M, Zuniga-Villanueva G, Streuli JC. Indicators Used to Assess the Impact of Specialized Pediatric Palliative Care: A Scoping Review. *J Palliat Med*. 2019 Feb;22(2):199–219.
184. Friedel M, Aujoulat I, Dubois AC, Degryse JM. Instruments to Measure Outcomes in Pediatric Palliative Care: A Systematic Review. *Pediatrics*. 2019 Jan;143(1):e20182379.
185. Feudtner C, Feinstein JA, Satchell M, Zhao H, Kang TI. Shifting place of death among children with complex chronic conditions in the United States, 1989-2003. *Jama*. 2007;297(24):2725–2732.
186. Martinson IM, Armstrong GD, Geis DP, et al. Home care for children dying of cancer. *Pediatrics*. 1978;62(1):106–113.
187. McIntosh J, Runciman P. Exploring the role of partnership in the home care of children with special health needs: Qualitative findings from two service evaluations. *Int J Nurs Stud*. 2008;45(5):714–726.
188. Leonard BJ, Brust JD, Nelson RP. Parental distress: Caring for medically fragile children at home. *J Pediatr Nurs*. 1993;8(1):22–30.
189. Stevens B, Croxford R, McKeever P, et al. Hospital and home chemotherapy for children with leukemia: A randomized cross-over study. *Pediatr Blood Cancer*. 2006;47(3):285–292.
190. Leonard BJ, Brust JD, Sielaff BH. Determinants of home care nursing hours for technology-assisted children. *Public Health Nurs*. 1991;8(4):239–244.
191. Teague BR, Fleming JW, Castle A, et al. "High-tech" home care for children with chronic health conditions: A pilot study. *J Pediatr Nurs*. 1993;8(4):226–232.
192. Knapp CA, Shenkman EA, Marcu MI, Madden VL, Terza JV. Pediatric palliative care: Describing hospice users and identifying factors that affect hospice expenditures. *J Palliat Med*. 2009;12(3):223–229.
193. Fowler K, Poehling K, Billheimer D, et al. Hospice referral practices for children with cancer: A survey of pediatric oncologists. *J Clin Oncol*. 2006;24(7):1099–1104.
194. Dickens DS. Comparing pediatric deaths with and without hospice support. *Pediatr Blood Cancer*. 2010;54(5):746–750.
195. Feudtner C, DiGiuseppe DL, Neff JM. Hospital care for children and young adults in the last year of life: A population-based study. *BMC Med*. 2003;1:3.
196. Lantos JD, Berger AC, Zucker AR. Do-not-resuscitate orders in a children's hospital. *Crit Care Med*. 1993;21(1):52–55.
197. Ashby MA, Kosky RJ, Laver HT, Sims EB. An enquiry into death and dying at the Adelaide Children's Hospital: A useful model? *Med J Austral*. 1991;154(3):165–170.
198. van der Wal ME, Renfurm LN, van Vught AJ, Gemke RJ. Circumstances of dying in hospitalized children. *Eur J Pediatr*. 1999;158(7):560–565.
199. McCallum DE, Byrne P, Bruera E. How children die in hospital. *J Pain Symptom Manage*. 2000;20(6):417–423.
200. Ramnarayan P, Craig F, Petros A, Pierce C. Characteristics of deaths occurring in hospitalised children: Changing trends. *J Med Ethics*. 2007;33(5):255–260.
201. Widger K, Seow H, Rapoport A, Chalifoux M, Tanuseputro P. Children's end-of-life health care use and cost. *Pediatrics*. 2017;139(4):e20162956.
202. Wolfe J, Hammel JF, Edwards KE, et al. Easing of suffering in children with cancer at the end of life: Is care changing? *J Clin Oncol*. 2008;26(10):1717–1723.
203. Wolff J, Robert R, Sommerer A, Volz-Fleckenstein M. Impact of a pediatric palliative care program. *Pediatr Blood Cancer*. 2010;54(2):279–283.
204. Cheng BT, Rost M, De Clercq E, Arnold L, Elger BS, Wangmo T. Palliative care initiation in pediatric oncology patients: A systematic review. *Cancer Med*. 2019;8(1):3–12.
205. MacDonald H, Callery P. Different meanings of respite: A study of parents, nurses and social workers caring for children with complex needs. *Child Care, Health Develop*. 2004;30(3):279–288; discussion 289.
206. Damiani G, Rosenbaum P, Swinton M, Russell D. Frequency and determinants of formal respite service use among caregivers of children with cerebral palsy in Ontario. *Child Care, Health Develop*. 2004;30(1):77–86.
207. Sutton D, Stanley P, Babl FE, Phillips F. Preventing or accelerating emergency care for children with complex healthcare needs. *Arch Dis Child*. 2008;93(1):17–22.
208. Steele R, Derman S, Cadell S, Davies B, Siden H, Straatman L. Families' transition to a Canadian paediatric hospice. Part two: Results of a pilot study. *Int J Palliat Nurs*. 2008;14(6):287–295.
209. Feudtner C, Rosenberg AR, Boss RD, Wiener L, Lyon ME, Hinds PS, Bluebond-Langner M, Wolfe J. Challenges and priorities for pediatric palliative care research in the U.S. and similar practice settings: Report from a pediatric palliative care research network workshop. *J Pain Symptom Manage*. 2019 Nov;58(5):909–917.e3.

3 | CHILDREN'S VOICES

The Experience of Patients and Their Siblings

ANNA C. MURIEL, ABBY R. ROSENBERG, AND BARBARA M. SOURKES

> Life is so strange. Sometimes you feel it's like a book with chapters to fill, never ending.
> Sometimes it's like a chess game where you have to make each move so carefully.
> Other times it's like a mystery where each hidden chamber reveals its secrets. It is even a war, where to live it is to win it.[1(p. 131)]
>
> KAREN BETH JOSEPHSON, AGE 10

> It's no privilege having someone with cancer in your family. Of all the things I ever could have chosen, having my brother get cancer is not one of them.[2(p. 38)]
>
> 8-YEAR-OLD SIBLING

In order to alleviate suffering and improve quality of life among children with serious illness and their families, it is necessary first to listen to their stories and observe their lived experiences. Most of the symptoms addressed by palliative care clinicians can only be addressed by soliciting and attending closely to patient and family perspectives. As pediatric palliative care develops into an interdisciplinary field, it is crucial to recognize the role of mental health and other multidisciplinary professionals in furthering our understanding of children's psychological responses to life-threatening illness.

Children with serious chronic illness experience high burdens of symptoms which can only be identified by asking. For example, physical symptoms like fatigue, pain, shortness of breath, and nausea, and emotional symptoms like anxiety, sadness, and irritability are common in children with medical illness. Poorly managed symptoms affect quality of life, satisfaction with care, and parent and family well-being both during the child's illness experience and thereafter.[3–7] Furthermore, the utility of colloquial questions like "how are you feeling" is limited; the answer to this question is not consistently associated with measurable patient- or parent-reported symptom burden.[8] Rather, pediatric palliative care clinicians must understand not only the developmental and disease-based communication needs and norms of different patients, but they must also be familiar with various techniques of connecting with patients and assessing their needs.

A few weeks before her death, Evangeline, age 13, spontaneously drew a pot of three flowers: two similar blooms nestled into one another, the other flower of a different kind leaning away. She was an only child who worried about how her parents would manage without her after her death (Figure 3.1). She mused, "What will I call this drawing? 'Flowers on a Journey' . . . No . . . 'Flowers Forever' . . . No. I think I will call it 'Magnificent Flower.'" She moved away from the title that reflected her vulnerability and instead chose the least-threatening option.

While much of our clinical literature and training focuses on the patient, we must not ignore their siblings. Although healthy siblings live the illness experience with the same intensity as the patient and parents, historically, they have stood outside the spotlight of attention and care.[9–10] Many of these children demonstrate positive growth in their maturity and empathy. Yet their distress can be significant, including elevated rates of anxiety and depression, symptoms of posttraumatic stress, few peer activities, lower cognitive development scores and school difficulties, diminished parental attention, and overall ratings of a poor quality of life.[11–12] Sibling relationships are a crucial axis within the family system, and the children's mutual caring and devotion can be enhanced rather than overlooked (Figure 3.2).

A group of siblings were asked: "Imagine that you are doing a campaign on behalf of siblings of seriously ill children. Draw a poster to illustrate your cause." The children drew an ill child in a hospital bed, surrounded by medical equipment, the parents at bedside. No siblings are present. They entitled their poster: "Don't brothers and sisters count, too??"[13] (Figure 3.2).

A 6-year-old sibling of a child who had been hospitalized for months spontaneously drew a smiling person—then

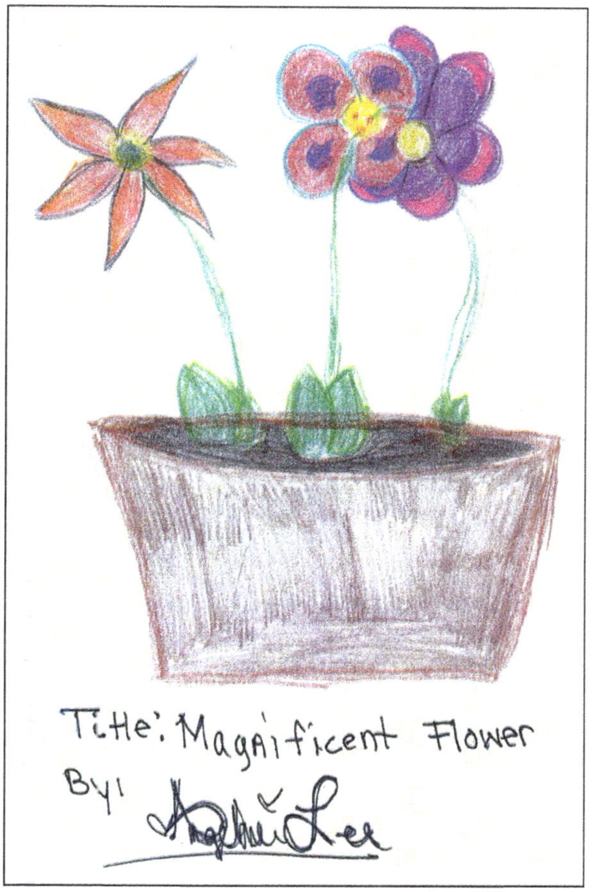

Figure 3.1 *Magnificent flower.*

changed the smile into a downturned mouth and said: "This is me. I am crying because I want my brother to be with me (Figure 3.3).

In many ways, the patient and his or her siblings live the illness in mirror-image fashion: while the patient endures the physicality of the illness in all its relentless and insistent

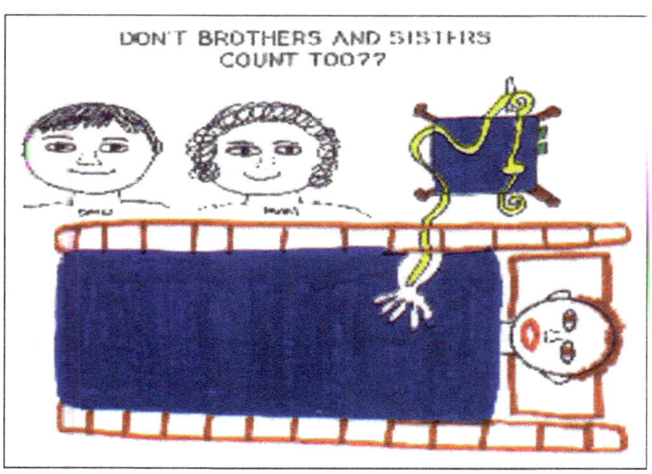

Figure 3.2 *Don't brothers and sisters count too??* Reprinted with permission from Sourkes B, et al. Food, toys, and love: Pediatric palliative care. *Curr Probl Pediatr Adolesc Health Care.* 2005;35(9):345–392.

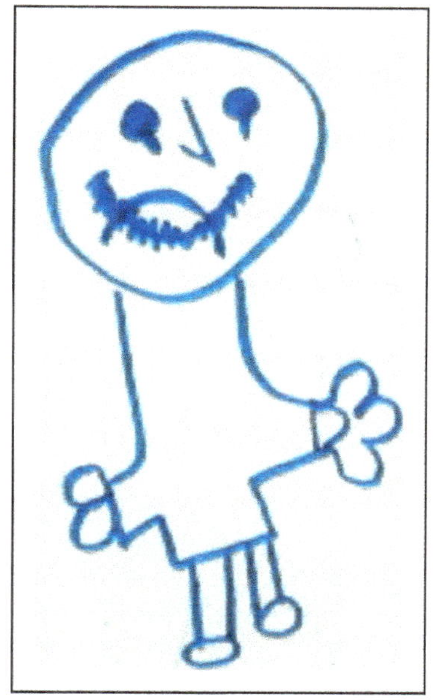

Figure 3.3 *This is me. I am crying because I want my brother to be with me.* Reprinted with permission from Sourkes B, et al. Food, toys, and love: Pediatric palliative care. *Curr Probl Pediatr Adolesc Health Care.* 2005;35(9):345–392.

presence, the siblings are witness to its ravages. All the children must cope with great uncertainty, confronted with the threat, if not the actuality, of premature separation, loss, and death.

Certain psychological themes are universal for both patients and siblings, although the mode of expression will depend on the child's level of cognitive and emotional development. These factors determine how he or she understands and integrates the illness itself as well as the responses of close family and friends. Also significant is the nature of the illness—its manifestations, its overall time course, and the particular phase at a given time.

This chapter provides a portrait, through the voices of both patients and siblings, of the experience of living with life-threatening illness. The words and images of children are essential touchstones for understanding pediatric palliative care. A conceptual overview of developmental considerations can frame the discussion of selected clinical themes: the impact of the illness itself, the children's awareness of their condition (or their sibling's), and anticipatory grief. The experiences of the children in this chapter are universal; however, the degree of openness and candor of their expression is a function of individual and family psychology, cognitive competence, and cultural background. The impact of culture emerges particularly in the discussion of the voice of the child in decision-making. The unique contributions of health professionals who provide mental health interventions such as child psychology, psychiatry, and social work, as well as the contributions of health professionals who provide other therapeutic supportive care, such as child life and art/music therapy, are all part of truly interdisciplinary pediatric palliative care.

DEVELOPMENTAL CONSIDERATIONS

The experience of children who are ill and their siblings is necessarily mediated by their age and stage of development, as well as by their individual temperament and sociocultural background. We review key characteristics of each developmental stage in order to set the stage for how children may understand and cope with illness. Physical, cognitive, and emotional development may vary in their paces, and each child deserves attention to their own unique trajectories.

INFANTS AND TODDLERS (AGES 0–3)

The earliest years are crucial for children's development of attachment and trust through their relationship to the primary caregiver, often, though not always the mother. At 6 to 12 months of age, infants go through a phase of stranger anxiety, mitigated by the proximity to the primary caregiver. Separation anxiety, which emerges between about 10 and 18 months, is a response to discrepancy: the more regular the presence of the caregiver, the earlier this anxiety manifests. By toddlerhood, the infant "becomes" a child with advances in motor, language, and social development.

The implications of serious illness, hospitalization, and pain for such young patients and siblings are enormous. At a critically formative time, the ill child may be overwhelmed with pain, strange people and situations, and separation. Nursing or feeding in infants is often disrupted, if not precluded. Parents caring for an ill child may be incapable of adapting to the cues of infant siblings. Toddlers, too young to fully comprehend verbal explanations, lack the means to make sense of crisis and unpredictability. Parents of such young children may be young themselves, or first-time parents. They are thrust into the medical world, often without experience of "normal" parenting. Much of the intervention with infants and toddlers (both patients and siblings) is to help the parents reestablish a secure routine and framework to enable the resumption of developmental progress.

Two-year-old Jimmy had been hospitalized for 6 months and had undergone many traumatic medical procedures. He was withdrawn; fearful of noises, sudden movements, and new people who entered his room; and disinterested in food or toys. Prior to his discharge home, the parents requested strategies from the psychologist to "get him back" to his prehospitalization level of functioning. Recommendations to the parents included

- Take a gradual and consistent approach with Jimmy in all areas. The 6-month disruption in his development will not be righted overnight; he needs to refamiliarize himself with his family, room, house, and toys.
- It is fine if he wants you within sight at all times. After all the coming and goings of the hospital, he will crave your presence. The intensity will abate with time. Very gradually, once he re-engages with toys, try to move away from him as he plays (first in the same room, then out of the room). Initially, do so for only moments at a time.
- Jimmy has to relearn how to play and have fun. Start with a few toys that he can get to know over the first few weeks, such as blocks to build up and knock down, a cloth for peek-a-boo, pull toys that encourage crawling, and cuddly stuffed animals. Keep the toys around him and do several play sessions with him each day.
- As much as possible, have him on the floor or in his playpen rather than in your arms. Put him into the playpen for as little as 10 seconds and gradually increase the time. Reinforce him with hugs and verbal praise for being a "big boy." Put toys or food slightly out of reach to tempt him to crawl and to stand to reach them.
- Jimmy should eat all his meals in his high chair, always in the same location. Put only a bite of each kind of food out at a time. Because he seemed to eat more in the hospital when he was playing, use small toys as both distraction and enjoyment.
- It is important that Jimmy begin to use his words again. When he points to an object, give him its name and develop a back-and-forth language game with him.

PRESCHOOL CHILDREN (AGES 3–5)

Natural egocentricity, magical thinking, and associative logic all characterize preschool children's thinking. They are therefore prone to interpret illness and suffering in terms of their own thoughts and actions and to have misconceptions about the cause of the illness or the reasons for medical treatment. Temporal coincidences may be interpreted as causal, and they may experience illness or treatment as punishment. While most of these children cannot yet express abstract concepts of time or the permanence of death, they are acutely aware of the emotional climate around them, particularly separation from caregivers and changes in routine.

Young children's reporting of symptoms is usually situation-specific, and they rarely can report their experience of physical or emotional symptoms over time. Thus, for example, responses about how they feel today as compared with yesterday, or concepts of better or worse may not be accurate indicators. However, these young children can readily express, through words and actions, their fears or dislike of specific sensations and circumstances.

Irritability may be a generalized response to physical discomfort or to the disruptions in routines. The behavior of a child with delays in language or cognitive development may appear particularly regressed and out of control, with disorganized or potentially aggressive responses to distress and frustration.

Similarly, while brothers and sisters may not report their sibling's symptoms accurately, they often resort to catastrophic images, often involving themselves, to express that something is drastically wrong. Symbolic play, stories, and drawing may be the most accessible expression of their experiences.

Matthew, 4, who was receiving palliative care for a brain tumor, told the psychologist: "I'm not sick anymore" and

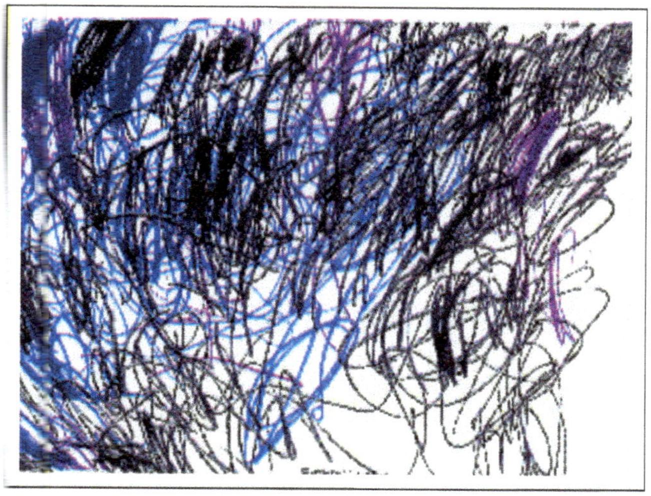

Figure 3.4 *Batman tunnel.* Reprinted with permission from Sourkes B: "Psychological impact of life-limiting conditions on the child." In Goldman, Haines, Liben, eds., *Oxford Textbook of Palliative Care for Children*. Oxford University Press, 2006.

adamantly denied any discomfort. His response to most queries by his parents or the medical team was "I'm OK" or "I'm fine" even when it was obvious that he was not. In fact, his non- or underreporting of symptoms made it difficult for his mother to administer pain medication effectively. The psychologist introduced Matthew to a rabbit puppet that he promptly named Donald Bunny. She used the puppet to model the reporting of symptoms (e.g., Donald Bunny has a headache, his eyes hurt when it is too bright, etc.). Matthew watched and listened with some interest. The psychologist left the puppet with him. At the next session, his mother said Matthew had begun reporting symptoms attributed "through the voice" of Donald Bunny. He still would not verbally acknowledge that he had any of these problems; however, his drawing of a dark and threatening "batman tunnel" (Figure 3.4) connoted distress and pain and contrasted with his earlier bright image (Figure 3.5). By the next session, while Matthew still would not initially mention any of what had been "bad" during the week, he did allow his mother to list some of his symptoms and would nod affirmatively to them. He then added spontaneously for the first time: "I don't like when I cough."[14]

A 3-year-old sibling manifested intense anxiety both at home and at preschool during his sister's long hospitalization. He drew a picture of the hospital with the following commentary: "A building with only three windows because some fell out and broke on the street. People have to be careful or their toes could get cut off. Nobody is in the hospital—they were all in a meeting. But you were there and were happy to see us and then everyone else came back. I was born and I got poison ivy and I died in the car. My sister was scared" (Figure 3.6).

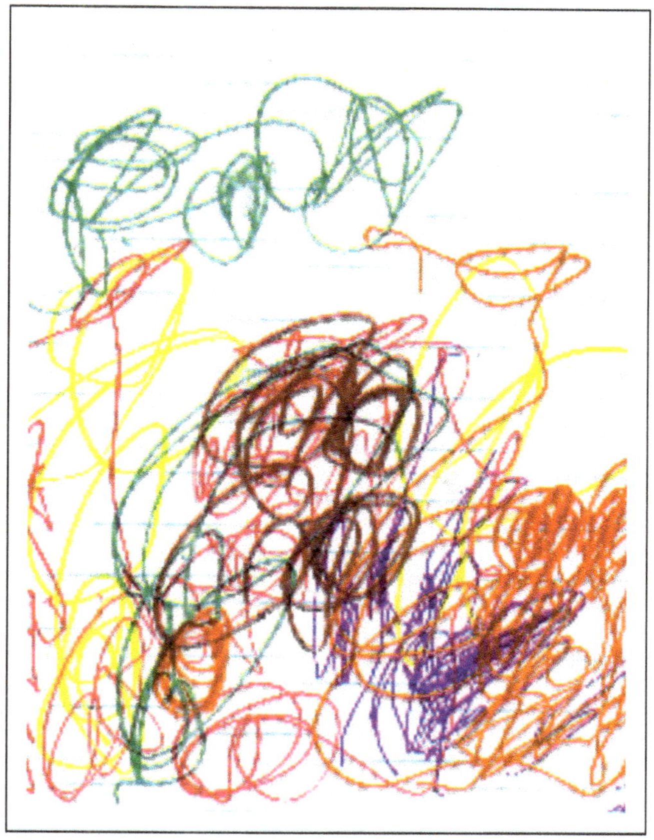

Figure 3.5 *Untitled early image.* Reprinted with permission from Sourkes B. Psychological impact of life-limiting conditions on the child. In Goldman, Haines, Liben, eds., *Oxford Textbook of Palliative Care for Children*. Oxford University Press, 2006.

SCHOOL-AGE CHILDREN (AGES 6–12)

Children in these middle years are ordinarily consumed with mastering skills in a range of physical, intellectual, and social activities. They are invested in fitting in with peers and with the social norms of their immediate community. Children struggling with illness are set apart by physical changes and loss of bodily integrity, absence from their usual activities, and, overwhelmingly, the ramifications of the diagnosis. They may experience the loss of friends and changes in their relationships with family members. Thinking patterns are characterized by relatively concrete cause and effect with an

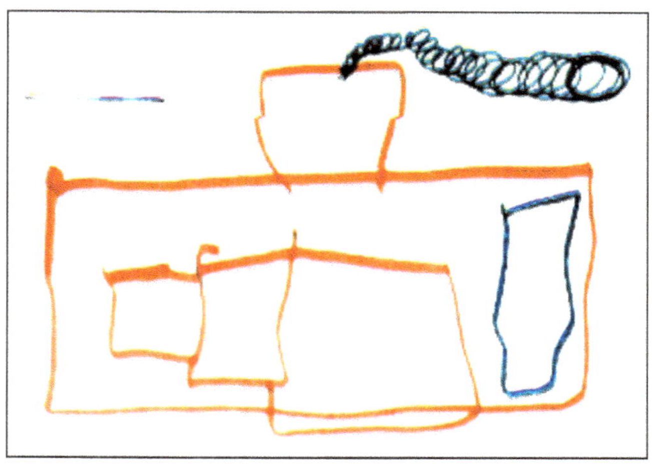

Figure 3.6 *Hospital picture.*

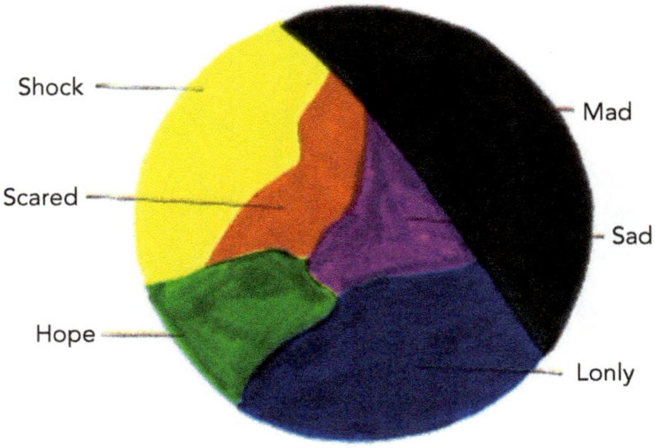

Figure 3.7 *How I felt when I heard that I had leukemia.* Reprinted and adapted with permission from Sourkes BM. *Armfuls of Time: The Psychological Experience of the Child with a Life-Threatening Illness.* University of Pittsburgh Press, 1996.

interest in bodily functions and factual information. They have an understanding of the permanence of death and yet may not always integrate that it is universal. There may be less direct expression of emotion and more coping by using cognition, activity, and distraction.

School-age children are aware of the impact of their illness and distress on others and may amplify or minimize their communication based on others' reactions. These children may not consciously change their behavior or be aware of the interplay between their emotions and their physical experiences. While children in this age group may use words more effectively than younger children, they may also need encouragement and normalization of experiences to freely describe their physical symptoms or emotional experience. Drawing and displacement through play or storytelling may continue to be important methods for expression.

Through a drawing (Figure 3.7), an 8-year-old boy captured the immediacy of his response to the diagnosis of a life-threatening illness: "When I heard that I had leukemia, I turned pale with shock. That's why I chose yellow—it's a pale color. Scared is red—for blood. I was scared of needles, of seeing all the doctors, of what was going to happen to me. I was MAD [black] about a lot of things: staying in the hospital, taking medicines, bone marrows, spinal taps, IVs, being awakened in the middle of the night. I was sad [purple] that I didn't have my toys and that I was missing out on everything. I chose blue for lonely because I was crying about not being at home and not being able to go outside. Green is for hope: getting better, going home, eating food from home, and seeing my friends." He has articulated the shock; the fear of everything from the concrete medical procedures to the sudden possibility of an altered future ("what was going to happen to me"); the constellation of sadness, grief, and loneliness of separation; and the absence from his normal life. Accompanying all these feelings is a forthright statement of hope.[1(p. 31)]

Tim, an 11-year-old boy, had struggled with recurrent cancer since the age of 4. He was troubled by insomnia and anxiety during an inpatient stay in isolation for intensive treatment. Upon discharge, he continued to have significant anxiety, avoiding school and playing with friends. His medical team had cleared him for all activity, and he did not report pain or side effects of his medication. Tim had been using escalating doses of benzodiazepines at bedtime, as well as when needed during the day. When interviewed alone by the psychiatrist, he reported feeling "nervous and worried."

PSYCHIATRIST: About what?
TIM: About dying.
PSYCHIATRIST: Which part?
TIM: Just being dead.

When questioned further, Tim articulated specific worries about many issues: dying suddenly while away from his parents; wondering what dying will feel like and what the afterlife holds; not being able to "come back as a ghost" to visit his family if they were to move away from their current house. He denied worry about pain: "I have been sick so long and had lots of pain." The discussion continued on a spectrum from the current stable status of his illness to his feelings about God and spirituality. Following this session, Tim engaged in the most direct conversation with his medical team ever: about his illness, the stability of his scan results, and the fact that death was not imminent. The team reassured him that there would be time to talk more when death was closer at hand. Over the next few months, Tim returned to active play with peers, engaged in video games and early romantic interests, prepared for the next school year, and articulated future plans to go to college and get a job.

Siblings also experience a sense of "apartness," of being different or stigmatized by having a seriously ill brother or sister. These children often live in fear of becoming sick themselves, along with suffering a complicated mix of guilt at having escaped the illness and shame at feeling this relief. They are exceedingly conscious of the physical exigencies of the illness, as well as the impact on the child's functioning. Private theories about what caused the illness are common, and the siblings frequently implicate themselves in the explanation. They often express a fervent wish to understand and be more involved.[9–10]

Bobby, 10, reported his version of the sequence of events that led to his sister's diagnosis of osteosarcoma and amputation: "She hurt her leg on the chain of her bike. She didn't even notice it until I pointed it out to her. I don't even ride my bike anymore. One night I went out and broke the chain so I couldn't ride it. I told my mother it broke by itself, but I broke it."[9(p. 55)] He wrote a story: "This is my sister (drew a one-legged stick figure) and this is me (drew a two-legged stick figure). There is a difference. But I still think that this is the same Cindy and I know that she is not the same to you and I think that she is beautiful." He then drew a picture of Cindy, stressing her very short hair and her stump. He expressed much concern about how the stump would look[3(p. 57)] (Figure 3.8). In a subsequent session, Bobby admitted to nightmares of "the same thing" happening to him (Figure 3.9).

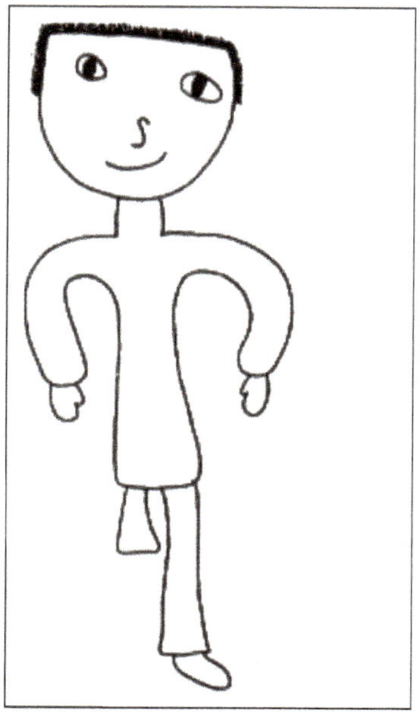

Figure 3.8 *Bobby's portrait of Cindy.* Reprinted with permission from Kellerman J. *Psychological Aspects of Childhood Cancer.* Charles C. Thomas, 1980.

A 10-year-old sibling spoke about her brother's diagnosis of a brain tumor: (Figure 3.10) "I feel scared (green)—I feel as if I don't really know what is happening. Sad is blue—at first my parents just told me that my brother needed an operation. They didn't say it was cancer. Confused is yellow—just all mixed feelings—I don't know what to think. Hopeful is purple—bright—I don't really have a lot of hope, but maybe just a little. Angry is red because that is a mad color. Why him? What did it have to happen to him? My drawing is called Mixed Messages' because I have all of these different feelings and everyone is telling me different things. Like they say mostly that he is going to be OK, but they—and I—don't really believe it."[15]

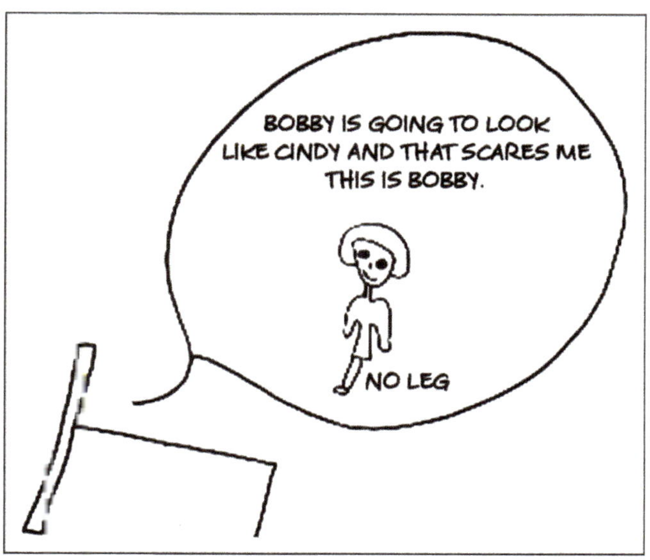
BOBBY IS GOING TO LOOK
LIKE CINDY AND THAT SCARES ME
THIS IS BOBBY.
NO LEG

Figure 3.9 *Bobby's nightmare.* Reprinted with permission from Kellerman J. *Psychological Aspects of Childhood Cancer.* Charles C. Thomas, 1980.

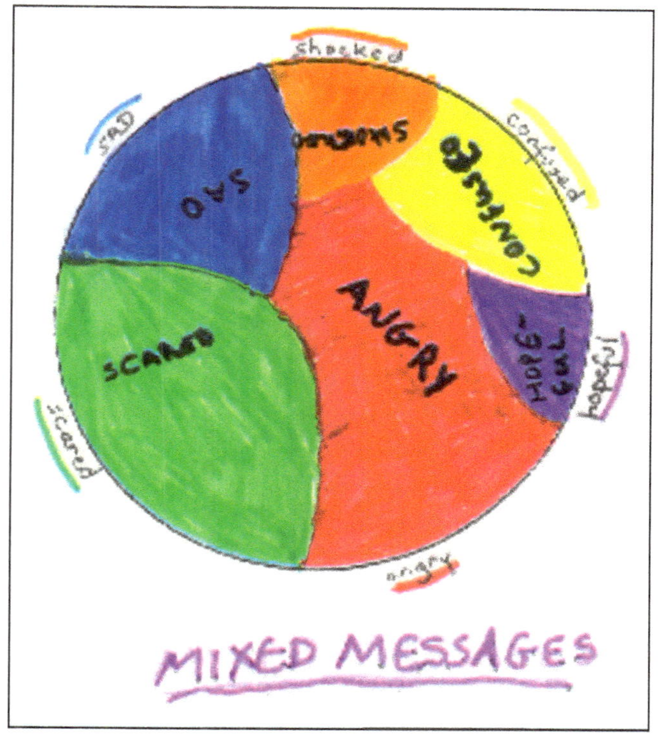

Figure 3.10 *Mixed messages.* Reprinted with permission from Pizzo P. *Principles and Practice of Pediatric Oncology*, 5th ed. Lippincott Williams, and Wilkins, 2006.

ADOLESCENTS (13–18 YEARS)

Adolescence is characterized by an evolving process of identity formation, appreciation of abstract concepts, and increasing sophistication in both intellectual and emotional understanding of situations and relationships. Future orientation is paramount in the areas of educational and career goals and the development of intimate relationships. Just as these young people are struggling to establish separation and autonomy from family, they must contend with the enforced dependence and vulnerability imposed by the illness. While adolescents understand the permanence and universality of death, they may still feel personally and emotionally invincible. Offering adolescents a role in decision-making is always important, whether or not they accept. They may need assistance from the medical team or mental health clinician to distinguish their preferences from those of their family. Because many adolescents try to protect their parents from their own distress, it can be a frightening prospect to make their own needs known. Peer relationships and activities and self-directed symptom management are critical components of quality of life for adolescents. Written expression, music, media, and web-based activities can provide windows into the impact of the illness on their life and how it has impinged on their sense of self.

In the words of Katherine (age 18):

> Younger children are not developed in themselves yet, in their own persons, in their own individualism. They can still be with their mother. Older people are away from their mother; they're detached, more adult. When you're in the middle, parents don't want

to let you go. You want to be set free a little bit, but you want to be able to come back. I just felt that I was denied any sort of chance. . . . Instead, it was decided for me: You are going to mature very fast right now. You have to make life-and-death decisions. You have to accept things that children who are young adults between the ages of 13 and 19 don't normally have to face." It's like: "Grow up right now and become what you have to become to deal with this." I never had the chance to be sweet 16. I never had the chance to be gay old 17. I had to automatically be an adult, and it was very hard.[2(p. 101)]

Adolescent siblings are caught in a similar web: just as they are beginning to develop their individual identity and negotiate their own independence, they are pulled back into the family. They are preoccupied and worried. These young people have difficulty sorting out their role and needs from that of being another parental figure.

Joanne fell on the stairs at school and split her lip open on the day before her sister's surgery. She explained: "I was walking in flat heels on the stairs. I thought of my sister's operation. That's why I fell."[9(p. 63)]

In response to the question: "What has been especially hard for you during your brother's illness?" an adolescent sibling responded: "Waiting while he is in the OR and worrying about what they are finding."

EMERGING ADULTS (18–29 YEARS)

Emerging adulthood is characterized by two sometimes divergent experiences. One is the establishment of education and early vocational goals, and the other is the existential search for meaning and purpose in life. Interestingly, this distinct period of identity exploration may be limited to industrialized nations and Western cultures where there is time, if not an expectation, for emerging adults to travel, pursue graduate-level education, or trial various career options.[16] Subjectively, emerging adults do not identify as adults or adolescents. They exist in an "in between" where there is no characteristic physical transition but, instead, a focus on solidifying an individual's love, work, and worldview identities. The goal of this age is self-sufficiency. Emerging young adults endeavor to be responsible for themselves and to achieve financial and decision-making independence.

Imagine the impact of serious illness on this age-group:

Family Reflection

Micah had left home for college and stayed in his new city to start an internship at a tech company. He had an active social life and shared apartment chores with two roommates. When he was diagnosed with leukemia, he first tried to manage his own medical needs and intermittently asked his roommates for help. Over time, he worried he was burdening his friends. When they were not at home, he felt lonely and sometimes afraid of what would happen if he had an emergency.

As Micah's needs escalated and his cancer persisted despite treatment, he moved home so that his parents could help care for him. "I felt like I was going in reverse," he said. "The goals I had, the things I wanted to do . . . they were suddenly out of my reach and I had no control."

Micah shared with his palliative care team that he was not done living. "The say my cancer can't be cured. But, what am I supposed to do? I want to have *lived*, and I haven't had enough time to leave my mark on the world." In response, Micah's palliative care team helped him navigate his values and goals through the end of his life, including setting up a legacy fund to support other young adults with cancer.

Meanwhile, Micah's sister, who was 27 when he was diagnosed, had her own struggles. "I was supposed to be moving on and starting my life and family. When Micah got sick, I felt divided. I wanted to be home with him, and I wanted to be very far away. In the end, I decided to be with him because that is the kind of person I want to be."

CHILDREN WITH DEVELOPMENTAL DELAYS

Children with developmental delays may need clinicians to pay particular attention to their parent's observations of their symptoms and individualized expressions of pain or distress. As these young people grow beyond their 18th birthdays, decisions about legal guardianship and medical decision-making must also be considered.

Youth with autism spectrum disorders may present unique concerns in the palliative care setting. Their level of impairment may be very variable, with more high functioning children having well-developed verbal and cognitive capacities, though with intense sensory sensitivities, rigid thinking, social challenges, and needs for routine that can be difficult to manage in the context of illness. They may have difficulty articulating specific aspects of their experience, areas of pain etc., becoming globally distressed, dysregulated, or shut down.

A 12-year-old with high-functioning autism spectrum disorder had a long-standing phobia of medical settings. As his cystic fibrosis progressed and he required frequent hospitalizations, he had a lot of difficulty managing even routine and nonpainful procedures. It was difficult for him to articulate his specific symptoms, and he had spiraling anxiety and dyspnea. Child life and psychology helped develop care routines and instructions for medical and nursing staff about speaking directly and clearly to him about what to expect, in what order to do vitals, etc. He was able to learn concrete coping skills for distraction with video games, slowing his breathing, and brief phrases about his preferences "call me Gabe not Gabriel, or sweetie."

CHILDREN WITH SEVERE NEUROLOGICAL IMPAIRMENT

Children who are severely neurologically impaired, nonverbal, with extremely limited capacity for interaction or awareness, pose enormous challenges for the team. How to understand their wants and needs? How to recognize distress or pain?[17]

As difficult as it is for professionals to "read" these children, their families, both parents and siblings, are truly the experts. Over and beyond the relentless reality of their physical care, families know their children psychologically. They can judge their well-being as well as identify the source and degree of a child's distress by subtle cues that would elude the professional team. Even young siblings become astute observers and reporters. The families' interpretation of their child's expressions or behavior is what defines their judgments about quality of life in decision-making.

The family of a teenager with lissencephaly who was nonverbal and confined to a wheelchair included him in all their activities, even camping. His mother explained that, despite his limitations, she can see that he "finds joy" in his life. She stated: "My son's condition will probably deteriorate at some point, but I hope he will live for as long as he's enjoying it."[18] During a difficult hospitalization, she reflected back on her words: "When he no longer has times of finding joy, then my decisions about prolonging his life will have to change."

Although psychotherapy or child life activities may play a relatively minor role in the direct care of these children, the interventions can be extremely important for their siblings. The issues that all healthy siblings confront are complicated by the double stress of having a brother or sister who is both chronically ill and developmentally devastated.

The medical team see these neurologically impaired children primarily in the hospital, at their most compromised. Many professionals express difficulty in both imagining and accepting that these children can have a reasonable, even good, quality of life. Despite the children's extreme limitations and the inordinate hardship in caring for them over months, years, and decades, they are an integral part of their families. Given this reality, it is important to respect families' considerations in decision-making and support them in their choices for their child.[17]

* * *

CLINICAL THEMES

THE ILLNESS EXPERIENCE

The patient experiences the illness both physically and emotionally through symptoms, changes in appearance and body image, and also the intrusion of technology. These traumatic aspects reverberate for siblings as well and may become a source of great distress because they often go unacknowledged.

PSYCHOLOGIST: If you could choose one word to describe the time since your diagnosis, what would it be?
PATIENT: PAIN—once I felt as if the IV was exploding in my arm!

The child went on to describe the excruciating pain he had felt amid the chaos of his IV pole falling over and crashing (Figure 3.11).[13(p. 365)]

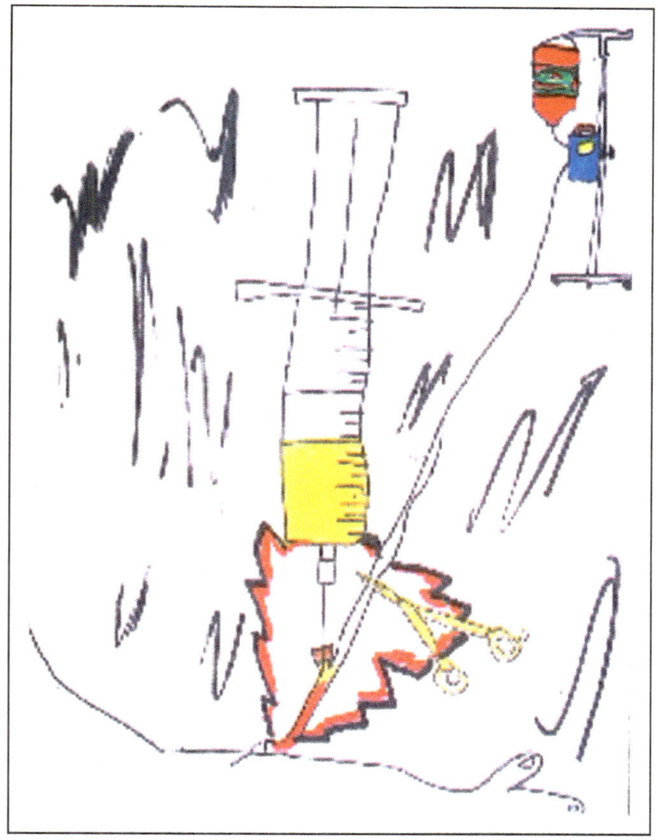

Figure 3.11 *IV exploding in my arm.* Reprinted with permission from Sourkes B, et al. Food, toys, and love: Pediatric palliative care. *Curr Probl Pediatr Adolesc Health Care.* 2005;35(9):345–392.

In response to the question: "What is the scariest feeling, thought, or experience you have had since your sister became ill?" a child drew her response: "Dreaming of my sister in pain." She depicted herself as a diminutive brown figure in a small bed, overwhelmed by the dream image of her sister in bright orange screaming "OW" (Figure 3.12).

A 12-year-old child with end-stage renal disease depicted his absolute dependence on hemodialysis to live. He entitled

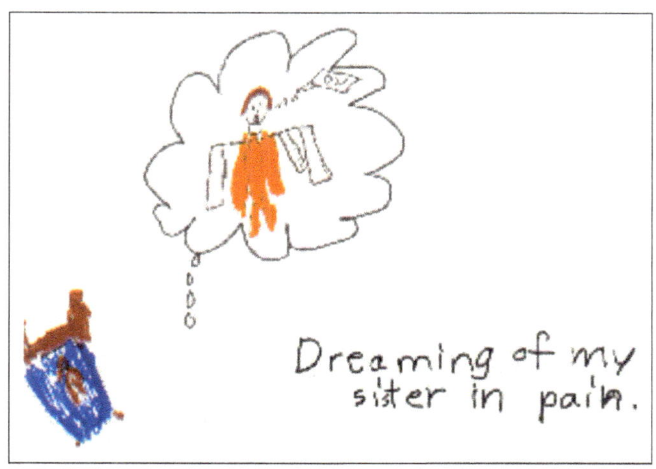

Figure 3.12 *Dreaming of my sister in pain.*

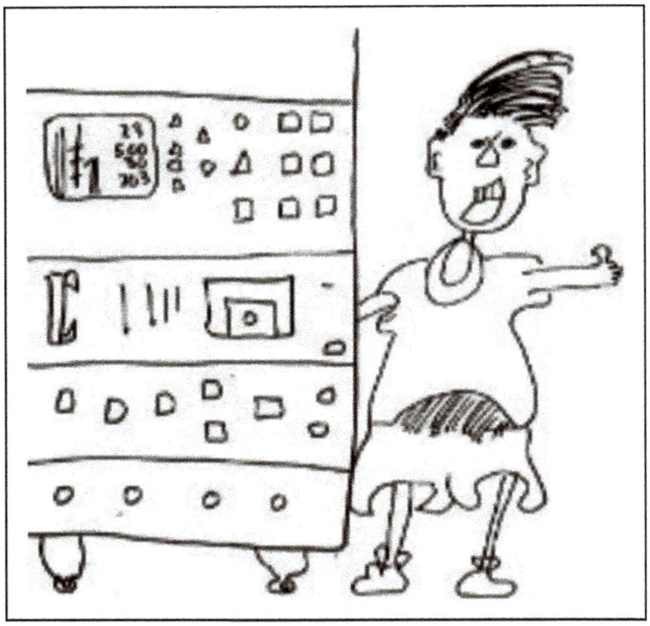

Figure 3.13 My machine.

his drawing "MY machine." One hand is literally plugged into the machine while the other is in a "thumbs up" gesture. His facial expression is ambiguous—triumph, horror, or a combination of the two (Figure 3.13).

A sibling's drawing of his brother hooked up to multiple wires and monitors communicates his fear at what he has witnessed (Figure 3.14).

Concerns about sexuality can be quite pronounced in children living with serious illness. Sexuality in all its facets represents a life force, which is exactly the struggle in which these children are engaged. Furthermore, the body is the focus of illness, and sexuality is an integral part of that same body. Sexual identity, functioning, and fertility—and the potential or actual losses thereof—loom particularly large for adolescents and young adults, although younger children may also harbor worries about immediate and long-term effects of illness and treatment.[19]

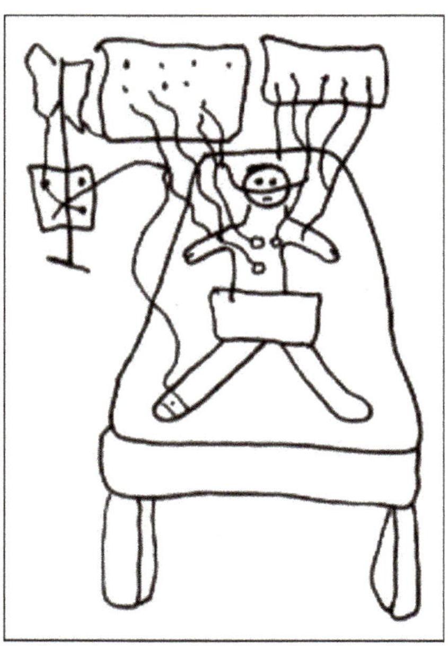

Figure 3.14 My brother in the hospital.

An 18-year-old boy who had had his leg amputated expressed fears about his sexual functioning and how his girlfriend would react. On a clinic visit shortly after surgery, he greeted the psychologist: "You'll be glad to know I still work! I was glad too!"[19]

A 12-year-old girl insisted on reading the informed consent for her bone marrow transplant. When she asked what "sterility" meant, her physician replied: "It means you can't have babies." She retorted quickly and with spirit: "Then I'll adopt!" However, following this discussion, she spoke frequently about her sadness at the loss of fertility.[19]

An 8-year-old sibling talked about her adolescent sister's hair loss secondary to chemotherapy. With some embarrassment, she admitted that she had glimpsed her sister in the shower and only then realized that she had lost her pubic hair as well. She was disturbed at seeing her sister's body looking like that of a young child again.

For all the children, their longing to return to their "normal life" or their "life from before" (or, in situations where a child has a congenital condition, "life without sickness") is counterbalanced by the recognition that the presence of illness in the family cannot be erased, nor its impact reversed.[1] Rather, the children are confronted with the extraordinary challenge of pursuing the developmental tasks of childhood and adolescence while negotiating the illness experience.

AWARENESS OF THE LIFE-THREATENING NATURE OF THE ILLNESS

Children's awareness is a fluid process, not a static state, and it depends on factors including their current medical status and knowledge about the illness (or that of the sibling's), their "wisdom of the body," the urgency and intensity of treatment, the emotions of family and caregivers, the family communication style, and encounters with other children who are ill.[1,20] These issues are particularly poignant when more than one child in the family has the illness. References to death may be somewhat veiled and allusive, or direct and explicit.

During a psychotherapy session in the last few months of her life, 13-year-old Evangeline drew a picture entitled "My Lungs." She portrayed herself as a heart with a sad face between (and connected to) two lungs: "One of my lungs is sad because it has disease in it; the other lung is smiling because it is still OK" (Figure 3.15). Her use of the word "still" expressed her qualified confidence in its current state.

A 4-year-old child had always done medical play with a stuffed Curious George monkey, giving him shots and bandages. In a session close to her death, she methodically covered him with tissues and taped them in place. By the end of her play, he appeared to be buried under a shroud. She was very quiet during her activity and made no comment about her play (Figure 3.16).[14]

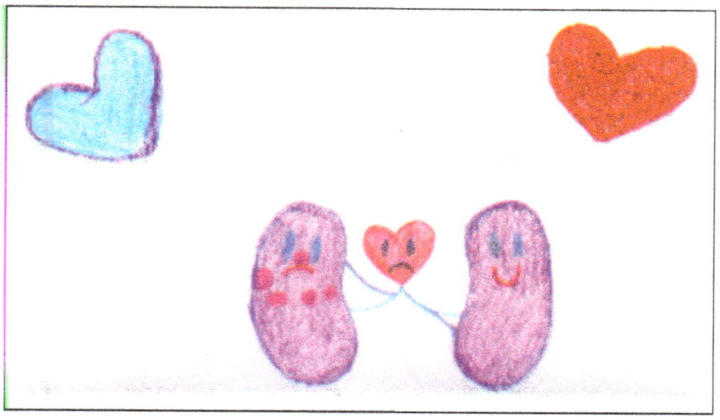

Figure 3.15 *My lungs.*

An 8-year-old boy with muscular dystrophy was tripping and falling constantly, but adamantly refused to use a wheelchair, protesting that he did not need it. His older brother with the same disease was already severely compromised. In a family drawing, the child portrayed himself jumping and smiling; he drew his brother as an incomplete almost ghost-like figure at the computer. The extremities of all four family members are distorted or missing. This child's awareness—and attempted denial—of his own progressive deterioration as well as his brother's status (and thus his own in the future) are embedded in the drawing (Figure 3.17).

A 14- year-old boy with hemophilia who had just been informed that he was HIV-positive graphically described the experience: "Before hearing the news, I was just thinking: I hope they are not going to tell me I have HIV" (on a "happy" purple background). After hearing the news, he depicted himself in a coffin against a black background saying: "I hope I'll be alive when they get the cure" (Figure 3.18).

An 8-year-old sibling said his biggest worry was that his brother might die of his illness. He drew a somber picture of two faceless black figures lowering a coffin into the ground, next to a tombstone inscribed "RIP" [Rest in peace] and a pile of dirt. Anxious scribbling filled part of the page (Figure 3.19).

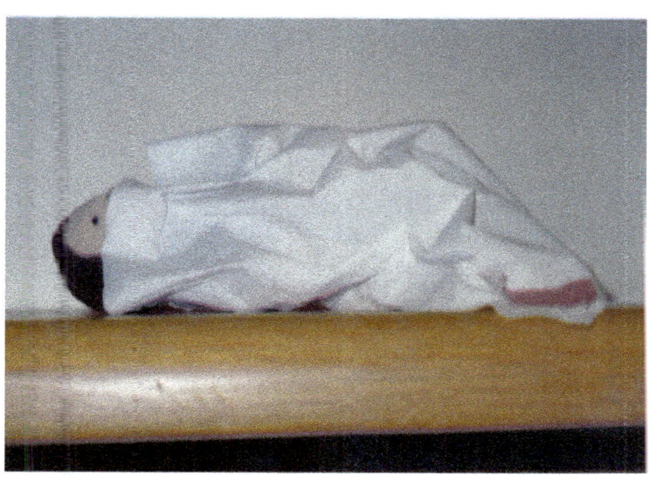

Figure 3.16 *Curious George under a shroud.* Reprinted with permission from Sourkes B. Psychological impact of life-limiting conditions on the child. In Goldman, Haines, Liben, eds., *Oxford Textbook of Palliative Care for Children*. Oxford University Press, 2006.

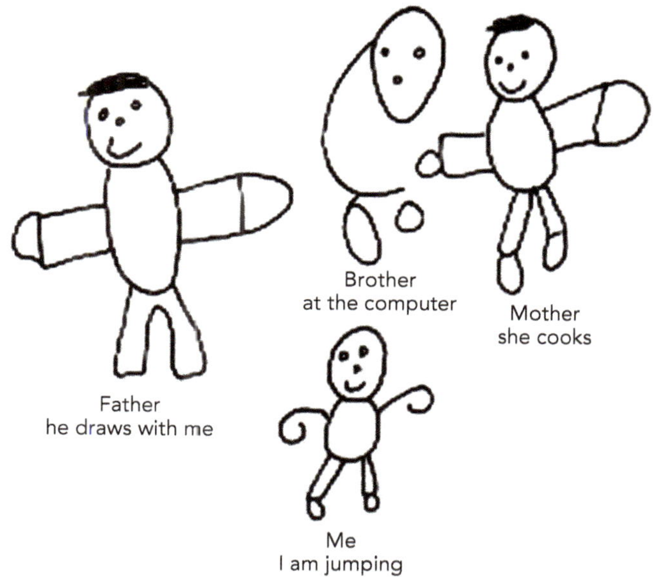
Brother
at the computer
Mother
she cooks
Father
he draws with me
Me
I am jumping

Figure 3.17 *I am jumping.*

ANTICIPATORY GRIEF

PSYCHOLOGIST: "Are you in any pain? Does anything hurt?"
JENNY: "My heart."
THERAPIST: "Your heart?"
JENNY: "My heart is broken . . . I miss everybody."[1(p. 153)]

Children's expressions of anticipatory grief—for many cumulative losses—accompany their awareness of the implications of the illness.[1–2,21] Patients grieve the loss of control over their body and disease, the loss of identity of what

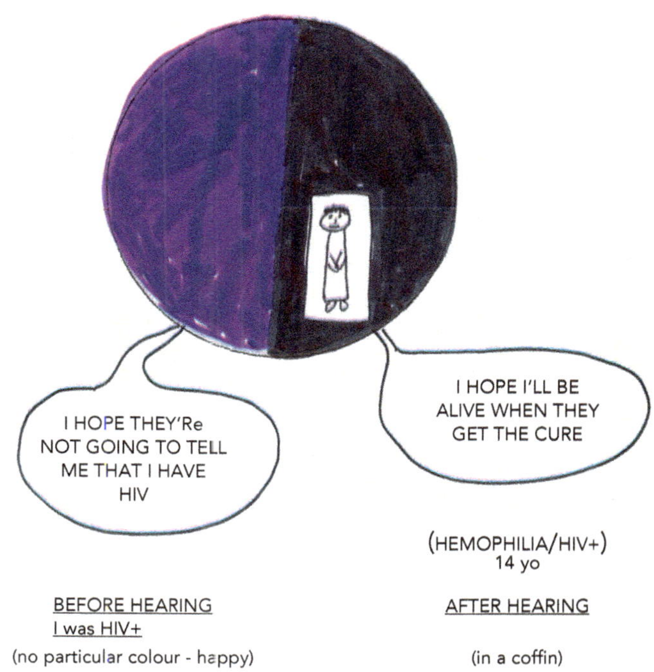

Figure 3.18 *Before and after.*

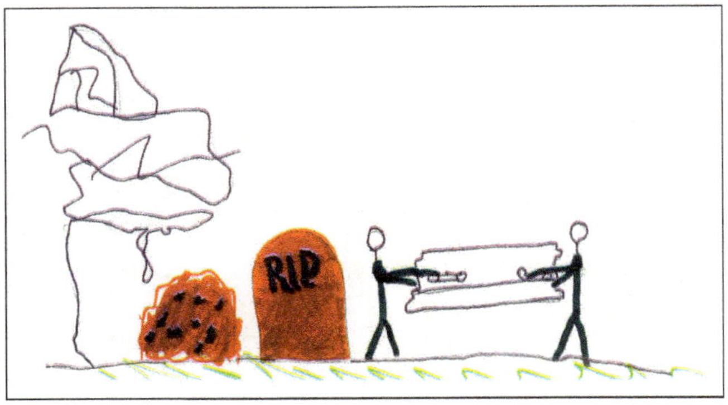

Figure 3.19 *Rest in peace.*

had been their roles and functions in the family and in the outside world, and the foregoing of future goals. The children face the ultimate leave-taking, the departure from all that is familiar and loved. Loss of relationships—expressed through fears of separation, absence, and, ultimately, death itself—is paramount and is the dimension shared with the siblings.

An interchange between Mariesa, 16, and Mikaela, her 10-year-old sister with a brain tumor:

MARIESA: We've always been really close. I just hate to think of . . . just too many scary thoughts and too many feelings. . . . I just know one thing: I just want everything to be OK and everything to go away and hopefully it will work out.
MIKAELA: Same with me.
MARIESA: And she knows that I love her no matter what.

An adolescent with thalassemia, whose brother had died in infancy of the same disease, drew a cemetery image: (Figure 3.20). "My parents and friends are surrounding me [the large cross]. Others who passed away are buried there—especially my little brother—actually, he was my oldest brother. It's raining—sad and depressing. Rain means that something has happened or will happen. I would like people to remember who I am. I don't want any enemies around my grave—or to visit me."

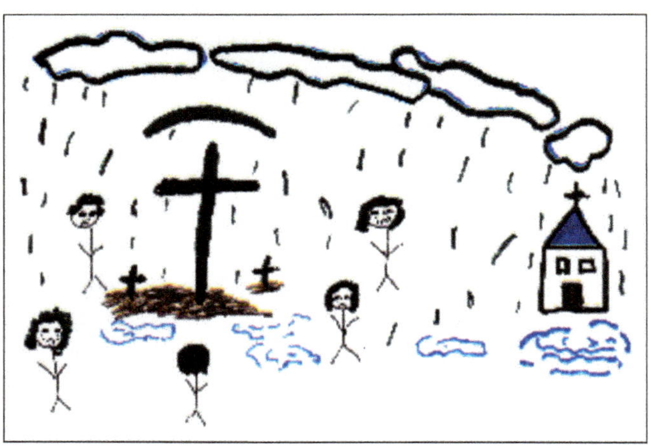

Figure 3.20 *Cemetery.*

A 7-year-old girl had a recurrent dream: "In the dream, I want to be with my mother, and I can never quite get to her." The girl recounted the dream in a joint psychotherapy session with her mother. Whereas the mother found the dream "excruciating," her daughter articulated that "even though the dream is very sad, it's not a nightmare." The dream eventually provided the focal image for mother and child to work through the anticipatory grief process.[2(p. 70)]

The distillation of anticipatory grief to its essence marks the imminence of death. At times imperceptibly, at other times dramatically, children often turn inward as they pull back from the external world. Cognitive and emotional horizons narrow because all energy is needed simply for physical survival. A generalized irritability is not uncommon. Children may talk very little and may even retreat from physical contact. Although such withdrawal is not universal, a certain degree of quietness is almost always in evidence. This behavior is a normal and expected precursor to death.[1]

THE VOICE OF THE CHILD IN DECISION-MAKING

Mikaela drew a picture entitled "This or This" (Figure 3.21) when she found out that her disease had recurred. On one side of a doughnut she depicted tumor cells, on the other side she drew a needle for spinal taps. In the middle of the doughnut is a little stick figure of a person. At the time of drawing the picture, Mikaela said: "I hate needles and spinal taps, but I also don't want my tumor to come back. If I don't have all the needles, then more tumor cells will grow. So if I don't want them to grow, I have to have all those awful needles. That's why I feel as if I am stuck in the middle of a doughnut." Reflecting on the drawing months later, Mikaela elaborated more explicitly: "What I mean by 'I was stuck in a doughnut' is that I had two choices and I didn't want to take either of them. One of the choices was to get needles and pokes and all that stuff and make the tumor go away. My other choice was letting my tumor get bigger and bigger and I would just go away up to heaven. . . . My mom wanted me to get needles and pokes. But I felt like I just had had too much—too much for

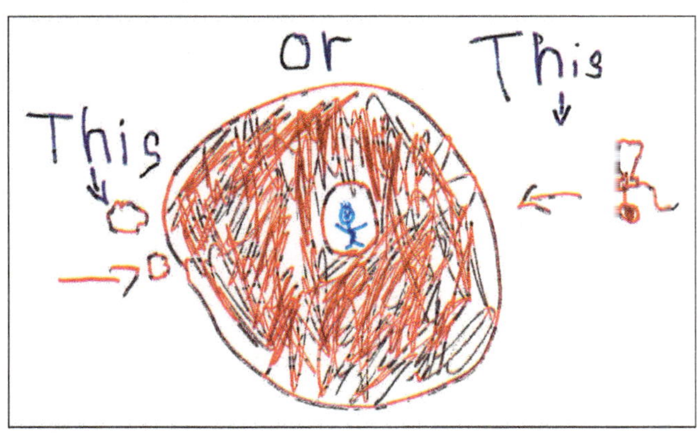

Figure 3.21 *This or this.* Reprinted with permission from Sourkes B, et al. Food, toys, and love: Pediatric palliative care. *Curr Probl Pediatr Adolesc Health Care.* 2005;35(9):345–392.

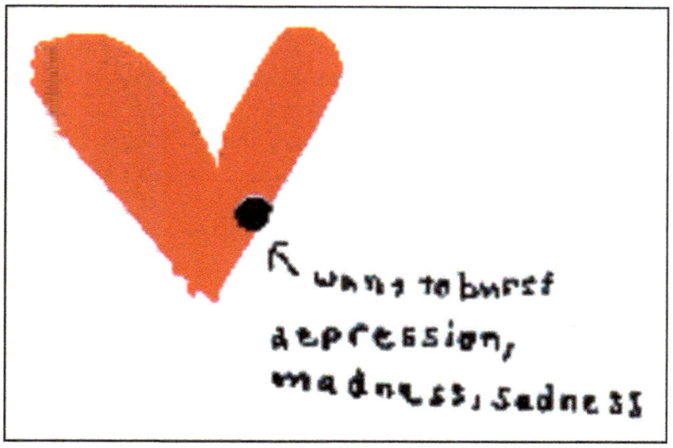

Figure 3.22 *A heart that wants to burst.*

my body—too much for me. . . . So I kind of wanted to go up to heaven that time. . . . But then I thought about how much my whole entire family would miss me and so just then I was kind of like stuck in a doughnut."[13]

A 10-year-old sibling whose sister was critically ill stated intensely: "I am mad at all the doctors. I think that they are giving up too soon. I KNOW that my sister will not die, I just know it. But I feel like it's only me who feels that way and no one listens to my opinion." She then drew a heart called "wants to burst" with a black dot of "depression, madness and sadness" (Figure 3.22).

Over the past decade, there has been increased recognition of children's participation in making treatment decisions. Attention to children's experience of their illness is essential not only to enhance their quality of life, but also as a guide to clinical decisions and goals of care. This may become more challenging as an illness progresses, especially if the family and clinicians are reticent to discuss death with children. A landmark study showed that bereaved parents who had talked with their child about death had no regrets about doing so, whereas those who had not engaged in such discussions were sometimes left with regret.[23] While younger children may not be able to take an abstract or time-based perspective, their expressed fears, concerns, and specific preferences can provide the basis for decisions. Older children and adolescents who have more capacity to plan over time can engage in complex end-of-life decisions that may be driven by interpersonal relationships.[24,25] However, because standardized assessment tools are still in development,[26] clinicians are often left to rely on their own judgment to assess children's understanding of the contingencies they face. (See Chapter 9 for an additional discussion of decision-making.)

Children are often aware of the diminishing curative or life-prolonging options available. It is at this time that they may ask anxiously: "What if this medicine doesn't work? What will you give me next?"[1] Input from members of the interdisciplinary team can be crucial at this juncture: children often express their understanding, awareness, and thoughts about treatment options and living or dying to individuals other than their parents or primary physician. Frequently, their most candid disclosures evolve within the context of psychotherapy.

The ethnic and spiritual culture of the family is a significant factor in how the child's voice is incorporated into the decision-making process. It is especially critical for clinicians to understand how a family's culture defines the construct of "childhood" in terms of protectiveness (e.g., if to tell, how much to tell a child, should a child be an active participant in planning?). A child's expressions about the illness experience must be understood within this framework. The current emphasis in mainstream American culture on the "rights" of children to have access to information and participate in decisions is far from universal. Furthermore, the zeal to include children may inadvertently create a burden on the child that he or she does not feel equipped to manage.

The following vignettes illustrate a spectrum of children's involvement in decision-making.

Child's voice is instrumental in determining plan.

> A 7-year-old girl told her parents that she was too tired to fight anymore and that she wanted to give up. She added: "If I have to continue suffering, I would rather be in heaven." She repeated this statement to the medical team. The parents acknowledged that their child's statements were major determinants in their shifting to a palliative care plan.[1(p. 156)]

An adolescent is comfortable within his family culture of noninvolvement in decision-making:

> A 16-year-old boy from the Middle East had HIV disease secondary to hemophilia. His parents were adamant that he not be told his diagnosis of HIV or the prognosis: "No child of any age should be burdened with such things." The boy politely and repeatedly declined staff's queries about whether he wanted more information about his condition or whether he had any opinions that he wished to express about treatment options. His knowledge, however "veiled," was nonetheless accurate: he stated that he had a serious immune condition in addition to the hemophilia, that he was aware of body fluid precautions including safer sex, and that he fully trusted his parents' decisions about treatment. Working within culturally and family determined norms, he was making an autonomous decision not to have further direct communication and functioned well, maintaining active involvement in school and with friends until his death.

The inadvertent burden of decision-making on a child:

> An 11-year-old child had been through many remission-relapse cycles and had been informed and involved in all aspects of her treatment from the beginning. When she was offered radiation therapy for palliative symptom control, she confided to her psychologist: "I'm scared because I'm not so good at making decisions. My parents want me to have radiation, but a little voice in me tells me not to. . . . My mother always said that if I die, she

wants me to die happy and at home. If I had radiation, I'd have to come into the hospital every day. And I don't know if radiation will really help, or if I would die anyway." Despite what had been her clear understanding of the reason for radiation therapy (exclusively for palliative symptom management), her intense emotion and hope overrode her intellectual grasp as she wondered whether the radiation would help her to live longer ("or would I die anyway").[1(p. 156)]

ROLE OF MENTAL HEALTH AND OTHER THERAPEUTIC PROFESSIONALS

Palliative care clinicians must rely on many sources to understand and relieve children's distress and strive to address the child as a whole, including their physical, emotional, and spiritual distress. Medically trained palliative care clinicians may not have the full range of training to work with more complex emotional and psychological symptoms and may need to collaborate with multidisciplinary clinicians with overlapping expertise.[27] These clinicians can help with differential diagnosis of symptoms and use a range of therapeutic modalities to address them. The etiology of psychological symptoms in children are multifactorial and responsive to a host of physical and situational variables. For younger children, physical complaints and irritable or withdrawn behavior may be the most common expressions of emotional distress. The differential for depression or anxiety syndromes includes delirium and encephalopathy, medication side effects, and pain or other physical symptoms such as dyspnea or fatigue. Anxiety may be generalized or specific to separation, procedures, or the anticipation of pain. Medical trauma and terror can also present in a variety of ways in both children and their parents. (See Chapter 17 for a full review of psychological symptoms and psychiatric syndromes.) Uncertainty around the illness, misconceptions, and lack of communication or secrets surrounding the illness can also fuel distress and changes in behavior. Mental health clinicians, and the entire medical team, need to pay close attention to the history provided by the parents. They also have a specific role, in the course of an evaluation or psychotherapy, to uncover the individual child's or adolescent's perceptions of the illness and its implications.

Because children's experiences are so intertwined with those of their parents and the professional team, it is essential to clarify whose distress is being reported. There are often discrepancies in parent and child assessment of symptoms of depression, for example, with parents both over- and underreporting as compared with their child's self-reports.[28] Children and, adolescents in particular, try to protect their parents from the extent of their distress.[29] Clinicians who care for these children must be vigilant about the influence of past personal or professional experiences, especially those involving loss, on their assessment of a particular situation.

In pediatric oncology, Standards of Psychosocial Care have been defined and include a range of interventions around psychosocial, spiritual, cultural, and palliative care needs. Mental health professionals, child life specialists, and art and music therapists focus on children's subjective experience of the illness. Their expertise lies in eliciting and understanding children's language, images, and play. As such, they often serve as interpreters of the child's experiences and needs to the medical team and the parents.

PSYCHOLOGICAL TREATMENT

A 6-year-old child stated: I felt much better because I knew that I had somebody to talk to all the time. Every boy needs a psychologist! To see his feelings![1(p. 3)]

You don't look at me like other people do and judge my behavior. Instead you analyze my behavior and try to get to the root of it. Mostly you helped me get to the root of it, and helped me handle it on my own. You can ask for your family's support, wisdom, experience; but it's not fair to burden them. I have an older sister whom I talk to, but at the same time, I don't want to upset her. I don't want to make her cry for me, I know that when I first met you, I didn't want to talk about it. I wanted to handle it on my own. But that faded so quickly because you're so helpless. You really do need somebody that can come in and help you.[2](p. 113)

Ideally, the psychological status of each child receiving palliative care should be evaluated in order to plan for optimal care, in the same way that medical and nursing assessments are carried out. The contribution of child psychology and psychiatry, as well as other mental health disciplines, provides specialized knowledge and skills. The specific and unique interventions include evaluation of the child's psychological status, diagnosis of psychological/psychiatric symptoms and disturbance, psychotherapy and psychotropic medication, and consultation to families and the team. The healthy siblings are included within this network of care.[14]

Reasons for referral for psychological treatment include

- Diagnosis of depression, anxiety, or traumatic responses in the child or sibling,
- Generalized distress in coping with the exigencies of the illness, as perceived by the child, parents, and/or team,
- Preexisting stressors or vulnerabilities in the child's life that are now exacerbated by the illness (e.g., psychiatric history in child or family member; recent geographical move, loss of employment, divorce, death of family member),
- Dilemmas in decision-making,
- Requests by parents who want their child to have all possible avenues of intervention and support.[30]

Children and their families respond best to referrals for psychological intervention when key team members explain it as recommended and routine and something that "other families we have treated have found helpful." Children's anxiety can be allayed when they hear the simple, nonthreatening explanation: "All children who are ill, or who have siblings who are ill, have worries." Terms such as the "talking doctor" or the "feelings doctor" provide a functional description that clearly distinguishes the mental health clinician from others on the team. The concept of confidentiality, or privacy, should be introduced early, with a definition of its meaning and boundaries. Over time, even if not articulated, children come to understand the mental health clinician's role in their care. For older children and adolescents, the concept of the "psych person" as a team member, albeit with special bounds of confidentiality, helps to diminish any sense of stigma.

Psychotherapy is the treatment modality unique to the mental health clinician and can add a crucial dimension to a child's comprehensive care. It facilitates psychological adjustment by providing a protected framework for the expression of profound grief and for the integration of all that he or she has lived, albeit in an abbreviated life span. The child conveys the experience of living with uncertainty and the threat of loss through words, drawings, and play and transforms the essence of his or her reality into expression. Furthermore, even for a young child, considerations about remaining quality of life may be discussed.[1,13] Psychotherapy may be the sole intervention or may be combined with psychotropic medication and behavioral symptom management techniques.

With the intrusion of the illness, the relationship between children and their parents organizes around the pivot of potential loss. Thus, it is critical that the mental health clinician not intercede as a divisive wedge between them. From the outset, an ongoing alliance diminishes this threat and optimizes the outcome of the work. Such collaboration is an essential part of the process. Because the parents must sustain the therapeutic work in the child's day-to-day encounters with both physical and emotional stresses, their role cannot be underestimated.[1]

The availability of psychological consultation in pediatric palliative care is often limited. While it is true that psychological treatment is not universally necessary, the opportunity to identify "high-risk" children and intervene in a timely fashion is often missed. The challenge, under these circumstances, is to provide thoughtful emotional support for the child in a carefully planned manner. Such support comes in many forms, from a willingness to listen and answer questions, to regular visits at expected times, to creative art and play that allow the child to express feelings and concerns. If a child has demonstrated particular comfort or closeness with one particular individual on the team, that person may be designated as a resource for the child, with efforts to ensure consistent contact between them. On a cautionary note, there are risks when unskilled or inadequately trained personnel attempt to undertake a psychotherapeutic role. These risks include opening up too much vulnerability in the child and then not knowing how to contain the emotion; interpreting—beyond simply clarifying—the child's disclosures; promising confidentiality that may set up competition, rather than collaboration, with the parents; and becoming involved with the child beyond appropriate boundaries.[14]

CHILD LIFE AND EXPRESSIVE THERAPIES

Child life specialists play a vital role in reducing the impact of stressful and traumatic events on children in medical settings.[31] They work with children and adolescents individually and in groups and develop the programs in hospital playrooms. They provide both therapeutic intervention and social recreation, framed by their understanding of children's responses to illness. Some settings also have art or music therapists who work in these specific modalities to help children cope with their experience through distracting or pleasurable activities. They also provide unique ways for youth to express their experience and manage emotion through activities like art, photography, creating playlists, or playing instruments. Their insights are integral to the team's understanding of a child's adjustment to the overall experience. They are often a source of emotional support to the siblings and parents as well.

Child life specialists use developmentally appropriate and enjoyable techniques with patients and their siblings to familiarize children with aspects of the medical experience and to provide outlets for their feelings. They prepare the children for medical procedures and teach them coping techniques to alleviate distress while at the same time enhancing their sense of control and mastery. Their encouragement of children's social interaction, both in the hospital and at home, as well as their liaison with school reentry programs, mitigates the children's sense of isolation. Importantly, child life specialists assist children in the process of decision-making by encouraging and facilitating communication with their parents and their medical team. Guiding parents in helping the child live as fully as possible, even when close to death, as well as in talking with and involving the siblings during the illness and in bereavement, is another aspect of the child life specialist's role. They are also often instrumental in initiating "legacy activities" with children, siblings, and parents to create lasting memories.

> A 5-year-boy who could not have visits from his little sister because he was being prepared for transplant missed her intensely. When it turned out that the transplant could not be done, plans were put in motion to transfer him to home hospice. During that week, he refused to get out of bed or play. When discharge was imminent, his mother asked the child life specialist how to engage him in play at home with his sister. The child life specialist gave the mother many suggestions and also put together a bag including fun objects such as silly string and serious materials including a handprint kit. The family was deeply appreciative and reported that the ideas and the materials had helped them interact and play as well as build memories.

> A 16-year-old girl who spoke only Vietnamese was hospitalized for a long period. The week before she died, a nurse asked the child life specialist to bring in a project that would be enjoyable for the child and that the mother could then keep as a memory. The child life specialist brought an example of spin art into the girl's room and, through an interpreter asked

whether she wanted to do it. The girl nodded. She had engaged in very little over the past few weeks. The child life specialist returned later in the day with the spin art materials and demonstrated how to do it. It was a magical moment: the child and her mother laughed together as she grabbed the paints and glitter. The child life specialist kept asking her if she wanted to make another, and she nodded yes over and over again. At the end of the afternoon, the mother showed the grandmother all the pictures that were lined up on display. The art project had brought enjoyment to the girl in the company of her mother, gave a sense of control as she wielded the spinner, and left good memories for the family.

CONCLUSION

The children who speak in this chapter articulate the concerns of patients and siblings who live in the shadow of life-threatening illness. Children who are not verbal, or who are developmentally delayed, also experience many of these issues, albeit in different ways. As children, adolescents, young adults, and families negotiate an illness through its progressive losses and the anticipation of death, palliative care clinicians, in their individual roles and as a team, are their unique companions.

ACKNOWLEDGMENTS

Portions of this chapter are reprinted with permission from Brandell, J. (ed.)*Countertransference in Psychotherapy with Children and Adolescents.* Jason Aronson Publishing Company, 1992. Additional portions are reprinted with permission from Sourkes, B. *The Deepening Shade: Psychological Aspects of Life-Threatening Illness,* University of Pittsburgh Press, 1992.

REFERENCES

1. Sourkes B. *Armfuls of Time: The Psychological Experience of the Child with a Life-Threatening Illness.* Pittsburgh: University of Pittsburgh Press; 1995.
2. Sourkes B. *The Deepening Shade: Psychological Aspects of Life-Threatening Illness.* Pittsburgh: University of Pittsburgh Press; 1982.
3. Van der Geest IMM, Darlington A-SE, Streng IC, et al. Parents' experiences of pediatric palliative care and the impact on long-term parental grief. *J Pain Symptom Manag.* 2014;47:1043–1053.
4. Vollenbroich R, Borasio GD, Duroux A, et al. Listening to parents: The role of symptom perception in pediatric palliative home care. *Palliat Support Care.* 2016;14:13–19.
5. Rosenberg AR, Orellana L, Ullrich C, et al. Quality of life in children with advanced cancer: A report from the PediQUEST Study. *J Pain Symptom Manag.* 2016;52:243–253.
6. Jalmsell L, Kreicbergs U, Onelöv E, et al. Anxiety is contagious: Symptoms of anxiety in the terminally ill child affect long-term psychological well-being in bereaved parents. *Pediatr Blood Cancer.* 2010;54:751–757.
7. Kreicbergs U, Valdimarsdóttir U, Onelöv E, et al. Care-related distress: A nationwide study of parents who lost their child to cancer. *J Clin Oncol.* 2005;23:9162–9171.
8. Rosenberg AR, Orellana L, Wolfe J, Dussel V. The limitations of "how are you feeling?" *J Pain Symptom Manag.* 2018;55(3):e6–e7. PMID 29169994.
9. Sourkes B. Siblings of the pediatric cancer patient. In Kellerman J, ed. *Psychological Aspects of Childhood Cancer.* Springfield, IL: Charles C. Thomas; 1980: 47–69.
10. Sourkes B. Siblings of the child with a life-threatening illness. *J Child Contemp Soc.* 1987;19:159–184.
11. Sharpe D, Rossiter L. Siblings of children with a chronic illness: A meta-analysis. *J Pediatr Psychol.* 2002;27(8):699–710.
12. Alderfer MA, Long KA, et al. Psychosocial adjustment of siblings of children with cancer: a systematic review. *Psychooncology.* 2009 October 27: Epub.
13. Sourkes B, Frankel L, Brown M, et al. Food, toys, and love: Pediatric palliative care. *Curr Probl Pediatr Adolesc Health Care.* 2005;35(9):345–392.
14. Sourkes B. Psychological impact of life-limiting conditions on the child. In Goldman A, Haines R, and Liben S, eds. *Oxford Textbook of Palliative Care for Children.* Oxford: Oxford University Press; 2006:95–107.
15. Wolfe J, Sourkes B. Palliative care for the child with advanced cancer. In Pizzo P, Poplack D, ed. *Principles and Practice of Pediatric Oncology,* 5th ed. Philadelphia: Lippincott; 2006:1531–1555.
16. Arnett JJ. Emerging adulthood. A theory of development from the late teens through the twenties. *Am Psychol.* 2000 May;55(5):469–480.
17. Hauer, J. *Caring for Children Who Have Severe Neurological Impairment: A Life with Grace.* Baltimore: Johns Hopkins; 2013.
18. Semeria J, Lucia A. A new vision for palliative care: Partners for hope. Stanford Children's Health Blog. November 23, 2016. https://healthier.stanfordchildrens.org/en/palliative-care-partners-for-hope/
19. Sourkes B. The child with a life-threatening illness. In Brandell J, ed. *Countertransference in Child and Adolescent Psychotherapy.* New York: Jason Aronson; 1992:267–284.
20. Bluebond-Langner M., ed. *The Private Worlds of Dying Children.* Princeton, NJ: Princeton University Press; 1978.
21. Sourkes B. The broken heart: Anticipatory grief in the child facing death. *J Palliat Care.* 1996;12(3):56–59.
22. Kuttner L. *Making Every Moment Count: Pediatric Palliative Care.* Documentary film. National Film Board of Canada; 2003.
23. Kreicbergs U, Valdimarsdóttir U, Onelöv E, et al. Talking about death with children who have severe malignant disease. *JAMA.* 2004;351(12):1175–1186.
24. Hinds PS, Schum L, Baker JN, Wolfe J. Key factors affecting dying children and their families. *J Palliat Med.* 2005;8(Suppl 1):S70–S78.
25. Hinds PS, Drew D, Oakes LL, et al. End-of-life preferences of pediatric patients with cancer. *J Clin Oncol.* 2005;23(36):9146–9154.
26. Friedel M, Aujoulat I, Dubois AC, Degryse JM. Instruments to measure outcomes in pediatric palliative care: A systematic review. *Pediatrics.* 2019 Jan;143(1). pii: e20182379. doi: 10.1542/peds.2018-2379.
27. Muriel AC, Wolfe J, Block SD. Pediatric palliative care and child psychiatry: A model for enhancing practice and collaboration. *J Palliat Med.* 2016 October;19(10):1032–1038
28. DeJong M, Fombonne E. Depression in pediatric cancer: An overview. *Psychooncology.* 2006;15:553–566.
29. Stuber ML, Gonzalez S, Benjamin H, et al. Fighting for recovery: Group interventions for adolescents with cancer and their parents. *J Psychother Pract Res.* 1995;4(4):286–296.
30. Sourkes B, Kazak A, Wiener L. Psychotherapeutic interventions. In Kazak A, Kupst M, Pao M, et al., eds. *Quick Reference for Pediatric Oncology Clinicians: The Psychiatric and Psychological Dimensions of Pediatric Cancer Symptom Management.* Charlottesville VA: International Psycho-Oncology Society Press; 2009:169–178.
31. Munn E, Robison K. Palliative care and the role of child life. *Child Life Council.* 2004;22(3):4–6.

4 | SETTINGS OF CARE

MOSHE COHN, EMILY JOHNSTON, AND JULIA MCBEE

Know from whence you came
And where you are headed
And before Whom you are destined to stand.
ETHICS OF THE FATHERS

Peace unto you
Peace unto your home
Peace unto all that is yours!
THE BOOK OF SAMUEL

INTRODUCTION

This chapter explores the settings in which children with serious, life-limiting conditions and their families receive palliative and end-of-life care. At varying times in the illness trajectory, patients may be treated at different sites such as acute care hospitals, home care facilities and agencies, and chronic care facilities, with different teams of clinicians in each setting. Care also extends to hospice, schools, and other community venues where the children continue to live their lives. The concept of *medical home*, as described by the American Academy of Pediatrics (AAP), has particular relevance for these children. The aim of a medical home is to support the needs of children through collaboration among families, clinicians, and community providers, extending "beyond the four walls of clinical practice."[1] Pediatric palliative care (PPC) clinicians strive daily to achieve this aim for the most complex and seriously ill children, wherever they are located. This requires varied roles by a large team capable of providing both primary and specialty palliative care. However, roles and team members involved varies between sites (and programs) as listed in Table 4.1. Successful integration of palliative care and hospice care teams across all settings in the continuum of care is in keeping with the Core Commitments set out by the AAP and the National Hospice and Palliative Care Organization (NHPCO).[2,3] This integration of palliative care across settings can have tremendous impact on children and their families, as highlighted in one family's experience with PPC (see family reflection).

Family Reflection

Last October, we brought our 14-month-old daughter to the emergency room after she stopped walking, talking, and eating. We heard the word "cancer." During those first 2 weeks, her oncologist suggested we speak with the palliative care team.

Upon hearing the word "palliative," we panicked, but she assured us they would be able to help.

With our fears palpable, we were introduced to the palliative nurse practitioner and quickly found a compassionate and astute medical professional who became an advocate for not only our daughter, but for us as well.

She checked in daily, became a treasured resource, a compassionate listener we could talk to about our fears and concerns. Along with our palliative doctors, Drs. A, Z, and L, she worked with the pediatric intensive care unit (PICU), the 9-East team, and oncology to manage our daughter's persistent discomfort.

Six months after it all started, our greatest fears became reality. She went into septic shock. Her liver failed, and it was only a matter of time before her heart would stop. That night, the NP and Dr. A met us in the PICU to discuss next steps and provide the emotional support we needed in our darkest hour. They carefully and caringly walked us through every option and assured us that any decision we made, they would support. We met the wonderful bereavement specialist, dedicated and caring.

We were scared and devastated, trying to process losing our beloved daughter, and these incredible people never left us. Their professionalism, knowledge, and,

TABLE 4.1 Who provides pediatric palliative care (PPC) in different settings of care?

CARE TEAM MEMBERS THAT PROVIDE PALLIATIVE CARE	LOCATIONS WHERE CHILDREN RECEIVE PALLIATIVE CARE				
	PEDIATRIC FLOOR	NICU	PICU	HOME	HOSPICE
Pediatrician or subspecialty pediatrician	xxx	x	x	xxx	x
Intensivist		xxx	xxx		
PPC physician	xx–xxx	xx–xxx	xx–xxx	Depends on PPC outpatient availability and structure	Depends on what services local hospice agencies provides versus PPC
PPC nurse practitioner	xx–xxx	xx–xxx	xx–xxx		
PPC clinical social worker	xx–xxx	xx–xxx	xx–xxx		
PPC child life specialist	xx	xx	xx		
PPC chaplain	xx	xx	xx		
PPC psychologist or psychiatrist	xx	xx	xx		

Degree of involvement: x, little involvement; xx, moderate involvement; xxx, extensive involvement.

above all, their compassion, was exemplary, and for this bereaved couple, we will always have the highest gratitude for them.

To help those providing palliative and end-of-life care understand where the children they care for live and die, this chapter addresses

- Epidemiological factors in children receiving palliative and end-of-life care services related to where they live and die
- Inpatient settings: the general pediatrics ward, intensive care units, and the emergency department. Community settings: home hospice, long-term care facilities, free-standing palliative and respite facilities, school, outpatient clinic, and telehealth.

WHERE ARE CHILDREN RECEIVING PALLIATIVE CARE?

PPC takes on many forms, locations, and patients. While the landscape of life-threatening illness has spread beyond oncology, trauma, and perinatal events, the commitments of PPC remain firm. Along with a growing population of children with complex chronic conditions (CCCs) comes a growing call for a palliative approach to their care from the time of diagnosis.[3] However, deciding who should receive specialty versus primary palliative and end-of-life care and when and where it should happen is challenging. Children receiving palliative care live far longer than their adult counterparts.[4] Unfortunately, despite tremendous medical and surgical advances, some children die from serious illness. End-of-life care is therefore an essential aspect of both primary and specialty PPC. In order to understand where children are receiving palliative care we need to know where children with complex, chronic, and life-threatening illnesses are living and where children are dying.

WHERE CHILDREN WITH COMPLEX CHRONIC CONDITIONS ARE LIVING

Children with CCCs spend a significant amount of time in the hospital. According to one report, these children spend an average of 27 days in the hospital in their last year of life, with 7 of those days in the intensive care unit.[5] On the other hand, they are spending 338 days, or 48 weeks, out of the hospital, during that same year. Additionally, children with CCCs are at high risk for readmission to the hospital.[6] Therefore, out-of-hospital care, or community-based care that incorporates palliative care is essential for children with CCCs to (1) ensure their medical needs are being met and (2) try to prevent admissions. In the community, these children will be spending time at home, in clinics, in schools, and in care facilities—all of which provide opportunities for delivery of PPC.

WHERE CHILDREN ARE DYING

More than 60% of children with CCCs die in the hospital,[7–9] with the majority of those deaths occurring in the intensive care unit (ICU).[8,10] Other locations of death include the emergency room or out in the field—typically after an acute event or severe trauma. Hospital length of stay is variable: while some children are hospitalized for just a few days before death, there are many who die after prolonged admissions lasting weeks or even months.[11] Although more children with a CCC die in the hospital than at home, and the majority of those hospital deaths occur in the ICU, the distribution varies significantly depending on admitting diagnosis, underlying condition, and number of existing CCCs.[8,9] In the early 2000s, there was a slight trend toward death at home for children with CCCs,[7] but in-hospital death remains more common. Given that most pediatric deaths occur in the hospital, the emergency department, and in the field, hospice services are uncommon in pediatrics: only 26% of children who died and were insured by Medicaid ever accessed hospice or home health services.[12]

PEDIATRIC PALLIATIVE CARE IN THE INPATIENT SETTING

THE HOSPITAL FLOOR

WHO IS CARED FOR ON THE FLOOR?

Due to advances in medical technology, children with CCCs are living for longer periods of time.[13] The life-sustaining devices on which they depend increases the educational and daily care burden on parents and caregivers, complicating discharge processes, and may be a significant factor in prolonged hospitalizations. In the past, a prolonged admission was defined as greater than 1 week. However, over the past decade this has changed to time measured in months and sometimes years.[14] These children are in effect *living* in the hospital for protracted periods of time. In the inpatient setting, children with CCCs will receive services from a multitude of subspecialists and interdisciplinary professionals including the PPC team.[15] According to the 2011 prospective cohort study of children cared for by six hospital-based PPC teams in the United States and Canada, the inpatient PPC team was most commonly consulted for patients with genetic/congenital conditions (40.8%), neuromuscular disorders (39.2%), oncologic diagnoses (19.8%), respiratory disorders (12.8%), gastrointestinal conditions (10.7%), cardiovascular conditions (8.3%), metabolic disorders (7.2%), renal diseases (2.7%), and immunologic conditions (2.6%).[4] Children from this cohort often required at least one type of assistive medical device, most commonly a feeding tube (68.2%) followed by a central venous catheter (22.3%), tracheostomy (10.1%), and 13% requiring assisted respiration with NIPPV.[4]

WHAT ARE THEIR SYMPTOMS?

Children with CCCs experience a high symptom burden throughout their disease trajectory, and management of their constellation of symptoms is a growing area of clinical research. On the ward the PPC team should take an active role in identifying and treating symptoms, which may be refractory to standard medical therapies. Children with CCCs, especially those with severe neurological impairment, may suffer from symptoms which are commonly underrecognized and undertreated, such as pain, disordered sleep, and feeding intolerance.[16] Among pediatric oncology patients, the involvement of a PPC team has been associated with parental perception of a decrease in distressing symptoms, such as pain, dyspnea, and anxiety, especially at the end of life, a time when overall symptom burden is likely to intensify.[17] Symptoms can be difficult to manage on the ward, sometimes due to institutional policies regarding opioid administration and use of adjuvant medication, as well as the level of monitoring available. This may be true especially for patients without the documentation of an advance directive. It is not uncommon for children to require ICU-level care for improved symptom management, especially during end-of-life care. Policies regarding palliative sedation, use of patient-controlled analgesia (PCA), and other related issues vary significantly between hospitals. The PPC team is uniquely situated to navigate these policies to ensure seamless care across hospital units and advocate for change if the local policies do not reflect best practices.

DO THEY SURVIVE? ARE THEY RECEIVING PALLIATIVE CARE?

Unlike the adult population, children receiving PPC live for more than a year after the initial inpatient palliative care consultation.[4] PPC involvement and team composition differ throughout children's hospitals across the United States, as demonstrated in a 2013 study.[18] Approximately 50% of hospitals surveyed reported having a PPC team.[18] Staff composition of the PPC teams typically includes a physician, nurse practitioner or other advanced practice provider, and a social worker. Psychologists, child life specialists, and chaplains may also be dedicated members of the interdisciplinary PPC team. The budgetary commitment to each of these disciplines, as a percentage of a full-time equivalent (FTE) is highly variable.[18] Of note, while the Joint Commission certifies palliative care programs at the institutional level, it is currently developing distinct regulations for pediatric programs, which could lead to standardization of PPC team composition and services.

PPC consultations in the hospital were most often for assistance with symptom management, followed by facilitating communication, aid in decision-making and discharge planning, and, less often, discussions regarding resuscitation status.[6] It should not be overlooked that specialty palliative care clinicians are not the only providers delivering PPC in the inpatient setting. Long before the initial PPC consultation is placed, hospitalists, bedside nurses, social workers, hematologists, and oncologists, among other specialists, such as mental health professionals, often employ primary palliative care skills when caring for children with CCCs. On the ward, the PPC team works alongside the primary clinical team to establish a lasting rapport with patients and families and provide goal-concordant care. The involvement of the PPC team is often longitudinal as the team follows the child and family through lengthy hospital stays and transitions across care settings.

CHALLENGES AND STRATEGIES FOR DELIVERING PALLIATIVE CARE ON THE HOSPITAL FLOOR

There are numerous hospital teams that will consult PPC, which presents many challenges for PPC teams. First, many team will introduce the idea of PPC prior to the team's arrival, which will vary considerably from team to team. PPC may be introduced as the end-of-life team, people to help with symptom management, or as an extra layer of support for families. Second, some teams will only want the PPC team to address the initial consult question, whereas others are happy to have the team explore other issues as they arrive. Third, each team in the hospital may have different level of social work, chaplain, psychology, and child life support, which may affect how the PPC teams plan is best enacted. Fourth, some teams will provide regular medical updates to the PPC and others will not. Finally, some teams will enact all of the PPC's teams recommendations and others will not. Essential to addressing many of these issues is clear communication with the primary team—from asking them what the family understands about PPC to exactly what the team wants out of the PPC consult to regularly touching base with the team about patient updates.

THE PEDIATRIC INTENSIVE CARE UNIT

WHO IS CARED FOR IN THE PEDIATRIC INTENSIVE CARE UNIT?

In most US hospitals, children with (or at-risk for developing) acute life-threatening illness are cared for in a single pediatric intensive care unit (PICU). Larger children's hospitals have specialized ICUs for children with critical cardiac or neurologic illness, analogous to similar units for adult patients. Children in the PICU typically suffer from failure of one or more organ or homeostatic systems, with a wide spectrum of presentations and acuity. Tertiary- and quaternary-care PICUs must therefore provide a range of medical care, from short-term postoperative stabilization to multisystem trauma, as well as mechanical organ support, such as continuous renal replacement therapy and extracorporeal membrane oxygenation (ECMO).[19]

An increasing percentage of PICU admissions is comprised of children with CCCs, many of whom develop "chronic critical illness," are assisted by medical technology, and experience prolonged ICU stays.[20,21] These children often have neurologic impairment resulting from hypoxic-ischemic injury in the perinatal and/or neonatal periods, trauma, and congenital/genetic disorders.

Given the dearth of inpatient hospice facilities for children, the PICU may serve as a surrogate "hospice" in caring for children at the end of life, although this varies significantly by underlying diagnosis. The availability of an inpatient PPC team is recommended for a PICU to provide high-quality end-of-life care.[19]

WHAT ARE THEIR SYMPTOMS?

As varied as the ages, diagnoses, and prognoses are in the PICU, so are the constellation of symptomatologies. The full gamut of symptom categories typically treated by a PPC team are encountered in the PICU: pain, psychiatric, gastrointestinal, neurologic, and respiratory. Specific management of these symptoms and symptom categories is discussed in Section III of this book. Children with CCC are more likely to have a higher overall symptom burden—in particular, acute-on-chronic pain, as well as gastrointestinal symptoms due to exacerbated dysfunction in the setting of critical illness. Acute delirium is prevalent in more than 25% of PICU patients in some studies and is likely underrecognized and poorly managed; symptoms of delirium, such as hallucination and catatonia, are quite distressing to both children and their families.[22,23] Along with delirium, disordered sleep is a particularly burdensome symptom in the pediatric setting, and both are amplified in the PICU by the associated and inconsistent use of sedatives, analgesics, and anxiolytics.[24]

For children receiving palliative care, the concept of a "total symptom" (such as total pain or total dyspnea) takes on unique characteristics in pediatrics and is amplified further in the PICU. In children with intact cognitive function, discomfort in any category may be exacerbated by exposure to their parents' emotions of anxiety, sadness, and fear.

DO THEY SURVIVE?

The overall mortality in PICUs has declined steadily in recent decades, although this varies by admitting diagnosis.[25,26] Mortality risk prediction in the PICU is a relatively young science, with several models being studied and refined.[27,28] While mortality may be strongly predicted for patients admitted with severe, multisystem trauma, such that trauma-related deaths would be expected to occur in the PICU or emergency department, this is not the case for surgical, oncologic, and other serious illnesses. Moreover, among children receiving palliative care services, those with a terminal prognosis whose death is not expected during a particular hospital stay may nevertheless become overwhelmed by an acute and irreversible clinical decline. Parent and child preference for a particular location for end-of-life care is being recognized as a potential factor in where children die.[29] At the same time, a 2013 study found that PPC involvement reduced deaths in the PICU by 25%.[30] In contradistinction to adults, it cannot be assumed that dying at home is the preferred option for most pediatric patients.[31]

ARE THEY RECEIVING PALLIATIVE CARE?

According to CAPC National Registry data, more than 25% of PPC referrals come from the PICU. If the neonatal ICU (NICU) is included in the tally, the total is more than 50%.[32] However, at present, it is unknown how many PICU patients are seen by palliative care specialists. This is an area of much needed research, but there is little, if any published data. An important area of ongoing research is how to best identify children who would benefit from a palliative care consult and, of those, whether or not they were seen by a PPC team.[31]

WHAT DOES PALLIATIVE CARE LOOK LIKE IN THE PICU?

The limited data from the National Registry suggests that the PICU is a location where PPC services are highly utilized. The involvement of the pediatric intensivist is a major factor that differentiates palliative care in the PICU from the hospital ward. While hospitalist pediatricians may have some education or experience with providing primary palliative care and basic medical decision-making, children with life-limiting illness or CCCs admitted to the general pediatrics ward are often followed closely by the relevant "primary" subspecialty, such as oncology, neurology, or nephrology. Such subspecialists are assumed to be in the best position to prognosticate and assist with medical decisions for their patients. In contrast, children with critical illness require an additional layer of clinical expertise.[19] Pediatric intensivists are trained to take a more clinically "holistic" approach to prognostication, in the sense that all organ systems are considered in contributing to the assessment of the ultimate outcome for the patient.

The pediatric intensivist may thus play the role of "gatekeeper" to life-sustaining, life-prolonging, or even heroic life-saving measures. The intensivist is a key participant in discussions regarding resuscitation, dialysis, or ECMO, as well as palliative extubation and limiting artificial nutrition and hydration. At the same time, involvement of a PPC team appears to be a factor in whether invasive interventions are utilized, especially at the end of life.[30] Perimortem decision-making such as determination of death by neurologic criteria, autopsy, and organ or tissue donation frequently involve intensivists as well.[33]

Urgency of care is an additional characteristic of PPC in the PICU setting. As critically ill patients are at higher risk for sudden or acute decline, the availability of an on-call PPC team is crucial to providing timely PPC services and should include social workers, child-life specialists, chaplains, and mental health professionals. In the PICU, members of the interdisciplinary PPC team provide a more "intense" level of service than they do elsewhere. For example, a dying child may be attended by a large family group, including siblings and grandparents. Emotions and stress levels are heightened among family and clinical staff. The presence of social workers and other psychosocial professionals, palliative care nurses, and child-life specialists is vital to facilitating communication, privacy, respite, and bereavement in this scenario.

Improving the quality of palliative care in the PICU has become a major focus of the Society for Critical Care Medicine, especially around end-of-life care.[34] In several published reports between 2010 and 2016, the Improving Palliative Care in the ICU (IPAL-ICU) Project describes several levels of palliative care education and provision in the PICU.[35–37] Models of care delivery, such as consultative and integrated models, are currently being studied,[38–40] and clinician education and resilience support have been identified as key components of quality care.[41] A recent qualitative analysis of speech used by pediatric intensivists and palliative clinicians suggests that the addition of a palliative care team to family meetings may improve communication with families.[42,43] Standardization of family meetings and decreasing PICU readmissions are stated goals of a recent program of the American Academy of Pediatrics, partnering PPC and intensive care clincians.[44] The crucial role of palliative care "champion" is most often played by the PICU nurse, who serves as the daily liaison between the child, the family, and all other clinical and nonclinical team members. The model of a palliative care "champion" may also be formalized in an effort to enhance quality of palliative care provision in the PICU.[45]

CHALLENGES AND STRATEGIES FOR DELIVERING PALLIATIVE CARE IN THE PEDIATRIC INTENSIVE CARE UNIT

In addition to the challenges of working with diverse teams on the floor, PPC teams in PICU face the additional challenges of working with families during an extremely stressful time. During PICU admissions, families may or may not be receptive to additional team involvement and may or may not have the emotional bandwidth to consider critical decisions that need to be made. Therefore, when possible, it can be beneficial to have someone familiar with the family introduce the PPC team, work with the family to identify the best time for discussions with PPC, and include the child and families' key support people when possible (these can be family members or people such as their primary oncologist or social worker). Finally, as mentioned earlier, not all PICU teams are equally receptive to PPC. Therefore, working to develop a PICU "champion" can be beneficial to all involved.

THE NEONATAL INTENSIVE CARE UNIT

WHO IS CARED FOR IN THE NICU?

There has been an increased admission rate to high-acuity NICUs in the past two decades, for reasons that are unclear.[46] Hospital policies vary about whether only newborns are admitted to the NICU or if neonates, once discharged, are "readmitted" to the NICU rather than the PICU. Regardless, NICU admissions include preterm and term infants requiring ICU-level care. As of 2012, 77.9 neonates out of every 1,000 live births were admitted to the NICU.[47] Preterm infants born at less than 31 weeks' gestation make up only 1.5% of the admissions, with up to 90.4% of NICU admissions having been born full-term.[47] Full-term infants in the NICU suffer from a variety of conditions, including respiratory failure, pulmonary hypertension, congenital anomalies, birth trauma, and infection.[46] The length of stay in the NICU can vary, from less than 1 day for certain conditions to an average of 43 days for babies weighing less than 1,500 g at birth.[48]

WHAT ARE THEIR SYMPTOMS?

Neonates regularly undergo painful procedures, such as IV catheter placement and frequent blood draws, along with major and minor surgeries. Evaluating the pain elicited from these procedures is challenging due to gestational age-related differences in pain physiology. Pain responses can be atypical, altered, or abnormal—phenomena such as hyperalgesia and neuropathic pain are not uncommon. Babies admitted to the NICU frequently require tube feedings and invasive respiratory support, which are nonphysiologic, and both are associated with distress. Environmental stimuli such as excessive ambient noise are particularly noxious to neonates, as enclosed isolettes amplify decibel levels reaching premature ears. An extensive discussion of these symptoms can be found in Chapter 28 of this book. Palliative care can not only be critical in managing these symptoms, but there is also pressing need for PPC services for parents of babies in the NICU. In addition to the challenges faced by all parents in the intensive care setting, those in the NICU face the added stress of early separation from their newborn child during a period critical for early attachment and parent–child bonding, and when mothers are often exhausted from childbirth.[49]

DO THEY SURVIVE?

The majority of neonates admitted to the NICU survive. At the same time, the majority of childhood deaths occur in the first year after birth, and particularly in the first 30 days of life.[50] Therefore, the NICU is a common location for death to occur in the inpatient setting.[51]

ARE THEY RECEIVING PALLIATIVE CARE?

There is a growing specialty of neonatal palliative care, which can even begin when diagnosis of a life-threatening condition is made during a prenatal visit.[52] Many programs have been developed to encourage primary and specialty PPC in the NICU for terminally and non–terminally ill patients. Many surviving neonates face a variety of long-term medical challenges including developmental delays, the need for supplemental oxygen, and the inability to feed by mouth. Decision-making around surgeries and the use of medical technology, such as tracheostomies and gastrostomies, may present an opportunity for the PPC team to become involved. Once a relationship is established, the PPC team can then support these neonates and their parents in the transition from hospital to home and can facilitate continuity between the NICU and outpatient care.

CHALLENGES AND STRATEGIES FOR DELIVERING PALLIATIVE CARE IN THE NICU

The PPC team in the NICU faces the same challenges mentioned on the floor and in the PICU. However, these challenges are compounded by recent childbirth and long admissions. Parents, particularly mothers after complicated pregnancies and deliveries, may not be available at the bedside. Other parents will have to decide if they want to be present at the bedside during the NICU stay or save their parental leave for when their child is discharged home. Therefore, working with the family to find appropriate times to talk (potentially utilizing telehealth or visits to the mother's hospital room) is essential.

PALLIATIVE TRANSPORT HOME FOR COMPASSIONATE EXTUBATION

There are children intubated in the NICU and PICU who would only survive a short period after extubation. Some families will chose to withdraw care and have their child pass away in the hospital. However, other families want their child to die at home—including parents whose neonate has spent their entire life in the hospital. Some facilities are equipped to provide palliative transport home, which is defined as "the medical transport to home or inpatient hospice of children with levels of life-sustaining support demanding a critical care team, with the expectation of death within minutes to days after the cessation of that support."[53] Such transport requires active participation by the ambulance company, nurses, respiratory therapy, and the PPC team. When families have chosen palliative transport home, they have reported that the ride home is stressful but that they were extremely grateful for the opportunity for their child to die at home.[53] Therefore, when available, palliative transport home may be a unique location for provision of PPC.

EMERGENCY DEPARTMENT

PPC has two potential areas of integration in the emergency department setting. Children with CCCs who are already followed by palliative care may present to the emergency department.[54] They constitute a unique group that may benefit from the availability PPC in the emergency department, which can serve as a point of contact and continuity. There is evidence that children with a higher number of CCCs have a greater likelihood of visiting the emergency department but without requiring inpatient admission.[55] As outpatient pediatric palliative programs are not ubiquitous, the emergency department may be an opportune setting for a PPC team to connect with patients with whom they have a long-standing relationship. A second group of patients consists of previously healthy children who experience sudden life-threatening events such as drowning, severe trauma, sudden infant death syndrome (SIDS), or sudden unexpected childhood death (SUCD). Some of these children will die in the emergency room while others will begin a long medical journey—and both may benefit from palliative care involvement. Unintentional injury remains the leading cause of mortality among children age 1–19 years, accounting for 44% of deaths.[39–41] From an epidemiologic perspective, the dominant trajectory of childhood death is sudden and, therefore, unexpected.[26,39,41] An estimated 20% of childhood deaths actually occur in the emergency medical services (EMS) environment.[42–44]

These two groups have vastly different needs and require different approaches to provide them with the PPC services they could benefit from in the emergency room. For children with CCCs, establishing new relationships with on-call palliative care providers in the emergency setting is not ideal. Therefore, if there are palliative care needs in the emergency setting, the emergency room team might reach out to the primary palliative care clinician already known to the family, if one exists. For those children who present in extremis following a trauma, a PPC clinician will not always be available. Therefore, it is essential that (1) emergency room physicians receive primary palliative care training and (2) chaplains, social workers, and other supportive care staff are available.[46]

PEDIATRIC PALLIATIVE CARE IN THE COMMUNITY

HOME

LIVING AT HOME

There is a large and growing population of children with CCCs living at home and requiring substantial caregiver support. A study of caregivers of children with special healthcare needs showed the average caregiver spent 11–20 hours per week providing direct care for their children and an additional 2 hours per week of care coordination.[57] Not surprisingly, 57% of these families face financial difficulties because of their child's health.[58] It is evident that these children and their families could benefit greatly from home-based palliative care or hospice. However, the life expectancy requirement for hospice enrollment, which is less than 6 months, limits which children can enroll in hospice. Some states in the US, such as California, have adopted hospice waiver programs to allow children with life expectancies greater than 6 months to receive hospice services. Other states, such as Massachusetts, have developed statewide programs to meet the PPC needs of children living at home. The Massachusetts program was developed in 2006 to provide statewide community-based palliative care.[59] As of 2010, they were caring for more than 200 children annually, and the most common services provided were psychosocial and case management.[59] For states without such programs, families frequently have to work with multiple agencies to get their home care needs met—from durable medical equipment to home nursing to transportation to appointments. Unfortunately, these agencies do not always have interagency collaborations, creating additional work for families and case managers.[60,61] The type of home care that is more commonly available to children is home nursing, but there is a significant shortage of providers for these children.[62] Additionally, there are disparities in access to these critically important resources, with minorities, those from poorer areas, and children with behavioral problems having the most difficulties.[63] These factors contribute to delays in discharge when children with CCCs are admitted and to the high care burden at home, and they highlight the critical role of case managers in maximizing home resources and coordinating delivery of needed services.

HOME HOSPICE

While the majority of children with CCCs die in the hospital, a growing minority dies at home and would derive significant benefit from hospice services. Hospice is intended to provide high-quality medical and psychosocial care for people with a life expectancy of less than 6 months. Traditionally, the hospice benefit provides for care related to end-of-life needs, including medications, durable medical equipment, nursing, and social work; curative or disease-directed treatment of the underlying disease is not typically covered. Hospice agencies will receive a fixed amount to cover all expenses for each day of hospice-related services provided.

Although some adult hospices and programs have an interest and willingness to care for pediatric patients, adult-focused programs and staff may be unprepared for the occasional pediatric referral and lack connections to pediatric-trained clinicians to assist them in providing safe, effective, and age-appropriate hospice care.[64,65] Adult-focused hospice agencies vary in the amount of pediatric experience among staff. The 2007 survey of hospice agencies by the National Hospice and Palliative Care Organization showed that 78% of hospice agencies report caring for children, but the majority see fewer than 10 children per year.[64] Given this low volume it is not surprising that many hospice agencies lack personnel trained to care for children: only 14% of hospice agencies report formal pediatric services, and only 37% report formal training in pediatric hospice care.[64] The Concurrent Care Provision of the Affordable Care Act allows children with Medicaid coverage to receive disease-directed therapies while enrolled in hospice. This scenario may be confusing to hospice agencies that are most familiar with adult patients, for whom curative treatment is not a covered benefit.

Clinician attitudes toward and education in palliative and hospice care create a ground-level barrier to children receiving these services. Physicians and other healthcare workers in the community may be unaware of or uncomfortable with the specialized services that pediatric hospice and palliative care programs have to offer and may be reluctant to make referrals.[55,56] Inadequate formal training in the fundamentals of PPC[57–60] can in turn have clinical ramifications, in that the children may not receive services that would otherwise enhance their quality of life even if they are enrolled in hospice. One such consequence is that some families report negative experiences with hospice. In a study of 12 parents of children with cancer who enrolled in hospice, 5 out of 12 (42%) revoked hospice because of poor symptom management and another child died in uncontrollable pain because the parents did not realize they could return to the hospital.[66] This is consistent with findings from a qualitative study about palliative care experiences that included 17 children who died at home with a variety of conditions, albeit predominately cancer.[67] Parents expressed frustrations with hospice and home health agency scheduling and staffing, particularly staff that explicitly stated they were unprepared to care for children.[67] With inadequate care at home, many parents wanted services that would have been provided in the hospital but were not available to them through hospice.[67] Another qualitative study of bereaved parents of children with cancer found similar frustrations with staffing that led to inadequate symptom management.[68] Others reported feeling abandoned by their pediatric oncology team when they enrolled in hospice.[68] These problems with hospice and home care are supported by a study of 95 patients with cancer who enrolled in hospice at a single institution: 41% of families withdrew from hospice before the child died.[69] It can be beneficial for families to have their primary teams continue to follow them while they are on hospice to ensure that their needs are being met, to remind them that they are always welcome to return to their hospital if their needs cannot be met at home, and to ensure continuity of care if families choose to return to the hospital.

HOME AWAY FROM HOME: A CLINICAL VIGNETTE

At large academic institutions with multiple subspecialists, it is not uncommon to find children who have traveled with their families from across the country and around the world for second opinions, novel surgical procedures, and clinical trials.

These children often need a "home away from home," which may mean living in the hospital where they are being treated. This clinical vignette describes the journey of a young woman and her mother who traveled to the United States for a second opinion after receiving a devastating oncologic diagnosis.

Team Reflection

JN was a previously healthy 15-year-old young woman with a history of constitutional mismatch repair deficiency, a cancer predisposition syndrome. Due to her genetic disease, she developed two distinct neoplasms: widely metastatic adenocarcinoma of the colon and a glioblastoma multiforme in her occipital lobe. JN was originally diagnosed with metastatic colon cancer in the Dominican Republic, where she lived with her siblings, mother, and father. After an extensive bowel resection in the Dominican Republic, her mother brought JN to the United States for further treatment of both oncologic diagnoses. Following resection of her brain tumor in the United States, JN was readmitted to the hospital with severe pain in her pelvis, legs, and shoulders due to rapid progression of her disease. The goals of the patient and her parents were clear: initiate all disease-directed therapy including chemotherapy, surgery, and radiation therapy while optimizing quality of life and focusing on intensive symptom relief. There were no limitations placed on resuscitation.

Shortly after arriving in the United States, JN and her mother found that their relatives here could not accommodate their needs, and they moved to the local Ronald McDonald House. She was treated on an outpatient basis for a short time, but, unfortunately, she suffered from severe, unrelenting bone pain. As a result, JN and her mother spent most days in the inpatient setting. Initiating hospice care proved difficult because there were concerns regarding emergency Medicaid coverage and the lack of a stable place of residence in the United States.

While hospitalized, JN was shuttled back and forth between the pediatric ward and the PICU because her clinical condition and her pain were constantly in flux. JN required high doses of both opioids and anxiolytics to remain comfortable. This was a source of distress to the staff on the pediatric ward. Without a do-no-resuscitate (DNR) order in place, fear of oversedation and respiratory compromise ultimately brought JN back to the PICU, where she could be monitored more closely. Due to her rapidly progressing disease and attendant symptom burden, JN required near-constant nursing care, and so she spent the last few months of her life in the PICU. While she continued to receive chemotherapy, her overall care shifted to focus on her comfort.

Yet there was tension during those last months. The PICU is a setting of extremes, where clinical staff may perform emergency resuscitation in one room and compassionate extubation in the next. It is not, however, a hospice. The prospect of caring for a child and her family during a slow and painful dying process caused great distress to the PICU team. There were many discussions around finding a better setting for JN to receive end-of-life care. The pediatric ward might be comfortable, with some of the recommended pain management strategies, but would not be able to staff her care appropriately. Returning to the Dominican Republic was impossible—the family explained they would not have access even to basic pain management at home, and JN's symptoms were refractory such that she required simultaneous intravenous and intrathecal opioid infusions, at high doses. And with the lack of free-standing pediatric inpatient hospice facilities, end-of-life care in the hospital was the only suitable option. The PPC team became a welcome presence on daily rounds in the PICU, educating the bedside nurses, social workers, and house staff, and they worked in close collaboration with all caregivers to create an inpatient hospice-like atmosphere. At the direction of JN and her mother, a DNAR/DNAI order was placed in her chart, with detailed instructions reflecting their wishes. Palliative sedation was initiated, and JN died peacefully in the PICU surrounded by her mother, aunt, and grandmother.

LONG-TERM CARE FACILITIES

As discussed previously, children with CCCs may live for many years with the assistance of medical technology. After spending a period of time on the ward or in the ICU, children with medical technology, such as gastrostomy tubes, central venous access, tracheostomies, and respiratory support (e.g., mechanical ventilators, bilevel positive airway pressure [BiPAP] machines), may require a stay at a subacute rehabilitation center or a long-term care facility as a bridge to home. It is often difficult for families to care for their children at home without access to around-the-clock shift nursing and the specialized support necessary to run a "miniature ICU" out of their living room. Long-term care facilities may also provide respite care for families who need time for self-care and resilience. Primary palliative care as well as end-of-life care can be delivered at subacute rehabilitation centers or long-term care facilities by physicians, advanced practice providers, nurses, clinical social workers, psychologist/psychiatrists, and clinical child life specialists. The hospital-based PPC team may provide continuity of care as patients and families transition from acute care to long-term care environments. The PPC team can provide the receiving clinical team with the context and history of the family's goals of care for their child, including important details from advance care planning discussions and symptom management preferences. It is not uncommon for the inpatient PPC team to continue following the patient and family via phone calls and emails and in person around appointments with other subspecialty providers.

FREE-STANDING HOSPICE FACILITIES

As of 2020, there are only three facilities in the United States that offer inpatient palliative and end-of-life care services for children and their families: the George Mark Children's

House in San Leandro, California; Exceptional Care for Children in Newark, Delaware; and Crescent Cover in Brooklyn Center, Minnesota. All three facilities offer respite care for families caring for seriously ill children as well as traditional inpatient hospice services for those children who have a life expectancy of less than 6 months when the family is unable to provide adequate end-of-life care at home or does not want either a hospital or home death for their child. The goal of respite care is to provide temporary relief or rest for the caregivers of the seriously ill child, either in or outside the home, for hours, days, or even weeks at a time.[70] Respite care provides caregivers the opportunity to take a break from their extensive duties and challenges of caring for their child. Respite care may be offered voluntarily by the facilities or on a fee-for-service basis as a benefit with some insurance plans. Although a free-standing hospice can be an invaluable resource for those who desire such a setting of care, in a study of preferences for location of death among bereaved parents of children with cancer, only 7% of parents felt a free-standing hospice would be a preferred location of death.[71] Added to this, the expense of operating such facilities and their reliance on donations for funding are likely reasons for these facilities to remain a rarity in the United States.

SCHOOL AS A LOCATION OF CARE

Appreciating the context of the child's life, understanding what makes it meaningful, and respecting the relationships that are central to it are essential in PPC.[72] For the child who wishes to attend school, crucial issues must be considered in preparation. Although the Individual with Disabilities Act requires that schools provide education for children with special healthcare needs, which includes the physical, occupational, and speech therapy necessary to meet learning goals, it does not require that schools provide medical care.[73] Does the school have a nurse or other designated personnel available to accommodate the child's medical needs? Is there a need for an out-of-hospital DNR order? What is the plan for managing issues in the child's care that might arise during the school day? What is the responsibility of the administration to the other students regarding the possibility of a child dying at school? Frequently parents decide that it is easier to have their child home-schooled rather than deal with these many and often controversial issues. However, under the Education for All Handicapped Children Act (Public Law 94-142), all children are guaranteed the right to be in the classroom. The question of "What is in the best interest of the individual child?" must be balanced against the interests of others in the situation, such as the school community.

In 2000, the American Academy of Pediatrics (AAP) Committees on Bioethics and School Health issued the policy statement that "parents have a legal right to forego cardiopulmonary resuscitation and to ask the school to respect that decision.[74] Rushton says DNR orders are simply an extension of the right of families to make decisions about medical treatment or nontreatment. However, school officials argue that medically untrained staff may misinterpret DNR order, thereby doing more harm than good for the child. Administrators are concerned that failing to act could make the school and/or school district liable.

The DNR order is usually honored without reservation in the hospital or hospice setting but is rarely supported for children in school or other community settings. Although 43 out of 50 states and the District of Columbia have enacted out-of-hospital DNR orders, only five would extend legal protection to school personnel for honoring such decisions.[75] Only 17 of these states and the District of Columbia permit advance healthcare decisions for minors. These ill-defined laws obviously create problems for parents and legal guardians of children who choose to attend school.

Hospital teams and community agencies can collaborate with the school for the child's care. Establishing a relationship with the school team early and sorting out dilemmas prior to the child's return to class will assure a better outcome. The school team should be included in discharge planning discussions, particularly about an out-of-hospital DNR. In anticipation of a life-threatening event occurring at school, the parents, school administrators, and clinicians, in conjunction with the local EMS system, need to delineate a plan that would invoke comfort care for the child rather than life-sustaining measures. The school nurse is a crucial part of this collaborative effort to assure that the best interests of the child are upheld, but school nurses are becoming less common and, when they do exist, are frequently covering multiple school. A proactive, coordinated plan that is communicated to the appropriate school personnel can go a long way in relieving their anxiety.

CLINIC AS A LOCATION OF PEDIATRIC PALLIATIVE CARE

Dedicated outpatient clinics providing PPC services are not common. In one statewide survey, fewer than 20% of pediatric palliative programs had outpatient clinics, seeing an average of only 10 new patients per year.[76] In contrast, despite the fact that most pediatric palliative programs are focused on the inpatient setting, for pediatric oncology patients, nearly all the components of care typically provided by a palliative team take place in the outpatient oncology clinic.[77] This is not surprising, as children with cancer are the largest group receiving PPC as outpatients. Successful models for outpatient palliative care at pediatric cancer centers have been demonstrated and may serve as templates, in modified form, for other pediatric subspecialties and programs.[78] Palliative care teams without their own specialty clinic may have opportunities to see patients during their visits to other subspecialists, their primary care pediatrician, or even other venues such as rehabilitation centers and hospice facilities. A recent, modern example of this is the "pop-up" model, which uses a mobile, on-call specialist PPC team to bring primary palliative care education to the clinic and other outpatient settings while ensuring availability of specialist-level palliative care in all care settings and transitions between them.[79] In any clinic-based model, a specialist pediatric palliative advanced practice nurse plays a key role in providing high-level continuity of care.[80]

TELEHEALTH TO DELIVER PEDIATRIC PALLIATIVE CARE TO DIVERSE LOCATIONS

Telehealth, or telemedicine, is a field that is growing rapidly as a model of healthcare delivery across many subspecialties, and hospice and palliative medicine is no exception. With respect to palliative care, it is the use of communications technology to bridge the institution-based team with the "real-world" setting in which patients spend most of their time. As with many innovations in healthcare, the most of literature supporting this intervention is adult-focused, with limited studies specific to pediatrics. A 2013 systematic review by Bradford et al. noted that there are multiple limitations to effective research in this field, making it difficult to ascertain the success of telehealth interventions.[81] However, more recent literature suggests that utilizing telehealth allows clinicians to reach children and families in rural and other remote areas that would not otherwise have access to specialty PPC.[82,83] These studies show that children and families often view telemedicine-based care as a positive intervention, allowing them to keep in regular contact with the multidisciplinary team.[82,83]

CHALLENGES AND STRATEGIES FOR DELIVERING PALLIATIVE CARE IN THE COMMUNITY

There are numerous settings for PPC delivery in the community, each with its own strengths and limitations with respect to providing quality PPC. Therefore, a major challenge to care delivery is that it cannot be normalized across these settings. What community resources are available and what care is possible varies greatly based on local healthcare agencies, telehealth capabilities, policies about medical care on school premises, and state policies or programs regarding hospice waivers or PPC provision. It is essential that PPC teams remain familiar with local healthcare, educational, and social service institutions, their policies, and regulations in order to deliver care across diverse settings and advocate for changes needed to meet the needs of their patients.

CONCLUSION

The changing landscape of PPC is dotted with newer and different types of patients and their diagnoses and life spans, as well as settings in which children experience life and death. The PPC team must be vigilant in surveying this landscape in order to succeed in optimizing continuity of high-quality palliative care wherever children who need it may be found.

REFERENCES

1. American Academy of Pediatrics. National Research Center for Patient/Family Centered Medical Home. https://medicalhomeinfo.aap.org/
2. National Hospice and Palliative Care Organization. Standards of Practice for Pediatric Palliative Care. https://www.nhpco.org/standards-of-practice-for-pediatric-palliative-care
3. Section on Hospice and Palliative Medicine and Committee on Hospital Care. Pediatric palliative care and hospice care commitments guidelines, and recommendations. *Pediatrics*. 2013;132(5):966–972. doi:10.1542/peds.2013-2731
4. Feudtner C, Kang TI, Hexem KR, et al. Pediatric palliative care patients: A prospective multicenter cohort study. *Pediatrics*. 2011;127(6):1094–1101. doi:10.1542/peds.2010-3225
5. Ananth P, Melvin P, Feudtner C, Wolfe J, Berry JG. Hospital use in the last year of life for children with life-threatening complex chronic conditions. *Pediatrics*. 2015;136(5):938–946. doi:10 1542/peds.2015-0260
6. Berry JG, Hall DE, Kuo DZ, et al. Hospital utilization and characteristics of patients experiencing recurrent readmissions within children's hospitals. *JAMA*. 2011;305(7):682–690. doi:10.1001/jama.2011.122
7. Feudtner C, Feinstein JA, Satchell M, Zhao H, Kang TI. Shifting place of death among children with complex chronic conditions in the United States, 1989-2003. *JAMA J Am Med Assoc*. 2007;297(24):2725–2732. doi:10.1001/jama.297.24.2725
8. DeCourcey DD, Silverman M, Oladunjoye A, Balkin EM, Wolfe J. Patterns of care at the end of life for children and young adults with life-threatening complex chronic conditions. *J Pediatr*. 2018;193:196–203.e2. doi:10.1016/j.jpeds.2017.09.078
9. Johnston EE, Bogetz J, Saynina O, Chamberlain LJ, Bhatia S, Sanders L. Disparities in inpatient intensity of end-of-life care for complex chronic conditions. *Pediatrics*. 2019;143(5). doi:10.1542/peds.2018-2228
10. Brandon D, Docherty SL, Thorpe J. Infant and child deaths in acute care settings: Implications for palliative care. *J Palliat Med*. 2007;10(4):910–918. doi:10.1089/jpm.2006.0236
11. Feudtner C, Christakis DA, Zimmerman FJ, Muldoon JH, Neff JM, Koepsell TD. Characteristics of deaths occurring in children's hospitals: Implications for supportive care services. *Pediatrics*. 2002;109(5):887–893.
12. Lindley LC, Lyon ME. A profile of children with complex chronic conditions at end of life among Medicaid beneficiaries: Implications for health care reform. *J Palliat Med*. 2013;16(11):1388–1393. doi:10.1089/jpm.2013.0099
13. Yu JA, Schenker Y, Maurer SH, Cook SC, Kavlieratos D, Houtrow A. Pediatric palliative care in the medical neighborhood for children with medical complexity. *Fam Syst Health J Collab Fam Healthc*. 2019;37(2):107–119. doi:10.1037/fsh0000414
14. Davies D, Hartfield D, Wren T. Children who "grow up" in hospital: Inpatient stays of six months or longer. *Paediatr Child Health*. 2014;19(10):533–536.
15. Drake R. Palliative care for children in hospital: Essential roles. *Children*. 2018;5(2). doi:10.3390/children5020026
16. Hauer J, Houtrow AJ, Section on Hospice and Palliative Medicine Council on Children with Disabilities. Pain assessment and treatment in children with significant impairment of the central nervous system. *Pediatrics*. 2017;139(6). doi:10.1542/peds.2017-1002
17. Osenga K, Postier A, Dreyfus J, Foster L, Teeple W, Friedrichsdorf SJ. A comparison of circumstances at the end of life in a hospital setting for children with palliative care involvement versus those without. *J Pain Symptom Manage*. 2016;52(5):673–680. doi:10.1016/j.jpainsymman.2016.05.024
18. Feudtner C, Womer J, Augustin R, et al. Pediatric palliative care programs in children's hospitals: A cross-sectional national survey. *Pediatrics*. 2013;132(6):1063–1070. doi:10.1542/peds.2013-1286
19. Hsu BS, Hill V, Frankel LR, et al. Executive summary: Criteria for critical care of infants and children: PICU admission, discharge, and triage practice statement and levels of care guidance. *Pediatrics*. 2019;144(4):e20192433. doi:10.1542/peds.2019-2433
20. Henderson CM, Williams EP, Shapiro MC, et al. "Stuck in the ICU": Caring for children with chronic critical illness. *Pediatr Crit Care Med*. 2017;18(11):e561–e568. doi:10.1097/PCC.0000000000001332
21. Namachivayam P, Taylor A, Montague T, et al. Long-stay children in intensive care: Long-term functional outcome and quality of life from

a 20-yr institutional study. *Pediatr Crit Care Med.* 2012;13(5):520–528. doi:10.1097/PCC.0b013e31824fb989

22. Patel AK, Bell MJ, Traube C. Delirium in pediatric critical care. *Pediatr Clin North Am.* 2017;64(5):1117–1132. doi:10.1016/j.pcl.2017.06.009
23. Silver G, Kearney J, Traube C, Hertzig M. Delirium screening anchored in child development: The Cornell Assessment for Pediatric Delirium. *Palliat Support Care.* 2015;13(4):1005–1011. doi:10.1017/S1478951514000947
24. Kudchadkar SR, Yaster M, Punjabi NM. Sedation, sleep promotion, and delirium screening practices in the care of mechanically ventilated children: A wake-up call for the pediatric critical care community. *Crit Care Med.* 2014;42(7):1592–1600. doi:10.1097/CCM.0000000000000326
25. Namachivayam P, Shann F, Shekerdemian L, et al. Three decades of pediatric intensive care: Who was admitted, what happened in intensive care, and what happened afterward: *Pediatr Crit Care Med.* 2010;11(5):549–555. doi:10.1097/PCC.0b013e3181ce7427
26. Burns JP, Sellers DE, Meyer EC, Lewis-Newby M, Truog RD. Epidemiology of death in the PICU at five U.S. teaching hospitals. *Crit Care Med.* 2014;42(9):2101–2108. doi:10.1097/CCM.0000000000000498
27. Jacobs A, Flechet M, Vanhorebeek I, et al. Performance of pediatric mortality prediction scores for PICU mortality and 90-day mortality. *Pediatr Crit Care Med.* 2019;20(2):113–119. doi:10.1097/PCC.0000000000001764
28. Pollack MM, Holubkov R, Funai T, et al. Simultaneous prediction of new morbidity, mortality, and survival without new morbidity from pediatric intensive care: A new paradigm for outcomes assessment. *Crit Care Med.* 2015;43(8):1699–1709. doi:10.1097/CCM.0000000000001081
29. Johnston EE, Martinez I, Currie E, Brock KE, Wolfe J. Hospital or home? Where should children die and how do we make that a reality? *J Pain Symptom Manage.* December 2019. doi:10.1016/j.jpainsymman.2019.12.370
30. Keele L, Keenan HT, Sheetz J, Bratton SL. Differences in characteristics of dying children who receive and do not receive palliative care. *Pediatrics.* 2013;132(1):72–78. doi:10.1542/peds.2013-0470
31. Bluebond-Langner M, Beecham E, Candy B, Langner R, Jones L. Preferred place of death for children and young people with life-limiting and life-threatening conditions: A systematic review of the literature and recommendations for future inquiry and policy. *Palliat Med.* 2013;27(8):705–713. doi:10.1177/0269216313483186
32. National Palliative Registry. Summary data. https://registry.capc.org/metrics-resources/summary-data/
33. Nakagawa T, Shemie S, Dryden-Palmer K, Parshuram C, Brierley J. Organ donation following neurologic and circulatory determination of death. *Pediatr Crit Care Med.* 2018;19(8S). doi:10.1097/PCC.0000000000001518
34. Parshuram C, Dryden-Palmer K. Practice in pediatric intensive care: Death and dying. *Pediatr Crit Care Med.* 2018;19:S1–S3. doi:10.1097/PCC.0000000000001595
35. Nelson JE, Bassett R, Boss RD, et al. Models for structuring a clinical initiative to enhance palliative care in the intensive care unit: A report from the IPAL-ICU Project (Improving Palliative Care in the ICU). *Crit Care Med.* 2010;38(9):1765–1772. doi:10.1097/CCM.0b013e3181e8ad23
36. Boss R, Nelson J, Weissman D, et al. Integrating palliative care into the PICU: A report from the Improving Palliative Care in the ICU Advisory Board. *Pediatr Crit Care Med.* 2014;15(8):762–767. doi:10.1097/PCC.0000000000000209
37. Lutmer JE, Humphrey L, Kempton TM, Moore-Clingenpeel M, Ayad O. Screening criteria improve access to palliative care in the PICU. *Pediatr Crit Care Med.* 2016;17(8):e335–e342. doi:10.1097/PCC.0000000000000848
38. Leading Causes of Death and Injury—PDFs|Injury Center|CDC. National Center for Injury Prevention and Control, Centers for Disease Control and Prevention, 2019.
39. Heron M, Sutton PD, Xu J, et al. Annual summary of vital statistics. *Pediatrics.* 2010;125:4–15.
40. Michelson KN, Steinhorn DM. Pediatric end-of-life issues and palliative care. *Clin Pediatr Emerg Med.* 2007;8:212–219.
41. Lunney JR, Lynn J, Foley, DJ, et al. Patterns of functional death at the end of life. *JAMA.* 2003;289:2387–2392.
42. Institute of Medicine, Committee on Palliative and End-of-Life Care for Children and Their Families. In: Field MJ, Behrman RE, eds. *When Children Die: Improving Palliative and End-of-Life Care for Children and Their Families.* Washington, DC: National Academy Press; 2003.
43. Wright J, Johns C, Joseph J. End-of-life care in EMS for children. In: Field M, ed. *When children die, Institute of Medicine.* Washington: National Academy Press; 2003:580–589.
44. Knapp J, Mulligan-Smith D, the Committee on Pediatric Emergency Medicine. Death of a child in the emergency department. *Pediatrics.* 2005;115:1432–1437.
45. Moynihan KM, Snaman JM, Kaye EC, et al. Integration of pediatric palliative care into cardiac intensive care: A champion-based model. *Pediatrics.* 2019;144(2). doi:10.1542/peds.2019-0160
46. Schulman J, Braun D, Lee HC, et al. Association between neonatal intensive care unit admission rates and illness acuity. *JAMA Pediatr.* 2018;172(1):17–23. doi:10.1001/jamapediatrics.2017.3913
47. Harrison, W, Goodman D. Epidemiologic trends in neonatal intensive care, 2007-2012. *JAMA Pediatrics.* 2015: 169(9): 855–862. doi:10.1001/jamapediatrics.2015.1305
48. Kowlessar NM. Healthcare Cost and Utilization Project (HCUP) statistical briefs: Hospital stays for newborns, 2011;#163.
49. Obeidat HM, Bond EA, Callister LC. The parental experience of having an infant in the newborn intensive care unit. *J Perinat Educ.* 2009;18(3):23–29. doi:10.1624/105812409X461199
50. Matthews T, MacDorman M, Thoma M. National Vital Statistics Report: Infant mortality statistics from the 2013 period linked birth/infant death data set. https://www.cdc.gov/nchs/data/nvsr/nvsr64/nvsr64_09.pdf
51. Trowbridge A, Walter JK, McConathey E, Morrison W, Feudtner C. Modes of death within a children's hospital. *Pediatrics.* 2018;142(4):e20174182. doi:10.1542/peds.2017-4182
52. Carter BS. Pediatric palliative care in infants and neonates. *Children.* 2018;5(2). doi:10.3390/children5020021
53. Nelson H, Mott S, Kleinman ME, Goldstein RD. Parents' experiences of pediatric palliative transports: A qualitative case series. *J Pain Symptom Manage.* 2015;50(3):375–380. doi:10.1016/j.jpainsymman.2015.04.004
54. Gaucher N, Humbert N, Gauvin F. What do we know about pediatric palliative care patients consulting to the pediatric emergency department? *Pediatr Emerg Care.* September 2018. doi:10.1097/PEC.0000000000001620
55. Carroll JM, Torkildson C, Winsness JS. Issues related to providing quality pediatric palliative care in the community. *Pediatr Clin North Am.* 2007;54(5):813–827.
56. Armstrong-Daily A, Zarbock S, eds. *Hospice care for children*, 3rd edn. New York: Oxford University; 2008.
57. Contro NA, Larson J, Scofield S, et al. Hospital staff and family perspectives regarding quality of pediatric palliative care. *Pediatrics.* 2004;114(5):1248–1252.
58. Allshouse C, Comeau M, Rodgers R, Wells N. Families of children with medical complexity: A view from the front lines. *Pediatrics.* 2018;141(Supplement 3):S195–S201. doi:10.1542/peds.2017-1284D
59. Bona K, Bates J, Wolfe J. Massachusetts' Pediatric Palliative Care Network: Successful implementation of a novel state-funded pediatric palliative care program. *J Palliat Med.* 2011;14(11):1217–1223. doi:10.1089/jpm.2011.0070
60. Nageswaran S, Ip EH, Golden SL, O'Shea TM, Easterling D. Inter-agency collaboration in the care of children with complex chronic conditions. *Acad Pediatr.* 2012;12(3):189–197. doi:10.1016/j.acap.2012.02.007

61. Golden SL, Nageswaran S. Caregiver voices: Coordinating care for children with complex chronic conditions. *Clin Pediatr (Phila).* 2012;51(8):723–729. doi:10.1177/0009922812445920
62. Maynard R, Christensen E, Cady R, et al. Home health care availability and discharge delays in children with medical complexity. *Pediatrics.* 2019;143(1). doi:10.1542/peds.2018-1951
63. Rosen-Reynoso M, Porche MV, Kwan N, et al. Disparities in access to easy-to-use services for children with special health care needs. *Matern Child Health J.* 2016;20(5):1041–1053. doi:10.1007/s10995-015-1890-z
64. National Hospice and Palliative Care Organization. HPCO's Facts and Figures Pediatric Palliative & Hospice Care in America 2015 Edition. 2015. http://www.nhpco.org/sites/default/files/public/quality/Pediatric_Facts-Figures.pdf
65. Sumner L. Pediatric care: the hospice perspective. In: Ferrell B, Coyle N, eds. *Textbook of Palliative Nursing*, 2nd edn. Oxford University Press: New York; 2006:916.
66. Thienprayoon R, Marks E, Funes M, Martinez-Puente LM, Winick N, Lee SC. Perceptions of the pediatric hospice experience among English- and Spanish-speaking families. *J Palliat Med.* 2015;19(1):30–41. doi:10.1089/jpm.2015.0137
67. Contro N, Larson J, Scofield S, Sourkes B, Cohen H. Family perspectives on the quality of pediatric palliative care. *Arch Pediatr Adolesc Med.* 2002;156(1):14–19.
68. Johnston E, Molina J, Martinez I, et al. Bereaved parents' perspectives on end-of-life care for children with cancer: Implications for quality markers. *Cancer.* 2020 Jul 15;126(14):3352–3359.
69. Thienprayoon R, Lee SC, Leonard D, Winick N. Racial and ethnic differences in hospice enrollment among children with cancer. *Pediatr Blood Cancer.* 2013;60(10):1662–1666. doi:10.1002/pbc.24590
70. American Academy of Pediatrics. Committee on Bioethics and Committee on Hospital Care. Palliative care for children. *Pediatrics.* 2000;106(2 Pt 1):351–357.
71. Kassam A, Skiadaresis J, Alexander S, Wolfe J. Parent and clinician preferences for location of end-of-life care: Home, hospital or freestanding hospice? *Pediatr Blood Cancer.* 2014;61(5):859–864. doi:10.1002/pbc.24872
72. Rushton CH, Will JC, Murray MG. To honor and obey: DNR orders and the school. *Pediatr Nurs.* 1994;20(6):581–585.
73. Individuals with Disabilities Education Act (IDEA). Individuals with Disabilities Education Act. https://sites.ed.gov/idea/
74. American Academy of Pediatrics Committee on School Health and Committee on Bioethics. Do not resuscitate orders in schools. *Pediatrics.* 200:105(4):878–879.
75. Kimberly MB, Forte AL, Carroll JM, Feudtner C. Pediatric do-not-attempt-resuscitation orders and public schools: A national assessment of policies and laws. *Am J Bioeth AJOB.* 2005;5(1):59–65. doi:10.1080/15265160590900605
76. Rabow MW, O'Riordan DL, Pantilat SZ. A statewide survey of adult and pediatric outpatient palliative care services. *J Palliat Med.* 2014;17(12):1311–1316. doi:10.1089/jpm.2014.0144
77. Brock KE, Snaman JM, Kaye EC, et al. Models of pediatric palliative oncology outpatient care: Benefits, challenges, and opportunities. *J Oncol Pract.* 2019;15(9):476–487. doi:10.1200/JOP.19.00100
78. Levine DR, Johnson L-M, Snyder A, et al. Integrating palliative care in pediatric oncology: Evidence for an evolving paradigm for comprehensive cancer care. *J Natl Compr Cancer Netw JNCCN.* 2016;14(6):741–748. doi:10.6004/jnccn.2016.0076
79. Mherekumombe MF. From inpatient to clinic to home to hospice and back: Using the "pop up" pediatric palliative model of care. *Children.* 2018;5(5). doi:10.3390/children5050055
80. Mauricio RV, Okhuysen-Cawley R. The caring continuum: Role of the pediatric critical care advanced practice nurse in palliative care program development. *Crit Care Nurs Q.* 2010;33(3):292–297. doi:10.1097/CNQ.0b013e3181ecd5a2
81. Bradford N, Armfield NR, Young J, Smith AC. The case for home based telehealth in pediatric palliative care: A systematic review. *BMC Palliat Care.* 2013;12:4. doi:10.1186/1472-684X-12-4
82. Weaver MS, Robinson JE, Shostrom VK, Hinds PS. Telehealth acceptability for children, family, and adult hospice nurses when integrating the pediatric palliative inpatient provider during sequential rural home hospice visits. *J Palliat Med.* December 2019. doi:10.1089/jpm.2019.0450
83. Winegard B, Miller EG, Slamon NB. Use of telehealth in pediatric palliative care. *Telemed J E-Health Off J Am Telemed Assoc.* 2017;23(11):938–940. doi:10.1089/tmj.2016.0251

5 | CULTURAL HUMILITY, SOCIAL DETERMINANTS, AND DISPARITIES IN PEDIATRIC PALLIATIVE CARE

DANIELLE JONAS, ALEXIS MORVANT, AND SARA MUNOZ-BLANCO

My humanity is bound up in yours for we can only be human together. We are different precisely in order to realize our need of one another.

DESMOND TUTU

INTRODUCTION

Pediatric palliative care (PPC) is known for its holistic approach in the care of patients and families facing a serious illness. Diversity is recognized by the Institute of Medicine as a core value in healthcare.[1] Human identity is complex, nuanced, and diverse, and it may include such factors as race and ethnicity, cultural values and norms, religious or spiritual beliefs, cumulative personal or familial experiences, and social environment.[1] As is the case in the adult world, various studies across pediatrics have elucidated the ways in which social disparities in healthcare directly impact access to critical aspects of PPC such as goals of care conversations, continuity in care, symptom management, resources, end-of-life care, and bereavement support.[2–5] For example, in their study out of California, Johnston and colleagues found that pediatric patients with complex chronic conditions (CCCs) who identified as Hispanic, as well as teenage/young adult patients, were two populations that were more likely to die in the hospital as compared to other children.[5] Further research is needed to understand if dying in the hospital was in line with these patients' goals or if they died in the hospital because of barriers to accessing alternative resources.[3,5]

Recognition of each patient's and family's human identity is a central part of high-quality PPC; it allows us to optimize relational building and trust and align family identity to goals of care and interventions. It is important to recognize that many human identity factors are also sources of disparities in healthcare, whereby families from minority ethnic and/or religious backgrounds and economically disadvantaged communities receive lower quality care. PPC is not exempt from these disparities in care. In addition, power imbalance and differences between providers' and families' values and social environment can be a source of conflict that can negatively affect the provider–family relationship. The practice of *cultural humility* invites us to reflect on our beliefs and biases and exercise genuine openness with and curiosity about learning about "the other." This can be applied within the culture of medicine with the hope of addressing factors that contribute to disparities in care.

In this chapter, we provide suggestions for how to assess communication preferences of pediatric patients and families, a framework on how to be culturally humble and curious, practical tips regarding the clinical PPC role, factors that contribute to disparities in PPC access, and an exploration of the concept of cultural humility within the social context of PPC. Figure 5.1 illustrates how social disparities and cultural humility impact provider care of patients and families, incorporating the identity factors of all parties involved.

COMMUNICATION IN THE CONTEXT OF SOCIAL/CULTURAL NORMS

In considering communication with families that is socially and culturally informed, it is crucial to remember that children exist within the context of a social system and within unique world paradigms. These paradigms may include cultural, religious, spiritual, or linguistic norms that inform the lens through which families view and accept their individual and group experience with the child's illness. While family-centered care should universally consist of relationship building, trust, and shared decision-making, differing familial backgrounds will result in differing communication preferences and needs from providers throughout the disease trajectory. Assessing and factoring in the individual and unique needs of families is a crucial component of providing ethical and compassionate PPC.

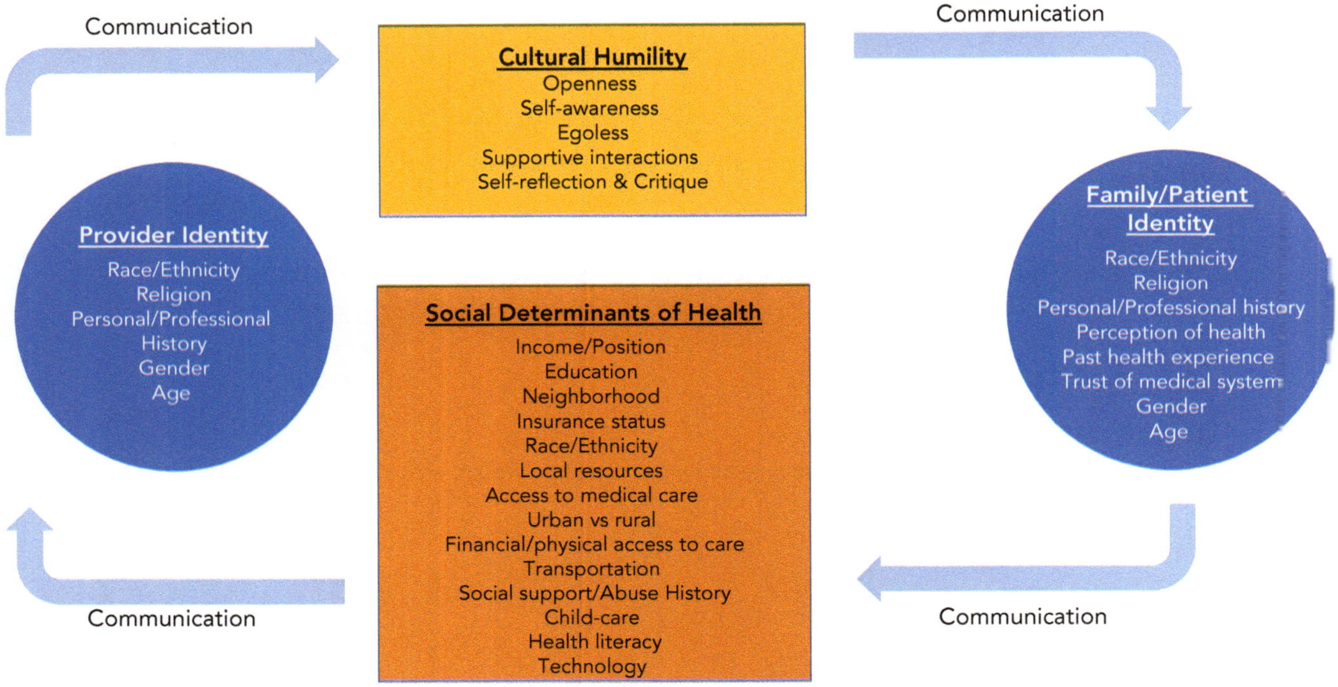

Figure 5.1 *Cultural humility, communication, provider/patient identity and social determinants of health in Pediatric Palliative Care (PPC).*

COMMUNICATION AS A PILLAR OF PEDIATRIC PALLIATIVE CARE

Communication is a pillar of palliative care. Breakdowns in communication due to language barriers can have detrimental effects on patient care. Awareness of our communication style, verbal and nonverbal, as well as being present during patient/family encounters is key to minimizing communication barriers. Being present, for instance, can prompt us to check in with families for understanding or when clarifications are needed. For example, many Latino parents nod while listening to providers. This nodding can be misinterpreted as agreeing with and/or understanding the information being provided, when in reality, it is often a sign of respect based on the cultural value of *respeto*, which emphasizes deferential behavior based on a person's authority, such as a physician. Nodding may be used by the family to let the provider know they're listening as opposed to understanding all or agreeing with the content.

Assumptions can influence the way we share and present information to patients and families and other medical providers. Furthermore, if inquiry and assessment of information are not carried out, misinterpretation of diagnosis, prognosis, interpretation of symptom burden, miscommunication, and misunderstanding of families' beliefs and values can occur. It is imperative that providers also consider the power structures at play, recognizing that parents may feel ashamed or embarrassed to ask questions, especially when they perceive that the provider assumes that they know or understand terminology and/or basic physiology. Providers should err on the side of overexplaining as opposed to assuming knowledge and understanding.

Assessment of communication preferences regarding the transmitting of information is crucial. For example, does the family prefer to talk about the big picture, or are they more detail-oriented? For some families, learning the details can provide the opportunity for anticipatory guidance and thus promote coping, preparation, and planning, as families focus on day-to-day changes or signs of disease progression. However, for other families, listening to the specific details of the care plan may promote anxiety, and, therefore, they may prefer to focus on more long-term factors and may appreciate the opportunity to talk through potential scenarios regarding how their child's disease may progress and/or consideration of larger medical decisions that may need to be made in the future.

Exploring families' preferences about the timing, manner, and place for receiving information is important; for example, visual learning via pictures or verbal communication, family-centered rounds, detailed care plans, or big picture synthesis. Attending to patient and family preferences can promote rapport-building, trust, and shared decision-making over time. Optimization of communication is a critical component when providing culturally tailored, family-centered care.

THE ROLE OF MEDICAL INTERPRETERS IN THE DELIVERY OF CULTURALLY SENSITIVE CARE

Optimizing communication between providers and families in the context of social/cultural norms can also include the use of medical interpreters. Language barriers can hinder shared decision-making, rapport-building with patients and families, health quality, symptom management, utilization of services, and end-of-life outcomes.[6] Effective medical interpretation in the hospital is a crucial aspect of culturally sensitive care for patients and families with limited English proficiency.[7] A systematic review of the literature found that patients with limited English proficiency had poorer discussions regarding quality goals of care and end-of-life care when professional medical interpreters were not used.[6]

Furthermore, several studies suggest that pre-meetings between providers and interpreters during which topics and terminology could be discussed and explained were important in optimizing goals-of-care conversations during encounters with patients and families.[6] Including medical interpreters along the care continuum can help to ensure that their perspective is fully informed to the nuances of the patient's condition, as well as the patient and family's framework, needs, and goals. Some studies have illuminated how interpreters may filter prognostic information at times, which may be due to cultural norms and/or fear of upsetting families or taking away hope.[7] Clarification of how prognostic information as well as other sensitive topics are interpreted within the social/cultural constructs of the family can improve medical interpretation and overall patient care. At the conclusion of meetings, it may also be helpful to debrief with the medical interpreter to gain insight into their own experiences and exchange feedback. For instance, an interpreter could point out, "when you said X, it did not really translate well." The debrief could also be an opportunity to check in on the interpreter's well-being and offer support if it was a particularly challenging or emotional meeting. This debrief can facilitate emotional processing and acknowledgment of their own pain in being the messenger delivering difficult news.

ASSESSING COMMUNICATION PREFERENCES AND EXPECTATIONS IN PEDIATRIC PALLIATIVE CARE

Patient and family communication preferences in PPC can be influenced by a variety of factors including culture of decision-making, religious or spiritual beliefs, ideas around communication about death with children and as a family, as well as global notions about suffering, pain, and the meaning of death.[8] One study found that a majority of parents of children with cancer preferred detailed, longitudinal prognostic information and verbalized a preference for more information rather than less.[9] Another study found that pediatric organ failure and transplant physicians do not regularly discuss end-of-life and prognostic information and that further research is needed to better understand how to optimize compassionate and honest information with patients and families within this population.[10]

Concise clinical assessment and rapport-building over time are crucial components for determining how each family system and each individual family member makes decisions. For example, some families may feel that it is best for the parents to receive all information before any information is shared with their child; whereas some families may prefer that providers be the ones to update the child about their condition. Adolescents and young adults (AYA) may or may not want to receive all information, even serious information, alone and some may want to receive all information even before their parents. It is important to assess this dynamic in the AYA population.

DECISION-MAKING STYLES

Decision-making style can be influenced by culture and religious/spiritual beliefs as well as by familial norms and/or past life experiences. Styles are likely to be unique to each family or individual and can vary depending on the magnitude and type of decision. Assessing a family's decision-making style early on in the relationship can foster trust, as the family will likely appreciate that their preferences and needs are being considered. Trust has been shown to influence decision-making style in adults, with low-level trust resulting in more autonomous decision-making preference (i.e., less shared decision-making).[11] Providers should carefully assess who the patient and family consider to be part of their decision-making "team." It is generally accepted that in Western culture the family unit tends to consist of immediate family members. Decision-making, therefore, may be up to the family nucleus, usually the parents and/or primary caregiver. In other cultures, this is not always the case. For example, *Familismo*, a Latino cultural construct, emphasizes the commitment and loyalty to family, immediate as well as extended.[12] Thus, some Latino families may prefer to consult with multiple family members to reach consensus before making a medical decision, which, if not known beforehand, can lead to delays in care and decision-making.[12] On the other hand, for some families of Latino or Asian descent, decision-making relies on the primary caregiver, usually the mother.[8] It is important to maintain a sense of cultural curiosity and avoid assumptions based on culture/ethnic background alone and clarify with the family who is/are key decision-maker(s). This can allow for timely planning of family meetings and goals of care setting, ensuring that all key players are present for important discussions.

Various factors may influence family engagement in medical decision-making, such as the opinions or preferences of a religious leader or past familial experiences with medical decision-making and/or end-of-life care. It may be helpful to assess if the family has had to make other difficult decisions for their child or another loved one in the past and to understand what was most supportive to them as they were faced with that decision or what was problematic in the past. It may be helpful to understand if they preferred a concrete medical recommendation or if there were other stakeholders who were involved in the process, such as extended family members or a religious leader.

In addition, some families may oppose involving the child in decision-making, which can cause significant distress among providers, especially for those patients able to participate in decision-making from a developmental standpoint. Generally speaking, pediatricians and other pediatric professionals tend to assume that children who function cognitively as a 7-year-old or higher should be given the opportunity to be included in their care and assent to medical decisions if they desire to do so. However, some families are resistant to involving their child in information-sharing, particularly when their child has a life-limiting illness. This resistance to involve the child can be due to cultural factors (children are not involved in decision-making, period) or to religious/spiritual beliefs, where speaking the truth out loud may cause the child to give up or the sickness to worsen.[13] Assessing decision-making style can result in better quality of care, family satisfaction, and trust. When tensions are particularly high around how and when to include the patient in the decision-making process, it may be helpful to consult additional resources such as the ethics committee, patient relations, or the hospital-based legal department.

CONSIDERING AND ASSESSING HEALTH LITERACY

In considering how to most effectively communicate with patients and families in a culturally and socially sensitive manner, providers must consider health literacy and developmental stages. *Health literacy* is defined as "the degree to which individuals have the capacity to obtain, process and understand basic health information and services needed to make appropriate health decisions."[14] The literature highlights that risk factors for low rates of health literacy include lower socioeconomic status (SES), limited English-language proficiency, and identification with minority racial/ethnic groups.[14] One comprehensive national study found that a significant portion of parents in the United States have limited health literacy and recommended that efforts to reduce literacy demand on parents would improve overall healthcare for children.[14]

In practicing culturally sensitive PPC, providers must be aware of individual health literacy levels and be willing and able to tailor communication given variations in literacy level. For example, providers commonly assume that parents know the name and function of each human organ system. Anecdotally, authors of this chapter have encountered parents who do not understand the basic functions of some organ systems affected by their child's illness. This was uncovered by explicitly asking parents if they knew what *x* organ did in the body; this anecdotal discovery has been a consistent experience across several diverse institutions. Therefore, when communicating the severity of a child's illness, a careful explanation regarding how and why the child's organ is not functioning properly may help to bridge communication and facilitate shared medical decision-making. Routinely including such explanations in discussions may help to ameliorate feelings of shame and embarrassment for parents who may be hesitant to ask questions regarding information that they are assumed to know. Child life specialists, child psychologists, and social workers can be particularly helpful in explaining serious illness to children and adolescents.

FUTURE CLINICAL DEVELOPMENT OF CULTURALLY SENSITIVE COMMUNICATION IN PEDIATRIC PALLIATIVE CARE

In recent years there has been a shift in medicine from cultural competency to cultural humility. *Cultural competency* is focused on learning specifics about different cultures and then applying that generalized knowledge to culturally diverse healthcare encounters. However, some argue that this lends itself to stereotyping and ignoring the diversity of individuals within cultures.[15] Cultural humility, on the other hand, invites providers to reflect on individual beliefs and biases (i.e., personal culture) and exercise genuine openness with and curiosity about the "other" (i.e., our patient/family). Within the culture of medicine this is referred to as *culturally humble care* or *cultural humility*.[16] There is limited information in the literature regarding how to best practice cultural and social humility and curiosity within the field of PPC. Further development of interventions and clinical practices that support patients of diverse backgrounds is needed.[7] This is especially pertinent in this field, as prognostic communication, the balance of hope and medical information, and end-of-life care are influenced by culture and religion. The tendency toward medical Western values and ethics does not always meet the needs of diverse patient populations.[7] If possible and as appropriate, it may also be beneficial to involve a clinician from the family's cultural background or consult with a provider or community member who may serve as a cultural ambassador to help navigate the clinical situation.

CULTURAL HUMILITY

Palliative care as a specialty aims to provide culturally humble care to all patients and their families. Recently, the term "cultural humility" has almost universally replaced "cultural competency," though at times the terms are mistakenly used interchangeably. So, what *is* cultural humility, exactly? Foronda and colleagues performed a concept analysis on the term "cultural humility" and described it as a life-long process with attributes of (1) openness (being open to new ideas, including interacting with others from different cultural backgrounds), (2) self-awareness ("What do I think/believe/feel about x-y-z? What are my implicit biases?"), (3) being egoless (being humble, neutral, and viewing everyone as equals), (4) embracing supportive interactions (having positive human interactions), and (5) self-reflection and critique ("What went well in that interaction, and what can I improve on?").[16]

Some providers suggest that cultural differences frequently present barriers to providing quality palliative care.[17] Cultural, religious, and spiritual norms, values, and beliefs, as well as our social environment and past experiences shape human perceptions of the world, including what happens to individuals and their families. These factors influence how individuals make decisions and perceive quality care as opposed to care that does not feel helpful or therapeutic. Therefore, working with, instead of against, these differences is imperative in optimizing the care of seriously ill children. Because cultural humility discourages overgeneralization in clinical care, suggested language is highlighted in Table 5.1.

TABLE 5.1 Suggested language for culturally humble encounters

OPEN-ENDED QUESTIONS	PURPOSE OF QUESTION
How would you prefer that information is shared with your family?	Communication preferences, rapport-building
How does your family make medical decisions? Who would you like to be present for larger discussions?	Medical decision making, rapport-building
Has your family had to make big medical decisions in the past? What was helpful during that time?	Medical decision making/communication preferences
What gives you strength?	Sources of support/faith
How does your family think about your loved one's illness? What words does your family use when discussing your loved one's illness?	Language about illness, meaning of illness
We know that medical information can be confusing and overwhelming, especially when you're hearing a lot of information at once. What clarifying questions do you have about what is happening in your child's body?	Health literacy, communication preferences, rapport-building
How would you describe your identity? (For child or family)	Cultural awareness, identity formation
How does your family think about the idea of suffering? What does suffering mean to you?	Cultural awareness, language about illness
Have you ever heard of palliative care before? What was the context?	Health literacy, cultural awareness
How does your family talk about what happens to a person after they die?	Cultural awareness, communication preferences
How has your child's illness impacted your life outside of the hospital?	Whole-person care, rapport-building
How are you managing the day to day?	Whole-person care, rapport-building
Tell me about your life/your child's life outside of the hospital?	Identity formation, rapport-building
What are you hoping for at this time?	Sources of support/faith, cultural awareness, rapport-building, health literacy
What are you most worried about right now?	Sources of support/faith, cultural awareness, rapport-building, health literacy
Does it feel helpful to talk about what could happen after your loved one dies? What would be important to you and your family during that time? Who would you want to be there?	Sources of support/faith, cultural awareness
How has your family been communicating about your child's illness? Would you like your child to be included within serious discussions with their healthcare team?	Communication preferences, rapport-building

PATIENT AND FAMILY INTERPRETATION OF ILLNESS

The interpretation of illness also varies between families and is usually rooted in culture, past life experiences, and religious or spiritual beliefs. In some traditions, families may believe that illness, suffering, pain, or even death are the result of bad karma (an imbalance of energies within us, as well as with others) or are consequences of a past sin. It is important for the clinical team to inquire about the patient's and family's understanding and interpretation of illness, symptoms, and death. Providers could consider asking a question like, "how do you think about your loved one's illness?" Or "how does your family talk about what happens to someone after they die?" It is equally important to validate and affirm these perceptions even if the clinical team does not share the same belief system because it helps the family feel heard and understood.

Having this information can aid providers in tailoring care and information to a family's specific needs. This is particularly helpful when interacting with pediatric patients and/or siblings as it is crucial to offer information or services that align with family language and beliefs. For instance, a family may be more accepting of chaplaincy services if their interpretation of their child's illness, symptoms, or death has deep spiritual roots or themes. However, there are some families who identify as highly religious but prefer the presence of their own religious leaders. A critical piece of this assessment is to explore the experience of suffering and create opportunity for patients and their families to communicate their subjective experience of suffering and the meaning behind it. Some patients and families may be focused on physical suffering in the form of symptoms, whereas others may express existential suffering about losses related to illness or spiritual suffering in the form of anger or disappointment that their god has allowed them to be sick. Additionally, some pediatric patients may be selective in how they express their physical symptoms depending on family dynamics and beliefs as well as what suffering represents within their family system.

Interpretation of illness, coping, and bereavement can also be influenced by individual family factors. Families with prior loss or previous hospice experience may be more or less amenable to palliative care services depending on their history. Some families who have had previous hospice experience may have a challenging time differentiating between palliative care and hospice, worrying that palliative care may carry the same prognostic implications as hospice did previously. Parents who have lost another child because of a genetic condition may be familiar with the interdisciplinary team approach and/or the trajectory/prognosis of their child's condition. Parents may have access to external resources, such as online support groups or relationships with other parents who have a child with the same or a similar diagnosis. Ensuring a full bio-psycho-social-spiritual assessment early in the care process can be helpful in assessing the family's experience of services and access to support systems. Palliative care providers are trained to compassionately ask about previous loss and offer families opportunity to reflect on these past experiences and process how their grief or trauma may be influencing their current illness experience. Interdisciplinary providers should be aware of how past experiences with loss and/or trauma may impact individual and family coping with serious illness.

PILLARS OF CULTURAL HUMILITY

When aiming to optimize rapport-building, it is best to ask questions in a compassionate and curious manner, free of judgment or assumptions. Understanding general notions regarding specific cultures/ethnic groups can be helpful in creating awareness of important differences. Asking questions guided by past experience in caring for patients and families of diverse backgrounds can enrich clinical understanding of general cultural constructs, thus promoting cultural competency. Using this general knowledge in conjunction with cultural curiosity can aid in avoiding stereotyping while also maintaining openness and awareness to diverse patient and family care needs throughout the illness trajectory and into bereavement.

Cultural humility not only applies to potential cultural, religious, and social differences between providers and families; it also applies to the inherent power imbalance of the provider–patient/family relationship as most people consider physicians to be highly educated, power leaders in society. The pillars of cultural humility—self-reflection of our beliefs, values, and biases and openness toward the other—allows providers to forgo some control, creating opportunity to optimize rapport-building. This approach will enhance family involvement in care, decrease the power imbalance, and maximize shared decision-making and overall communication.

In summary, cultural humility entails personal reflection regarding one's own ideas, beliefs, implicit and explicit biases, and cultural constructs, as well as those observed through experience and exposure. Cultural humility is likely to improve the quality of PPC for vulnerable patients who are living with serious illness and their families.

PRACTICAL PEARLS FOR THE PPC PROVIDER

SITTING WITH SUFFERING AND UNCERTAINTY

PPC interventions often entail intangible interactions such as sitting with suffering or being present with the patient and family in the processing of their grief. PPC providers are able to acknowledge the uniqueness of each experience as a means of tending to clinical and existential needs with the goal of optimizing quality of life in a patient-centered manner.

For some patients and families, optimization of quality of life may include the opportunity for story-sharing of past experiences from life before an illness or hospitalization. Some individuals may benefit from feeling as though their providers are informed of their child's or sibling's identity outside of the hospital. Some patients may themselves benefit from describing their life, skills, experiences, relationships, and abilities from before their illness as a way of sharing other aspects of their identity and purpose to their providers and loved ones. For some families, it can be helpful for care teams to meet and interact with people from their personal lives. However, for others, it may feel important to keep their medical team and personal lives completely separate as means of preserving dignity and privacy. The best way to know what is most helpful to families with regards to rapport-building is to ask how the clinical team can be most helpful in their involvement.

Relationship-building between PPC providers and patients and their families is unique in that these relationships can last for months or years at a time as the team follows the child throughout the course of their disease trajectory. As PPC providers engage with the patient and family throughout the illness experience, they often become an integral part of the care, decision-making, and overall medical experience, getting to know family friends and extended family members. Cultural factors may influence how and when patients and families are open to this relationship-building over time as some families may be more vulnerable in their openness and desire for support, whereas others may perceive the relationship to be invasive or representative of poor prognosis. It is imperative that PPC providers be aware of and flexible with the differences in desire for support and how this need can ebb and flow over time. Families may find palliative care services more or less helpful throughout the course of the child's illness trajectory.

Providers should consider that the definition of "family" is according to the family. It may also be the case that family members may not be helpful in their ability to offer support during highly stressful times or may have estranged relationships from the patient and/or their family, situations that may in fact add to the level of stress. Providers should be diligent about documenting, communicating, and respecting who each individual family considers to be part of their family and support structure, regardless of biological relationship.

MEDICAL VERSUS SPIRITUAL COPING

Another crucial role for the palliative care team is to support discussions of medical information that exist alongside spiritual beliefs and coping. Often, families cope with difficult news by balancing their processing of medical information with enhanced religious faith and belief in a Greater Being and the power of prayer. The ability to balance worries with some semblance of hope and faith is nuanced. Expressions of faith and hope in the face of a terminal medical diagnosis can often be confused with a lack of understanding regarding the provider's assessment.[18] Furthermore, providers may feel inclined to reinforce their prognostic indications in the face of hope in the form of badgering or repeating information multiple times to "ensure" the family has heard a prognosis, which some family members may perceive as unhelpful or even disrespectful.

Communicating permission for continued parental hope is crucial for parental functioning. When difficult information is being shared or processed, the optimal provider response is to sit with suffering and reflect a position of comfort and presence during moments of silence. In some cultures, the ability to be present with expressions of grief is considered to be supportive and helpful. However, in other cultures, individuals prefer to express their grief privately. Palliative care providers can explicitly ask how to be most helpful during these moments if they are unsure of family or individual preference.

END-OF-LIFE CARE AND BEREAVEMENT: CLINICAL IMPLICATIONS

When a child dies it is reported to be the "worst loss" that a human being can experience.[19] Culturally sensitive care and decision-making support is imperative in optimizing parental and family bereavement outcomes.[19] The literature highlights how parental demographics can affect the grief experience and overall bereavement outcomes.

Given the high risk for poor grief outcomes and prevalence of posttraumatic stress disorder, bereavement support is particularly important.[19] The majority of children die in hospitals, and, unfortunately, very few hospitals offer quality bereavement programs that are institutionally funded, meaning that families must turn to their own communities, resulting in the secondary loss of a connection with familiar hospital-based teams and longitudinal relationships.[19] Future prospective studies looking at this particular patient population could be helpful in fully grasping the nuances of this complexity.

In a similar manner, culture and religious/spiritual practices can also have a meaningful influence on how families process grief and bereavement. For some families, performing certain spiritual or religious rituals prior to the death of the child may be important. Burial within 24–48 hours of death is preferred, and cremation is usually forbidden in Islamic and Jewish traditions, for example. Catholic families may want their loved one to receive the sacrament of the sick and Holy Communion by a Catholic priest. In addition, autopsies, which are often valued by providers, may not be acceptable for some families due to cultural or religious beliefs, as in Hinduism or Jehovah's Witnesses religions. The information we may obtain from an autopsy, which can support healing or even genetic information that could influence future children of an affected family, must be balanced with respect for that family's cultural or religious/spiritual beliefs.

Organ donation can help some families find purpose and meaning in their loved one's death, which can aid the bereavement process. However, anecdotal experience highlights how discussion about organ donation may result in an added layer of distrust of the medical system, as some minority groups worry that their care may be compromised for the sake of saving the lives of more advantaged groups. In general, facilitation of religious and spiritual rituals that are important to the family can be enhanced by providers remaining culturally curious, asking questions about familial needs as end of life approaches, and making accommodations on visitation policies, presence of particular religious/spiritual leaders, or expedited burial arrangements when needed.

Team Reflection

Jocelyn was a 12-week-old baby girl of Guatemalan origin with Trisomy 18 who was intubated with an advance care plan protecting her from cardiac resuscitation and indicating comfort-focused care. Her mother spoke Spanish as her primary language and was unable to finish high school because of financial strain. Her mother immigrated to the United States about 1 year ago. Jocelyn's father was also involved in her life; he worked 90 hours per week to support his family and largely deferred to Jocelyn's mother for medical decision-making and caretaking. After multiple goals-of-care conversations with the pediatric intensive care unit team and the PPC team, they learned that her mother viewed a life supported by machines as suffering and wished to protect her daughter from this experience. Given her goals, the teams and her mother worked together to make the loving decision to intensively focus on comfort while discontinuing life-sustaining therapies, allowing a natural death. However, over the following 2 weeks, Jocelyn's mother repeatedly express hesitation about the timing of extubation. The palliative care team continued to meet with Jocelyn and her mother daily to ensure that her symptoms were being managed during this interim period. The palliative care social worker helped Jocelyn's mother with funeral arrangements and communication with other family members regarding the plan of care. Nonetheless, her mother continued to express hesitation about setting a time for extubation. Eventually, the providers felt frustrated with the mother, expressing concern that Jocelyn's suffering was being prolonged. After careful communication, including further discussion and active listening, Jocelyn's mother was able to voice an unspoken fear. Specifically, she had heard rumors from friends that Jocelyn's ashes would be mixed with other people's remains following cremation and that she would not be able to keep the remains of her child. She also expressed worries that her child's organs would be used to save the lives of "wealthy Americans." Her mother expressed feelings of embarrassment regarding her fears to the provider and communicated gratitude for the opportunity to disclose and work through her concerns. The palliative care team collaborated closely with the funeral home to ensure that all of the mother's concerns were addressed. Ultimately, while intensively focusing on Jocelyn's comfort, life-sustaining therapies were discontinued, and she died peacefully, surrounded by her loving family. Her mother later notified the team that she was able to be present while Jocelyn was cremated and that she keeps her daughter's remains at her bedside.

DISPARITIES IN ACCESS TO PPC SERVICES

Parents of a child with serious illness can rarely plan for the financial, psychosocial, and spiritual impact on their child and the rest of their family. Furthermore, a family's geographic location, race, and financial security complicate the overall experience of serious illness extending into the intensity of treatment at end of life, access to PPC, morbidity, and mortality.[5,20–22] Children facing serious illness, whether cancer or other CCCs, are among the most vulnerable of human beings at high risk for suffering.[23] PPC then becomes an integral aspect of the care for any child living with serious illness to anticipate, prevent, and mitigate suffering in all its forms. Even though more research is imperative to understand complicated intricacies that go into delivering equitable and just healthcare, especially for serious illness, PPC must continue to make strides in understanding the experiences of serious illness through the lens of all stakeholders and how these experiences relate to communication, delivery of equitable healthcare, and familial goal concordance.[20]

WHERE IS PPC AS IT RELATES TO DISPARITIES IN CARE?

Overall access to PPC has generally improved over the past few decades; however, more advances are needed to create equitable access for all families living with serious illness. In 2013, Feudnter et al. reported that about 50% of children's hospitals in the United States had PPC programs which were mostly inpatient-only, available during traditional business hours, and with variable team structure.[24] While the PPC workforce is growing, evidence shows that we must continue the growth trajectory in outpatient and community-based services, 24/7 coverage, and bereavement services to provide quality care.[24,25] Currently, PPC programs are mostly located within teaching hospitals and are in urban areas, meaning that access to care in rural areas is still a challenge for various geographic regions of the United States. According to 2018 data from the Center to Advance Palliative Care (CAPC) most PPC programs have the following likelihoods of certain disciplines being included: a physician (97%), advance practice nurse (74%), social worker (67%), and chaplain (48%).[26] Only 37% of PPC services have the full interdisciplinary team of a nurse, physician, social worker, and chaplain.[26] Regarding global PPC, one study from 2011 showed that 65.6% of countries had no known PPC, and the highest need for PPC is in low- to middle-income countries.[27,28]

In many areas of the United States, PPC is inadequately funded and therefore ineffectively delivered, especially in more rural areas of the country, thus indicating that further development of community PPC is needed.[22,24] Given the scarcity of PPC services in US rural areas, patients hailing from these regions are especially disadvantaged when it comes to access to quality PPC.[22] Access to hospice and bereavement services for pediatric families continues to improve and must continue on this trajectory for equitable access to quality in-home care with hospice and home-based PPC.[29]

While training opportunities are expanding, there is still a lack of prioritization of educational curricula on primary palliative care skills, which may undermine addressing suffering for children with serious illness. The same is true regarding specialty palliative care training for interdisciplinary team members such as social work and nursing.

ACCESSING PPC

There are four important realms to consider when discussing access and disparities within PPC: policy and payment, health systems, organizations, and individual relationships among providers, patients, and families (see Figure 5.2).[25] A major contributor to geographic and socioeconomic disparities in

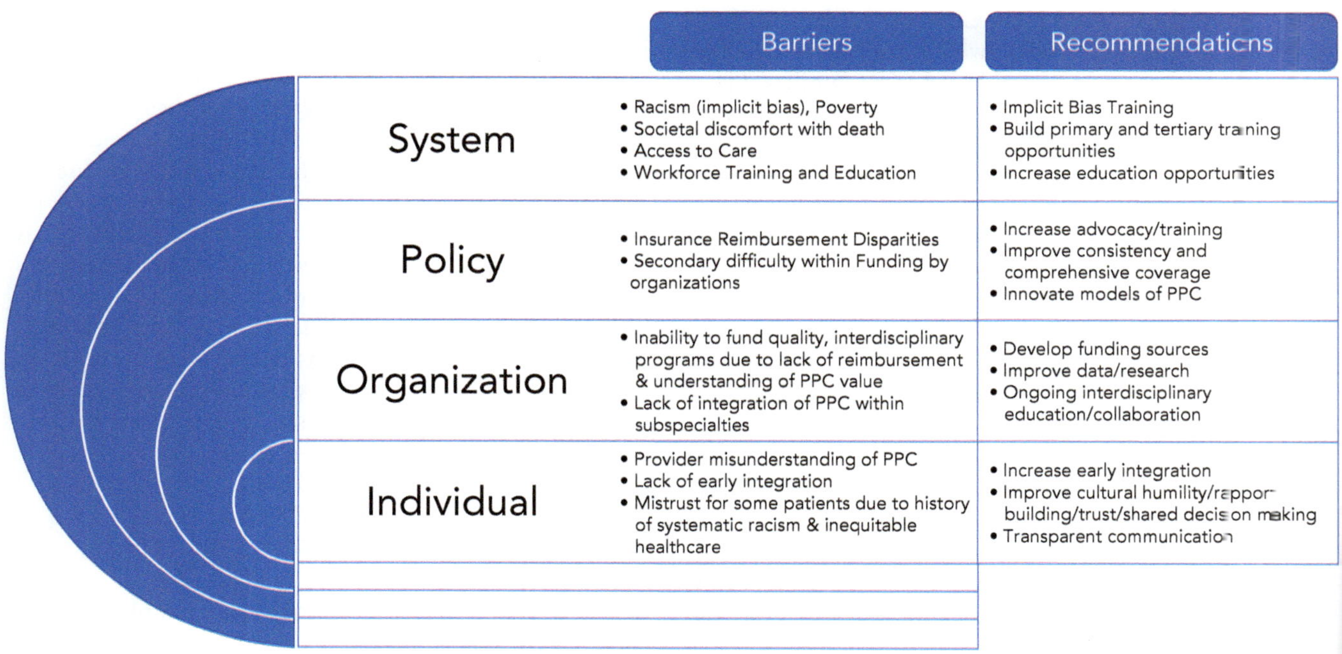

Figure 5.2 Barriers and recommendations to access pediatric palliative care services.

PPC is how coverage of services varies state to state.[25] In addition, Medicaid programs also differ in coverage from private insurance companies within the same state. Furthermore, disparities within reimbursement for team members such as psychologists, chaplains, social workers, nurses, and bereavement coordinators also exist.[22] Within health systems, PPC program models can vary dramatically by institution. Some PPC programs have ineffective coverage; others have a volunteer-based team, where physicians, nurses, and social workers have limited to no protected time within their full-time occupation to dedicate to PPC.[24] These suboptimal programs may be the result of an organization's lack of understanding of what PPC can offer or an issue with funding. This leads to the inability to provide sustainable service coverage, which can also impact team resiliency. Smaller programs may especially be at risk of being understaffed and/or may lack formally trained interdisciplinary teams due to disparities in reimbursement and hospital funding.[22,24] Because of difficulties in financing teams, investing in educational resources and training for the PPC workforce is challenging, especially for staff in safety net hospitals.[24,25]

Finally, relationships between the PPC team and other medical teams is often influenced by the general view and understanding of what palliative care is and its value. Often, PPC services are not consistently utilized, and, when PPC is utilized, it is not always within an early integration model.[22] As education about what palliative care is continues to develop and improve across institutions, some disease-specific providers continue to experience resistance to palliative care referrals. Depending on the political dynamics and power structures within an institution, this resistance can further impede access to optimal palliative care services.

BARRIERS TO HOSPICE ACCESS

Parents' decision to pursue hospice care is personal and challenging. Hospice provides an interdisciplinary healthcare team in the home for children and adults who have a 6-month or shorter prognosis. Hospice care includes all aspects of serious illness including improving quality of life and mitigating suffering in all its forms: spiritual, existential, psychosocial, and physical. According to the Andersen Behavioral Healthcare Utilization Model, there are three determinants of healthcare service utilization, and Lindley et al. compare this model to determinants of access to pediatric hospice.[30,31]

- *Predisposing factors* (demographics; position within social structure; and health knowledge, beliefs, and values)
- *Enabling factors* (financial and physical access to healthcare services)
- *Need factors* (evaluated and self-perceived health status)

According to Lindley et al. and taking these different factors into account, a family may not access hospice because there is no hospice program within their area.[30] In addition, existing hospices in the area may not feel comfortable accepting a pediatric patient.[32] Many adult hospice providers may worry about such factors as how to dose opioids for infants or young children at the end of life. There are also some instances where hospices will accept pediatric patients even though their staff lack adequate training or expertise, which can cause decreased quality of care despite having access.[33–35] Studies have also shown access to hospice correlates with geographic distance from services. A study from 2010 showed that most Americans live within 30 minutes of a hospice agency, indicating an increasing access to hospice from 2000 to 2010.[32] However, there are still approximately 35 million Americans who are greater than 30 minutes from a hospice agency and approximately 6 million Americans who are greater than 60 minutes from a hospice agency.[32] Carlson et al. also found that lower income and lower education areas were more than 30 minutes from a hospice, showing concern for disparities.[32] In contrast, in predominately African American communities, there is a higher correlation with geographic access to hospices even though the African American community is less likely to utilize hospice services.[32] This relationship may be more related to system bias than to geographic access disparities.

Access to hospice and other in-home palliative care services can be further complicated by documentation status and/or housing status. For example, many hospices are not able to provide services at temporary housing sites such as shelters or Ronald McDonald Houses. Additionally, many families who do not have proper documentation are unable to access resources and/or may be hesitant to allow providers into their home out of fear of exposure or deportation.

The field of PPC has proved its value over time for children and families living with serious illness, but it has work to do to deliver equitable care to all in need.[25] Lack of access to PPC points toward families not being fully supported within the physical, psychosocial, and spiritual pillars of serious illness, likely leading to suffering.

SOLUTIONS FOR DISPARITIES IN ACCESS TO PPC

Solutions proposed in various studies are to create more consistent, equitable, and comprehensive coverage of PPC services both in the hospital and in the home, in addition to innovative state models.[25] The American Academy of Pediatrics (AAP) has called for improved reimbursement and coverage for PPC services, including but not limited to advance care planning, goals-of-care discussions, family meetings, and added psychosocial support or care coordination.[36] As a solution to disparities in access to PPC, some states such as Florida, Colorado, Massachusetts, and Washington have created high-quality community-based PPC systems. One specific example is the Massachusetts Pediatric Palliative Care Network (PPCN), which is a state-funded community-based PPC program for all children living with serious illness regardless of insurance type.[25]

An example at the federal level is the Medicaid Concurrent Care for Children Requirement from the Affordable Care

Act in 2010.[25] The Concurrent Care hospice benefit ensures that seriously ill children under 21 years of age and evaluated as likely to have a 6-month or less prognosis are entitled to receive a hospice benefit in addition to all necessary disease-directed therapies with the goal of providing access to comprehensive care to live as long and as well as possible. Medicaid continues to pay for disease-directed therapies in addition to the hospice benefit (i.e., providing comfort-directed therapies). This benefit ensures parents are never forced to decide to stop life-prolonging therapies in order to receive quality care at home from an interdisciplinary hospice team focused on comfort. The hope in the future is to expand the prognosis barrier to greater than 6 months for earlier integration and to extend this benefit to non–Medicaid-supported families.[25]

Additionally, the PPC workforce should continue to improve availability of care through continued efforts for programmatic expansion. Enhanced training opportunities for primary and specialty palliative care skills within the curricula for students, residents, and fellows would also increase PPC access for all families.

In conclusion, leaders and members of the field must continue impactful advocacy work and training to change reimbursement, funding, and availability of PPC at tertiary hospitals within the community and in the home. Leaders must continue to strive to cultivate a compelling, unified marketing strategy to promote access on the provider level in addition to advocating for appropriate reimbursement and funding. In general, the human reaction is to lean away when bearing witness to suffering; furthermore, some of the answers to access and barriers to PPC services may lie within PPC's ability to tell our stories compassionately, honestly, and passionately.

SOCIAL CONTEXT OF PPC AS IT RELATES TO DISPARITIES

IMPACT OF SOCIODEMOGRAPHIC FACTORS

Sociodemographic factors such as race, English language proficiency, and SES, impact families' access to and quality of care in PPC and hospice services throughout the nation.[22] Traditionally social determinants of health can include geographic location, access to transportation, food security, job security, and health insurance, among others, and can positively or negatively impact access to care.[22] In addition, racist and discriminatory experiences, especially in the healthcare setting, can foster mistrust and have detrimental effects on patients' and families' experience of care.[37,38] For example, Mexican Spanish-speaking families whose child had a serious illness reported discriminatory experiences in the inpatient setting, which remained painful memories months to years after the child's death.[39] Such discriminatory experiences can have a negative impact on families' bereavement and long-term psychological effects. Furthermore, infamous historical events such as the Tuskegee Study can make it challenging for people of minority groups to trust that the medical system has their best interests in mind.[40] As a result, members of minority groups report feelings of mistrust or skepticism of the medical system, especially with regards to end-of-life care. Culturally humble care includes inquiring in a compassionate and safe manner about social determinants of health, including attitudes and belief toward the medical system as well as prior discriminatory experiences in the healthcare setting.

When it comes to opioid access in serious illness, studies show that pharmacies located in predominant black or Hispanic neighborhoods will have minimally equipped storage of opioids compared to pharmacies in non-Hispanic white neighborhoods.[41] This is an important factor to consider as the fallout from the recent opioid epidemic will likely continue to impact opioid access for different populations to varying degrees.

ECONOMIC EXPERIENCE OF SERIOUS ILLNESS

Parents of patients receiving PPC face many hardships within the experience of serious illness, especially related to financial challenges. In the United States, 1 in 5 children live in poverty, exacerbating the experience of serious illness.[42] One study showed that, regardless of SES, 94% of families with advanced cancer report work disruptions; families with lower SES were disproportionately impacted.[43] Disadvantaged families tend to experience longer length of stays, higher rates of unplanned readmissions, and, ultimately, higher mortality and morbidity.[44] In general, access to quality healthcare is closely related to SES, which causes disparities in the overall experience of serious illness with regards to quality of life, morbidity, and mortality.[2,43]

A quarter of bereaved families within the United States report a great deal of financial hardship.[43] About three-quarters of families face work disruptions in the first year after a diagnosis of cancer, and up to one-third of parents must quit work, as reported by bereaved families of children who died from cancer.[45] As a coping strategy, many families attempt fundraising, and poor families tend to participate in more fundraising than more affluent families.[45] Not surprisingly, young single bereaved parents report having experienced the worst hardships.[44]

The importance of an interdisciplinary team, one specifically having a trained social worker, comes to fruition in attempting to compassionately screen patients for economic hardships. An assessment during an initial palliative care consultation can be initiated by asking such questions as, "How are you managing day to day?" This type of question poses an open-ended, safe evaluation of the psychosocial experience of serious illness. Assessment of goals of care can be difficult if the family is hungry or feeling unsafe or if they do not have Maslow's basic hierarchy of needs met.[46] Other assessment questions could include, "Aside from your child's illness, what is worrying you most today?", "Are there other responsibilities that you feel have been challenging to tend to as a result of this hospitalization?" "Is there anything else that our team can help you to think about right now?"

Another approach would be to incorporate compassionate screening tools such as the Beaune et al. screening questions.[44]

- Do you have trouble making ends meet?
- Do you have trouble feeding you family?
- Do you have trouble paying for medications?
- Do you have a safe place to live?
- Do you have enough help caring for your child and other children?

In addition to these questions, psychosocial providers should be aware of available resources within the hospital, community, and state as well as who is eligible for these resources and how to access them. Available resources vary by state. Therefore, psychosocial providers can assist families in navigating and optimizing government support programs such as Medicaid benefits, social security, governmental nutrition programs, and private insurance. Psychosocial clinicians can also assist in advocating for community support and resources through formal letters and communication articulating the family's circumstances and needs (i.e., Family Medical Leave Act [FMLA] or writing letters to the siblings' schools).
Other questions to consider:

- Has your work been supportive and understanding of you needing to miss work?
- Does your child's teacher/school know what your child is experiencing?
- Is your child supported with medical insurance?
- Do you need assistance with navigating government assistance programs (i.e., forms/documentation)?

PPC teams may consider initiating collaborative relationships with hospital development and philanthropic offices with the purpose of creating *quality-of-life funds*. Quality of life funds can be given to families to use toward concrete resources such as electricity bills, transportation, food, and cellphones. This fund may also be used toward legacy building such as family gatherings, celebrations, funeral expenses, and other creative/celebratory entities that improve quality of life for children and their families. In general, access to quality healthcare is closely related to SES, which causes disparities in the overall experience of serious illness with regards to quality of life, morbidity, and mortality.[2,43]

DISPARITIES AT END OF LIFE

Minority and low SES families with child members who have CCCs have a greater likelihood that these children will experience more intensive interventions and a hospital death than do wealthy white patients with CCCs.[5] African Americans are more likely to die after an unsuccessful resuscitation as opposed to discontinuation of intensive intervention.[5,47] Some of these outcomes may be driven by family goals, and it is unknown whether equitable access to PPC would change these outcomes.[20] Additionally, highly intensive interventions at end of life are associated with worse bereavement outcomes such as prolonged/complicated bereavement in an already vulnerable population. Further studies looking at variations in end-of-life interventions in a prospective manner would be helpful in fully grasping the nuances of this complexity.[5]

The assumption in American society has historically been that a death at home is considered to be "good death."[48,49] However, what a good death may mean varies by certain factors, including consideration of culture, SES, spirituality and ethnicity. Increased deaths at home are linked to greater availability of hospice providers, caregivers, and greater local wealth.[22] Anecdotally, if family members do not feel that they are able to maintain adequate levels of comfort and support in the home, they may be more likely to bring their loved one back to the hospital. Some barriers within this context may be hospice's inability to take on pediatric patients or the discomfort of providers in caring for pediatric patients, as previously discussed. Furthermore, the literature elucidates that areas where there is low or no hospice availability are linked with disadvantaged socioeconomic areas, and, according to Linton et al., this finding suggests fundamental structural and socioeconomic barriers to the establishment of hospice programs.[22]

CONTRIBUTION OF BIAS TO DISPARITIES

Over the past decade, studies in healthcare have shown that implicit bias is the root cause of many healthcare disparities, especially within minority populations. Whether it is opioid prescription writing, access to hospice services, maternal–fetal health, access to quality PPC, morbidity and mortality, or highly intensive intervention at end of life, racial identity continues to be associated with disparities in healthcare.[41] These commonalities point toward a higher experience of suffering within serious illness for non-white families from low SES backgrounds. PPC is not immune to these findings, and implicit or systemic bias could be a contributing explanation for the disparities found within the healthcare experiences for minorities facing serious illness.

More studies are needed in PPC to more fully understand the nuances of trust, provider race concordance, access to palliative/hospice/bereavement care, and PPC's implicit biases. Additionally, more information is needed to better understand how the goal concordance of families facing serious illness affects bereavement experiences.[20–22] It is important to consider both the individual and the health system's implicit bias within PPC and how this may affect minorities' overall experience with serious illness and interactions with PPC, as well as how these interactions impact overall bereavement outcomes for parents, siblings, and extended family members.

Other contributing factors to consider according to Linton et al. are provider bias, prejudice, and stereotypes within the PPC field.[22] Research has shown that race concordance between providers and patients allows for more positive perceptions of the care received.[22] In other words, in general, patients and families representing minority populations feel more confident in the care they receive when their providers look like them and/or have similar cultural or religious identities. While this concept needs to be studied more to better understand the full implications, one may wonder whether or not implicit bias training could also increase diversity in the field. Linton et al. also discuss quality of information exchanged and how studies have shown that communication tends to be worse for minorities.[22] This work found that, in particular, Hispanic, Asian American, and African American patients are more likely to report communication barriers.[22] Importantly in the literature review by Linton et al., the authors mention trust as a fundamental component of the patient–clinician relationship, highlighting how the black community has historically experienced neglect and exploitation in the US healthcare system resulting in inherent fear of receiving inferior care.[22]

Understanding why disparities exist, especially within the context of families living with serious illness, is necessary to unveil solutions to mitigating suffering for the most vulnerable of society. Incorporating a stance of humility and an awareness that the field of PPC is not immune to implicit bias may be a piece of the puzzle in moving our field forward to equitably prevent, anticipate, and mitigate suffering in all its forms without regard to race, ethnicity, socioeconomic advantage, religion, or culture.

SUMMARY

The field of PPC has made great strides in advancing its pillars of improving communication, incorporating cultural humility, bearing witness to and mitigating suffering in all its forms at all stages of serious illness, and improving disparities as they relate to the care of minorities and access to quality PPC. At the same time, specialty PPC providers should learn more about their own implicit and explicit biases, how to mitigate these biases, and how to further optimize care for all seriously ill children and their families.

REFERENCES

1. Institute of Medicine. *The Future of Nursing: Leading Change, Advancing Health.* Washington, DC: National Academies Press; 2010.
2. Ilowite MF, Al-Sayegh H, Ma C, Dussel V, Rosenberg AR, Feudtner C, Kang TI, Wolfe J, Bona K. The relationship between household income and patient-reported symptom distress and quality of life in children with advanced cancer: A report from the Pediquest study. *Cancer.* 2018 Oct 1;124(19):3934–41.
3. Boss RD. Social disparities and death among children with complex chronic conditions. *Pediatrics.* 2019 May 1;143(5):e20190511.
4. Cawkwell PB, Gardner SL, Weitzman M. Persistent racial and ethnic differences in location of death for children with cancer. *Pediatr Blood Cancer.* 2015 Aug;62(8):1403–1408.
5. Johnston EE, Bogetz J, Saynina O, Chamberlain LJ, Bhatia S, Sanders L. Disparities in inpatient intensity of end-of-life care for complex chronic conditions. *Pediatrics.* 2019;143(5). doi:10.1542/peds.2018-2228.
6. Silva MD, Genoff M, Zaballa A, Jewell S, Stabler S, Gany FM, Diamond LC. Interpreting at the end of life: A systematic review of the impact of interpreters on the delivery of palliative care services to cancer patients with limited English proficiency. *J Pain Symptom Manage.* 2016 Mar 1;51(3):569–580.
7. Butow PN, Sze M, Eisenbruch M, Bell ML, Aldridge LJ, Abdo S, Tanious M, Dong S, Iedema R, Vardy J, Hui R. Should culture affect practice? A comparison of prognostic discussions in consultations with immigrant versus native-born cancer patients. *Patient Education Counseling.* 2013 Aug 1;92(2):246–252.
8. Wiener L, McConnell DG, Latella L, Ludi E. Cultural and religious considerations in pediatric palliative care. *Palliat Support Care.* 2013 Feb;11(1):47–67.
9. Sisk BA, Kang TI, Mack JW. Prognostic disclosures over time: Parental preferences and physician practices. *Cancer.* 2017 Oct 15;123(20):4031–4038.
10. Cousino MK, Schumacher KR, Magee JC, Wolfe J, Yu S, Eder SJ, Fredericks EM. Communication about prognosis and end-of-life in pediatric organ failure and transplantation. *Pediatric Transplant.* 2019 May;23(3):e13373.
11. Kraetschmer N, Sharpe N, Urowitz S, Deber RB. How does trust affect patient preferences for participation in decision-making? *Health Expectations.* 2004 Dec;7(4):317–326.
12. Muñoz-Blanco S, Raisanen J, Donohue P, Boss R. Enhancing pediatric palliative care for Latino children and their families: A review of the literature and recommendations for research and practice in the United States. *Children.* 2018 Jan;5(1):2.
13. Mazanec P, Tyler MK. Cultural considerations in end-of-life care: How ethnicity, age, and spirituality affect decisions when death is imminent. *AJN.* 2003 Mar 1;103(3):50–58.
14. Yin HS, Johnson M, Mendelsohn AL, Abrams MA, Sanders LM, Dreyer BP. The health literacy of parents in the United States: A nationally representative study. *Pediatrics.* 2009 Nov 1;124(Supplement 3):S289–98.
15. MacKenzie and Hatala. Addressing culture within healthcare settings: The limits of cultural competence and the power of humility. *CMEJ* 2019, 10(1): e124–e127.
16. Foronda C, Baptiste DL, Reinholdt MM, Ousman K. Cultural humility: A concept analysis. *J Transcult Nurs.* 2016 May;27(3):210–217.
17. Davies B, Sehring SA, Partridge JC, Cooper BA, Hughes A, Philp JC, Amidi-Nouri A, Kramer RF. Barriers to palliative care for children: Perceptions of pediatric health care providers. *Pediatrics.* 2008 Feb 1;121(2):282–288.
18. Mack JW, Cronin AM, Kang TI. Decisional regret among parents of children with cancer. *J Clin Oncol.* 2016 Sep 12;34(33):4023–4029.
19. Morris SE, Dole OR, Joselow M, Duncan J, Renaud K, Branowicki P. The development of a hospital-wide bereavement program: Ensuring bereavement care for all families of pediatric patients. *J Pediatr Health Care.* 2017;31(1):88–95. doi:10.1016/j.pedhc.2016.04.013
20. Bona K, Wolfe J. Disparities in pediatric palliative care: An opportunity to strive for equity. *Pediatrics.* 2017;140(4). doi:10.1542/peds.2017–1662
21. Hall WJ, Chapman MV, Lee KM, Merino YM, Thomas TW, Payne BK, Eng E, Day SH, Coyne-Beasley T. Implicit racial/ethnic bias among health care professionals and its influence on health care outcomes: A systematic review. *Am J Public Health.* 2015 Dec;105(12):e60–76.
22. Linton JM, Feudtner C. What accounts for differences or disparities in pediatric palliative and end-of-life care? A systematic review focusing on possible multilevel mechanisms. *Pediatrics.* 2008;122(3):574–582. doi:10.1542/peds.2007-3042

23. Wolfe J, Grier HE, Klar N, Levin SB, Ellenbogen JM, Salem-Schatz S, Emanuel EJ, Weeks JC. Symptoms and suffering at the end of life in children with cancer. *N Engl J Med.* 2000 Feb 3;342(5):326–333.
24. Feudtner C, Womer J, Augustin R, Remke S, Wolfe J, Friebert S, Weissman D. Pediatric palliative care programs in children's hospitals: A cross-sectional national survey. *Pediatrics.* 2013 Dec;132(6):1063–1070. http://www.ncbi.nlm.nih.gov/pubmed/24190689
25. Haines ER, Frost AC, Kane HL, Rokoske FS. Barriers to accessing palliative care for pediatric patients with cancer: A review of the literature. *Cancer.* 2018;124(11):2278–2288. doi:10.1002/cncr.31265
26. Center to Advance Palliative Care. National Registry Data. 2018. registry.capc.org
27. Knapp C, Woodworth L, Wright M, Downing J, Drake R, Fowler-Kerry S, Hain R, Marston J. Pediatric palliative care provision around the world: A systematic review. *Pediatric Blood Cancer.* 2011 Sep;57(3):361–368.
28. Connor SR, Downing J, Marston J. Estimating the global need for palliative care for children: A cross-sectional analysis. *J Pain Symptom Manage.* 2017 Feb 1;53(2):171–177.
29. Mooney-Doyle K, Keim-Malpass J, Lindley LC. The ethics of concurrent care for children: A social justice perspective. *Nursing Ethics.* 2018;26(5):1518–1527. doi:10.1177/0969733018765308
30. Lindley LC. Determinants of access to pediatric hospice care: A conceptual model. *J Hospice Palliat Nurs.* 2015 Apr;17(2):113–118.
31. Andersen R, Newman JF. Societal and individual determinants of medical care utilization in the United States. The Milbank Memorial Fund Quarterly. *Health Society.* 1973 Jan 1:95–124.
32. Carlson MD, Bradley EH, Du Q, Morrison RS. Geographic access to hospice in the United States. *J Palliat Med.* 2010 Nov 1;13(11):1331–1338.
33. Kaye EC, Gattas M, Kiefer A, et al. Provision of palliative and hospice care to children in the community: A population study of hospice nurses. *J Pain Symptom Manage.* 2019;57(2):241–250.
34. Kaye EC, Applegarth J, Gattas M, et al. Hospice nurses request paediatric-specific educational resources and training programs to improve care for children and families in the community: Qualitative data analysis from a population-level survey. *Palliat Med.* 2020;34(3):403–412.
35. Kaye EC, Gattas M, Kiefer A, et al. Investigation of modifiable variables to increase hospice nurse comfort with care provision to children and families in the community: A population-level study across Tennessee, Mississippi, and Arkansas *J Pain Symptom Manage.* 2020;S0885-3924(20)30580-7.
36. American Academy of Pediatrics, Committee on bioethics and Committee on Hospital Care. Palliative care for children. *Pediatrics.* 2000;106(2):351–357
37. Born W, Greiner KA, Sylvia E, Butler J, Ahluwalia JS. Knowledge, attitudes, and beliefs about end-of-life care among inner-city African Americans and Latinos. *J Palliat Med.* 2004 Apr 1;7(2):247–256.
38. Contro, N.; Davies, B.; Larson, J.; Sourkes, B. Away from home: Experiences of Mexican American families in pediatric palliative care. *J Soc Work End Life Palliat Care.* 2010;6(3–4):185–204.
39. Davies B, Larson J, Contro N, Cabrera AP. perceptions of discrimination among Mexican American families of seriously ill children. *J Palliat Med.* 2011;14(1):71–76.
40. Freimuth VS, Quinn SC, Thomas SB, Cole G, Zook E, Duncan T. African Americans' views on research and the Tuskegee Syphilis Study. *Soc Sci Med.* 2001 Mar 1;52(5):797–808.
41. Morrison RS, Wallenstein S, Natale DK, Senzel RS, Huang LL. "We don't carry that": Failure of pharmacies in predominantly nonwhite neighborhoods to stock opioid analgesics. *N Engl J Med.* 2000 Apr 6;342(14):1023–1026.
42. Macartney SE. Child poverty in the United States 2009 and 2010: Selected race groups and Hispanic origin. US Department of Commerce, Economics and Statistics Administration, US Census Bureau. 2011. https://www.census.gov/library/publications/2011/acs/acsbr10-05.html
43. Bona K, Dussel V, Orellana L, et al. Economic impact of advanced pediatric cancer on families. *J Pain Symptom Manage.* 2014;47(3):594–603. doi:10.1016/j.jpainsymman.2013.04.003
44. Beaune L, Leavens A, Muskat B, et al. Poverty and pediatric palliative care: What can we do? *J Soc Work End of Life Palliat Care.* 2014;10(2):170–185. doi:10.1080/15524256.2014.906375
45. Dussel V, Bona K, Heath JA, Hilden JM, Weeks JC, Wolfe J. Unmeasured costs of a childs death: Perceived financial burden, work disruptions, and economic coping strategies used by American and Australian families who lost children to cancer. *J Clin Oncol.* 2011;29(8):1007–1013. doi:10.1200/jco.2009.27.8960
46. Trowbridge A, Walter JK, McConathey E, Morrison W, Feudtner C. Modes of death within a children's hospital. *Pediatrics.* 2018 Oct 1;142(4):e20174182.
47. Maslow AH. A theory of human motivation. *Psychological Rev.* 1943 Jul;50(4):370.
48. Walter T. Historical and cultural variants on the good death. *BMJ.* 2003 Jul 24;327(7408):218–220.
49. Payne SA, Langley-Evans A, Hillier R. Perceptions of a "good" death: A comparative study of the views of hospice staff and patients. *Palliat Med.* 1996 Oct;10(4):307–312.

6 | PROGRAM DEVELOPMENT

TAMMY I. KANG, DANIEL P. MAHONEY, MEAGHANN S. WEAVER, AND STACY S. REMKE

Great things are done by a series of small things brought together.

VINCENT VAN GOGH

Family Reflection

"The members of the pediatric palliative care team worked together to support our daughter and our family. We talked openly about hopes with the team members. The chaplain, the social worker, the doctors, and the nurses all knew about our hopes and our goals, and they worked together to foster our hopes even when the medical situations were getting worse. No matter where we were, whether home or in the intensive care unit or at the skilled nursing facility or even when transitioning back to a final week at home, they just kept showing up and they never left until we had a hope to help focus and sustain us. Even now, in grief, we are still working together with our palliative care team to maintain new hopes as a bereaved family. We could sum them up as the "work together, show up often" team. Even when the days feels very long or very hard or risk feeling even lonely, the team reminds us that we were never alone, and we never will be alone because they were always our daughter's team and they are still our family's team."

Paige's Family, Hand-in-Hand Care Recipients

INTRODUCTION

The field of pediatric palliative care (PPC) has evolved over the past two decades in response to an escalating acknowledgment of need and a call to action by the Institute of Medicine (IOM) report *When Children Die*.[1] A nationwide survey in 2013 showed that 112 of 162 children's hospitals in the United States had PPC programs and many more were developing them.[2] Developing and implementing a PPC program requires not only an understanding of the principles and practice of good PPC, but also a familiarity with business and design principles.

Palliative care program development is not a fixed, linear process; rather, it unfolds and takes shape over time. There are opportunities to address needed changes in organizations in each phase of program evolution. Incorporating input and fostering ownership longitudinally among all stakeholders, including patients and families, cannot be overestimated. The goal of program development is to change the culture of the healthcare organization to one that anticipates and provides for palliative care needs of children, ideally from the time of their diagnoses.

The majority of children with life-threatening conditions are referred to a regionalized medical center with expertise in complex pediatric health problems. Most childhood deaths occur in hospitals. These same hospitals may provide care for an additional estimated 10-fold number of children who have chronic, complex conditions that may shorten lifespan or impact wellness. It is crucial for these institutions to make palliative care available to children and their families.

This chapter outlines phases of program development, including suggestions for tasks or important work to be done, challenges, and strategies to promote buy-in and generate small successes that facilitate bigger change. Change is an ongoing process that requires focused, consistent efforts and responsiveness to emerging obstacles and needs. Shifting the culture of an institution requires both flexibility and tenacity (grit!) in achieving the goal of excellent interdisciplinary palliative care for children.

Although this chapter focuses on development of a PPC program in the hospital, the phases of growth and the challenges of each stage share commonalities across diverse settings. The strategies offered here can be extrapolated and adapted to other circumstances. One exception to this is program development in limited resource settings, such as global low- and middle-income countries, which deserves special consideration and will be addressed separately. No hospital-based program would be complete without the ability to coordinate with the community resources that serve these same children and their families. Through such reciprocal relationships continuity of care can occur.

The phases of program development described are neither rigid nor self-contained. Certain tasks, such as ensuring alignment with institutional goals and priorities, should be repeated in each phase. Some tasks that drive organizational change may prove too difficult to be completed within one phase and thus stages may blur. Nevertheless, it is useful to have a structure that facilitates planning the requisite steps for change and addresses challenges proactively as the program evolves.

PHASE I: PLANNING

Comprehensive preparation and planning from the earliest stages is essential (see Box 6.1). No PPC program will develop at an institution without the buy-in and support from institutional leadership. It is therefore important to make the case to leadership, as with many palliative care interventions, in the target audience's language. In the case of institutional leadership and administration, this is frequently the language of business plans and design strategies. The Center to Advance Palliative Care (CAPC) offers comprehensive resources to assist those looking to establish palliative care programs using the "target language" of institutional leadership [CAPC]. Successful planners should identify areas where palliative care program goals can overlap with or support institution-wide goals, incorporate local champions and stakeholders to include family champions, conduct a thorough top-down needs assessment, and plan for stepwise growth and implementation conscious of the new team's capacity and operating costs.

IDENTIFY AND ALIGN WITH INSTITUTIONAL GOALS

In 1962, Everett Rogers published *Diffusion of Innovation*,[3] which has been widely applied to a variety of economic and development topics. PPC is an innovation that has established itself as an integral part of the care of seriously ill children, growing from innovative and "early adopter" institutions to now include much of the "early and late majorities" as described by Rogers. This is worth considering when brainstorming strategies for developing new PPC programs as institutions (and the individuals that comprise them) have their own traits that will impact the likelihood of adopting this innovation. Identifying the institution's values helps early champions and stakeholders focus on goals and strategies most likely to be effective within their target organization. Consider the recommendations of Friedrichsdorf and Bruera, which help planners anticipate institutional challenges and myths related to PPC that frequently must be addressed in the course of program development.[4]

Good planning examines how the palliative care program will fit into the institution and whether its goals are compatible with the overall mission of the institution. The receptivity of hospital administrators is enhanced not only through adherence to organizational priorities, but also through meeting national standards of excellence for palliative care. These standards are recommended by influential organizations such as the American Academy of Pediatrics (AAP), the Joint Commission (TJC), the National Hospice and Palliative Care Organization (NHPCO), the American Academy of Hospice and Palliative Medicine (AAHPM), the CAPC, and the National Quality Forum (NQF).

> **BOX 6.1 HELPFUL PLANNING QUESTIONS**
>
> - Is this institution welcoming or skeptical of innovation?
> - Are there specific motivations that will increase the likelihood that this innovation will be adopted (such as social recognition by peers, accreditation bodies, or educational communities)?
> - Can this innovation complement or facilitate preexisting goals or activities?
> - Can this innovation be adopted in a stepwise fashion, with specific levels or areas of testing for observation of impact?

ENLIST EARLY CHAMPIONS

Everyone feels a greater sense of ownership in projects in which they feel personally vested. It is from this observation that participatory action research (PAR[5]) has grown in both popularity and efficacy for scholarly work addressing health and social needs of a variety of groups. Similarly, the Institute for Healthcare Improvement (IHI) recommends inclusion of relevant and diverse champions[6] and stakeholders, inclusive of patient and family members, when working to improve the quality of any process or system within a healthcare setting. Early champions will be able to communicate a cohesive and consistent message that substantiates the need for improved palliative care at the institution. Creating a team of interdisciplinary champions from the start is fundamental to establishing a balanced program. It is strategic to include a well-respected physician who will advocate for inclusion of the interdisciplinary team. Whether or not this individual eventually assumes the medical directorship, they can help advance early planning efforts. In many settings, particularly within an academic hospital, a physician and a clinician from another discipline share leadership responsibilities. The leader or leaders should be clearly defined for the development team as well as for the larger hospital community.

The development team should expand over the first several months to include respected *champions*[6]—individuals within the institution who have demonstrated a special interest and expertise in palliative care. The central work of this group is to communicate what is needed, generate institutional support, identify possible solutions, and organize improvements in the delivery of care. To succeed at transformative program development,[7] it is imperative to assemble individuals who are respected as achievers, experts, innovators, and leaders. They will be key spokespeople in creating a coalition for change.[7,8] Recruitment focuses on individuals who have power within the institution through their influence and reputation, the skill to leverage organizational resources, and the clinical expertise to advance program development effectively.

SECURE STAKEHOLDER SUPPORT

Securing institutional stakeholder support begins by consulting with and recruiting key administrative and clinical stakeholders for their opinions and support. This purposeful effort includes seizing every informal or formal opportunity to influence stakeholders by publicizing the program's vision while building collegiality around a common purpose and including families in the core mission and message.[7,8] In this effort, education is marketing, and marketing is education. Partnering with existing familiar venues within the organization for communication and education, such as Grand Rounds, interdisciplinary staff meetings, clinical rounding, and resident conferences, successfully reaches staff without asking them to attend extra meetings. Participating in these educational initiatives fosters team cohesion and promotes consistency of the PPC vision among the development team as well as throughout the organization. The team should be ready to communicate a compelling case for the program within the context of an informed understanding of the organization. Ultimately, the goal is to obtain endorsement of the endeavor; doing so secures essential buy-in and paves the way for access to tangible resources needed to establish the program.

Creating a small advisory council of administrative and clinical leaders can foster their ongoing investment in the program. This group's involvement validates the importance of PPC and helps sanction quality improvement efforts in this area. This phase also includes soliciting constructive feedback from potential antagonists of palliative care program development, as well as from staunch supporters. Individuals from both groups can be recruited as advocates for the program, and they should be given options for their involvement.

NEEDS ASSESSMENTS

New programs or programs wishing to expand often begin by conducting a needs assessment. Typically, programs focus on a detailed clinical needs assessment, which can uncover the concerns of patients, families, and staff in addition to the circumstances and practices that affect the provision of care. The assessment generally describes current clinical metrics, such as the documentation of pain scores and the numbers and locations of hospital deaths, which can validate the program's necessity and scope. The data identify strengths and weaknesses as well as challenges and opportunities for quality improvement initiatives—all critical for program development. This type of needs assessment can also serve as a baseline for comparison of metrics once the program is established: what progress is being made, where changes are still needed, and whether services are making a difference. Thus, planning efforts are designed to integrate data, service delivery strategies, and goals from the outset, facilitating an ongoing process of evaluation and improvement.

Another helpful approach may be to consider incorporating a top-down needs assessment. This is a way to structure the assessment by prioritizing needs. While organizational priorities are driven by patient needs and community factors, including a top-down approach highlights the importance of incorporating organizational needs and priorities at the onset, particularly if programs are seeking organization funding. A first step for the needs assessment is to consider the needs of the organization—what are the immediate, mid-range, and long-term priorities? How can palliative care assist with achieving some of these goals? A next step is to study the priorities of high-level clinical leadership including chief medical officers, department chairs, and service chiefs. In what ways could palliative care assist with their priorities? Considering these higher level needs early can tailor a detailed clinical needs assessment which typically involves providers, patients, and families. For new programs, the needs identified are often broad and numerous. Beginning with a few key metrics that are important to organizational leadership can build credibility and narrow the scope of initial work to be done. A potential downside to this approach is lack of buy-in from a broader range of individuals who may have an interest in or be affected by the evaluation and results. This can be mitigated with strategic communication and engagement.

For programs ready to engage in a comprehensive clinical needs assessment, there are several avenues to pursue, including reviewing the literature, contacting other institutions for advice, sharing tools that can be modified to address unique institutional questions, and enlisting the assistance of other departments within the organization. The quality improvement (QI) staff may already have relevant information or may be able to help with data collection. Other areas, such as strategic support, may be able to analyze pertinent hospital statistics including length of stay (LOS) in intensive care settings prior to death, days on the ventilator, and costs associated with the last days of life. Needs assessments may also include a chart audit, a staff survey, a parent survey, focus groups with providers or family members,[9,10] or the results from applicable metrics already collected at the institution, such as Press Ganey Satisfaction with Care scores. A broad-based understanding of organizational issues and opinions is important. Clinicians and administrators surveyed should represent various disciplines and levels of experience; families should represent different backgrounds and have children with different ages and diagnoses. A needs assessment can turn into a labor-intensive endeavor, so adequate time and resources should be allocated. A realistic option is to pilot a needs assessment in one or two areas (such as the pediatric intensive care unit [PICU], neonatal ICU [NICU], or hematology oncology service) and then eventually expand to other areas.

A representative appraisal also seeks opinions from clinicians who may be less receptive to program development efforts. Resistance may come from those who are uncomfortable with limiting intensive medical interventions for personal or moral reasons, from those who lack familiarity with clinical practice standards in PPC, or from those concerned about either redundancy of services or infringement of their relationships with children and families. The needs assessment often uncovers the belief that a separate program for PPC is unnecessary because it is already done well enough within the institution. A better understanding of the principles of PPC can mitigate many of these objections, and staff education is often a result of the assessment itself.

Comparing the institution's palliative care program efforts with those of other local, regional, and national institutions is also valuable. Ultimately, the data from benchmarking, the systems assessment, and the needs assessment will comprise the evidence that makes a solid case for program support to the institution and potential funding sources. The information also contributes to the development of a strategic business plan and focuses clinical resources where they are most needed.[11]

Strategies should be well-thought out for communicating the assessment results, together with program recommendations, to all leadership groups. Emotionally charged, real-life clinical stories, both positive and negative, can highlight critical points and carry the important message of family-centered care. All of this initial information identifies a clear direction for the program's development and promotes the acceptance necessary to move into the next phase.

A helpful assessment activity is the *strengths, weaknesses, opportunities, and threats* (SWOT) analysis,[12] which can reveal the overt and covert power dynamics of the organization. This type of introspection prepares the planning team for difficulties that may arise in program implementation, and it allows them to develop proactive strategies to avoid or minimize barriers. This activity should include an examination of how existing resources within the institution and community might interface with the PPC program.

MISSION, VISION, AND IMPLEMENTATION PLAN

Within the first few months, the development team must begin to articulate the program goals[13] which will eventually lead to a mission or vision statement, as well as an implementation plan.[7,8,14] A well-articulated *mission statement* clearly defines PPC[7] and reveals core objectives that guide program planning. By contrast, a *vision statement* should describe the future role of palliative care within the organization as envisioned by the development team. These two statements will serve as the foundation of the business plan and executive summary,[15] which will be described in more detail later in this chapter.

The implementation plan will explain the range of services that the program plans to offer. The start-up paths of programs can vary. For example, programs have begun with a primary focus on staff support and education,[16] on advanced care planning and care coordination,[17] or on services within the pediatric oncology population.[18] Each team's start-up path will depend on the local goals, values, and needs of their institution or organization. The authors recommend starting with a comprehensive palliative care service that is implemented in a stepwise, modular fashion to address the assessed organizational needs according to their priority as determined by the development team and organization leadership. To paraphrase a famous concept, it is better to do one thing well and build on success than to do several things poorly and lose momentum. It is the positive experience of participating in high-quality PPC that will drive the satisfaction and implementation of the team within the institution.[19] In addition to the implementation plan, create a concurrent implementation risk table (Table 6.1). This a way to organize potential implementation challenges, identify the impact of the challenge, and develop potential strategies to mitigate the challenges.

Building a program is a daunting endeavor. Helpful steps include outlining small, manageable steps; using resources that already exist, and establishing a realistic timeline. The CAPC has designed a training methodology for programs at any stage of development. Expert guidance and written worksheets are combined with year-long mentoring. The CAPC website, www.capc.org, also offers extensive program development resources.[20]

CREATE AN IDENTITY: CHOOSING A PROGRAM NAME

The program's name should be selected by the time Phase II begins. Consistently using a name helps to brand and market the program within the institution and the community. Administrators and clinicians, as well as patients and their families, appreciate being able to identify the program and understand its focus for services. Clear identification makes it easier for those who need help to seek assistance from the program and for those who appreciate the program's efforts to give credit where credit is due. Some programs have chosen succinct, medical-based names, with or without reference to palliative care, such as pediatric advanced care team (PACT), pediatric advanced comfort care team (PACCT), and pain and palliative care team. Others have chosen a name that is associated with metaphoric imagery such as Palette of Care, Bridges, Footprints, Compass Care, the Butterfly Program, and Hand in Hand. Parents have emphasized how an identified program name improves access to services. Some believe, however, that including palliative care in the name can be associated with diminished hope[21,22] and associated with hospice. Other opinions focus on the importance of calling it what it is and then working to dispel misunderstandings in the broader community. Either naming approach means the team must be prepared for the ongoing challenge of addressing misperceptions around the term "palliative care" until the term is better understood by society.[21]

PHASE II: CREATING THE FOUNDATION: PROGRAM IMPLEMENTATION

The tasks during this phase are to delineate both the scope and components of the PPC services that are to be offered and to elucidate the logistics involved in service delivery and program marketing (see Table 6.2). Helpful steps include making a site visit to learn from other successful programs and building collaborative relationships with key personnel

TABLE 6.1 Implementation risk table example

IMPLEMENTATION RISK	DESCRIPTION	MANAGEMENT STRATEGY
Lower than estimated penetrance	Many physicians and families believe that palliative care is equivalent to "giving up" This belief may limit the number of consultations	• An intensive education program targeting nursing and physician staff emphasizing the benefits of providing comprehensive palliative care services to all patients with life-limiting or life-threatening diseases • Team members will participate in care planning rounds for high need areas
Less than expected reimbursement for billable services	Third-party payers and institution billing team may not be familiar with billing codes most appropriate for palliative care services	• Targeted and ongoing evaluations with billing/coding team will help maximize potential billing revenue
Higher than expected patient care burden	There are potentially hundreds of children in the system that may be eligible for palliative care services. A larger than expected consult service and outpatient follow-up service may overwhelm the allocated resources	• Provide a service based on collaborative consultations. The primary physicians will maintain an active role in the patient's care • Target inpatient consultations initially with a plan to grow outpatient services
Expectation of palliative care service line to meet other unmet related needs including acute and chronic pain, mental health services, complex patient care coordination	Many patients suffering from acute and chronic pain have illnesses qualifying them for palliative care services. Primarily managing pain both inpatient and outpatient will require a much more robust clinical team	• Develop clear protocols for patient enrollment and clear guidance regarding service palliative care and reasonably offer consistently
Staffing model which incorporates existing psychosocial staff (i.e., child life); spiritual care may not be sufficient	The model above which utilizes in part existing psychosocial, spiritual services may not be adequate depending on consult volume and patient and family needs	• Develop clear treatment plans and document services provided and gaps which are identified

from departments within the hospital. Take time to learn the options; carefully consider what may work well in the organization, what may present unforeseen barriers, and how internal resources might be used to support program efforts. Throughout this phase, it will also be important to constantly analyze services given ongoing needs, gaps, strengths, and priorities, culminating in a multiyear business plan to ensure sustainability. Building a comprehensive program also includes developing expertise at interfacing effectively with community agencies and optimizing palliative care services across settings. It will also be important for the service to learn from its own experience as it accumulates (e.g., by assessing success and sustainability after adding a new population of consults) and be prepared to constantly refine the operations within their own healthcare system and community context.

CREATING A BUSINESS AND FINANCIAL PLAN

A business plan (Box 6.2) is a formal document that makes a solid case for program operations and strategic propositions. Producing a business plan can be instrumental in securing institutional support for dedicated resources allocated to PPC services. Some hospital-based programs have initiated a business plan early on in their evolution while others launched the program, collected data, and then developed a business plan. The timing reflects a combination of factors, including attention to planning, institutional politics, financial considerations, and the level of strategic guidance provided at the institution. For clinicians without experience in writing business plans, collaboration with helpful institutional partners, including senior leadership and finance staff, is recommended.

There are core elements included in a business plan that can be tailored to meet specific needs at various stages of program development. The introduction provides supporting background information, outlining the needs and rationale for the program. For this section, the team carefully selects and expands on the data from the systems and needs assessments. The document explains how the program shares and builds on existing resources. The central message emphasizes the value added to the institution and the breadth and depth

TABLE 6.2 Program development

MARSHAL RESOURCES FOR CHANGE	DEFINE AND PROMOTE THE PROGRAM	EDUCATE
• Carefully select task force/ planning committee members • Engage stakeholders, inclusive of patient and family champions • Investigate start-up funding possibilities • Create an action plan to initiate change	• Align mission and goals with those of the organization • Solicit input from proponents and antagonists • Uncover strengths and weaknesses • Convey clear, consistent program message	• Communicate needs and plans • Hone expertise and skill of planning committee • Use every opportunity, formal and informa • Extend awareness of PPC principles • Reinforce the message

BOX 6.2 BUSINESS PLAN COMPONENTS

- Executive summary: Synthesizes content of overall plan
- Context for the proposal
- Identified need to be addressed; how proposed plan will create improvements
- Key program features
- Funding requirements
- Expected impact and measures
- Statement of need and rationale for proposed program
- System and needs assessment data
- Pertinent clinical patient data: Number and locations of deaths, average LOS, pain scores; current or improved with pediatric palliative care involvement
- Family and staff input/satisfaction with care data
- Financial implications as appropriate
- Competing local/regional initiatives
- Operational plan for implementation
- Description of program goals and services
- Program model and structure; clinical care, education, research, community involvement
- Collaboration with other programs in the hospital and community
- Target patient population, estimated patient volume, and capacity projections over time
- Staffing requirements and roles
- Space and equipment needs; additional operational resources requested
- Basic policies and procedures for program operations
- Evaluation plan and expected impact: clinical, operations, financial metrics
- Marketing plan
- Financial/budget summary with projections over multiple years
- Appendices
- Documents, data, and other supporting information

Adapted with permission from CAPC resources on business plan development: The Business Plan (Level I: Worksheets; Appendix 3.6: PowerPoint—Business Plan Basics; Module 2: Creating Compelling Business and Financial Plan; http://www.capc.org/building-a-hospital-based-palliative-care-program/designing/presenting-plan/index_html (Building a Palliative Care Program-Presenting the Business Plan).

BOX 6.3 MAKING THE CASE FOR A HOSPITAL-BASED PALLIATIVE CARE PROGRAM

- Coordinates services from diverse hospital departments for safe, effective, and efficient family-centered care of patients with serious illnesses
- Facilitates high-quality, well-planned treatments that address current needs as well as anticipated needs
- Advances quality of care and pain management standards used to accredit and/or evaluate services by the Joint Commission and *U.S. News and World Report* annual rankings
- Facilitates care coordination, case management, and referrals to appropriate care settings as indicated
- Improves quality of care and services, which can help strengthen ratings of family satisfaction with care
- Provides staff support to ease the stress in caring for the most emotionally and time-intensive patients and their families, which can strengthen staff satisfaction and retention
- Increases visibility of the institution in the community as being responsive to the holistic needs of patients with advanced illness and their families
- Maintains or increases capacity by matching resources to needs and preferences
- Promotes goals-of-care discussions, honoring the needs and wishes of patients and/or families, which can help avoid futile and burdensome treatments when medically advisable.

Adapted with permission from "The Case for Hospital-Based Palliative Care" Center to Advance Palliative care. https://www.capc.org/tools-for-making-the-case/

of services provided by the PPC program. The CAPC has outlined compelling points that are useful in justifying program development (Box 6.3). These points can be personalized to address institution-specific data and resource-specific design (Box 6.4) when presented to hospital administrators and community members.

The plan should include a detailed, multiyear program budget, indicating direct program expenses, such as salaries with benefits, marketing costs, equipment and supplies, staff education, and specific program resources (e.g., memorials, educational literature, and comfort carts). The financial analysis includes all revenue streams, such as medical center support for salaries and/or operations, as well as income from consult billing, philanthropy, and grants. The business plan also presents outcome data that the team will track to demonstrate program impact. Typical categories include operational, customer, clinical, and financial metrics.[11,20]

The business plan should speak the language of its intended audience: institutional leadership. It should reflect their goals and their priorities, be fiscally responsible and sustainable, and promote the necessary changes to fuel the growth of interdisciplinary palliative care. Do not ask for unlimited resources and financial support but rather demonstrate how the program uses its budget to advance institutional goals.[25] The business plan makes the case for action, clearly stating what is needed from the institution to develop or expand the palliative care program.[26] Be careful to match expected workload to allocated resources, avoiding the precedent of giving away services without adequate institutional support at the expense of practitioners. A business plan is not a static document; it should be reviewed and revised repeatedly as the program changes and expands. The business plan should be able to reflect lessons learned in practice, during growth, and in integration into the institution. Business plans should include resources for the professional development of the team as individuals as well as the team as a whole. Many organizations provide professional development funds for physicians and nurse practitioners but not other disciplines. It is prudent for palliative care teams to consider how to

BOX 6.4 PEDIATRIC PALLIATIVE CARE (PPC) PROGRAM DEVELOPMENT IN LOW-RESOURCE SETTINGS[23,24]

The Need:

Estimated 21 million children in low- to middle-income countries (LMIC) with serious illness needing access to PPC
65% of LMIC had no known PPC activity as of 2011
The World Health Organization (WHO) considers access to PPC and pain management an imperative

The Challenges:

High and growing burden of serious noncommunicable illness in LMIC
Policy and resource issues limit access to analgesics such as oral morphine
Perpetuation of myths and lack of PPC education among clinical workforce
Coordination of outpatient or home-based PPC can be challenging in LMIC

Overcoming Barriers:

Advocacy and public awareness at all levels of health system
Education for clinical workforce about primary and specialist PPC
Partner with governments and nongovernmental organizations to address access to essential medications
Design novel PPC care delivery models unique to local context

Measure Quality and Outcomes:

Ensures quality and efficacy of care provided
Informs local and national health policy
Success builds on documented success

Adapted with permission from Downing J, Boucher S, Daniels A, Nkosi B. Paediatric palliative care in resource-poor countries. *Children (Basel, Switzerland).* 2018;5(2); and Downing J, Namisango E, Harding R. Outcome measurement in paediatric palliative care: Lessons from the past and future developments. *Annals of Palliative Medicine.* 2018;7(Suppl 3):S151–S163.

support the education and development needs of all interdisciplinary team members.

BUILDING A BUSINESS CASE

Building a business case with cost-saving financial metrics is a significant challenge for PPC programs trying to start, grow, or sustain their services.[27] Pediatric programs have not achieved the same financial model of cost neutrality and cost avoidance that exists in the Diagnostic Related Groups–driven adult palliative healthcare environment. Rather, the most compelling value proposition lies in aligning with the priorities, needs, and challenges of the institution.[27] For example, growing evidence suggests palliative care contributes to greater satisfaction from families and referring clinicians and achieves better bereavement outcomes.[28–30] Although similar work is being done in pediatrics to create reliable cost accounting methods and templates to calculate appropriate staffing, volume, and projected income, pediatric programs are still forced to secure financial support from their institutions and outside sources.[27]

Programs should work closely with finance staff, including billers and coders, to maximize revenues given the constraints and payer mix at the institution. One important step is to purposefully learn if other specialty services bill for symptom management; if they do not, the PPC team should do so when appropriate. Specifically learning about billing from other adult and PPC programs is quite instructive, as well as from internal and external educational resources for understanding finances.[20] PPC programs can demonstrate their roles in maximizing efficient, coordinated care that optimizes quality of life despite intense medical and practical needs.[27] More analysis needs to be done within the pediatric community to determine the financial impact of providing PPC and end-of-life services to children in the hospital and home.

FOSTERING PHILANTHROPIC PARTNERSHIPS

Philanthropic financial support provides not only direct payment to the institution, but also recognition and valuable community public relations. Most administrations look favorably on these contributions to the overall budget[25] and to the institution's reputation. Allocating time to work closely with the development office, ensuring it understands program objectives and services, and advocate fundraising for specific aspects of the program are steps that invest in the immediate and future foundations for the program. Prepare talking points, fundraising proposals, patient impact stories, and a wish list of both small and large program items so that both development officers and PPC team members are always ready to meet with potential donors.

Part of a program's fiscal responsibility includes participation in regional and state advocacy efforts with other healthcare institutions to improve access and reimbursement for quality pediatric palliative and hospice care services.

FUNDAMENTAL PROGRAM COMPONENTS

There are fundamental program components that serve as the building blocks of PPC program development. These components include the team, the practice model, coverage and referral practices, and program operations. The specific characteristics and infrastructure for implementation may vary considerably from program to program. Yet through the significant growth of the field over the past decades, there now exist clear lessons learned and guidelines for programs to follow.[31]

SERVICE DELIVERY: THE INTERDISCIPLINARY CARE TEAM

The current state of the art of PPC requires the effective, collaborative efforts of an interdisciplinary team, which includes the child, as appropriate, and the family.[1,32,33] Team members may be selected from the original planning group. However, these individuals will need approval from their departments and the organization to allocate time in their current roles to provide palliative services throughout the hospital. This sanction for their work is critical to success. Once assembled, the interdisciplinary PPC team will work closely with a larger advisory group and/or task force to continue to direct the program's growth. Members of the team will need to be highly visible and receptive to a wide range of staff, patients, and families. When feasible, select team members who represent practice areas where specific needs have been uncovered or where program receptivity is anticipated, such as pediatric oncology or pediatric intensive care, is highly recommended. Clinical proficiency, leadership abilities, excellent interpersonal and diplomacy skills, and a capacity to influence others are qualities desired in each team member. Consultation etiquette expectations should be clearly defined and discussed within the team to ensure consistent behavior across the service.

In addition to palliative care–specific competencies, interprofessional team-based competencies have been described to ensure effective collaborative practice. The Interprofessional Professional Education Consortium has identified four competencies for team effectiveness (IPEC, 2011).

- Values and ethics for interprofessional practice
- Understanding roles and responsibilities
- Interprofessional communication
- Understanding teams and teamwork

Successful teams will attend not only to palliative care knowledge and skills, but also to their group process as a team. Shared goals, understanding of roles and responsibilities as well as scopes of practice, attention to stress management, conflict mediation, and effective communication will all enhance team functioning and set an important foundation for growth and sustainability.[34] The CAPC website has resources to help calculate team staffing requirements, including projected needs based on program growth over the next several years.[20] More about team structure and dynamics is discussed in Chapter 11.

Team Reflection

Strategic Inclusion of Interdisciplinary Team Members

A seasoned palliative care physician had started up a new service at his hospital 3 years prior. He told a colleague:

> We made a decision to have an MD [physician] and NP [nurse practitioner] at the start for budget reasons and planned to use unit-based social workers as needed. That was a mistake. Now, looking back, I see that as the NP and I developed our palliative care skills and service, we missed the opportunity to have a social worker grow in that team with us. Now it is really apparent how much time and energy we spend trying to compensate for that gap on our team. The unit staff just don't have the same shared perspectives and skills.

A social worker or chaplain focused exclusively on palliative care is likely to develop greater expertise than someone who practices palliative care as only occasionally as a part of their clinical assignment. Teams that learn and grow together often develop greater capacity than a group of individual practitioners operating in parallel. As this story illustrates, teams develop by bringing roles into relationship to one another. Issues like shared or co-located office space and meeting opportunities to discuss patient care, but also team process, are essential. This happens both formally, as in team rounds, and also informally, as when working at adjacent desks and overhearing a description of a critical incident and offering input in the moment. Good planning should advocate for these essential building blocks of team effectiveness.

PRACTICE MODEL: CONSULTATIVE OR INTEGRATED

Many programs use a structure that resembles a medical *consultation service model*, wherein a formal consult request is made to the PPC team. Institutional protocols for a formal consult often require that a physician make the request and specify a reason for the referral and that the consult be completed within a specific time frame. In some institutions, this request may be for a particular problem such as pain control or for transfer to the palliative care team for end-of-life management. The consult team, generally led by a physician or an advanced practice nurse (APN), is typically identified as a distinct service having additional training, skills, and, in an increasing number of programs, formal credentialing or certification in palliative care appropriate to their discipline.

In the consultative model, the primary team acknowledges a need for outside assistance. Without the primary team's acknowledgment of need and request for services, PPC may not be available to all children and families who would benefit, or access may come only at the end of life. Ongoing provider education, which reiterates the principles of palliative care and clarifies the distinction between palliative, end-of-life, and hospice care, is crucial for promoting provider acceptance and the timely initiation of services.

An alternative to a consultative model is an *integrated model*, where the interdisciplinary team supports and educates providers in developing basic competencies in pediatric primary palliative care as appropriate to their disciplines. This approach incorporates palliative care core values throughout the institution. The primary team, guided by the PPC team, ensures the delivery and continuity of palliative care through recovery or death. The integrated model also has the advantage that it maintains continuity with familiar and trusted care providers at the most trying times for families and supports the primary team to introduce palliative care resources early in the illness. Policy and procedure guidelines may be needed in this model to facilitate buy-in from the larger system. The PPC team may mentor the primary team in having difficult conversations or challenging symptom management cases, and it can also identify helpful practices being used in some parts of the hospital that could be more widely disseminated for the benefit of patients in other areas. The team's involvement could also come via suggestions at interdisciplinary unit rounds, through the charge or bedside nurse, or when the social worker from the primary team requests additional resources or clinical support. This model helps to raise the bar of clinical practice in the hospital by providing ongoing education at the bedside.

Consultative and integrated models are not mutually exclusive. In practice, features of both models are often found together in institutions with successful programs. The goal is to couple broad-based institutional understanding and acceptance with the expertise of the interdisciplinary palliative care team to address the most complex needs. As in any other specialty, providers get better and more efficient as they practice. This capacity development sets the skills of the PPC team apart over time and helps define their expertise to the organization.

COVERAGE AND REFERRAL CONSIDERATIONS

Ideally, regardless of the program model, team members with training in palliative care should be available to provide round-the-clock assistance to hospital staff.[32,35] Program size, demand, and allocated resources will dictate team availability. Coverage needs to be realistically planned, both to manage expectations and avoid burnout. Many programs provide on-site consults Monday through Friday and offer phone consultation during off-hours. This model can help staff contend with patient needs while protecting team members' time off, an important consideration for team sustainability over time. With a consult model, the practical aspects of staffing require a larger, more formal commitment of dedicated physician or APN full-time equivalent (FTE) work hours to fulfill the clinical demands of a separate service. This expense can be partially offset by billing for eligible clinical services. State agencies, and even the institution itself, can have different rules specifying who can bill for care, so it is important to know these rules.

The benefits of early palliative care referral, such as at the time of diagnosis with a life-threatening condition, are widely advocated.[1,32,36,37] From a practical standpoint, the biggest challenges are initiating these discussions and gaining entry from providers or family members for early palliative care team involvement. Teams can prepare marketing materials and educational talking points to address myths and misunderstandings about palliative care with providers and families to effect culture change. This is a gradual process. Programs should also recognize that the kinds of services needed at the time of diagnosis may differ considerably from the services required at the end of life.[27,38]

A number of resources offer suggestions as to how and when palliative care should be discussed.[17,27] These guides often identify significant medical events or diagnoses, such as the need for a bone marrow transplant or the placement of a nonurgent tracheostomy, that serve as automatic triggers for a consult. With these triggers in place, clinicians may be more inclined to initiate PPC earlier, thereby conforming to best practice standards. Triggers should be developed in collaboration with referring specialty teams to ensure buy-in.

In addition to the timing of the team's involvement, the mechanism by which its input is requested should be defined. The palliative care team will need to decide if a formal order from a physician is required to initiate services or if any staff or family member can request assistance. How a request for team involvement is initiated may be dictated in part by hospital policy and by whether the services will be billed to insurance, as in a formal consult.

PROGRAM OPERATIONS AND INTERNAL MARKETING

Program operations are the practical, day-to-day reality of running a fledgling PPC team as if it were a start-up business within a larger organization's business model. Operations should be defined as clearly as possible in the business and financial plans. Aspects of operations that should be addressed include securing consultation and office space, setting up program contact information, ensuring provider credentialing, access to emergency medical response (EMR), and compensation.

When marketing the program to administrators, clinicians, foundations, and the community, it is imperative that the team be able to clearly describe the various services it can provide. The range of services (see Box 6.1) may change as resources are added and programs become more established. Services may expand to include outpatient PPC consults, co-management for hospice care, perinatal palliative care, or a chronic pain clinic. The marketing aim is to effectively communicate the value added for accessing both palliative care resources and team members to help with time-intensive, challenging care. The message to clinicians is that these extra measures enhance interdisciplinary care while continuing to involve the primary team(s).[25,32]

In addition to responding to referrals, the team should take advantage of the many ways to influence care. For example, team members can conduct educational sessions at staff or division meetings and participate on the hospital pain or ethics committee. Another approach is to offer pilot activities in clinical areas where greater acceptance is anticipated, relying on the support of the so-called early adopters. Many units have routine, interdisciplinary meetings to review important patient issues, and perhaps certain PPC team members might be able to attend.

Increased visibility is an effective method for marketing the program. Take every opportunity to talk to staff members from various units, disciplines, departments, and community agencies about the new services. Trust and acceptance will evolve as staff and families experience positive collaborative relationships with palliative care team members.

CONTRIBUTING TO THE SYSTEM: EDUCATION

Education, training, and engaged practice experience form the foundation for collaborative practice. Education takes several forms, all of which contribute to the mission and value added to the institution. These include education and professional development training for the entire interdisciplinary PPC team, education of other clinicians at the institution, and education of hospital administrators and others making financial decisions that could impact the team.

The definition of interprofessional education (IPE) is that which occurs "when two or more professions learn with, from and about each other to improve collaboration and the quality of care" (CAIPE, 2002). Many palliative care practitioners have learned "on the job," as a member of a team[39] or through professional development opportunities. Too often educational opportunities are uniprofessional. In palliative care, interprofessional education should be the rule more than the exception. Beyond clinically focused training, the core team must also acquire program-building skills including managing program operations, creating a business plan, philanthropic fundraising, and developing quality improvement projects. Interdisciplinary education and training are discussed in more detail in Chapter 11.

An ongoing step is to educate generalist and specialty teams about the ways that they already provide services under the domain of palliative care.[25] This awareness and use of PPC resources raise the profile of the program and thus become an effective internal marketing strategy. Efforts to establish a range of clinical care and educational resources should be directed at making "the right way the easy way."[14] This includes responding to the everyday practice needs of busy clinical staff and managers. It also requires a cooperative approach when redesigning operations so that these resources can incorporate palliative care practices into daily routines.[14] For example, because most PICU deaths involve withdrawal of life-sustaining treatments, it may be useful to collaborate on Compassionate Extubation Guidelines with staff in the intensive care areas. Make a point to investigate the tension points or gaps that develop around policies and procedures, which are difficult and confusing to staff: these are areas of opportunity.

PPC curricular content, including national practice standards, should be widely disseminated both in the institution and in the wider healthcare community. Teaching must also include program information on appropriate criteria for referrals, as well as what services can and will be provided to patients, families, and staff by the team and other clinicians at the institution. Perhaps most importantly, education initiatives can highlight how good PPC helps the institution meet its goals.

Extensive expertise in specifically defined skill sets that PPC team members demonstrate enables them to be highly effective practitioners. These core competencies have been delineated by several groups, including the CAPC and the ACGME (www.acgme.org). Discipline-specific competency guidelines are also emerging as the field advances, for example, in social work.[40] Although these competencies will overlap with those of colleagues who practice in other specialty areas, they also include certain skills and perspectives that particularly belong to PPC. This combination of strengths will help establish the value added by the palliative care service to their colleagues and to patient and family consumers.

Education may also take the form of clinical care resources, which make a difference at the point of care and include such tangible items as a comfort care room or comfort care cart and baskets of nonperishable food delivered to a child's room during family vigils at the end of life. End-of-life bedside practices can be standardized throughout the hospital by providing each unit with disposable cameras, memory boxes, and keepsake supplies to make handprints or footprints, to clip a lock of hair, and to measure the child's height using decorative ribbon (Figure 6.1). Rather than attempting to create resources from scratch, staff can seek examples from colleagues that can be adapted to program needs. This will save time, money, and frustration as established tools will be more readily implemented. Many programs maintain resource libraries of anticipatory grief and bereavement literature for staff to give to families. Promoting varied resources and providing the necessary educational support puts consistent palliative care into action throughout the institution.

Clinicians are not the only group that should be targeted for education. Hospital administrators, including those responsible for financial decisions, institutional strategic development, quality improvement, information systems, philanthropic or grant fundraising, and community relations, will all need to understand palliative care. Ongoing conversations help administrators understand that death, or the possibility of death, is a significant aspect of providing care to children with complex medical problems, and, as such, palliative care is an obligation of the institutions that provide care to these children and their families.

SCOPE OF SERVICES

THE ROLE OF COMMUNICATION

Effective, collaborative communication is indispensable when striving for the highest quality of palliative care. In fact, communication has been described as one of the most common procedures in medicine, and the most important.[9,10,22,37,41-43] When performed well, communication conveys both reciprocal information and compassion, justifying its importance as a core competency for the PPC team. Effective communication is also paramount to building a cohesive team and promoting positive, collaborative exchanges with referring staff, which ultimately facilitates both continuity and quality of care.

A core function of the PPC program is to foster and enhance interdisciplinary and family communication. Another critical use of communication, especially early on, is "consult etiquette": the ability to turn every communication opportunity into a positive relationship-building encounter, whether with families, referring providers, interdisciplinary team members, or hospital administrators.

Many palliative care teams introduce documentation tools to facilitate communication, decision-making, and continuity of care, such as the Five Wishes advanced illness/directive booklets (available at www.agingwithdignity.org/index.php).[32] As EMR use expands, some teams have collaborated with EMR developers to incorporate PPC documents and screening tools into the EMR, such as the Epic Userweb PPC Navigator. Effective written communication is essential and should be designed with multiple aims in mind, including clear communication of the medical plan to other clinicians, recognizing its use as a medical, legal, and billing document, and documentation of the patient narrative.

Routine interdisciplinary palliative care team (IDT) meetings, adapted from the hospice model of care, have come to be regarded as an essential requirement for team communication and program functioning. Meeting agendas are focused on reviewing cases, solving problems, collaborating on quality improvement initiatives, and handling important administrative issues. (see Chapter 13 for in-depth information regarding Communication in PPC).

THE ROLE OF PAIN AND SYMPTOM MANAGEMENT

Developing pain and symptom management skills is a pivotal component of building a successful PPC program.[33,35] Some institutions already have pain teams prior to the adoption of palliative care programs. However, not all pain services, especially if they are primarily focused on adults, are equipped to address the range of needs commonly found in PPC. Even if the institution has a separate pain service, it remains crucial that PPC team members receive rigorous training to acquire specialist-level proficiency in symptom identification and management. Integrating pain teams and palliative care programs, or at minimum establishing a formal, collaborative working relationship between them, helps ensure relief of suffering and optimizes quality of life throughout the continuum of care.[44] Addressing pain and symptom management is the focus of Section III of this textbook.

THE ROLE OF BEREAVEMENT CARE

Services to help ill children and their families cope with anticipatory grief, the end-of-life experience, and the ensuing bereavement are integral to PPC and hospice programs. A growing body of literature suggests that the grief experienced when a child dies is more protracted and complex than the grief associated with adult death (this will be discussed further in Chapter 15).[45,46] Providing bereavement care is unique among hospital services rendered because much of the support offered occurs when the actual patient is deceased. The family then becomes the focus of care.

When building bereavement services, programs should[47] start simple, plan realistically, and access community organizations, collaborating whenever possible and expanding as resources allow. In the hospice model of care, bereavement support is built into the payment structure. However, this is not the case for hospitals, and funding for bereavement services can be limited. Many hospitals rely on philanthropy to fund bereavement support, which may be administered through the spiritual care department, social work department, or PPC program. In some settings, bereavement services may be a separate program within the hospital. Establishing a collaborative relationship, even allocating a portion of the PPC team's time and funding, enhances the spectrum of interventions that includes care through death and bereavement. The program planning and budgeting process should include resources for staff time, supplies, publications, space requirements, and other bereavement support resources. Bereavement support, activities, and roles of PPC team members is discussed further in Chapter 15.

THE ROLE OF STAFF SUPPORT

Addressing staff support and team wellness is widely recognized as an essential endeavor.[32,48] The intensity of care and emotional demands experienced by staff place them at risk for compassion fatigue, moral distress, and burnout. Promoting staff support and self-care is vital in preserving effective functioning for the palliative care team, as well as for the staff who provide bedside care. Taking the time to process the intense and highly

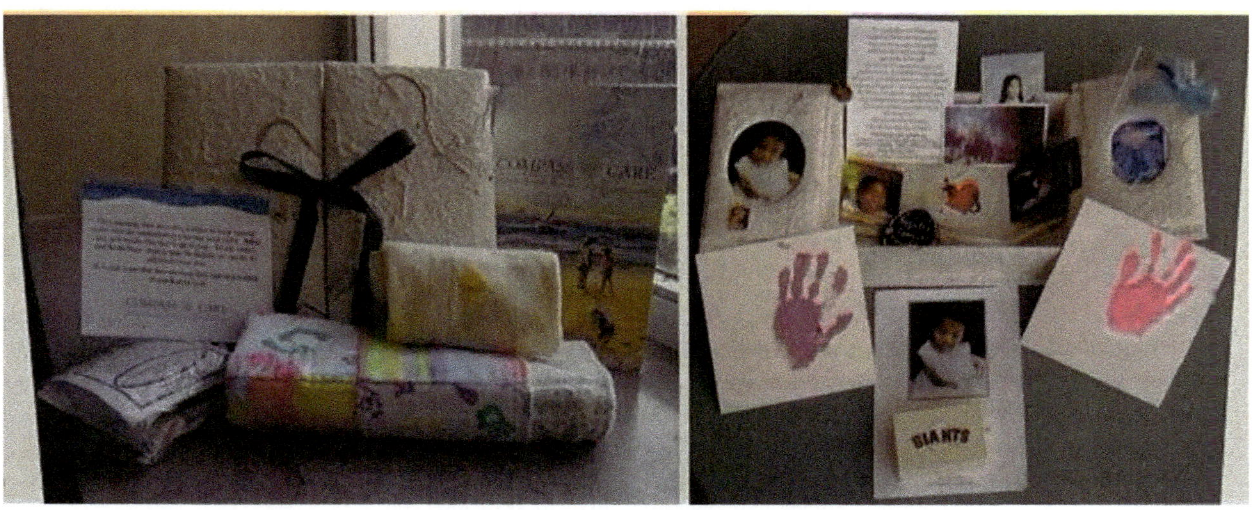

Figure 6.1 Examples of bereavement and legacy packets for families

emotional clinician-patient-family experiences recognizes the humanistic and compassionate nature of this work. This potential impact on care providers can be framed as secondary trauma: the consequences of witnessing the suffering of others.[49–51]

The impact of services to support staff in their caregiving role may be difficult to accurately measure with quantitative data (such as turnover, sick days, apathy) but it is an inherent function of a palliative care program. Ongoing staff-support activities offered by the palliative care team help build trusting relationships with clinicians, facilitating program acceptance, collaboration, and referrals. For the team itself, both formal and informal mechanisms for reflection and renewal are advised. Annual retreats for professional development and renewal, "project time" as breaks from direct care, flextime, monthly meetings with a designated counselor, and periodic memorial observances are practices that programs have employed. While team and self-care practices are essential, they are not enough to ensure resilient practitioners and teams. To ensure resilience, planning for reasonable workload expectations, adequate resources to manage patient care demands, and ongoing measures to identify needs and address team support are required. No amount of self-care can compensate for unreasonable expectations, chronic unacknowledged uncompensated overtime, and unmanageable workloads. Administrative acknowledgment of this important area, coupled with policy-level planning for staff support, can go a long way toward developing a strong and stable workforce.[49]

INTERFACING WITH COMMUNITY PARTNERS: UNDERSTANDING UNIQUE CONSTRAINTS

Children with complex, life-threatening conditions have spent significant amounts of time in hospitals because of limitations in community-based services. Children and their families can feel an immense sense of support from hospital clinicians, often believing that the hospital represents a haven. That said, the hospital remains an unnatural and distorted place to live out one's childhood. Research and practice experience validates that a child's development and the family's coping are best served at home with adequate resources.[52] It is therefore important that PPC teams develop strategic partnerships to enable safe, coordinated, and continuous care between the hospital and community.

Advances in science and technology, along with children's resiliency, mean that children are living longer with complex therapies that mimic ICU care at home. However, it can be extremely difficult to find this level of pediatric technology support and clinical expertise needed, particularly in rural areas. The reality is that parents usually have the primary responsibility for around-the-clock complex care at home. In these cases, respite care is an important consideration. While families initially may not be comfortable using community-based options, especially if they have not had the opportunity to establish trust in alternative caregivers, they will need encouragement to make long-term plans and develop relationships with respite providers. Those relationships are important and underscore the importance of effective collaboration between home-based and hospital-based services.

Overall, the number of children requiring PPC is significantly less than the number of adults using home care and hospice services. The challenge to community agencies is to acquire adequate experience to develop and sustain the knowledge, skills, and confidence necessary for providing care to children. Some adult providers describe the emotional burden of caring for children as prohibitive. With expert help, many adult home care or hospice programs have been open to pediatric training, consultative support, and education to help develop competencies and greater comfort in caring for pediatric patients and their families.

One of the more challenging goals of an inpatient PPC program is to develop a seamless interface with community-based home care and hospice programs that serve these same children. For home-based pediatric palliative and end of-life care programs to be truly successful, they should embrace a concurrent model of care. Philosophically, this concurrent approach is more acceptable to families who are not focused on end-of-life care, but who are still interested in receiving supportive measures focused on enhancing quality of life, such as expert symptom management and psychosocial care. These kinds of services have traditionally been available in the home through community hospice programs. However, the hospice movement has developed around a different philosophy of care based on the more predictable disease trajectories of many common adult diseases with an emphasis on end-of-life care for patients expected to live 6 months or less. The adult hospice model typically abides by rules and regulations that require patients to give up life-prolonging treatments. Financial reimbursement tied to these restrictions is usually based on Medicare guidelines, which leads to a philosophy and practice not suitable for children with life-threatening conditions. Fortunately, in recent years, federal support for concurrent care through reimbursement avenues has helped bridge this gap. Now PPC practitioners can partner with hospice services to develop appropriate plans for children and families.[53]

Adult hospice medical directors and clinicians may not be comfortable with the prognostic uncertainty and complex care plans characteristic of PPC patients. Costs for PPC can be much greater than those of the typical adult hospice patient; children often receive life-prolonging therapies such as home total parenteral nutrition (TPN), repeated transfusions, palliative chemotherapy, and home IV antibiotics, which are not conventionally allowed under the hospice benefit. Most hospices, which operate on daily reimbursement, cannot provide this costly care unless they have sufficient philanthropic funds to offset expenses associated with pediatric cases. Significant financial and resource limitations cause many community-based providers to pursue both home care and hospice licensure, allowing greater flexibility for reimbursement based on patient acuity. A fee-for-service billing model, used by home care agencies, can offer a more financially solvent approach, particularly when caring for PPC patients. Additionally, some hospices are willing to work with insurance companies to develop individual agreements to carve out a fee for service for certain therapies in order to be able to provide concurrent care. Understanding these intricacies allows the PPC team to be more effective in discharge planning and advocating with payers.

Team Reflection

Interfacing with Community Partners

An identified children's hospital has formal partnerships with several home-based adult hospice programs that cover different geographic areas. These hospice programs have agreed to care for children with support from the hospital staff. Hospital physicians are available to consult with the agency staff around unexpected clinical challenges. The hospital PPC team provides quarterly education, case consultation, and training to the home-based team. Standardized communication forms between the two agencies have been created to facilitate transfer of healthcare information and treatment plans. Families are asked to sign Releases of Information to enable effective coordination of care. A Discharge Checklist accompanies the child when they go home from the hospital. A Home Update Form accompanies the child to all outpatient clinic appointments and admissions to the hospital to document changes in the treatment plan. An Advanced Care Planning Form describes child and family preferences and goals for care and is shared with the child's team. The inpatient team appreciates improved communication about what is going on at home, and the home-based team's work benefits from improved communication around changes in the child's condition, orders, and updates from the hospital team. The hospice team is challenged by the need to be more flexible about procedures and interventions, which are not usually authorized within a strict hospice plan of care. They are learning how to utilize the benefits of concurrent care. It has taken some time to come to understand what each partner can expect from another. The community-based service is now more willing to care for children in their community with complex healthcare needs. The hospital-based team has promoted the partnership as a strategy for greater stability in home-based care, and, while it requires some staff time, it is well worth it to avoid crises and allow improved responses for unexpected care challenges.

PHASE III: ENSURING SUSTAINABILITY

During Phase III, program development is focused on sustainability. Palliative care programs need time to reach a level of maturity where benefits for patients, families, the hospital, and the community are perceived as indispensable. For full and ongoing impact, a palliative care program must be able to sustain its activities, organizational practices, community partnerships, and core mission salience to ensure durability of benefits to children and families.[54] Thinking only of program implementation risks wasting valuable resources, damaging trust, and limiting goal achievement; whereas thinking about longer term sustainability early and often is a way to think of program protection. Sustainability "is the ability to maintain programming and its benefits over time."[55]

Sustainability capacity includes the processes, partnerships, and structures that allow a palliative care program to survive and even thrive long-term. PPC programs must be able to leverage resources to not only effectively plan, design, and implement a program but to then also effectively maintain evidence-based services longitudinally.[56] Pacing program development and service reach in a stepwise or modular manner is a way to set the program up for long-term success.

Sustainability requires ongoing stepwise goal-setting with timelines for implementation of goals to maintain the larger programmatic mission. Sustainability goals warrant addressing goal development and then systematically readdressing goal outcomes. Evaluation of whether the goals were reached is an important team process not just for program startup, but also for mid- and long-term program survival. Sustainability goals may be considered according to Table 6.3.

Critical features of a successful, sustainable PPC program include fostering attitudes of acceptance among referring providers, families, and the community; acquiring ongoing financial support; ensuring efficient use of resources; and promoting expert skill development throughout the institution.

Referring clinicians will recognize that the PPC service is helpful to them as well as to patients and their families. In this sense, these clinicians are also clients of the PPC team. If the team does not support and affirm the relationship the primary provider has with the child and family, or if the primary clinician feels challenged or criticized by the team's actions, then future referrals can be threatened. By taking time to address the needs of all parties, the team demonstrates effectiveness and becomes an important part of the care delivery system. Aligning interventions to the stated goals of referring physicians, families, and others invested in the outcomes is important to program survival. This intricate communication process also serves the palliative care program by inviting ongoing feedback that helps refine and refocus the team's efforts.

A mature team takes feedback seriously, reflects on its practice, and makes the necessary changes. Provider and family satisfaction surveys provide metrics indicative of program impact. If the team considers that all stakeholders are clients from the outset, then the customer service attitude has the added benefit of creating allies and reducing potential conflict. When palliative care teams experience particular "buy-in" or heavy volume from a subspecialty that feels difficult to sustain with current staffing, the team may create training programs in primary palliative care practices for the providers[57] or identify an embedded palliative champion within that subspecialty.[58]

Reevaluation of priorities and adjustment to new needs point to areas for expansion. The team must determine if it is meeting its own, as well as the institution's, expectations and goals. Additional information may be gained through focus groups with clinicians and/or family members. Chart audits

TABLE 6.3 Palliative care program sustainability dimensions and definitions

SUSTAINABILITY DIMENSION	DEFINITION	ANNUAL GOAL EXAMPLE
Supportive engagement	The tangible indicators of organizational and community support (engagement of leaders, institutional receptivity to palliative interventions, shared prioritization of palliative care)	• Create quarterly information graphics to demonstrate the palliative care program's impact on patients satisfaction ratings to share with senior leadership and external partners to leverage additional service opportunities
Program evaluation	Collection and analysis of program's activities, characteristics, and outcomes	• Review the palliative care cohort's rural zip codes to consider adaptation of consult availability for oncology patients receiving care at satellite clinic
Funding stability	Secure and sustainable economic support for the longitudinal wellness of the palliative care program with opportunity for growth	• Develop multimedia success story vignettes to share with donors with goal to increase annual benevolence fund by 10% in the coming year
Strategic partnerships	Relationship between palliative care and community partners in collaborative work	• Formalize a partnership contract with a trusted local hospice agency to together extend hospice home health services for children
Organizational capacity	The social architecture and leadership which fosters the ability of palliative care to achieve a measurable improvement in mission	• Introduce a Bereavement Coordinator role on the team to assist with bereavement phone calls and mailings to expand programmatic mission
Communication	The formal and informal webs of information-sharing	• Develop an integrated communications plan to update community physicians on the palliative program's new process for referrals
Ongoing strategic planning	Processes to guide the program's directions, goals, and strategies	• Establish a Palliative Advisory Council to meet quarterly to determine goals, objectives, and strategies for the coming year

comparing patients with similar diagnoses who have and who have not had PPC team consultation may also be valuable, as could identifying reasons for patient readmissions within a week after discharge.

Another approach the team can take to embed itself in the system is to adopt tasks important to the organization's mission or operational requirements. For example, the team can take a lead role in policy and procedure development, such as revising Withdrawal of Artificial Life Sustaining Therapy or Patient Controlled Analgesia or Opioid Use Agreements. Team members might also serve on ethics, residency training, resiliency, or family advisory committees. PPC teams may also be able to identify emerging patterns or trends and so address potential problems before they escalate. Helping the organization meet its regulatory requirements, quality standards, and other tasks validates the team's breadth of expertise and worth. The presence of a strong PPC program presents marketing opportunities for the institution, particularly if community or regional organizations do not have similar programs serving seriously ill children.

Many programs start with funding for a limited time, receiving small grants from organizations or philanthropic sources. Over time, that funding may dry up, or new criteria for continuation may be established. It is very important to consider these initial sources of support and consider how the program's activities meet the funder's expectations. However, it is critical that each revision of the business plan addresses the need for ongoing funding that keeps up with expanding program demands. Philanthropic goals are necessary to achieve sustainability. Fundraising events and corporate contributions engage community support and increase institutional visibility, as does inviting the input of community representatives as advisory council members. Families who appreciated the care their child received from the team can be wonderful spokespeople for the program. When one home-based hospice program cared for a child in their community, they operated at a loss during the acute care phase of providing end-of-life care. The community responded with significant donations because they applauded the agency's willingness to care for children. Over time, philanthropy, grants, patient-care revenue, and cost-saving or cost-avoiding formulas can assist programs in developing a financial argument that supports their operations. Broad-based financial support can help programs move from start-up to self-sustaining.

PPC team leadership should provide formal and informal program updates to the administrative and clinical leadership on a regular basis. Palliative care programs may consider creating an advisory council consisting of the palliative care team members, administrators, hospital leaders, parent and patient stakeholders, and community members with quarterly meetings. At these meetings, demonstration of palliative care programmatic involvement in multiple quality improvement initiatives that have advanced more efficient, effective, consistent, and coordinated care helps to integrate the program within the institution. Sources of data for quality improvement should include measurements of patient outcomes and activities that reflect organizational priorities, including numbers of referrals changing over time, pain and symptom management needs identified and successfully treated, trends in patient satisfaction scores, and improved practices at the end of life.

Through initiatives and partnerships that are focused on sustainability, the program achieves credibility, accomplishes good work, and is well accepted by administrative, clinician, and family members.[59] The program has matured in its capability to offer services with depth of knowledge, skills, and resources, serving needs in many if not all areas where children and families are cared for within the organization. By the end of this phase, the program clearly will be able to validate that it makes a significant difference in many arenas, that successful practices have been adopted throughout the institution, and that palliative care has been woven into the fabric of the institution.

PHASE IV: SURVIVING SUCCESS

Surviving success requires effective and forward-thinking management of program growth, increased patient care volume, and competing priorities (see Table 6.4). As experience grows, staff members and the team develop expertise, economies of scale, and greater efficiency. With this increased capacity the same number of staff members can provide more services—up to a point.

How many providers does it take to deliver excellent care, especially as programs mature? The CAPC has developed some formulas to address this question, but setting and practice patterns are likely to affect these numbers. It is important not to promise more than can be delivered and to communicate barriers to achieving goals as this information becomes apparent. As the field evolves, patterns of practice and expectations for productivity need to be studied so that benchmarks can be developed.

Monitoring growth while planning for current and future needs requires not only attention to data but also attention to how the team is functioning. In such a stressful area of practice, personal coping and team effectiveness go hand in hand. Self-care practices translate into healthy work habits and positive contributions to the team. Conversely, when burnout begins to surface, it can become increasingly difficult to deliver the quality of care desired. Each individual has his or her own needs and capacities, so formulaic responses are likely to have only limited success. Members of well-established, seasoned teams agree that they have succeeded, at least in part, by managing the personal stresses associated with their work, which helps maintain professional vitality.

TABLE 6.4 Program development Phase IV: Surviving success

STRIVE FOR CONTINUED EXCELLENCE	MAINTAIN PROFESSIONAL VITALITY
• Analyze areas still in need of improvement • Implement strategies to achieve new goals • Report needs, challenges, and contributions to administration • Establish a mechanism to keep up with advances in pediatric palliative care • Incorporate structure for ongoing program evaluation	Balance professional demands with self-care Celebrate accomplishments Support educational growth of staff and palliative care team Create regular opportunities for self-reflection

One opportunity for regular self-care check-ins is the IDT meeting. These meetings can "take the temperature" of how the team is functioning. Regular check-ins and application of standardized tools that measure team functioning, burnout risks, and vicarious trauma, for example, can help teams notice when they are encountering greater stress. Early identification of needs and introduction of relief measures can be critical to success and resilience over time.

One of the challenges of having a successful program is recognizing that the work is never done. A program that does not evolve will not continue to be successful, or at the least, it risks sliding into mediocrity without periodic readjustment. Research contributes to new knowledge and therapies. There are always areas that could be improved or new services that would address unmet needs. The sense of never being finished is real and adds a compelling motive to incorporate reflection and development of new goals into the team's plans. At the same time, acknowledging past accomplishments can lend a heartening perspective on the great strides that have been made and an appreciation for the distance already traveled.

REMAINING TRUE TO THE CORE TEAM VALUES

Palliative care team member well-being and collective team health must be central priorities to sustain an excellent future. Programs need to nurture the teams' growth curve by carefully planning for continual team development. When volume grows and staff attrition occurs, it becomes necessary to bring on new team members. The team should reevaluate training and mentorship needs regularly so that the newest staff members have time and support to become successful on the team. Effective team functioning can improve staff recruitment and retention and facilitates greater capacity to address patient care needs. Encouraging staff to participate in nonclinical activities such as advocacy, education, and research allows intermittent respite from the intensity of care delivery.

As programs mature, teams encounter developmental issues in clinical expertise, collaboration, and productivity. Individual practitioners come into the team with variations in their knowledge, skills, and practice abilities. Over time, each develops greater capacity to manage patient volume efficiently and with proficiency. Pacing program growth to allow protected onboarding time and orientation training for newer team members retains the team's core identity while allowing incoming colleagues to ease into the team culture. The team as a whole can accomplish more than the sum of its parts, but this requires attentiveness to team identity and team unity. Teams eventually establish a common set of terms and practices, allowing a healthy synergistic interdisciplinary care model to take hold. When a consistent practice occurs across the team's members, an interdisciplinary approach emerges.

In the sustainability model, teams are wise to name and maintain the principles and values that continue to identify their purpose as a team. Teams may consider identifying their daily core purpose such as "quality care for children and families" which they will uphold as unwavering and as core to their purpose and mission throughout seasons of programmatic changes or growth.

CONSIDERING GLOBAL PARTNERS

While focusing on local care, PPC teams may consider recognizing the opportunity for global partnerships and collaborations. Whether in the form of teleconferences, shared education, learning exchanges, or quality improvement partnerships, palliative care teams may consider deliberate opportunities to learn with and from international palliative care partners. The opportunity for collaborations and communication across PPC settings is an opportunity to enhance worldview and appreciation for the diversity of palliative care application across settings.

CONCLUSION

PPC members have moved from initial development phase to now focusing on sustainability and recognizing the phase of surviving success. This translates into a deliberate attentiveness to remain true to the initial guiding core team values of quality patient-centered, family-focused, interdisciplinary care while adapting to exponential growth and ongoing care needs. Programs are now primed to evolve into academic divisions within hospitals and to advance the science of PPC, expand the research base, and still remain committed to competent care of children and families. The initial vision and mission statements of compassionate care and strong interdisciplinary collaborations remain central to the sustainability of this maturing field.

REFERENCES

1. Field MJ. *When Children Die: Improving Palliative and End-of-Life Care for Children and Their Families: Summary.* Washington, DC: National Academies Press; 2003.
2. Feudtner C, Womer J, Augustin R, et al. Pediatric palliative care programs in children's hospitals: A cross-sectional national survey. *Pediatrics.* 2013;132(6):1063.
3. Rogers EM. *Diffusion of Innovations* (4th edition). New York: Free Press; 2010.
4. Friedrichsdorf SJ, Bruera E. Delivering pediatric palliative care From denial, palliphobia, pallilalia to palliactive. *Children (Basel Switzerland).* 2018;5(9) .
5. Nitsch M, Waldherr K, Denk E, Griebler U, Marent B, Forster R Participation by different stakeholders in participatory evaluation of health promotion: A literature review. *Eval Program Plann.* 2013;40:42–54.
6. Meier DE. Ten steps to growing palliative care referrals. *J Palliat Med.* 2005;8(4):706–708.
7. Kotter J. Leading change: Why transformation efforts fail. *Engineering Management Review, IEEE.* 2007;37.
8. Perrakoil VS. Change management: The secret sauce of successful program building. *J Palliat Med.* 2009;12(4):329–330.
9. Contro NA Larson J, Scofield S, Sourkes B, Cohen HJ. Hospital staff and family perspectives regarding quality of pediatric palliative care. *Pediatrics.* 2004;114(5):1248–1252.
10. Contro N, Larson J, Scofield S, Sourkes B, Cohen H. Family perspectives on the quality of pediatric palliative care. *Arch Pediatr Adolesc Med.* 2002;156(1):14–19.
11. Weissman DE, Meier DE. Operational features for hospital palliative care programs: Consensus recommendations. *J Palliat Med.* 2008;11(9):1189–1194.
12. Learned EP. *Business Policy: Text and Cases.* Homewood, IL: R. D. Irwin; 1969.
13. Radwany S, Mason H, Clarke JS, Clough L, Sims L, Albanese T. Optimizing the success of a palliative care consult service: How to average over 110 consults per month. *J Pain Symptom Manage.* 2009;37(5):873–883.
14. Byock I, Twohig JS, Merriman M, Collins K. Promoting excellence in end-of-life care: A report on innovative models of palliative care. *J Palliat Med.* 2006;9(1):137.
15. Spragens LH. Developing a business plan for your outpatient palliative care program: A technical assistance monograph from the IPAL-OP Project.
16. Meier DE, Beresford L. Pediatric palliative care offers opportunities for collaboration. *J Palliat Med.* 2007;10(2):284–289.
17. Toce S, Collins MA. The FOOTPRINTS model of pediatric palliative care. *J Palliat Med.* 2003;6(6):989–1000.
18. Duncan J, Spengler E, Wolfe J. Providing pediatric palliative care: PACT in action. *MCN, The American Journal of Maternal/Child Nursing.* 2007;32(5):279–287.
19. Verberne LM, Kars MC, Schepers SA, Schouten-van Meeteren AYN, Grootenhuis MA, van Delden JJM. Barriers and facilitators to the implementation of a paediatric palliative care team. *BMC Palliat Care.* 2018;17(1):23.
20. Care CtAP. Building a hospital based palliative care program: Implementation and staffing. 2020.
21. Morstad Boldt A, Yusuf F, Himelstein BP. Perceptions of the term palliative care. *J Palliat Med.* 2006;9(5):1128–1136.
22. Zhukovsky DS, Herzog CE, Kaur G, Palmer JL, Bruera E. The impact of palliative care consultation on symptom assessment, communication needs, and palliative interventions in pediatric patients with cancer. *J Palliat Med.* 2009;12(4):343–349.
23. Downing J, Boucher S, Daniels A, Nkosi B. Paediatric palliative care in resource-poor countries. *Children (Basel, Switzerland).* 2018;5 (2).
24. Downing J, Namisango E, Harding R. Outcome measurement in paediatric palliative care: Lessons from the past and future developments. *Ann Palliat Med.* 2018;7(Suppl 3):S151–S163.
25. Portenoy R, Heller KS. Developing an integrated Department of Pain and Palliative Medicine. *J Palliat Med.* 2002;5(4):623.
26. Care CtAP. Financing a Palliative Care Program. 2015. https://www.capc.org/toolkits/funding-a-palliative-care-program/
27. *Pediatric Palliative Care Field Guide.* 2019.
28. Hinds PS, Schum L, Baker JN, Wolfe J. Key factors affecting dying children and their families. *J Palliat Med.* 2005;8 Suppl 1:S70–78.
29. Kassam A, Skiadaresis J, Alexander S, Wolfe J. Parent and clinician preferences for location of end-of-life care: Home, hospital or free-standing hospice? *Pediatric Blood Cancer.* 2014;61(5):859–864.
30. Thrane SE, Maurer SH, Cohen SM, May C, Sereika SM. Pediatric palliative care: A five-year retrospective chart review study. *J Palliat Med.* 2017;20(10):1104–1111.
31. Sisk BA, Feudtner C, Bluebond-Langner M, Sourkes B, Hinds PS, Wolfe J. Response to suffering of the seriously ill child: A history of palliative care for children. *Pediatrics.* 2020;145(1).
32. American Academy of Pediatrics. Committee on Bioethics and Committee on Hospital Care. Palliative care for children. *Pediatrics.* 2000;106(2 Pt 1):351–357.
33. Organization NHaPC. *Standards of Practice for Pediatric Palliative Care and Hospice.* In. Alexandria, Virginia2019:31.
34. Altilio T, Dahlin C, Remke S, Tucker R, Weisman D. Strategies for maximizing the health / function of palliative care teams: A resource monograph from the Center to Advance Palliative Care. 2013.

35. *A National Framework and Preferrred Practices for Palliative and Hospice Care Quality.* Washington DC: 2006.
36. Frager G. Pediatric palliative care: Building the model, bridging the gaps. *J Palliat Care.* 1996;12(3):9–12.
37. Mack JW, Hilden JM, Watterson J, et al. Parent and physician perspectives on quality of care at the end of life in children with cancer. *J Clin Oncol.* 2005;23(36):9155–9161.
38. Thompson LA, Knapp C, Madden V, Shenkman E. Pediatricians' perceptions of and preferred timing for pediatric palliative care. *Pediatrics.* 2009;123(5):e777–782.
39. Sumser B, Remke S, Leimena M, Altilio T, Otis-Green S. The Serendipitous Survey: A look at primary and specialist palliative social work practice, preparation, and competence. *J Palliat Med.* 2015;18(10):881–883.
40. Gwyther LP, Altilio T, Blacker S, et al. Social work competencies in palliative and end-of-life care. *J Soc Work End-of-Life Palliat Care.* 2005;1(1):87–120.
41. Hinds PS, Drew D, Oakes LL, et al. End-of-life care preferences of pediatric patients with cancer. *J Clin Oncol.* 2005;23(36):9146–9154.
42. Hsiao JL, Evan EE, Zeltzer LK. Parent and child perspectives on physician communication in pediatric palliative care. *Palliat Support Care.* 2007;5(4):355–365.
43. Meyer EC, Ritholz MD, Burns JP, Truog RD. Improving the quality of end-of-life care in the pediatric intensive care unit: Parents' priorities and recommendations. *Pediatrics.* 2006;117(3):649–657.
44. Friedrichsdorf SJ, Remke S, Symalla B, Gibbon C, Chrastek J. Developing a pain and palliative care programme at a US children's hospital. *Int J Palliat Nurs.* 2007;13(11):534–542.
45. Jonas D, Scanlon C, Rusch R, Ito J, Joselow M. Bereavement after a child's death. *Child Adolesc Psychiatr Clin N Am.* 2018;27(4):579–590.
46. Snaman J, Morris SE, Rosenberg AR, Holder R, Baker J, Wolfe J. Reconsidering early parental grief following the death of a child from cancer: A new framework for future research and bereavement support. *Support Care Cancer.* 2019.
47. Contro N, Sourkes BM. Opportunities for quality improvement in bereavement care at a children's hospital: Assessment of interdisciplinary staff perspectives. *J Palliat Care.* 2012;28(1):28–35.
48. Care NCfHaP. Clinical Practice Guidelines for Quality Palliative Care 4th Ed. In:2019.
49. Jones BaRS. Self care for pediatric oncology professionals. In Abrams A, Muriel, N and Weiner, L., eds. *Pediatric Psychosocial Oncology: Textbook for Multidisciplinary Care.* New York: Springer; 2016:367–377.
50. Lipsky LvD. *Trauma Stewardship: An Everyday Guide to Caring for Self While Caring for Others.* 2009.
51. Renee SK, Therese AJ. *When Professionals Weep: Emotional and Countertransference Responses in Palliative and End-of-Life Care.* New York: Taylor and Francis; 2016.
52. Dussel V, Kreicbergs U, Hilden JM, et al. Looking beyond where children die: Determinants and effects of planning a child's location of death. *J Pain Symptom Manage.* 2009;37(1):33–43.
53. Center TNCfMHIatC. Your child's health care and the Affordable Care Act (ACA): Concurrent care for children. 2014. https:// medicalhomeinfo.aap.org/tools-resources/Documents/ACA-ConcurrentCare%20FINAL.pdf
54. Schell SF, Luke DA, Schooley MW, et al. Public health program capacity for sustainability: A new framework. *Implement Sci.* 2013;8:15.
55. Scheirer MA, Dearing JW. An agenda for research on the sustainability of public health programs. *Am J Public Health.* 2011;101(11):2059–2067.
56. Savaya R, Elsworth G, Rogers P. Projected sustainability of innovative social programs. *Eval Rev.* 2009;33(2):189–205.
57. Marc-Aurele KL, English NK. Primary palliative care in neonatal intensive care. *Semin Perinatol.* 2017;41(2):133–139.
58. Moynihan KM, Snaman JM, Kaye EC, et al. Integration of pediatric palliative care into cardiac intensive care: A champion-based model. *Pediatrics.* 2019;144(2).
59. Bruera E. The development of a palliative care culture. *J Palliat Care.* 2004;20(4):316–319.

7 | INTERDISCIPLINARY EDUCATION AND TRAINING

KATHARINE E. BROCK, JENNIFER HWANG, MARSHA JOSELOW, BLYTH LORD, JANET DUNCAN, AND DEBORAH A. LAFOND

There is only one way to see things until someone shows us how to look at them with different eyes.

PABLO PICASSO

INTERDISCIPLINARY EDUCATION AND TRAINING

LANGUAGE

In the literature, online collaboratives, curriculum repositories, evaluation tools, and fellowship training programs, two terms are used: "interdisciplinary" and "interprofessional." These are often used interchangeably, with *interdisciplinary* the preferred convention for referring to two or more disciplines in pediatric palliative care, and *interprofessional* more common in education, evaluation methods, teamwork, and policy literature. For the purpose of this chapter, we will use the term "interdisciplinary" except when "interprofessional" is included as a formal title, policy, survey assessment tool, or direct quote.

PRINCIPLES OF ADULT EDUCATION

Much of the day-to-day learning in the healthcare environment happens organically in the process of caring for children and their families. That said, it is valuable to think about the educational principles that can make this experience most successful, whether the learning environment is the ward, clinic, or classroom. The experiential learning of clinical training in all disciplines can be described through the work of David Kolb.[1,2]

Kolb described a cycle in which a learner has an experience. The experience leads to reflection. The reflection leads to formulation of abstract concepts and congruent generalizations. These concepts and generalizations are then applied during a new situation which permits learners to test their new understanding. This testing in another clinical encounter is followed by another cycle of reflection, abstraction/generalization, and application which perpetuates the cycle.[1,2]

Palliative care providers will recognize that this cycle plays out in their own clinical practice multiple times per day. Every patient we meet generates reflection on the part of a palliative care provider (e.g., Why is the patient's pain refractory to opioids?). This leads to a formulation of concepts and generalizations (Perhaps the pain is a manifestation of non-physical factors?). In the next clinical encounter, this hypothesis leads to additional exploration which unveils additional information (i.e., the patient also has deep spiritual and psychological stressors).

Beyond recognizing the constant cycles of experiential learning in clinical training and practice, considerable work has been done over the past 30 years to characterize adult learning or andragogy. Initially described by Malcolm Knowles and adapted and refined by many others, adult learners are described as having six unique needs for learning.[3]

1. Adults need to understand why they need to know something.
2. Adults have knowledge of how they learn and need flexibility to learn in their own way.
3. Adults come to learning with previous experiences which they value and which educators should acknowledge and respect.
4. Adults seek learning when they are ready to learn, as they respond to changing circumstances in their environment.
5. Adults are ready to learn because they see learning as a way to help them respond to a challenge they perceive in their current or future setting.
6. Adults' motivation to learn is internally motivated.[2]

When learners seek out palliative care training, their justification often reveals Knowles's principles of *andragogy*. They have had experiences or anticipate experiences in patients with refractory symptoms, complex communication, or care for patients with life-limiting illnesses which motivate them to seek additional knowledge and skills. There is no learner more motivated than practitioners who anticipate they will need knowledge they do not possess during their upcoming clinical shift. The just-in-time training provided by palliative care teams to primary teams every day reflects this reality. Similarly, learners who seek additional training through lectures, seminars, conferences, clinical rotations, or advanced fellowship typically come to these experiences with personal life experiences and motivations that define the lens through which they view palliative care education.

PRINCIPLES OF INTERDISCIPLINARY EDUCATION

INTERDISCIPLINARY VERSUS MULTIDISCIPLINARY

The World Health Organization (WHO) defines palliative care for children as "the active total care of the child's body, mind and spirit, and also defines giving support to the family."[4] This charge to care for body, mind, spirit, and family, by definition, requires an interdisciplinary team. While multidisciplinary teams are created simply by putting health professionals with different professional backgrounds together to care for the same patient, interdisciplinary teams are defined by the collaboration over time of health professionals with different professional backgrounds to care for the patient (see Figure 7.1).[5] Body, mind, spirit, and family are integrated in the patient and thus require the integrated and collaborative practice of an interdisciplinary team.

Team leadership is another place where multidisciplinary and interdisciplinary teams often differ. Multidisciplinary teams tend to have a single leader who gathers input from team members prior to making a decision. Interdisciplinary teams have more fluid leadership in which all members may lead the team in the care of specific children and their families based on the needs of the patient and the unique skills of each team member. Multidisciplinary teams have a clear "head of the table" whereas interdisciplinary teams sit at a round table where leadership may come from any team member and may even change between different members of the interdisciplinary team depending on the unique needs of the patient, family, and/or clinical situation.

Interdisciplinary team practice is a learned skill that has only recently gained attention in the education of medical professionals. Much of the focus has been on interdisciplinary education during training in recognition that these skills are easier to cultivate in novice learners. According to the WHO, interprofessional education (IPE) is an experience that "occurs when students from two or more professions learn about, from, and with each other" (see Figure 7.2).[6]

Experiential learning, either in simulated settings or direct patient care, is the primary element of interdisciplinary education. Thibault explains experiential learning as students entering a practice environment to gain understanding in how to work collaboratively in "real-life" situations. Thibault also highlighted that true interdisciplinary education "requires purposeful integration and collaboration among the disciplines."[7]

UNIQUE DYNAMICS OF PEDIATRIC PALLIATIVE CARE

Pediatric palliative care (PPC) presents unique challenges in educating clinicians from different disciplines and varied levels of experience. Some of these unique dynamics to be considered include

- Death is not "normal" in pediatrics, as compared to the relative normalcy of expected death in adulthood, particularly in the geriatric population.
- Children have a wide variety of serious, often chronic, medical conditions that are amenable to integration of

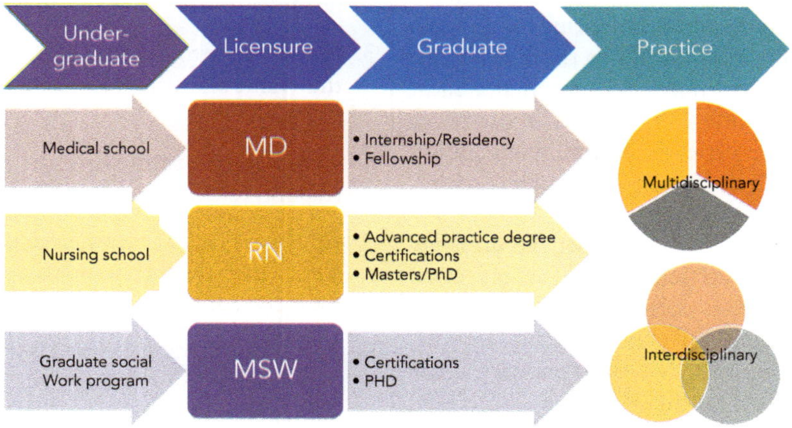

Figure 7.1 Educational silos can foster disciplinary distance. Differing educational systems and training models can foster disciplinary distance and lead to multidisciplinary teams in which each member performs separate and distinct functions. However, through the addition of interdisciplinary training and education, it is possible to foster interdisciplinary healthcare teams. Abbreviations: MSW, Master of Social Work; RN, registered nurse; MD, medical doctor. Reprinted with permission from Rabinowitz E, et al. Finding strengths in our differences: How interprofessional training prepares clinicians for collaborative practice (SA507). *J Pain Symptom Manag.* 2019;57(2):444–445.[83]

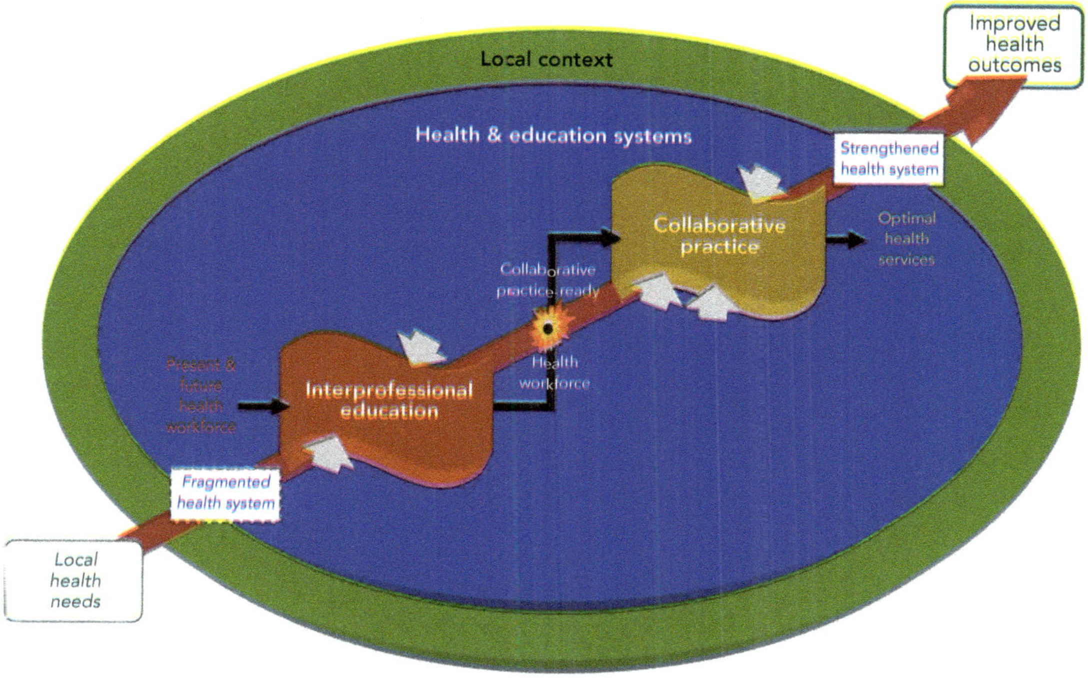

Figure 7.2 Framework for action on interprofessional education (IPE) and collaborative practice. Interprofessional education is more than just learning together in the same environment. True IPE encompasses the dynamic elements of learning about each other and from each other. It requires relational interactions and opportunities for each discipline to contribute to group learning. IPE is necessary to produce a workforce that is ready for collaborative practice. It enhances learner outcomes, which in turn should lead to improved collaborative practice and enhanced clinical outcomes. Reprinted with permission from World Health Organization (WHO), *Framework for Action on Interprofessional Education & Collaborative Practice*. WHO; 2010. https://www.who.int/hrh/resources/framework_action/en/

palliative care.[8,9] In the adult population, cancer and chronic cardiorespiratory illnesses are common entry points for palliative care.[10,11]

- The trajectory of serious illness in pediatrics may be over years, while the average length of enrollment for adults in hospice is just 76.1 days.[12]
- PPC crosses developmental stages, from perinatal to young adults, contributing to challenges in assessment. Self-report measures for pain and nonpain symptoms often cannot be used or may not be appropriate.[10,11]
- Pediatric care is often cure- or disease-directed, even when quality of life may be compromised. Children have increased use of medical technology, as compared to adults, often under the provision of concurrent care.[13]
- Parents or legal guardians serve as surrogate decision-makers for children under the legal age of majority or for those with developmental/cognitive delays.
- There is a lack of evidence-based pharmacokinetic and pharmacodynamic data in prescribing medications for the pediatric population.
- Pediatric patients often continue care by multiple medical specialties while enrolled with concurrent palliative care services, while adults most often receive their primary care from the hospice team once enrolled.
- As a child ages into young adulthood, transition of care from pediatric providers to adult providers may be challenging when adult providers lack expertise in childhood-related serious illnesses.
- There are substantially fewer trained pediatric home care, palliative care, and hospice clinicians as compared to those who care for the adult population.

When designing and implementing interdisciplinary education and training, one must consider these unique challenges so that care can be provided by clinicians who can implement an appropriate plan.

PEDIATRIC COMPETENCIES, CURRICULAR MILESTONES, AND ENTRUSTABLE PROFESSIONAL ACTIVITIES

When hospice and palliative medicine became an official medical subspecialty in 2006, a group of clinician-educators was asked to create a list of competency-based outcomes for fellowship training by the Accreditation Council of Graduate Medical Education (ACGME). These competencies were to inform the Next Accreditation System of the ACGME, which uses competency-based outcomes to assess trainees. These competencies did not take into account the unique needs of PPC and so a new list of pediatric competencies was developed based on the original competencies document (http://aahpm.org/competencies/ped-competencies).[14]

In 2014, the American Academy of Hospice and Palliative Medicine (AAHPM) brought together a group of hospice and palliative medicine (HPM) fellowship directors to create the Entrustable Professional Activities that define the work of a hospice and palliative care physician (http://aahpm.org/uploads/HPM_EPAs_Final_110315.pdf). Entrustable Professional Activities (EPAs) define the key tasks of a subspecialty and require a combination of knowledge, skills, and attitudes.[15] This group went on to create Curricular Milestones to help program directors organize curriculum and create a standard for what should be taught as part of an HPM medical fellowship (http://aahpm.org/uploads/HPM_Curricular_Milestones.pdf).[16] Both the EPAs and the Curricular Milestones were designed to address the comprehensive needs of both pediatric and adult hospice and palliative care patients across the life span. Finally, Reporting Milestones were created as a tool to provide semi-annual feedback to the ACGME about the developmental skill acquisition of fellows over the course of their fellowship.

Competencies, EPAs, and milestones all evolved from the ACGMEs transition to a competency-based model of accreditation. While the ACGME is specifically focused on postgraduate medical training, these documents still offer guidance for the nonphysician members of an interdisciplinary team. As previously described in this chapter, the day-to-day clinical roles of nurse practitioners and physicians often are very similar. This means that these documents can offer guidance in the training of advanced practice providers.

TEAM INTERDISCIPLINARY EDUCATION AND TRAINING

Clinicians in PPC must develop an exemplary individual toolkit of knowledge and skills in caring for pediatric patients with serious illness and their family, yet the highest quality of care is best provided by an interdisciplinary team to address all domains of suffering: physical, psychosocial, spiritual, and environmental. Education of interdisciplinary teams may take several approaches to foster the development of knowledge, attitudes, and skills in PPC. Formal education methods, such as didactic lectures, serve as a basis of knowledge acquisition. Simulation provides practice and adoption of skill-based learning. Mentoring serves as a path for attitude change. Use of these strategies is a catalyst for team interdisciplinary education and training.[17,18]

STRATEGIES

KNOWLEDGE

Team knowledge is often based on didactic learning in either in person or online education through programs such as the End-of-Life Nursing Education Curriculum–Pediatrics (ELNEC-PPC), Education in Palliative and End-of-Life Care–Pediatrics (EPEC-Peds), Palliative Care Education and Practice-Pediatric Track (PCEP-Peds), Pediatric Pain Master Class, concurrent and preconference sessions at the American Academy of Hospice and Palliative Medicine/Hospice and Palliative Care Nurses Association Annual Assembly (AAHPM/HPNA), the Center to Advance Palliative Care (CAPC) and the National Hospice and Palliative Care Organization (NHPCO), International Children's Palliative Care Network (ICPCN), various state coalition webinars, and other local, regional, and national conferences (Table 7.1). Appropriate for individual learning, these offerings encourage team participation and cooperative group learning.

SKILLS

Simulation is the hallmark of skill-based learning and can be actualized as high- or low-fidelity simulation, role-play, prescribing exercises, and case-based discussion.[19,20] In addition, simulation can be used for ongoing learning, to maintain and improve competencies through quality improvement and break down barriers of departmental and discipline silos.[21] Specifically in palliative care, interdisciplinary communication has been demonstrated to be positively impacted by simulation.[22,23] Simulation is described in more detail in the section, "Models of Training."

ATTITUDES

Attitudes can be influenced by knowledge and skill-based learning, however, mentoring often serves as the catalyst for lasting adoption of attitude change and helps facilitate adaptive coping skills, potentially mitigating the emotional aspects of caring for children with serious illness. While this can be positive or negative adoption, engaging in nurturing teamwork can improve patient safety, communication, staff support, situational awareness, and leadership style. Team STEPPS, developed by the Agency for Health Care Quality (AHRQ) and the Department of Defense (DOD) (https://www.ahrq.gov/teamstepps/instructor/index.html), is an example of team-based learning and mentoring that has demonstrated impact on team attitudes.[24] Mentoring across disciplines embraces the interdisciplinary nature of palliative care, where clinicians are often faced with addressing physical, psychosocial, spiritual, and environmental aspects of suffering.[25] Engaging in interdisciplinary mentoring encourages collaboration and partnerships in care.[26]

MODELS OF TRAINING

One size does not fill all teams. The purpose, dynamics, and structure of teams vary. Finding the training model that works best for each unique team, from novice to expert, is essential to success.[24,27] Utilizing an interdisciplinary team approach to learning provides opportunities for members to learn from one another and appreciate differing perspectives.[28,29] This section outlines several models of interdisciplinary training in PPC but is not all inclusive.

TABLE 7.1 Sample of pediatric palliative care interdisciplinary education opportunities

NAME OF PROGRAM	DESCRIPTION	WEBSITE
American Association of Hospice and Palliative Medicine/ Hospice and Palliative Nurses Association Annual Assembly	This annual convening of palliative and hospice care professionals from across all disciplines offers a wide variety of educational and interactive opportunities addressing the state of the science in caring for children, adolescents, and adults with serious, advanced illness. Pediatric specific sessions are available.	http://apps.aahpm.org/meeting?productid=30925426
California State University Shiley Institute for Palliative Care Certificate program	The Shiley Institute for Palliative Care at California State University offers both a certificate in pediatric palliative care for physicians, advanced practice nurses, physician assistants, and registered nurses, as well as a multidisciplinary certificate for social workers, chaplains, and other providers. The programs are comprised of self-paced, online modules which can be purchased individually for continuing education or in total for the certificate.	https://csupalliativecare.org/programs/pediatrics/
Canadian Network for Palliative Care for Children	This network offers a variety of online and certificate learning programs for healthcare professionals.	https://www.chpca.net/professionals/canadian-network-of-palliative-care-for-children.aspx
Center to Advance Palliative Care (CAPC)	A variety of resources are available to CAPC members. CAPC sponsors Palliative Care Leadership Centers (PCLC) for specialized training and mentorship, including pediatric Centers of Excellence.	https://www.capc.org/palliative-care-leadership-centers/
Children's Hospice International	Children's Hospice International has multiple publications available to purchase that address pediatric palliative and hospice care, including *Interdisciplinary Clinical Manual for Pediatric Hospice and Palliative Care, Home Care for Seriously Ill Children: A Manual for Parents*, and the ChiPACC Implementation Manual.	Http://www.chionline.org/helpful-resources/
Cure4Kids – Sponsored by St. Jude's Children's Research Hospital	Cure4Kids is an online resource for healthcare professionals dedicated to enhancing the care of children who have cancer and other life-threatening diseases in countries around the globe. Cure4Kids offers online education and collaboration tools that are freely available to registered users.	https://www.cure4kids.org/
Education in Palliative and End of Life Care – Pediatrics (EPEC- Pediatrics)	EPEC–Pediatrics is a comprehensive adaptation of the EPEC curriculum designed to address the needs of children, their families, and pediatric oncology providers and other pediatric clinicians. It was developed by and continues to receive input from experts in several pediatric disciplines as well as parent advocate advisors. It consists of 24 modules in pain and symptom management in palliative care. These topics are taught as a combination of 20 distance learning modules and 6 in-person conference sessions. This in-person conference is offered annually.[93]	https://www.bioethics.northwestern.edu/programs/epec/curricula/pediatrics.html
End of Life Nursing Education Curriculum Pediatric Palliative Care (ELNEC- PPC)	ELNEC–Pediatric Palliative Care was designed and developed by 20 pediatric palliative care experts and piloted in 2003. Each year, at least three national train-the-trainer pediatric palliative care courses are offered across the US. The curriculum also includes perinatal and neonatal content. Originally designed by and targeted to nurses, these courses are appropriate for and encourage interdisciplinary education and collaboration.	https://www.aacnnursing.org/ELNEC/About/ELNEC-Curricula
International Children's Palliative Care Network (ICPCN)	ICPCN has an online e-learning platform with multiple courses helpful for professional and lay people working with children who have serious illness. Courses are available in multiple languages. The courses have both a theoretical and clinical component.	http://www.icpcn.org/icpcns-elearning-programme/
National Hospice and Palliative Care (NHPCO)	NHPCO has a variety of educational materials, including the ChiPPS e-journal. This quarterly electronic journal is available free of charge with registration. Other NHPCO free pediatric resources include information on concurrent care and pediatric standards of practice. Additional resources are available with NHPCO membership.	https://www.nhpco.org/palliative-care-overview/pediatric-palliative-and-hospice-care/chipps-pediatric-e-journal
Palliative Care Education and Practice (PCEP)	A comprehensive course delivered in two parts on an adult or pediatric track. PCEP provides physicians, nurses, and social workers a structure in which to efficiently acquire the competencies necessary to influence our current changing healthcare environment. Held in two parts, this course uses experiential learning, training, and consolidation.	https://pallcare.hms.harvard.edu/courses
Pediatric Pain Master Class	The Pediatric Pain Master Class offers state of the art education in pain management for the pediatric patient from a holistic and interdisciplinary perspective. The program covers pharmacological, medical, psychosocial, and integrative therapies in the management of children's acute, procedural, and complex/chronic pain. The Master Class is primarily designed for physicians and advanced practice nurses to develop their expertise in the field of pediatric pain medicine in a highly interactive seminar format. This course is also open to other individuals who work within the field of pediatric pain.	https://www.childrensmn.org/events/12th-annual-pediatric-pain-master-class/

(continued)

TABLE 7.1 Continued

NAME OF PROGRAM	DESCRIPTION	WEBSITE
Together for Short Lives	Developed in the United Kingdom, this organizational website has resources for health care professionals and families. Care pathways are available.	https://www.togetherforshortlives.org.uk/
University of Washington Graduate Certificate in Palliative Care – Pediatric Track	The University of Washington offers a graduate certificate in palliative care, including a pediatric track. This interdisciplinary curriculum is designed for practicing healthcare professionals from nursing, medicine, social work, spiritual care, and other disciplines. seeking specialty training in palliative care. The 9-month graduate certificate includes three 5-credit courses taken sequentially in the Autumn, Winter, and Spring quarters. This is a hybrid program with both in-person and online learning.	http://uwpctc.org/
VitalTalk	This interdisciplinary, evidence-based, communications training utilizes an engaging curriculum available at in-person and online courses, as well as providing a variety of clinician resources available online and in the Vital Talk app. Vital Talk provides training in communication about serious illness in a culturally sensitive and patient-centered manner. Currently there is not a pediatric specialty track within Vital Talk, however, this interactive communication training is quite applicable to the pediatric population.	https://www.vitaltalk.org/about-us/

AN INTERDISCIPLINARY PALLIATIVE CARE TRAINING MODEL: TRI-DISCIPLINE APPROACH

Training of future clinicians and leaders in the field of PPC should be offered in the model in which care is delivered. This model of training is exemplified in the Boston Children's Hospital/Dana-Farber Cancer Institute Pediatric Advanced Care Team's *tri-discipline fellowship training program.* Physicians, nurse practitioners, and social workers train side by side as PPC fellows in this unique learning experience.[30] Fellowship is 1 year, and fellows are each salaried with benefits.

Each clinician learner brings to the fellowship his or her own discipline-specific training and experience. By the end of the fellowship, the goal is that all clinicians will have gained core palliative care knowledge, begin to master interdisciplinary teamwork, and hone their skills in their unique disciplines to contribute fully to the caregiving team.

All fellows participate in core curriculum didactic training, both alone and with the adult palliative care fellows (physicians, nurse practitioners, and pharmacists). The core curriculum includes intensive training in communication, pain and symptom management, ethics, bereavement, and processing moral distress. Here, "moral distress" is defined as the cognitive-emotional dissonance that arises when one feels compelled to act against one's moral requirements.[31] As a result, pediatric fellows learn from each other and have the added value and perspective gained from their adult palliative care counterparts. The multiple perspectives of interdisciplinary learners and instructors contribute to the deep understanding of these didactic offerings.

The vast majority of training occurs in the clinical field under the guidance of highly skilled interdisciplinary clinicians who model best care and communication practices. Fellows move toward independent clinical work, ultimately leading rounds, new consults, and directing patient care under the watchful mentorship of experienced discipline-specific clinicians with feedback from the entire interdisciplinary team.

This fellowship aims to have learners leave with advanced practice training and clinical experience. The goal is to prepare fellow graduates to move on to independent clinical practice and program leadership and position them to become leaders in research and education. They also leave with a deep understanding and appreciation of the value of interdisciplinary care in caring for children with serious illnesses and their families.

MULTIDISCIPLINARY PSYCHOSOCIAL FELLOWSHIP

While the core triad of a palliative care interdisciplinary team is a nurse, a physician, and a social worker, there are many other disciplines that deeply enrich the care provided. Psychosocial team members, which may include chaplains, child life specialists, psychologists, psychiatrists, and creative/expressive arts therapists, often provide extensive support to a patient and family before, during, and after death. While their contributions are invaluable, the ability for psychosocial providers to access advanced training with an interdisciplinary PPC team is rare. The Y.C. Ho/Helen & Michael Chiang Foundation has funded the Multidisciplinary Psychosocial Fellowship at the Children's Hospital of Philadelphia and the social work fellowship at Boston Children's Hospital/Dana-Farber Cancer Institute.

Social workers, chaplains, child life specialists, and creative/expressive arts therapists are all eligible to apply to this 1-year funded fellowship for one psychosocial provider. Formal supervision is provided by the whole psychosocial team, with added support from the team member who shares the primary discipline of the psychosocial fellow. Fellows participate in the care of inpatient, outpatient, and home hospice patients with a focus on psychosocial support provided in the home environment. The psychosocial fellow joins the medical fellowship cohort for didactics and support. Mentored educational scholarship, including presenting at palliative care grand rounds, is required in hopes of encouraging interdisciplinary teaching. This fellowship aims to have psychosocial providers develop skills and comfort in providing psychosocial support to patients, siblings, and their families as well as bereavement support for siblings and families after the child's death.

SIMULATION-BASED INTERDISCIPLINARY EDUCATION

Interdisciplinary education simulation enables learners of all levels and disciplines to gain an appreciation for one another's role, improve teamwork, and perform hands-on skills.[32] Students in interdisciplinary simulations experience cognitive and behavioral changes after learning about the core principles and concepts that contribute to other disciplines.[33]

Simulated experiences prepare healthcare workers for clinical situations and contribute to safe and efficient care of patients.[34] While most interdisciplinary simulations have focused on acute events such as resuscitation, a growing number are using high-fidelity (highly realistic, often using actors) simulations in the palliative care field, including those focusing on spiritual assessments, discontinuation of life-sustaining technology, disclosure of death, and palliative care communication with interpreters.[20,22,35–42] Interdisciplinary education occurs in two places: (1) during the simulation scenario, in the form of combining two or more disciplines (physician, nurse, social worker, interpreter, pharmacist, psychologist, or chaplain), and (2) during the debrief, which can also include actor/parent and clinician participation. Participants can portray their own discipline or another to better understand the unique challenges of others' roles. TeamTalk, an interdisciplinary adaptation of VitalTalk, utilizes physicians, nurses, chaplains, and/or social workers and can be adapted to include interpreters, physical therapists, and other disciplines.[37]

In its most advanced form, interdisciplinary education is built into the health education system itself, blending interdisciplinary teaching with a multidisciplinary audience of learners.[39,42–45] The Institute for Professionalism and Ethical Practice (IPEP) conducts programs focusing on difficult conversations among clinicians, patients, and families.[46] IPEP, which has trained more than 6,000 individuals, uses a validated approach to hands-on learning, the Program to Enhance Relational & Communication Skills (PERCS). PERCS incorporates ethics and practice, simulation using skilled actors, and patient and family voices. Workshops bring together interdisciplinary participants including patients, family members, staff, and facilitators in a model that dissolves barriers and models team communication.[47–49] This model was adapted for busy hospital-based practices by moving sessions into the hospital.[49]

MedEdPORTAL INTERPROFESSIONAL EDUCATION COLLECTION

The Interprofessional Education Collaboration (IPEC) was founded in 2009, by representatives from medical, nursing, pharmacy, osteopathic medicine, dentistry, and public health.[50] Core competencies focus on four domains: values and ethics, roles and responsibilities, interprofessional communication, and teams and teamwork.[51] IPEC partnered with MedEdPORTAL, the American Psychological Association, Physician Assistant Education Association and American Physical Therapy Association, to create the Interprofessional Education Collection.[52] One palliative care example is "Incorporation of an Interprofessional Palliative Care-Ethics Experience Into a Required Critical Care Acting Internship." The collection fosters the identification, development, and deployment of educational resources aimed at supporting the team-based care essential to training an interdisciplinary workforce.[52] The collection creates a national repository of curriculum resources for interdisciplinary education.

MOCK NO CODES

Mock code training has been a standard in medical and nursing education since the 1990s and has improved survival outcomes.[53] Yet there is little training on how to respond to requests for code interventions when the clinical situation does not warrant intensive, life-sustaining interventions. Clinicians may have differing education on resuscitation in these complex scenarios, which may impact team cohesiveness and family education.[54] Nurses and respiratory therapists often report little to no education on do-not-resuscitate (DNR) orders.[55] While physicians and advanced practice nurses report some education, only 44% of medical students report retaining knowledge regarding DNR and advance care planning, with only 16% retaining knowledge of how to respond to religious and cultural issues surrounding death and dying.[56] In other studies, graduating pediatric residents reported not feeling adequately trained to fulfill the responsibilities associated with providing palliative and end-of-life care for children.[57,58]

One method of addressing these complex issues is to consider "mock no-code" simulation. Similar to communication skill–based simulation training, this approach utilizes pediatric cases that illustrate how not intervening with intensive, life-sustaining interventions may be in the patient's best interest to promote comfort and optimize quality of life given the advanced nature of the underlying serious illness. Utilizing skilled critical care and palliative care clinicians as facilitators aids bedside clinicians in addressing requests for resuscitation interventions in various simulated situations. Examples include but are not limited to

- When previously the family and/or patient stated their wishes to have a do not attempt resuscitation order in place
- The clinical situation no longer warrants intensive, life-sustaining interventions, as agreed upon by the primary and specialty teams involved
- Stopping ventilatory or circulatory support that is no longer clinically indicated
- Family members have conflicting goals of care
- Addressing religious and/or cultural norms
- Ethical situations that impact resuscitation
- Death pronouncement

Further research is needed to validate this approach; however, use of mock no code clinical simulation scenarios may improve clinician knowledge, attitudes, and skills regarding challenging end-of-life situations in PPC.

PRIMARY PALLIATIVE CARE

Specialty PPC is a well-established model of care delivery; however, access to specialty PPC teams may be limited by geographic availably, hours of service, team members, and confusion with multiple medical teams involved in care and decision-making. The specialty PPC team is used for complex cases or refractory pain and symptom management. Primary PPC is defined as training bedside clinicians in the basic tenets of PPC. Primary PPC education and training improves access to care, mitigates symptom distress, and reduces moral distress for clinicians.[59,60] In addition to the models described in this chapter, one such model at Children's National Hospital utilizes a 12-month education and mentorship program comprised of didactic interdisciplinary group learning, self-directed learning, mentoring, and unit-based quality improvement projects to address knowledge acquisition, changing the culture of PPC within the unit or organization, and skill-based workshops to improve attitudes and skills. This program has trained 271 interdisciplinary clinicians, in four cohorts, and has demonstrated significant increases ($p < 0.001$) in self-reported confidence in introducing PPC, pain and symptom management, communication, end-of-life care, and accessing resources. In addition, nearly 100% of participants stated the training was valuable, and they have made significant changes in their own clinical practice to integrate palliative care earlier for children with advanced, serious illness. Self-reported moral distress decreased by 33% across all four cohorts. Findings have been sustained over 2 years to date.[59] This model has been replicated in several other healthcare systems across the United States with similar preliminary findings.

In this curriculum, the quality improvement projects and mentoring were key to changing culture and sustaining impact. Engaging participants in what matters most to them in their clinical work prompted change in policy and procedures in caring for children with serious illness and their families. One example is integrating PPC into a specialty neuro-oncology clinic, which increased early hospice referrals, demonstrated increase in advance care planning, and improved communication between specialty teams.[61] Opportunities for rounding with the specialty PPC team also provided opportunities for interdisciplinary mentoring, while one-on-one or small-group mentoring by one or two PPC leaders provided opportunities for exploring moral distress and initiatives to promote resilience.[62]

HOSPICE TEAM EDUCATION

There are few stand-alone PPC programs, most likely due to patient volumes. Although many adult hospices have pediatric specialty teams, their volume is often low, and, as a result, professionals may lack confidence in their care of children.[63–65] Several approaches for educating hospice providers may be helpful. Hospices may partner with local tertiary care pediatric centers, especially those with specialty PPC teams, to join in collaborative education programs.[66] The primary PPC program illustrated in the previous section includes community hospice partners in this education program. This has improved communication and collaboration across care settings. Shared interdisciplinary education programs improve understanding of roles, sharing of resources, and collaboration in care.

Other options for education for hospice providers include offering PPC training within their local hospice, such as ELNEC-PPC or EPEC-Peds, or inviting members from the local tertiary care center specialty PPC teams to present in-services and workshops. Given the limited staffing and not-for-profit nature of the financial structure of hospices, it may be difficult for hospice providers to be relieved of patient care duties to attend all-day or multiday conferences. Another option to address this issue includes self-directed or online learning curriculums for PPC. One such program is available through the California State University and offers online education toward a certificate in PPC for nurses and other interdisciplinary team members and includes a team education option.[67] Several other programs are in development, and ELNEC-PPC and EPEC-Pediatrics have online learning options that can be adapted for the hospice audience. AAHPM and HPNA also host pediatric webinar learning opportunities. The NHPCO and the CAPC have online pediatric learning opportunities. There are several state PPC coalitions that provide educational opportunities such as webinars and conferences. Other examples of educational resources are included in Table 7.1, although this is not an exhaustive list.

PROJECT ECHO: "MOVING KNOWLEDGE, NOT PEOPLE"

Project ECHO (Extension for Community Healthcare Outcomes) is a telementoring medical education program designed to disseminate knowledge and increase the capacity of local clinical teams to provide best practice care. Founded in 2003, at the University of New Mexico,[68] it is now an international program, serving more than 70,000 learners in 37+ countries and all 50 states.[69] Project ECHO uses video-conferencing and virtual clinics to allow specialist teams to mentor local community providers and staff. There is no direct patient care. Instead, a community of healthcare professionals share knowledge, experience, and best practices to work on specific clinical cases and future cases. The standardized ECHO clinic methodology includes an "interdisciplinary analysis of the case conducted in a participatory manner."[70]

Project ECHO is being used in more than 49 programs across 10 countries to foster exceptional palliative and hospice care.[70–72] Within pediatric palliative and hospice care, programs are located in Canada, Northern Ireland, Uruguay,

India, and England.[72–74] Programs have included medical staff nurses, students, healthcare attendants, social workers, chaplains, and administrative staff. ECHO Palliative Care programs have demonstrated improved nursing and staff confidence and self-efficacy.[75,76]

PARENTS AND FAMILIES AS TEACHERS

BEREAVED PARENT EDUCATORS IN INTERDISCIPLINARY EDUCATION

> The experience was so formed, enhanced, and illuminated by the parents' presence, generosity, input, and sharing. I was truly blessed by what they brought to our learning. I'm blown away and [as a physician] will never be or teach the same.[77]

Team Reflection

Kathe was a 7-year-old, born premature at 26 weeks, female with cerebral palsy secondary to an intercranial hemorrhage shortly after birth. She was the light of her family, which included both parents and her three siblings, ages 17, 13, and 3 years. She developed a volvulus at the age of 3 years, which required resection of a large portion of her bowel and creation of an ileostomy. Kathe eventually developed short gut syndrome and was not tolerating full enteral feeds, requiring long-term total parental nutrition (TPN). Multiple attempts were made to slowly reintroduce enteral feeds, but she was admitted approximately every 3–4 weeks over the period of a year for feeding intolerance. Her parents noted that Kathe had lost that sparkle and joy that seemed to radiate from her when she was feeling well. They watched her for several months while intensive symptom management was tried, but Kathe did not recover to her former quality of life. Although she was alert, she did not seem to enjoy even the simple things such as being with her family and her room decorated with her favorite sparkling Christmas lights, which she normally enjoyed all year long. Kathe's parents requested to stop enteral and TPN, as they felt she was clearly showing them that her quality of life had diminished and that, despite intensive symptom management, she was suffering. The primary team was not in agreement with the family to stop artificial fluids and nutrition. They requested a meeting with the palliative care team and the primary team to discuss goals of care. Kathe's parents were eloquent in describing her normal quality of life and how they had watched her decline over the past 3–4 years, with more abrupt decline in the past year. They shared that their faith traditions supported a natural death without artificial fluids and nutrition and point blank asked the medical teams if her underlying gut failure could be fixed. The medical team shared that they felt they could prolong Kathe's life for months to years, however, they could not fix the underlying problem. They asked that Kathe be allowed to feed for comfort but to stop TPN and attempts to increase enteral feeds and allow a natural death with intensive supportive care. The medical team agreed to this plan and Kathe was discharged with home hospice. She died 3 months later, peacefully at home, surrounded by her family and her sparkling Christmas lights with a smile on her face. In this case, the palliative care team was not the educators; it was the family who eloquently shared their definitions of quality of life and supported the primary medical team in coming to terms with stopping artificial fluids and hydration.

Understanding the patient and family perspective and communicating effectively with families is at the heart of pediatric practice, and harnessing the voices of patients and families as catalysts for learning outside the clinical setting can be incredibly powerful for adult learners. The intimacy and eloquence of personal stories recounted by parents and families who have had time to reflect on their experience has enormous impact on professional training and development, as attested to by the clinicians themselves. Hospitals have begun including family members in new resident orientation, grand rounds presentations, and advisory councils. Palliative care programs and hospices are creating novel ways to involve families in educational initiatives, institutional trainings, and conferences. Some curricula are also encouraging clinicians to involve family members in institutional change.

Inviting parents to teach alongside clinicians has been identified as a critical element of the educational experience.[77,78] Parents, families, and, notably, bereaved parents can be valued members of the interdisciplinary team whose perspectives cannot be obtained from any other team member. Through their experiences, they have developed expertise and insights into the medical world from a unique perspective. This may be especially true of medical decision-making, where parents of seriously ill children are often expected to understand medical therapies and potential outcomes with no clear indication of the "best choice." Parents, bereaved or otherwise, have lived through the emotional upheaval and are able to articulate the priorities that are most important and meaningful to them. By hearing from parents, learners can gain invaluable insight into the family experience and thereby increase their knowledge, empathy and understanding which in turn improves communication, builds trust, and allows for concordant goals of care.

The experience is also beneficial to parents. Parents feel empowered, affirmed, and experience benefits such as an improved sense of purpose, fulfillment with giving back, meaning-making, and appreciating "the depth of caring and commitment that clinicians feel toward the children and families they serve."[77,78] Moreover, for many bereaved parents, they often see this as part of their responsibility to their child's memory and find that participating in activities that honor their child is actively therapeutic.

Clinicians are responsible for screening, selecting, training, and protecting the emotional integrity of families who participate in educational initiatives. Careful selection of individuals is needed; families need to be able to share their story and "manage the upsurge of intense emotion without being overwhelmed."[78] Educational programs should identify a clinical team member who is available for support and follow-up to the family.[78]

At St. Jude Children's Research Hospital, bereaved parent educators have been successfully integrated into PPC educational conferences and pediatric oncology fellowship education, benefitting both the participants and the bereaved parents.[79–81] Parents who are at least 2 years out from the death of their child, have demonstrated emotional and behavioral stability throughout their child's treatment and end-of-life course, had good interpersonal skills, an ability to "tell their story" without displaced anger, and no evidence of complicated grief are eligible to participate. Prospective parent volunteers participate in a screening phone call. Parent volunteers attend a full-day bereaved parent mentor program training that involves role-playing, didactic education, and resources for additional support. Involvement of trained parent educators in interdisciplinary educational forums is feasible and effectively improves attendee comfort in communication with and caring for patients and families with serious illness.[79–81]

COURAGEOUS PARENTS NETWORK

Courageous Parents Network offers another way to bring the parent voice into the educational setting through web-based videos. Courageous Parents Network's open digital platform—easily accessible on web, mobile phones, and tablets and available 24/7 (www.courageousparentsnetwork.org)—features hundreds of professionally produced and curated short videos of parents—some still actively parenting their child, some bereaved—talking about their lived experience of caring for their child from point of diagnosis through end-of-life and bereavement.[82] Topics include anticipatory grief, decision-making about medical interventions such as spinal fusion surgery and tracheostomy, working with the medical team, finding palliative care, fear of regrets, and transitioning to the child's end of life. These videos are a way for learners to hear from families without the logistical element of facilitators having to identify and prepare live parents to participate in person. In addition, because the parents are not in-person, the videos provide a safe learning modality for exploring the perspective of families free of worries about hurting feelings, offending, or sounding unprofessional, thus opening space for learners to be more open and vulnerable. Finally, the videos provide a depth to the feelings and thinking of parents that is rarely heard in a planned parent/clinician meeting: for example, the agony of a mother as she deliberates whether her son should receive a tracheostomy or parents on their intense feelings leaving the neonatal intensive care unit after their baby has died (Box 7.1)

BOX 7.1 THE PATIENT AND FAMILY PERSPECTIVE

From a couple who has participated as parent educators in multiple medical education settings:

Mother: My husband and I have three children. Our youngest daughter had a very severe neurological disease called Aicardi-Goutières syndrome, and she passed away before her seventh birthday. It is very important for us to work with the medical community to continue to improve communication.

- She ultimately presented the experience of her daughter's end of life at home, including what went well and what was difficult, to the Massachusetts Pediatric Palliative Care Network consisting of community-based pediatric palliative care providers (Fall 2019) and wrote about this experience for the American Academy of Pediatrics' Section on Hospice and Palliative Medicine newsletter (Fall 2019)

Father: While we are interested in medical advancements and always helping people in need, what's really important to us—and why we want to be a part of these efforts—is connecting with the medical team from an emotional standpoint [having them] hear what is on our minds, understand our goals and objectives. It just makes this whole journey just a little bit better along the way.

- As a couple, they participated as themselves and as "actors" in a video simulation of a parent–provider office visit and conversation for the American Academy of Pediatrics' Education in Quality Improvement for Pediatric Practice (EQIPP) course "Talking About Serious Illness" (2020) and shared their story on Courageous Parents Network (2015).

Written by family member.

BENEFITS AND CHALLENGES OF INTERDISCIPLINARY PEDIATRIC PALLIATIVE CARE EDUCATION

The interdisciplinary training model has numerous benefits and some unique challenges. The interdisciplinary training model promotes a less hierarchical system and dialogue among clinicians rather than silos of learning. This gives team members a shared educational experience, deeper respect for roles and perspectives, and the ability to work together to provide comprehensive patient care. This understanding commonly leads to better triaging of team resources, utilization of colleagues' talents, and greater sustainability in the work as there is natural system for debriefing.[83] In a survey of former fellows, more than 90% noted that the advantages of interdisciplinary education outweigh the disadvantages.[84] One former fellow noted "Being on an interprofessional team allows the opportunity to formulate modalities and develop clinical approaches that are more nuanced, more dynamic, and ultimately more complete given the complex systems in which all families function."[84]

There are several challenges to interdisciplinary training, including complex team dynamics and inefficiency as interdisciplinary care is often more time-consuming. Trainees arrive with very different training, both in intensity and length, and have different educational needs (Figure 7.1). Physicians may have completed 3–6 years of prior residency and fellowship training, whereas nurse practitioners and social workers may have variable lengths of education and work history. Role overlap and role uncertainty occur due to the cross-training mentality. During palliative care training, a nurse practitioner's clinical responsibilities almost entirely overlap with the physician's (documentation, prescribing, on-call coverage) even though their clinical training and prescribing experience may differ. Accommodations need to be made to support new nurse practitioners in the early stages of training as their skill set advances. In addition, fellowships may have differing clinical requirements of physicians, nurse practitioners, and social workers, leading to varying time on inpatient consultative services. Last, because medical providers on a PPC team are attuned to psychosocial, spiritual, and sibling/family stressors, the psychologists, chaplains, child life specialists, and social workers may be especially prone to feelings of role uncertainty.

Practical challenges include different recruiting, hiring, and matching processes for obtaining palliative care fellows. Once trainees have arrived, there are different competencies across disciplines and often different salary, vacation, and benefits across specialties. One significant challenge is funding for interdisciplinary fellowships, which often comes from philanthropic sources or grants that can vary from year to year. Program sustainability is difficult in the face of funding insecurity.

FUTURE DIRECTIONS

MOVING INTERDISCIPLINARY EDUCATION INTO PRACTICE AND RESEARCH STUDIES

Research evaluating the effect of interdisciplinary education is needed. While this is happening more at the undergraduate and graduate medical education levels, some investigators are also assessing whether interdisciplinary education and practice improves patient and family outcomes in PPC. One such example is the Communication Plan: Early through End of Life Intervention (COMPLETE) study.[85,86] The aim of COMPLETE was to train an interdisciplinary (physician/registered nurse) dyad in palliative care and end-of-life communication, and, ultimately, describe parental perspectives. COMPLETE nurtured realistic hope and meaningful dialogue for parents connecting with healthcare providers as a dyad and helped parents to make informed decisions.[85]

EVALUATION TOOLS

In addition to discipline-specific competency evaluation, numerous tools evaluate different aspects of interdisciplinary education and interdisciplinary collaboration.[87,88] However, little is published specific to PPC. For example, although the Readiness for Interprofessional Learning Scale (RIPLS) and the Assessment of Interprofessional Team Collaboration Scale (AITCS-II) are available, neither has been applied to PPC-related education.[89,90] The Interprofessional Education Collaborative (IPEC) survey measures interprofessional competencies in four domains: values and ethics, roles and responsibilities, interprofessional communication, and teams and teamwork.[91] Currently available tools may need to be extrapolated or modified to assess for interdisciplinary education and collaboration among the interdisciplinary team within the hospital and community. For example, medical and social work students who received interdisciplinary education demonstrated a significantly better ability to lead family conferences in palliative care than did the control group.[92]

CONCLUSION

Interdisciplinary care is the hallmark of caring for children with serious illness and their families. Education is key to empowering clinicians from all disciplines to provide the highest quality of care. Children are not just small adults, and clinicians require specialized training to improve outcomes, foster comfort, and optimize quality of life for children with serious illness. Utilizing principles of adult learning with creative pediatric-specific educational opportunities, including simulation, fellowship training, primary palliative care education, and mentoring through interdisciplinary methods, fosters improved knowledge, skills, and attitudes, with the ultimate goals of improved patient and family outcomes.

REFERENCES

1. Kolb D. *Experiential Learning: Experience as the Source of Learning and Development.* Prentice Hall, Englewood Cliffs NJ. 1984.
2. Taylor DCM, Hamdy H. Adult learning theories: Implications for learning and teaching in medical education: AMEE Guide No. 83. *Med Teacher.* 2013;35(11):e1561–e1572.
3. Knowles M, Holton E, Swanson R. *The Adult Learner: The Definitive Classic in Adult Education and Human Resource Development* (8th ed.) New York: Routledge; 2015.
4. Catalyst center. Financing pediatric palliative and hospice care programs: An important but underutilized service for children with life-limiting conditions. 2011. http://cahpp.org/wp-content/uploads/2015/04/palliativecare.pdf
5. Chamberlain-Salaun J, Mills, Usher K. Terminology used to describe health care teams: An integrative review of the literature. *J Multidisc Healthc.* 2013:65.
6. World Health Organization. *Framework for Action on Interprofessional Education & Collaborative Practice.* Geneva: WHO; 2010.

7. Institute of Medicine (IOM). *Interprofessional Education for Collaboration: Learning How to Improve Health from Interprofessional Models Across the Continuum of Education To Practice: Workshop Summary.* Washington, DC: National Academies Press; 2013.
8. DeCourcey DD, Silverman M, Oladunjoye A, Balkin EM, Wolfe J. Patterns of care at the end of life for children and young adults with life-threatening complex chronic conditions. *J Pediatri.* 2018;193:196–203 e192.
9. Johnston EE, Rosenberg AR. Better understanding the importance of palliative care for pediatric patients. *JAMA Oncol.* 2020 Jun 1;6(6):817–818.
10. Groh G, Feddersen B, Fuhrer M, Borasio GD. Specialized home palliative care for adults and children: Differences and similarities. *J Palliat Med.* 2014;17(7):803–810.
11. Hill JD, Cuthel AM, Grudzen CR. Access to home and community health services for older adults with serious, life-limiting illness: A study protocol. *Am J Hospice Palliat Care.* 2021;38(1):12–18.
12. 2020 Edition: Hospice Facts and Figures. Alexandria, VA: National Hospice and Palliative Care Organization. August 2020. www.nhpco.org/factsfigures.
13. Snaman JM, Kaye EC, Lu JJ, Sykes A, Baker JN. Palliative care involvement is associated with less intensive end-of-life care in adolescent and young adult oncology patients. *J Palliat Med.* 2017;20(5):509–516.
14. Klick JC, Friebert S, Hutton N, et al. Developing competencies for pediatric hospice and palliative medicine. *Pediatrics.* 2014;134(6):e1670–1677.
15. Landzaat LH, Barnett MD, Buckholz GT, et al. Development of entrustable professional activities for hospice and palliative medicine fellowship training in the United States. *J Pain Symptom Manage.* 2017;54(4):609–616 e601.
16. Gustin JL, Yang HB, Radwany SM, et al. Development of curricular milestones for hospice and palliative medicine fellowship training in the U.S. *J Pain Symptom Manage.* 2019;57(5):1009–1017 e1006.
17. Bressler T, Persico L. Interprofessional education: Partnerships in the educational proc. *Nurse Educ Pract.* 2016;16(1):144–147.
18. Murdoch NL, Epp S, Vinek J. Teaching and learning activities to educate nursing students for interprofessional collaboration: A scoping review. *J Interprof Care.* 2017;31(6):744–753.
19. McGaghie WC, Issenberg SB, Cohen ER, Barsuk JH, Wayne DB. Does simulation-based medical education with deliberate practice yield better results than traditional clinical education? A meta-analytic comparative review of the evidence. *Acad Med.* 2011;86(6):706–711.
20. Brock KE, Cohen HJ, Sourkes BM, Good JJ, Halamek LP. Training pediatric fellows in palliative care: A pilot comparison of simulation training and didactic education. *J Palliat Med.* 2017;20(10):1074–1084.
21. Boysen PG, 2nd, Daste L, Northern T. Multigenerational challenges and the future of graduate medical education. *Ochsner J.* 2016;16(1):101–107.
22. Bradway C, Cotter VT, Darrah NJ, et al. An interprofessional education simulation workshop: Health professions learning palliative care communication. *J Nurs Educ.* 2018;57(8):493–497.
23. Smith MB, Macieira TGR, Bumbach MD, et al. The use of simulation to teach nursing students and clinicians palliative care and end-of-life communication: A systematic review. *Am J Hospice Palliat Med.* 2018;35(8):1140–1154.
24. Vertino KA. Evaluation of a teamstepps(c) initiative on staff attitudes toward teamwork. *J Nurs Adm.* 2014;44(2):97–102.
25. Cheng YH, Chen CH, Chen FJ, et al. The training in SHARE communication course by physicians increases the signing of do-not-resuscitate orders for critical patients in the emergency room (cross-sectional study). *Int J Surg.* 2019;68:20–26.
26. Fox L, Onders R, Hermansen-Kobulnicky CJ, et al. Teaching interprofessional teamwork skills to health professional students: A scoping review. *J Interprof Care.* 2018;32(2):127–135.
27. Mazanec P, Lamb G, Haas S, Dahlin C, Mooney A, LaFond D. Palliative nursing summit: Nurses leading change and transforming care: The nurse's role in coordination of care and transition management. *J Hosp Palliat Nurs.* 2018;20(1):15–22.
28. Hellier S, Davidson L. Team teaching in nursing education. *J Contin Educ Nurs.* 2018;49(4):186–192.
29. Lie DA, Forest CP, Kysh L, Sinclair L. Interprofessional education and practice guide No. 5: Interprofessional teaching for prequalification students in clinical settings. *J Interprof Care.* 2016;30(3):324–330.
30. Duncan J, Spengler E, Wolfe J. Providing pediatric palliative care: PACT in action. *MCN Am J Matern Child Nurs.* 2007;32(5):279–287.
31. Berger JT. Moral distress in medical education and training. *J Gen Intern Med.* 2014;29(2):395–398.
32. Pardue KT. A framework for the design, implementation, and evaluation of interprofessional education. *Nurse Educ.* 2015;40(1):10–15.
33. Decker S, Fey M, Sideras S, et al. Standards of best practice: Simulation Standard VI: The debriefing process. *Clin Simulation Nurs.* 2013;9(6):S26–S29.
34. Committee on Measuring the Impact of Interprofessional Education on Collaborative Practice and Patient Outcomes; Board on Global Health; Institute of Medicine. *Measuring the Impact of Interprofessional Education on Collaborative Practice and Patient Outcomes.* Washington (DC): National Academies Press (US); 2015 Dec 15: https://www.ncbi.nlm.nih.gov/books/NBK338360/.
35. Bays AM, Engelberg RA, Back AL, et al. Interprofessional communication skills training for serious illness: Evaluation of a small-group, simulated patient intervention. *J Palliat Med.* 2014;17(2):159–166.
36. Brock KE, Tracewski M, Allen KE, Klick J, Petrillo T, Hebbar KB. Simulation-based palliative care communication for pediatric critical care fellows. *Am J Hospice Palliat Care.* 2019;36(9):820–830
37. Donesky D, Anderson WG, Joseph RD, Sumser B, Reid TT. Teamtalk: Interprofessional team development and communication skills training. *J Palliat Med.* 2020 Jan;23(1):40–47.
38. Gilliland I, Frei BL, McNeill J, Stovall J. Use of high-fidelity simulation to teach end-of-life care to pharmacy students in an interdisciplinary course. *Am J Pharm Educ.* 2012;76(4):66.
39. Ellman MS, Schulman-Green D, Blatt L, et al. Using online learning and interactive simulation to teach spiritual and cultural aspects of palliative care to interprofessional students. *J Palliat Med.* 2012;15(11):1240–1247.
40. Smith MB, Macieira TGR, Bumbach MD, et al. The use of simulation to teach nursing students and clinicians palliative care and end-of-life communication: A systematic review. *Am J Hospice Palliat Care.* 2018;35(8):1140–1154.
41. Stout-Aguilar J, Pittman A, Bentley R, Livingston J, Watzak B. The effects of interprofessional pediatric end-of-life simulation on communication and role understanding in health professions students. *Nurs Educ Perspect.* 2018;39(6):360–362.
42. Lippe M, Stanley A, Ricamato A, Halli-Tierney A, McKinney R. Exploring end-of-life care team communication: An interprofessional simulation study. *Am J Hospice Palliat Care.* 2020;37(1):65–71.
43. Schulz C, Wenzel-Meyburg U, Karger A, et al. Implementation of palliative care as a mandatory cross-disciplinary subject (QB13) at the Medical Faculty of the Heinrich-Heine-University Düsseldorf, Germany. *GMS Z Med Ausbild.* 2015;32(1):1–22.
44. Gadoud A, Lu WH, Strano-Paul L, Lane S, Boland JW. A pilot study of interprofessional palliative care education of medical students in the UK and USA. *BMJ Support Palliat Care.* 2018;8(1):67–72.
45. Koffman J, Higginson IJ. Assessing the effectiveness and acceptability of interprofessional palliative care education. *J Palliat Care.* 2005;21(4):262–269.
46. Institute for Professionalism & Ethical Practice. Skilled communications for difficult conversations and better care. http://ipepweb.org/
47. Institute for Professionalism & Ethical Practice. Difficult conversations in healthcare. http://ipepweb.org/workshop-schedule/difficult-conversations-in-healthcare/
48. Institute for Professionalism & Ethical Practice. Palliative care conversationsacrossthespectrumofcare.http://ipepweb.org/workshop-schedule/palliative-care-conversations-across-the-spectrum-of-care/

49. Rachwal CM, Langer T, Trainor BP, Bell MA, Browning DM, Meyer EC. Navigating communication challenges in clinical practice: A new approach to team education. *Crit Care Nurse.* 2018;38(6):15–22.
50. Association of American Medical Colleges. Interprofessional education. https://www.aamc.org/what-we-do/mission-areas/medical-education/interprofessional-education
51. Interprofessional Education Collaborative. *Core Competencies for Interprofessional Collaborative Practice: 2016 Update.* Washington, DC: Interprofessional Education Collaborative; 2016. https://www.ipecollaborative.org/ipec-core-competencies
52. Interprofessional Education MedEdPORTAL. https://www.mededportal.org/collection/interprofessional-education/
53. Moreira RA, Tibbetts LM. Pediatric mock codes: An evidence-informed focused pediatric resuscitation program. *J Emerg Nurs.* 2015;41(4):337–339.
54. Hepps JH, Yu CE, Calaman S. Simulation in medical education for the hospitalist: Moving beyond the mock code. *Pediatr Clin North Am.* 2019;66(4):855–866.
55. Arzuaga BH, Wraight CL, Cummings CL, Mao W, Miedema D, Brodsky DD. Do-not-resuscitate orders in the neonatal ICU: Experiences and beliefs among staff. *Pediatr Crit Care Med.* 2018;19(7):635–642.
56. Parikh PP, White MT, Buckingham L, Tchorz KM. Evaluation of palliative care training and skills retention by medical students. *J Surg Res.* 2017;211:172–177.
57. Faung B, Soliman A, Kabani A, Siswanto L, Mohamed A. Self-assessment for competency and educational needs of physician trainees regarding pediatric palliative care. *J Pediatr Palliat Care.* 2019;2(2):6–10.
58. McCabe ME, Hunt EA, Serwint JR. Pediatric residents' clinical and educational experiences with end-of-life care. *Pediatrics.* 2008;121(4):e731–e737.
59. Lafond DA, Bowling S, Fortkiewicz JM, Reggio C, Hinds PS. Integrating the comfort theory into pediatric primary palliative care to improve access to care. *J Hosp Palliat Nurs.* 2019;21(5):382–389.
60. National Academies of Sciences, Engineering and Medicine; Health and Medicine Division; Board on Health Sciences Policy; Board on Health Care Services; Roundtable on Quality Care for People with Serious Illness. *Models and Strategies to Integrate Palliative Care Principles into Care for People with Serious Illness: Proceedings of a Workshop.* Washington, DC: The National Academies Press (US); 2017 Oct 24.
61. Lafond D, Hancock L, Rodriquez Y. Overcoming barriers and challenges in integrating palliative care for children with brain tumors: A primary palliative care approach. *Neuro-Oncology.* 2016;18(suppl 3):iii135.133–iii135.
62. Rossfeld ZM, Tumin D, Humphrey LM. Self-assessment of skills and competencies among residents participating in a pediatric hospice and palliative medicine elective rotation. *J Palliat Med.* 2018;21(2):229–235.
63. Kaye EC, Gattas M, Kiefer A, et al. Provision of palliative and hospice care to children in the community: A population study of hospice nurses. *J Pain Symptom Manage.* 2019;57(2):241–250.
64. Kaye EC, Applegarth J, Gattas M, et al. Hospice nurses request paediatric-specific educational resources and training programs to improve care for children and families in the community: Qualitative data analysis from a population-level survey. *Palliat Med.* 2020 Mar;34(3):403–412.
65. Weaver MS, Jenkins R, Wichman C, et al. Sowing across a state: Development and delivery of a grassroots pediatric palliative care nursing curriculum. *J Palliat Care.* 2021 Jan;36(1):22–28.
66. Perko K, Lafond D. Primary Pediatric Palliative Care: Teaching and learning from the bedside to the community (SA521). *J Pain Symptom Manage.* 2017;53(2):404–405.
67. Shiley Institute for Palliative Care. Pediatric palliative care education. California State University. https://csupalliativecare.org/programs/pediatrics/
68. Arora S, Thornton K, Murata G, et al. Outcomes of treatment for hepatitis C virus infection by primary care providers. *N Engl J Med.* 2011;364(23):2199–2207.
69. ECHO Program. U.S. Reach and impact overview. https://echo.unm.edu/doc/factsheets/ECHO%20US%20Reach%20and%20Impact%20Infographic.pdf
70. Piriz Alvarez G. Technology for improving accessibility of end-of-life care: Extension for Community Healthcare Outcomes Project. *Curr Opin Support Palliat Care.* 2018;12(4):466–471.
71. Arora S, Smith T, Snead J, et al. Project ECHO: An effective means of increasing palliative care capacity. *Am J Manag Care.* 2017;23(7 Spec No.):SP267–SP271.
72. ECHO Program. ECHO hubs and programs: Global. https://echo.unm.edu/locations/global. Updated December 2019
73. The Hospital for Sick Children. Paediatric Project Echo. http://www.sickkids.ca/ProjectECHO/. Published 2019
74. McCloskey S. *Project ECHO: Creating a community of practice in children's palliative care.* Maruzza Congress on Paediatric Palliative Care. Rome, 2018.
75. Dowling MJ, Payne C, Larkin P, Ryan DJ. Does an interactive, teleconference-delivered, palliative care lecture series improve nursing home staff confidence? *J Palliat Med.* 2020 Feb;23(2):179–183.
76. White C, McIlfatrick S, Dunwoody L, Watson M. Supporting and improving community health services: A prospective evaluation of ECHO technology in community palliative care nursing teams. *BMJ Support Palliat Care.* 2019;9(2):202–208.
77. Solomon MZ, Browning DM, Dokken DL, Merriman MP, Rushton CH. Learning that leads to action: Impact and characteristics of a professional education approach to improve the care of critically ill children and their families. *Arch Pediatr Adolesc Med.* 2010;164(4):315–322.
78. Adams G, Green A, Towe S, Huett A. Bereaved caregivers as educators in pediatric palliative care: Their experiences and impact. *J Palliat Med.* 2013;16(6):609–615.
79. Snaman JM, Kaye EC, Spraker-Perlman H, et al. Incorporating bereaved parents as faculty facilitators and educators in teaching principles of palliative and end-of-life care. *Am J Hospice Palliat Care.* 2018;35(12):1518–1525.
80. Snaman JM, Kaye EC, Levine DR, et al. Empowering bereaved parents through the development of a comprehensive bereavement program. *J Pain Symptom Manage.* 2017;53(4):767–775.
81. Snaman JM, Kaye EC, Cunningham MJ, et al. Going straight to the source: A pilot study of bereaved parent-facilitated communication training for pediatric subspecialty fellows. *Pediatr Blood Cancer.* 2017;64(1):156–162.
82. Courageous Parents Network. www.courageousparentsnetwork.org.
83. Rabinowitz E, Brock K, Freitas J, Scanlon C, Liaw S-N, deLima Thomas J. Finding strengths in our differences: How interprofessional training prepares clinicians for collaborative practice (SA507). *J Pain Symptom Manage.* 2019;57(2):444–445.
84. Liaw S-N. Interprofessional education for our interprofessional world. Paper presented at Pediatric Advanced Care Team (PACT) Rounds. Boston, 2018.
85. Hendricks-Ferguson VL, Haase JE. Parent perspectives of receiving early information about palliative and end-of-life care options from their child's pediatric providers. *Cancer Nurs.* 2019;42(4):E22–E30.
86. Hendricks-Ferguson VL, Kane JR, Pradhan KR, et al. Evaluation of physician and nurse dyad training procedures to deliver a palliative and end-of-life communication intervention to parents of children with a brain tumor. *J Pediatr Oncol Nurs.* 2015;32(5):337–347.
87. Walters SJ, Stern C, Robertson-Malt S. The measurement of collaboration within healthcare settings: A systematic review of measurement properties of instruments. *JBI Database System Rev Implement Rep.* 2016;14(4):138–197.
88. National Center for Interprofessional Practice and Education. Assessment and Evaluation. 2019. https://nexusipe.org/advancing/assessment-evaluation-start
89. McFadyen AK, Webster VS, Maclaren WM. The test-retest reliability of a revised version of the Readiness for Interprofessional Learning Scale (RIPLS). *J Interprof Care.* 2006;20(6):633–639.

90. Orchard C, Pederson LL, Read E, Mahler C, Laschinger H. Assessment of Interprofessional Team Collaboration Scale (AITCS): Further testing and instrument revision. *J Contin Educ Health Prof.* 2018;38(1):11–18.
91. Dow AW, Diazgranados D, Mazmanian PE, Retchin SM. An exploratory study of an assessment tool derived from the competencies of the interprofessional education collaborative. *J Interprofessional Care.* 2014;28(4):299–304.
92. Fineberg IC. Preparing professionals for family conferences in palliative care: Evaluation results of an interdisciplinary approach. *J Palliat Med.* 2005;8(4):857–866.
93. Friedrichsdorf SJ, Remke S, Hauser J, et al. Development of a pediatric palliative care curriculum and dissemination model: Education in Palliative and End-of-Life Care (EPEC) pediatrics. *J Pain Symptom Manage.* 2019;58(4):707–720 e703.

8 | QUALITY IN PEDIATRIC PALLIATIVE CARE

CONRAD WILLIAMS IV, AMANDA L. THOMPSON, AND KATHIE KOBLER

Quality is never an accident. It is always the result of intelligent effort.

JOHN RUSKIN

INTRODUCTION

Across all healthcare settings and specialties, clinicians are charged with providing care that exemplifies the National Academy of Medicine's quality aims of safe, effective, patient-centered, timely, efficient, and equitable care.[1] Pediatric palliative care (PPC) provision inherently incorporates the Institute for Healthcare Improvement's quadruple aim for optimizing care: enhancing the patient experience, improving health outcomes, reducing healthcare costs, and enhancing healthcare professionals' experiences.[2] Measurement of healthcare quality is often framed in the Donabedian model,[3] as teams evaluate the structures, processes, and outcomes of their care.[4] Implementing quality measures and reporting health outcome data are increasingly important in the current climate of healthcare accountability, accreditation, and reimbursement.[4,5]

As the field of PPC matures, interdisciplinary PPC teams are called to draw from the growing evidence base and deepen their quality-focused efforts to optimize care for children with serious illness. Quality in healthcare is grounded in providing effective, safe care that results in optimal or desired health and is reflected by a culture of excellence.[6] Quality in PPC embodies and extends this definition by addressing and optimizing the well-being of both the child and family in an interdisciplinary fashion. In this chapter, we explore quality in PPC from the child/family, individual clinician, and team perspectives, and we provide a review of national quality-focused organizations and initiatives currently advancing PPC. Practical strategies are offered from an interdisciplinary perspective to encourage PPC teams to incorporate quality measurement and improvement initiatives into their clinical practice.

IMPORTANCE OF QUALITY IN PPC

PPC clinicians strive to provide quality care with integrity and in a manner that honors the preferences and goals of children with serious illness and their families. Core PPC tasks include providing effective interventions that enhance well-being, coordinating care throughout the child's trajectory and across all settings, and supporting problem-solving and decision-making for all involved in the child's care.[7] Quality-focused initiatives to evaluate how such core tasks are provided and to measure their outcomes are vital to optimize access, reduce variation in services delivered, and build evidence about the impact of PPC. Contributions from quality improvement initiatives allow PPC clinicians to nimbly address time-sensitive issues impacting a child or family. New comprehensive, evidence-based clinical practice guidelines provide a sound framework for PPC teams to engage in quality assurance activities and evaluate how they are achieving their goals and intended level of care delivery.

QUALITY CHALLENGES AND GAPS IN PEDIATRIC PALLIATIVE CARE

From an individual program level, high-quality PPC provision depends on team structure and staffing, costs and resource availability, and individual clinicians' level of education, expertise, and competency in quality improvement (QI) methodology. Any strain on these essential components impacts both team members' capacity to optimally meet the needs of the children in their care and their ability to engage in quality measurement activities.[8]

In the field as a whole, most existing palliative quality measurement initiatives are adult-care oriented and not fully applicable to the unique needs of children with serious illness.[9] The PPC community is significantly challenged in developing pediatric-focused measures to capture the complexities and nuances inherent when managing symptoms, optimizing communication, and coordinating care for a vast spectrum of neonatal, pediatric, and young adult conditions and care trajectories. The dearth of evidence-based literature, relatively small population served, and lack of time and funding to develop quality measures are current quality-related hurdles encountered by PPC teams. The variability of PPC program structure and delivery models further complicates the field's ability to benchmark quality and productivity.[10] While PPC research continues to deepen, clinicians are challenged by the relative dearth of high-quality, psychometrically sound instruments to assess the impact of PPC interventions.[11]

PPC-focused research leads to the development of new knowledge, which is critical to QI initiatives that implement such new knowledge. Although the PPC literature has grown substantially over the past two decades, significant gaps remain in the current research base. Identifying these gaps will encourage investigators to engage in collaborative and interdisciplinary PPC scholarship efforts. Research priorities may be distinct from adult palliative care[9] and include pediatric-specific palliative and end-of-life quality and outcomes measures, along with evidence-based intervention trials.

In a multidisciplinary workshop conducted by the Pediatric Palliative Care Research Network, PPC experts and rising investigators in the field identified five crucial research topics for the growth of PPC: (1) advance symptom and outcomes measurement; (2) improved symptom management and quality of life interventions; (3) improvement of communication, elicitation of goals of care, and decision-making; (4) understanding of family impact and improvement of family adaptation and coping; and (5) analysis and improvement of systems of care, policy, and education.[12] These five areas line up well with important quality initiatives in PPC that might ensure the implementation of developing evidence-based practice in these five topics. Workshop attendees also emphasized the importance of enhancing the early career training and ongoing professional development of PPC investigators, along with developing core PPC research resources, such as large administrative databases and valid and reliable measures.[12]

Initiatives in PPC that are focused on fostering increased attention to research and quality efforts are crucial to support sustained and efficient development of evidence-based and high-quality PPC practice. Such initiatives also are able to support those who choose a career path focused on PPC research or quality.

PERSPECTIVES ON QUALITY IN PEDIATRIC PALLIATIVE CARE

Quality PPC provision depends on an awareness of the experiences and perspectives of all involved in a child's care, followed by a willingness to tailor interventions and support to meet the preferences and goals of each family. This section explores considerations on quality from the perspectives of those actively receiving or providing PPC.

CHILD AND FAMILY

Listening and attending to the individualized needs of a child with serious illness and his or her family is perhaps the purest form of quality in PPC. PPC teams are encouraged to reflect on and remember ways in which they actively seek to identify, acknowledge, and honor a child's perspective amid a complex care situation. Ensuring that team members have the time and space in their schedules to engage thoughtfully with a child and family is a necessity in quality PPC care provision. In Box 8.1, Mattie's parents, Victoria and Peter Brown, offer their reflections on what quality in PPC means to their family, and how their experiences are now shaping quality care for others.

Research teams have created innovative methods to evaluate a child's experiences during treatment in order to enhance quality symptom management[13] and to better assess child/parental needs at the start of PPC provision.[14] Researchers also explored what it means for parents to be a "good parent" during their child's serious illness to further enhance strategies to support parents during decision-making.[15] In their research to understand parents' perspectives as their child received home-based hospice or PPC, Thienprayoon and colleagues[16] identified that parents prioritized compassionate care as a key domain for quality PPC. This new knowledge sets the stage for the development and selection of child-/family-centered quality measures.

INDIVIDUAL CLINICIAN AND TEAM REFLECTION ON PRACTICE

In addition to understanding the child/family perspective, PPC clinicians should be mindful of how quality is reflected in their daily practice. Incorporating strategies for both individual clinician and PPC team reflection on practice is imperative to ensuring quality of care for individual children, as well as identifying avenues for QI within a PPC program. Box 8.2 offers examples of self-inventory questions to assist with fostering a culture of honest inquiry and process improvement orientation, which can ultimately lead to team members collaborating in QI projects.

SETTING THE STAGE FOR QUALITY MEASUREMENT

Creating effective methods to measure quality in palliative care for children and adults is recognized as a vital need for the entire field.[4,7,17] On a national level, palliative care–focused quality initiatives and organizations have been established to foster collaboration and a standardized approach to quality-related efforts. While many of these quality initiatives are adult-care oriented, PPC teams are encouraged to familiarize themselves with these organizations and initiatives because the resources and guidance they offer may be adapted by PPC teams to meet their quality measurement and QI needs. What follows is a synthesis of such resources, with attention to PPC team applicability. Table 8.1 provides a summary of how to access each, with notation of PPC-specific resources.

NATIONAL QUALITY

Organizations National Quality Forum (NQF) is a nationwide membership organization devoted to improving healthcare through quality measurement. The NQF is recognized as the leader in setting the standards for healthcare measurement; NQF members have access to a wide range of QI resources and tools. The

BOX 8.1 PARENTS' REFLECTIONS ON QUALITY IN PPC

Victoria Sardi-Brown, PhD, LPC (Co-Founder and President) and Peter J. Brown, MBA (Co-Founder and CEO)

Mattie Miracle Cancer Foundation

Mattie Brown was our little engineer. He was precocious, vivacious, and was fascinated by how things around him worked. At the age of 6, he was diagnosed with multifocal synchronous osteosarcoma with four primary tumor sites. Mattie's 14 months of treatment included high-dosage chemotherapies, experimental immunotherapy, three limb-salvaging surgeries, and a bone graft. Eleven months after his diagnosis, Mattie underwent a sternotomy to remove nine tumors found in his lungs. Six weeks off treatment, Mattie's cancer spread to his lungs and liver, and we were faced with end-of-life decisions.

Cancer treatment left Mattie with profound functional impairments that affected his quality of life. He could no longer walk, run, dress, or toilet himself, and we faced the reality that Mattie not only had cancer but also had significant impairments. Despite the physical suffering, the psychosocial toll of diagnosis and treatment was overwhelming and resulted in Mattie being diagnosed with clinical depression, anxiety, and medical traumatic stress.

Palliative care was never discussed with us. Instead, symptom management was handled by the treatment team as it arose, rather than proactively addressing our family's concerns, needs, and issues before they reached a critical level. We had no advance care or end-of-life planning in place and instead made these difficult decisions while actively watching Mattie die. Seeing Mattie suffer will remain with us always, but why did it have to be this way?

Our experience taught us: quality PPC must be integrated into the treatment plan starting on Day 1 of a pediatric cancer or life-threatening illness diagnosis, with a focus not just on physical symptoms but psychological ones as well. PPC and psychosocial providers, then, are a crucial part of the multidisciplinary team, and I believe if such a team had been in place for Mattie, his physical, social, and emotional experiences would have been managed more effectively, and he would have been relieved of his pain, isolation, and fear about treatment. Since childhood cancer is a family disease, both the voice of the child and the family must be included when assessing and treating physical, psychological, social, and spiritual issues.

In 2009, 2 months after Mattie died, we created the Mattie Miracle Cancer Foundation. We are the only national nonprofit dedicated to psychosocial awareness, advocacy, support, and research of childhood cancer. Based on Mattie's cancer journey, we know that childhood cancer is not just about the medicine. Therefore, we advocated for the creation of evidence-based psychosocial standards of care so that children and their families have access to optimal psychosocial care throughout the cancer trajectory. The Standards were published in *Pediatric Blood and Cancer* in 2015, with Standard 13 devoted to PPC and Standard 14 devoted to bereavement follow-up care.

When children are suffering, the health and well-being of the entire family are impacted. Healthcare providers have a responsibility to address that suffering through quality palliative care efforts. Psychosocial and palliative providers are an essential part of the healthcare team because they understand that parents entrust their child's care to the team with the hope that the needs of whole child will be honored and respected.

NQF has robust adult-oriented palliative and end-of-life measures,[18] which are used as the framework for many adult-focused quality initiatives. However, these NQF palliative measures have not been updated since their original creation. The NQF Healthcare Coordination Measures initiative may be of interest to PPC clinicians who coordinate care for children across settings.

BOX 8.2 REFLECTION ON PRACTICE FOR PPC CLINICIANS AND TEAMS

- What went well today as I engaged with children and their families?
- What was different than I expected?
- What did I learn from each child/family today?
- What mattered most?
- Did our team accomplish what we set out to do today?
- What components of our practice are grounded and evidence-based?
- What do we wish could be enhanced or changed?
- Where are opportunities for improvement?

Measuring What Matters (MWM) is a consensus project of the American Academy of Hospice and Palliative Medicine (AAHPM) and Hospice and Palliative Nurses Association (HPNA), with a focus on developing quality measures related to current palliative care guidelines and standards. MWM investigators identified potential quality indicators that mapped onto the National Consensus Project's (NCP) Clinical Practice Guideline domains.[19] Using a Delphi process with key stakeholders, the list was narrowed to 10 quality palliative measures: one in the NCP domain Structure and Process (Comprehensive Assessment), three in Physical Aspects (Screening for Physical Symptoms, Pain Treatment, and Dyspnea Screening and Management), one in Psychological and Psychiatric Aspects (Discussion of Emotional or Psychological Needs), one in Spiritual and Existential Aspects (Discussion of Spiritual/Religious Concerns), and three in Ethical and Legal Aspects (Documentation of Surrogate, Treatment Preferences, and Care Consistency with Documented Care Preferences). While MWM measures are primarily adult-care focused, reviewing them will inspire PPC teams to consider how

TABLE 8.1 National quality organizations and initiatives

NAME	WEBSITE
National Quality Forum	http://www.qualityforum.org/Topics/Palliative_Care_and_End-of-Life_Care.aspx
Measuring What Matters	http://aahpm.org/quality/measuring-what-matters
MACRA Palliative Care Quality Measures Project	https://www.nationalcoalitionhpc.org/macra/
Global Palliative Care Quality Alliance (GPCQA)	http://www.gpcqa.org/
Palliative Care Quality Network	https://www.pcqn.org/ (Includes pediatric-focused resources)
National Palliative Care Registry™	https://registry.capc.org/ (Includes pediatric-focused data collection criteria)
Palliative Care Quality Collaborative	https://www.capc.org/collaborations/palliative-care-quality-collaborative/
National Consensus Project (NCP) Clinical Practice Guidelines for Quality Palliative Care, 4th edition	https://www.nationalcoalitionhpc.org/ncp/ (4th Edition includes PPC specific criteria, clinical exemplars, and resources)
NHPCO Standards of Practice for Pediatric Palliative Care Programs	https://www.nhpco.org/hospice-care-overview/hospice-standards-of-practice
Standards for Psychosocial Care for Children with Cancer and their Families	https://www.mattiemiracle.com/standards

similar measures could be adapted to their current program and patient needs.

Medicare Access and CHIP (Children's Health Insurance Program) Reauthorization Act (MACRA) Palliative Care Quality Measures Project is a joint effort of the AAHPM, the National Coalition for Hospice and Palliative Care, and RAND Health as directed by the Center for Medicare and Medicaid Services (CMS). Funded in 2018, this project will develop two patient-reported outcome measures for adults with serious illness and their families receiving care in community settings. This initiative is engaging a broad range of key stakeholders and clinical experts in the development of these outcome measures. PPC clinicians providing care in community settings may be interested in following the progress of this project.

NATIONAL QUALITY MEASUREMENT COLLABORATIVES

For the pursuit of high-quality palliative to be successful, it is crucial that programs participate in quality data collection and analysis collaboratives. Historically, each individual program has developed its own unique methods for tracking and analyzing data that are not easily translatable outside of that specific organization. As a result, much of the quality work exists in individual silos.[20] There have been exciting developments regarding facilitating collaborative quality work that PPC clinicians should explore.

The *Global Palliative Care Quality Alliance* (GPCQA) was developed in 2007, as a quality assessment and improvement collaboration initially focused on a single state and inclusive of academic and community care settings. Originating at Duke University, GPCQA developed into a fee-based membership collaborative with national and even global scope.[21] While GPCQA has established an overall palliative care outcome registry, there have been no specific efforts focused on pediatrics within this alliance. In 2020, GPCQA became one of the founding partners of the Palliative Care Quality Collaborative (PCQC) and no longer functions independently.

The *Palliative Care Quality Network* (PCQN), established in 2009 at the University of California-San Francisco, also was focused initially within a single state and then expanded nationally with a fee-based membership structure. PCQN's stated goal is to help sustain and grow palliative care by providing teams with all the tools, data, and support they need to demonstrate value, build strong teams, and promote resilience in their clinicians. The core dataset focuses on care processes and patient-level outcomes in addition to metrics around financial outcomes of palliative care. Like GPCQA, data are entered in a registry, and custom reports are produced for both individual member programs and the whole collaborative.[22] PCQN has also focused on the unique needs of PPC.[23] Along with GPCQA, the PCQN serves as a founding partner of the PCQC and no longer functions independently.

National Palliative Care Registry. While GPCQA and PCQN have primarily emphasized patient-level outcomes, the National Palliative Care Registry is focused on the structural and programmatic delivery of high-quality palliative care across all healthcare settings. A joint effort of the Center to Advance Palliative Care and the National Palliative Care Research Center, the registry aims to provide data that programs can use to secure, expand, and retain resources for delivery of high-quality palliative care and to support the establishment of new palliative care programs where none exists. The Registry collects data on all service settings across the continuum of care, including hospital, long-term care, office/clinic, and home-based palliative care. The Registry formatting was recently updated to further meet the unique needs of pediatric programs, and PPC clinicians are encouraged to submit their team's data to both support their program's measurement needs and contribute to the national PPC dialogue.

The *PCQC* is a recently established 501c3 effort that combines GPCQA, PCQN, and the National Palliative Care Registry into one organization to collect program-level data on structure and process and patient-level data. The goal of PCQC is to improve the care and well-being of people with serious illness and their caregivers by delivering timely and useful patient- and program-centered data that identifies and promotes best practices through QI research and supports accreditation, accountability, and benchmarking. A PPC physician serves on the PCQC Board of Directors. A significant investment in the PCQC infrastructure will ensure integration with electronic health record (EHR) systems and real-time access to data analysis and visualization.[24] All adult and pediatric palliative programs are strongly encouraged to commit to participating in the PCQC collaborative registries. Participation in the program-level data and reporting comes at no cost. There is a fee associated with the patient-level data entry and reporting.

Pediatric Palliative Improvement Network. Specifically, within the field of PPC, the Pediatric Palliative Improvement Network has formed as a loose association of interdisciplinary professionals from pediatric programs across the country that span care settings. The network has focused on QI education mainly through holding regular conferences and online collaboration. Additionally, members have participated in a collaborative QI project focused on pain assessment. The group used the American Academy of Pediatrics Quality Improvement Data Aggregator to collect, analyze, and report data.[25]

PEDIATRIC-SPECIFIC COLLABORATIVE EFFORTS, GUIDELINES, STANDARDS

The growth of a more robust evidence base in PPC allows for the ongoing development and revision of clinical care guidelines (i.e., practice recommendations) and standards of care (i.e., best practices) that lay the blueprint for quality clinical care of patients and their families within and across institutions. Several organizations and multidisciplinary efforts, to date, have outlined standards or guidelines for palliative care, each including a focus on PPC.

The National Consensus Project (NCP) *Clinical Practice Guidelines for Quality Palliative Care*, 4th edition. The latest edition of the NCP guidelines for quality palliative care outlines core concepts, structures, and processes necessary for quality palliative care, with an emphasis on access to quality care for all people with serious illness regardless of setting, diagnosis, prognosis, or age.[26] Developed by 16 national organizations with experts representing all disciplines in hospice and palliative care and endorsed by more than 80 national organizations, the NCP guidelines outline criteria across eight domains for quality palliative care provision. Each domain is supported by a systematic review of evidence[27] and includes an emphasis on assessment, care coordination, culturally inclusive care, and communication. Operational implications are now outlined for each domain, including a description of essential skills needed by all PPC clinicians for each domain.[26] Domain 1, Guideline 1.9 emphasizes the importance of continuous QI work for all palliative care teams.[26]

The PPC community was actively engaged in the writing and review of the fourth edition, resulting in deepened perinatal-, neonatal-, and pediatric-focused criteria in each domain, along with pediatric case examples, program exemplars, and PPC evidence and resources. PPC clinicians can use the NCP Guidelines to enhance their existing program and identify opportunities for quality care measurement and QI improvement activities.

National Hospice and Palliative Care Organization's (NHPCO) Standards of Practice. NHPCO's *Standards of Practice for Hospice Programs* (revised in 2019) are organized around core components of quality hospice care and thereby provide a method for organizations to perform quality self-assessments and/or set performance benchmarks. The NHPCO Standards include pediatric-specific criteria[28] that serve as a supplement for palliative and/or hospice programs providing care to children, adolescents, and young adults, whether that care is delivered in the home, hospital, long-term care, or respite facility.

STANDARDS FOR PSYCHOSOCIAL CARE FOR CHILDREN WITH CANCER AND THEIR FAMILIES

Models of standardized quality palliative care are also emerging within specific pediatric illness groups, like childhood cancer, via collaborative and multidisciplinary efforts. Recognizing the significant variability in psychosocial services offered to patients in different pediatric oncology settings and the lack of published, comprehensive, evidence-based standards for pediatric psycho-oncology care, pediatric oncology psychosocial professionals collaborated with an interdisciplinary group of experts and stakeholders to develop the first evidence- and consensus-based standards for pediatric psychosocial care.[29] As described by the Browns (Box 8.1), this set of 15 Standards for Psychosocial Care for Children with Cancer and Their Families, endorsed by more than 15 professional organizations, was based on a systematic review of relevant literature and rigorous evaluation of the evidence quality.

Standard 13 addresses PPC specifically and recommends (1) early introduction of palliative care concepts regardless of disease status and (2) developmentally appropriate end-of-life care.[30] Standard 14, addressing bereavement follow-up care, recommends contact by a member of the family's healthcare team after a child's death to assess family needs, identify those at risk for negative psychosocial sequelae, continue care, and provide resources for bereavement support.[31] These established standards help to ensure that all children with cancer receive essential psychosocial care.

INTEGRATING NATIONAL STANDARDS/ GUIDELINES FROM A QUALITY PERSPECTIVE

The guidelines just described are not quality measures in and of themselves, yet they provide a valuable foundation and framework for developing such measures and can be a useful tool in QI initiatives for both national projects and individual programs.

While the *Standards for Psychosocial Care for Children with Cancer and Their Families*[29] are a valuable blueprint for clinicians and organizations, additional guidance was needed on best practices regarding how to adopt and implement the standards, with consideration for the heterogeneity of program size and resource availability. As a result, the multidisciplinary working group has provided implementation toolkits for individual cancer site use and guidance on how to evaluate both quality of care and systems change. Accompanying each standard is (1) a Matrix (Institutional Assessment Tool), utilizing a scoring system of 1–5, with 1 reflecting lack of implementation of the standard and 5 reflecting the gold standard (comprehensive care and complete implementation), and (2) Guidelines, providing specific guidance on "how to" improve implementation of each standard (i.e., action items with strategies, along with useful tools and resources) and thus improve each center's score. These additions have been developed as tools for individual program self-assessment and setting of benchmarks and therefore lay the foundation for QI projects, regardless of treatment setting.[32]

For the palliative care standard, for example, the guidelines recommend, among a number of specific strategies, the use of standardized advance care planning (ACP) tools to facilitate early discussions with children and families about goals of care. As such, PPC programs may initiate QI projects to increase the percentage of adolescents undergoing bone marrow transplantation who participate in ACP and who have decisions documented in the EHR. Similarly, the guideline for this standard recommends close collaboration with community-based palliative and hospice providers to honor family preference for location of end-of-life care and to ensure ongoing symptom management. This standard could also inspire QI initiatives to evaluate percentages of patients who die in their preferred location.

QUALITY MEASURES IN PPC

Moving beyond clinical guidelines or best practices, the PPC community must also identify and validate quality measures specific to PPC and then monitor and assess the quality of care provided to children with life-threatening conditions and their families using those indicators. Quality measures provide definitions of the eligible populations (denominator), rules for determining when the care aligns with the best practices (numerator), and rules for exclusions and outcome interpretation (risk adjustment).[9] Quality indicators, for example, may include availability of specialized PPC services (including bereavement care), proportion of children suffering from a variety of symptoms, proportion of families with documented discussion of goals of care, proportion of children dying in their preferred location, and proportion of parents satisfied with PPC services.[33]

PPC QUALITY MEASURE EVOLUTION

Recognizing the need for pediatric-specific quality measures, especially in the domain of end-of-life care, Johnston and colleagues[9] utilized the NCP Guidelines and the framework from MWM to suggest modifications to quality measures that better meet the needs of dying children and their families. These include measuring death in the preferred location rather than only home versus hospital, developmental and age-appropriate symptom assessment, sibling support training for palliative care programs, and assessment of bereaved parent outcomes. These authors also advocate for establishment of a task force to develop pediatric-appropriate end-of-life measures.

Similarly, other research teams are exploring how and where the existing NCP Guideline domains and criteria should be translated to pediatric-specific measurements of quality. Thienprayoon and colleagues' research, for example, focused on defining provider priority domains of quality in home-based pediatric hospice and palliative care. Their work recommended the addition of new domains for quality criteria and measurement development, that of Coordination of Care and Coordination of Bereavement.[34] Most importantly, there is growing recognition of the need to focus on the development of person-centered measures that ensure that patients and families are key stakeholders in the identification of such measures.[35–37]

CALL TO ACTION: IMPLEMENTING QUALITY MEASURES IN PPC PROGRAMS

Overcoming the inertia of starting a QI initiative is a significant challenge. The barriers are many: lack of QI knowledge and expertise, overwhelming clinical demands, small team size, inability to identify a project, and insufficient evidence base.[38] An important initial step is to ensure the PPC team places value on delivering high-quality care as a core objective of their service. Establishing a culture focused on providing high-quality services will help to set the stage for establishing an effective QI structure in the team. When focused on getting a structure established and starting an initial project, PPC clinicians should consider the following:

Learn the Basics of QI Methodology. A key initial step is to assess the knowledge level of team members in QI methodology. If there is little prior experience or knowledge, then teams should consider identifying an individual who can pursue further education and training in primary QI methodology. Such training might be available through internal institutional quality experts, national organizations such as the Institute for Healthcare Improvements Open School,[39] or groups specific to PPC such as the Pediatric Palliative Improvement Network. One individual with specific interest or expertise in QI methodology can serve as the quality champion for the program. Consideration should also be given to regular interdisciplinary team education on QI methodologies.[40]

Think Small and Relevant. QI projects need not be intimidating. Projects that are narrow and specific in scope can be fairly easy to implement. For PPC teams with limited capacity outside of clinical work, it is important to focus on a very specific project. Identification of a tension point in the team or a perceived weakness that concerns a team member may aid in considering a project focused around this issue.

An ideal initial QI project is one that aligns closely with the core focus of the team and also will not require significant changes in workflow or unnecessary additional burden to the interdisciplinary team. This is especially true for smaller programs that may fear a lack of bandwidth to accomplish a QI project. Focus should be on a population that is currently being served by the team.

Think Interdisciplinary. As the Brown's story reminds us, a core feature of PPC is the interdisciplinary nature of the service. QI work is not possible without drawing on the skills and expertise of all disciplines on the PPC team. Box 8.3 outlines examples of potential QI structure, process, and outcome projects and the opportunity for PPC interdisicplinary team members' participation.

A PPC team's quality work should include evaluating medical, psychosocial, and spiritual aspects of palliative care delivery, along with strongly considering input from children/families to inform individual projects and global QI strategy. Child and family input provide unique perspectives to help identify specific areas of improvement, and their perspectives also add to the imperative of why high-quality PPC is crucial—it is impacting human beings in very vulnerable moments.[16] Child and family perspectives deepen the breadth, scope, and impact of continuous quality improvement.

Know the Evidence Base. Research informs evidence-based practice, which informs QI initiatives. Once a potential project has been identified and implementation planning begins, teams should take the time to determine what, if any, research and evidence-based practices are available to inform the project. QI at its essence is the implementation and utilization of healthcare processes that have been established by the best evidence available.

Don't Reinvent the Wheel. There are several available resources and examples of palliative care QI projects that can help to inform a team's decision on individual QI projects. The NCP Guidelines for Quality Palliative Care (4th ed.)[26] and MWM[19] initiative are helpful to provide a framework for developing quality measures. Collaboration is crucial. No one individual program can produce high-quality care that is universally generalizable. Possibilities for collaboration include other PPC programs delivering similar services within the same state as well as programs across the country. Teams may consider accessing the Pediatric Palliative Improvement Network to enhance their QI methodology knowledge and

BOX 8.3 QUALITY IMPROVEMENT (QI) PROJECT IDENTIFICATION BY AN INTERDISCIPLINARY PEDIATRIC PALLIATIVE CARE (PPC) TEAM

Case Presentation: Brianna is a 16-year-old girl with osteosarcoma diagnosed 15 months ago, now with metastatic disease to her lungs and brain discovered 6 months prior. She is admitted to the intensive care (ICU) with progressive respiratory distress and failure due to disease burden. She is on mechanical ventilatory support, and attempts at weaning from support have not been successful. The PPC team was consulted for end-of-life care.

The PPC team has some difficulty establishing a therapeutic relationship with Brianna's family, who are overwhelmed with her sudden deterioration. Because of her condition, she is unable to participate in the consultation process. The PPC team works closely with Brianna's family and the intensive care unit and oncology teams to make plans for her extubation with a focus on end-of-life care.

Following Brianna's death, the PPC team reflects on the experience in hope of identifying opportunities to enhance future care for children and families in similar situations. The following team members share ideas for potential QI projects:

Team Leadership/Medical Director: The director was concerned about the late timing of the PPC consult. The suggestion is made that it would be best to receive a consult around the time that a relapse or progression of malignancy has occurred.

Physicians/Advanced Practice Providers: These clinicians shared their concern about the high burden of Brianna's end-of-life symptoms specifically related to pain and dyspnea. They recommend exploring ways for frequent assessment of patient reported outcomes.

PPC Nurses: The nurses shared their concern for Brianna's level of end-of-life comfort and also wondered how their care might have been different if they had established an earlier relationship prior to her deterioration.

Social Worker and Psychologist: Both clinicians were distressed that no advance care planning or discussion of Brianna's general wishes for her medical care were completed or documented. They jointly suggested an initiative focused on advance care planning for adolescents on the oncology service, with increased documentation of goals of care in the electronic health record.

Child Life Specialist: The child life specialist expressed concern that Brianna's siblings, ages 8 and 6, did not have an opportunity for developmentally appropriate education related to their sister's disease progression and, ultimately, death. She wondered about options for better sibling support in the ICU.

Chaplain: The hospital chaplain discovered after Brianna's death that her family had a strong Christian faith. He feels that there was a missed opportunity to provide spiritual support and is interested in improving referrals to pastoral care either at the time of diagnosis or concurrent with PPC referral.

After deliberation, this interdisciplinary team determined that the common thread in their concerns was that of timely PPC consultation and establishment of therapeutic relationship by all members of the team with Brianna and her family. Box 8.4 outlines the next steps taken by the team to implement their QI project.

join in collaborative QI projects. Teams should also prioritize participation in the PCQC.

Connect with Institutional Resources. Every healthcare organization has some form of QI infrastructure and expertise. PPC teams should familiarize themselves with such resources in their local institution. With the growing focus on value, quality care, and patient-focused outcomes, PPC is uniquely situated to flourish in an evolving health system. Institution leadership, when aware of this potential, may be willing to support PPC quality infrastructure and measurement. Such resources can aid in education and likely support the development and implementation of the team's QI initiatives and specific projects.

For those working in academic medical centers especially, programs should consider partnering with local professional schools (medical, nursing, social work, etc.). Many curriculums require QI experience. Students also interested in PPC might be willing to participate in quality projects. The same is true for graduate medical education, as residents and fellows are often required to focus on a QI project during their training. Additionally, physicians should be mindful of eligibility of quality projects to satisfy maintenance of certification requirements for continued board certification.

A focus on interacting with bedside nurses and house staff can benefit the PPC team in ways beyond the implementation of QI projects. Such emphasis on education can lead to an increase in consults and utilization of specialty PPC services while also enhancing the primary PPC skills of professionals throughout an organization.[41]

Consider the Role of the EHR. The reality of QI projects is that they can often be labor intense, placing an additional stress on an already overburdened PPC team. Efficiency in project design and implementation is crucial. There is opportunity to enhance efficiency through capabilities of the EHR. Meeting early and often with information technology experts at the PPC team's institution can help to build a framework for more efficient management of QI projects.

Ideally, clinical documentation would contribute to quality data collection simultaneously, limiting need for time-intense data extraction and allowing for real-time data collection and reporting that provides immediate value to individuals and programs.[20] Additionally, PPC clinicians could work with their EHR teams to contribute data directly from the EHR to a national PPC registry, such as that being developed by the PCQC.

Working with institutional information technology/EHR can lead to the creation of dashboards or scorecards[42] that can be used to provide real-time feedback and reporting on the PPC's chosen specific quality measures. Such real-time feedback can also ensure continued motivated engagement in QI initiatives by team members.

QI PROJECT IMPLEMENTATION AND TEAM COLLABORATION

Implementation of a QI project is a team effort. Consideration for involvement of individuals should include interdisciplinary backgrounds, familiarity with QI processes, influence to effect change, and project leadership. Each project should have a goal or aim statement, "What are we trying to accomplish?" Such statements should be specific, measurable, achievable, relevant, and time-limited.[43] Once an aim has been established, attention should turn to establishing quality measures that answer the question, "How will we know if an improvement has occurred?" The team must then focus on identifying changes to practice that might help to achieve the aim. The next step in project implementation is to continually test changes. One such method for testing that is commonly used is the Plan-Do-Study-Act (PDSA) cycle. PDSA is an iterative process involving four steps:[44]

- *Plan*: In this phase, the team must determine action needed to achieve the aim, develop a plan to test the change, predict the results, and prepare to implement the change.
- *Do*: The team then must implement the change, document issues and observations, and ensure data are collected.
- *Study*: The team then must make time to analyze the data, compare the results to predicted outcomes, and summarize learning points.
- *Act*: In this stage, the team then takes action based on the results by refining the change needed for continued improvement leading into the next cycle. Attention must also be given to dissemination of the results and lessons learned.

An important component of QI projects is for the PPC team to share the knowledge gained from the process with both internal (PC team, hospital leadership) and external (journals, conferences, collaboratives) audiences. Box 8.4 provides a clinical exemplar of a PPC team identifying a QI project, highlighting the unique perspectives that each clinician/discipline brings to such a project. Box 8.5 describes how the PPC team implements their chosen QI project.

QUALITY AND ADVOCACY

Barriers to accessing palliative care are important quality targets, and therefore it is crucial that attention is paid to legislative and policy efforts that ensure access to high-quality palliative care for all children with serious illness. Section 2302 of the 2010 Patient Protection and Affordable Care Act enhanced access to hospice services by allowing children with Medicaid or Children's Health Insurance Program to receive hospice benefits concurrently with insurance payment for treatments focused on cure or disease modification.[45] While federal policy is key, more emphasis is needed on state policy. Several states have developed innovative programs aimed at enhancing access to home-based PPC services and ensuring delivery of such services closer to the point of diagnosis than death.[46] In Florida, for example, a collaboration between state-employed base managers and hospices provided home-based

BOX 8.4 QUALITY IMPROVEMENT (QI) PROJECT IMPLEMENTATION BY A PEDIATRIC PALLIATIVE CARE (PPC) TEAM

The PPC team reviewed important strategies before launching into their QI project:

- *Learn the Basics*: The medical director and social worker had previous advanced expertise in QI methodology, so they were designated project leads and mentored the team. The psychologist attended a QI workshop and assisted with the project.
- *Think Small and Relevant*: The team agreed on an aim of receiving timely referrals from the oncology service for children with a diagnosis of relapsed or progressive malignancy. The team felt they could handle this potential increase in consult volume.
- *Think Interdisciplinary Team*: All team members reflected on their experiences together and collaborated to determine the QI project topic. As the team learned from this early referral project, they set a goal to focus on discipline-specific projects in the near future.
- *Know the Evidence Base*: The team reviews the evidence in favor of timely referrals to PPC and the impact of PPC in the oncology population. Standard 13 of the *Psychosocial Standards of Care for Children with Cancer and their Families*[27] supports early integration of PPC.
- *Don't Reinvent the Wheel*: The team reached out through the PPC QI Network to learn from other teams. One of the PPC nurses learns of a similar process implemented at another hospital and brings that information back to the team to review and consider.
- *Connect with Institutional Resources*: The project leaders connect with the hospital's QI infrastructure experts and also receive feedback from the hospital's quality committee. A hospital leader offers to advocate for the team's planned QI work at an upcoming meeting with oncology and ICU leadership.
- *Role of Electronic Health Records*: In order to gather baseline data, the medical director worked with IT services to perform a retrospective EHR review, with these findings: of the 45 diagnoses of relapse or progression of cancer in the past 2 years, 40% of those patients received a PPC consult at the time of relapse diagnosis. The PPC team then works with the EHR team to identify potentially eligible patients and to build in reminders to trigger PPC consults.

Chosen SMART Aim for the project: 80% of children diagnosed with relapse or progression of malignancy will receive a PPC consult at the time that relapse or progression is first diagnosed. This goal will be attained within 12 months of implementation.

Chosen QI Process: The team collaborated to complete the QI project using the Plan-Do-Study-Act model, implementing the EHR triggers, which were challenging to build and required a full 6 months of effort to ensure timely PPC consultations.

Project Outcome: The PPC collected data on their QI outcome, finding that 82% of targeted children received a PPC consult at the time of relapse, meeting the initial goal.

Project Dissemination: The QI team shared their results with the internal quality committee and submitted a QI manuscript to a palliative journal for publication.

PPC services to eligible children. Results showed high levels of satisfaction among those parents whose children received services.[47]

A similar program was developed in California, with demonstrated reduced healthcare costs of $3,331 per enrollee per month. Such cost reductions were realized from decreased number of inpatient days, reduced length of stay for hospital admissions, and care focus shifted to less expensive outpatient care.[48] A home-based PPC and hospice care program in Minnesota demonstrated that patients with noncancer diagnoses in the program for at least 6 months had a significantly decreased average length of stay in the hospital and an average decrease in hospital charges of $275,000 when compared with time prior to enrollment in the program.[49] Such data can provide compelling motivation for state Medicaid offices and private payers to consider supporting such programs. Further evaluation of impact is needed.

CONCLUSION

As the field of PPC grows, there is an increasing need to emphasize the delivery of high-quality, evidence-based interdisciplinary services to all children with serious illness and their families. PPC programs of all types must enhance efforts focused on improving the quality of care delivered. With growth of availability and acceptance of PPC services comes enhanced internal and external scrutiny on those providing such services to ensure they are of the highest quality and consistent with national practices.

PPC programs must focus on strengthening internal QI infrastructure. They must also focus on collaborating with other programs to identify quality gaps and standardize measure development and data collection, analysis, and reporting. As stressed by Mattie's parents, quality efforts should include both the child and family voice and a focus on improvement of both physical and psychological symptoms. PPC teams' QI activities should also include varied patient populations, interdisciplinary services, and healthcare settings.

The content of each chapter in this book highlights current PPC evidence and best practice, serving as an excellent resource for PPC teams willing to either initiate engagement in or extend their commitment to quality in PPC provision. It is our hope that PPC teams in all settings will be encouraged by the tremendous efforts in place to embed PPC

BOX 8.5 EXAMPLES OF QUALITY IMPROVEMENT PROJECTS FOR INTERDISCIPLINARY PEDIATRIC PALLIATIVE CARE (PPC) TEAMS

QUALITY CONCEPT

Structure

- What should be the minimal composition of a team in order to be considered an interdisciplinary palliative care program?
- What percentage of team members should maintain maximal PC certification in respective discipline, if available?
- What is the ideal staffing model based on consult volume?
- What should be the availability of pediatric expertise within an adult-focused hospice organization?[50]
- How does one best measure productivity of a palliative care program?

Process

- On admission, what percentage of palliative care patients are screened for symptom distress using validated scales?
- What percentage of patients received a spirituality screen upon initial clinical evaluation? What percentage of those include an appropriate trigger for a spirituality assessment based on result of the screen?

Outcome

- What proportion of patient families received care concordant with stated goals of patient?
- At end of life, did the use of life-sustaining therapies align with stated goals of child and family?
- Does early integration of PPC services impact patient/family satisfaction?
- What percentage of adolescents participate in advance care planning and have decisions documented in the EHR?
- What percentage of patients die in their preferred location?
- Impact of care coordination on healthcare system utilization (e.g., emergency department visits, admissions, lengths of stay, costs)?

Implementation of a QI project is a team effort, and interdisciplinary collaboration is critical. Depending on the project, team members who should be considered as key stakeholders in design and implementation include physicians, advance practice professionals (NPs, PAs,), psychologists, social workers, nurses, child life specialists, chaplains, dieticians, occupational and physical therapists, and art and music therapists.

quality measurement, outcome evaluation, and QI projects as key components to optimizing their teams' work.

REFERENCES

1. Institute of Medicine. *Crossing the Quality Chasm: A New Health System for the 21st Century.* Washington, DC: National Academy Press; 2001.
2. Bogetz JF, Friebert S. Defining success in pediatric palliative care while tackling the quadruple aim. *J Palliat Med.* 2017;20(2):116–119.
3. Donabedian A. Evaluating the quality of medical care. *Milbank Memorial Fund Q.* 1966;44(3 suppl):166–206. Reprinted in *Milbank Q.* 2005;83(4):691–729.
4. National Academies of Sciences, Engineering, and Medicine. *Implementing Quality Measures for Accountability in Community-Based Care for People with Serious Illness: Proceedings of a Workshop.* Washington, DC: National Academies Press; 2018.
5. Valuk T, Montgomery R. Data needs for serious illness care accountability system: A framework and recommendations. *J Palliat Med.* 2018;21(S2):S1–S6.
6. Allen-Duck A, Robinson JC, Stewart MW. Healthcare quality: A concept analysis. *Nurs Forum.* 2017;52(4):377–386.
7. Feudtner C, Zhong W, Faerber J, Dai D, Feinstein J. Pediatric end-of-life and palliative care: Epidemiology and health service use. In Institute of Medicine Committee on Approaching Death: Addressing Key End-of-Life Issues. *Dying in America: Improving Quality and Honoring Individual Preferences Near End of Life.* Washington, DC: National Academies Press; 2015: 533–572.
8. Kane JR, Baker JN. Quality improvement. In Goldman A, Hain R, Liben S, ed. *Oxford Textbook of Palliative Care for Children.* 2nd ed. New York: Oxford University Press; 2012: 430–440.
9. Johnston EE, Rosenberg AR, Kamal AH. Pediatric-specific end-of-life care quality measures: An unmet need of a vulnerable population. *J Oncol Pract.* 2017;12(10):e874–880.
10. Kaye EC, Abramson ZR, Snaman JM, Friebert SE, Baker JN. Productivity in pediatric palliative care: Measuring an elusive metric. *J Pain Symptom Manage.* 2017;53(5):952–961.
11. Friedel M, Aujoulat I, Dubois AC, Degryse JM. Instruments to measure outcomes in pediatric palliative care: A systematic review. *Pediatrics.* 2019;143(1):1–22.
12. Feudtner C, Rosenberg AR, Boss RD, et al. Challenges and priorities for pediatric palliative care research in the US and similar practice settings: Report from a pediatric palliative care research network workshop. *J Pain Symptom Manage.* 2019;58(5):909–917.
13. Rosenberg AR, Orellana L, Ullrich C, et al. Quality of life in children with advanced cancer: A report from the PediQUEST Study. *J Pain Symptom Manage.* 2016;52(2):243–253.
14. Donnelly JP, Downing K, Cloen J, et al. Development and assessment of a measure of parent and child needs in pediatric palliative care. *J Pain Symptom Manage.* 2018;55(4):1077–1084.
15. Feudtner C, Walter JK, Faerber JA, et al. Good-Parent beliefs of parents of seriously ill children. *JAMA Pediatr.* 2015;169(1):39–47.
16. Thienprayoon R, Grossoehme D, Humphrey L, et al. "There's just no way to help, and they did." Parents name compassionate care as a new domain of quality in pediatric home-based hospice and palliative care. *J Palliat Med.* 2019 Dec 27.
17. Meier DE, Back AL, Berman A, Block SD, Corrigan JM, Morrison RS. A national strategy for palliative care. *Health Aff (Millwood).* 2017;36(7):1265–1273.
18. National Quality Forum. *National Voluntary Consensus Standards: Palliative Care and End-of-Life Care: A Consensus Report.* Washington, DC: National Quality Forum; 2012.
19. Dy SM, Kiley KB, Ast K, et al. Measuring What Matters: Top-ranked quality indicators for hospice and palliative care from the American Academy of Hospice and Palliative Medicine and Hospice and Palliative Nurses Association. *J Pain Symptom Manage.* 2015;49(4):773–781.
20. Kamal AH, Hanson LC, Casarett DJ, et al. The quality imperative for palliative care. *J Pain Symptom Manage.* 2015;49(2):243–253.

21. Kamal AH, Harrison KL, Bakitas M, et al. Improving the quality of palliative care through national and regional collaboration efforts. *Cancer Control.* 2015 Oct;22(4):396–402.
22. Pantilat SZ, Marks AK, Bischoff KE, et al. The Palliative Care Quality Network: Improving the quality of caring. *J Palliat Med.* 2017 Aug;20(8):862–868.
23. Bogetz JF, Marks A, Root MC, et al. Development of the Pediatric Palliative Care Quality Network. *J Palliat Med.* 2019 Jul;22(7):747–748.
24. American Academy of Hospice and Palliative Medicine. Registries in Hospice and Palliative Medicine. http://aahpm.org/quality/registries-in-hpm
25. Jones E, Thienprayoon R, Humphrey L, Ragsdale L. Creation of a QI collaborative learning network for pediatric palliative care utilizing the AAP Quality Improvement Data Aggregator (QIDA). *Pediatrics.* Aug 2019;144(2 Meeting Abstract):441.
26. National Consensus Project for Quality Palliative Care. *Clinical Practice Guidelines for Quality Palliative Care.* 4th ed. Richmond, VA: National Coalition for Hospice and Palliative Care; 2018.
27. Ahluwalia SC, Chen C, Raaen L, et al. A systematic review in support of the National Consensus Project Clinical Practice Guidelines for Quality Palliative Care, fourth edition. *J Pain Symptom Manage.* 2018;56(6):831–870.
28. National Hospice and Palliative Care Organization. *Standards of Practice for Pediatric Palliative Care.* Alexandria VA: National Hospice and Palliative Care Organization; 2019.
29. Wiener L, Kazak AE, Noll RB, Patenaude AF, Kupst MJ. Standards for the psychosocial care of children with cancer and their families: An introduction to the special issue. *Pediatr Blood Cancer.* 2015;62:S419–424.
30. Weaver MS, Heinze KE, Kelly KP, et al. Palliative care as a standard of care in pediatric oncology. *Pediatr Blood Cancer.* 2015;62:S829–S833.
31. Lichtenthal WG, Sweeney CR, Roberts KE, et al. Bereavement follow-up after the death of a child as a standard of care in pediatric oncology. *Pediatr Blood Cancer.* 2015:62(S5):S834–869.
32. Wiener L Kupst MJ, Pelletier W, Kazak AE, Thompson AL. Tools to guide the identification and implementation of care consistent with the psychosocial Standards of care. *Pediatric Blood & Cancer.* 2020 Sep;67(9):e28586.
33. Duc J, Widger K, Johnston K, Rapoport A, Siden H, Feudtner C, Wolfe J. Identifying indicators of quality pediatric palliative care: A systematic review. *J Pain Symptom Manage.* 2016 Dec 1;52(6):e133–134.
34. Thienprayoon R, Alessandrini E, Frimpong-Manso M, Grossoehme D. Defining provider-prioritized domains of quality in pediatric home-based hospice and palliative care: A study of the Ohio Pediatric Palliative Care and End-of-Life Network. *J Palliat Med.* 2018;21(10):1414–1435.
35. Ananth P, Mun S, Reffat N, et al. A stakeholder-driven qualitative study to define high quality end-of-life care for children with cancer. *J Pain Symptom Manage.* 2021. https://doi.org/10.1016/j.jpainsymman.2021.01.134
36. Johnston EE, Molina J, Martinez I, Dionne-Odom JN, Currie ER, Crowl T, Butterworth L, Chamberlain LJ, Bhatia S, Rosenberg AR. Bereaved parents' views on end-of-life care for children with cancer: Quality marker implications. *Cancer.* 2020 Jul 15;126(14):3352–3359.
37. Johnston EE, Martinez I, Bhatia S, Asch S. Expert panel endorsed quality metrics for end-of-life care for children with cancer: Results of a modified delphi panel. *Oral Presentations: American Academy of Hospice and Palliative Medicine State of the Science,* 2020.
38. Dixon-Woods M, McNicol S, Martin G. Ten challenges in improving quality in healthcare: Lessons from the Health Foundation's programme evaluations and relevant literature. *BMJ Qual Saf.* 2012 Oct;21(10):876–884.
39. Institute for Health Care Improvement Open School. http://www.ihi.org/education/IHIOpenSchool/Pages/default.aspx
40. Lakin JR, Brannen EN, Bernacki RE, Jones E. A curriculum in quality improvement for interprofessional palliative care trainees. *Am J Hosp Palliat Care.* 2020;37(1):41–45.
41. Lafond DA, Bowling S, Fortkiewicz JM, Reggio C, Hinds PS. Integrating the Comfort Theory into primary pediatric palliative care to improve access to care. *J Hosp Palliat Nurs.* 2019;21(5):382–389.
42. Kittleson S, Pierce R, Youngwerth J. Palliative Care Scorecard. *J Palliat Med.* 2017 May;20(5):517–527.
43. Doran GT. There's a S.M.A.R.T. way to write management's goals and objectives. *Management Rev.* 1981;70(11):35–36.
44. Institute for Health Care Improvement. Science of improvement: Testing changes. http://www.ihi.org/resources/Pages/HowtoImprove/ScienceofImprovementTestingChanges.aspx
45. National Hospice and Palliative Care Organization. *Concurrent Care for Children Implementation Toolkit.* https://www.nhpco.org/wp-content/uploads/2019/06/CCCR_Toolkit.pdf
46. Kaye EC, Rubenstein J, Levine D, et al. Pediatric palliative care in the community. *CA Cancer J Clin.* 2015 Jul-Aug;65(4):316–333.
47. Knapp CA, Madden VL, Curtis CM, et al. Partners in care: Together for kids: Florida's model of pediatric palliative care. *J Palliat Med.* 2008 Nov;11(9):1212–1220.
48. Gans D, Hadler MW, Chen X, et al. Cost analysis and policy implications of a pediatric palliative care program. *J Pain Symptom Manage.* 2016;52(3):329–335.
49. Postier A, Chrastek J, Nugent S, et al. Exposure to home-based pediatric palliative and hospice care and its impact on hospital and emergency care charges at a single institution. *J Palliat Med.* 2014;17:183–188.
50. Weaver MS, Jenkins R, Wichman C, et al. Sowing across a state: Development and delivery of a grassroots pediatric palliative care nursing curriculum. *J Palliat Care.* 2019 Nov 26;1–7.

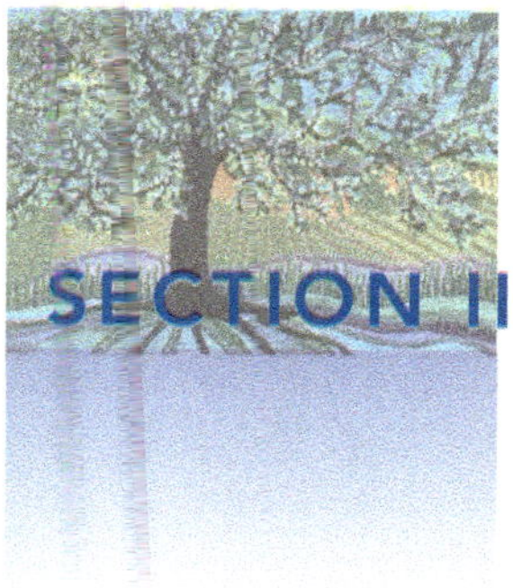

SECTION II | RELATIONSHIPS AND COMMUNICATION

Everyone here loves me . . .
Mommy, Daddy, all the nurses and my doctor love me.
And I know you do.

SIX-YEAR-OLD CHILD TO HIS PSYCHOLOGIST[1]

The chapters in this section provide perspectives on the complex and deeply meaningful relationships among children, families, clinicians, and teams in the field of pediatric palliative care (PPC). A relationship-centered view illuminates the experiences, dynamics, and influences that develop within the context of the care setting. Sociocultural and spiritual-religious factors, inextricable from these relationships, can have powerful impact. Communication is foundational in all relationships and emerges as the connecting thread throughout these chapters.

Chapter 9, "Relationships with Children and Ensuring Their Voices in Decision-Making," opens this section. As the field of PPC has evolved, the crucial importance of "listening to" the child's voice has emerged. Although many children do not have the ability (for age-related, developmental, or clinical reasons) to articulate their experience, there is nonetheless increasing acknowledgment of taking the child into account as the subject rather than the object of plans and decisions. This chapter provides a conceptual framework with strategies and tools to enable families and clinicians to integrate the child's perspective.

Each child is embedded within a family, and the impact of a seriously ill child reverberates throughout the family system. Chapter 10, "Family Experience and Relationships," describes the experiences of families along the illness trajectory, with implications for the delivery of PPC. Conceptual models (social-ecology, systems, and traumatic stress) provide the framework for understanding how individual members, as well as the family as a collective, are affected. The chapter focuses on the reorganization of family roles and responsibilities to accommodate the "extensive intensive care" of the child, with the ensuing impact on parents and siblings.

Through interdisciplinary teamwork, palliative care strives to meet the unique needs of individual children and their families. Chapter 11, "Team Relationships," presents conceptual underpinnings for the creation, growth, and sustainability of a highly functional team. Its basic structure and the composition of its members influence relationships, and ongoing attention to overall team dynamics is essential. The chapter describes processes (what teams do) and relational states (how teams feel) that are critical for optimal functioning—both within and between teams. Strategies to support the well-being of the team and its individual members are presented.

Clinicians in PPC enter the world of children living with life-threatening conditions and their families. They repeatedly come face to face with the relentlessness of illness, the uncertainty of prognosis, and, at times, the inevitability of death. Chapter 12, "Witness to Suffering: The Clinician Experience," examines the nature of clinicians' suffering and addresses the challenge of "preserving oneself" while sustaining the ability to be effective and empathic with children and families. Building resilience and engaging in self-care are critical, both for the integration of clinicians' own experience and for the provision of optimal care.

In Chapter 13, "Practical Aspects of Palliative Care Communication," the focus is on how clinicians can adapt their mode of communication to "match" the capacity of the child and the dynamics of the family within the context of their cultural beliefs. Communication skills are crucial in the establishment and maintenance of a therapeutic alliance. Specific tools to guide conversations, including a structure for effective family conferences, are presented. The central theme is how to balance the delivery of difficult information with emotional support, both necessary components to facilitate families' decision-making.

Advance care planning is now considered standard of care in PPC. In Chapter 14, "Advance Care Planning Along the Care Continuum," these discussions are conceptualized as an extension of goals-of-care conversations. Advance care planning addresses future-oriented topics and imagines the child in a worse state of health, along an expected or possible trajectory. These discussions afford the opportunity for children and families to plan for end-of-life care, including location of care, preferences for resuscitation, use of medical technologies and potential life-extending interventions, and legacy-making. The chapter also includes discussion of organ donation and autopsy.

Chapter 15, "Anticipatory Grief and Bereavement," describes the universal grieving process of children and families, from the time of diagnosis through the illness trajectory, and—when a child dies—into bereavement. The swath of grief encompasses parents, siblings, extended family members, friends, members of the care team, and the wider community. There are complex psychological, spiritual, and physical manifestations of grief, deeply influenced by cultural, spiritual, and religious dimensions. It is important that all clinicians be aware of factors associated with anticipatory grief and bereavement, as well as with supportive interventions that can be integrated into the child and family's care.

The last chapter in the section, Chapter 16, "Resolving Conflicts in Pediatric Palliative Care," addresses situations in which relationships are in jeopardy and restoration may ultimately depend on the acuity and sensitivity of clinicians' communication. These include conflicts between families and teams, between pediatric patients and their parents, and intrateam disagreements. When conflict is ignored, trust is compromised, and a minor disagreement can devolve into a fracturing of relationships. Conversely, when addressed constructively, conflicts can lead to deeper understanding and cohesion among children, families, and clinicians. Approaches to resolution, including a discussion of legal and ethical paradigms, are presented.

The overlap in content among the chapters in this section represents the unified mission and commitment of interdisciplinary PPC. Along with such commonality, each topic is also viewed through multiple distinctive lenses. The varied layers and perspectives that emerge are testimony to the wisdom and richness of the field.

AUTHOR'S NOTE

Many of the themes in this section continue into the first chapters of Section III: "Psychological Symptoms" and "Existential Distress and Suffering."

REFERENCE

1. Sourkes, B. *Armfuls of Time: The Psychological Experience of the Child with a Life-Threatening Illness*. Pittsburgh, University of Pittsburgh Press, 1995.

9 | RELATIONSHIPS WITH CHILDREN AND ENSURING THEIR VOICES IN DECISION-MAKING

KAREN RON-LI LIAW, BECKY LOIS, JULIA MCBEE, AND ERIN COLLINS

I do have a voice. So let me enjoy it until I can't any longer, until all of my options are gone.

FAITH, a young adult living with cystic fibrosis

We couldn't protect our son from all the ways his body would eventually fail him but we could choose providers and treatments that allowed him to thrive as himself.

JEN, mother of Alex, a 3-year-old with leukodystrophy

CHILD DEVELOPMENT: CONSIDERATIONS FOR ENGAGEMENT AND COMMUNICATION

Diagnostic disclosure to children matters because it improves overall understanding and cooperation with procedures as well as adherence to treatment.[1] Furthermore, disclosure may decrease uncertainty, improve quality of life, and set the course for active participation and advocacy in care decisions.[1] However, when engaging children in medical decision-making, consideration should be paid to several important factors: developmental level, cognitive and language development, and emotional development and capacity for coping.

DEVELOPMENTAL LEVEL

Children's understanding of illness and death changes as they progress through normal developmental stages, moving from concrete understanding to grasping more abstract, nuanced ideas. Children under the age of 5 experience distress when separated from primary caregivers; the concept of separation is an important first step in the eventual understanding of death as a permanent form of separation. By the age of 5, children can understand that death is final and irreversible.[2] Later stages involve an awareness that death can apply to oneself and that death can be unpredictable. Research and clinical consensus indicate that by the age of 9, children can fully comprehend the complex nature and idea of death.[1]

Understanding of what causes illness is also related to developmental level, as children between the ages of 4 and 7 may rely on magical thinking (e.g., my thoughts or wishes can "cause" illness in myself or others) and subsequently develop a sense of guilt or blame. This type of thinking leads to a misunderstanding of how illness is spread and requires clarification and developmentally appropriate, concrete teaching on the part of the treatment team to ensure that information about diagnosis and treatment is appropriately conveyed. Children become more capable of understanding key biological concepts and utilizing reasoning skills as they age. For instance, children between the ages of 7 and 11 can understand changes related to their illness, like weight gain or hair loss, as these changes are easily observable and tangible. Over time, more abstract concepts (e.g., the effect of chemotherapy on my internal system; how my medication works inside my body to help me, the long-term side effects of my medication regimen) can be understood.[3] Last, while these age "norms" may be true for children in general, seriously ill children often demonstrate understanding of the concepts of illness and death at a much earlier time.

The ability to *understand* proposed medical treatment options and the choice at hand requires the interrelated skills of attention, orientation, intelligence, language, and memory to take in and integrate relevant information. The foundational brain architecture for these skills and neurocircuits are laid down during early childhood and mature from age 6–12 and then through adolescence and young adulthood.[4] Similarly, the ability to logically *reason* and weigh risks, benefits, and consequences of treatment options develops between the ages of 8 to 11 and accelerates in accuracy, speed, and complexity during adolescence.[4] Yet many adolescents still struggle to understand the long-term nature of decision-making and thus may make choices that can appear short-sighted or more focused on instant gratification or avoidance of significant consequences. The executive functioning system, which controls our ability to plan, self-regulate, multitask, and focus attention, is not fully developed until the mid-20s.[5] Thus, the *appreciation* of the nature of a situation and personal relevance of the decision at hand requires abstract, higher order thinking, which develops through adolescence and at different rates and potential for different people even into adulthood.

COGNITIVE AND LANGUAGE DEVELOPMENT

Regardless of developmental level, children's ability to process information and communicate effectively about their emotions, concerns, and questions may vary and requires assessment. For instance, young children commonly engage in magical thinking (e.g., "I got cancer because I was bad"). To understand complex and at times confusing information and conversations, treatment teams need to engage children with concrete, clear language when discussing diagnosis, causes, physical symptoms, and physical consequences to the external body and internal systems.

It is crucial that the treatment team find innovative ways to communicate information that accommodates for and builds on children's cognitive strengths and limitations. Consultation with the family as "experts" can be invaluable in understanding what works best when communicating with their child. Partnership with interdisciplinary psychosocial team members can also help ensure that communication is clear and that the child is processing the information correctly. Cognitive limitations, challenges, or differences are not an excuse to refrain from informing; rather, they should be assessed, understood, and factored in when engaging children's voices in decision-making.

EMOTIONAL DEVELOPMENT AND CAPACITY FOR COPING

Emotional challenges may complicate processing and reception of information, regardless of clarity of content. Furthermore, patients may struggle to share their concerns in a clear or appropriate way due to a sense of overwhelming panic or distress. Emotionality that is externalized (e.g., crying, irritability, excessive anxiety) is often easiest to see and adjust for; however, an apparent lack of an emotional response does not necessarily indicate a lack of distress. Instead, these patients may be emotionally numb, withdrawn, or not fully aware of the significance of their prognosis or treatment plan. In these instances, the need to assess their emotional state and understanding of their medical status is extremely important.

Mental health issues frequently emerge during adolescence: 50% percent of adults who present with a mental health condition had that condition first emerge during adolescence.[6] Assessment of emotional distress and normalization of the emotional challenges that seriously ill patients face are important in order to address these concerns head-on and manage their impact on quality-of-life, engagement in care, and adherence.

The team should check in with the patient and family about the child's baseline level of coping and typical strategies that might be employed around any challenging or upsetting communication during treatment. Psychosocial team members (e.g., clinical social workers. child psychologists and psychiatrists, child life specialists) have expertise in conducting assessments that can aid the interdisciplinary team in understanding whether the level of coping in a patient is adequate, effective, or not adaptive to their current environment. Patients may benefit from creative strategies to come to terms with their current physical limitations while approximating their favorite activity. For example, a patient who typically goes for a run to reduce stress is not able to employ that strategy during a medical admission or during periods of physical deconditioning. Alternatives could include walking around the medical unit to "get the body moving" or listening to a favorite running music mix while engaging in guided imagery of running through the woods by their house.

Last, the coping of close and extended family should be included in any assessment. The family's overall coping style and capabilities, as well as each individual's, are important considerations.[7] One person's struggle can impact the coping of everyone in the family. Factors that may influence family coping include socioeconomic status and financial stressors, level of education and health literacy, degree of social support, and general emotional health and well-being. See Figure 9.1 for an illustration of these factors and how the medical team, children, and families may communicate with one another when children are faced with a life-threatening condition.[1] Of note, healthcare professional factors also have an influence on patient and family coping and will be discussed further later.

CHILDREN AND RELATIONSHIPS

When a child is diagnosed with a life-threatening illness it is important to consider the impact of their relationships with family and their medical team on medical decision-making. Parents may be anxious or fearful about sharing prognostic information with their child and may experience a strong urge to protect them from upsetting information. Medical teams can provide education to parents on how disclosure is associated with improved outcomes[1] and can reassure parents that interdisciplinary team supports can be in place to support the family through the disclosure process and beyond. Parents may be eager to serve as communicators to their children but may need coaching and education from the team to serve that role well. Furthermore, consideration should be paid to the multiple and complex roles that parents may play in the communication process: "facilitators of conversation; go-between for the child and the medical team; human database for all incoming information; buffer or filter for upsetting questions or updates; communication broker to repeat or clarify potentially confusing communication; confidante for the child's private opinions or fears; ally to support expression of child preferences; and general emotional safety and support."[1] Siblings can also play an important role, with literature indicating a preference for involvement in decision-making.[7,8] Last, friends, same-aged peers, and school staff benefit from communication and sharing of information because it can

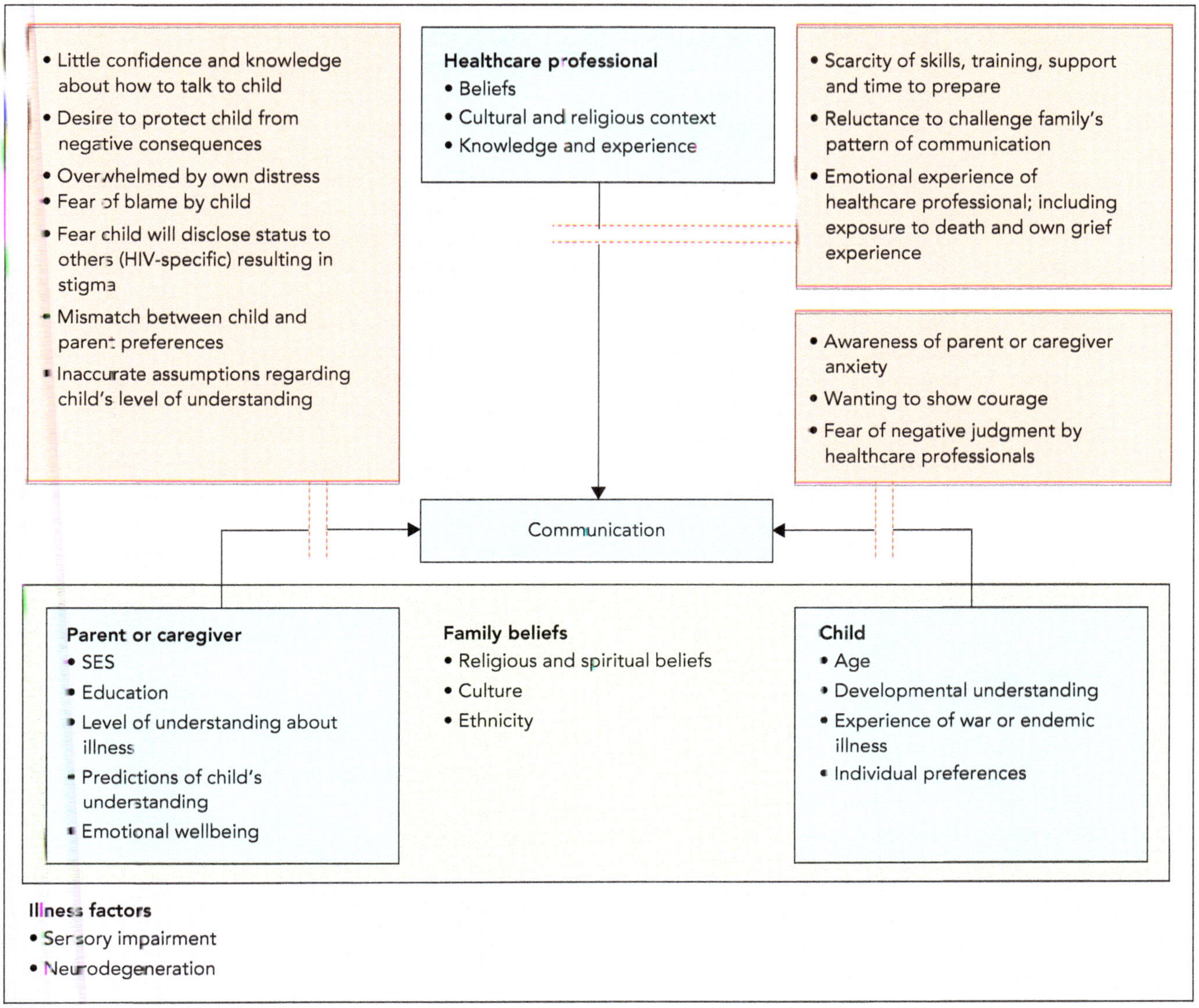

Figure 9.1 *Factors influencing communication with children about their own life-threatening condition.*

Reproduced with permission from Stein A, Dalton L, Rapa E, et al. Communication with children and adolescents about the diagnosis of their own life-threatening condition. *Lancet.* 2019;393(10175):1150–1163.

increase compassion and decrease the likelihood of future bullying of the ill child or anxiety about their own health.[9]

In addition to the child's family, friends, and community members, the medical team undoubtedly plays a transactional role in a child's and family's engagement and partnership in medical decision making. Pediatric palliative care (PPC) may be delivered by a specialty PPC team or by the child's primary medical team. The interdisciplinary PPC team is uniquely suited to work with families and children when discussing prognosis, medical decision-making, and end-of-life care. Early involvement in care alongside the primary team ensures time to build rapport, address goals, and provide support throughout the disease trajectory.

Clinicians' beliefs about disclosure to children, anxiety about how to present difficult or upsetting information, management of their own distress as care providers, and challenges when children and their parents desire differing levels of information are only a few of the factors that can lead to complication. They may take comfort in knowing that families prefer open communication; families have rated trust, honesty, and empathy as the most important traits in their medical providers when their child has been diagnosed with a life-threatening condition.[1]

CHILDREN'S VOICES, FAMILIES, AND DECISION-MAKING: ETHICAL AND PRACTICAL CONSIDERATIONS

Children's decision-making capacity is a dynamic construct. How might we develop strategies and practices to best incorporate children's voices, perspectives, and what matters most to them throughout the process of healthcare decision-making? How might we tailor our approach to engagement, information sharing, decisional scaffolding and coaching based on our understanding of human development and emerging, maturing capabilities?

The United Nations Convention on the Rights of the Child recognizes children's rights to protection, the promotion of their well-being, and participation in matters that affect their lives.[10] In 2001, the National Academy of Medicine defined patient-centered care as "care that is respectful of and responsive to individual patient preferences, needs, and values" and that ensures "that patient values guide all clinical decisions."[11] International laws and guidelines emphasize the importance of respecting the evolving capabilities and autonomy of children. Bartholome stated, "the experience, perspective and power of children" in collaboration with pediatric interdisciplinary teams and families remains a foundational guide for pediatric care.[12] Decision-making science and practice continue to evolve in response to technology, discovery, and legal rulings.[12] However, an evidence base to guide best practices in engaging children, adolescents, and young adults and integrating their voices and values in healthcare decision-making is scarce.

THE CLINICIAN-PATIENT-PARENT RELATIONSHIP AND ETHICAL PRINCIPLES

The clinician-patient-parent triadic relationship is a unique aspect of pediatric care. This triadic relationship impacts the application of foundational, universally accepted principles of medical ethics: autonomy, beneficence, nonmaleficence, and justice. The principle of *autonomy* refers to an individual's right to make decisions and act on them freely and without interference.[13] A person has a right to control what is done to his or her body and to refuse treatment, and healthcare teams have an obligation to respect patient integrity and wishes. The term *capacity* refers to the "degree to which an individual has the ability to understand a proposed therapy or procedure, including its risks, benefits, and alternatives; to communicate relevant questions; and to arrive at a decision consistent with his or her values."[14] In general, children are not believed to have capacity to make significant medical decisions, such as undergoing surgery or starting medication. However, depending on developmental stage and the particular situation, children should be invited to participate in discussions about their health and care, "recognizing and respecting the child's developing ability to participate and where appropriate, to assent."[14] Assent should be offered in situations when a child will truly have a choice in what is being proposed as all too often their opinion is solicited yet not followed. *Assent* includes the following components: helping patients achieve a developmentally appropriate awareness of the nature of his or her condition, what can be expected with tests or treatments, assessing understanding of the situation and influencing factors, and soliciting an expression of willingness to accept proposed care.[12]

The principle of *beneficence* refers to a healthcare team's obligation to act in the patient's best interest to maximize benefits and minimize burdens, such as pain and suffering. Within pediatrics, beneficence applies to both pediatric patients and their families. The principle of *nonmaleficence* holds that there is an obligation for healthcare teams to not inflict harm on others and is closely associated with the maxim *primum non nocere* ("first do no harm"). The principle of *justice* obligates us to equitably distribute healthcare-related benefits, risks, costs, and resources.[13] Within PPC, there are circumstances when the principles of beneficence, nonmaleficence, and autonomy can come into conflict.

The provider-patient-parent triadic relationship means that *surrogate decision-making* is generally the rule in pediatrics. The role of surrogate decision-maker nearly always falls to parents (or legal guardians) based on an understanding of their right to speak for and determine what is done to their child. Parental decision-making is best understood as parents' responsibility to support the interests and well-being of their child and preserve family relationships. [12] In pediatric care, the *best-interest standard* is most commonly applied and refers to a surrogate's aim to maximize benefits and minimize harms to the patient while using a holistic view of the patient's interests. The words of Jen, mother of a child with leukodystrophy, portray the complexity of parental surrogate decision-making, with the overarching goal of optimizing a child's quality of life.

Family Reflection

A Mother's Story: Jen, Mother of Alex, 3 Years Old

Two years after Alex's leukodystrophy diagnosis, he was getting some skills back and starting to learn new ones. Alex was exceeding all our expectations and that of his practitioners. He was the happiest child. He even had been managing to stay out of the hospital for a long time. Our family had focused on Alex having quality of life over quantity from the very beginning. We did things that made our family feel normal and happy like taking trips to Disney World and apple picking. We went through in vitro fertilization with preimplantation genetic diagnosis so we could expand our family and give Alex a chance to be a big brother. We were working closely with our palliative care team as well as his doctors and therapists to allow Alex to reach his potential and keep him as healthy and happy as possible.

We then took Alex to a specialized leukodystrophy center for an interdisciplinary appointment to help manage his syndrome. It was our second appointment at that clinic. These appointments were long, devastating appointments where specialist after specialist would come in the room delivering worst-case scenarios and focusing on all the things that didn't feel right for our family. When we tried to talk about our goals and hopes for our son's life and death, they were different from what the providers wanted for Alex.

After this visit, we decided we wanted to exclusively focus on care that would meet our ultimate goal of making Alex happy. We couldn't protect our son from all the ways his body would eventually fail him, but we could choose providers and treatments that allowed him to thrive as himself. We could all work together as a team to ensure that every day he had an opportunity to still smile, laugh, and be a toddler instead of a medical experiment.

It was important for our family to find its voice about how Alex would live. We followed Alex's lead, which gave him some control. We focused on treatments and therapy he enjoyed and thrived at like aqua and hippo (equestrian) therapies. We had difficult conversations with our palliative care team about Alex unexpectedly dying. We worked with our palliative care team to finalize paperwork for donating Alex's brain and lungs. We repeatedly made sure that all of Alex's providers were focusing on our family's goals for him. We are careful that interventions meet our family's goals and do not harm Alex. This has become even more important over the last year as Alex has started to decline with seizures, increased tone and spasticity, chronic pain, fevers, chilblains, and unexplained neurological events.

We have continued to work closely with our palliative care team inpatient and outpatient to make sure we are managing symptoms to allow Alex to be happy and comfortable. I believe that Alex has lived a longer and happier life than expected because we have put his palliative care at the forefront of his medical care. No matter how Alex's story ends, we know he was able to live a meaningful life filled with love and happiness.

In adult care, *substituted judgment* is the most common standard for decision-making and refers to a surrogate's aim to put a patient's stated wishes into action (regardless of whether the medical team or family considers those wishes to be "best interest"). Substituted judgment is not commonly used in pediatric care except in cases when mature adolescents have expressed wishes about goals of care, which should be respected by parents and healthcare teams.

Based on ethical theory and the law, the current concept of *informed consent* in medical practice consists of three duties: (1) providing information about the nature of the illness or condition, proposed diagnostic steps and/or treatments, and potential risks, benefits, uncertainties, and alternatives to patients and their surrogates; (2) assessment of understanding and capacity for medical decision-making, assuring time for questions by patient and surrogate; and (3) obtaining informed consent and ensuring voluntary agreement with the plan.[12] An individual must be deemed to have decision-making capacity to be able to provide informed consent for diagnostic assessments, interventions, and treatment.

SHARED DECISION-MAKING IN PEDIATRIC CARE

Shared decision-making (SDM) is foundational to patient- and family-centered care and improves knowledge, experience, adherence, and, outcomes.[15,16] Within pediatric care, SDM has been defined as a process in which patients, families, and interdisciplinary healthcare teams "simultaneously participate in all phases of the decision-making process and together arrive at a treatment plan to be implemented."[16] The SDM process is particularly challenging in pediatric care given the dynamic, complex relationship triad that "encompasses the autonomy of the patient, legal authority of the parent, and beneficence," the clinical expertise of the interdisciplinary team, and the evolving nature of these relationships as children grow and mature.[17] Eliciting, navigating, and integrating the at times conflicting perspectives and priorities of the child, parent, and clinician can be difficult, especially when few established effective, practical frameworks, tools, and interventions exist to include children and family voices within medical decision-making. (See Chapter 16, "Resolving Conflicts," for further discussion.)

A qualitative study on child and parental perspectives on communication and decision-making in pediatric chronic kidney disease (CKD) revealed four themes: (1) feeling disempowered by knowledge imbalance (unprepared and ill-informed, suspicion of censorship), (2) recognizing one's own expertise (intuition and instinct unique to parental bond, emerging wisdom and confidence, identifying opportunities for control and inclusion, and empowering participation in children), (3) striving to assert one's own priorities (negotiating broader life impacts, choosing to defer decisional burden, overprotected and overruled, and struggling to voice own preferences), and (4) managing child's involvement (respecting child's expertise, attributing "risky" behaviors to rebellion, and protecting children from illness burden) (see Figure 9.2).[17]

Fostering children's involvement in decision-making encompasses sharing information about choices and their potential impact, eliciting their voices and priorities, respecting their experience and expertise, and supporting and scaffolding their incremental involvement in decision-making as they mature. Younger children wanted to be involved in their care and decisions, particularly when choices had the potential to constrain their social freedoms and participating in normal childhood activities.[17] Adolescents and young adults had better clinical understanding and could take on more responsibilities, independence, and autonomy.[17]

There continues to be a lag in developing effective strategies and frameworks to elicit and integrate the child's perspective in decision-making. Decision aids and *coaching*, which refers to individualized facilitated discussion to prepare the patient for upcoming decision-making, have had moderate effects in improving the decision process, alignment, and satisfaction regarding information shared about options.[18,19] Visual aids, role playing, and journaling, and online and mobile applications all show promise in better engaging children in expressing their preferences, reporting symptoms, describing their feelings, accessing decision supports, and sharing information with their parents and healthcare team.[17] Snaman et al.[20] developed the *MyPref* tool for adolescents and young adult (AYA) patients with cancer to facilitate decision-making and optimize communication among stakeholders

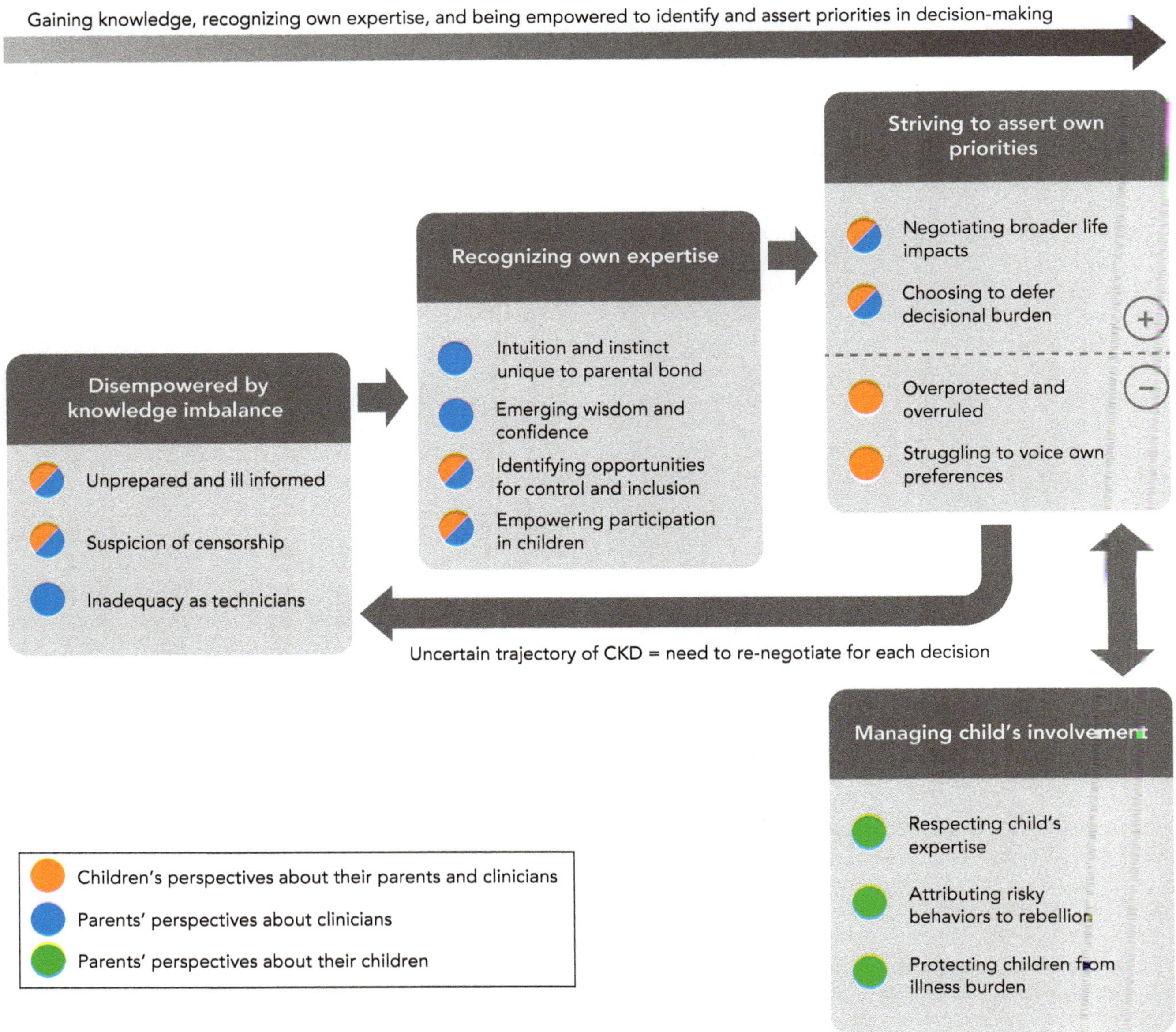

Figure 9.2 Thematic schema: Child and parent perspectives on communication and decision-making in pediatric chronic kidney disease (CKD).

Reproduced with permission from Gutman T, Hanson CS, Bernays S, et al. Child and parental perspectives on communication and decision making in pediatric CKD: A focus group study. *Am J Kidney Dis.* 2018;72(4):547–559.

to ensure delivery of goal-concordant care. *MyPref* tool, which factors in treatment considerations, quality of life, symptoms and side effects, and survival, provides an opportunity for AYA patients and their parents/trusted persons to "clarify their preferences in an objective way and empowers them to actively participate in decision-making." Children, adolescents, young adults, parents, families, and interdisciplinary healthcare teams must come together to design the next generation of innovative, effective SDM strategies, frameworks, and tools.

CULTURE, DIVERSITY AND DECISION-MAKING

Families' core values, beliefs, communication, relational dynamics, and other aspects of culture influence the decision-making process. Culture can be defined as "a dynamic, adaptive, ecologically based multilevel and multidimensional system for a population group that creates a social structure, which provides its members a set of beliefs, expectations, and tangible means to achieve a sense of safety, identity, and meaning of and for life."[21] Through an integrative review of palliative care literature, Cain et al. demonstrate how culture matters in the provision of high-quality palliative care in four areas: (1) preferences for care, (2) communication patterns, (3) meanings of suffering, and (4) decision-making processes.[21] With respect to decision-making, differences arise across cultures in their orientation toward individualism or communalism and how individuals express or suppress their autonomy. US laws concerning decision-making prioritize autonomy as the most important principle. Yong's clinical vignette highlights how cultural and family factors impact preferences, communication patterns, and decision-making.

Differences in decision-making processes and preferences are seen in the completion of formal advance directives. However, some families prefer to communicate their wishes verbally, are reluctant to discuss advance directives, and place their trust in caring relationships with clinicians. Religious and spiritual beliefs also affect decision-making through the belief that a higher power makes the ultimate decisions. Clinicians should be aware of implicit bias and become skilled in eliciting diverse beliefs, values, and having difficult conversations with an emphasis on humility and openness rather than on overgeneralizations and stereotypes.[21] From a societal health disparities perspective, research indicates that racial and ethnic minorities are less likely than non-Hispanic whites to have access to quality care, including standard medical, experimental, and palliative care, and suffer higher morbidity and lower quality of life in comparison.[22,23]

Yong's story illustrates how medical decision-making is impacted by the critical role of culture, a child or adolescent's emotional state, and the family system.

Team Reflection

Yong, 18 Years Old

Yong is a Chinese American 18-year-old with a history of Duchenne muscular dystrophy (DMD), profound scoliosis, paraplegia, restrictive lung disease with obstructive sleep apnea, cardiomyopathy, dysphagia, malnutrition, and major depressive disorder. Yong had been receiving interdisciplinary care at the muscular dystrophy clinic since the age of 11 years. He lived at home in a one-bedroom apartment with his father, mother, and two younger siblings. Yong's parents were Mandarin-speaking only and frequently declined interpreters. Throughout the years, Yong's general health deteriorated. His weakness worsened, and he was unable to feed himself, leading to significant weight loss. He became dependent on his parents for bladder and bowel care, and most notably he required rectal stimulation for all passage of stool. His lung function slowly deteriorated, and he required nighttime noninvasive positive pressure ventilation (NIPPV), an intervention he was generally not amenable to. Yong had once enjoyed going to school, playing video games, and interacting with friends and family; however, over time he became ashamed of his condition and started missing school and medical appointments.

When Yong was able to come to clinic, it was frequently with his father, as his mother was home caring for his siblings and worked part time in a restaurant. Clinic visits were distressing for Yong as his father insisted on speaking to the team alone regarding the progressive nature of his son's disease. His father often noted that he wished to protect his son from discussions regarding medical decision-making and prognosis as "Yong would give up hope if he knew how bad his disease is" and "what's the point of telling him all these details. He probably doesn't understand anyway." When clinical providers asked if they could disclose facts about Yong's diagnosis, his parents shared that in their culture it was uncommon for family members to know all the details about their illness.

At age 16, Yong confided in his social worker and expressed his understanding regarding DMD from his own independent online research. He presented with depressed mood, anhedonia, and a general sense of hopelessness in relation to his decreased function and poor prognosis. Yong often expressed passive suicidal ideations and explained, "What's the point of living now when I know what's in store for me." Due to insurance issues and limited access to mental health providers in the area, Yong was unable to establish longitudinal outpatient care with a mental health provider.

Over time, Yong lost the ability to use a motorized wheelchair, which had devastating consequences to his quality of life and mobility outside the house. Both parents valued their privacy and were hesitant to allow medical staff into the home due to limited space. Yong was home schooled for a period of time; however, due to his significant depressive symptoms he would frequently sleep through sessions and choose not to engage with teachers. His father often stated that his son would receive better care at a facility; however, Yong said that he would rather "die than live in a nursing home" and enjoyed the company of his siblings and parents.

After a pediatric intensive care unit (PICU) admission for pneumonia requiring intubation, two medical interventions were discussed with the family, and, at the team's request, Yong was included. A tracheostomy and gastrostomy tube were offered to prolong his life. Yong was vehemently against either recommendation and frequently asked "to die" instead. He expressed concerns about his current quality of life and how he could not imagine living with the aid of medical technology. Yong would have to live at a long-term care (LTC) facility with a tracheostomy and mechanical ventilation because his family's apartment was too small to accommodate the extensive equipment required. However, after much discussion with his primary providers and PICU staff, the decision was made to proceed with tracheostomy and gastrostomy placement as his parents felt this was the only option that matched their goals to improve and extend Yong's life. Due to Yong's depressive symptoms, which impacted his decision-making capacity, it was also determined that he could not make decisions for himself.

A tracheostomy and gastrostomy tube were placed, and Yong spent approximately 6 months in the hospital due to complications and limited availability of LTC facilities capable of caring for patients with tracheostomies and ventilators. Yong frequently stated that he would rather be at home than in a facility, which created great distress for his inpatient interdisciplinary caregivers. He was eventually transferred to a LTC facility, where he lived for about a year. At 18 years old, Yong was readmitted to the hospital for a respiratory infection, and upon discussion with the palliative care team, a do-not-resuscitate (DNR) order was placed in the chart reflecting his wishes. The palliative care team further explored his choices regarding being placed back on the ventilator or not being treated with antibiotics. Yong's parents continued to remain involved in decision-making for their son, with the hope that he would choose life-prolonging measures.

Yong's situation is not uncommon and highlights a frequent experience for clinicians as they attempt to simultaneously respect complex family and cultural systems while focusing on quality of life and child well-being.

IMPACT OF ILLNESS ACROSS THE CONTINUUM: CHILDREN, FAMILIES AND THE INTERDISCIPLINARY HEALTHCARE TEAM

DIAGNOSIS AND PROGNOSIS

As discussed previously, parents often refrain from delivering bad news in an effort to protect their children. This basic parental instinct should not be overlooked. Parents experience profound grief when hearing their child has a life-threatening illness, which is compounded by the idea of disclosing the diagnosis. A mother of a teen with a newly diagnosed diffuse intrinsic pontine glioma (DIPG) once tearfully stated, "I can barely comprehend what lies ahead; it makes me sick to imagine telling my son he has a year to live." Families agonize over what information should be shared and by whom. Barriers to parents disclosing poor prognosis to their child (as described through self-report) include emotional distress and information overload, inadequate knowledge on how to disclose, and worry over burdening their children with bad news.[24]

There is an extensive history of clinicians also feeling uncomfortable engaging in difficult discussions regarding diagnosis and prognosis for fear of taking away hope and causing distress.[25,26] For physicians, this fear frequently comes from a lack of training in medical schools and residency programs on how to communicate difficult news.[26] The hesitancy of clinicians to discuss a poor prognosis can lead to patients misjudging their chance of cure or life prolongation, which may impact their decision-making.[25] In an effort to avoid openly discussing poor prognosis, clinicians often use optimistic language and frequently wait for patients and families to ask specific questions directed at prognosis.[27]

A recent study of adolescents and young adults with cystic fibrosis (CF) revealed that patients with CF want their parents to be involved in discussions regarding prognosis and believe that their physician should be the one to initiate such disclosures.[28] Approximately one-third of the study participants reported learning of their prognosis and clinical trajectory from their CF healthcare providers, one-third deduced the progressive nature of CF from their own health decline, and the rest gleaned this knowledge from their parents or from online sources.[28] The patient participants often felt that prognosis was "sugar-coated" by whomever disclosed the information, be it providers or parents. Interestingly, when patients learned of their prognosis, 62% reported no impact on future CF treatments and 38% reported a positive impact on their attitude. None of the study participants reported that disclosure had a negative impact on their emotional state or adherence to treatment regimens. The majority (77%) of patients reported that learning of their prognosis had no effect on their overall goals of care and life plans, and, if it did, it was positive.[28]

Although the evidence-base supports developmentally appropriate, open, and honest disclosure of diagnosis and prognosis, the matter is complex and case-dependent.[26] In the field of PPC (and pediatrics in general), it is imperative to view the child as part of a larger family infrastructure influenced by history, values, culture, and religion. In particular, culture and religion may weigh heavily on a parent's willingness to disclose diagnosis and prognosis.[26] In some cases, parents may instruct medical personnel to omit facts regarding a diagnosis and, in rare cases, to even lie. In these cases, clinicians can offer a "compromise" that strikes a balance between respecting a family's wishes and maintaining trust and alliance with their patient. Helpful phrasing may include "we will honor your communication preferences with your adolescent, however if they ask us direct questions regarding their disease and prognosis, we cannot lie." This compromise will most often require several back-and-forth negotiations—the concept of "shuttle diplomacy"[29]—toward an approach that feels more comfortable for everyone. Unfortunately, these negotiations are often fraught with distress from the interdisciplinary healthcare team, especially in cases involving adolescents. Clinicians may feel that a family's cultural or religious traditions clash with ethical standards of medical care and that they are not able "to do what's right by their patient." In these instances, it is helpful to further explore the family's values and belief systems with a focus on respecting these beliefs.[26] Discussion with parents and children regarding prognosis may evolve and shift over time as an illness progresses.[26] It is also important to note that for some families who are disinclined to open communication and prognostication, repetitive attempts at disclosure can cause undue distress to the patient and family. In these cases, the risk of negatively impacting a family's experience with illness and grief may outweigh the benefit of total disclosure. Maintaining the treatment alliance and trust, openness to compromise when required, and honesty when questions are posed directly are all of paramount importance.

As discussed, every family system functions differently and has its own unique communication preferences.[26] To build trust and rapport, clinicians must respect the framework and preferences of the family first and foremost. After receiving permission from the family to disclose diagnosis, medical information, and prognosis, finding the right time, environment, interdisciplinary team members, and developmentally appropriate language is imperative for effective communication.[30] Once the stage is set, it is crucial to address the child's goals, hopes, worries, understanding of illness, and coping mechanisms.

The *Five Cardinal Questions* listed here[31] explore goals of care with patients and families before addressing medical decision-making. Once the patient and family's goals of care are established, treatment decisions are more likely to fall into place. Many initial PPC team consults start with these five questions and often include the additional questions listed. When addressing an adolescent or young adult, these five questions will also help build rapport and trust with the interdisciplinary clinical team. The end result ideally represents the adolescent's voice as a person rather than as a patient. The PPC team frequently utilizes some of these questions throughout the illness trajectory. For instance, the answer to "What are your hopes?" may shift significantly as the patient's disease progresses. It is encouraged that all providers integrate these questions into their routine practice, especially when establishing a new relationship with a patient and family.

1. Tell me about yourself as a person. What do you like to do when you're outside the hospital? What does a good day look like?
2. What has your healthcare team been telling you about your illness/diagnosis? What's your understanding?
3. Knowing what you know about your illness, what's most important to you? What are you hoping for? Big hopes and little ones.
4. What are you worried about most? What are your fears?
5. What gives you strength? How well is that working for you?
6. How are you/your family managing day to day?
7. How do you make decisions? Do you involve your parents, grandparents, friends?
8. How do you like to receive information? Visuals, literature, discussion?
9. How are you managing day-to-day?

DECISION-MAKING AROUND TREATMENT INITIATION AND ADHERENCE

There is evidence to suggest that involving pediatric patients in medical decision-making enhances their coping with illness and allows them to maintain a sense of control.[32,33] For young children, this may amount to small decisions in their care, such as offering choice around when to take a medication or where to place an IV.[33] Engaging child life specialists, bedside nurses, and the family can be helpful in creating choices for children, who often lose a sense of control, especially in the inpatient setting.

Ensuring the child's voice in medical decision-making should be standard of care; however, for the reasons discussed earlier, this is not always feasible. Mack et al. note that adolescents and young adults with oncologic diagnoses frequently wish to be active participants in decision-making; however, they are not always given the chance.[34] In their 2019 study, 58% of adolescents and young adults hoped to share cancer treatment decision-making with their oncologists, and 51% favored limited involvement from their parents.[34] Unfortunately, a quarter of that cohort expressed decisional regret frequently linked to limited trust and mutual understanding with their oncologist. As noted previously, Farber et al. found that patients with CF expressed that disclosure of prognosis had limited effect on their adherence to treatment.[28] This further validates the notion that disclosing poor prognosis and involving children in treatment decisions does not equate to the pediatric patient losing hope, "giving up," or discontinuing treatment.

In the following account, a young adult with CF illustrates the complex interplay of knowledge of prognosis and adherence to treatment.

Family Reflection

Finding My Voice: Faith, 23 Years Old

I have been lucky to find my voice over the years through my cystic fibrosis journey; however, it has its costs. Guilt, shame, and even worry are only some of the costs I pay for my autonomy. Because I have a beautiful relationship with my healthcare team, I don't want to disappoint them. And I often feel ashamed for not following through with the regimen that has been set forth; I am labeled as "noncompliant." I feel guilty when I make decisions to do things differently, because I may have another option when other patients may not. Sometimes I feel guilty when I can afford these medications and let them expire while other people would die for my health status or financial security. Knowing that I'm "one of the lucky ones" because I have my health doesn't mean I'm free of hospitalizations or mandatory medications; even when I'm healthy, I am still sick. I am worried that I've taken my health for granted just as everyone has warned. I worry when I'm really sick if I've pushed myself too far. I worry even when something goes right. I will say that even these emotions could not take away the importance of freedom for me. I do have my health, and I do have a voice. So let me enjoy it until I can't any longer, until all of my options are gone. Working through these feelings with the help of interdisciplinary care has completely changed my outlook on my diagnosis. Every aspect of my health is being considered, and cystic fibrosis is no longer all that I am in the hospital environment. I would give a lot of credit for my health status to the interdisciplinary part of my team. Without them, the transition into adult care would be unbearable. This is my team, and I'm the head coach.

Faith, 23 years old, diagnosed at 8 months old

APPROACHING DEATH

Discussing the dying process with a pediatric patient can induce significant anxiety and distress for the patient, parent, and interdisciplinary team. As with disclosing poor prognosis, parents and clinicians seek to protect their patients from distressing information and generally wait until death is imminent to initiate this difficult conversation.[35] Kreicbergs et al.'s 2004 study of 429 Swedish parents who had a child die of cancer found that, overall, no family who had talked to their child about dying regretted sharing that information. However, 27% of parents who did not talk to their child about dying regretted not sharing that information.[36] At first glance, these findings support a recommendation for parents to discuss dying with their child to prevent decisional regret. However, it is important to note that while 27% of parents who did not talk to their child about dying experienced regret, the other 73% of parents in this cohort did not feel regret. Furthermore, and as discussed previously, culture and religion influence a family's ability to engage is such discussion.

Before starting the conversation, it is again imperative to partner with the family to address their views on disclosure. After addressing communication preferences, asking permission from the adolescent or young adult to discuss this difficult topic allows them the choice to engage or not. It is generally assumed that, similar to their desired involvement in decision-making and understanding prognosis, adolescents and young adults wish to engage in conversations regarding death and dying. Interestingly, Jacobs et al. noted that 75% of adolescents wished to discuss end-of-life decisions; however, 12% were not comfortable at all. [37] Interdisciplinary teams should continually reassess pediatric patient's readiness and willingness to discuss death and dying, as this may shift over time. It is best practice to follow patients' lead and respect their decision if they do not wish to engage in such discussions.[26] It is important to know that even when children do not "appear" to know that they are at the end of life, many do, in fact, have that understanding.[26] They may act as if they do not know in order to protect their parents.[38]

When the decision has been made to discuss dying and death with a pediatric patient, the PPC team can recommend helpful strategies and language to prepare families for difficult questions while respecting their wishes. A child may ask the question: "Am I dying?" which can catch a parent and clinician off guard. A parent's instinct may be to immediately offer reassurance by answering: "No, we are going to get through this." Instead, it is suggested that the parent pause and ask the question: "Why are you asking me this right now?" which can help guide their answer. Children may then express their worries about symptoms, timing, and fear of the unknown. Parents can then respond with these example phases: "You are very sick right now and the team is worried that you won't get better and will die. But you are not dying right now. Would you want to know if you are closer to dying?" Or "You are very sick and will soon be dying, however you will never be alone and the team will help you feel as comfortable as possible." Parents and clinicians should receive frequent guidance and support surrounding these very difficult discussions.

Team Reflection

Mateo, 19 Years Old

Mateo was diagnosed with osteosarcoma 3 months after moving to the United States from Guatemala. Along with his three young adult cousins, Mateo left his parents and three younger siblings to work in the United States and send money back home. As he adjusted to life in New York City, he began to feel a dull pain in his leg and found himself struggling to keep up with his cousins on the soccer field. Soccer was his passion and outlet, and while playing he felt closest to home. His pain persisted. His cousins first noticed that his leg was dragging, then he was limping, and eventually Mateo was not able to bear any weight. His cousins carried him into the emergency room.

The osteosarcoma was quickly diagnosed. He underwent initial surgery to remove the tumor and began intensive rounds of chemotherapy and radiation, followed by an above-the-knee amputation. Secondary to the demands of treatment, Mateo was no longer able to work and spent most of his days alone while his cousins continued to work to support him and his family. During his first meeting with his outpatient social worker, Mateo described himself as "hopeful, lonely, and in desperate need of help." He had difficulty with his inferior living conditions. Furthermore, his limited psychosocial support and his parent's inability to travel to the United States forced Mateo to be his own advocate to make decisions about his treatment.

During his 2 ½ years of treatment, Mateo forged a strong bond with his two social workers (inpatient and outpatient), who, in partnership with his oncologist and eventually the PPC team, diligently guided him through each of his care decisions. Paramount were decisions about how to proceed following recurrence of disease and subsequent pulmonary metastasis (more surgery and chemotherapy) and further exploration into ways to optimize his quality of life. Mateo had excellent insight into the severity of his disease, the significance of the recurrence, and that, sadly, he would not be cured. He expressed fear of suffering, both physical and emotional; despite that fear, he focused on making decisions that "came from my heart." The sicker he became, the more he sought out opportunities to discuss his complex feelings and thoughts around dying, stating "I am not afraid to die" and affirming that his spiritually and faith in God would guide him.

Throughout the course of his illness journey, Mateo was steadfast in his capacity and ability to choose happiness over sadness, believing that embracing moments of joy through painting, laughing with his cousins, playing music, talking with his social workers, and prayer made him feel better. Indeed, these moments of joy gave him hope that he could still have control despite his ongoing pain, chronic coughing, extended hospitalizations, and, ultimately, his death.

The PPC team and Mateo's social worker began having advance care planning conversations with him and his cousins, and he remained committed to wanting to be comfortable, safe, and surrounded by love. Shortly after his medical orders for life-sustaining treatment (MOLST) was completed and in the chart, Mateo's social worker introduced the advance care planning guide, Five Wishes (see later discussion). Five Wishes helped Mateo to describe what good end-of-life care would look like to him and allowed him to make decisions about his death. This was important as he also expressed that he did not want to burden his cousins or family back home in Guatemala with making decisions for him. He also specified that he did not want to suffer or experience pain as he transitioned through end of life. He understood that, even in death, he had choices about where he wanted to die. Most importantly, Five Wishes allowed him to make decisions about his funeral, which meant that he could finally return home. After his death, Mateo's social workers were able to secure funding to cover the cost of his funeral as well as the costs to transfer his body back to Guatemala for burial. In the end, Mateo's interdisciplinary care team felt humbled and honored that they were able to help him make decisions that "came from his heart."

DECISION-MAKING TOOLS: FIVE WISHES AND VOICING MY CHOICES, VOICING MY WISHES, AND FAMILY-CENTERED PEDIATRIC ADVANCE CARE PLANNING

Five Wishes[39] was created by Aging with Dignity, in partnership with the American Bar Association's Commission on Law and Aging. It is a simple and easy to use living will, written in plain language to help patients express their wishes in the areas that matter most: the personal, spiritual, medical, and legal. The document is published in 27 languages and contains check boxes and spaces for the patient to write their own thoughts.

Voicing My Choices[40] A Planning Guide for Adolescents and Young Adults and Voicing My Wishes for younger children are also created by Aging with Dignity in partnership with the Pediatric Oncology Branch, National Cancer Institute, and the National Institutes of Mental Health at the National Institute of Heath. Both Voicing My Choices and Voicing My Wishes are easy to use workbooks that are meant to help young children, teens, and young adults express their voice/wishes for when they are living with a serious, life-threatening illness. Similar to the Five Wishes, both are valuable therapeutic guides to help children and teens think through how they want to be supported and remembered while giving them the opportunity to decide how they want to live during the dying process. Both tools allow children, teens, and young adults the opportunity to complete as many sections as they choose, and each section has check boxes and space to write their own narrative. For example, the first section in My Wishes is entitled *Wish #1 My Wish for How I Want People to Treat Me* very clearly and simply invites the child to check as many boxes they want:

- I wish to be cared for with kindness and cheerfulness.
- I wish to have my hand held and to be talked to whenever possible.
- I wish people would pray for me.
- I wish to have my favorite things with me if possible. My favorite things are: ______________________________

____

Family/Adolescent-Centered Pediatric Advance Care Planning (FACE)[41] is a structured advance care planning guide that helps providers facilitate advance care planning discussions with teenage patients and their families with the aim of better understanding and honoring the adolescent patient's wishes. FACE has been utilized with adolescents with a variety of life-limiting conditions, such as cancer, HIV, and rare diseases. This highly structured intervention is comprised of three 60-minute sessions with a trained/certified interviewer. In a multisite randomized, controlled trial, FACE was conducted when the patient was medically stable; the instrument was found to respect individual differences, acknowledging those who prefer to have their doctor or family make these decisions for them or who are interested but not ready and promote SDM. It is conducted by certified/trained facilitators utilizing a structured curriculum.

CONCLUSION

In summary, when children are diagnosed with a life-threatening or life-limiting condition, it is important to ensure that both their voice and the voice of their family are heard at the outset of diagnosis, during discussion of prognosis and treatment options, and through the process of end of life. Consideration should be paid to developmental, cognitive, and learning levels of the child and family, as well as to the values, beliefs, emotional states, and coping capacity of all involved. Interdisciplinary PPC care teams play a crucial role in providing developmentally tailored, family-centered information about conditions and choices, helping children and their families find their voices in decision-making, navigating conflicts and challenges in treatment and advance care planning, and improving the experience and outcome of care for everyone involved. Children, adolescents, young adults, families, and interdisciplinary healthcare teams must come together to develop the next generation of innovative, effective SDM strategies, frameworks, skills, and tools.

REFERENCES

1. Stein A, Dalton L, Rapa E, et al. Communication with children and adolescents about the diagnosis of their own life-threatening condition. *Lancet.* 2019;393(10176):1150–1163.
2. Slaughter V. Young children's understanding of death. *Aust Psychol.* 2005;40:179–186.
3. Eiser C. Children's concepts of illness: Towards an alternative to the "stage" approach. *Psychol Health* 1989;3:93–101.

4. Grootens-Wiegers P, Hein IM, van den Broek JM, de Vries MC. Medical decision-making in children and adolescents: Developmental and neuroscientific aspects. *BMC Pediatrics*. 2017;17:120.
5. Taylor SJ, Barker LA, Heavey L, McHale S. The longitudinal development of social and executive functions in late adolescence and early adulthood. *Front Behav Neurosci*. 2015 Sept 15;9:252.
6. Kessler RC, Angermeyer M, Anthony JC, et al. Lifetime prevalence and age-of-onset distributions of mental disorders in the World Health Organization's World Mental Health Survey Initiative. *World Psychiatry*. 2007;6:168–176.
7. Wiener L, McConnell D, Latella L, Ludi E. Cultural and religious considerations in pediatric palliative care. *Palliat Support Care*. 2013;11(1), 47–67.
8. Gaab EM, Owens GR, MacLeod RD. Siblings caring for and about pediatric palliative care patients. *J Palliat Med*. 2014 Jan;17(1):62–67.
9. Hay GH, Nabors ML, Sullivan A, Zygmund A. Students with pediatric cancer: A prescription for school success. *Phys Disabil Educ Related Serv*. 2015, 34(2):1–13.
10. United Nations. *Convention on the Rights of the Child*. London: UNICEF; 1989.
11. Institute of Medicine (IOM). *Crossing the Quality Chasm: A New Health System for the 21st Century*. Washington, DC: National Academies Press; 2001.
12. AAP Committee on Bioethics. Informed consent in decision-making in pediatric practice. *Pediatrics*. 2016 Aug;138(2): e20161484
13. Beauchamp TL, Childress JF. *Principles of Biomedical Ethics*. 6th ed. Oxford: Oxford University Press; 2009.
14. Cummings CL, Mercurio MR. Ethics for the pediatrician: Autonomy, beneficence, and rights. *Pediatr Rev*. 2010 Jun;31(6):252–255.
15. Fiks AG, Localio AR, Alessandrini EA, Asch DA, Guevara JP. Shared decision-making in pediatrics: A national perspective. *Pediatrics*. 2010 Aug;126(2):306–314.
16. Adams RC, Levy SE. AAP Council on Children with Disabilities. Shared decision-making and children with disabilities: Pathways to consensus. *Pediatrics*. 2017;139(6): e20170956.
17. Gutman T, Hanson CS, Bernays S, et al. Child and parental perspectives on communication and decision making in pediatric CKD: A focus group study. *Am J Kidney Dis*. 2018;72(4):547–559.
18. Feenstra B, Boland L, Lawson ML, et al. Interventions to support children's engagement in health-related decisions: A systematic review. *BMC Pediatrics*. 2014;14:109.
19. Malone H, Biggar S, Javadpour S, Edworthy Z, Sheaf G, Coyne I. Interventions for promoting participation in shared decision-making for children and adolescents with cystic fibrosis. *Cochrane Database Syst Rev*. 2019;Issue 5.
20. Snaman JM, Blazin L, Holder RL, Wolfe J, Baker JN. Identifying and Quantifying Adolescent and Young Adult Patient Preferences in Cancer Care: Development of a Conjoint Analysis-Based Decision-Making Tool. *J Adolesc Young Adult Oncol*. 2019 Apr;8(2):212–216. Epub 2018 Oct 25.
21. Cain C, Surbone A, Elk R, Kagawa-Singer M. Culture and palliative care: Preferences, communication, meaning, and mutual decision making. *J Pain Symptom Manage*. 2018 May;55(5):1408–1419.
22. Institute of Medicine. *Unequal Treatment: Confronting Racial and Ethnic Disparities in Health Care*. Washington, DC: National Academies Press; 2003. https://doi.org/10.17226/10260
23. Institute of Medicine. *Dying in America: Improving Quality and Honoring Individual Preferences Near the End of Life*. Washington, DC: National Academies Press; 2015.
24. Badarau DO, Wangmo T, Ruhe KM, et al. Parents' challenges and physicians' tasks in disclosing cancer to children: A qualitative interview study and reflections on professional duties in pediatric oncology. *Pediatr Blood Cancer*. 2015;62(12):2177–2182.
25. Mack JW, Fasciano KM, Block SD. Communication about prognosis with adolescent and young adult patients with cancer: Information needs, prognostic awareness, and outcomes of disclosure. *J Clin Oncol*. 2018;*36*(18):1861–1867.
26. Sisk BA, Bluebond-Langner M, Wiener L, Mack J, Wolfe J. Prognostic disclosures to children: An historical perspective. *Pediatrics*. 2016;138(3):e20161278.
27. Mack JW, Joffe S. Communicating about prognosis: Ethical responsibilities of pediatricians and parents. *Pediatrics*. 2014;133(suppl 1): S24–S30.
28. Farber JG, Prieur MG, Roach C, et al. Difficult conversations: Discussing prognosis with children with cystic fibrosis. *Pediatr Pulmonol*. 2018;53(5):592–598.
29. Bluebond-Langner M, Cico A, Belasco J. Involving children with life shortening illness in discussion about participation in clinical research: A proposal for shuttle diplomacy and negotiation. *Ethics Res Child*. 2005;323–343.
30. Olszewski AE, Goldkind SF. The default position: Optimizing pediatric participation in medical decision making. *Am J Bioethics*. 2018;18(3):4–9.
31. Waldman E, Wolfe J. Palliative care for children with cancer. *Nature Rev Clin Oncol*. 2013;*10*(2):100–107. doi:10.1038/nrclinonc.2012.23
32. Knopf JM, Hornung RW, Slap GB, DeVellis RF, Britto MT. Views of treatment decision making from adolescents with chronic illnesses and their parents: A pilot study. *Health Expect*. 2008;11:343–354
33. Gumidyala AP, Plevinsky JM, Poulopoulos N, Kahn SA, Walkiewicz, R, Greenley N. What teens do not know can hurt them: An assessment of disease knowledge in adolescents and young adults with IBD. *Inflam Bowel Dis*. 2017;23(1):89–96.
34. Mack JW, Fasciano KM, Block SD. Adolescent and young adult cancer patients' experiences with treatment decision-making. *Pediatrics*, 2019;143(5):1–10.
35. Marsac ML, Kindler C. Weiss D, Ragsdale L. Lets talk about Ii: Supporting family communication during end-of-life care of pediatric patients. *J Palliat Med*. 2018;21(6), 862–878.
36. Kreicbergs U Valdimarsdóttir U Onelöv E Henter J.-I Steineck G. Talking about death with children who have severe malignant disease. *N Engl J Med*. 2014;351(12):1175–1186.
37. Jacobs S, Perez J, Cheng YI, Sill A, Wang J, Lyon ME. Adolescent end of life preferences and congruence with their parents' preferences: Results of a survey of adolescents with cancer. *Pediatr Blood Cancer*. 2015;62(4):710–771.
38. Bluebond-Langner M, Belasco JB, DeMesquita Wander M. "I want to live, until I don't want to live anymore": Involving children with life-threatening and life-shortening illnesses in decision making about care and treatment. *Nurs Clin North Am*. 2010;45(3):329–343.
39. Five Wishes Organization. Learn about advance care planning: Five Wishes. 2019. https://fivewishes.org/five-wishes/individuals-families/individuals-and-families/advance-care-planning.
40. Five Wishes Organization. Children and young adults: Five Wishes. 2019. https://fivewishes.org/five-wishes/individuals families/individuals-and-families/children-and-adolescents
41. Lyon ME, Garvie PA, Briggs L, He J, McCarter R, D'Angelo LJ. Development, feasibility, and acceptability of the Family/Adolescent-Centered (FACE) Advance Care Planning intervention for adolescents with HIV. *J Palliat Med*. 2009;12(4):363–372.

10 | FAMILY EXPERIENCE AND RELATIONSHIPS

KIM MOONEY-DOYLE, MEGHAN L. MARSAC, ELISSA G. MILLER, JANET A. DEATRICK, AND MELISSA A. ALDERFER

> We all come from families. Families are big, small, extended, nuclear; multigenerational, with one parent, two parents and grandparents. We live under one roof or many. A family can be as temporary as a few weeks, as permanent as forever. We become part of a family by birth, adoption, marriage, or from a desire for mutual support. As family members, we nurture, protect and influence one another. Families are dynamic and are cultures unto themselves, with different values and unique ways of realizing dreams. Together, our families become the source of our rich cultural heritage and spiritual diversity. Each family has strengths and qualities that flow from individual members and from the family as a unit. Our families create neighborhoods, communities, states, and nations.
>
> Attributed to the New Mexico's Memorial Task Force on Children and Families and the Coalition for Children (p. 394)[1]

Families are crucial to the development, well-being, and health of children. When a child is diagnosed with a serious medical condition, all members of the family, as well as the overall functioning of the family, are affected. The delivery of effective family-centered pediatric palliative care requires attention to the family experience of the diagnosis, treatment, and course of the medical condition, as well as the impact of these factors on family relationships and functioning.

The initial diagnosis of a serious illness is often shocking and especially devastating when the prognosis is poor. Everyone within the family interprets and reacts in his or her own way to such news. Family members' reactions are dynamic and interdependent and affect their relationships with one another, both in the moment and over time. Reactions grow and change as family members incorporate the reality of their situation, garner resources, confront new challenges, and adapt and readjust their lives. Suddenly, parents may need to make life-altering medical decisions and must incorporate the illness and treatment into ongoing family life. Parents may also need to learn how to prioritize critical child-rearing responsibilities for both their ill child and their well children. They may need to renegotiate their roles and responsibilities with their partners and others in the family system. Siblings of the child with the medical condition may be confused about what is happening to their brother or sister. They may experience changes in their routines, including repeated or extended separations from immediate family. Along with their concern and caring, they may also struggle with difficult emotions of anger, jealousy, and guilt. Furthermore, the family must interface with a new system—the healthcare system—which can be confusing and difficult to navigate.

While the role of the family may shift and change over time, seriously ill children generally depend on their family for physical care, medical decision-making, implementation of treatment plans, and emotional support. As a result, the ways in which a family responds to a serious pediatric health condition affects the ill child's experience with healthcare and health outcomes.[2,3] Stable and secure family environments support behaviors needed for appropriate management of the condition, help buffer negative emotional reactions to the illness and treatment, and ensure that normative developmental goals are accomplished by the family and its members. For example, adherence to treatment and medical outcomes are better for children with serious illnesses when families function well.[4] Red flags in family functioning include difficulty problem-solving and/or managing and integrating the treatment regimen into daily routines; poor communication, oversight, and monitoring; and family relationships characterized by conflict, hostility, and emotional overinvolvement.[5–9] In short, the health and well-being of children with serious illness are inextricably woven into the functioning of the family system while the child's medical condition and its treatment impacts the functioning of the family.

The overall purpose of this chapter is to describe the experiences of families throughout their child's illness trajectory and to outline the implications of these experiences for the delivery of pediatric palliative care (PPC). The chapter begins by describing three guiding frameworks that can help conceptualize the experience of the family at different levels. First, the social ecology model provides an overarching framework for understanding the various social systems within which a developing child is embedded and with which their family interacts. How this framework applies specifically to children with serious illness and their families is explained. Second, family systems theory is described with reference to specific models of family functioning in the context of serious pediatric illness. These models provide guidance regarding important aspects of family functioning and describe patterns of family-system level responses across time. The third model places the focus on individual family members and their relationships with one another within the frameworks of loss and traumatic stress. While presenting these conceptual models, the chapter presents examples from the empirical literature illustrating the impact of serious pediatric health conditions on the family members and the family system. Finally, the chapter concludes by presenting implications of these models and the empirical evidence for the delivery of trauma-informed, family-centered PPC.

CONCEPTUALIZING THE FAMILY IN CONTEXT: THE SOCIAL ECOLOGY MODEL

A substantial body of literature supports the value of using the social ecology model to organize our understanding of the experiences of families of children with serious medical conditions.[10,11] This model provides a theory-based framework for understanding how different layers of social systems impact the everyday lives of children and their families. According to the social ecological model, the development of every child is influenced by personal characteristics (e.g., gender, biological predispositions, thoughts, beliefs, and behaviors), social settings, and contexts in which they are embedded.[12] Bronfenbrenner's model defines four layers of social systems that impact the developing child differentially across time and the child's life span. These systems are referred to as the macrosystem, exosystem, mesosystems, and microsystems (Figure 10.1).

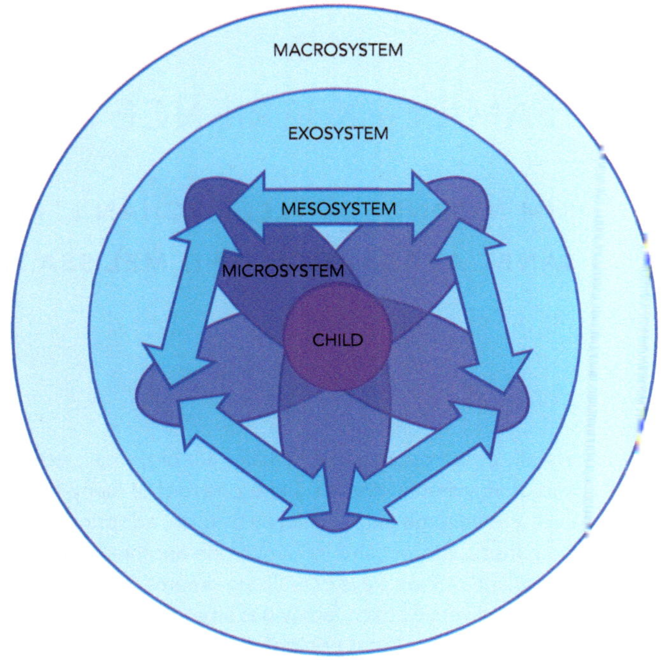

Figure 10.1 *Components of the social ecology model.*

The broadest context in which the child is embedded is termed the *macrosystem* and is defined by the society and culture in which the child lives. Examples of macrosystem influences include cultural and ideological values and forces (e.g., individualism, systemic racism), the global and national economy, health, housing, education and public policy (e.g., universality of healthcare), and governmental regulations and law. Of special concern for children with serious medical conditions are the social determinants of health and the structural impediments (e.g., health policy, racism, health inequities) that influence the health outcomes of children.[13] More proximal to the developing child is the *exosystem*, those social systems with which the child may not have direct day-to-day contact but that impact the child in a broader way. For example, these social systems include the parent's workplace (e.g., benefits, leave policies), mass media, and community resources (e.g., local economics, availability of fresh food, neighborhood safety). Recent attention to the social determinants of health (Figure 10.2)[13] focuses on factors acting on the health of individuals arising from the macro- and exosystems. There is increased awareness of these forces and the belief by some that they may be of equal or greater importance than biological mechanisms for preventing and treating disease.[14]

The *microsystems* most proximal to children (i.e., the ones in which children are embedded and interact regularly with) include their family, school, and peer group, among others. These *microsystems* and the individuals within them influence and are influenced by the developing child in a reciprocal fashion. When a child has a serious illness, the hospital or healthcare team becomes a microsystem within which the child develops.[10,11] Finally, *mesosystems* are conceptualized as linkages between microsystems. Examples of mesosystems include the extent to which the family and school communicate and work together to foster the child's development or the degree to which the healthcare team and family work together in a family-centered way to meet the needs of the ill child. These connections between microsystems are important in the coordination of efforts to promote better child outcomes.

The following vignette provides an account of a family's experience after the birth of a child with a severe form of congenital heart disease. The case illustrates that as a child with a serious illness grows and develops, changes happen within the child (e.g., desire for autonomy, failing health) and within their environments.[12] Individuals who have a direct influence on the child and who are influenced by the child exist within microsystems. The family system (e.g., JJ's mother and sibling), school setting and peer network (e.g., JJ's teacher and friend), religious/community organizations (e.g., JJ's family pastor), and healthcare teams are examples of these microsystem environments. Mesosystems are important in the coordination of efforts to promote better outcomes (e.g., family and home hospice regarding symptom management). Finally, aspects of the exosystem (e.g., closest major hospital 2 hours away) and macrosystem (e.g., health insurance tied

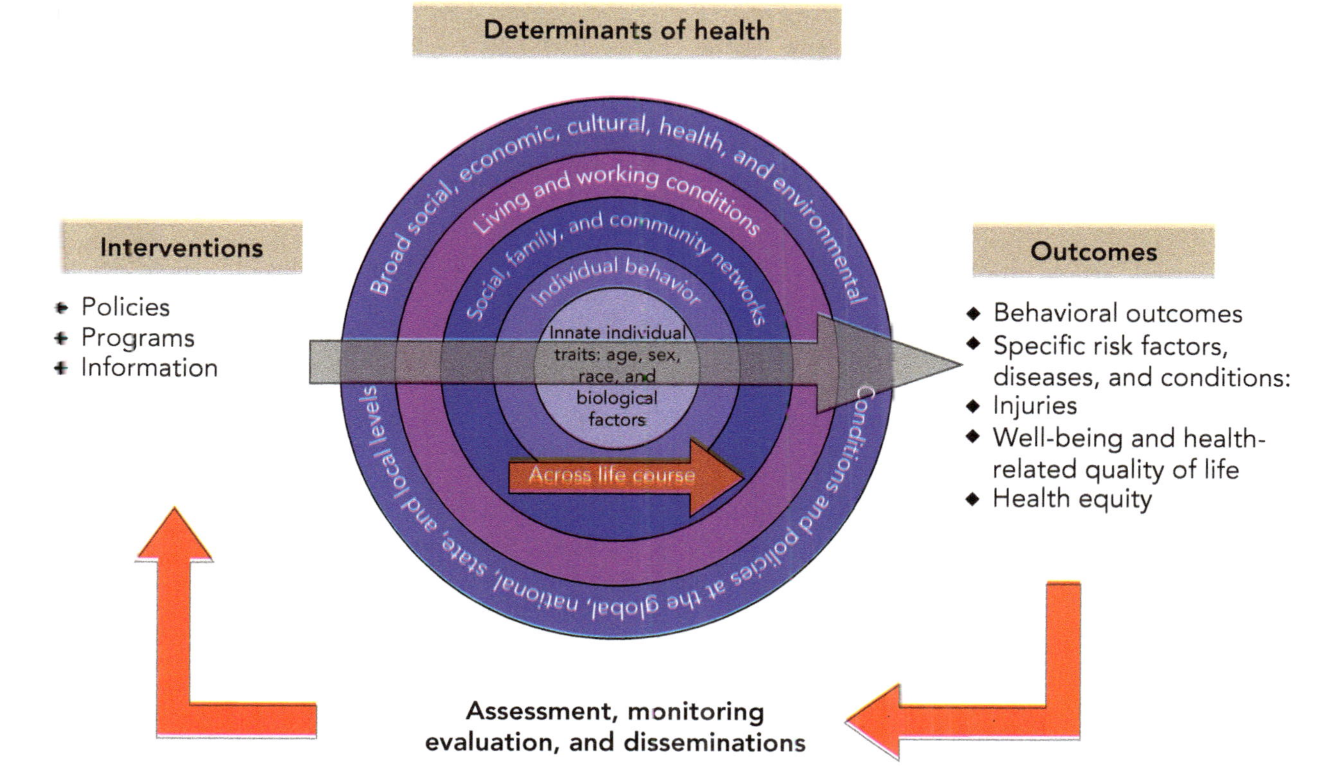

Figure 1[illegible].2 *Action model to achieve Healthy People 2020 overarching goals.* Healthy People 2020 [Internet]. Washington, DC: U.S. Department of Health and Human Services, Office of Disease Prevention and Health Promotion [cited [March9, 2020]. OBJECTIVES FOR 2020 PHASE I REPORT RECOMMENDATIONS FOR THE FRAMEWORK AND FORMAT OF HEALTHY PEOPLE 2020 (2008). Action model to achieve Healthy People 2020 overarching goals. Pg. 7.
Available from: https://www.healthypeople.gov/sites/default/files/PhaseI_0.pdf

to employment; high healthcare cost) also have a significant impact on families.

Team Reflection

JJ, an Adolescent with Congenital Heart Disease

Shortly after he was born, JJ was diagnosed with hypoplastic left heart syndrome, a severe form of congenital heart disease. He underwent a three-stage surgical palliation (procedures to extend life when total corrective surgical repair is not possible) as an infant and young child. During each of his hospitalizations, some of which lasted for many weeks, his older brother stayed with an aunt so that their single mother could be with JJ at the closest major hospital, 2 hours away.

Now, at 17 years of age, JJ is becoming increasingly ill from his underlying heart condition and a Fontan procedure. His mother relies on her sister for medical decision-making support. At almost 18 years of age, however, JJ is eager to exert his decisional autonomy despite having baseline mild cognitive deficits. He asked a friend to help make his "Bucket List"—things that he wants to accomplish before he dies. (He got the idea from watching the 2007 movie of the same name.) He reached out to a teacher at school to help him accomplish some of the goals on the list. He does not want to talk to his mother about his Bucket List because he thinks it will make her sad. He knows if he talks to his aunt about it, she will tell his mother. Therefore, he hides the list from his family and tries to meet his goals on his own with the help of friends.

As JJ gets sicker, he becomes more and more physically dependent on his family. Shortly after his 18th birthday he was hospitalized with worsening heart failure. During his hospital stay, his family's pastor visited from their local church. The pastor noted that JJ and his mother were not talking about his worsening disease, and he facilitated a conversation between the two. Through tears, JJ was able to ask his mother to help him achieve the last item on his Bucket List: to die at home with his puppy in bed with him. With intensive symptom management, JJ was able to enjoy a few more weeks at home, supported by home hospice. After his death, his high school planted a garden in his memory, which his mother continues to visit years after his death.

CONCEPTUALIZING THE FAMILY MICROSYSTEM: FAMILY SYSTEMS THEORY

As illustrated by the quotation that opens this chapter, family microsystems can vary greatly. The composition and structure may vary substantially from one family to the next or within a family over time. In addition to biological, adopted, extended, and step relatives, families may include friends and "created" relatives including important community members such as religious leaders or educators. Families may also be termed multigenerational or transracial; parents may be termed single or partnered; partners may be cisgender, same-sex, or nonbinary.[15,16] The composition and structure of the family may change day to day, depending on the challenges they face and the resources that they need to meet those challenges. When caring for children with serious illness, it is important not to make assumptions about who is considered family or how the family is organized. Each child and caregiver should be asked who they consider to be family.

Family systems theory views families as operating like biological systems: organized units with component parts (members), interacting in relation to one another in rule-governed patterns. Families are comprised of a collection of individuals, each with his or her own biological predispositions, attitudes, characteristics, and personal histories. These individuals interact with one another in specific subsystems within the family defined by specific roles. Each individual has a specific role within each subsystem and may hold multiple roles simultaneously (e.g., partner and parent; son and sibling). Individual family members are interdependent, such that a change in one family member has an impact on all other family members and the family system. As with any system, families self-regulate to maintain stability while also accommodating changes in individuals.[17–19] The process of altering the composition, organization, and/or structure of the family requires flexibility, open, clear communication, renegotiation of roles and responsibilities, and effective management of the emotional turmoil that these changes can produce. To understand the family experience of serious medical conditions, it is important to conceptualize the impact on individual family members, their relationships, and the functioning of the family as a whole.

SERIOUS ILLNESS IN CHILDREN: A NEED TO REORGANIZE THE FAMILY SYSTEM

The impact on roles, responsibilities, relationships, and the structure of the family when a child is seriously ill has been well-documented in the qualitative literature. The most obvious change to the structure of the family is the need to fulfill a new role: medical caregiver. Often a responsibility of parents, medical caregiving includes a range of responsibilities from learning about the condition, making medical decisions, scheduling and attending medical appointments, negotiating with healthcare providers, managing treatment, considering treatment pathways, ensuring adherence, arranging ancillary services (e.g., therapies, educational plans), and optimizing physical and psychosocial outcomes. Some aspects of medical caregiving may be spread across family members and fall to siblings[20] or extended family members. Of note, families comprised of single parents or lone caregivers (those with no secondary caregiver or support) face particularly great difficulties in fulfilling the medical caregiver role.[21]

Other organizational changes within the family may include expanding the family to help manage the increased needs resulting from a new serious illness. Families may enlist extended family to care for sibling and friends and community members to provide meals or help with other tasks. Modifications to household rules such as laxer parenting, and changes in relationship patterns such as closer bonds being formed between the primary caregiver and the patient may also occur.[20,22,23] The qualitative studies that produce such findings attest to the need for families to adjust daily life to accommodate the demands of a child's illness and treatment.

Quantitative research has found that roles are less clear and more difficult to establish and maintain when a family member is ill. These patterns have been documented in families of children with diabetes,[24] spina bifida,[25] and pediatric cancer.[26] Some evidence suggests that families managing illness are likely to be dysregulated in terms of their flexibility. Families of children with cancer are more likely than those with healthy children to be either chaotic (very high in flexibility) or rigid (very low in flexibility).[27,28] Families of children with diabetes have been found to be more rigid than is the norm[29] and to become less flexible across the first few months after diagnosis.[30] What remains unclear is whether these differences are truly "dysfunctional" or if they are adaptive in the process of ensuring that the medical needs of the child are being met.

SERIOUS ILLNESS IN CHILDREN: IMPACT ON THE EMOTIONAL CLIMATE OF THE FAMILY

The emotional climate of the family refers to the degree of their connectedness and emotional closeness (cohesion), the extent of emotional expression and responsiveness (affective involvement), and the amount of conflict. Many families affected by childhood serious illness report a sense of increased emotional closeness and cohesion. That being said, family reactions to illness are actually quite variable, both within and across families; reports of increased sibling rivalry and family conflict have also emerged.[20,31] For example, Blair, Freeman, and Cull found that families of children with cystic fibrosis were more emotionally involved compared to families with healthy children.[32] Families of children with diabetes[33] and cancer[34] show higher than average levels of cohesion shortly after diagnosis and throughout the illness. Increased cohesion is a common theme in qualitative studies of families of children with cancer.[35] A meta-analysis of the influence of pediatric cancer on family functioning revealed higher levels of maternal-reported conflict in these families compared to those families with healthy children.[36] Similarly, Liakopoulou and colleagues observed mothers of children with diabetes to express more critical comments, hostility, and overinvolvement with their children.[37] Greater difficulties in affect management, affective responsiveness, and affective involvement have been reported for families of children with diabetes[24] and adolescent cancer survivors.[26] It is important to pay attention to the family's emotional climate (i.e., conflict, cohesion, and emotional expressiveness) as it has a demonstrated effect on child psychological health.[38,39] In sum, although families of children with illness seem to be more emotionally connected, they may also experience difficulties managing appropriate levels of affective involvement and responsiveness and may be prone to conflict.

SERIOUS ILLNESS IN CHILDREN: THE IMPORTANCE OF FAMILY COMMUNICATION

Communication is a key component of family functioning.[40] Communication, both verbal and nonverbal, is the means through which roles and responsibilities are negotiated and agreed upon; relationships are established, maintained, and changed; emotional needs are expressed; and support is provided. Overall, difficulties with communication within the family impact the health and well-being of all family members.[38,41] The way a family communicates about a child's serious illness can impact the formation of goals of care, decisions regarding care, and how they survive the threatened or actual death of the child. In the following quote, we see how a sibling's understanding of a child's illness and prognosis unfolds and is shaped by parents' nonverbal communication.

> I said suddenly, "I wish Molly were here." My mother made a small noise and when I looked at her, she was crying. I looked back at Dad in bewilderment, and there were tears on his face, too, the first time I'd seen him cry. . . . I knew then what they hadn't wanted to tell me. Molly wouldn't be coming home again, that Molly was going to die. (Lowry, 1977/2015)[42]

While children and adolescents describe wanting honest communication about their disease or their sibling's disease,[43-44] many families face barriers to this disclosure. Families may have unofficial rules about what topics are taboos (e.g., death) and with whom such topics can be discussed (e.g., discussion limited with children). These rules can become barriers to important conversations because particular topics may be disallowed for fear of diminishing hope, increasing burden, or fueling conflict.[45] Other barriers to communication may arise out of specific challenges related to the child's illness.[46] For example, the physical separation engendered by extended hospitalizations may impact the opportunity for family conversations. Finally, family may have limited knowledge about children's developmental understanding of serious illness and death. They may not know what to say in such a conversation with their children.

LOSS AND TRAUMATIC STRESS: IMPACT ON INDIVIDUAL FAMILY MEMBERS AND ON THE FAMILY AS A WHOLE

A wealth of research shows that the diagnosis of a medical problem in a child causes enormous distress for family members and that the death of a child is one of the most difficult experiences a family can face.[47] Generally, distress is greatest at the times of diagnosis and then at the child's death. This distress typically diminishes with time,[30,48] although for some individuals, it may persist long term.[49] Those individuals who experience more anger and negative appraisals may be more at risk for persistent distress; additional factors that are associated with increased long-term distress include ongoing health and financial challenges.[50] Central to the experience of individual family members are the concepts of loss and traumatic stress.

When a child is seriously ill, the threat of loss becomes the defining framework for the family's experience (as well as for the child's). Day-to-day losses may include loss of perceived "normalcy," loss of family and child developmental milestones, and loss of feelings of security. Such ongoing losses, both small and large, impose a cumulative burden that gradually erodes hope and shapes worries. The story of Baby S highlights a few of the many losses the family had to grieve, including their birth plan and expectations for their child.

Family Reflection

My Baby S: Renegotiating Expectations

My wife and I struggled for years to get pregnant. We had both dreamed of becoming parents, and, when we married, raising a family was a priority for us. When my wife finally became pregnant, we were ecstatic.

We were then shocked when a prenatal diagnosis of Down syndrome was made, and we again had to renegotiate our expectations for our child. We also had to change our expectations about her birth because of the danger of her health problems. Instead of delivering in our local hospital, we had to travel to the city and deliver at a center equipped to deliver high-risk babies. We understood the importance of embracing new expectations about her birth because they would not only be best for our baby but also for my wife.

Armed with these expectations we traveled to the city for the delivery only having to change our expectations again and again. After our baby's S birth, she had to be admitted to the neonatal intensive care unit. Discharge dates came and went, and we began to understand them as somewhat arbitrary times when we might hope to bring our baby home. As time went on, our hopes for the future eroded and worries predominated. Once we met with the palliative care team, however, they helped us reframe our current situation and start to garner local resources so we could take our baby home to our family and community.

When a child dies, the family faces the ultimate loss—as well as their image for the future of their family.[51] Grief becomes a defining emotion, pivotal to their experience. Although loss and grief impact the family as a unit, they are also experienced individually by its members within the context of family relationships.

Some families, or individual members, may seek to make sense of and find meaning in their child's death. This process may result in positive understanding (e.g., posttraumatic growth, benefit finding), negative understanding (e.g., non-benefit finding; "this is an insurmountable tragedy"), or neutral understanding (e.g., "brain tumors just happen") of their family's new realities.[52]

There is growing recognition of the potentially traumatic impact of life-threatening illness on the child and family. Models of traumatic stress have emerged as useful frameworks for capturing the range of their responses. *Pediatric medical traumatic stress* (PMTS) is defined as "a set of psychological and physiological responses of children and their family members to pain, injury, serious illness, medical procedures, and invasive or frightening treatment experiences."[53] PMTS symptoms include intrusive thoughts, hyperarousal, avoidance of trauma-related stimuli, and negative thoughts or feelings. More specifically, PMTS may include negative emotional reactions (e.g., guilt, sadness, anger, complicated grief), physical symptoms (somatic complaints, sleep difficulties), cognitive disturbances (intrusive thoughts or memories, dissociation, difficulty concentrating), and behavioral issues (poor school or work performance, risky actions). It can also involve difficulties within social or interpersonal relationships.[54]

The latest revision of the Integrative (Trajectory) Model of PMTS illustrates and emphasizes different trajectories of PMTS response over time.[55,56] Informed by recent longitudinal studies, the updated model proposes four possible trajectories of PMTS: Resilient, Recovery, Chronic, and Escalating (Box 10.1).

It is important to note that this model was not developed specifically for those individuals and families facing the unique challenges of life-threatening illness. Thus, while it may elucidate some of the child and family's emotional reactions, it does not fully account for the depth of anticipatory grief, including the child's, or the long-term grief that becomes part of a family's journey.

BOX 10.1 TRAJECTORIES OF PEDIATRIC MEDICAL TRAUMATIC STRESS

Resilient: Individuals categorized as resilient are those who have minimal traumatic stress symptoms in context of the child's medical diagnosis and treatment.

Recovery: Individuals in the recovery trajectory present with trauma symptoms in the early aftermath of a medical condition, but their symptoms resolve fairly quickly (1–3 months).

Chronic: Those individuals who fall within the chronic trajectory category present with consistently elevated trauma symptoms for a longer duration (e.g., 6–24 months).

Escalating: Those in the escalating condition present with traumatic stress symptoms early in the course of the child's medical condition, and these symptoms worsen over time.

From Price J, et al. (2015).[55]

THE IMPACT OF A CHILD'S SERIOUS ILLNESS ON PARENTS/CAREGIVERS

When a child has a serious medical condition, the stress of supporting the child, worrying about the child's health, managing complex medical regiments, maintaining typical caregiving roles, and making medical decisions can take a toll on caregivers. Although research that focuses specifically on families who have a child who is currently receiving palliative care services is somewhat limited, PMTS symptoms have been documented within family members of patients experiencing a range of serious medical conditions (e.g., cancer, injury, diabetes, asthma, and congenital heart disease). Across these diagnoses, approximately 30% of caregivers experience moderate to severe PMTS,[55] with higher rates near the time of diagnosis. For example, within 1 month of diagnosis, about 60% of parents of children with diabetes meet clinical cutoffs for depression and anxiety,[57] and 40–50% of parents of children with cancer qualify for a diagnosis of acute stress disorder.[58]

Many parents report long-term effects of losing a child, regardless of the cause. For example, parents may experience posttraumatic stress (PTS) reactions,[59,60]depressive symptoms, diminished overall well-being, and health problems.[61] In a study of 872 parents, 59% reported high levels of complicated grief symptoms 6 months after their child's death in the pediatric intensive care unit (PICU).[62] However, some parents may experience posttraumatic growth following the loss of a child in a recent systematic review of 13 articles, Waugh and colleagues concluded that mothers identify more growth than fathers, that culture may play a role in the experience of growth, and that growth is often identified after some time has passed. Domains of posttraumatic growth included changes in self-perception, relationships, recognizing new possibilities, an appreciation for life, and existential views (i.e., "changes in how living in the world is viewed and understood")[63] (see Chapter 15).

When a child has a serious illness, the roles and responsibilities of being a parent change. Parents describe a new definition of "Being a Good Parent" when their child is seriously ill and strive to achieve this definition.[51,64–67] For example, parents of children with advanced cancer described that a "good parent makes informed, unselfish decisions in the child's best interest; provides the basics of food, shelter, and clothing; remains at the child's side regardless of circumstances; shows the child that he or she is cherished; tries to prevent suffering and protect health; teaches the child to make good choices, to respect and have sympathy for others, and know God; advocates for the child with medical staff; and promotes the child's health."[66(p. 5982)] Parents also talk about the need for "intense parenting:" the evolving, laborious roles that parents assume at home in caring for their ill child, including the ability to be ready to provide care at a moment's notice.[68] This provision of extensive, intensive care means that parents have less time to address other important facets of life, such as their own health, relationships with partners, and a social life. They devote their time and energy to ensure their child's health, safety, and quality of life while acting in the role of nurse, case manager, teacher, and advocate in addition to loving parent.

When the family has multiple children, as parents learn to parent the seriously ill child, they are simultaneously adjusting and relearning their approach to parent the healthy siblings. Parents may have similar overall goals or beliefs about what is important in being a parent to both their seriously ill and healthy children. For example, parents describe that it is most important that all their children know they are loved; in particular, they do not want healthy siblings to feel neglected. They also want to minimize disruption for the siblings, maintain normalcy, and promote their health.[51] Parents describe trying to juggle competing demands as a process of trading-off one child's needs over those of another, with those of the ill child frequently taking precedence. For example, a parent may want to attend a sibling's sporting event but fears leaving the ill child unattended. The discrepancy between what parents *want to* do and what they *can* do may be a source of significant distress.[69–71]

In families with two adults in a partner relationship, the child's illness impacts their identity and functioning as a couple. While not broadly studied, a systematic review of couples' functioning after a diagnosis of pediatric cancer indicated that most couples adapt well across domains such as emotional closeness, marital support, marital satisfaction, and general marital adjustment. However, they can be challenged by issues related to marital conflict, communication, and sexual intimacy.[72] In exploring family functioning and risks to the couple relationship in families caring for a child with serious congenital malformations, Brenner and colleagues found that families do not seem to be at greater risk for dysfunction or separation over the first several years of the child's life. However, couples experienced greater challenge and risk when the child with the congenital malformation was a second or subsequent child.[73] Thus, factors internal and external to the relationship can impact the health of the couple's relationship. Research suggests that it is important to address the couple's dyadic coping with stressors, given the potential impact on overall family health and care of the ill child and siblings.[74–76] Such assessment is called for in recent standards for psychosocial assessment.[77,78]

In two-parent families, both parents are often involved in the medical caregiving of the child. The quality of the relationship between parents is of vital importance as they negotiate the challenge. Typical areas of discordance include differences of opinion about the child's care, worries about the child's care in the future, and how past interpersonal conflicts or unfulfilled needs complicate the present situation.[79] At their child's end of life, parents in medical caregiving roles may have different goals. While it is common for goals to change between the time of illness diagnosis and end of life, the relationship between parent caregivers becomes complicated when one parent changes their goals and the other parent does not[80] (see Chapter 15).

THE IMPACT OF A CHILD'S SERIOUS ILLNESS ON SIBLINGS

Recent estimates indicate that more than two-thirds of children receiving palliative care services have at least one sibling.[81] Thus, if there are nearly 400,000 children who would benefit from palliative care, there are at least 250,000 children facing the possible death of their brother or sister.[82] A recent meta-analysis found that siblings of children with chronic health conditions are at greater risk for emotional and behavioral problems than siblings of healthy brothers and sisters.[83] These negative effects were more pronounced for siblings of children with life-threatening or highly intrusive conditions than for siblings of children with less severe conditions.[83] Systematic reviews of the literature regarding siblings of children with cancer[84,85] reveal that siblings may experience poor quality of life in emotional, family, and social domains; school problems including poorer academic functioning and more absenteeism; and strong negative emotions (e.g., shock, fear, worry, sadness, helplessness, anger, and guilt). While rates of psychiatric disorders such as generalized anxiety disorder and major depression are not usually elevated, symptoms of worry and sadness are common, and many siblings report high rates of cancer-related PTS. In one study, two-thirds of siblings of children with cancer within 3 years of diagnosis reported moderate to severe levels of cancer-related PTS, and a quarter met diagnostic criteria for posttraumatic stress disorder.[86] A recent review of the literature regarding siblings of children with congenital heart disease also documented parent reports of increased symptoms of anxiety, depression, anger, and behavioral problems in siblings, along with declines in school performance.[87] However, despite the challenges that siblings of children with serious medical conditions may face, new research has highlighted some potential positive outcomes: one pilot study found that approximately 75% of siblings of children with cancer exhibited a resilient or recovery trajectory of PMTS, with 25% experiencing chronic or escalating symptoms.[88]

Studies of bereaved siblings indicate that up to 50% can have prolonged grief disorder, and 10–50% meet criteria for posttraumatic stress disorder.[89,90] Furthermore, bereaved siblings experience particular physical,[91,92] psychological, and social risks including anxiety, depression, substance abuse, academic performance concerns, and emotional distress.[93,94] These risks increase when the seriously ill child's life is at grave risk or when illness management strains family time and routines.[95] Adolescent and young adult (AYA) siblings in particular may opt to engage in risky behavior, withdraw from peer and family relationships, and decline sharing concerns with parents whom they perceive to be overburdened.[45]

Siblings of children with serious illness can experience a range of role changes. Some take on aspects of medical caregiving such as helping administer medication or treatment components[20] or take on a designated role of treatment companion, entertainer, or source of distraction. These new roles are added at a time when rules that once governed that relationship may be changing. In qualitative studies, for example, siblings of children with cancer have discussed how they struggle to know how to appropriately interact with their brother or sister. Rough and tumble play may be restricted, or infectious disease precautions may place greater distance between siblings. Additionally, feelings of jealousy, anger, and guilt may complicate the sibling relationship.[20] As described by a teenager who lost her twin at age 7, feelings about a sibling's illness and death can be intense and long-lasting and can also lead to post-traumatic growth over time.

Family Reflection

A Sibling's Story

One of the best things that can happen in life is you can be gifted a sibling or in my case, a twin sister. You get to grow up together, share gentle moments, and fight endlessly. Having a sibling is a different kind of relationship in that you always have a friend, a protector, and a confidant in the best and worst of times. But what if you saw your sibling in pain every day while you had to sit back and helplessly watch. That was my life as the sibling of a terminally ill sister.

There were many times I saw my sister in pain and so desperately wanted to take the hurt away, protect her from everything bad. The sister I once knew seemed to slowly fade away until at some points I didn't know who she was. My sister died, and I could not fix it. Her death affected every part of my life. As a 7-year-old kid, I never expected my world to fall apart. The days of uncertainty affected every part of me to the point where I could barely make it through the day, never knowing what would happen to my sister and scared of what was to come.

It's not a normal thing to have a sick sibling and to be sat down by your parents to learn that soon your beloved sister, your twin, would die. All I ever wanted was normalcy and routine—the life I had once enjoyed—playing and fighting with my sister. An experience like this is scary for adults, let alone kids. I felt very lonely and isolated as none of my friends or classmates could relate. I often went to bed wondering why all of this was happening to me. I've wondered that every night for many years.

To this day, I wish I knew why this happened to my family. The loss of my twin sister changed who I am as a person because it led me to see that life is fragile and death can happen, even to kids. One of the moments that has stuck with me is the moment I found out my sister was going to die in a few short hours. That was the moment where I knew my life would never be the same, my new normal was going to be different in every way. That was when I knew that life would be full of times when even a simple question like "How many siblings do you have?" would always take me back to my life with a sister and the fact that she is now only a distant memory.

Everyday I remember my sister. I remember the pain and hurt. All that I went through will always stick with me. But what I have learned from all of this is that every day I must wake up, work hard to live my life to the fullest while honoring my sister, and live the life she never got to experience.

Kaitlyn Dunne, age 15

Roles and relationships of healthy siblings with parents are also affected. This may be particularly challenging because parents are an important source of support, guidance, and information for the siblings. At times, their absence may be perceived as a form of neglect or rejection. Research indicates that when a sibling perceives they are not accepted by their parents, they are at greater risk for psychosocial distress,[35] and, as family-level difficulties accumulate (e.g., relationship quality, satisfaction, problem-solving ability, affection), the threat to sibling adjustment multiplies.[96] Sometimes grandparents provide key support in maintaining some sense of stability for the healthy siblings.[51,64,97]

Communication between parents and healthy siblings is an important component of nurturing relationships. Few studies focus on communication between parents and seriously ill children, and even fewer focus on communication between parents and the healthy siblings of these children. Siblings often report troubling gaps in key areas of communication leaving them to feel excluded from discussions,[98] misled,[99] and unprepared for their brother or sister's illness and death.[43,93,100] These gaps may strain family relationships and perpetuate distress and diminished sense of well-being.[101] Siblings who report poorer communication have the highest psychological distress.[43] As with the ill child, the desire to protect children from difficult emotions becomes a barrier in open communication with siblings.[102] The hesitancy to openly communicate is not only initiated by parents; adolescent and young adult siblings often do not share their distress with their parents so as to not add the burden their parents are experiencing.[45]

BEING A GRANDPARENT WHEN GRANDCHILDREN ARE SERIOUSLY ILL

Approximately 7 million grandparents in the United States live with at least one of their grandchildren.[103] Across the globe, grandparents play a pivotal part in the lives of families in the ways that they shape family practices and social networks.[104] Grandparents around the world vary in how they enact the grandparenting roles as teacher, caregiver, supporter of cultural values, and source of knowledge. A recent systematic review suggests that grandparents affect physical and psychological health outcomes in their grandchildren, especially around feeding behaviors, safety, and illness management.[104] During serious illness, grandparents play various roles and can provide many different types and levels of support, including financial, practical, and emotional assistance.[104]

Although research on grandparents of children with serious illnesses is just beginning to be developed, evidence suggests that grandparents also experience elevated anxiety, depression, anger, uncertainty, and helplessness. For example, Wakefield and colleagues found that grandparents of children with cancer experience psychological distress at increased rates compared with grandparents of children without cancer.[105] Mendes-Castillo and Bousso describe grandparent distress as "multiplied and muted."[106] They see their own children, their healthy grandchildren, and their ill grandchild suffer but hesitate to share their own distress because they perceive it as less important than that of their children and grandchildren.[106] Youngblut and colleagues compared mothers' and grandmothers' grief symptoms and experiences.[107] They found mothers and grandmothers both experienced negative effects from the death of the child, but mothers experienced the loss with greater intensity and with more negative emotions. Both mothers and grandmothers experienced rates of depressive symptoms significantly higher than the US population (though mothers' rates were higher than grandmothers). Both mothers and grandmothers of seriously ill children also reported low levels of personal growth. Indeed, serious illness and associated caregiving can take a toll on grandparents.[108]

IMPLICATIONS FOR CLINICAL CAREGIVERS: FAMILY-CENTERED TRAUMA-INFORMED PEDIATRIC PALLIATIVE CARE

The conceptual models and empirical evidence that we have presented culminate in our recommendation that PPC be both family-centered and trauma-informed. Figure 10.3 depicts how such a model of care (the inner rectangle) encompasses the child and family living their experience of loss and trauma and spans the various social ecological systems in which the child and family are embedded (the concentric circles).

Care based on these models recognizes the importance of helping the family restructure their roles and responsibilities, recognizing the emotional toll of this trauma, providing trauma-informed care, and engaging in and fostering open communication within the family.

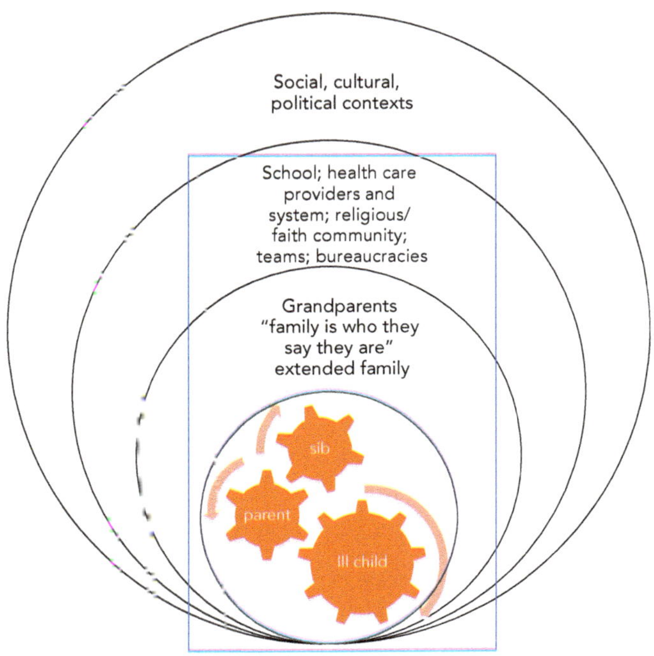

Figure 10.3 *Ecological Understanding of Pediatric Medical Traumatic Stress.*

To recognize these goals, it can be helpful to implement family-centered care. Family-centered care has been the standard of care for children for more than 40 years and is now integrated into the accreditation of most institutions and organizations.[109] It prioritizes developing partnerships with families to provide programs and services that are consistent with the following core concepts: promoting dignity and respect; integrating patient and family values, beliefs, knowledge and cultural backgrounds into the planning and delivery of care; sharing information with patients and families in ways that are affirming and useful in decision-making; encouraging and supporting patient and family participation in care and decision-making at the level they choose; and collaborating with patients and families in all aspects of healthcare program and policy development, implementation, and evaluation including facility design, research, and professional education. (See the Institute for Family-Centered Care for more information and resources. https://www.ipfcc.org/.) Family-centered care is based on research about the importance of the family in all parts of children's lives including healthcare and about the quality of life for every member of the family. Considering each family's unique experiences and reactions is central to the delivery of family-centered care and PPC.[110] Determining the needs, strengths, and current challenges for key family members of an ill child (as previously described) can be a first step in establishing family-centered care.

Care must also be trauma-informed in order to minimize the potential for medical care to become traumatic and address trauma-related family and child distress.[111] In the case of PPC this could include prevention of trauma during a range of procedures and treatment experiences that could be traumatic (e.g., needles, taking medications, magnetic resonance imaging, surgeries, peer teasing) and screening and referring any child or family for more support when needed (e.g., significant impairing symptoms, difficulty with bereavement). Healthcare organizations can provide general training for all providers and support staff, and specialized training for each patient population, thereby ensuring that trauma-informed practices are implemented by *all* individuals across the pediatric healthcare network. Such approaches are complementary to family-centered care and enhance quality of care.

Barriers exist to routine integration of trauma-informed approaches into pediatric care and PPC, including a lack of available training and unclear best-practice guidelines. Training in trauma-informed practices includes the prevalence of trauma in patients and staff, the impact of trauma, and trauma-informed practices to prevent retraumatization or new trauma. The Center for Pediatric Traumatic Stress (CPTS), a multidisciplinary intervention development center within the National Child Traumatic Stress Network (NCTSN), developed HealthCareToolBox.org, provides evidence-based resources including videos, continuing education courses, and handouts for children and parents.

The interdisciplinary PPC team is central to the delivery of specialty palliative care across inpatient, ambulatory, community, home, and hospice care settings, according to the National Consensus Project guidelines.[78] Members of the team can include chaplains, nurses, physicians, social workers, child life specialists, advanced practice registered nurses (APRN), psychologists, and bereavement coordinators. Teams may also include expressive therapists, case managers, pharmacists, and volunteers. Table 10.1 provides descriptions of these roles.

Ideally, all clinicians have strengths from which to offer primary PPC. Primary team members often have established long-standing trusting relationships with patients and families. Primary PPC includes attending to communication between the medical team and family and within the family; providing anticipatory guidance; clarifying family goals, and initiating advance care planning discussions. All clinicians can support pain and symptoms management in primary PPC through comprehensive assessments and understanding safe prescribing and monitoring practices. Finally, all clinicians can support families by attending to family member distress and providing education and referral or connection to supportive services in their communities.[112]

Specialty PPC teams can often partner with the primary team to provide more targeted, expert-level care through consultation or co-management with the primary team. The specialty PPC team can approach care by working with the family and primary team to maximize quality of life across the child's physical, psychological, social, and spiritual domains of health. They can offer expert management of challenging symptoms across settings, as well as facilitate communication with child and family.[112]

If medical teams expect families to communicate with their family members, it can be helpful to role model how to communicate with each other. Furthermore, based on the premise that healthcare providers aspire to professional and ethical obligations to provide the best possible care for their patients, care that is not only safe but also effective, and that the nature of their "best care" changes over time as goals of care change, communication about changes in goals and treatment must be ongoing. For instance, child-centered goals may change for many reasons, including protocolized treatments that may not be available or appropriate, ongoing treatments that may no longer achieve the desired outcome, or children who may become vocal about their wishes. We also can role model that involvement of the child and their siblings requires careful consideration by discussing them with parents. These factors include the child's present physical condition and the age and cognitive capacity of the child and their siblings as well as the family's cultural beliefs and mode of communication about the illness. These factors may complicate or modify how the child and their siblings are involved but should not automatically exclude their early and ongoing involvement.

Across roles as palliative care providers, it is important to help families identify and build on their strengths and capabilities as well as support their problem-solving when they address challenges and demands by providing the necessary psychosocial support and by connecting them to resources across all parts of their ecological system.[113] With a

TABLE 10.1 Description of interdisciplinary palliative care team member roles[124]

SPECIALTY TEAM MEMBER	FUNCTION
Chaplain	• Support spiritual beliefs of patient, family, staff across cultures and faith traditions • Address religious (e.g., sacramental) or nonreligious needs • Spiritual or existential symptoms assessment • Assist with goals or care, advance care planning, and decision-making discussion
Child life specialist	• Expertise in child emotional and developmental needs • Support in bereavement and coping skills
Nurse: RN and APRN	• Holistic support of physical, psychosocial, spiritual health • Enhanced communication skills • Pain and symptom management: knowledge of pharm and nonpharm approaches and evaluate their efficacy • Coordination of care • Patient and family education • Debriefing with staff around challenges in care For APRN: as above, plus: • Determine and order appropriate diagnostic testing and pharmacologic treatments • Advance care planning discussions
Physician	• Expertise of medical diagnoses, disease trajectory, prognostication • Goals of care conversation expertise • Pain and symptom management • Assist primary team by clarifying information and advocating for patient and family wishes • Assist with discharge planning: assess fit of community or home placement
Psychologist	• Assess for psychological and emotional distress • Assessment of developmental level and cognitive ability • Psychoeducation/neuropsychological testing • Counseling for child, adolescent/young adults, siblings
Social worker	• Assess patient and family needs, strengths, and resources • Connect to resources to meet emotional, legal, and financial needs • Work with case managers to support continuity in care • Expertise in understanding family dynamics, weaving cultural considerations into care for patient and family • Advocacy for patient and family wishes
Palliative bereavement coordinator	• Follow-up with families • Assess for complicated grief • Send notes and resources to grieving families • Maintain contact with bereaved family members • Coordinate memorial services for families and staff

comprehensive understanding of the nature of traumatic experience, it behooves the palliative care community to adapt communication and care strategies to every individual patient and their family (www.ipfcc.org). The implementation of trauma-informed family-centered care has the potential to improve patient outcomes and satisfaction with healthcare and is the responsibility of all members of the specialty interdisciplinary PPC team. As shown in Figure 10.4, family-centered and trauma-informed care share many components and can be effectively integrated.

The interdisciplinary PPC team is uniquely positioned to model the integration of trauma-informed and family-centered care for other members of the healthcare team. Relationships with family members should be based on their areas of strength and our respect for their knowledge of their children, their cultural beliefs, and the multiple roles that they try to balance. When providing care, it is essential that family members be viewed as experts in their child's care and that professionals collaborate with them when planning the way that care is provided. This includes using trauma-informed, family-centered approaches at the bedside to minimize the potentially distressing and painful aspects of treatment as well as the impact of treatment on the child, parents, and other members of the family. Family members and other caregivers can be encouraged and supported to participate and be involved in the child's care as much as they are able to and to the degree desired by the child and parents. Healthcare providers are responsible for giving families accurate and up-to-date information and that communication should continue throughout the child's illness. In addition, it is important that care providers, both family and professionals, care for themselves so they care best care for seriously ill children.

The child, families, and healthcare providers should collaborate in decisions about goals of care and in strategies to reach those goals—an approach that defines ideal interdisciplinary palliative care. Families may need assistance in having difficult conversations.[46] Openness and honesty in communication require willingness to take risks and be vulnerable, especially if the information to be shared is sensitive or difficult for families to discuss. The lack of time and physical absence may be barriers to having conversations when some family members are at the hospital and others are at home. This can be addressed through establishing new technology-assisted routines (e.g., video chat with siblings after school)

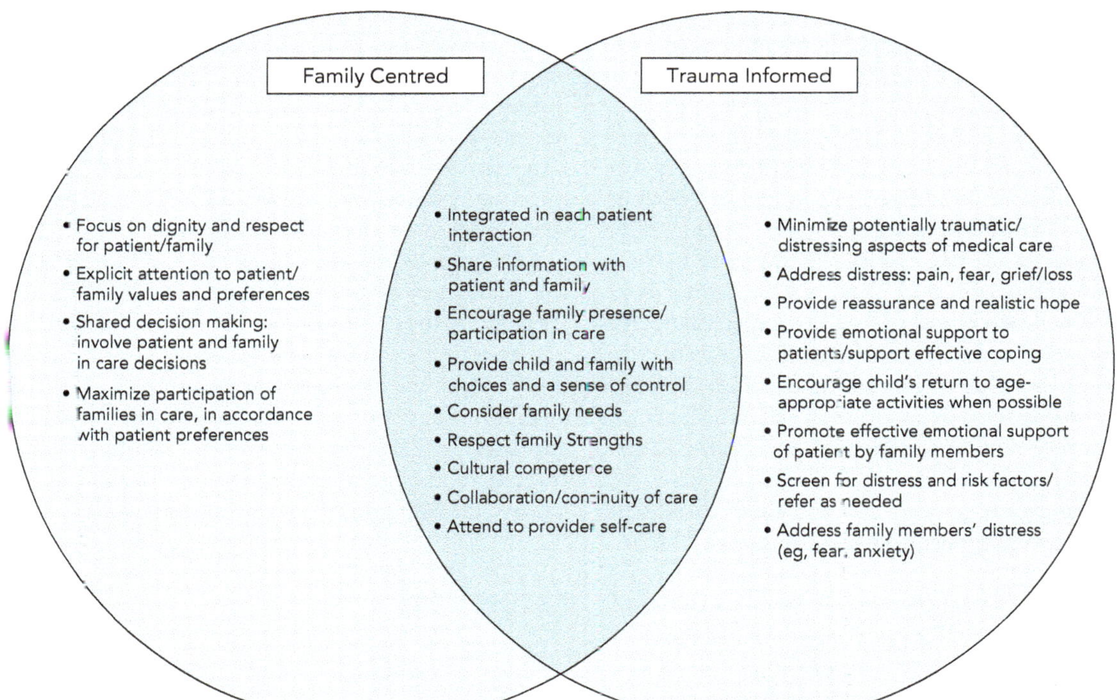

The overlapping circles highlight shared elements of the family-centered and trauma-informed care approaches. Unique complementary elements of family-centered and trauma-informed care are displayed in the non-overlapping portions of the circles. Adapted with permission from HealthcareToolBox.org

Figure 10.4 Unique and overlapping elements of family-centered and trauma-informed pediatric care. The overlapping circles highlight shared elements of the family-centered and trauma-informed care approaches. Unique complementary elements of family-centered and trauma-informed care are displayed in the non-overlapping portions of the circles. Adapted with permission from HealthcareToolBox.org and Marsac ML, Kassam-Adams N, Hildenbrand AK, et al. Implementing a trauma-informed approach in pediatric health care networks. *JAMA Pediatr.* 2016;170(1):70–77. doi:10.1001/jamapediatrics.2015.2206

or by engaging others in the family to help with these tough conversations. Family members and healthcare providers may need to develop sensitivity to nonverbal gestures and cues for support to know when a child or family members need more or less information. Attention to important barriers to and facilitators of communication is part of an important foundation for collaborative decision-making.

In families caring for a seriously ill child, day-to-day decision-making may be done by the adult who is providing the most hands-on care for the child. Most complex medical decisions, however, are made by a core group of family members in partnership with the healthcare team.[114] It is important for parent-partners or family decision-making partners to discuss their own hopes for the child, the family, and themselves before making serious treatment-related decisions. The decision-making partners may have different goals of care and may identify or prioritize concerns differently from the parents. All team members, those on the specialty palliative care team and those on the primary team, can promote open, productive communication among decision-making partners. Team members can talk in smaller groups with family members who are dominating or critical of others to problem-solve more productive ways to communicate their concerns. Teams can ask family members as individuals, dyads, or groups about their usual functioning, their values, and expectations. The team can then better understand and provide support to the family in making difficult decisions, coming to consensus on goals, and providing needed care.

Parents and family caregivers may need guidance on how to have important conversations with their children and support in doing so. Parents who describe being more religious, whose seriously ill children are older, or who perceive their child already understands their condition are more likely to have discussions with their child. Parents who discuss death with seriously ill children report a desire to prepare their children, help them cope, and attend to their wishes. Parents who do not engage their children in conversations about death typically report doing so to maintain their relationship status quo and protect the children and themselves from the pain of acknowledging the child will die.[115,116]

The following exchange illustrates the types of difficult conversations parents may need to have with their children:

> He said, "Pop-pop, you always know how to fix things and get something done. Can you do something about this cancer?" I said, "I can do a lot of things, but this is how it's going to work. We're going to pray about this situation here. But I can guarantee you one thing for sure. If Jesus come along and want to take you by the hand and tell you to come on and walk with me, you go ahead and walk because he's going to make sure everything is going to be all right. You just go along with him."[117]

The desire to protect family members from difficult emotions may stifle efforts to engage children and their parents in important conversations as early as possible in the course of the child's illness. These early conversations lay a foundation for ongoing conversations and may be especially important if the child becomes too sick to communicate later in their illness course. For instance, adolescents and young adults with advanced cancer experience great symptom burden, including emotional and psychological symptoms,[118,119] sadness, fear, and loneliness.[120] The quality of family communication (i.e., supportive; conflictual) can influence the intensity of how those symptoms are experienced.[121] Healthcare providers can help parents accept the importance of such conversations and prepare them by offering prompts, role play, and advice. Through such discussions, the parents and healthcare team may be able to provide care consistent with the wishes of the adolescent and young adult, appropriate palliative care services, advance care planning, goal-setting, and decision-making.[122]

Reframing or relabeling challenges to cast problems in a new light can help to shift patterns of thinking, normalize family experiences, and build on family strengths. Optimally, the team initiates these discussions and assures the family that they will have time to contemplate and make decisions without feeling immediate pressure. This often helps individuals within the family system to interact and process what they have experienced and make decisions with less regret.[123] Alternatively, when families feel pressured with directives from care providers, they can freeze and become dysfunctional. Creating room for families to engage in vital conversations helps them become true members of the team during the child's serious illness; this inclusion can be important to enhancing their child's well-being and their own long-term functioning. The role of the PPC team may most importantly be to advocate for the family to have the time and space in which to make decisions.

Accompanying and supporting families as they manage the challenges of living with a seriously ill child can help them along the continuum of the illness. No matter if a team is supporting a family through a child's death into bereavement or into the long-term survivorship of a child, we cannot abandon them. Through a trauma-informed, family-centered approach to PPC, we can support families so they can, in turn, help their children with life-threatening illnesses to achieve the best possible, goal-directed quality of life.

REFERENCES

1. American Academy of Pediatrics Committee on Hospital Care and Institute for Patient- and Family-Centered Care. Patient- and family-centered care and the pediatrician's role. *Pediatrics.* 2012;129(2):394–404.
2. Alderfer M, Stanley C, Baum A, Revenson TA, Singer J. Health and illness in the context of the family. In: Baum A, Revenson TA, Singer JE, *Handbook of Health Psychology.* 2nd ed. New York: Psychology Press; 2012: 493–518.
3. Weihs K, Fisher L, Baird M. Families, health, and behavior: A section of the commissioned report by the Committee on Health and Behavior: Research, Practice, and Policy Division of Neuroscience and Behavioral Health and Division of Health Promotion and Disease Prevention Institute of Medicine, National Academy of Sciences. *Families, Systems, Health.* 2002;20(1):7–46.

4. Psihogios AM, Fellmeth H, Schwartz LA, Barakat LP. Family functioning and medical adherence across children and adolescents with chronic health conditions: A meta-Analysis. *J Pediatr Psychol.* 2018;44(1):84–97.
5. Butcher JL, Nasr SZ. Direct observation of respiratory treatments in cystic fibrosis: Parent-child interactions relate to medical regimen adherence. *J Pediatr Psychol.* 2015;40:8–17.
6. Ehrlich KB, Miller GE, Chen E. Family functioning, eosinophil activity, and symptoms in children with asthma. *J Pediatr Psychol* 2015;40:781–789.
7. Fiese BH, Wamboldt FS, Anbar RD. Family asthma management routines: Connections to medical adherence and quality of life. *J Pediatr.* 2005;146(2):171–176.
8. Iskander JM, Rohan JM, Pendley JS, Delamater A, Drotar D. A 3-year prospective study of parent-child communication in early adolescents with type 1 diabetes: Relationship to adherence and glycemic control. *J Pediatr Psychol.* 2015;40:109–120.
9. Wood BL, Lim J, Miller BD, et al. Testing the biobehavioral family model in pediatric asthma: Pathways of effect. *Family Process.* 2008;47(1):21–40.
10. Eriksson M, Ghazinour M, Hammarström A. Different uses of Bronfenbrenner's ecological theory in public mental health research: What is their value for guiding public mental health policy and practice? *Social Theory.* 2018;16(4):414–433.
11. Kazak AE. Families of chronically ill children: A systems and social-ecological model of adaptation and challenge. *J Consult Clin Psychol.* 1989;57(1):25–30.
12. Bronfenbrenner U. *The Ecology of Human Development: Experiments by Nature and Design.* Cambridge, MA: Harvard University Press; 2009.
13. World Health Organization. Social Determinants of Health. 2017. http //www.who.int/social_determinants/en/
14. Deatrick JA. Where is "family" in the social determinants of health? Implications for family nursing practice, research, education, and policy. *J Family Nurs.* 2017;23(4):423–433.
15. Meyer C. *Can Social Work Keep Up with the Changing Family.* Columbus: Ohio State University College of Social Work; 1990.
16. Hepworth DH, Rooney RH, Larsen JA, Strom-Gottfried K, Rooney GD. *Direct Social Work Practice: Theory and Skills.* 8th ed. Belmont, CA: Brooks Cole; 2009.
17. Hoffman L. *Foundations of Family Therapy: A Conceptual Framework for Systems Change.* New York: Basic Books; 1981.
18. Nichols MP, Schwarts RC. *The Essentials of Family Therapy.* Boston, MA: Allyn & Bacon; 1981.
19. Wynne LC. Systems theory and the biopsychosocial approach. In Frankel RM, Quill TE, McDaniel SH, eds. *The Biopsychosocial Approach.* Rochester, NY: University of Rochester Press; 2003: 219–230.
20. Christofferson J, Stenman K, Kazak AE, Pierce J, Kelly C, Schifano E, Sciola J, Deatrick J, Alderfer MA. Family consequences of potentially traumatic pediatric medical events: Implications for trauma-informed care. *J Family Psychology.* 2020;34(2):237–246.
21. Brown RT, Wiener L, Kupst MJ, et al. Single parents of children with chronic illness: An understudied phenomenon. *J Pediatric Psychology.* 2008;33(4):408–421.
22. Pollock KGJ, Duncan E, Cowden JM. Emotional and behavioral changes in parents of children affected by hemolytic-uremic syndrome associated with verocytotoxin-producing escherichia coli: A qualitative analysis. *Psychosomatics.* 2009;50(3):263–269.
23. Trollvik A, Severinsson E. Parents' experiences of asthma: Process from chaos to coping. *Nurs Health Sci.* 2004;6(2):93–99.
24. Piazza-Waggoner CC, Modi WA, Powers BS, Williams ML, Dolan RL, Patton RS. Observational assessment of family functioning in families with children who have type 1 diabetes mellitus. *J Develop Behav Pediatr.* 2008;29(2):101–105.
25. Ammerman RT, Kane VR, Slomka GT, Reigel DH, Franzen MD, Gadow KD. Psychiatric symptomatology and family functioning in children and adolescents with spina bifida. *J Clin Psychol Med Settings.* 1998;5(4):449–465.
26. Alderfer MA, Navsaria N, Kazak AE. Family functioning and posttraumatic stress disorder in adolescent survivors of childhood cancer. *J Fam Psychol.* 2009;23(5):717–725.
27. Horowitz WA, Kazak AE. Family adaptation to childhood cancer: Sibling and family systems variables. *J Clin Child Psychol.* 1990;19(3):221–228.
28. Madanswain A, Brown R, Sexson SB, Baldwin K, Pais R, Ragab A. Adolescent cancer survivors: Psychosocial and familial adaptation. *Psychosomatics.* 1994;35(5):453–459.
29. Lawler MK, Volk R, Viviani N, Mengel MB. Individual and family factors impacting diabetic control in the adolescent: A preliminary study. *Matern Child Nurs J.* 1990;19(4):331–345. PMID: 2136583.
30. Northam E, Anderson P, Adler R, Werther G, Warne G. Psychosocial and family functioning in children with insulin-dependent diabetes at diagnosis and one year later. *J Pediatr Psychol.* 1996;21(5):699–717.
31. Brown C, Pikler VI, Lavish LA, Keune KM, Hutto CJ. Surviving childhood leukemia: Career, family, and future expectations. *Qualit Health Res.* 2008;18(1):19–30.
32. Blair C, Freeman C, Cull A. The families of anorexia nervosa and cystic fibrosis patients. *Psychol Med.* 1995;25(5):985–993.
33. Dashiff CJ. Parents' perceptions of diabetes in adolescent daughters and its impact on the family. *J Pediatr Nurs.* 1993;8(6):361–369.
34. Varni JW, Katz ER, Jr RC, Dolgin M. Family functioning predictors of adjustment in children with newly diagnosed cancer: A prospective analysis. *J Child Psychol Psychiatry.* 1996;37(3):321–328.
35. Wiener LS, Steffen-Smith E, Battles HB, Wayne A, Love CP, Fry T. Sibling stem cell donor experiences at a single institution. *Psycho-oncology.* 2008;17(3):304–307.
36. Pai ALH, Greenley RN, Lewandowski A, Drotar D, Youngstrom E, Peterson CC. A meta-analytic review of the influence of pediatric cancer on parent and family functioning. *J Family Psychol.* 2007;21(3):407–415.
37. Liakopoulou M, Alifieraki T, Katideniou A, et al. Maternal expressed emotion and metabolic control of children and adolescents with diabetes mellitus. *Psychotherapy Psychosomatics.* 2001;70(2):78–85.
38. Leeman J, Crandell JL, Lee A, Bai J, Sandelowski M, Knafl K. Family functioning and the well-being of children with chronic conditions: A meta-analysis. *Res Nurs Health.* 2016;39(4):229–243.
39. Van Schoors M, Caes L, Knoble N, Verhofstadt LL, Goubert L, Alderfer MA. Associations between family functioning and child adjustment after pediatric cancer diagnosis: A meta-analysis. *J Pediatr Psychol.* 2017;42:6–18.
40. Olson DH, Russell CS, Sprenkle DH. Circumplex model of marital and family systems: VI. Theoretical update. *Fam Process.* 1983;22(1):69–83.
41. Svavarsdottir EK, Gisladottir M. How do Family Strengths-Oriented Therapeutic Conversations (FAM-SOTC) advance psychiatric nursing practice? *J Nurs Scholar.* 2019;51(2):214–224.
42. Lowry L. *A Summer to Die.* 2nd ed. New York: Houghton Mifflin Harcourt; 2015.
43. Rosenberg AR, Postier A, Osenga K, et al. Long-term psychosocial outcomes among bereaved siblings of children with cancer. *J Pain Symptom Manage.* 2015;49(1):55–65.
44. Marsac ML, Kindler C, Weiss D, Ragsdale L. Let's talk about it: Supporting family communication during end-of-life care of pediatric patients. *J Palliat Med.* 2018;21(6):862–878.
45. Wilkins KL, Woodgate RL. A review of qualitative research on the childhood cancer experience from the perspective of siblings: A need to give them a voice. *J Pediatr Oncol Nurs.* 2005;22(6):305–319.
46. Mack JW, Hilden JM, Watterson J, et al. Parent and physician perspectives on quality of care at the end of life in children with cancer. *J Clin Oncol.* 2005;23:9155–9161.
47. Hooyman NR, Kramer, BJ. *Living Through Loss: Interventions Across the Life Span.* New York: Columbia Press; 2006.
48. Alderfer MA, Kazak AE. Family issues when a child is on treatment for cancer. In: Brown RT, ed. *Comprehensive Handbook of Childhood Cancer and Sickle Cell Disease: A Biopsychosocial Approach.* New York: Oxford University Press; 2006: 53–74.

49. Kazak AE, Alderfer M, Rourke MT, Simms S, Streisand R, Grossman JR. Posttraumatic stress disorder (PTSD) and posttraumatic stress symptoms (PTSS) in families of adolescent childhood cancer survivors. *J Pediatr Psychol.* 2004;29(3):211–219.
50. Mayou RA, Ehlers A, Bryant B. Posttraumatic stress disorder after motor vehicle accidents: 3-year follow-up of a prospective longitudinal study. *Behav Res Ther.* 2002;40(6):665–675.
51. Mooney-Doyle K, Deatrick JA, Ulrich CM, Meghani SH, Feudtner C. Parenting in childhood life-threatening illness: A mixed-methods study. *J Palliat Med.* 2018;21(2):208–215.
52. Rabelais E, Jones NL, Ulrich CM, Deatrick JA. Meaning making and religious engagement among survivors of childhood brain tumors and their caregivers. *Oncol Nurs Forum.* 2019;46(2):170–184.
53. National Child Traumatic Stress Network. *Definition of Pediatric Medical Traumatic Stress.* Medical Traumatic Stress Working Group Meeting, September 2003.
54. Landolt MA, Buehlmann C, Maag T, Schiestl C. Brief report: Quality of life is impaired in pediatric burn survivors with posttraumatic stress disorder. *J Pediatr Psychol.* 2007;34(1):14–21.
55. Price J, Kassam-Adams N, Alderfer MA, Christofferson J, Kazak AE. Systematic review: A reevaluation and update of the integrative (trajectory) model of pediatric medical traumatic stress. *J Pediatr Psychol.* 2015;41(1):86–97.
56. Kazak AE, Kassam-Adams N, Schneider S, Zelikovsky N, Alderfer MA, Rourke M. An integrative model of pediatric medical traumatic stress. *J Pediatr Psychol.* 2005;31(4):343–355.
57. Streisand R, Mackey ER, Elliot BM, et al. Parental anxiety and depression associated with caring for a child newly diagnosed with type 1 diabetes: Opportunities for education and counseling. *Patient Educ Counsel.* 2008;73(2):333–338.
58. Patiño-Fernández AM, Pai ALH, Alderfer M, Hwang WT, Reilly A, Kazak AE. Acute stress in parents of children newly diagnosed with cancer. *Pediatr Blood Cancer.* 2008;50(2):289–292.
59. Murphy SA, Braun T, Tillery L. et al. PTSD among bereaved parents following the violent deaths of their 12- to 28-year-old children: A longitudinal prospective analysis. *J Trauma Stress.* 1999;12:273–291.
60. Christiansen DM. Posttraumatic stress disorder in parents following infant death: A systematic review. *Clin Psychol Rev.* 2017;51:60–74.
61. Rogers CH, Floyd FJ, Seltzer MM, Greenberg J, Hong J. Long-term effects of the death of a child on parents' adjustment in midlife. *J Family Psychol.* 2008;22:203–211.
62. Meert KL, Donaldson AE, Newth CJ, Harrison R, Berger J, Zimmerman J, Anand KJ, Carcillo J, Dean JM, Willson DF, Nicholson C, Shear K, Eunice Kennedy Shriver National Institute of Child Health and Human Development Collaborative Pediatric Critical Care Research Network. Complicated grief and associated risk factors among parents following a child's death in the pediatric intensive care unit. *Arch Pediatr Adolesc Med.* 2010;164(11):1045–1051.
63. Waugh A, Kiemle G, Slade P. What aspects of post-traumatic growth are experienced by bereaved parents? A systematic review. *Eur J Psychotraumatol.* 2018;9:1.
64. Mooney-Doyle K, Deatrick JA. Parenting in the face of childhood life-threatening conditions: The ordinary in the context of the extraordinary. *Palliat Support Care.* 2015;14(3):187–198.
65. Feudtner C, Walter JK, Faerber JA, et al. Good-parent beliefs of parents of seriously ill children. *JAMA Pediatr.* 2015;169(1):39–47.
66. Hinds PS, Oakes LL, Hicks J, et al. "Trying to be a good parent" as defined by interviews with parents who made phase I, terminal care, and resuscitation decisions for their children. *J Clin Oncol.* 2009;27(35):5979.
67. October TW, Fisher KR, Feudtner C, Hinds PS. The parent perspective: "being a good parent" when making critical decisions in the PICU. *Pediatr Crit Care Med.* 2014;15(4):291–298.
68. Woodgate RL, Edwards M, Ripat JD, Borton B, Rempel G. Intense parenting: A qualitative study detailing the experiences of parenting children with complex care needs. *BMC Pediatr.* 2015;15(1):197–197.
69. Carnevale FA, Alexander E, Davis M, Rennick J, Troini R. Daily living with distress and enrichment: The moral experience of families with ventilator-assisted children at home. *Pediatrics.* 2006;117(1):e48.
70. Mooney-Doyle K, Ulrich CM. Parent moral distress in serious pediatric illness: A dimensional analysis. *Nurs Ethics.* 2020:969733019878838.
71. Walsh JP. *Care, Committment and Moral Distress.* New York: *Springer Nature*; 2018.
72. Van Schoors M, Caes L, Alderfer MA, Goubert L, Verhofstadt L. Couple functioning after pediatric cancer diagnosis: A systematic review. *Psycho-Oncology.* 2017;26:608–616.
73. Brenner M, Côté SM, Boivin M, Tremblay RE. Severe congenital malformations, family functioning and parents' separation/divorce: A longitudinal study. *Child Care Health Dev.* 2016;42(1):16–24. doi:10.1111/cch.12269
74. Long KA, Marsland AL. Family adjustment to childhood cancer: A systematic review. *Clin Child Fam Psychol Rev.* 2011;14(1):57–88. doi:10.1007/s10567-010-0082-z
75. Wijnberg-Williams BJ, Van de Wiel HB, Kamps W, Hoekstra-Weebers JE. Effects of communication styles on marital satisfaction and distress of parents of pediatric cancer patients: A prospective longitudinal study. *Psychooncology.* 2015;24(1):106–112. doi:10.1002/pon.3617
76. Arruda-Colli MNF, Bedoya SZ, Muriel A, Pelletier W, Wiener L. In good times and in bad: What strengthens or challenges a parental relationship during a child's cancer trajectory?. *J Psychosoc Oncol.* 2018;36(5):635–648. doi:10.1080/07347332.2018.1485813
77. Kearney JA, Salley CG, Muriel AC. Standards of psychosocial care for parents of children with cancer. *Pediatr Blood Cancer.* 2015;62 Suppl 5(Suppl 5):S632–S683. doi:10.1002/pbc.25761
78. National Consensus Project for Quality Palliative Care. *Clinical Practice Guidelines for Quality Palliative Care*, 4th edition. Richmond, VA: National Coalition for Hospice and Palliative Care; 2018. https://www.nationalcoalitionhpc.org/ncp
79. Deatrick JA, Barakat LP, Knafl GJ, Hobbie W, Ogle S, Ginsberg JP, Fisher MJ, Hardie T, Reilly M, Broden E, Toth J, SanGiacomo N, Knafl KA. Patterns of family management for adolescent and young adult brain tumor survivors. *J Fam Psychol.* 2018;32(3):321–332.
80. Edwards KE, Neville BA, Cook EF, Aldridge SH, Dussel V, Wolfe J. Understanding of prognosis and goals of care among couples whose child died of cancer. *J Clin Oncol.* 2008;26(8):1310–1315.
81. Feudtner C, Kang TI, Hexem KR, et al. Pediatric palliative care patients: A prospective multicenter cohort study. *Pediatrics.* 2011;127(6):1094.
82. Institute of Medicine. Dying in America: Improving quality and honoring individual preferences near the end of life. *Military Med.* 2015;180(4):365–367.
83. Vermaes IP, van Susante AM, van Bakel HJ. Psychological functioning of siblings in families of children with chronic health conditions: A meta-analysis. *J Pediatr Psychol.* 2012;37(2):166–184.
84. Alderfer MA, Long KA, Lown EA, Marsland AL, Ostrowski NL, Hock JM, Ewing LJ. Psychosocial adjustment of siblings of children with cancer: A systematic review. *Psycho-Oncology.* 2010 Aug;19(8):789–805.
85. Long KA, Lehmann V, Gerhardt CA, Carpenter AL, Marsland AL, Alderfer MA. Psychosocial functioning and risk factors among siblings of children with cancer: An updated systematic review. *Psycho-Oncology.* 2018;27(6):1467–1479.
86. Kaplan LM, Kaal KJ, Bradley L, Alderfer MA. Cancer-related traumatic stress reactions in siblings of children with cancer. *Fam Syst Health.* 2013;31(2):205–217.
87. Parker R, McKeever S, Houghton S, Bichard E. Impact of congenital heart disease on siblings: A review. *J Child Health Care.* 2020:1–20.
88. Alderfer MA, Logan BA, DiDonato S, Jackson L, Hayes MJ, Sigmon ST. Change across time in cancer-related traumatic stress symptoms of siblings of children with cancer: A preliminary investigation. *J Clin Psychol Med Settings.* 2020;27(1):48–53.

89. Brooten D, Youngblut JM. School aged children's experiences 7 and 13 months following a sibling's death. *J Child Fam Studies.* 2017;26(4):1112–1123.
90. Youngblut JM, Brooten D. Parents' report of child's response to sibling's death in a neonatal or pediatric intensive care unit. *Am J Crit Care.* 2013;22(6):474–481.
91. Rostila M, Berg L, Saarela J, Kawachi I, Hjern A. Experience of sibling death in childhood and risk of death in adulthood: A national cohort study from Sweden. *Am J Epidemiol.* 2017;185(12):1247–1254.
92. Yu Y, Liew Z, Cnattingius S, et al. Association of mortality with the death of a sibling in childhood. *JAMA Pediatr.* 2017;171(6):538–545.
93. Eilertsen M, Eilegard A, Steineck G, Nyberg T, Kreicbergs U. Impact of social support on bereaved siblings' anxiety: A nationwide follow-up. *Pediatr Blood Cancer.* 2014;61:S156–S156.
94. Fullerton JM, Totsika V, Hain R, Hastings RP. Siblings of children with life-limiting conditions: Psychological adjustment and sibling relationships. *Child Care Health Devel.* 2017;43(3):393–400.
95. Limbers CA, Skipper S. Health-related quality of life measurement in siblings of children with physical chronic illness: A systematic review. *Families Systems Health.* 2014;32(4):408–415.
96. Long KA, Alderfer MA, Ewing LJ, Marsland AL. The role of contextual threat in predicting self-reported distress among siblings of children with cancer. *J Clin Psychol Med Settings.* 2013;20(2):199–208.
97. Moules N, Strother D, Laing C, Tapp D. Doubled and silenced: Grandparents experiences of childhood cancer. *Pediatr Blood Cancer.* 2010;55(5):845–845.
98. Eilegård A, Steineck G, Nyberg T, Kreicbergs U. Psychological health in siblings who lost a brother or sister to cancer 2 to 9 years earlier. *Psycho-Oncology.* 2013;22(3):683–691.
99. Sveen J, Eilegård A, Steineck G, Kreicbergs U. They still grieve: A nationwide follow-up of young adults 2–9 years after losing a sibling to cancer. *Psycho-Oncology.* 2014;23(6):658–664.
100. Labay LE, Walco GA. Brief report: Empathy and psychological adjustment in siblings of children with cancer. *J Pediatr Psychol.* 2004;29(4) 309–314.
101. Wallin AE, Steineck G, Nyberg T, Kreicbergs U. Insufficient communication and anxiety in cancer-bereaved siblings: A nationwide long-term follow-up. *Palliat Support Care.* 2016;14(5) 488–494.
102. Malcolm C, Gibson F, Adams S, Anderson G, Forbat L. A relational understanding of sibling experiences of children with rare life-limiting conditions: Findings from a qualitative study. *J Child Health Care.* 2014;18(3):230–240.
103. Ellis RR, Simmons T. Coresident grandparents and their grandchildren: 2012. 2014. http://www.census.gov/content/dam/Census/library/publications/2014/demo/p20-576.pdf
104. Pulgaron ER, Marchante AN, Agosto Y, Lebron CN, Delamater AM. Grandparent involvement and children's health outcomes: The current state of the literature. *Fam Syst Health.* 2016;34(3):260–269. doi:10.1037/fsh0000212
105. Wakefield CE, Fardell JE, Doolan EL, et al. Grandparents of children with cancer: Quality of life, medication and hospitalizations. *Pediatr Blood Cancer.* 2017;64(1):163–171.
106. Mendes-Castillo AMC, Bousso RS. The experience of grandmothers of children with cancer. *Revista brasileira de enfermagem.* 2016;69(3):559–565.
107. Youngblut JM, Brooten D. Comparison of mothers and grandmothers physical and mental health and functioning within 6 months after child NICU/PICU death. *Ital J Pediatr.* 2018;44(1):89. doi:10.1186/s13052-018-0531-8
108. Reinhard S, Levine C. Home alone: Family caregivers providing complex care. *Gerontologist.* 2016;56(Suppl3):636–636.
109. Committee on Hospital, Institute for Patient- and Family-Centered Care. Patient-and family-centered care and the pediatrician's role. *Pediatrics. 2012;*129(2)::394–404.
110. Section on Hospice and Palliative Medicine and Committee on Hospital Care. Pediatric palliative care and hospice care commitments, guidelines, and recommendations. *Pediatrics.* 2013;132(5):966–972.
111. Marsac ML, Kassam-Adams N, Hildenbrand AK, Nicholls E, Winston FK, Leff SS, Fein J. Implementing a trauma-informed approach in pediatric health care networks. *JAMA Pediatr.* 2016 Jan;170(1):70–77. doi:10.1001/jamapediatrics.2015.2206. PMID:26571032;PMCID: PMC4939592.
112. Sreedhar SS, Kraft C, Friebert S. Primary palliative care: Skills for all clinicians. *Curr Probl Pediatr Adolesc Health Care.* 2020;50(6):100814. doi:10.1016/j.cppeds.2020.100814
113. Kazak AE, Schneider S, Didonato S, Pai AL. Family psychosocial risk screening guided by the Pediatric Psychosocial Preventative Health Model (PPPHM) using the Psychosocial Assessment Tool (PAT). *Acta Oncol.* 2015;54(5):574–580.
114. Madrigal NV, Carroll WK, Hexem RK, Faerber AJ, Morrison EW, Feudtner EC. Parental decision-making preferences in the pediatric intensive care unit. *Crit Care Med.* 2012;40(10):2876–2882.
115. Niepage M GG, Shama W, Lucchetta S. Exploring adolescents' cancer journey through photovoice: A narrative synthesis. *J Adolesc Young Adult Oncol.* 2018;7(1):15–21.
116. Weaver MS, Baker JN, Gattuso JS, Gibson DV, Hinds PS. "Being a good patient" during times of illness as defined by adolescent patients with cancer. *Cancer.* 2016;122(14):2224–2233.
117. Hinds P. How parental constructs affect parent and family well-being after a child's death children's national medical center.
118. Bell C, Skiles J, Pradhan K, Champion V. End-of-life experiences in adolescents dying with cancer. *Support Care Cancer.* 2010;18(7):827–835.
119. Wolfe J, Hammel JF, Edwards KE, et al. Easing of suffering in children with cancer at the end of life: Is care changing? *J Clin Oncol.* 2008;26(10):1717–1723.
120. Theunissen JMJ, Hoogerbrugge PM, van Achterberg T, Prins JB, Vernooij-Dassen MJFJ, van den Ende CHM. Symptoms in the palliative phase of children with cancer. *Pediatr Blood Cancer.* 2007;49(2):160–165.
121. Kay JS, Juth V, Silver RC, Sender LS. Support and conflict in relationships and psychological health in adolescents and young adults with cancer. *J Health Psychol.* 2016;24(4):502–517.
122. Keim-Malpass J, Erickson JM, Malpass HC. End-of-life care characteristics for young adults with cancer who die in the hospital. *J Palliat Med.* 2014;17(12):1359–1364.
123. Wiegand D. In their own time: The family experience during the process of withdrawal of life-sustaining therapy. *J Palliat Med.* 2008;11(8):1115–1121. doi:10.1089/jpm.2008.0015
124. Mazanec P, Reimer R, Bullington J, et al. Interdisciplinary palliative care teams: Specialists in delivering palliative care. In Ferrell B, Paice J, eds. *Oxford Textbook of Palliative Nursing.* 5th ed. New York: Oxford University Press; 2019: 89–97.

11 | TEAM RELATIONSHIPS

MICHELLE R. BROWN, JODY CHRASTEK, AND KRIS CATRINE

If they don't have scars, they haven't worked on a team. Teams don't just happen. They slowly and painfully evolve. The process is never complete. The work involved is usually underestimated.

BALFOUR MOUNT[1]

By its very nature, and in fact by legislative decree in the case of hospice,[2] palliative care is a team endeavor. Through teamwork, palliative care is able to uniquely tailor care plans to the needs of children impacted by complex illnesses and their families. Through a cyclic process of "forming, storming, norming, and performing,"[3] teams are ever-evolving, with a flexibility that allows them to accommodate the changing needs of children and families as well as those of the care providers within the larger institution. The creation, ongoing growth, and sustainability of highly functional teams is not automatic; it requires sophisticated, multimodal skills. This chapter explores the basic types of teams, team processes, and relational states that support team performance; practical strategies to preserve and protect optimal team functioning; and common challenges of interdisciplinary teams.

TEAM STRUCTURE

Team relationships are influenced by the inherent structure of the team itself, which varies in degree of communication, collaboration, and integration. *Multidisciplinary* teams, the most traditional model, are comprised of individual practitioners who work side by side toward shared goals.[4] Professional identities are primary, while team membership is a secondary priority. Leadership is generally hierarchical, and practitioners function as "wedges in a pie,"[5] wherein roles and responsibilities remain fixed and circumscribed. Information is most often communicated via the patient's chart or in staff meetings or rounds where providers report their clinical findings. Their recommendations are added to, rather than integrated into, the plan of care for the child. The lack of integrated care increases burdens on families who become responsible for keeping their care providers apprised of changing symptoms and treatments,[6] thus making the multidisciplinary model a poor fit for palliative care.

Most palliative care teams, as is evident throughout this book, are self-described as *interdisciplinary*, a model that builds on and adds complexity to the multidisciplinary approach. In an interdisciplinary team, professionals from different disciplines come together through an interactive, collaborative process, creating a combined wisdom to deliver care that is far more than the sum of the individual discipline.[5,7] The identity of the overall team is set above individual professional identities. Yet it is the unique and varied perspectives from each team member that enables a comprehensive understanding of each patient and family and their specific needs. Treatment plans are developed together after considering input from all team members. Decisions are often made by consensus,[8] contributing to a sense of shared responsibility and accountability. This flexible working relationship enables interdisciplinary teams to approach patient care holistically, with the relevant providers attending to concerns as they arise and adapting the care plan as needs change over time.

Team Reflection

An inpatient palliative care team had met Alice, a now 16-year-old girl, when she was first diagnosed with rhabdomyosarcoma. Her disease had progressed despite treatment, and the palliative care team was reconsulted for medication recommendations to manage nausea. A physician and social worker from the palliative care team met Alice and her parents with her oncologist, who introduced them as a new addition to the care team. The palliative care providers addressed her nausea and also spent time understanding what the relapse meant to Alice and her family, along with their hopes and fears. Alice shared her anxiety about her health, her disappointment about missing out on spring break plans with friends, and her fears that her boyfriend would reject her after learning this news. Alice's father was concerned about how to inform her younger sister, who understood very little about the disease. At the weekly interdisciplinary meeting, Alice's case was discussed with the larger palliative care team. Although the initial consult request focused on medication management, the team engaged in an conversation regarding all aspects of her well-being. The psychologist noted that Alice's anxiety might be contributing to her intractable nausea and recommended individual psychotherapy to explore her fears about her uncertain prognosis as well as to provide training in self-hypnosis for symptom management. Music therapy was suggested as an additional way to help Alice channel her anxiety. The child life specialist offered to meet with the parents to facilitate discussions with Alice's sister. Spiritual care was available as the family explored their faith in the face of Alice's illness

Teams may also be referred to as *transdisciplinary*. In this model, team members learn basic knowledge and skills in disciplines other than their own. This allows for the enhanced sharing of responsibilities. For example, if the chaplain is not immediately available for a family, another team member may feel at least a modicum of comfort and competence in assessing and addressing their spiritual request. Thus, in a limited way, team members can provide what the patient or family needs at a given moment until the expert individual becomes available. While this approach has its advantages (e.g., conserving resources, expediting delivery of care), careful attention to mutual recognition of the boundaries in roles and effort is essential.

TEAM COMPOSITION

The composition of each specialty pediatric palliative care (PPC) team will vary depending on site, goals, and scope of services as well as available resources. Ideally, every team will include professionals representing the following fields: medicine, nursing, psychosocial (which may include social work, psychology/psychiatry, child life), and spiritual and bereavement care.[9,10] Even if not formal members, most palliative care teams have access to such providers within their institution, along with high-quality adjunct services including pharmacy, nutrition, case management, expressive therapies, rehabilitation, and education. When fully actualized, a PPC team is like a tapestry in which different colored threads are interwoven to produce a complete picture. At times one color—or one discipline—may be more prominent while others take a more background role. But the presence of each makes the tapestry complete when well-woven around the child and family's goals of care.

Within the hospital setting, there are a variety of specialty pediatric palliative team configurations. Some hospitals have a team whose members are exclusively dedicated to palliative care. In other hospitals, teams may be composed of designated providers from varied departments with a portion of their professional time formally allocated to the team. Alternatively, teams may assemble ad hoc professionals who have particular interest in palliative care. Specialty PPC teams will also collaborate with a range of other professionals as part of the child's broader care, including other medical subspecialists. When children are out of the hospital, their team expands to include providers in outpatient medical clinics and those who provide care at home and in the community (e.g., formal hospice and palliative care programs or partnerships with pediatric professionals who provide home-based care). The community-based team extends to services provided through the county (e.g., social workers, physiotherapists, child development workers, counselors), the school (e.g., teachers, aides, nurses, counselors), and the religious community.

Although each individual specialty offers a unique contribution to the complex needs of children and their families, the role that each team assumes may vary. Exactly who delivers which aspects of care will change over the course of the child's illness. For example, for a child with high-risk leukemia, an oncology team may be most prominent during early stages of treatment, while a stem cell transplant team and a palliative care team may become increasingly involved in the event of disease recurrence. Later, a home hospice team may play a primary role or work conjointly with hospital-based teams.

Family Reflection

Our time on hospice was a powerful experience. It was very scary in the beginning; we worried this meant we were giving up. We quickly learned that hospice was a wonderful support network. I wish we had it sooner. Navigating the road of a child with a terminal diagnosis is complex and involved the family as a whole. As the intensity of our daughter's condition increased, the support and resources each member of the team gave and the team as a whole became an invaluable resource for us. Although there were different roles, they were all very beneficial in different ways and together walked with us through this most difficult of times. They each validated the different care we were providing and helped guide us through the day- to-day challenges. Some of these were practical "hands-on"—like what medications to use—other times it was to help us step back and see the bigger picture. Although each team member had their own expertise, I felt safe to talk with any of them about a concern I had knowing they would support me and bring in the expertise I needed.

The involvement of multiple teams and the transitions among them can, at times, cause confusion or concern for families, particularly when collaboration is impaired by "competition" or possessiveness as to who best knows the patient. Yet, in optimal circumstances, families feel enormous support when their care is enhanced by rich, collaborative teamwork.

The composition of an interdisciplinary team differs for each patient and may change over time. Figure 11.1 illustrates the kaleidoscope of an interdisciplinary team, with roles at times overlapping and shifting to the meet the needs of the child and family. The specialty palliative care team serves as a bridge across the three settings, providing continuity of care for the patient and family. While some families prefer to minimize the overall number of providers involved in their care and reduce duplication of services, other families prefer the services that each team offers to continue simultaneously.

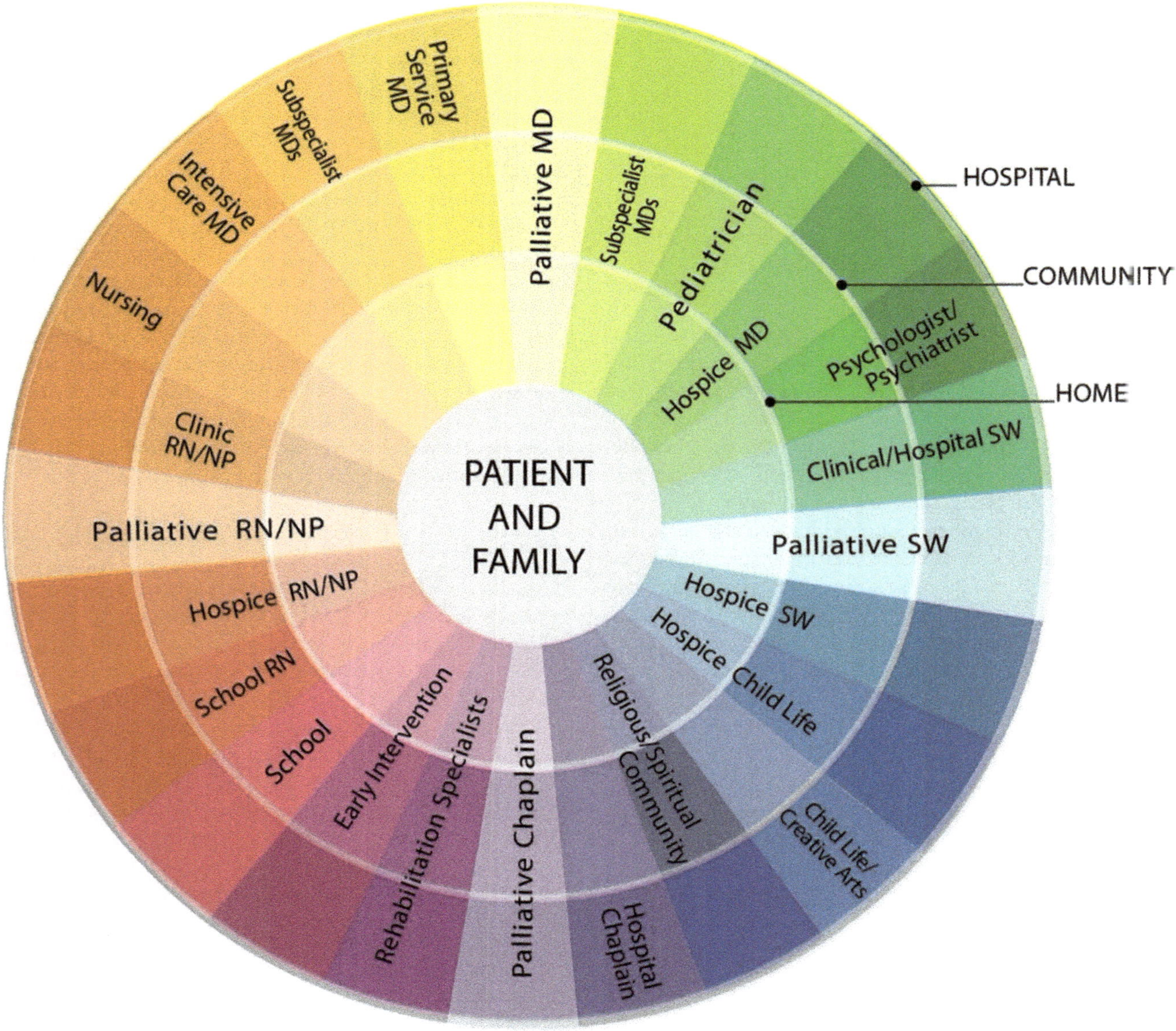

Figure 11.1 The interdisciplinary team in pediatric palliative care. The specialty palliative care team serves as a bridge across all three settings: hospital, community, and home. The community includes hospital-based clinics. MD, physician; NP, nurse practitioner; RN, registered nurse; SW, social worker.

Hence, it is essential that all teams involved in the care of these children and families commit to an agreed-upon philosophy that incorporates the families' choices and goals of care.

PARENTS AS PARTNERS IN CARE

Within the circle of care, the child and family reside in the center, as "partners" with the palliative care team in their own child's care. Yet, in partnering *with* the care team, the patient and family do not become members *of* the team. While absolutely critical in their child's care, parents do not share the team's history, its achievements and failures, its traumas and successes, or its trajectory through time. Nor do they necessarily have the same goals, values, and priorities that a team holds for itself and the families it serves. And, not insignificantly, to view parents and patients as members of the team is to demean the unique relationship not only between ill children and their parents, but also between teams and those they serve.[11]

FRAMEWORK OF TEAM FUNCTIONING

The very nature of the work in PPC necessitates a high level of attention to the dynamics and care of its individual members and the team as a whole. Every interdisciplinary PPC team has, at some point, engaged with families or providers who challenge the integrity of the team. Without careful maintenance, the cohesiveness of PPC teams can splinter, fragmenting the care provided to children and families. (See Chapter 16 on resolving intrateam conflict.) What enables an adaptive, well-functioning team? Models within the healthcare system have identified core processes—referred to as the *C's of team performance*—that are critical for optimal relationships both within and between teams.[12,13] Those especially relevant to palliative care include cognition, collaboration, coaching, and communication in addition to the relational states of cohesion, mutual trust, and psychological safety.

TEAM PROCESSES

COGNITION

Cognition refers to shared mental models,[12,14] identified as one of the critical mechanisms that undergird effective teamwork in general[15] as well as in healthcare specifically.[16–18] Within the palliative care team, shared mental models refer to a common understanding of the goals of patient care, the plan for treatment, and the roles and tasks of the individuals in the team. This is often described as the team being "on the same page."[19]

Most providers of palliative care hold a shared mental model regarding its philosophy, with common values and commitment to the approach. However, perceptions around strategies for accomplishing appropriate goals may vary widely. When team goals are poorly defined—or not defined at all—care providers may be uncertain of their professional role or specific value to the team. Such ambiguity can impair their sense of overall commitment. For example, a newly formed team in a pediatric hospital may identify the expansion of clinical services as a primary goal. Yet expansion can occur through various pathways. Should the team focus their limited resources on collaborating with a specific medical service, or would resources be better spent working with children from many different services who are admitted to the pediatric intensive care unit (PICU)? Should resources be allocated for a nurse practitioner or a clinical social worker? Without well-defined goals, discord can develop within the team as to the "right" action, and frustrations can arise from the perceptions of substandard care or limited progress of the program as a whole. In contrast, clearly defined goals orient team members to the collective purpose.

Teams may be further strained when agreed-upon goals lack specific outcome measures. For example, in an effort to "improve palliative care," a team may implement educational initiatives for nursing and increased clinical availability to various medical services. Outcome measures could be (for example) pre- and post-questionnaires to assess the educational intervention and satisfaction ratings from medical services. Without such measures, the effectiveness is unknown. Team members can be frustrated when, despite significant time and energy—and often the perception of positive impact—there is no evaluation of outcome in place. Without evidence of positive outcomes, these efforts may go unrecognized by the administrators who allocate financial and other resources to programs within the organization.

The delineation of roles and responsibilities is important to clarify each individual's contribution to the team. When team members believe that duties have been fairly distributed and that everyone is working for the greater good, a sense of commitment and cohesion is fostered. In contrast, when roles are not adequately delineated, diffusion of responsibility becomes more likely. Team members may blame one another for lack of progress, leading to hostility and ill will. Chronic unresolved conflict or dissatisfaction may lead to personal detachment or fractures within the team. A lack of clearly defined roles can precipitate the blurring of professional boundaries, whereby team members' engagement with patients and families can overextend into areas that are not their primary expertise nor typical for the culture of the broader team. The risk of this occurrence increases when team members distrust others' ability to provide optimal care in their defined role.

Team Reflection

Susan, a nurse practitioner, had connected immediately with a family with whom she shared many interests and background, Susan met with 6-year-old Poppy and her parents frequently, both in clinic and in their home; managing medications as symptoms worsened, offering emotional support to both parents, and even providing brief respite to afford them some time alone. The parents frequently noted how indebted they were to Susan; in turn she felt appreciated and needed. As Poppy's death neared, Susan provided the family with her personal cell phone number and encouraged them to call at any time. Susan was concerned that the on-call providers were not as skilled as she in palliative care. When Poppy died suddenly on a Saturday afternoon, the family tried desperately—and unsuccessfully—to reach Susan. Eventually, they called the 24-hour emergency number, but the delay caused them additional suffering.

In addition to the risk of causing greater challenges for families, clinicians who overextend their roles can set up other team members to be judged as less engaged in care. They also can cause confusion among consulting services, who may come to expect a higher degree of availability than what the palliative team can realistically offer. The risk of these situations occurring may be reduced by regular and ongoing review of team roles specific to each patient and family.

COLLABORATION

In addition to well-defined goals and roles, commitment to collaborative relationships is crucially important to healthy team functioning. While team goals orient actions, supportive and collaborative relationships help to achieve them.[20] In fact, the two may be considered interdependent because the more supportive the team, the more likely members are to commit to work tasks, meaningful goals, and to the development of compassionate relationships.[11]

Coordination and cooperation have been identified as two separate but related processes that synchronize team dynamics.[12] As such, collaboration requires team members both to recognize the unique roles and specific contribution of every other member and to integrate their work efforts to achieve team goals. Through this interdependence, the whole becomes greater than the sum of the individual parts. For a collaborative alliance to develop, care providers must spend time working together, sharing experiences, exploring different viewpoints, and developing a common language that does not exclude any member. It requires an open, reflective process that enables team members to challenge their own and others' thinking and share experiences with a receptiveness to potential change.[21] Together, teams can consider strategies for coping, implement new initiatives and change, enhance the ability to take risks, and, ultimately, grow as a team.

Collaborative relationships are sustained by mutual support. Studies indicate that one of the primary factors that contributes to professional burnout is not the team's confrontation with multiple child deaths, however distressing, but rather a team's inability to support its members.[22–24] Four essential types of support include informational support, instrumental support, emotional support, and support in the construction of meaning.[20] The specific form of support provided will vary at different times under different circumstances (see Box 11.1).

Informational support lays the foundation for collaboration. Teams often have structures in place to enable regular exchange of information (e.g., patient handoffs between team members, weekly team meetings). When fractures in team relationships exist, informational support can be easily overlooked, particularly during periods of high census and/or patient acuity. For example, a team member may forget to inform others of a scheduled care conference for a shared patient. Or the news of a patient's death is not relayed to other team members who had been closely involved. While such oversights may be innocent, their impact on collaboration can be significant.

Scarce financial resources may result in differences in how much dedicated time individuals actually have for their participation on the team. These differences are not always known or remembered by others. Conflict arises when workload expectations for individuals are greater than what would be reasonable for their time allocation. When they are less available than others to participate in certain activities, their professionalism may be questioned. In turn, these members may feel underappreciated or undervalued and, as a result, less committed to the team as a whole.

Collaboration is enhanced when support is responsive to the emotional needs of team members, as well as to the construction of meaning.

BOX 11.1 TYPES OF SUPPORT

Informational support: Involves the exchange of information about the people served and the team's mode of operation; it comprises mutual feedback about and evaluation of individual or team performance with opportunities to expand one's knowledge and skills.

Instrumental support: Involves helping each other with practical issues such as sharing the workload and the coordination of efforts toward the achievement of specific tasks. Shared goals, role clarity, and trust in each other's knowledge and skills enhance this form of support.

Emotional support: Involves opportunities for sharing personal feelings and thoughts in a safe environment in which one feels heard, understood, valued, and appreciated. Sometimes the presence of another colleague during stressful moments is all that is needed.

Support in meaning construction: Involves opportunities to reflect on and work through work-related experiences and invest individual and collective efforts with meaning. Care providers help each other understand their responses, correct distortions, and reframe situations in ways that make sense to them.

Adapted from Papadatou D. *In the face of death: Professionals who care for the dying and bereaved.* New York: Springer; 2009.

Team Reflection

In discussion with a recently bereaved mother, the team nurse practitioner felt troubled by the mother's doubt around her decision to forgo a second stem cell transplant for her child. The mother had declined further life-prolonging efforts in the hope that her child would be more comfortable. Yet, in the end, the child's last days were spent in an inordinate amount of pain and suffering. Upon reflection, the nurse practitioner worried that she had unwittingly influenced the mother to make the wrong decision. However, in a later discussion with the team, another member reminded her that the mother's questioning was a normal part of the grieving process. Without this opportunity to reframe her experience and receive both emotional and "meaning-making" support, the nurse practitioner may have carried a burden of guilt that could hinder her ability to fully engage with families in the future

Collaboration is impaired when a mismatch exists between the type of support provided by individual members and the needs of the team as a whole. For example, if one or more team members provide excellent informational support but do not respond to the emotional needs of others, the team may be less likely to debrief, problem-solve, or support one other when needed.

COACHING

Coaching, also referred to as *team leadership*, plays an important role in promoting team effectiveness[12] by setting the tone and guiding team members and the program as a whole. Team-centered leaders are visionary and proactive. They inspire constructive teamwork and mutual support, communicate clearly and frequently, are open to questions and feedback, consider problem-solving a team responsibility, and mediate the conflicts that inevitably arise. They honor their own commitments, expect the same in return, and recognize both individual and team accomplishments. These leaders focus on the effectiveness and well-being of the team above their own personal reputation. They recognize members' individual strengths, coach them to reach their full potential in their role, and distribute responsibilities to optimize these strengths for the advancement of the entire team.

COMMUNICATION

Communication is perhaps the single most important factor in team success.[12,25] It is important that teams commit to a regular meeting time to communicate about clinical issues in patient care as well as the team process. Open communication enables members to discuss difficult issues directly and respectfully, be receptive to differing opinions, and use these situations as learning experiences for the team as a whole. Furthermore, just as palliative providers facilitate debriefings with treatment teams around stressful or traumatic events, the same opportunity should be offered within the palliative care team itself.

How conflict is handled between individuals can either strengthen or damage the team as a whole. Not uncommonly, in a misguided effort to be collaborative, conflict is not acknowledged, as in the proverbial "elephant in the room."[26] With guidance from the leader, teams can draw upon their individual and collective skills to identify and address unspoken issues toward conflict resolution.

Team Reflection

Karo, Nurse Lead, and Keysha, Social Work Lead, had worked hard over years to develop the palliative care and hospice team. They were well respected as leaders of their program. Over time the program expanded, and they recruited a social worker with a decade of palliative care experience to join their team. The transition was seamless and both Karo and Keysha felt that Ana brought fresh ideas that enhanced the program. A year after Ana's arrival, the hospice program suffered three deaths in short succession that deeply affected everyone. Staff looked to Karo and Keysha for support and later acknowledged them in the institutional newsletter. Ana was hurt that she was not equally recognized. Soon thereafter, Ana began to make comments to other staff members that planted doubt in the team leadership. The whole team felt a change in atmosphere. In a private talk with the leaders, Ana shared that she did not feel her contribution to the team was appreciated. She also expressed a desire for a leadership role. As an outcome of this discussion, they developed a plan that addressed Ana's individual concerns as well as ways to focus on the team process and communication.

TEAM RELATIONAL STATES

Whereas team processes reflect what teams do, relational states, including cohesion, trust, and psychological safety, reflect how teams feel. These states are typically dynamic in nature and vary as a function of context, experiences, and outcomes. Their influence is bidirectional: how a team engages in communication and collaboration will affect the sense of team cohesion. Similarly, the more cohesive a team, the more engaged the members become in collaboration and open communication.[12]

COHESION

Cohesion refers to the creation and maintenance of ties among members of the team.[12] It fosters a sense of collective identity in which team goals are prioritized over those of the individual.[27] Sustaining cohesion demands an ongoing commitment of time and energy by each team member and by the team as a whole. Team members who are committed only to their own work may fail to value or develop genuine interest in the contribution of others. Relationships may be experienced as competitive or conflicted when individuals perceive their role as more central to a patient's care than others. Furthermore, because of the intensity of the clinical issues that team members face in their work with patients and families, some individuals may not want to devote time and energy to work on team building.

Teams with a poor sense of collective identity and cohesive organization also are more vulnerable to being "tested" by anxious patients and families. For example, parents may ask multiple staff members the same question in search of a unified response. When, in the absence of team cohesion, individual members provide different answers, they can inadvertently weaken the family's confidence in the team as a whole.

MUTUAL TRUST AND PSYCHOLOGICAL SAFETY

Mutual trust reflects the degree to which team members believe that they can rely on one another.[12,16] It evolves over time from confidence that team members can perform well in their roles, and it enables them to share opposing perspectives, admit mistakes, and accept feedback.

Trust is necessary for individuals to have the confidence that their feelings—and confidentiality—will be respected. Within a safe environment, care providers can acknowledge their vulnerability and suffering and lean temporarily on others who understand first-hand the strain of caring for children with life-threatening illnesses. The team as "shelter" is critical—when professionals feel supported by their colleagues, they can more effectively guide and support patients and their families.

Team Reflection

Maria was a hospice nurse caring for a family whose young son was nearing end of life. She was highly regarded by her team for her compassionate clinical care and exceptional work ethic. Over the past two interdisciplinary team meetings, Maria had arrived late and was unprepared to discuss her patients. Recognizing that this behavior was out of character for Maria, her team members gently noted their observations and asked how she was doing. Maria shared that her son attended the same school as her patient and that every time she cared for her patient, she thought of her son and felt her anxiety rise. She was even beginning to doubt her nursing skills. Her team reflected on her experience with her and provided validation and reassurance. The social worker offered to join Maria in future home visits, so that she would feel more able to preserve professional boundaries without compromising the emotional support provided to the child and his family.

In contrast, teams that strive to avoid suffering can handicap the team's overall development. If the expression of emotional distress is interpreted as a sign of weakness and incompetence, team members may withhold personal disclosure to avoid being judged as "too close" or "too invested" in their patients. Furthermore, in fear of receiving negative performance evaluations, they may refrain from seeking the support that would enable them to function more effectively.

As is evident, creating and maintaining teams is an extremely complex undertaking. Box 11.2 briefly operationalizes the processes described above as strategies for creating a well-functioning PPC team.

SELF-CARE

PPC can exact a heavy toll on professionals.[28] It is crucial to attend to the health and well-being of the team as a whole as well as its individual members. A *team covenant* is a valuable tool to address this need. This document lays out expectations for individual team members to acknowledge, with the goal of ensuring their shared understanding and commitment to the team as a whole. As circumstances and personnel change, the covenant can be updated to keep it relevant and beneficial to the team (see Box 11.3).

BOX 11.2 CREATING WELL-FUNCTIONING PPC TEAMS

- Cultivate time, space, and patience. Ensure that team members understand the definition and unique contributions of one another's roles to optimize collaboration.
- Establish clear policies and processes that value and support teamwork, including open discussion of challenging issues with reinforcement of boundaries.
- Maintain ongoing awareness of team functioning. Consider bringing in consultant for reexamination of team processes and goals as needed.
- Establish and practice conflict resolution strategies within the team.
- Focus on creation of a team environment with qualities that include optimism, personal recognition, respectful and empathic exchange of ideas, perceptions and feelings, openness and flexibility, egalitarianism, and mutual support.
- Establish procedures to evaluate effectiveness and quality of team efforts.
- Design, enact, and revisit team self-care plans.

BOX 11.3 TEAM COVENANT

I __________ (name), as part of our team, will:

- Take responsibility for my actions, personal well-being and health
- Respect the other team members and their varied perspectives
- Regularly review a self-care plan
- Thoughtfully bring important issues and conflicts to the team
- Consider whether conflicts are best addressed individually or at the team level
- Acknowledge to myself and my team when I am in need of added support
- Be honest when current circumstances limit me from providing additional support to team members
- Give and accept feedback—both positive and negative—in a constructive way
- Recognize the skills and strengths of each team member

________________ __________

Team Member Date

Self-care plans are a more personal method for individuals to help themselves maintain healthy lives while working so closely with loss and sadness (see Chapter 12). The concept of the self-care plan is not new, yet its formal development and practical use are recent. These are detailed, private documents that serve to remind members of how best to care for themselves, especially when under stress. It is essential to address the issues holistically; therefore, similar to all palliative care interventions, physical, emotional, social, and spiritual domains are included. As with the team covenant, ongoing evaluation—and reevaluation—of self-care plans is encouraged, particularly during stressful times.

WORKING WITH PRIMARY AND OTHER SUBSPECIALTY TEAMS

The same processes that support optimal functioning within the palliative care team are relevant to working with the child's primary and subspecialty teams as well.[13] While the collective wisdom of medical experts often enhances patient care, physical distance among clinical settings and limited in-person interaction between palliative team members and those from other services can make communication difficult. Conflicts may arise that in turn result in parental confusion, fractured trust, and reinforcement of rigid territorial boundaries among teams.

Cultural differences within teams in decision-making processes—on a spectrum from "democratic/consensus building" to "hierarchical/authoritarian"—may hinder optimal functioning between teams. Regularly scheduled care conferences, during which primary and subspecialty teams can share perspectives and together inform the treatment plan, help to prevent individuals or a single team from making unilateral decisions around patient care. Primary and/or subspecialty teams also vary in their expectations of the involvement of the specialty palliative care team. At times, these expectations may not align with the palliative care team's assessment of appropriate engagement. Conflict may arise among subspecialty teams when they differ in perspectives around the risks and benefits of particular interventions or in what they consider to be a reasonable quality of life.

Team Reflection

A pediatric intensivist requested a palliative care consult to facilitate a goals-of-care conversation with the parents of 1-year-old Angel, diagnosed with pulmonary hypertension. The PICU team felt that there was little likelihood for his long-term survival and expressed concern about the pain and suffering associated with ongoing invasive medical procedures. They were unaware of any children like Angel who had survived into later childhood. Angel's parents spoke to the importance of his quality of life and elected to transition his care to "comfort measures only" with a plan for compassionate extubation. The pulmonary hypertension specialist, however, had been unaware of the palliative care consult and was angered that he had not been included by the PICU team in the discussion. He strongly disagreed with the conclusion drawn by the PICU team. He had cared for many children with this condition over several years, and his prognosis for Angel was more optimistic. He shared his views in a subsequent meeting with Angel's parents, which led them to reverse their decision and request that all medical intervention be provided. The parents, who previously had felt strong sense of trust in the PICU team, now questioned their motivations. They feared that the recommendation to discontinue life-sustaining interventions was driven by a desire to reduce healthcare costs to the hospital

Many providers feel a deep emotional investment in their patients' well-being. They also develop their own beliefs regarding what is in the child's best interest, informed by knowledge of the patient and family as well as their own values. Significant distress may arise when care plans conflict with the provider's beliefs, as when they perceive that a treatment is causing more burden than benefit. Discussions that arise in palliative care consultations can assist all team members in understanding their own and the family's perspectives.

Team Reflection

Jamal, a 4-year-old boy awaiting heart transplant, suffered a stroke resulting from the ventricular assist device that was supporting him. At a care conference with his parents, the cardiovascular intensive care team shared the magnetic resonance imaging (MRI) results, which indicated profound neurologic injury. They recommended discontinuation of life-sustaining interventions, including deactivating the ventricular assist device. Although the parents understood that they had lost their son as they had known him, their religious beliefs prohibited their consent. Bedside nurses who were not present at the care conference nor updated about the conversation with parents reported significant distress in caring for Jamal, stating, "The parents just don't get it. He's not going to get better." It was only after a palliative care consult (requested by nursing staff) that the parent's understanding of Jamal's prognosis was clarified. With goals of care more clearly stated, nursing felt more comfortable delivering care to Jamal in the remaining days of his life.

In caring for critically ill children, particularly in the face of prognostic uncertainty, disagreements can emerge among primary and subspecialty teams. With open communication and respect for the perspectives of all team members, the PPC team can assist in reconciling differing opinions regarding goals of care and related treatment options. The setting of a care conference, at times providers only, at times including the parents, can be invaluable.

Team Reflection

Layla, 4, was born with complex cardiac disease and had spent nearly a year after birth in the cardiac ICU undergoing several surgeries. Her care team had often commented on how she "developed every possible complication," including an episode of fungemia from which she made an unexpectedly full recovery. The medical staff became quite attached to Layla and her parents. Despite all efforts, Layla's cardiac failure progressed, and she required a heart transplant. In what staff viewed as her "first lucky break," she received a heart after only a month of being listed. However, the night after her transplant she began having seizures and a brain MRI revealed a large intracranial bleed. She underwent emergency surgery but remained unresponsive.

As weeks went by without signs of significant neurologic recovery, differing opinions about Layla's prognosis emerged among teams, along with increasing tension. The intensive care physician and nurses felt that care should be redirected to focus on comfort, while the cardiac transplant team felt strongly that it was too soon to discontinue intervention. Neurology expressed doubt as to whether Layla could ever return to her baseline functioning. Layla's parents shared that she had "beaten the odds" before and that she had always taken many months to recover from complications.

The specialty palliative care team was invited to attend a care conference, with the goal of bringing about consensus for a plan for Layla's care. The palliative team suggested a 2-week trial of continuing all intervention, to be followed by reassessment. Everyone agreed with this plan. During this 2-week period, the palliative team met with the family jointly, first with the transplant team and then with intensive care, to provide a picture of what Layla's life might look like in both the best and worst outcomes. The team also partnered with spiritual care, social work, and the family's trusted primary care physician to explore with the parents what "quality of life" for Layla would mean. At the end of the trial, based on worsening MRI and electroencephalogram (EEG) results, the teams agreed to recommend that Layla's care be focused entirely on ensuring her comfort. After long and emotional discussion with the team, Layla's family elected compassionate extubation, with the proviso that should she be able to support her own breathing, they would take her home with hospice support.

Achieving such consensus across settings which hold disparate mental models for care can require more effort. This is especially evident when a child moves from the hospital into the community. Schools, for example, while expert in the education and socialization of children, understandably feel unprepared to manage the care of a medically fragile child. Yet, despite their different knowledge base and expertise, a focus on shared goals can enable teams to collaborate around a mutually agreeable plan.

Team Reflection

Callie, an 8-year-old child with glioblastoma, was cared for in a community-based home hospice program. Although her health was deteriorating quickly, the highlight of her days was to attend school and be with her friends. The school principal, aware that Callie was enrolled in hospice, had informed her parents that, despite the do-not-resuscitate (DNR) order in place, he would nonetheless be legally obligated to call 911, as for any child. Callie's parents felt conflicted, wanting both to allow her to continue to enjoy school and to die without unwanted interventions. The hospice team facilitated a discussion with Callie's parents and school staff to reach a plan acceptable to everyone. Callie would continue to attend class for a few hours each day, during which time her father would remain close by. The school agreed to call him and 911 if Callie had a sudden medical event so that he could present her Physician Orders For Life-Sustaining Treatment (POLST) form when emergency medical services arrived. Thus, Callie was able to continue in school while both her parents and the staff felt comfortable with a plan that addressed her needs and abided by legal obligations.

CONCLUSION

Interdisciplinary teamwork is vital to providing quality care for our most vulnerable children and families. Yet a team of experts does not, in itself, make an expert team.[29] To operate effectively, a team must know how to cooperate, coordinate, and communicate well together with attention paid to the dynamic processes that foster and maintain healthy relationships. Unlike other concepts in PPC, teamwork is not usually formally taught. Instead, most teams learn these important skills by modeling what they have observed in their clinical experience. Recently, training has been expanded to build team competencies across healthcare systems more broadly.[30] (For further discussion, see Chapter 7, Interdisciplinary Education and Training). Increased integration of these specific knowledge, skills, and attitudes into existing palliative care curricula will promote the creation and maintenance of effective interdisciplinary PPC teams.

REFERENCES

1. Mount BM, Voyer J. Staff stress in palliative/hospice care. In Ajemian I, Mount BM, eds. *The RVH Manual on Palliative/Hospice Care: A Resource Book.* Arno Press; 1980: 457–488.
2. Centers for Medicare and Medicaid Programs. Conditions of participation: Hospice care. https://www.cms.gov/Regulations-and-Guidance/Legislation/CFCsAndCoPs/Hospice
3. Tuckman B. Developmental sequence in small-groups. *Psychol Bull.* 1965;63(6):384–399. doi:10.1037/h0022100
4. Lee S. Interdisciplinary teaming in primary care: A process of evaluation and resolution. *Social Work Health Care.* 1980;5(3):237–244. doi:10.1300/J010v05n03_01
5. Crawford GB, Price SD. Team working: Palliative care as a model of interdisciplinary practice. *Med J Aust.* 2003;179(S6):S32–34.
6. Street A, Blackford J. Communication issues for the interdisciplinary community palliative care team. *J Clin Nurs.* 2001;10(5) 643–650. doi:10.1046/j.1365-2702.2001.00549.x
7. Rubin IM, Beckhard R. Factors influencing the effectiveness of health teams. *Milbank Mem Fund Q.* 1972;50(3):317–335.
8. Cummings I. The interdisciplinary team. In Doyle D, Hanks GWC, MacDonald N, eds. *Oxford Textbook of Palliative Medicine.* 2nd ed. Oxford University Press; 1998:19–30.
9. National Consensus Project for Quality Palliative Care. *Clinical Practice Guidelines for Quality Palliative Care.* 4th ed. National Consensus Project for Quality Palliative Care; 2018.
10. Section on Hospice and Palliative Medicine and Committee on Hospital Care. Pediatric palliative care and hospice care commitments, guidelines, and recommendations. *Pediatrics.* 2013;132(5):966–972. doi:10.1542/peds.2013-2731
11. Papadatou D, Bluebond-Langer M, Goldman A. The team. In Wolfe J, Hinds PS, Sourkes BM, eds. *Textbook of Interdisciplinary Pediatric Palliative Care.* Elsevier/Saunders; 2011:55–63.
12. Weaver SJ, Feitosa J, Salas E, Seddon R, Vozenilek JA. The theoretical drivers and models of team performance and effectiveness for patient safety. In Salas E, Frush K, eds. *Improving Patient Safety Through Teamwork and Team Training.* Oxford University Press; 2013 3–26.
13. DeChurch LA, Marks MA. Leadership in multiteam systems. *J Appl Psychol.* 2006;91(2):311–329. doi:10.1037/0021-9010.91.2.311
14. D'Ambruoso SF, Coscarelli A, Hurvitz S, et al. Use of a shared mental model by a team composed of oncology, palliative care, and supportive care clinicians to facilitate shared decision making in a patient with advanced cancer. *J Oncol Pract.* 2016;12(11) 1039–1045. doi:10.1200/JOP.2016.013722

15. Salas E, Cooke N, Rosen M. On teams, teamwork, and team performance: Discoveries and developments. *J Hum Fact Ergonom Soc.* 2008;50:540–547.
16. Salas E, Sims D, Burke C. Is there a "Big Five" in teamwork? *Small Group Res.* 2005;36(5):555–599.
17. Burtscher MJ, Kolbe M, Wacker J, Manser T. Interactions of team mental models and monitoring behaviors predict team performance in simulated anesthesia inductions. *J Exp Psychol Appl.* 2011;17(3):257–269. doi:10.1037/a0025148
18. Westli HK, Johnsen BH, Eid J, Rasten I, Brattebø G. Teamwork skills, shared mental models, and performance in simulated trauma teams: An independent group design. *Scand J Trauma Resusc Emerg Med.* 2010;18(47). doi:10.1186/1757-7241-18-47
19. Weller J, Boyd M, Cumin D. Teams, tribes and patient safety: Overcoming barriers to effective teamwork in healthcare. *Postgrad Med J.* 2014;90(1061):149–154. doi:10.1136/postgradmedj-2012-131168
20. Papadatou D. *In the Face of Death: Professionals Who Care for the Dying and the Bereaved.* Springer; 2009.
21. Larson DG. *The Helper's Journey.* 2nd ed. Research Press; 2019.
22. Vachon MLS. *Occupational Stress in the Care of the Critically Ill, the Dying, and the Bereaved.* Hemisphere Publishing; 1987.
23. Vachon M. Recent research into staff stress in palliative care. *Eur J Palliat Care.* 1997;4:99–103.
24. Papadatou D, Martinson IM, Chung PM. Caring for dying children: A comparative study of nurses' experiences in Greece and Hong Kong. *Cancer Nurs.* 2001;24(5):402–412. doi:10.1097/00002820-200110000-00013
25. Youngwerth J, Twaddle M. Cultures of interdisciplinary teams: How to foster good dynamics. *J Palliat Med.* 2011;14(5):650–654. doi:10.1089/jpm.2010.0395
26. Lencioni P. *The Five Dysfunctions of a Team: A Leadership Fable.* Jossey-Bass; 2002.
27. Leasure EL, Jones RR, Meade LB, et al. There is no "i" in teamwork in the patient-centered medical home: Defining teamwork competencies for academic practice. *Acad Med.* 2013;88(5):585–592. doi:10.1097/ACM.0b013e31828b0289
28. Sourkes B, Frankel L, Brown M, et al. Food, toys, and love: Pediatric palliative care. *Curr Probl Pediatr Adolesc Health Care.* 2005;35(9):350–386. doi:10.1016/j.cppeds.2005.09.002
29. Salas E, Reyes DL, McDaniel SH. The science of teamwork: Progress, reflections, and the road ahead. *Am Psychol.* 2018;73(4):593–600. doi:10.1037/amp0000334
30. Rosen MA, DiazGranados D, Dietz AS, et al. Teamwork in healthcare: Key discoveries enabling safer, high-quality care. *Am Psychol.* 2018;73(4):433–450. doi:10.1037/amp0000298

12 | WITNESS TO SUFFERING

The Clinician Experience

BARBARA M. SOURKES, STEPHEN LIBEN, AND DANAI PAPADATOU

Look long and hard at the things that please you,
even longer and harder at what causes you pain.

Colette[1]

To provide optimal care to children living with life-threatening conditions and their families, clinicians in pediatric palliative care (PPC) must be prepared to enter into their world: coming face to face with the relentlessness of illness, the uncertainty of prognosis, and, at times, the inevitability of death. Clinicians are often asked: "How can you do that work? It must be so depressing." In fact, depressing is one of the few things it *isn't*. Rather, it can be fulfilling and rich, arduous and frustrating, sad, poignant, and, ultimately, profoundly moving.[2] Clinicians must possess—or develop—a high threshold for witnessing the anguish of threatened separation and loss, inextricably linked with the harsh ravages of disease. To witness is not a passive process.[3] Every encounter offers clinicians the opportunity for a sense of connection and meaning that can, to some degree, counterbalance the suffering before their eyes and within themselves.

The core challenge for professionals in PPC who experience repeated cycles of attachment and loss is: "How do I preserve myself while, at the same time, sustain my ability to be an effective and empathic clinician?" This chapter examines relationship-centered care with a focus on the complex reciprocal influences among children, families, and clinicians. It describes the nature of clinicians' suffering, including the impact of a child's death. Building resilience and engaging in self-care are discussed as critical practices, both for the integration of clinicians' own experience and for the provision of optimal care of children and their families (see Figure 12.1).

A RELATIONSHIP-CENTERED APPROACH TO CARE

Papadatou[4] suggests that it is necessary to expand our view of the care of seriously ill children beyond the family-centered approach, with its limited focus on the patient and family. A relationship-centered approach provides a broader perspective. It illuminates the dynamics that develop among patients, families, clinicians, and teams, and it considers the larger organizational and sociocultural context in which care is provided. It explores the reciprocal influence among patients, families, and clinicians and sheds light on their experiences and interactions. In essence, the relationship-centered approach focuses on whatever transpires when the private and social worlds of ill children and their families interact with the private and social worlds of clinicians. To better understand the outcomes of such encounters, it is important to consider its basic components.

1. The subjective world of the child or family understood in light of his or her personal and family history and sociocultural background.
2. The subjective world of the clinician understood in light of his or her personal, family, and professional history and sociocultural background.
3. The culture of the team or organization that provides services to seriously ill children and their families.
4. The larger social, economic, and cultural context in which care is offered and received.
5. The intersubjective space that is formed when the child or parent meets and interacts with a clinician or team within a specific sociocultural context. This space belongs to their unique relationship (Figure 12.2).

The intersubjective space is defined as "the domain of feelings, thoughts, and knowledge that two (or more) people share about the nature of their current relationship."[5(p. 243)] When children, families, and clinicians are open to one another and to their respective worlds, then the intersubjective space enlarges to enable rich collaboration. It also offers opportunities for new learning, increased self-awareness, and growth in the midst of uncertainty. Such experiences render the process of care deeply meaningful. By contrast, when both

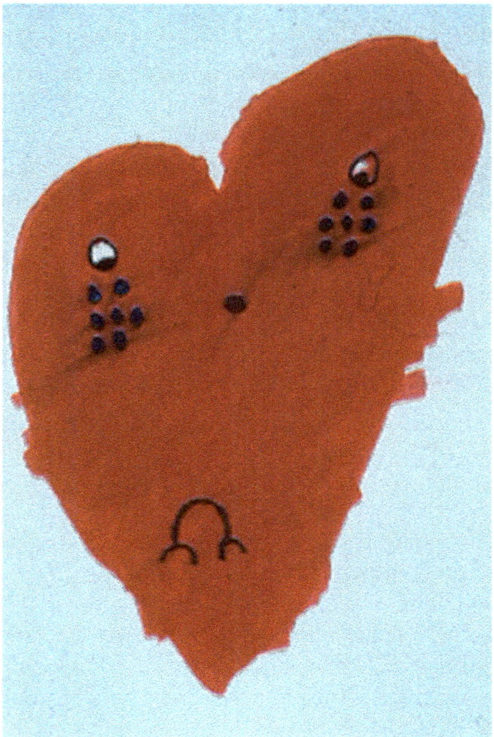

Figure 12.1 *A heart weeping (7-year-old child).*

clinicians and family members merely enact prescribed roles and focus solely on what needs to be done, then the intersubjective space narrows in its capacity to offer opportunities for genuine connection. It also limits the potential for viewing reality in new ways and for developing resilience in the midst of suffering and loss. Both perspectives are illustrated in the following family reflection.

Family Reflection

Both my daughters, Maria—and then 2 years later—Stella, were born with a rare, undiagnosed syndrome that resulted in severe developmental delay, neurological and motor problems, frequent seizures, and pulmonary infections. Each of them lived until age 9. My experience with the care they received during their last hospitalizations—in two different intensive care units—could not have been more different.

Maria's hospitalization lasted 10 days, and during those days, staff members did their duty. The care she received, from the first physician to the last nurse, was very professional, but what was missing was personal warmth and humanity. It was a physician who informed me that Maria's condition was critical and that it was uncertain whether she would survive. The way he imparted this information was so cold, so distant. . . . Some doctors avoid giving time to parents, and I fully understand it because they have to attend to several children besides our own. But we, the parents who have children with serious problems, have the right to clear information, to some compassion, to be treated as if we are their own people. The night Maria died, they told us that it would be a difficult night. But we, the parents, always hope for a miracle. What I remember is that when I squeezed her hand, she bit the breathing tube. When I saw the machines react, I ached. I realized that she was aware I was there. I was then asked to leave the intensive care unit because Maria was crying and the staff felt that my presence agitated her. And 10 minutes later she left [died]. . . .

Stella was admitted to another intensive care unit and was hospitalized for 40 days. From the moment we were

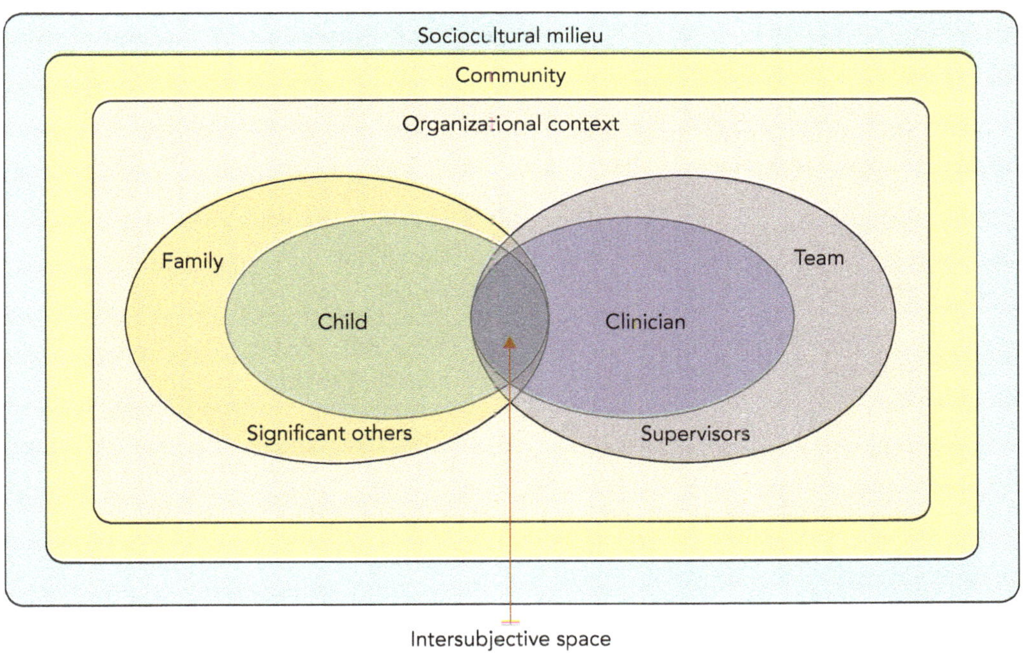

Figure 12.2 *The intersubjective space.*

admitted to the moment Stella left [died], we experienced a tremendous difference in our relationships with the staff as compared to our experience with Maria. The doctors outdid themselves; they were very human, warm, and made us feel as if we were their family. Yes, we were indeed their family. My child was also their child. There are no words to describe it. We just felt it. And to tell you the truth, Stella felt it, too. Although she was on a respirator, she felt the care, the concern, and the love that staff members communicated to her. I could see it in her face. She was content, happy. In this unit, professionals had a place for her and for us. They were interested in my concerns and discussed Stella's condition and what would be in her best interest. We did not want her to suffer. They gave us some choices.... And they respected our decisions, and I am deeply grateful for that. I remember it was Sunday when the physician on call informed us that Stella had developed arrhythmias and that, sadly, the end was close. Again, I did not want to believe it. I sat next to Stella until the moment she died. I expressed the desire to hug her one last time, which was difficult because she was on the respirator. The staff removed the respirator to help me take her in my arms for one last hug.

* * *

Mrs. L. acknowledges that the clinicians in both intensive care units had dealt with the physical aspects of their daughters' care with great competence and had informed the family when each child's death was imminent. Of note, however, is that Mrs. L's overall satisfaction with the care that each of her children and the family had received was directly related to the nature of their relationships with the clinicians. Whereas Maria's death was experienced as highly traumatic, Stella's death brought some comfort. These contrasting outcomes attest to the profound impact of the relationship between the family and the team.

THE PRIVATE WORLDS OF CLINICIANS

To engage in a process of self exploration and understanding, clinicians must first recognize misconceptions such as

- Clinicians do not and should not experience suffering. Suffering affects only seriously ill children and the people who are significant in their lives.
- Effective care is ensured through objectivity and specialized skills. Emotions are subjective and lead to bias and impaired clinical judgment.
- An attitude of detached emotional concern that involves an intellectualized interest and concern for others protects clinicians from occupational hazards such as burnout.

These beliefs prevent clinicians from developing authentic relationships in which they are fully present and aware of what unfolds in the intersubjective space. "Knowing oneself" is of equal importance to "knowing" the child and the family. Such self-knowledge is not limited to cognitive understanding, but also includes the integration of information gathered from one's emotional responses, physical senses, and bodily reactions. Openness is the antithesis of detachment and counteracts any attempt to identify a "correct" distance in clinical relationships. Remaining open to the child's and family's experiences, no matter how distressing, "permits us to meet the unknown in life, in others, or in ourselves.... This process requires time, energy, and commitment. When we are consumed by the everyday and rush from one activity . . to the next, we do not engage in a deep examination of our experiences and we restrict our capacity to provide effective care." p, 330 [4]

"BEING VULNERABLE ENOUGH"

"Being vulnerable enough"[4,6] is a strength that differs qualitatively from being either highly vulnerable or from projecting an image of invulnerability. When clinicians so overidentify with patients and families that they cannot differentiate their own experience, they develop enmeshed relationships in which they feel overwhelmed and thus highly vulnerable. In contrast, when clinicians feel threatened by the intense emotions engendered in work with seriously ill children, they may project an image of overcompetence and control to counteract their own anxiety. In striving to appear invulnerable, clinicians may build rigid boundaries and remain oblivious to the private worlds of children and parents, as well as to their own. Their focus narrows to their prescribed role and functions.

"Being vulnerable enough" involves an openness and permeability that enables clinicians to develop a deeper understanding of others, witness suffering without being threatened, and assist with the ongoing challenges of illness. It also involves clinicians' recognition of how they affect—and are affected by—encounters with children and their families, as well as the impact on other team members and on the team as a whole. Furthermore, "being vulnerable enough" acknowledges the crucial importance of clinicians attending to their own distress and grief. In this mandala[7] (Figure 12.3), a pediatric hospice nurse describes the richness of her commitment, her own suffering, and her reckoning with her own mortality:

> I always feel challenged (green) in the work—it surrounds everything and keeps my commitment going. Commitment (purple) is the core and affects all the other feelings. Feeling hopeful (yellow) and in control (orange) are important if you are going to keep doing this work. Anger (red) is the only feeling that doesn't touch on commitment in my drawing—so that it does not impinge on it. I have the anger embedded in control. Frustration is there (brown)—you always wish you could do more. And fear (black). . . . Hospice forces me to confront and come to terms with death. As children I work with go, I know that I will go too . . . Sadness (blue) is there, but it does not take over all my other feelings.

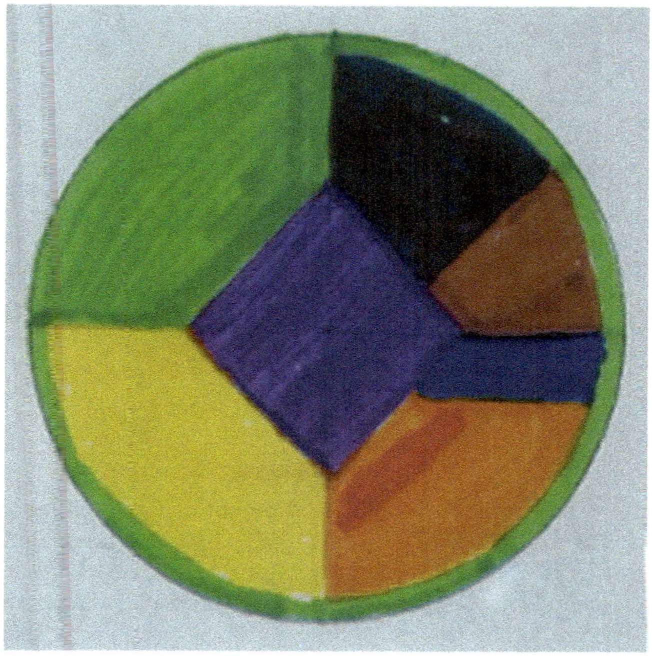

Figure 12.3 Mandala: "As children I work with go, I know that I will go too . . . ."

CLINICIANS' SUFFERING

It can be challenging to distinguish between normal, expected, and unavoidable suffering in clinicians who care for seriously ill children from the overwhelming suffering that is associated with anxiety, depression, and disillusionment. While the distinction is not always evident, the implications are important for clinicians' own well-being and for their relationships with patients, families, and their team.

SUFFERING THAT LEADS TO IMPAIRMENT

Common stress conditions which are associated with health and mental health problems are burnout and traumatization.[8–10] Suffering that leads to impairment in the provision of care may develop progressively, as in the case of burnout, or appear suddenly, as in traumatization. When clinicians suffer from burnout or are seriously traumatized by their involvement with seriously ill children and families, they may develop negative beliefs about themselves, their worldview, and the meaning of life. These inner transformations impact not only their own well-being, but also the nature of their relationships with those for whom they provide care.

Burnout

Burnout is "a state of physical, emotional, and mental exhaustion caused by long-term involvement in emotionally demanding situations."[11] Although described as a static state, burnout is actually more of a process that unfolds over time. The key dimensions of burnout are[12,13]:

- *Emotional exhaustion*: A sense of emotional depletion and lack of energy to meet professional demands.
- *Depersonalization*: A detached, negative, sometimes cynical response to children and families. Loss of interest and compassion leads to an impersonal quality in clinical relationships.
- *Sense of professional incompetence and lack of achievement*: Negative self-image leads to the belief that one can no longer work effectively; the professional may display indifference or apathy in his or her professional role.

Burnout is associated with frequent absences, the provision of poor quality of care, and high rates of job turnover. Clinicians feel overwhelmed and lack the resources to cope with distressing work conditions. They frequently hold high or unrealistic expectations for themselves or from others (e.g., to "save" seriously ill children, to always be in control). Without opportunities to process their experiences or find outlets for relief, feelings of disappointment, frustration, guilt, inadequacy, and distrust are common.

Traumatization

Clinicians may themselves experience trauma directly and may also be susceptible to vicarious traumatization through exposure to narratives recounted by children and families. Clinicians may manifest traumatic responses including

- *Reliving the traumatic event or narrative through intrusive thoughts and feelings, nightmares, and flashbacks*. Reexperiencing symptoms of physiological and psychological distress when exposed to reminders (particular child, family, clinical situation) associated with the trauma.
- *Avoidance of thoughts, feelings, settings, or circumstances that have been experienced as traumatic and bring back memories.*
- *Hypervigilance*—always on guard for other trauma—leads to difficulty concentrating, disrupted sleep patterns, irritability, and being easily startled.
- *Negative changes in cognition and mood.*

Traumatic stress responses usually subside after few days or weeks, when self-care practices are adopted or the clinician is supported by colleagues who do not minimize the impact of the event. However, with the cumulative effect of repeated exposure to trauma, basic needs for secure self-esteem, feeling safe, in control, and trusting others are shaken, leading in turn to the avoidance of intimacy in both personal and professional relationships.[14]

When a clinician's suffering from either burnout or traumatization becomes intense, prolonged, and pervasive, consultation with a mental health professional is indicated.

SUFFERING THAT IS NORMAL, EXPECTED, AND UNAVOIDABLE

> We all have to learn to live with loss, but the person who works in this sphere must confront it every day.
>
> Raphael[15(p. 401)]

Not all suffering is hazardous to clinicians' well-being or to the quality of their work. Some distress is normal and to be expected in PPC. Often it reflects a grieving process over losses that are anticipated and experienced in the clinical setting.[16–20] It is critical to be aware of the power of anticipatory grief, defined as "grief expressed in advance when the loss is perceived as inevitable."[21(p. 4)] Experientially, the process reflects the emotional response to the pain of separation prior to the actuality of loss as it charts a "subterranean course" along the illness trajectory.[22(p. 67)] Clinicians may not recognize anticipatory grief and thus can experience a sense of loneliness and confusion at the intensity of their emotion, not understanding its source.

While the death of a child represents the ultimate loss, there are many losses that may occur during the course of an illness. For example, when children with cancer first relapse and the possibility of "curing" the disease decreases, clinicians' expectations and hope adjust accordingly. Or, in the case of children with neurologically deteriorative conditions, witnessing the loss of each milestone invokes a sense of helplessness and grief. In both these instances, the current loss portends the threat of death, however distant in the future.

A loss may mean different things at different times for different clinicians.[4] For example, grief following the death of a child may be over a special bond that has been severed, or the inability to achieve the professional goal of cure, or over a personal loss that surfaces in the emotion of the present clinical situation. Most often such losses trigger a fluctuating process between experiencing the grief and avoiding or repressing it. This ebb and flow enables clinicians to both acknowledge their loss and set it aside in order to function. By contrast, a lack of such fluctuation may lead to manifestations of grief overload that can overwhelm clinicians and compromise the quality of care that they can provide.[6,4] Clinicians' suffering may be more intense or pervasive when there is a confluence of professional experiences with personal issues or situations, especially those involving loss. At these times, collegial support, mentoring, or psychological intervention can help them to reset their boundaries and identify ways to mitigate their suffering as they continue in their professional practice.

Suffering may also be caused or intensified by interpersonal or systems issues in the professional setting. These may include team conflict, feeling powerless to effect change due to organizational structure or limited resources, and a work culture that values rules and task achievement over vision and creative accomplishment (see Chapter 11, "Team Relationships").

BENEFITS TO CLINICIANS OF UNDERSTANDING THEIR PRIVATE WORLDS

- Reminds them that they are not immune to suffering; professional expertise does not guarantee immunity to pain, uncertainty, and loss.
- Offers opportunities to examine their reasons for caring for seriously ill children and families, recognize their limitations, and address personal anxieties in the face of suffering and loss.
- Motivates them to develop coping strategies to ease their distress, transform it in creative ways, and seek help when suffering is unbearable.
- Sensitizes them to aspects of suffering that may impair their provision of care.
- Incites them to ensure resources for themselves and their team that enhance resilience in the face of adversity.

THE DEATH OF A CHILD: IMPACT ON CLINICIANS

The impact of a child's death on clinicians of all disciplines is a relatively new focus, even in the palliative care world. Until recently, it was rarely addressed as an entity of its own rather it was simply "taken for granted" as a difficult part of clinical work. Early initiatives to address this impact have been with trainees, recognizing the intensity of their interactions with children and families at such an early stage of their professional development. The paucity of training until recently is revealed in reflections written by residents.[23–25] Educational goals over the past two decades have focused on residents "gaining insight into the impact of death on their own emotions and the importance of addressing [them]."[26(p. 278)] Identifying the kinds of deaths that residents find the most upsetting and factors that lead to their "positive" experiences in handling a child's death have been explored.[27] Residents value didactic and experiential sessions, the support of their peers and attendings, and opportunities for debriefings and psychological support.[23,28–31] The American Academy of Pediatrics (AAP) curriculum, *Resilience in the Face of Grief and Loss*,[32–33] developed for pediatric trainees, is actually relevant for pediatric clinicians of any discipline and at any level. The course was developed as a result of requests from the AAP Section on Medical Students, Residents, and Fellowship Trainees and the AAP Section on Hospice and Palliative Medicine.

Early studies with experienced clinicians examined cross-cultural perspectives on how the grief of nurses and physicians is expressed and supported.[34–35] For healthcare professionals in general,[36–37] the value of existing forms of support after a child's death (e.g., peer, colleague, or family/friend support) as well as what more is needed (e.g., debriefings, immediate and easier access to a psychologist) have been described. Members of different disciplines may experience varying levels of intensity of grief, raising the question of what general as well as discipline-specific training and support is needed. Studies have also focused on specific clinician groups, including, for example, pediatric oncologists[38–39] and acute care cardiovascular nurses.[40] The impact of a patient's death on both their personal and professional lives was considerable. Individuals' history of illness and loss, level of professional experience, and the support of colleagues were among many factors associated with their coping.

Understanding the complexity of clinicians' response to a child's death in terms of what facilitates or impedes optimal coping and then designing supportive interventions for individuals within and across disciplines offer both clinical and research challenges (Figure 12.4A,B).

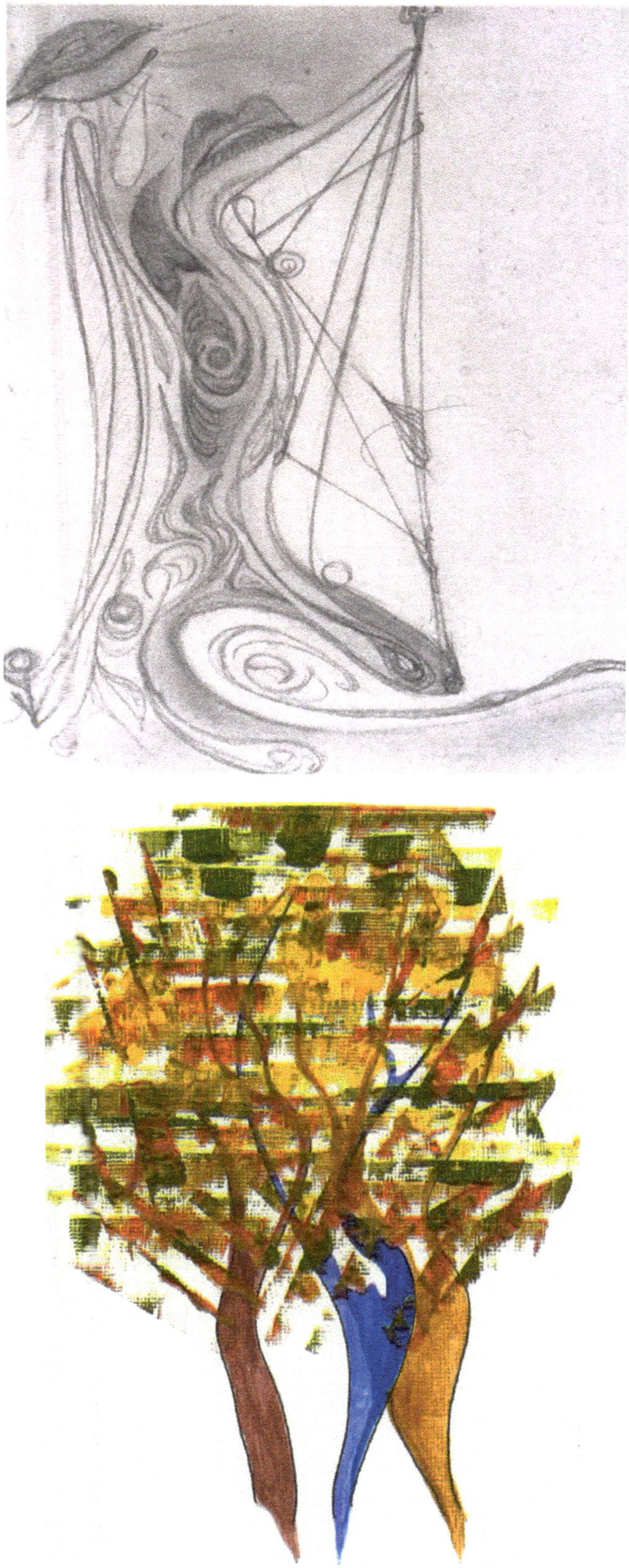

Figure 12.4 (A, B) From solitary grief to reconnection and reintegration.

A FRAMEWORK FOR UNDERSTANDING THE IMPACT OF A CHILD'S DEATH

> Am I going to die from this tumor?.
> And can I ask you a personal question: Are you going to cry when I die?
>
> Adolescent to her physician[22(p. 74)]

The death of a child is the endpoint of an illness continuum that extends from the child who is seriously ill, to a child who is living under the threat of death, to a child who is dying. Thus, consideration of the impact of a child's death on the individual clinician, as well as on the team as a whole, encompasses this spectrum in all its complexity. Caring for dying children and coping with the death of a child is an ongoing challenge for clinicians, both in personal and professional spheres.

For clinicians of any discipline who are new to a high-acuity pediatric setting, the death of a child often looms as a pivotal source of fear. At one level is the anxiety about what to do for the child and family in the immediacy of death. However, at a deeper level, they also wonder what to do for themselves to be able to cope in these circumstances. In clinical settings, it is not infrequent to hear statements such as: "I don't know why this child's death hit me so hard—more so than any of the others." Or, "I feel guilty because I hardly reacted at all to this child's death. I know it's sad and I feel for the family—but I don't have much emotion around it."

The following framework (Table 12.1) was initially developed to provide trainees with a structure within which to make sense of their experience of the impact of a child's death. It distills themes that emerged from small group sessions with pediatric residents and fellows, trainees from other disciplines, and staff at Lucile Packard Children's Hospital Stanford over a two-decade period. It offers scaffolding for the issues to consider when working with seriously ill children or following a child's death, whether in the immediate, short-, or long-term period thereafter. The underlying theme is that the focus, intensity, and quality of the impact of a child's death on an individual is affected by many intertwined factors: situational (e.g., nature of death), deeply personal (e.g., loss history), relational (relationship with the child and family), and systemic/sociocultural (e.g., structure of rotations, culture of the team).

NATURE OF THE CHILD'S DEATH

The nature of the death itself is fundamental to how it is experienced by an individual clinician.

EXPECTED OR UNEXPECTED DEATH

With an expected death, there is the potential opportunity to "prepare" oneself: cognitively, in terms of understanding the inexorable trajectory of the disease, and psychologically, through the process of anticipatory grief. However, when the course of a child's illness is protracted, or when parents insist on continuing disease-related therapy while the team considers such intervention to be "futile," clinicians may harbor the wish for it just to be "over." However understandable, guilt prevents them from articulating the feeling aloud or even acknowledging it to

TABLE 12.1 Death of a patient: Impact on YOU. A Framework*

Focus, intensity, and quality of impact depend on many factors ...

SITUATIONAL: NATURE OF CHILD'S DEATH	PERSONAL/PRIVATE: YOUR OWN PSYCHE	RELATIONAL: RELATIONSHIP WITH CHILD AND FAMILY	SYSTEMIC/SOCIOCULTURAL: OCCURRENCE OF DEATH AND AFTERMATH
Expected/unexpected	Current balance of resilience/vulnerability in personal/professional life	Close identification	At what point death occurs (in professional development)
Traumatic aspects	Loss history	"Favorite"	Series of deaths
Infrequently encountered deaths (previously healthy child/suicide / non-accidental trauma)	History of serious illness	Negative/problematic	Inclusion/support within the team
--- Disenfranchised grief --- Do I have the right to grieve?			
--- Cumulative grief --- A heavy toll			
--- How the PPC team can be of help to you ---			
Team meetings/debriefings; Individual confidential meetings; Access to mental health clinicians and chaplains; Referral to outside resources for psychotherapy; Educational resources (e.g., teaching sessions, readings); Hospital or unit-based memorial services			

Developed by Barbara M. Sourkes, PhD.

This framework distills themes that emerged from small group sessions co-led by Barbara Sourkes, PhD, and Harvey J. Cohen, MD, PhD, with pediatric residents and fellows, trainees from other disciplines, and staff at Lucile Packard Children's Hospital, Stanford, California, over a two-decade period.

themselves. Rather, clinicians may verbalize a more acceptable version in terms of "wishing the agony were over for the parent and family" while denying any impact on themselves.

In circumstances of an unexpected death, the shock is compounded by unanswered questions and, at times, a sense of guilt. Medical professionals in particular face the mystery of the unexplained cause, the fear that something may have been missed, and, perhaps most difficult of all, the possibility that the death was due to the very intervention they had implemented.

UNIQUELY TRAUMATIC ASPECTS OF THE DEATH

Over and above the intrinsic tragedy of a child's death, traumatic elements include a child who dies in intense and unrelieved suffering, whether physical or psychological; disturbing visual images (e.g., bleeding, seizures); family issues (e.g., conflict that erupts around the time of the child's death; or a parent or other close family member who could not be present for a myriad of reasons (including prohibitive immigration policies). Clinicians express that such traumatic images imprint deeply and endure.

LESS FREQUENTLY ENCOUNTERED DEATHS

New and experienced clinicians alike cite three categories of childhood death that they encounter infrequently, but that nonetheless cause intense distress.

The death of a previously healthy child heightens everyone's awareness of the fragility of life and the randomness of fate. Those who have healthy children are reminded that their good fortune can never be taken for granted. The impact on individuals who do not have children is often minimized or left unacknowledged. Yet those who may become parents in the future are just as shaken, often with a new thread of anxiety woven into their hopes.

When a child dies by suicide, clinicians' reactions are a complicated version of those to a "previously healthy child." In these instances, they grapple with how the usual definition of the "previously healthy child" often does not acknowledge—or minimizes—a history of mental health issues. They express confusion and anxiety about what unknown secrets and despair a child may have harbored or gone underrecognized by the family. Their fear reflects back on themselves as individuals.

The death of a child from nonaccidental trauma elicits devastation, complicated by a web of questions, judgments, and often fury about the family's active guilt or collusion in the abuse. Many clinicians cannot bring themselves to demonstrate any caring for family members who are known or suspected to have had any involvement. These deaths are experienced as "absolute tragedies" by clinicians at every stage of development.

YOUR PRIVATE PSYCHE

CURRENT BALANCE OF RESILIENCE/VULNERABILITY IN PERSONAL AND PROFESSIONAL LIFE

This balance is profoundly affected by an individual's preexisting inner resources. For example, strong personal relationships or a deeply integrated system of beliefs provide a grounding, a wellspring through emotionally arduous times.

Periods of resilience and vulnerability fluctuate in individuals' personal lives alongside, or intertwined with, all that unfolds in their professional world. Vulnerability may be exacerbated by something basic and identifiable (e.g., sleep deprivation) or complicated and distressing (e.g., depression, relationship problems, illness in a family member). There is often great reluctance to disclose these issues, which remain unspoken and unknown to colleagues and supervisors. Yet they can impinge significantly on professional functioning and particularly on the capacity to handle the death of a patient.

LOSS HISTORY

Current threatened or actual losses, both personal and professional, do not exist in a vacuum. In a parallel to identifying families' loss history as a context for understanding their coping with a seriously ill child, clinicians' personal history can significantly impact their work in PPC. Memories of loss—particularly from childhood—encompass not only death, but also illness/disability, divorce, geographical dislocation. Past experiences that are in some way similar to a current clinical situation can be particularly intense. Clinicians who have not yet encountered significant losses in their own lives often feel particularly unshielded in working with these children. In addition to the fear of a patient's death comes the fact that they do not have any "blueprint" as a starting point in anticipating their response. In addition, past clinical experiences, especially those involving children who have died, figure significantly. Reflecting back on such experiences identifies strengths and vulnerabilities, pessimism and optimism, unresolved losses—all of which can provide some guidance as to what might facilitate or impede their coping in the present.

HISTORY OF SERIOUS ILLNESS

Clinicians who have their own history of serious illness (e.g., long-term survivors of childhood cancer; chronic illness) bring with them a unique empathy—at times facilitative in their relationships with children and families, at other times disruptive in reigniting their own past or ongoing trauma.

QUALITY OF YOUR RELATIONSHIP WITH THE CHILD AND FAMILY

Clinicians' responses intensify when there is a strong identification with the child and family. Dimensions include being of a similar cultural background or having a child of the same age as the patient. Trainees in particular may express anguish in work with adolescents and young adults, recognizing that they are only a few years apart, and feel a sense of grief—even guilt—for what they have and for what their patient will not have the opportunity to experience. Clinicians often hesitate to acknowledge that a certain child or family has become "a favorite" for fear of being considered unprofessional. Yet in all relationships, including those in a clinical setting, certain affinities emerge. There is a particular richness and depth in these attachments, along with the attendant vulnerability when the child dies. However, the risk of these "special bonds" can be overidentification and overinvolvement in a way that may compromise the professional relationship. In contrast, clinicians may feel intense shame and guilt at their lack of response—or even relief—at the death of a child when they have found the relationship with the family to be problematic. Two areas of difficulty are frequently mentioned. (1) Parents who have pursued disease-related treatment beyond what the team has recommended. The individual clinician is (privately) critical of their decision in the belief that they subjected the child to needless suffering. (2) Families who have been disrespectful or hostile to the clinician. All clinicians, especially trainees, need support in recognizing that while the parents' behavior may be reflective of their stress, even profound suffering does not make abuse acceptable.

SYSTEMIC/SOCIOCULTURAL ISSUES

Systemic and sociocultural issues, both logistical and interpersonal, rather than individual psychological factors, can also have great impact on the response to the death of a child.

AT WHAT POINT THE DEATH OCCURS

The learning curve of training for health and mental health professionals is steep. Thus, the impact of a child's death can be quite different depending on when it occurs in clinicians' professional development and, perhaps even more importantly, whether they have already been through the experience. The point at which a child's death occurs during a specific rotation can also be significant. In both instances, "early" is often more challenging, as new professionals are still grappling with their clinical learning as well as attempting to discern the culture of the hospital or a particular unit or team. When these factors are compounded by their lack of experience in dealing with a patient's death, clinicians describe intense stress and challenge to their ability to cope.

A CHILD'S DEATH IN A "SERIES" OF DEATHS

Clinicians of all disciplines and at all levels articulate that while they are able to cope with a single death on the unit, a series of deaths over a brief period is overwhelming. Whereas they may find the time to reflect on one child's death in an attempt to absorb its impact, multiple deaths render that task impossible. They feel guilty and frustrated that they cannot give each family optimal care, nor can they attend to themselves. Their coping skills are frayed thin and—in the case of trainees—may lead them to question their choice of pediatrics or of a subspecialty that would involve seriously ill children.

INCLUSION AND SUPPORT WITHIN THE TEAM

Being included—as witness or participant—around the time of a child's death is crucial to clinical and experiential learning. Generally, it is assumed that the trainees will be present along with other team members, although their degree of involvement can vary. In some instances, an attending or supervisor gives trainees a choice, without judgment, as to their preference. At other times, in an attempt (potentially misguided) at protection, trainees are told that there is no need for their involvement, that they already have "enough on their plates." Some feel a great sense of relief at this permission (and guilt at that relief is rarely expressed openly). However, those who do want to be present can be unsure as to how much they can insist. In a harsh version of exclusion, trainees describe instances of team members ignoring them or even informing them that they are not to be present. This is especially unfortunate when they have been intensely involved with the child and family, and they are rendered invisible at this crucial time. Trainees talk of being "devastated" by the exclusion and may later reflect on the time as having been deeply traumatic.

Support around the time of a child's death, for each individual and for the team as a whole, can be profoundly comforting and strengthening. In the immediate aftermath, it is immensely important for a leader of the team to recognize the profundity of what has just occurred, acknowledge the experience of caring for the child and parents (referring to them by name), and express appreciation for everyone's contribution. This "pause," a time apart, even if brief, can be invaluable before moving on to the next task, the next patient. When this affirmation is supplanted by a strictly medical review of events, clinicians at all levels can leave deeply imprinted by the experience, yet they carry the experience alone. Also important is to offer the opportunity (whether on an individual or team basis) for further discussion, at the very time of the child's death (when feasible) or in the days ahead. For trainees, witnessing others' responses and sharing their own experience can be crucial in the development of their coping. What a team leader or mentor models in terms of dealing with stress and grief in the face of a child's death can be formative for trainees. They begin to identify, model, and integrate the strategies that "fit" for them and reject those that do not.

Whatever an individual's outside support of family and friends, a trusted colleague within the institution can provide refuge. In such relationships can be found a depth of understanding of the shared experience of this uniquely emotionally demanding work.

DISENFRANCHISED GRIEF

"Disenfranchised grief" is defined as "the grief that persons experience when they incur a loss that is not or cannot be openly acknowledged, publicly mourned, or socially supported."[41(p. 4)] Grief can be disenfranchised when the relationship, the griever, or the loss itself is not recognized.[42,43]

Disenfranchised relationships (Figure 12.5) are somehow deemed to have an insufficient or inappropriate basis for grief; disenfranchised grievers are individuals who "should not need" to grieve. Both aspects are expressed all too frequently by clinicians. The belief that somehow their grief is not legitimate is reflected in statements such as "I shouldn't be feeling such sadness. It's not like I'm the parent—it's not my child." It is critical to "enfranchise" clinicians early in their professional development: to point out that there are many types of relationships and many forms of grief, with neither competition nor hierarchy among them. Caring for a child and family, often over a long period, is its own unique relationship and can result in deeply felt attachment and loss.

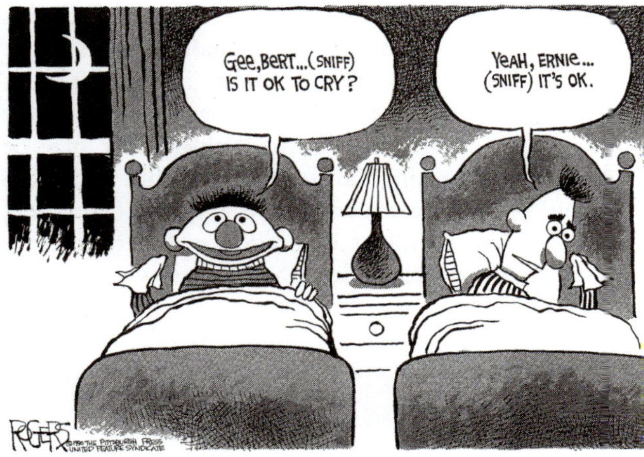
GEE, BERT...(SNIFF) IS IT OK TO CRY?
YEAH, ERNIE... (SNIFF) IT'S OK.

Figure 12.5 "Is it OK to cry?" (Rob Rogers). Reprinted with permission from Andrews McMeel Syndication. All rights reserved, 1990.

CUMULATIVE GRIEF

> Tears unwashed are stones upon the heart that choke the healing stream.
>
> Melville[44(p. 60)]

Cumulative grief in PPC is identified by clinicians of all disciplines and at all levels. It arises for a myriad of reasons including the challenge of integrating the impact of an individual child's death, the cascade of a series of deaths in a short period, and reluctance to let down self-protective defenses or a strategy to delay "dealing with" a death until there is time to process it. A sense of being a "disenfranchised griever" is a compounding factor. Cumulative grief can present in many guises and is often associated with burnout. Supervisors and colleagues may offer temporary accommodations in the work setting (e.g., reduced on-call schedule) to mitigate the distress. However, cumulative grief is a phenomenon of its own, and, when not identified as such, these work-related interventions may fail to address the individual's profound anguish (Figure 12.6).

INTERVENTIONS

Mental health professionals who have experience in PPC can provide important guidance for clinicians facing the death of a patient. Intrinsic to training in psychology, psychiatry, and social work is the focus on introspection and self-understanding within clinical situations. Furthermore, training in psychotherapy focuses on the complexity of others' actions and reactions and the ability to contextualize and interpret them. When faced with the suffering of colleagues, these tenets provide a framework for understanding their experience and guiding them through the overwhelming emotions that so often accompany loss.[2,22,45–46]

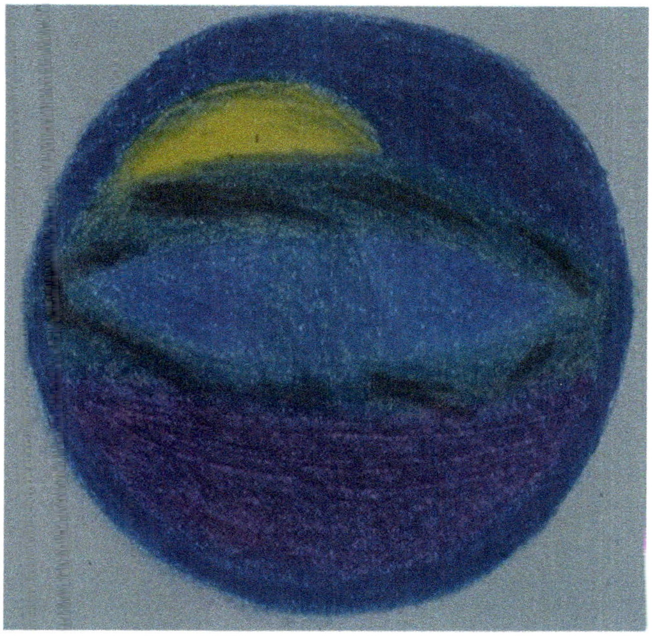

Figure 12.6 *After many losses, "the eye begins to see." Roethke "In a dark time the eye begins to see. I meet my shadow in the deepening shade . . . "* From Roethke T. The Collected Poems. Doubleday; 1975.

The palliative care specialty team is frequently called upon to provide support to trainees or staff around the time of a child's death or following a series of deaths on a unit. They in turn work closely in conjunction with services (that may not be represented on the team itself) to offer a range of interventions. While members of the primary team may themselves be skilled facilitators, it is important for them to be participants when the focus is on their patient. The role of the consultant is to facilitate emotional sharing among colleagues in a setting where each individual's experience is witnessed and heard. Some individuals may disclose quite private aspects of their response, while others may choose only to listen. Factors that have emerged as important through clinical experience include

- Attendance must be entirely voluntary.
- Recognize team preference for timing of a debriefing (as soon as possible in the immediacy of an event or at a later date). Once the session is scheduled, it is important to offer individual meetings for those whose "timing" differs from the group choice.
- Interdisciplinary leadership of a debriefing—particularly a "pairing" of a health and mental health clinician—can be invaluable. For example, a physician provides residents and fellows with a "same-discipline" role model, someone who has been through similar professional training and experiences. A mental health clinician offers a psychological perspective on the event as well as observation of the participants during the meeting. Of particular importance is the identification of and follow-up with any individual who appears particularly vulnerable or distressed.

Clinical staff and trainees appreciate the outlet afforded by confidential meetings (that they can request) with a palliative care specialty team member who is not in their direct line of reporting. A particularly poignant—and not infrequent—occurrence is when clinicians are confronting loss simultaneously in both their personal and professional lives. Consultations with the mental health clinician or chaplain on the team can be crucial to their sense of balance and self-preservation in their work. Referral for psychotherapy may also be indicated.

Memorial services to commemorate the children who have died, whether hospital-wide or unit-based, also pay tribute to the clinical staff who cared for them. These events can provide an important time for shared grieving "in community" with others and for the renewal of a sense of professional commitment.

A Clinician's Reflection

A Clinician's Reflection I think that when most physicians reflect back on their residency, they can identify certain formative experiences that had an everlasting impact on their training and in shaping the physicians they are now. I can recall my own experiences in dealing with death from my time as a pediatric resident working with oncology patients. Of all of the children I cared for during a month-long rotation, a few patients died while under my care and a total of 17 passed away within a year.

It was a lot to process. I did not have the tools to do so on my own, with working 80-hour weeks, keeping up with all that was expected of me as a trainee, not to mention the fact that I, too, had a personal life and a need to take care of myself. I developed different types of relationships with different patients and their families, and, as such, the impact their deaths had on me varied. I remember one family who chose to pursue life-prolonging treatments for their child, even though the child was making it very clear to the medical team that he was ready to die. The anger and frustration I felt toward them when I could see their child suffering was incredibly poignant. I remember another patient who I became very fond of; witnessing him dealing with his own illness and facing his own mortality was heartbreaking.

The PPC team was instrumental in helping me deal with all of the emotions and feelings I encountered. They provided a safe space where I was allowed to focus on myself; where it was OK to talk about the impact that patient deaths or difficult situations were having on me. To have my feelings validated—to share my doubts, my guilt, and my fears—was invaluable. In the many years of my practice since then, I do think that the framework I was given to process my own grief has allowed me to become a better, more compassionate pediatrician. And it has made me feel more equipped to help my patients and families when faced with death.

Veena Goel Jones, MD, Pediatric Hospitalist

BUILDING RESILIENCE

Resilience has traditionally been understood as the ability to rebound or recover after an adverse event or time period, the capacity to cope with and adapt to trauma and stress. An important corollary is the role of perception: "events are not traumatic until we experience them as traumatic"[47] and thus the term "potentially traumatic event."[48] Recent conceptualizations of resilience have broadened from the focus on adversity to a more positive valence. For example, resilience is "the process of harnessing the resources we need to sustain well-being."[49] A multifaceted view of "resilience resources" includes internal resources (identification of and optimizing one's own strengths), external resources (availability of supportive individuals, community), and existential resources (meaning of challenge, what can be learned).[50] This analysis provides clinicians a framework with which to assess their own resilience history, to identify what has worked or not worked for them in related situations in the past. Across all definitions, a common theme is that resilience is not a fixed state; rather, it is a flexible process that can be developed and strengthened. In PPC, resilience may also function as "the capacity to see each clinical encounter as a new opportunity to learn and be helpful to the self and others."[51]

DEATH ANXIETY AND AWARENESS

> As a prerequisite for asking patients to confront mortality, I have advised professionals first to confront their own.
>
> Weisman[52(p. 119)]

The exploration of personal attitudes about death, along with self-awareness about the reciprocal impact of our relationships with children and families have been identified as key educational objectives for professionals who specialize in PPC.[53–55]

Studies arising from Terror Management Theory,[56] particularly the concept of *mortality salience* (explicit reminders of one's own mortality), indicate that death anxiety can have powerful impact on behavior. Clinicians are often totally unaware that their death anxiety has consequences not only for their relationships with patients and families but also for the creation of bias in their clinical decision-making: thus, the critical importance during training of learning to identify one's own fears about death, cognitively and emotionally reframe them, and, as a result, avoid projecting those fears onto patients. In essence, the goal is to convert one's anxiety about death into a focused awareness of its omnipresence in the clinical setting of palliative care. In the following reflection, the supervisor sensitively provides the opportunity for this learning.

Clinical Vignette

Anna a trainee, was spending a month on the PPC service under the supervision of a senior clinician. On the third day of her rotation, the supervisor noted that A. had appeared increasingly distressed during a meeting with the mother of a 4-year-old child. Her daughter had a brain tumor that was unresponsive to all disease-directed treatments. The mother refused to discuss options for the location of her end-of-life care, stating that she could not accept even "the possibility of her death" and that to imagine that her daughter might not be cured was "unacceptable." The clinician acknowledged the mother's distress at approaching this topic and instead was able to engage her in exploring how to better control her daughter's pain and other symptoms. A. did not say anything.

In a debriefing meeting afterward, A. stated: "But there must be more we can do than just make her comfortable before she dies! I understand what the mother is saying because part of me also feels we can do better than just watching her die! I feel so mad that this is happening." A's supervisor understood her distress—her response to the confrontation with mortality, human fragility, and the limits of medical science. Rather than offer explanations or advice, he invited her to further explore her response: "Can you say more about what you are feeling?" to whatever degree she was comfortable.

REACTING AND RESPONDING

Both resilience and burnout) are processes that result not from what happens per se, but rather emerge from how we either react or respond to events. Reactions are automatic and "unchosen" and arise from preexisting biases and beliefs that do not require much time or cognitive effort to appear. In other words—acting on our initial impulses. Responses, in contrast, occur after a brief mental pause that allows for a reexamination of our initial reaction. Being responsive is not denying or suppressing the immediate reaction, but rather consciously deciding not to act while at the same time allowing the emotions of the initial reaction to remain as they are. The movement from an initial reaction to a considered response depends on having an "in the moment" (mindful) capacity to pause and reevaluate before taking action.[51]

MINDFULNESS

> If we consider the role of the doctor . . . it becomes especially important . . . to be in tune with . . . [our] own mental well-being as well as the impact of . . . [our] words and actions on others. To develop the ability to pause and reflect on our feeling before we act on them . . . requires a certain amount of self-awareness.
>
> Realizations include thinking more about my patients' point of view and trying to be there more in the moment.
>
> Medical students (anonymous)[51]

Kabat-Zinn has defined mindfulness as "paying attention in a particular way: on purpose, in the present moment, and nonjudgmentally"—and the awareness that arises thereof.[57] An attribute that is of particular relevance to PPC comes from the writing of Thich Nhat Hanh: "Mindfulness is the best way to be with our suffering without being overwhelmed by it"[58] and to be with others' suffering as well. Although a state of mindfulness can occur spontaneously, it can also be taught and cultivated with specific training that can be integrated into any belief system. The practice of mindfulness meditation simultaneously raises awareness of one's inner reality (physical, emotional, and cognitive) and of the external reality of interpersonal interactions and the environment.[51,59] Educational interventions that foster insight, improve attentional capacity, and build resilience focus on experiential learning practiced in small groups. Such learning may be discipline-specific (e.g., mindful medical practice, a required course for medical students)[51] or for individuals of any background (e.g., mindfulness-based stress reduction) as a way "to change our relationship to stress using mind and body awareness, to participate in our own self-care . . . growth and development as human beings."[60] The "resilient zone" model outlines the normal variability of in-the-moment mindful capacity.

THE RESILIENT ZONE

The concept of the "resilient zone"[61] illustrates how we function optimally, even in stressful situations, with normal fluctuations of energy, focus and attention (Figure 12.7).

The two straight horizontal lines serve as the upper and lower limits—or boundaries—of the zone, within which the autonomic nervous system is well-balanced and fluctuates between relaxation and alertness. (The sympathetic nervous system represents increased energy and the parasympathetic nervous system signifies rest.) At the upper limit we have more energy and mindful attention, which can transform into irritability and anxiety when that limit is exceeded. When we exceed the lower limit of the resilient zone (characterized by less energy and alertness), we feel overwhelmingly fatigued and drained of energy. This state can be associated with a clinical picture of burnout and depression. These boundaries are not fixed; rather, they are dynamic, change over time, and can be impacted by sleep deprivation, hunger, and other physiological needs.

The following reflection illustrates a clinician's responses when "outside and inside" the resilient zone.

Clinical Vignette

It is 4:30 PM on a Friday and you are thinking about your plans for the weekend when a neonatologist pages you with a new consult. A 3-day-old infant with extensive bihemispheric brain infarcts had been compassionately extubated that morning after the parents had agreed to a "do-not-resuscitate" order. While both the neonatal ICU (NICU) staff and the parents thought that he would die within minutes, he has continued to breathe on his own and it now seems possible that he might live for an indeterminate period. Parents are asking to leave with the infant to have as much time as possible with him at home before he dies. The NICU staff has agreed that "home is the best place" for him. They are asking you to see the parents and infant now so that they can leave "before rush hour tonight." You ask about home care support beyond the medical needs, and you realize even over the phone that this is not a simple discharge. To send the infant home safely will require a support system that is difficult to put in place in just a few hours. You have had a difficult week and the thought arises: "I just want to get out of here!"

When You Are Outside Your Resilient Zone

- What you think:
  "I can't believe they would call me for this completely unreasonable request on a late Friday afternoon. Especially because had they let us know earlier, we could have made arrangements more easily. This is going to take hours—I will get home so late—and I don't even think it will be possible to get this infant home tonight. Even worse, both the parents and NICU staff will be upset if I can't somehow make this unrealistic expectation work—I hate this!"
  [Your underlying focus is on the inconvenience that this situation creates for you in your life.]

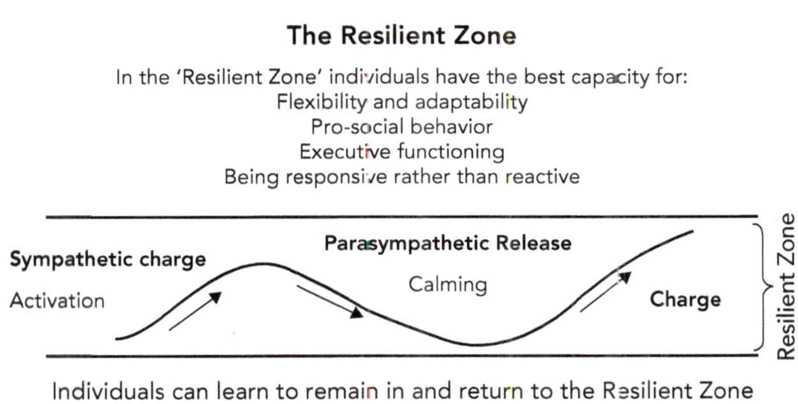

Figure 12.7 The resilient zone.

- What you say over the phone:
  "Why did you not call me earlier today? Do you know how hard it is to arrange a safe transfer home on a Friday afternoon? I hope you did not promise the parents that we would be able to make this happen."

When You Are Inside Your Resilient Zone

- What you think:
  "I wish they would have called me earlier, but I can imagine that they did not expect the infant to breathe on his own after extubation. It will take hours to work this all out. I better get something to eat and make a call home now. I hope we can somehow make this happen so late in the day."
  [Your underlying focus is both on the inconvenience that this situation creates for you as well as what the parents may be experiencing to lead to such an urgent request.]
- What you say:
  "I'll be there in 30 minutes to see what is possible at this late hour in the day. I hope we can find a way to make it work. Is that OK for you and the parents?"

SELF-CARE

Healing begets healing begets healing.

Mount and Kearney[61(p. 658)]

Clinicians in PPC sustain relationships with children and families whose lives are filled with suffering and uncertainty. Faced with this ongoing challenge, self-care is essential—yet what is actually meant by the term can be elusive. In a recent study of palliative care nurses and doctors, self-care was defined as a "proactive, holistic and personalized approach to the promotion of health and well-being."[62] The authors point out that, to a certain degree, the palliative care literature has "conflated" the terms "self-care strategy" and "coping strategy." Despite the conceptual understanding of self-care as promoting well-being (i.e., preventative and ongoing), the focus has in fact been on coping strategies in response to stress.

The following definition includes several critical elements: "Self-care is being *intentional* about caring for yourself. Self-care is the practice of setting aside time to invest in oneself and one's well-being"[63] In other words, self-care involves a conscious decision and plan for an ongoing commitment to maintaining one's own physical and mental health. It suggests the importance of finding a balance between clinical demands (on time, energy, and emotion) and the preservation of one's inner resources. Certainly the maintenance of well-being overlaps with the tasks of resilience-building. Self-care is multifaceted and includes drawing strength and love from personal relationships, finding enjoyment and creativity in interests and activities, turning inward to access one's own wellspring of spirituality and belief systems, and, at times, finding "escape" through periods away from work. Most profoundly, it involves care for one's own psyche. Clinicians "must engage in an ongoing, honest appraisal of . . . their capacity for repeated cycles of attachment and loss. An awareness of and respect for one's limitations is an integral part of such an assessment. Introspection must be . . . a constant companion, with the attendant willingness to acknowledge one's own vulnerability."[22(p. 121)]

PPC demands clinicians' "use of self to an extraordinary degree."[22(p.121)] Thus, self- care is neither a selfish undertaking nor a luxury.[64] Rather, self-care provides the crucial counterbalance that enables clinicians to maintain sensitive and effective involvement over time with children and their families.

REWARDS FOR CLINICIANS

PPC offers clinicians of all disciplines the potential for deeply meaningful work and rewards that may be experienced both professionally and personally.[4]

Professional rewards include:

- The richness of therapeutic relationships, often over many years, with children and families.
- The knowledge and creativity to identify, develop, and implement therapeutic options that enable children to live "as long as possible as well as possible."
- The satisfaction of providing an abiding presence and availability to children and families through what may be unspeakable suffering.
- The invaluable teamwork and collaboration with colleagues in the pursuit of shared goals.

Personal rewards include:

- Growth in self-perception. Increased awareness of and ability to acknowledge one's own strengths and vulnerabilities. Greater sense of confidence and competence in dealing with stress and suffering. • Growth in perception of and connection with others. Enhanced capacity for genuine relationships. Ability to remain open to others' experiences and to relate with greater compassion and respect.
- Growth in life perspective. The appreciation for life and the active desire to live in a way that is meaningful and enriching for oneself and loved ones. The recognition that prior choices and priorities may be changed in order to live life more meaningfully.[65] At the confluence of these professional and personal rewards is the opportunity to reflect on "lessons learned" and how these recognitions can transform the care of children and families.

CONCLUSION

Thank you for giving me aliveness.

Six-year-old child[7(p. 167)]

These words, spoken by a six-year-old child to his psychologist, express the essence of PPC. While life itself cannot be guaranteed, clinicians can "give aliveness" to a child, for however long their life may last. Clinicians in PPC commit to being an anchoring presence for children and families whose lives are filled with uncertainty. The responsibility for this commitment is intensified by the threat of separation and loss and the determination to live as meaningfully as possible.

REFERENCES

1. Colette S-G. *Lettres au Petit Corsaire*. Flammarion; 1963.
2. Sourkes B. The child with a life-threatening illness. In Brandell J, ed. *Countertransference in Child and Adolescent Psychotherapy*. Jason Aronson; 1992:279.
3. Sourkes B. Witness through time. *J Palliat Care*. 1990;6(1):55–56.
4. Papadatou D. *In the Face of Death: Professionals Who Care for the Dying and the Bereaved*. Springer; 2009.
5. Stern D. *The Present Moment in Psychotherapy and Everyday Life*. WW Norton; 2004.
6. Papadatou D. Healthcare providers' responses to the death of a child. In Hain R, Goldman A, Rappaport A, Meiring M, eds. *Oxford Textbook of Palliative Care for Children*. 3rd ed. Oxford University Press.
7. Sourkes B. *Armfuls of Time: The Psychological Experience of the Child with a Life-Threatening Illness*. University of Pittsburgh Press; 1995.
8. Bakker AB, Demerouti E. Towards a model of work engagement. *Career Development International*. 2008;13(3):209–223.
9. Bakker AB, Demerouti E. Multiple levels in job demands-resources theory: Implications for employee well-being and performance. In Diener E, Oishi S, & Tay L, eds. *Handbook of Wellbeing*. DEF Publishers; 2018.
10. Leka S, Jain A. Health impact of psychosocial hazards at work: An overview. 2010. https://apps.who.int/iris/bitstream/handle/10665/44428/9789241500272_eng.pdf;jsessionid=A9D665B24A57EAB5A59AC574754B8884?sequence=1
11. Pines A, Aronson E. *Career Burnout: Causes and Cures*. Free Press; 1988.
12. Maslach C, Jackson S. *Maslach Burnout Inventory Manual*. 2nd ed. Consulting Psychologists Press; 1986.
13. Maslach C. Job burnout: New directions in research and intervention. *Curr Dir Psychol Sci*. 2003;12(5):189–192.
14. Pearlman L, McCann L. *Understanding and Addressing Vicarious Trauma*. Headington Institute; 2008. https://headingtoninstitute.org/files/vtmoduletemplate2_ready_v2_85791.pdf
15. Raphael B. *The Anatomy of Bereavement*. Basic Books; 1983:401.
16. Davies B, et al. Caring for dying children: Nurses' experiences. *Pediatr Nurs*. 1996;22(6):500–507.
17. Hinds P, et al. The impact of a grief workshop for pediatric oncology nurses on their grief and perceived stress. *J Pediatr Nurs*. 1994;9(6):388–397.
18. Kaplan L. Toward a model of caregiver grief: Nurses' experiences of treating dying children. *Omega: J Death Dying*. 2000;41(3):187–206.
19. Rashotte J, Fothergill-Bourbonnais J, Chamberlain M. Pediatric intensive care nurses and their grief experiences: A phenomenological study. *Heart Lung*. 1997;26(5:372–386.
20. Shanfield S. The mourning of the health care professional: An important element in education about death and loss. *Death Educ*. 1981;4(4):385–395.
21. Aldrich C. Some dynamics of anticipatory grief. In Schoenberg B, Carr A, Kutscher A, Peretz D, Goldberg J, eds. *Anticipatory Grief*. Columbia University Press; 1974.
22. Sourkes B. *The Deepening Shade: Psychological Aspects of Life-Threatening Illness*. University of Pittsburgh Press; 1982.
23. Yang C, Leung J, Hunt E, Serwint J, Norvell M, Keene EA, Romer LH. Pediatric residents do not feel prepared for the most unsettling situations they face in the pediatric intensive care unit. *J Pall Med*. 2011;14(1):25–30. doi:10.1089/jpm.2010.0314. Epub 2010 Nov 6
24. Vohra S. Learning not to move forward. *JAMA* 2014;312(21):2215.
25. Gambill L. Doctors grieve too: A lesson I did not learn in medical school. 2016. https://www.kevinmd.com/blog/2016/01/doctors-grieve-lesson-not-learn-medical-school.html.
26. Serwint J, Rutherford L, Hutton N, Rowe, P, Barker S, Adamo, G. I learned that no death is routine: Description of a death and bereavement seminar for pediatrics residents. *Acad Med*. 2002;77(4):278–284.
27. Senthil K, Serwint J, Dawood, F. Patient end-of-life experiences for pediatric trainees: Spanning the educational curriculum. *Clin Pediatr*. 2016;55(9):811–818.
28. Serwint J. One method of coping: Resident debriefing after the death of a patient. *J Pediatr*. 2004;145(2):229–234. doi:10.1016/j.jpeds.2004.04.055
29. Serwint J, Rutherford LE, Hutton N. Personal and professional experiences of pediatric residents concerning death. *J Palliat Med*. 2006;9(1):70–81.
30. Bateman S, Dixon R, Trozzi M. The wrap-up: A unique forum to support pediatric residents when faced with the death of a child. *J Palliat Med*. 2012;15(12):1329–1334.
31. French-O'Carroll R, Feeley T, Crowe S, Doherty EM. Grief reactions and coping strategies of trainee doctors working in paediatric intensive care. *Br J Anaesth*. 2019;123(1):74–80. doi:10.1016/j.bja.2019.01.034. Epub 2019 Mar 6. PMID: 30916024.
32. American Academy of Pediatrics. Resilience curriculum: Resilience in the face of grief and loss: A curriculum for medical students, pediatric residents, and fellows. 2016. https://www.aap.org/en-us/advocacy-and-policy/aap-health-initiatives/hospice-palliative-care/Pages/Resilience-Curriculum.aspx
33. Serwint J, Bostwick S, Burke A, Church A, . . . Baldwin D. The AAP resilience in the face of grief and loss curriculum. *Pediatrics*. 2016;138; doi:10.1542/peds.2016-0791 [published online October 10, 2016].
34. Papadatou D, Martinson IM, Chung P. Caring for dying children: A comparative study of nurses' experiences in Greece and Hong Kong. *Cancer Nurs*. 2001;24(5):402–412.
35. Papadatou D, et al. Greek nurse and physician grief as a result of caring for children dying of cancer. *Pediatr Nurs*. 2002;28(4):345–353.
36. Keene E, Hutton N, Hall B, Rushton C. Bereavement debriefing sessions: An intervention to support health care professionals in managing their grief after the death of a patient. *Pediatr Nurs*. 2010;36(4):185–189.
37. Plante J, Cyr C. Health care professionals' grief after the death of a child. *Pediatr Child Health*. 2011;16(4):213–216. doi:10.1093/pch/16.4.213
38. Fanos J. Coming through the fog, coming over the Moors: The impact on pediatric oncologists of caring for seriously ill children. *J Cancer Ed*. 2007;22:119–123.
39. Granek L, Bartels U, Scheinemann K, Labrecque M, Barrera M. Grief reactions and impact of patient death on pediatric oncologists. *Pediatric Blood Cancer*. 2015;62(1):134–142. doi:10.1002/pbc.25228. Epub 2014 Sep 11.
40. Cook A, Mott S, Lawrence P, Jablonski J, . . . Connor J. Coping while caring for the dying child: Nurses' experiences in an acute care setting. *J Pediatr Nurs*. 2012;27(4):e11–21. doi:10.1016/j.pedn.2011.05.010. Epub 2011 Aug 5.
41. Doka K. Disenfranchised grief. In Doka K, ed. *Disenfranchised Grief: Recognizing Hidden Sorrow*. Lexington Books; 1989:3–11.
42. Corr C. Enhancing the concept of disenfranchised grief. *Omega*. 1999;38(1) 1–20.
43. Lathrop D. Disenfranchised grief and physician burnout. *Ann Family Med*. 2017;15(4):375–378.
44. Melville H. Source unknown. In Bertman S, ed. *Facing Death: Images, Insights and Interventions*. Hemisphere Publishing; 1991.
45. Strada E. *Palliative Psychology: Clinical Perspectives on an Emerging Specialty*. Oxford University Press; 2018.

46. Larson D. *The Helper's Journey*. 2nd ed. Research Press Publishers; 2020.
47. Konnikova M. How people learn to become resilient. *New Yorker*. Feb. 11, 2016. https://www.newyorker.com/science/maria-konnikova/the-secret-formula-for-resilience 11, 2016
48. Bonanno G, Mancini A. The human capacity to thrive in the face of potential trauma. *Pediatrics.* 2008;121;369. doi:10.1542/peds.2007-1648
49. Southwick S, Bonanno G, Masten A, Panter-Brick C, Yehuda R. Resilience definitions, theory, and challenges: Interdisciplinary perspectives. *Eur J Psychotraumatol.* 2014;5(10). 3402/ejpt.v5.25338. [Published online first Oct 1, 2014]. doi:10.3402/ejpt.v5.25338
50. Rosenberg A. Seeking professional resilience. *Pediatrics.* 2018; 141(3):e20172388. doi:https://doi.org/10.1542/peds.2017-2388
51. Liben S, Hutchinson T. *MD Aware: A Mindful Medical Course Guide.* Springer; 2020.
52. Weisman A. The psychiatrist and the inexorable. In Feifel H, ed. *New Meanings of Death*. McGraw Hill; 1977:119.
53. Downing J, Ling J, Benini F, Payne S, Papadatou D. A summary of the EAPC White Paper on core competencies for education in paediatric palliative care. *Eur J Palliat Care*. 2014;21(5):245–249.
54. Liben S, Papadatou D. Self-care: The foundation of caregiving. In Wolfe J, Hinds P, Sourkes B, eds. *Textbook of Interdisciplinary Pediatric Palliative Care.* Elsevier; 2010:168–178.
55. Papadatou D. Training of health professionals in caring for dying children and grieving families. *Death Studies*. 1997;21(6):575–600.
56. Solomon S, Greenberg J, Pyszczynski T. A terror management theory of social behavior: The psychological functions of self-esteem and cultural world views. In Zanna M, ed. *Advances in Experimental Social Psychology*. Academic Press; 1991:93–159.
57. Kabat-Zinn J. *Full Catastrophe Living: Using the Wisdom of Your Body and Mind to Face Stress, Pain, and Illness.* Delta; 2005.
58. Nhat Hanh T. 5 practices for nurturing happiness. 2020. Lion's Roar. https://www.lionsroar.com/5-practices-for-nurturing-happiness/
59 . Mount B, Kearney M. Healing and palliative care: Charting our way forward. *Palliat Med.* 2003;17(8):657–658.
60. University of Massachusetts Medical Center. Mindfulness based stress reduction (MBSR). https://www.umassmed.edu/cfm/mindfulness-based-programs/mbsr-courses/about-mbsr/history-of-mbsr/
61. Leitch L. Action steps using ACEs and trauma-informed care: A resilience model. *Health Justice.* 2017;5(5). https://doi.org/10.1186/s40352-017-0050-5
62. Mills J, Wand T, Fraser J, et al. Exploring the meaning and practice of self- care among palliative care nurses and doctors: A qualitative study. *BMC Palliative Care.* 2018;17(63). https://doi.org/10.1186/s12904-018-0318-0
63. Overbeck T. Putting on your own oxygen mask first. Pediatric e-Journal Workgroup: Pediatric e-Journal. *Pediatr Palliat Hospice Care*. Self-Care. 2020 Nov;61.
64. Kearney M, Weininger R, Vachon M, Harrison R, Mount B. Self-care of physicians caring for patients at the end of life: "Being connected . . . a key to my survival." *JAMA.* 2009;301(11):1155–1164. doi:10.1001/jama.2009.352
65. Yalom I. *Staring at the Sun: Overcoming the Terror of Death.* Jossey-Bass; 2008.
66. Roethke T. *The Collected Poems.* Doubleday; 1975.

13 | PRACTICAL ASPECTS OF PALLIATIVE CARE COMMUNICATION

LINDSAY RAGSDALE, TESSIE OCTOBER, AND CAITLIN SCANLON

The right word may be effective, but no word was ever as effective as a rightly timed pause.

MARK TWAIN[51]

Effective communication among children, their families, and the healthcare team is woven into the fabric of pediatric palliative care (PPC). PPC clinicians balance communication needs of the family with those of the child, as well as serving as interpreters of complex clinical information that the primary team has offered. Coordinating communication among multiple clinicians can be quite complex and requires a delicate balance between providing the that information families need to make decisions with the emotional support necessary for them to feel comforted in those decisions.[1] Adding to this complexity is the need to adapt the mode of communication to "match" the developmental age and capacity of the child, the dynamics of the family, and relevant cultural and religious dimensions. Balancing these "moving parts" requires skill. Communication is a learned skill that requires listening, openness, flexibility, and deliberate practice to achieve mastery. In this chapter we explore the importance of communication and provide useful tools to tackle these conversations empathetically. We also delve into communication about goals of care, prognosis, and managing hope. Clinicians can utilize these practical frameworks to improve communication and establish therapeutic alliances with patients and their families.

WHAT IS EFFECTIVE COMMUNICATION?

Effective communication is not defined solely by the words one uses; a successful communication event considers the context, timing, and even the absence of speech.[2] It requires a dialogue, an active passing of the baton where one speaker truly listens and responds to what is said and what is implied. It demands that the clinician actively track the conversation, decrypting the emotion behind the patient or family's question to determine if it is a cognitive inquiry or an emotional plea.[3] Communication in PPC, both verbal and nonverbal, is about establishing human and caring connections among a child, family, and healthcare team. The transmission of information, while essential, is by no means the only role of effective communication. The communication encounter can also serve as the foundation for a relationship that unfolds over time. The PPC clinician asks questions that provide the opportunity to learn about the child and family: who they are as people, their beliefs and sources of support, the meaning of the illness in their lives, their needs, their goals, their hopes, and their worries. Clinicians gather this information to ensure that recommendations are tailored to reflect a family's hopes and values. Clinicians who approach communication encounters with a sincere desire to listen and get to know the child and family are likely to be most successful in gathering important information.

Key concepts in effective communication in PPC are *vulnerability* and *empathy*. PPC clinicians are meeting patients and families at their most vulnerable time—when they are receiving a new, life-altering diagnosis; suffering through a painful experience; or looking toward a future that is uncertain or shortened. To communicate with a family living this experience requires the clinician to attempt to "leave the agenda at the door" and let the patient and family direct the path of the conversation. This shifting of the power dynamic can feel unsettling to clinicians, but it can also be rewarding. The patient and family are more likely to reveal their fears and worries when given the opportunity and some measure of control. At other times, the skilled clinician will need to gently probe and explore to guide patients and families walk down an uncertain path. Knowing which approach is warranted demands that the clinician rely on patience, empathy, and flexibility. As with any skill, mastery requires knowledge, feedback, and deliberate practice. Fortunately, as the field has evolved, there are some tools to help build the communication skill set.

PALLIATIVE CARE MISSION

Communicating about PPC to patients and their families should emphasize the ways that a palliative interdisciplinary team can provide an extra layer of support and address quality of life issues. At times the introduction of a specialty PPC team can be met with trepidation because many families and medical providers believe PPC is synonymous with end-of-life and/or hospice care. The first introduction of a PPC team should include clarifying the mission of PPC and address the potential misconceptions the patient and family may have. It may be useful to address the similarities and differences of PPC and hospice care up front. This initial conversation can highlight that PPC is woven into care of patients with serious illness all along the illness journey. Early introduction of PPC allows for more time to understand the patient and family's goals to optimize quality of life during treatment. Ensuring that patients and families have a clear idea of the purpose of PPC can set the stage for future honest conversations about their values and goals. Building a relationship based on mutual trust begins with a clear introduction to the meaning of palliative care.

BUILDING TRUST

Building trust with patients and families at the most vulnerable time of their life encompasses not only verbal, but nonverbal communication as well. When patients feel as though their team is both physically and emotionally present, they can begin to experience the sense of trust necessary for exploring end-of-life wishes.[4] Understanding which decisions are most important to families and engaging in shared decision-making can lead to better outcomes for them in the future. Families value empathic, supportive relationships with staff members throughout the illness course. Teams can deepen trust by providing families with the necessary information to make informed decisions about the things they can control—amid many which they cannot. The team thus empowers families to decide what constitutes the right choices for their child as well as share concerns and worries.[5–10]

DISCOVERING PREFERENCE AND VALUES

Delivering medical care that aligns with a patient and family's goals and values is what health systems strive to accomplish; however, the logistics of developing such plans can be challenging.[11] A shared decision-making model of care involves elucidating goals from the patient and family and melding them with recommendations and guidance from the medical team. The first component of this model involves assessing patient and family preferences, needs, and values.[12] A PPC interdisciplinary team can help to clarify these values and goals by exploring the patient and family's understanding of the illness, spiritual and cultural beliefs, social context, economic support, definition of good quality of life, hopes, and worries (please see Chapter 11, "Team Relationships," for a more in-depth analysis on team roles and functions, challenges, and more). These conversations can vary in duration and intensity and must be approached with humility, curiosity, and empathy. Attempting to understand the holistic context of a patient's background can help to hone the medical care. To approach these contextual issues, a provider can use queries that are open and nonjudgmental. For example, taking a spiritual assessment should avoid assumptions that every person has a spiritual belief or attends religious services. Asking about spiritual beliefs could be approached with a question such as, "Do you have spiritual or religious beliefs that are important to you?" This question avoids judgement in the language used and conveys honest curiosity about the patient's life. Table 13.1 outlines questions that can be helpful to explore the many facets that can inform a patient's goals and values. By viewing the patient "beyond" just a medical diagnosis, the PPC team acknowledges that each individual has impact on—and is impacted by—the many people and systems with which they interact.

Clarifying a family's nuanced values and beliefs is critical preparation for exploring how these thought patterns and lived experiences will affect future decision-making.[8] Understanding aspects of a family's culture can most efficiently be achieved through an attitude of curiosity and direct inquiry.[13] Culture is not simply one part of a family's life, but rather all of the pieces encompassed in their lives.[8] Cultural aspects will impact who the family prefers to receive important information and who they look to for assistance in decisions, including legal decisional authority. Clarifying the identity of the decision-makers early in the illness trajectory can prevent confusion at critical times. When interpersonal conflicts among family members impact their ability to make decisions in the best interest of the child, the care team may need to step in to assist.[14]

> The staff helped me a lot by explaining and answering questions and supporting me. As a parent I want to know everything. The team asked me how I wanted to receive information and then they practiced what they preached. It eased my stress when I had all the information. (Mother of a critically ill child)

The endeavor to find out more about a patient and family includes topics such as the unfairness of children having illness, parental guilt, worries about truth-telling sibling relationships, school disruption, and changes in the expectation for child's future. These conversations will be different depending on the age and developmental stage of the patient and involve different contexts from prenatal to young adult patients. For example, parents with an imperiled pregnancy or a prenatal diagnosis of a serious condition face unique challenges while trying to make plans and decisions for an unborn baby. Shared decision-making in these perinatal cases should acknowledge the baby as a meaningful part of the family unit, and decisions should be approached with respect and empathy.[15] Providers can use the baby's name (if already given) and acknowledge the emotional nature of the discussions. Families of older children may want to talk about the child's personality and understanding of illness. Engaging each patient and family with openness and flexibility can help to uncover their preferences, beliefs, and values. The goal of these discussions is to create a more complete depiction of the patient and family in order to guide discussion of their preferences and goals of care. Combining this holistic picture

TABLE 13.1 Questions to explore individual goals and values

Getting to know the child and family	Can you tell me about your child as a person? Can you describe what your child is like when feeling well outside of the hospital? How did you choose your baby's name? (for infants) Can you tell me about your family?
Spiritual context	Do you have spiritual faith or religious beliefs that are important to you? Would you share with me what gives you strength right now? What gives you strength to get through each day?
Cultural context	Are there beliefs about medicine or science that you grew up with? Are there family rituals or beliefs that are important to you?
Social context	Who do you look to in your life for support at this time? When there are medical decisions to discuss, who do you choose to discuss the options with? How are you managing day to day? How are you coping with this admission? What kind of self-care activities help you manage stress? Sometimes, in an effort to "protect" their parents, children may not share all their worries with them. Are there other trusted adults in your child's life who they may confide in *in addition to you?*
Understanding illness	What do you understand about what is happening to your child medically? What has the medical team told you about your child's illness? What is a good or bad day like for your child? Do you feel that your child has been experiencing more "good days" or more "difficult days" lately? How do you prefer to receive medical information? It is common for families to use internet resources to obtain extra information; have you found any that have been helpful to you? Have you had experience with medical care before or had sick loved ones?
Hopes and fears	What are your biggest hopes and worries? What do you worry the most about happening in the future? What do you think the medical team worries about?
Life goals	What do you see for your child in the future? What does your child want to do when they grow up? What are the things your child and family are hoping to accomplish in the coming days/ months/etc.? Anything tzhat you were hoping to accomplish? Does your family have any upcoming travel plans?
Quality of life	What does the expression quality of life mean to you? What does your child enjoy doing the most? What makes your child happy? How does your child show you that they are suffering or in pain? Are there things that would be a bad quality of life for your child?

of a patient and family with the medical recommendations provides an optimal alignment for person-centered care.

PPC teams can clarify goals with patients and families and then amplify and advocate for them during medical team discussions. PPC teams can also provide the context for the reasons behind a family's preferences. This information may decrease provider distress in challenging situations when the medical team and family have different ideas about what is in the child's best interest.[16] By highlighting the family's values that determine their decisions, the PPC team can facilitate more constructive and less adversarial conversations.[17] (See Chapter 16, "Resolving Conflicts.")

Family Reflection

Our son Anthony has had quite a journey with short gut syndrome over the past few years. The majority of that time has been at the Children's Hospital. To say this has been a difficult voyage would be a gross understatement. When a child is admitted into a hospital for critical illness and an extended stay, it is not only the patient along for the ride. The family members are passengers as well, not to mention trying to keep a semblance of normality in the home life that still must continue. The doctors and nurses, especially in the pediatric intensive care unit (PICU) were fantastic in their communication with us during our stay. What we didn't realize is that the hospital offered an advocate for the family on top of the great care for the patient.

From the moment we met the palliative team, we were blown away by how caring and genuine they are. They have mastered one of the most underrated techniques in this life: talking to someone and not just talking at them. The holistic approach to making sure we were doing all right was unexpected, but certainly welcomed. The palliative physician was able to elicit responses from my wife that no one else had because she was masterful at making her feel comfortable in a situation that is not the easiest to block out the anxiety. The nurse practitioner and the social worker have been phenomenal in their duties as well. I won't begin to list all of the kind things they have done, but the team has really done leg work that we could not during these events. The team helped us paint an overall picture of our family situation, and they work tirelessly to fill in the gaps where we need it most. The best part is they're able to sometimes just come in and talk to us. As parents, you get to hear a lot of reports about your child's health and the overall medical outlook. Sometimes it's nice when someone comes in and can talk to each of us about anything other than just the same cold hard facts of the situation.

It's so easy to feel isolated in a hospital, even though there are tons of people in the building. This team was able to come into the room and make us feel like they were there to see us, and for their visit we felt like we actually had a reprieve, even if for a little while. This is extremely crucial for the emotional side of the family. I realize it's hard to measure things like that, but every family in the hospital is going through something. One of the saddest parts to that is there are probably a few people who won't take advantage of what palliative care can do for them because they can't shake the feeling of acrimony over the circumstances.

Valerie and Jason Flanagan, parents of 3-year-old Anthony

COLLABORATION WITH INTERPRETERS

Knowledge of the family's culture of origin is important in discussions about preferences and values. Insight from interpreters, chaplains, and community elders into general standards of communication and areas that are particularly sensitive is crucial.[18] However, making generalized assumptions about the meaning of culture for a particular family should be avoided.[18,19] As valued members of the interdisciplinary team, interpreters can assist by being conscious of the clinician's tone when information is shared, as well as serving as a cultural "bridge" when there is no direct translation for a particular concept. The leader or facilitator can "preview" both the content and the actual words that will be used in the meeting. Interpreters may need time for debriefing after the meeting due to the emotional content discussed. They are often not trained in serious news disclosure and may lack the resources in their own department for support. By facilitating these discussions, the PPC team can make a significant contribution to their colleagues' well-being.[20]

GOALS OF CARE

ESTABLISHING GOALS OF CARE

Assessing and identifying a set of goals for a pediatric patient is a crucial part of PPC. The intricacies of verbalizing, refining, and revisiting these goals can be challenging for both providers and family. The following are practical steps and guidance about how to proceed as the clinical picture evolves.

Ideally, goals-of-care discussions should be initiated during calm periods. However, at times circumstances dictate that these discussions happen during a crisis when emotions are amplified for parents as well as for providers who need decisions to be made in the moment. During these pressured times, it is important to remember the human part of communication and take as much time with families as is realistically possible. Goals-of-care conversations are multifaceted and can involve personal experiences, beliefs, cultural considerations, and values which need to be elicited to come to a shared decision. Creating connections with families can help to provide a trusting environment to discuss their personal beliefs and values.

Conversations about goals of care begin by asking about the family's beliefs, values, and experiences and then allowing them sufficient time to express their thoughts. The meaning of quality of life is subjective; therefore exploring a family's definition is necessary to create a care plan. Many families can verbalize their definition of quality of life clearly and choose to create a plan with that exclusive focus. Some loving families may value longevity and place importance on the child being alive even if the required medical care is burdensome. Other loving families articulate the combined goal of "as long as possible" with careful attention to specific aspects of quality of life, such as the ability to breathe without technology or the ability to be awake and interact with the environment. Figure 13.1 illustrates the spectrum of goals of care through these concepts of the relationship between quality of life and longevity.

It is important to explore what factors (e.g., changes in the child's mental status, ability to interact, expressiveness, ambulation, and nutrition) might alter the family's decisions. Goals of care encompass a wide range of components including where the child would want to spend time, a special trip, birthdays, graduation, achieving a milestone, seeing a friend, or succeeding in a functional goal. These goals represent hope for the future and do not necessarily imply a lack of understanding of the child's current medical status. Parents may describe their hopes and dreams for their child while at the same time fully recognize the seriousness of the illness. PPC teams can assist the primary team in understanding that families can hold hopes and reality simultaneously.

In the process of decision-making, many families appreciate a recommendation from the medical team that is consistent with their own values and goals.[21] The palliative care team can play an important role by encouraging primary providers to offer their expert opinion. Parents often feel distress and guilt in making these significant decisions about their child on their own. Guidance and recommendations from the medical team can help them feel that the decision-making process is shouldered by all.[22,23] It is important to note that recommendations are offered with the proviso that a family has the autonomy to follow or not follow them.

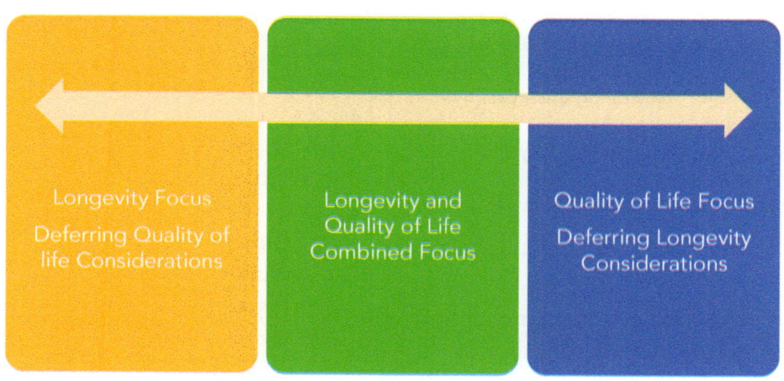

Figure 13.1 Spectrum of goals of care.

SHIFTING AND REFRAMING GOALS OF CARE

Goals of care can change for many reasons along the illness trajectory. Opportunities to revisit goals of care include changes in medical status, declining baseline, new diagnoses, admissions to the hospital, refractory symptoms, or changes in social structure or caregiver. For example, in the case of infants with neurological abnormalities, their differences from healthy peers may not be evident until the age when developmental milestones can be evaluated. Providers can use these opportunities to ask how the family perceives the child's development and reflect on their own observations. Another example is parents who may want to talk about goals of care for their child who has cerebral palsy and has had multiple hospital admissions for aspiration pneumonias. Helping them process their worry can provide an opportunity to explore and refocus on their goals, including improving quality of life. Working with families at a challenging time can serve as a pivot point toward the opportunity to align the plan of care with their newly refined goals.[24]

Some families are open to disengaging from a prior goal and connecting with a new goal that is more attainable.[24] This openness to "regoaling" has been associated with decreased depression and improved well-being.[25] However, some parents may choose to continue with their initial goal because they feel that it better represents their family values and beliefs. During times of transition, palliative care providers can facilitate a discussion with the parents about their child's current status and whether the current goal is still aligned with their values. The time frame of when parents may be open to changing goals will differ based on multiple factors including individual decision-making practices, clinical status, or immediacy of crisis. Allowing time for parents to readjust expectations and process new information is essential.

SETTING THE STAGE FOR A FAMILY CONFERENCE

A framework that is often used to discuss prognosis and goals of care involves a stepwise approach to ensure that all elements are addressed in a family-centered way. Figure 13.2 depicts the framework for prognostic disclosure including preparation, consensus building, delivery of news, pause, and follow-up.[26]

Thoughtful preparation for a conference with a patient and family begins with data gathering to understand current factors that may impact the conversation. A team member should inquire about whose presence would be beneficial to the family when receiving important information from the medical team. Preparation includes steps to ensure that all relevant individuals named by the parents are invited, including, for example, grandparents, friend, counselor, coach, spiritual guide, or community leader. Technology minimizes barriers and creates the opportunity for people to join the discussion remotely. Additionally, families may be asked "which providers do you most trust and look to for guidance in medical decision-making for your child?" Whenever possible, these individuals should be present. Given their importance to the family, it is ideal if they can arrange for coverage for the duration of the meeting. It should also be noted that some families prefer small meetings, and such preferences should be honored.

The presence of psychosocial team members at the conference is vital. Family meetings can be laden with intense emotions and fears which may not be noticed or fully addressed by the medical team members. Social workers, psychologists, chaplains, and child life specialists can aid in identifying and responding to emotions and highlight underlying hopes and fears. Many times, the family appreciates a team member staying after the meeting to debrief and further explore their feelings about what was discussed.

Many families have preferences for inclusion of their child or may wonder how to disclose their diagnosis or likely prognosis. Some teams approach the parents with an invitation for a family conference and explore how and if to include the child in the discussion. Honest disclosure of medical information that is tailored to the child's developmental stage—and taking into consideration the child's desire to know such information—is crucial.[27,28] Many families attempt to protect their child from difficult conversations by avoiding telling them medical information. While medical providers will respect the family's wishes for nondisclosure in some cases, it is strongly suggested that they be honest that they will not lie if the child asks the provider a direct question.[29,30] For example a provider could say, "I know you want to protect your son from the news about his cancer, however if he asks me directly if he has cancer I will not lie to him. I will explore with him why he is asking and what all he wants to know. If he wants to know, then I will tell him in a gentle way." This sets expectations with the family about the medical provider's responsibility for truth-telling and protecting trust in the relationship with the child.[31] If a child is present in family conference, explanation of the medical facts should be tailored to their developmental understanding, and the child can be asked about concerns or questions. Parents may request that they receive the information and have time to discuss it with the team prior to the child joining the meeting.

Setting the scene takes into account the location for the discussion. Choosing a quiet setting for an uninterrupted discussion is ideal, but it is also important to include the family in this preparation. For example, a parent of a critically ill child in the ICU may report anxiety when leaving their child's bedside. Similarly, a family may be hesitant to enter into certain meeting rooms if the room is associated with a previous conversation in which they received information that they considered difficult to hear. While it is ideal to have seating arranged so that all participants can see one another in a family meeting, this may not always be feasible due to time constraints, acuity, and facility barriers. PPC teams are in an optimal position to facilitate the staging of a family meeting and ensure that interdisciplinary team members are present.

Other considerations for a family meeting include anticipation of potential responses of the patient or family

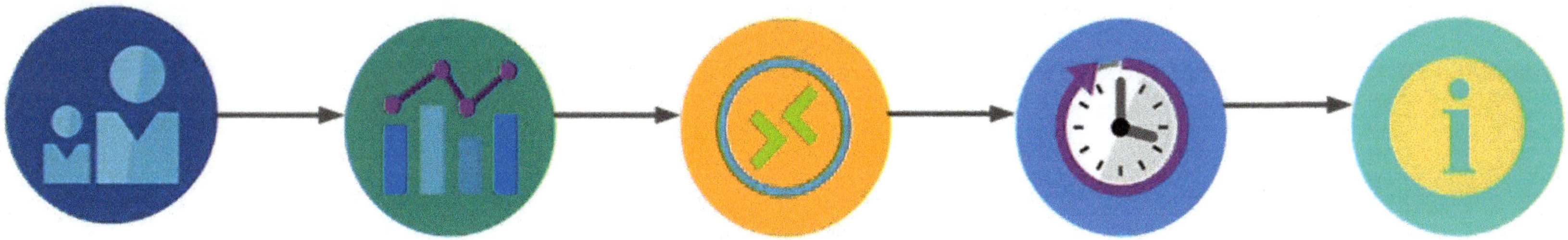

Preparation	Consensus	Delivery	Pause	Follow up
Select room, participants, and timing of discussion	Ensure consistent, succinct message before meeting with family	Give serious news clearly and with empathy	Allow time for silence and support emotional responses	Ensure follow up plan for communication and next steps
• *Arrange for the a private meeting space* • *Seating available for all participants*	• *Interdisciplinary team pre-meeting to ensure agreement on news to deliver* • *Work through disagreements* • *Agree on topics to cover*	• *Introduce all participants* • *Ask for suggestions from family to include in the discussion* • *Review agenda* • *Ask family for their perception of child's status*	• *Allow time for emotional response* • *Empathetic listening* • *Pause in talking*	• *If family ready to continue, outline next steps* • *Elicit questions and answer honestly* • *Have more information readily available, if requested*
• *Identify family members to be present* • *Identity health providers/interdisciplinary team members to be present* • *Identity support staff and/or spiritual leaders to be present*	• *Select leader of discussion* • *Role delineation for participants*	• *Use Ask-Tell-Ask to guide discussion* • *Can give "warning" that news in not what was hoped for*	• *Use body language to communicate caring* • *Observe for emotions* • *Can respond with empathetic statements* • *"I wish this wasn't the news we had to share"*	• *Reassurance that medical team will not abandon regardless of decision made* • *Reaffirm central goals* • *Outline when further communication* • *Follow through on communication plan*
• *Set meeting for an agreed upon time* • *Allow enough time for discussion*	• *Prepare images, reports graphs* • *Define potential choices, treatment options. recommendations* • *Anticipate potential questions and emotional responses*	• *Give serious news clearly* • *"The bone marrow biopsy shows that he has leukaemia"*	• *Anticipate strong emotions at times including disagreements among participants* • *Some family members may not be able to proceed at this time*	• *Empatethically address emotional responses* • *Arrange for additional emotional and/or spiritual support*

Figure 13.2 Framework for serious news disclosure.

and preparing the team for what to do should they occur. Emotional responses to difficult news can vary, but may include crying, anger, shock, vaso-vagal reactions such as passing out or vomiting, and people leaving the room abruptly. Given that crying can be a common response from families, having tissues available within reach is beneficial. In the team pre-meeting, one member should be identified to seek additional personnel to help should a family member experience syncope or other vaso-vagal responses.

COMMUNICATION TOOLS TO GUIDE THE CONVERSATION

Goals-of-care conversations can be challenging for providers for many reasons, including lack of specific training, discomfort with emotional content, and worries about the effects of these intense conversations on hope.[28,32] To help overcome the discomfort in these discussions, there are guides to help providers frame the conversation. No one framework will provide all the tools to successfully navigate a conversation; however, guidelines can give the clinician a foundation. Although several guides exist, three (SPIKES,[33] Ask-Tell-Ask,[34] and NURSE[35]) are paramount in framing how to navigate the conversation. While these frameworks are helpful, clinicians must recognize that children and families experience illness from within their cultural context, and medical communication should be sensitive to differences in informational needs and decision-making styles.

Introductions (including of the family members) should open the meeting, with participants introducing themselves and identifying their role on the team. After introductions, it is often helpful to gather information from the patient (if present) and family about their understanding of the current health status of the patient and questions they have for the healthcare team. All too often, clinicians enter a conversation with an agenda, thereby missing an opportunity to understand what is at the forefront in the mind of the patient and family. Utilizing Ask-Tell-Ask shifts the dynamic by first asking for understanding from the family. The data-gathering that occurs in the first Ask can help the clinician decide what should be said in the Tell and how it should be communicated, often using the family's language to describe the illness. Hearing the family's observations and concerns provides insight into their understanding of the current illness and highlights areas of focus. Asking the patient or family about their understanding should come from a place of curiosity and clarification, rather than testing their knowledge. Some families may feel intimidated by being asked to tell a room full of medical providers what their understanding is regarding the medical situation. A provider can ask, "So that we know where to begin, would you mind sharing with us what you have been told is going on with your child?" or "We want to ensure that we provide all of the information that you are hoping to receive today. It would be helpful to us if you can share what you have heard from the medical teams, so we know where to begin." "You've met so many doctors and the information can often be confusing. It would be helpful for us to know your understanding of what the doctors have told you about how [insert name of child] is doing." Asking is not just for the beginning of the conversation. Throughout the conversation, ask for permission—permission to enter their room, permission to share serious news, or permission to make a recommendation; ask for clarification; ask for additional details; and ask for a recap to ensure the patient and family heard what was said.

Communicating serious news is one of the most challenging aspects of medical care. Research suggests that clinicians feel unprepared and report inadequate training in communication techniques.[32] The most anxiety-provoking aspect of communication around serious illness is dealing with the heightened emotions of these intense conversations. The first step for clinicians is to anticipate that emotions will be present and appear in different forms—anger, sadness, anxiety, denial, or guilt. The key is to recognize them and respond with empathy. The NURSE mnemonic gives clinicians five types of responses to emotion: Naming, Understanding, Respecting, and Supporting or Exploring the emotion. These responses are not meant to be prescriptive; they are guides that use supportive language in response to emotion.

It is important to recognize that these conversations are not one-time events, and it often takes several discussions to understand a family's motivations, worries, and hopes. Creating opportunities for interaction with quiet presence on a regular basis, not just when there is medical news to be delivered, can help establish and foster rapport. The connections made between the larger family meetings may be rich with meaning that informs all interactions as well as creating a safe space where permission will likely be given to explore more sensitive topics in future. Presence sends a powerful message about the consistent care the clinician provides and the value of the child and family.

Team Reflection

Bobby was a 2-year-old boy diagnosed with cardiomyopathy due to history of treatment for cancer diagnosed at birth. He loved the color green, big trucks, and his large, adoring family. The oncology team consulted the PPC team at birth for ongoing support given Bobby's uncertain future. The PPC introduced themselves as "an additional layer of support offered to patients and families facing a serious illness." When asked "What is your major support that gives you strength?" The family replied that "they were rooted in their faith and that God would continue to give them strength." The PPC team aligned with the family's faith and offered spiritual support at each family meeting throughout Bobby's life.

In the first several months of his life, Bobby defied the odds, overcoming respiratory failure and showing tumor response to chemotherapy, permitting a full tumor resection. Throughout this time, PPC was able to establish a strong therapeutic relationship with the family, taking the time to understand their dynamics, beliefs, and values by delving deeply into questions such as "At this time, what do you fear most?" or "Who are the most important people for us to give information to about how Bobby is doing?" The PPC team used that information to ensure that at difficult treatment crossroads the important people were in the room.

Several months later Bobby suffered from a cardiac arrest at home. As a result he had severe injury to several organs, including his brain, and appeared to have minimal response, if any, to stimulation. Throughout several family meetings, the family expressed that their faith remained strong, citing that Bobby was a "fighter" and he had "proven the doctors wrong before." The PPC team supported the family by praising them for their role as advocate for Bobby, such as "We can see how much you care for Bobby" or by empathizing with them, such as "I cannot imagine how devastating it must feel to see Bobby this way."

As Bobby continued to worsen, the PPC team was able to sit with the family, reflecting on Bobby's previous hospital stays and alerting the family to "We're in a different place." Then asking, "Given that we're worried Bobby will have a life connected to machines, what is important to you now?" The PPC team was then able to convey the family's narrative to the PICU team in an effort to bridge gaps in communication. Together, the healthcare team met with the family several times to clarify wishes. Slowly, family members began to share their worries that "this time was different" and that they feared Bobby would not survive. The PPC team engaged in discussions with the family about their hopes for the days to come, as well as their worry and apprehension of the unknown. The family spoke about a desire for him to live until his second birthday (2 more days) and to have a big truck birthday party for him, after which they would discuss a plan to discontinue the use of life-sustaining therapies. The family decorated the room and had friends and extended family members, as well as team members come to celebrate his birthday. Child life specialists worked with the family to create memory-making items such as hand molds and prints.

The following week, the family spoke with the healthcare team about discontinuing ventilatory support. They posed thoughtful questions about obtaining a final blessing and asked about "the next steps." They identified the few family and healthcare team members to be present at time of death and asked that the remaining team members assist in keeping other family members in the lounge area. The team arranged for chaplaincy to be present to provide a blessing, and the social worker assisted the family in contacting a funeral home. PPC medical team members provided education and anticipatory guidance regarding what symptoms Bobby might experience and how they would be treated. They also invited the family to assist in bathing him after his death.

Several days after Bobby's death, the social worker followed up with family to explore further needs asking, "How best can we help you now?" and to inform them of available bereavement support both within the hospital and in the community. The social worker reinforced the parenting role by saying, "Throughout the time I've known you guys we have seen you show nothing but love for Bobby. He was lucky to have you guys as his advocates and parents." The PPC team also met with the PICU team to debrief on the life and death of Bobby and its effect on the healthcare team.

Through early and ongoing PPC involvement in Bobby's care, the team was able to provide thoughtful guidance and support for all domains of their and Bobby's suffering, as well as support for the primary PICU team.

SHARING SERIOUS NEWS

> In the family meeting the palliative care team used the least number of words, but they said so much. It was like they knew what the rest of us were thinking.
>
> Nurse caring for a critically ill child

Sharing serious medical news with families can be a stressful undertaking for providers.[36] There are numerous barriers that can prevent disclosure (or timely disclosure) of serious news to parents and patients. Providers may feel that the parents are not yet "ready" to hear the information when, in fact, it is they themselves who may not be personally or professionally "ready" to accept a poor prognosis. Some providers express worry that disclosing serious news may take away the patient or family's hope for the future. Research has shown that disclosing devastating medical information does not take away hope or fracture the relationship with providers. Evidence suggests that being honest about the medical facts gives patients the ability to plan, can decrease anxiety, and, in some families, can increase hope for other goals.[27,28,37,38]

Once the team is ready to share serious information with a family, the first phase includes specific attention to the way that the news is delivered, what news is being discussed, who is delivering the news, the setting in which the discussion will take place, who the family would like to be present, and follow-up after the news is shared. During this highly stressful time, some of these details can be overlooked and the discussion can be rushed without proper preparation. Successful disclosure of highly sensitive information, which may elicit emotionally laden responses from families, should include a thoughtful plan for how this news will be shared.

The second phase is the consensus phase, including a team pre-meeting to discuss the content of the meeting. This pre-meeting should include a selection of a leader for the family meeting. The goal of the pre-meeting is to have team members reach consensus on the medical facts and prognosis to form a cohesive and succinct message for the family.

TABLE 13.2 Communication tools to guide clinician-family conversations: SPIKES, Ask-Tell-Ask, NURSE

SPIKES	ASK-TELL-ASK	NURSE	RESPONSE STATEMENTS TO EMOTION
Setting up the interview	Ask—Ask for personal assessment and understanding Ask—Ask for permission	Name	"This situation is overwhelming."
Assessing the patient's Perception	Tell—Tell the news	Understand	"I can't imagine how hard this must be."
Obtaining the patient's Invitation	Ask—Ask for understanding and strategies for improvement	Respect	"I am impressed by what good care you've taken of your daughter."
Giving Knowledge and information to the patient		Support	"Our team will keep helping you sort out what the options might be."
Addressing the patient's emotions with Empathetic responses		Explore	"What's the hardest part of all of this for you?"
Summary and Strategy			

Additionally, the team can review previous conversations and determine their shared clinical recommendations for next steps in the child's medical plan. Last, the pre-meeting provides a space for psychosocial team members to voice family coping styles, barriers to care, psychosocial challenges, and family dynamics.[39]

The third phase is the delivery of the news during the family meeting. Using the Ask-Tell-Ask guideline can ensure involvement of the family in the discussion (Table 13.2). The medical status should be reviewed, including establishing the goal for the current meeting. Giving the family a warning that serious news is coming can be used to prepare them for what is about to be said, as well as allow space for a family to give permission to the team to share this information. It can be said as simply as, "the results of the test are not what we were hoping for." This warning can give the family a moment to catch their breath and prepare themselves, although current data are mixed on the effects of distress levels on family members.[40] The medical news should then be told clearly, with empathy and avoiding medical jargon. For example: "your daughter's lungs have continued to worsen, and, unfortunately, our treatments are not working." Pause to allow the family time to process the news, synthesize the information and respond to the team. The medical team can use a short empathetic statement such as, "I wish we had different news to share." Helpful phrases are listed in Table 13.3, as well as comments that should be avoided. After a pause the family may be ready to proceed (sometimes they need time before they are ready to go on with discussion), and team members should volunteer to answer any questions they have. Team members can then provide additional information that may be requested and discuss next steps. The conference leader can offer a choice, "would it be helpful to talk about what lies ahead, or should we take a break and meet again later today or tomorrow?" This follow-up phrase allows the team to emphasize that communication will continue and that the family will not be abandoned. Plans should be made with the family for subsequent discussions after they have had time to process the information presented and potential new questions emerge.

PARENTAL ROLE AND SENSE OF DUTY

Throughout the process of rethinking goals of care, parents should be involved in exploring their perspectives on their child's current medical status.[41] During these conversations, discussing how they define their role and obligations as a parent can be helpful in understanding their perspective. Parents may feel their duty is to continue to opt for all the medical interventions available and not "give up" until all options are exhausted. Other parents may be driven by the overriding sense of duty to protect their child and keep them safe, focusing on protecting their child from interventions that are harmful or painful and unlikely to result in alleviation of suffering. Intensive measures at end of life, including cardiopulmonary resuscitation (CPR), can be painful and parents may choose to forego these interventions in an effort to align with their duty to protect.

Medical teams can discuss the parental role in the context of daily care and also long-term goals of care. The daily care of their child should strive to provide parents with an opportunity to maintain their bond and uphold their parental role such as (when possible) allowing physical closeness, touch, and holding. If the goals of care are changing, the conversation may need to include how their parenting role may alter or evolve as the clinical status of their child changes. This anticipatory guidance can help parents maintain a feeling of being a "good parent" to their child. Medical providers can assist in this conversation by affirming and validating that the parent is acting out of love and upholding their parental duty. Addressing a parent's fear of their changing role can help facilitate the parent–child relationship during times of transition.[42] Providers can ask parents directly, "What would need to happen for you to feel you are being a good parent?"[42] For example, a mother may be worried that she would not be able to feed her child after the placement of a gastrostomy tube. Prior to the procedure, it would be important to address the mother's sense of her role in feeding and nutrition and how her nurturing may differ once her child receives the intervention. She may find new ways to care for her child with the improvement in nutritional status and ease of providing nutrition to her child in an alternate way. These parental roles

TABLE 13.3 Helpful phrases for effective communication

UTILIZE	AVOID
Treatment was not as successful as we had hoped	Patient failed treatment
Patient has a do-not-resuscitate (DNR) order in place	Patient is a DNR
Focus on intensive symptom management/maximize quality of life	Do nothing
Equally loving families make different decisions	"Need to" statements Example: "You need to follow our recommendations for a tracheostomy."
Would you like me or another member of the team to assist in calling additional important people? Would you like one of us to be present/stay with you when you make the calls?	You should consider the other people in your family who you need to think about when you make this decision.
Can we discuss the treatments and interventions we are providing that no longer seem to be helping and may be causing harm?	We should stop futile interventions.
Let's review the care we have provided so far, what results we have seen, and decide together where we should go from here.	There is nothing more we can do.
I can't imagine how difficult this must be.	I know how you feel.
What questions can I answer? If none comes to mind right now, write them down so that we can review the next time we meet. I can be available later today or tomorrow if you think of other questions or concerns.	Do you have any questions?
I worry that he may not reach this goal.	Your child will never be able to do that milestone.

and obligations should be intentionally addressed when discussing goals of care.

COMMUNICATING WITH CHILDREN

The complexity of communicating with children who are seriously ill is well recognized by clinicians and is underscored in their reported anxiety about discussions with these children and their families.[43,44] Parents vary in their preferences for who shares serious information with their child. Some prefer that a trusted clinician have these discussions alone with the child or in the presence of the parents, while others may not want the clinician to initiate certain discussions with their child, preferring to initiate the discussion themselves. In the latter case, there remain important roles for clinicians, including preparing parents for the discussion with their child or being present when the parents share information. Parents may experience a natural reluctance to share serious information with their child in hopes of protecting them.[45] Reluctance to disclose information likely stems from fear of the child's emotional reaction, loss of hope, or diminished willingness on the child's part to interact with the parents and others. While these fears may be common, evidence supports the honest disclosure of information to children on a level they will understand.[31] Honest disclosure has not been shown to reduce hope and may support reframing or regoaling.[28] Clinicians can help prepare parents for these discussions by exploring underlying reasons for concerns, offering suggestions for possible ways to share the information, or even role-playing with the parents in advance of the discussion. The medical team in conjunction with psychologists, social workers, child life specialists, and chaplains can prepare parents for what words they may say or questions they may ask based on the developmental stage and individual personality of the child. Some parents may want to rehearse what to say to prepare them for the conversation. Parents have indicated that after they or the clinicians have such conversations with their child, they want clinicians to treat their child the same way as they did before the child's condition became so serious.[46] Recognizing and honoring parental preferences around inclusion of their child in discussions is fundamental to opening the door to these discussions with children. If a parent asks for a clinician to withhold information from a child, a conversation about this approach should occur to outline some boundaries. Many clinicians will set expectations that if a child asks them a question directly, they will tell them the honest truth in a way the child will understand. The expectation of truth-telling will help to establish a trusting relationship with the clinician for future conversations. A clinician can ask more clarifying questions of the child if they are asking intense questions. For example, if a child asks, "Is it my fault that I got sick." A clinician can respond by asking, "Can you tell me more about your question? Have you been worried about it being someone's fault?" These clarifying questions can ensure that the root of the question is being uncovered instead of just simply saying, "No, It's not your fault, don't think that," which might cut off the conversation, not allow for the child's worries or hopes to be explored, and could lead to negative feelings or further isolation for the child. A young child may indulge in *magical thinking* that connects something they failed to do, like making their bed, with being sick as a side effect. It can be helpful to allow space for the child to express their worries and respond with patience and empathy.

After establishing parental preferences for the clinician sharing information with the child, the clinician is tasked with detecting clues from the child about information needs. The clinician should begin by gently inviting the child to engage in sharing information, thoughts, and feelings. Some clinicians use games, books, or metaphors as a vehicle to engage with children.[47] Other forms of media which can also be very helpful in sharing information and feelings between clinicians and children include drawings, pictures, or diagrams.[48] Perhaps one of the most powerful communication tools that a clinician can use is silence, using the quiet time to listen to the child. Clinicians must be able to quiet their own thoughts and not try to plan their next comment, but instead listen with the intention of discovering insight about this child, family, situation, and about themselves.[49]

The importance of the interdisciplinary team cannot be overstated. Psychosocial team members may be most effective in engaging children in discussions. For example, a psychologist may address the child's emotional needs as an important component of the meeting, or a child life specialist may help clarify a child's fears. Both professions rely not only on verbal interactions, but also on the children's expression through their words and play. In addition to providing the family with the opportunity to reflect on the conversation afterward, interdisciplinary team members may actively participate by observing interactions carefully, recognizing and attending to emotional content, and being alert to miscommunications. When communicating with a child and his or her family, having individual professionals specifically assigned to each dimension of care may be the best way to ensure cues are not ignored and the needs of all participants are addressed.

COMMUNICATION WITH THE ADOLESCENT AND YOUNG ADULT PATIENT

Tailoring communication strategies to meet the needs of each patient should be the goal of each encounter. While there may be a reluctance on behalf of clinicians and families to disclose serious news to adolescents and young adults (AYA, research suggests that this patient population desires clear communication and increasing autonomy in decision-making.[28] Developmentally, this is a time in an individual's life when they have emerging autonomy, but, due to medical illness, they are now likely having to rely more frequently on caregivers for daily needs. Honest disclosure with AYA patients can give them time to process the information and form new goals, thereby creating opportunities for autonomy and self-advocacy. For example, in the context of telling a 17-year-old patient that he is dying from his disease, the opportunity opens for clinicians to explore with the AYA what is most important to him. This adolescent may want to prioritize attending significant life events over other treatment options that keep him in the hospital. Without including the AYA patient in these discussions, these individual goals may be overlooked or underrecognized. Professionals in social work, psychology, child life, and chaplaincy are specifically trained in navigating these conversations and can facilitate exploration of and advocacy for the patient's goals and wishes. Many AYA patients are used to expressing their emotions by text or online and may choose to explore their thoughts through these modalities.[50] Electronic communication (that protects health information) can sometimes be a more comfortable way for them to communicate. Additionally, AYA patients may seek support and advice in online forums or groups with peers who are experiencing similar life circumstances. For all of these reasons, it is beneficial for clinicians to ask these young people about their preferred method of communication and collaborate to meet their preferences.

CONCLUSION

Effective palliative communication with patients and families requires team preparation, attention to patient and family needs, responding to emotions, and patiently assisting families as they cope and readjust over time. This chapter outlined practical advice for primary teams to introduce PPC into the treatment team and suggestions on how to introduce PPC to families. PPC can assist in disclosure of serious medical news and also help when goals of care need to be established. Clinicians can work on improving their communication skills by adapting a collaborative communication strategy and learning more about a patient and family's goals and preferences. An interdisciplinary approach to these challenging situations is best practice to address the full spectrum of family needs.

REFERENCES

1. October TW, Hinds PS, Wang J, Dizon ZB, Cheng YI, Roter DL. Parent satisfaction with communication is associated with physician's patient-centered communication patterns during family conferences. *Pediatr Crit Care Med.* 2016;17(6):490–497.
2. October TW, Dizon ZB, Arnold RM, Rosenberg AR. Characteristics of physician empathetic statements during pediatric intensive care conferences with family members: A qualitative study. *JAMA Network Open.* 2018;1(3):e180351.
3. October TW, Dizon ZB, Roter DL. Is it my turn to speak? An analysis of the dialogue in the family-physician intensive care unit conference. *Patient Educ Couns.* 2018;101(4):647–652.
4. Benbenishty JS, Hannink JR. Non-verbal communication to restore patient-provider trust. *Intensive Care Med.* 2015;41(7):1359–1360.
5. Meyer EC, Ritholz MD, Burns JP, Truog RD. Improving the quality of end-of-life care in the pediatric intensive care unit: Parents' priorities and recommendations. *Pediatrics.* 2006;117(3):649–657.
6. Postier A, Catrine K, Remke S. Interdisciplinary pediatric palliative care team involvement in compassionate extubation at home: From shared decision-making to bereavement. *Children (Basel).* 2018;5(3):37.
7. Falkenburg JL, Tibboel D, Ganzevoort RR, Gischler SJ, van Dijk M. The importance of parental connectedness and relationships with healthcare professionals in end-of-life care in the PICU. *Pediatr Crit Care Med.* 2018;19(3):e157–e163.
8. Chrastek JJR, Goloff N, Moore T. A case study in cross-cultural health care and ethics: Who decides what is in the child's "best interest"? *J Hosp Palliat Nurs.* 2019;21(1):8–13.
9. Longden JV, Mayer AP. Family involvement in end-of-life care in a paediatric intensive care unit. *Nurs Crit Care.* 2007;12(4):181–187.
10. Aldridge J, Shimmon K, Miller M, Fraser LK, Wright B. "I can't tell my child they are dying." Helping parents have conversations with their child. *Arch Dis Child Educ Pract Ed.* 2017;102(4):182–187.

11. Barry MJ, Edgman-Levitan S. Shared decision making--pinnacle of patient-centered care. *N Engl J Med.* 2012;366(9):780–781.
12. Institute of Medicine Committee on Quality of Health Care in America. *Crossing the Quality Chasm: A New Health System for the 21st Century.* National Academies Press; 2001.
13. Macdonald ME, Carnevale FA, Razack S. Understanding what residents want and what residents need: The challenge of cultural training in pediatrics. *Med Teach.* 2007;29(5):444–451.
14. Cornfield DN, Kahn JP. Decisions about life-sustaining measures in children: In whose best interests? *Acta Paediatr.* 2012;101(4):333–336.
15. Côté-Arsenault D, Denney-Koelsch E. "My baby is a person": Parents' experiences with life-threatening fetal diagnosis. *J Palliat Med.* 2011;14(12):1302–1308.
16. Cavinder C. The relationship between providing neonatal palliative care and nurses' moral distress: An integrative review. 2014;14(5):322–328.
17. Sannino P, Giannì ML, Carini M, et al. Moral distress in the pediatric intensive care unit: An Italian study. *Front Pediatr.* 2019;7:338.
18. Surbone A. Cultural aspects of communication in cancer care. *Supportive Care Cancer.* 2008;16(3):235–240.
19. De Trill M, Kovalcik R. The child with cancer. Influence of culture on truth-telling and patient care. *Ann N Y Acad Sci.* 1997;809:197–210.
20. Prentice J, Nelson A, Baillie J, Osborn H, Noble S. "Don't blame the middle man": An exploratory qualitative study to explore the experiences of translators breaking bad news. *JRSM.* 2014;107(7):271–276.
21. Childers JW, Back AL, Tulsky JA, Arnold RM. REMAP: A framework for goals of care conversations. *J Oncol Pract.* 2017;13(10):e844–e850.
22. Sharman M, Meert KL, Sarnaik AP. What influences parents' decisions to limit or withdraw life support? *Pediatr Crit Care Med.* 2005;6(5):513–518.
23. Kirsch RE, Coronado J, Roeleveld PP, Tweddell J, Mott AM, Roth SJ. The burdens of offering: Ethical and practical considerations. *World J Pediatr Congenit Heart Surg.* 2017;8(6):715–720.
24. Hill DL, Miller V, Walter JK, et al. Regoaling: A conceptual model of how parents of children with serious illness change medical care goals. *BMC Palliat Care.* 2014;13(1):9.
25. Wrosch C, Scheier MF, Miller GE, Schulz R, Carver CS. Adaptive self-regulation of unattainable goals: Goal disengagement, goal reengagement, and subjective well-being. *Pers Soc Psychol Bull.* 2003;29(12):1494–1508.
26. Feudtner C. Collaborative communication in pediatric palliative care: A foundation for problem-solving and decision-making. *Pediatr Clin North Am.* 2007;54(5):583–607.
27. Ghoshal A, Salins N, Damani A, et al. To tell or not to tell: Exploring the preferences and attitudes of patients and family caregivers on disclosure of a cancer-related diagnosis and prognosis. *J Glob Oncol.* 2019;5:1–12.
28. Mack JW, Wolfe J, Cook EF, Grier HE, Cleary PD, Weeks JC. Hope and prognostic disclosure. *J Clin Oncol.* 2007;25(35):5636–5642.
29. Rosenberg AR, Wolfe J, Wiener L, Lyon M, Feudtner C. Ethics, emotions, and the skills of talking about progressing disease with terminally ill adolescents: A review. *JAMA Pediatr.* 2016;170(12):1216–1223.
30. Rosenberg AR, Starks H, Unguru Y, Feudtner C, Diekema D. Truth telling in the setting of cultural differences and incurable pediatric illness: A review. *JAMA Pediatr.* 2017;171(11):1113–1119.
31. Hudson N, Spriggs M, Gillam L. Telling the truth to young children: Ethical reasons for information disclosure in paediatrics. *J Paediatr Child Health.* 2019;55(1):13–17.
32. Back AL, Arnold RM. "Yes it's sad, but what should I do?" Moving from empathy to action in discussing goals of care. *J Palliat Med.* 2014;17(2):141–144.
33. Baile WF, Buckman R, Lenzi R, Glober G, Beale EA, Kudelka AP. SPIKES-A six-step protocol for delivering bad news: Application to the patient with cancer. *Oncologist.* 2000;5(4):302–311.
34. Back AL, Arnold RM, Baile WF, Tulsky JA, Fryer-Edwards K. Approaching difficult communication tasks in oncology. *CA Cancer J Clin.* 2005;55(3):164–177.
35. Smith RC, Hoppe RB. The patient's story: Integrating the patient- and physician-centered approaches to interviewing. *Ann Intern Med.* 1991;115(6):470–477.
36. Studer RK, Danuser B, Gomez P. Physicians' psychophysiological stress reaction in medical communication of bad news: A critical literature review. *Int J Psychophysiol.* 2017;120:14–22.
37. Matthews T, Baken D, Ross K, Ogilvie E, Kent L. The experiences of patients and their family members when receiving bad news about cancer: A qualitative meta-synthesis. *Psychooncology.* 2019;28(12):2286–2294.
38. Kamihara J, Nyborn JA, Olcese ME, Nickerson T, Mack JW. Parental hope for children with advanced cancer. *Pediatrics.* 2015;135(5):868–874.
39. Jonas D, Scanlon C, Schmidt L, Bogetz J. Creating a seat at the table: How family meetings elucidate the palliative care social work role. *J Palliat Med.* 2020;(12):1688–1691.
40. Porensky EK, Carpenter BD. Breaking bad news: Effects of forecasting diagnosis and framing prognosis. *Patient Educ Couns.* 2016;99(1):68–76.
41. Zaal-Schuller IH, de Vos MA, Ewals FV, van Goudoever JB, Willems DL. End-of-life decision-making for children with severe developmental disabilities: The parental perspective. *Res Dev Disabil.* 2016;49–50:235–246.
42. Feudtner C, Walter JK, Faerber JA, et al. Good-parent beliefs of parents of seriously ill children. *JAMA Pediatr.* 2015;169(1):39–47.
43. Masera G, Chesler MA, Jankovic M, et al. SIOP Working Committee on psychosocial issues in pediatric oncology: Guidelines for communication of the diagnosis. *Med Pediatric Oncol.* 1997;28(5):382–385.
44. Feudtner C, Santucci G, Feinstein JA, Snyder CR, Rourke MT, Kang TI. Hopeful thinking and level of comfort regarding providing pediatric palliative care: A survey of hospital nurses. *Pediatrics.* 2007;119(1):e186–192.
45. Mack JW, Wolfe J. Early integration of pediatric palliative care: For some children, palliative care starts at diagnosis. *Curr Opin Pediatr.* 2006;18(1):10–14.
46. Barrera M, D'Agostino N, Gammon J, Spencer L, Baruchel S. Health-related quality of life and enrollment in phase 1 trials in children with incurable cancer. *Palliat Support Care.* 2005;3(3):191–196.
47. Wiener L, Battles H, Mamalian C, Zadeh S. ShopTalk: A pilot study of the feasibility and utility of a therapeutic board game for youth living with cancer. *Supportive Care Cancer.* 2011;19(7):1049–1054.
48. Rollins JA. Tell me about it: Drawing as a communication tool for children with cancer. *J Pediatr Oncol Nurs.* 2005;22(4):203–221.
49. Rushton CH. A framework for integrated pediatric palliative care: Being with dying. *J Pediatr Nurs.* 2005;20(5):311–325.
50. Hausmann JS, Touloumtzis C, White MT, Colbert JA, Gooding HC. Adolescent and young adult use of social media for health and its implications. *J Adolesc Health.* 2017;60(6):714–719.
51. Twain M. Autobiographical dictation, 11 October 1907. In *Autobiography of Mark Twain.* Vol. 3. University of California Press; 2015.

14 | ADVANCE CARE PLANNING ALONG THE CARE CONTINUUM

JONATHAN MULLIN, RACHAEL BURGESS, AND JUSTIN BAKER

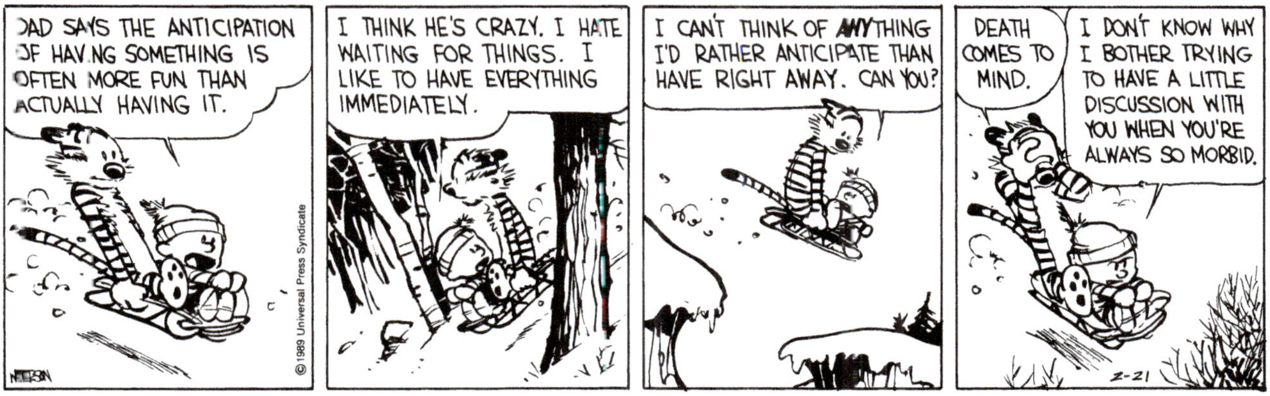
DAD SAYS THE ANTICIPATION OF HAVING SOMETHING IS OFTEN MORE FUN THAN ACTUALLY HAVING IT.
I THINK HE'S CRAZY. I HATE WAITING FOR THINGS. I LIKE TO HAVE EVERYTHING IMMEDIATELY.
I CAN'T THINK OF ANYTHING I'D RATHER ANTICIPATE THAN HAVE RIGHT AWAY. CAN YOU?
DEATH COMES TO MIND.
I DON'T KNOW WHY I BOTHER TRYING TO HAVE A LITTLE DISCUSSION WITH YOU WHEN YOU'RE ALWAYS SO MORBID.
© 1989 Universal Press Syndicate
2-21

ADVANCE CARE PLANNING

Advance care planning in adult medicine has been defined as a process of understanding and sharing values, goals, and preferences regarding current and future medical care, which occurs among patient, family, and healthcare providers.[1,2] As the field of pediatric palliative care (PPC) has emerged, advance care planning has grown to include children, adolescents, and young adults with serious illness and is now considered standard of care.[3] In pediatrics, the child is legally presumed to lack decision-making capacity, which falls to a parent or surrogate on the basis of parental authority—a responsibility to make decisions on behalf of the child, acting in their best interest.[4] However, best practices include involving children in any decision-making process, including advance care planning, to the extent that their age and development allow, to the degree they desire/are willing, and when consistent with family values, including assent when appropriate.[4] Box 14.1 provides examples of specific language to use for advance care planning topics throughout this chapter.

ADVANCE CARE PLANNING IN PEDIATRICS

The American Academy of Pediatrics (AAP) Policy Statement on Pediatric Palliative Care and Hospice Care Commitments, Guideline, and Recommendations emphasizes the importance of the process of advance care planning over time, stating "at a minimum, goals of care and treatment choices should be revisited whenever requested by the patient or family, with every hospitalization or with any significant change in treatment course or prognosis, and at least annually for children with complex chronic conditions."[5] Practically, this includes assessing a child and family's understanding and information preferences and incorporating the child into the advance care planning process as able. It is crucial to elicit input from a child who is involved in the decision-making process so that their goals and values can be understood and documented (while *they can have such conversations*). As with adults, advance care planning in pediatrics can capture the child's voice and wishes prior to the child losing the ability to participate in discussions. However, many pediatric patients are unable to participate in advance care planning discussions because of age, developmental level (including children with developmental delays), or because of child and family preference. In these situations, advance care planning often becomes less about understanding or documenting preferences (prior *to capacity being lost*) and instead helping surrogate decision-makers, typically parents, think and plan ahead about decisions they may need to make in the future. Unlike with adults, surrogates often have to make decisions for children who have never been and will never be able to participate in decision-making. This can increase the burden and emotional weight of advance care planning for children.

Benefits of advance care planning in pediatrics include preparation for end-of-life care, such as choosing the location

BOX 14.1 COMMUNICATION STRATEGIES FOR ADVANCE CARE PLANNING

INTRODUCING ADVANCE CARE PLANNING

Would it be helpful for us to talk about if things don't go as we all hope?

I wonder if we should think together about how to care for Allison if her condition continues to worsen.

In situations like this, many families wonder about what the future holds and can find comfort in planning ahead, including worst-case scenarios.

Honestly, I'd recommend that we continue to hope for the best and start to prepare for anything. Can we talk about what that means?

DISCUSSING RESUSCITATION PREFERENCES

In light of your goals to focus on comfort, if José's heart would stop, I'd recommend that we not attempt CPR or other interventions to restart the heart, recognizing that José has reached the natural end of his life.

MEDICAL TECHNOLOGIES AND POTENTIAL LIFE-EXTENDING INTERVENTIONS

As children approach the end of their life, we often have to have difficult conversations about tradeoffs. Specifically, there may be medical interventions offered that can prolong your child's life and also have implications about your child's quality of life and level of care. Would it be okay to talk about this?

DISCUSSING LOCATION

As we prepare for the end of Leah's life, have you discussed details? Sometimes children and their families have a preference about where they would want to spend the rest of their life if they knew time was short. Would it be helpful to think about this together?

DISCUSSING POLST FORMS

Given what we have just discussed about not performing CPR, should Max's heart stop, I'd recommend we make sure this preference can be honored outside of the hospital. This means that together we complete a form that documents these decisions and protects Max from undergoing these interventions no matter where he is.

---

of death; a decreased perception of suffering; and a better experience of end-of-life care.[6–8] Children and families value advance care planning,[3,8,9] including the ability to make good decisions, prepare, and facilitate coping.[3] Parents identify feelings of lack of readiness and the burdensome nature of thinking about the future as barriers to advance care planning[3] despite studies showing that advance care planning does not cause significant distress for children and their families.[3,10] Clinicians cite the biggest barriers as unrealistic parental expectations, differences in understanding of prognosis, lack of parental readiness for discussions, worry about taking away hope, uncertainty about prognosis, and ability to have these discussions.[3,11] These perceived barriers often lead to lack of discussions with children and their families,[3,12,13] and discussions occur later in the course of illness despite parental and provider opinions that they should occur much earlier.[8,11]

Advance care planning discussions are often perceived as "high stakes" and can be emotionally challenging for patients, families, and clinicians. Parents differ in preferences on who should initiate these discussions[8] but voice their desire for partnering with clinicians in a sensitive manner, with some degree of their child's involvement.[3] Involvement of the child can include explicit conversations and use of advance care planning tools, direct statements from the child about nonparticipation, and parental assessment of child's preferences that have been established throughout the child's life and illness. An additional factor is that clinician training and experience with advance care planning discussions may be limited and/or variable.[3]

ADVANCE CARE PLANNING AS GOALS-OF-CARE CONVERSATIONS

Advance care planning discussions are best thought of as an extension of goals-of-care conversations that address future-oriented topics and imagine the child in a worse state of health along an expected or possible trajectory, including at end of life. These discussions can be approached through the process of shared decision-making. Broadly, shared medical decision-making includes decisions made by more than one party, each aware of treatment options and implications, jointly contributing their expertise, knowledge, and values to the decision-making process.[14] This method is most commonly used when multiple medically reasonable treatment options with variable benefit-to-burden ratios exist.[15] (For further information about goals-of-care conversations, see Chapter 12: "Practical Aspects of Palliative Care Communication.")

Advance care planning discussions often include discussions about worsening health and end-of-life care and are best preceded by honest disclosures of prognosis. Given the emotional weight of discussing poor prognosis, advance care planning discussions may be best preceded by conversations about their nature and process. Often referred to as "talking about talking about it," discussing the logistics, advantages, disadvantages, and information preferences about advance care planning can be helpful to reach a shared understanding with children and their families about the specifics of these conversations before they happen.[16] Once aware of child and family information preferences, providers can tailor conversations to the individual needs of children and their families. Discussions about prognosis may need to include multiple providers from palliative care, primary care, and other medical subspecialties, with the goal of having the necessary expertise to provide the medical information and answer any questions that might arise. These discussions can then include a review of testing and treatments provided, with clear, unambiguous explanations of negative outcomes. For children with chronic complex conditions, discussing trajectory of illness, comparing it to known natural histories, and discussing child, family, and provider perceptions of progression can help children and their families align their understanding with that of the medical teams. Uncertainty will always exist in prognostication; however, discussing "best case, worst case, and most likely" can allow for the uncertainty to be contained within the reasonable expected range of outcomes and can avoid mistrust that can arise when the disclosed prognosis does not match the child's actual prognosis. Additionally, providers must use clear language, including the words "death" and "dying" and avoid the temptation to provide reassurance about the prognosis *itself*, as this may obfuscate the message.[17]

Barriers to discussing a poor prognosis include the belief that sharing a poor prognosis will cause psychological harm and lead to a loss of hope and the belief that children and their families do not want to know what is ahead,[18,19] which can cause providers to avoid or delay discussing prognoses or deliver prognoses in an overly vague manner.[18,20] In fact, parents usually want to know as much prognostic information as possible to allow them to make good decisions,[21,22] and disclosure of poor prognosis does not cause parental distress or depression but decreases anxiety, increases satisfaction, and, perhaps counterintuitively, allows parents to feel hopeful.[22–26]

Even when prognosis is poor and the child is at the end of life, families remain hopeful.[23] When hope for a cure or hope for a full and meaningful life is taken away by illness, the hopes of a child and family often expand to include hope for comfort, meaning, time, and love.[27] Still, children and families may continue to hope for positive outcomes that they know will not occur. Openly labeling these hopes as unrealistic or implying that children and their families are in denial or do not understand the prognosis risks isolating families or causing more distress. Aligning with hopes by using phrases such as "We will join you in hoping for a miracle," or "I wish that were possible," can offer support and show empathy without providing any misleading or false statements.[28]

Advance care planning discussions can then typically include honest, thorough, and relevant medical information, followed by discussions of goals, hopes, and values. These conversations can include discussing alternative care options, examining risks and benefits of proposed treatment options, exploring tradeoffs, and formulating a plan, which may or may not include formal and/or legal documentation.[29] Historical focus on advance directives and misconceptions that advance care planning is equivalent to discussions about do-not-resuscitate (DNR) orders may unduly shift the focus of advance care planning discussions to documentation and/or orders to limit medical interventions. Best practices include multiple conversations over time, recognizing that goals and preferences may change and that plans of care are often more complex than what can be formally documented.[30] Special attention must also be paid to provider education in advance care planning conversations and provider self-care.

ADVANCE CARE PLANNING AS END OF LIFE APPROACHES

As a child approaches end of life, advance care planning can afford the opportunity for children and their families to prepare and plan for end-of-life care, including location of care, preferences for resuscitation, use of medical technologies, and use of life-extending interventions. As mentioned, best practices include an individualized and family-centered approach incorporating family values and beliefs. This involves developing and mobilizing provider–patient and provider–parent relationships.[31] This approach optimally results in direct, honest, open, and compassionate delivery of information using neutral language to describe possible options and offering recommendations based on shared understanding of the illness trajectory. Providers should be aware of factors that influence decision-making across the spectrum of PPC.[32–35] Parents are motivated to be "good parents," which involves allowing the child to be as healthy as possible while being present and advocating for their child.[33] As discussions turn to end-of-life care, family decision-making is influenced by the likelihood of improvement or treatment success, perception of the child's suffering and will to live, and quality of life.[32–35]

Providers approach advance care planning at end-of-life in a family-centered manner, individualized to the needs and preferences of each family, looking to achieve shared decision-making. This can be best achieved through collaborative communication: establishing a common goal or set of goals, exhibiting mutual respect and compassion, developing an understanding of differing perspectives, assuring maximum clarity and correctness in communication, and managing interpersonal and intrapersonal processes that affect how information is sent, received, and processed.[36] In the setting of advance care planning, the provider must take the responsibility to seek and attempt to understand the patient and family perspective. Attunement to one's own beliefs and values is crucial in mitigating the impact of bias on questions asked, language used, and recommendations given.

At times, despite everyone's best intentions/efforts, advance care planning can lead to conflict or disagreement about medical decision-making and future plans of care. These disagreements can be between providers, between providers and the patient and/or family, between patient and family, or between joint surrogate decision-makers (e.g., between two parents). Providers should pay special attention to disagreements between themselves or their teams. These disagreements can foster mixed messages and lapses in communication that can spur other conflicts. Providers should, through introspection, seek to understand their own perspectives and values and how those may be contributing to any existing conflicts, especially as they relate to the perspectives and values of other providers (for further information, see Chapter 16, "Resolving Conflicts in Pediatric Palliative Care").

PREFERENCES FOR RESUSCITATION

Despite best practices that advocate for advance care planning to include multifaceted goals and preferences for care *as a whole*, including a discussion of a patient's preferences for resuscitation is appropriate. Cardiopulmonary resuscitation (CPR) is unique in that an order is required to forgo it, as it is presumed to be desired unless there is an explicit order or statement of refusal.[37] When treatment preferences include forgoing CPR, an order indicating this preference is documented in the appropriate place. Terminology may vary, including DNR, do-not-attempt-resuscitation (DNAR), and allow natural death (AND). DNR is most frequently used in the United States and instructs providers to not do CPR in the setting of a cardiopulmonary arrest. Other terms have been proposed to clarify these orders' meanings. For example, DNAR attempts to negate, or at least attenuate, the underlying assumption that CPR will be successful if performed. AND has been recommended as a more favorable term from the patient's perspective, although this has not been studied with children and their families.[38] Regardless of terminology used, any orders for limitations of resuscitation should indicate what has been discussed, recommended, and/or agreed upon, recognizing that having a DNR order in place and/or placing limitations around other life-sustaining therapies are often the most difficult decisions for parents to make.[39]

Discussions about preferences for resuscitation are an important part of advance care planning as these interventions can significantly affect other stated goals of care, including location of care, quality of life, comfort, perceptions of suffering, and timing of the dying process. As in all goals-of-care discussions, providers should seek to understand patient goals and perspectives, discuss potential options, and offer recommendations that align with these goals. Provider-led, goal-concordant recommendations or options enable decisions around resuscitation to be consistent with best resuscitative practices. This also helps to avoid the "menu approach," where components of a resuscitation may be discussed or offered separately, devoid of context and relationship to goals. For example,

> Based on our discussion and your goals, we recommend that if your child's heart should stop, this would indicate that she has reached the end of her life and it would not make sense for her to undergo CPR or be placed on a breathing machine. In order to make sure we are all on the same page about this, we will put an order in the chart that will protect her from these interventions. Does this make sense?

In the absence of a cardiopulmonary arrest, having a DNR order in place should not alter a child's overall care, and medically appropriate treatment should be provided.[40,41] Providers should avoid making a false assumption that a DNR order signifies that only comfort-focused interventions should be offered or performed. Providers should avoid the term "comfort measures only" (CMO), which is subjective and nonstandardized. This term can be used to signify the forgoing of laboratory testing, monitoring, respiratory support, medications, artificial fluids and nutrition, and/or nursing interventions. Providers may have different understandings about the specific interventions to which this term refers, which can generate confusion. Additionally, decisions around interventions at end-of-life merit clear and explicit discussions and an individualized approach. (For further information, see Chapter 27, "Easing Distress when Death Is Near.") Language used in discussing preferences for resuscitation can significantly affect delivery of care. Reducing a child to their resuscitation status by using phrases such as "he is a DNR" or "we just made her a DNR" may lead to missed opportunities to provide high-quality, goal-concordant care during the end-of-life period.

ORDERS FOR LIFE-SUSTAINING TREATMENT

Medical, Physician, Provider, or Clinician Orders for Life-Sustaining Treatment (MOLST, POLST, or COLST) are forms that document medical orders for life-sustaining medical treatment, which includes CPR (chest compressions, vasoactive medications, and defibrillation or cardioversion), respiratory support (invasive and noninvasive), artificial nutrition and hydration, dialysis, and antibiotics, and can include information about preferred level of medical intervention.[42] These forms were designed for use in adults but can be completed by the parent or guardian of a minor. In adults, these forms have led to a decreased incidence of unwanted resuscitation and are now being used more in pediatric practice.[43] Once completed, POLST forms are transferrable across settings and allow preferences to be known at home, work, or school and by emergency medical personnel and healthcare providers in the out-of-hospital setting or emergency room. Additionally, POLST forms can serve as a reference for hospital-based providers when confirming inpatient resuscitation preferences when children with completed POLST forms are cared for in the hospital setting. For children with a POLST form, the AAP recommends a collaborative approach, whereby schools, parents, clinicians, emergency medical services (EMS), and legal counsel review goals of care and POLST forms on a semi-annual basis.[44] This collaboration can help to ensure that the preferences on these forms is respected.

Similar to other advance care planning documents, these forms are tools to document and ensure that the medical care being provided matches the goals of children and their families. When discussing POLST forms with children and their families, it is important to highlight that these forms may be necessary legally to protect the child from unwanted resuscitation because emergency medicine personnel are required to provide resuscitative efforts without such forms and that these orders can be reversed or altered at any time.

USE OF MEDICAL TECHNOLOGIES AND POTENTIAL LIFE-EXTENDING INTERVENTIONS

Advance care planning affords the opportunity to discuss preferences surrounding medical technologies and potential life-extending interventions, specifically not initiating or discontinuing these interventions. These can include, but are not limited to, disease-directed therapies, antibiotics, blood products, mechanical ventilation (via endotracheal tube or tracheostomy), noninvasive respiratory support, and artificial nutrition and hydration. Similar to other aspects of advance care planning, these interventions can substantially affect goals of care and impact length and quality of life. Consensus statements and ethical precedent supports the withholding or discontinuation of medical interventions should the burden outweigh the benefit.[45] Preferences for these interventions may be related to the interventions themselves; children's and their families' assessments of the impact of these interventions on quality of life, location of care, and comfort; and the symbolism tied to the interventions. Some families may feel that non-initiation or discontinuation of medical interventions is equivalent to actively participating in the child's death, which may require support and reframing. Specific attention should be paid to the non-initiation or discontinuation of respiratory support and artificial nutrition and hydration to support families through their concerns that they are "suffocating" or "starving" their child. Additionally, as children and their families imagine themselves or their child in a worse state of health, providers may have the opportunity to provide guidance about benefits and burdens associated with specific interventions, enabling informed and individualized advance care plans to be made.

LOCATION OF END-OF-LIFE CARE

The goal of advance care planning around location of end-of-life care is to allow the child and family the opportunity to make an informed decision about which setting best coincides with their goals and values and that their preference is not driven by provider or societal expectations about where a "good death" might occur. Sudden unexpected events, changes in trajectory, and how available resources match child and family preference are all challenges in coordinating location of death. These challenges mean that, despite planning ahead, at times, a child's death may not happen at the preferred location. At the least, advance care planning allows for discussions about tradeoffs related to location of end-of-life care and other family goals and preferences. Additionally, the process of planning for (a hoped-for) location of death itself brings significant meaning to a child and family, and preparedness is a key factor in parental perception of end-of-life care.[46] In addition to presenting options to children and their families, providers should be aware of available resources for care and support regardless of location, with the focus on matching the location of care and services with larger goals such as time, comfort, and familiarity with caregivers. Having these discussions well before a child is nearing the end of life provides maximal time for clinicians to organize resources and make proper arrangements to honor the wishes of the patient and family.

LEGACY-MAKING

Legacy-making can be defined as doing or saying something that can be remembered, either intentionally or serendipitously.[47] At the end of their lives, children and adolescents often feel a strong need and want to be remembered.[42] Legacy-making can help children prepare for their own deaths, influence others' lives, and inspire and comfort family members.[47] Legacy projects can be activities completed by the child with or without a parent, including artwork, writing, poetry, songs, videos, and scrapbooking, or activities completed on behalf of the child and parent, such as photographs, hand and foot prints and molds, and a lock of hair. Additionally, seeing family members, taking a meaningful trip, and bequeathing belongings also constitute legacy-making, as might the ability to participate in research or be an organ or tissue donor. Providers from many different disciplines, including child life specialists, art and expressive therapists, psychologists, chaplains, and social workers may have unique relationships and specialized skills to assist in meaningful legacy-making as a part of advance care planning. Legacy-making can evoke difficult or painful emotions and may be interpreted as meaning that death is near and, therefore, these efforts can be met with resistance from children themselves.[48] Discussions around starting legacy-making should be approached in a sensitive and respectful manner and can often be as simple as allowing children and their families to revisit and celebrate the good times in their lives, which itself can facilitate positive coping.[16]

INCORPORATING THE CHILD INTO ADVANCE CARE PLANNING

Research supports involving adolescents and young adults in their healthcare decision-making, including advance care planning; these patients' concerns and needs differ from those of adults or patients' family members.[49] Medical decision-making in the adolescent and young adult population is often influenced by immediate family, peers, social media, a lack of experience with healthcare, and concerns about confidentiality, which should all be considered.[50] These patients want to share their values, beliefs, and preferences about end-of-life care[49,51–53] and have developmentally specific needs, including hope for a legacy and being remembered, a greater emphasis on connection with others, and a growing need for both independence and autonomy.[51,53,54] Advance care planning in adolescents and young adults can help meet these needs, prevent emotional and social isolation toward the end of life, and support parental decision-making (for adolescents who are not legal decision-makers).

Children of all ages should be incorporated into advance care planning. There is not a one-size-fits-all approach for providers. As mentioned, discussing the logistics, advantages, disadvantages, and information preferences about advance care planning with the child and family can be useful to develop an individualized approach. Providers need to balance being respectful of child and family preferences and consider making recommendations to children and their families about the process of advance care planning. Respectful and collaborative provider guidance can help direct children and their families toward best practices.

Family Reflection

"What's worse than death?" It's a question we had to discuss openly with our 19-year-old son as he battled a slowly incapacitating and mysterious neurological disease that left him deaf and paralyzed from the shoulders down. It was also a question gently raised by the palliative care team at the hospital where our son was receiving treatment. Even though we had been enduring this difficult medical situation for years, we were not prepared to handle the end-of-life decisions that were foisted on us by his declining situation. Thankfully, the palliative care team was there to raise the issues that needed to be discussed in a way that blended personal care and professional tact. The team engaged our son directly, as a legal adult, helping him face sad realities. They forged an emotional bond with him that allowed him to feel more cared for in an otherwise scary and sterile hospital environment. The team also spoke with us as parents and with all of us as a family, helping us move forward together, as a family unit going through one of the worst crises imaginable. With our son's condition rapidly deteriorating, we never did get a signed medical directive, despite our efforts. In the early stages of his illness, he was understandably reluctant to make such grave decisions in such an official way. He left the medical documents unsigned, sitting by his bedside. And, as his disease progressed, communication became difficult, and his mental and physical faculties were too compromised to complete the directive despite the increased value of having one finished. Knowing what we know now about his fate, we wish we had been more intentional about having those conversations earlier—while, of course, respecting his freedom not to have them if he wasn't ready. But the conversations facilitated by the palliative care team were nonetheless invaluable in helping us understand our son's wishes when we needed to have that information. His answer to the worse-than-death question was clear: "To me, being unable to engage the world and loved ones is worse than death. Being 'locked-in' [fully conscious but unable to communicate with the outside world] is worse than death." While it was unimaginably difficult to hear our beloved son confront his own death like that, it was reassuring knowing what his wishes were. And when he slipped into a permanent and unresponsive neurological state, we were able to make the painful decision to end life support with the confidence of knowing it was the decision he wanted. To be sure, these conversations with the palliative care team were almost unbearable to have. But they saved us added grief and confusion in what was an already tragic and confusing time.

Matt and Michele H.

PROVIDER CONSIDERATIONS

Most children with serious illness will be cared for by a variety of providers from different disciplines, which may include primary care providers, subspecialists, psychosocial providers, and members of an interdisciplinary palliative care team. When the need for advance care planning arises, the question also often arises: Who should initiate and discuss advance care planning? Again, there is not a one-size-fits-all approach, and an individualized approach is warranted. Factors to consider include relationship and rapport of the provider with the child and family, provider experience and comfort with advance care planning, and role and discipline of the provider. Some children and families may want to discuss advance care planning with their primary care or long-standing subspecialists, others with psychosocial providers, others with members of the palliative care team.

Providers should approach advance care planning as a process that unfolds over time and covers an array of topics. This can allow for multiple providers to participate in different aspects of advance care planning that match providers expertise, experience, and comfort with child and family comfort and presence. For example, primary care providers or subspecialists can discuss disease-directed therapies, palliative care providers can discuss resuscitation preferences and life-extending interventions, chaplains and social workers can discuss anticipatory grief and provide information about ceremonies after death and bereavement, child life specialists can partner with children and their families for meaningful legacy work. However, providers should avoid restricting providers to discussing only portions of advance care planning based on stereotypes of roles and experience, as this can miss opportunities to best meet child and family needs. For example, a child with significant mood or anxiety issues may benefit from having conversations about life-extending interventions with a psychosocial provider present, or a child and family may each want to have conversations about resuscitation preferences with different providers based on rapport and relationships. Providers also need to have frequent, open communication about the nature of discussions and consider joint discussions to avoid mixed-messaging and protect children and their families from unnecessarily repeating conversations.

ADVANCE CARE PLANNING TOOLS

Advance care planning is documented in the form of *advance directives*. In adults, advance directives can be statutory documents, such as a durable power of attorney or a living will, or nonstatutory documents, which identify a healthcare proxy or healthcare preferences.[55] These directives serve to designate surrogate decision-makers and document preferences for medical care in specific situations. Patients of legal age who have decision-making capacity and are cared for by pediatric providers may benefit from discussing and completing statutory advance directives. This point merits special attention because providers at pediatric institutions are often less familiar with advance directives than their colleagues in adult settings. Additionally, many young adults live with illnesses that span from childhood into their adult years: when these children become legal adults, there may be no practical change in how advance care planning or medical decision-making occurs; however, new or additional documents may be legally required or beneficial. Documents in these situations include a durable power of attorney for healthcare (often referred to as a *healthcare proxy*), which authorizes a surrogate to make decisions about healthcare on the patient's behalf, and a living will, which can specify medical treatment preferences in certain situations that may arise when the patient is unable to participate in decision-making. Palliative care providers should be familiar with the legal documents available in the area in which they practice.

Children not yet of legal age can also use tools to participate in the advance care planning process and to provide guidance for the surrogate (parent, guardian, or other) making decisions on their behalf. Examples of advance care planning tools include the pediatric-specific tools Voicing My CHOiCES and My Wishes and the adult advance care planning document Five Wishes. Even prior to completing an advance care planning document, providers can introduce an "Advance Care Planning Readiness Assessment" by asking children (1) whether talking about what would happen if treatments were no longer effective would be helpful, (2) whether talking about medical care plans ahead of time would be upsetting, and (3) whether they would be comfortable writing down/discussing what would happen if treatments were no longer effective.[56] Advance care planning documents can be selected based on the child's age and developmental level and provider assessment, experience, and preference. Specific for pediatric populations, Voicing My CHOiCES was designed through feedback from adolescents and young adults about how they would want to document their wishes and how they would want to be cared for, supported, and remembered.[49]

Once a document has been selected, it can be filled out by children with or without their families, with provider assistance and collaboration as needed or desired. These documents may be completed during multiple discussions over time or at a pacing that matches the child's and family's abilities and preferences. Some children and their families may want to complete the tool in its entirety to minimize the need for to revisit these topics. Some may want to think through the document and discuss choices without putting preferences into writing. Others may want to complete different portions of the tool at different times or not at all. Any advance care planning document is only a tool in the difficult yet important process of advance care planning and can occur alongside ongoing goals of care discussions. As such, provider involvement can be critical to help support children and their family in thinking through and completing emotionally challenging portions of the document and to clarify questions about medical treatment options. When used in a family-centered fashion, these tools can enhance preparation, improve communication, increase understanding of child and family goals, and reduce the burden of surrogate decision-making.[57]

HOME-BASED PALLIATIVE CARE AND HOSPICE

As discussed in detail in Chapter 4, "Settings of Care," a majority of children who die in the United States do not die at home. Nearly three-fourths of pediatric deaths occur in the hospital, mostly in intensive care units (ICUs) where intensive, life-sustaining medical therapy is typically provided.[58] Home-based palliative care and hospice programs, funded through usual insurance mechanisms of hospice insurance benefits, serve children in the home setting, including at end of life. The number of children who die at home as a result of complex chronic conditions has been steadily increasing and has been cited as a justification to expand the capacity for pediatric home-based hospice and home-nursing care.[59] Home-based palliative care and hospice for children may improve end-of-life care and bereavement;[46] allow the child's death to occur in the preferred location;[46,60] improve the child's symptom management, comfort, and quality of life and the family's quality of life;[61,62] and improve resource utilization and increase cost savings.[60]

Despite the benefits home-based services provide, they are often underused.[63] Providers must first understand barriers to hospice and home-based care, embrace the uncertainty of the time course of the end-of-life period in pediatrics, and use available resources to manage transitions of care, both logistically and emotionally. Providers will then be able to make appropriate referrals, thus maximizing the benefit children and their families receive. Understanding the benefits and barriers allows for thoughtful communication with children and their families.

BARRIERS TO HOME-BASED PALLIATIVE CARE AND HOSPICE

The barriers to introducing palliative care and hospice for children often differ from those identified for adult hospice referrals. They may include barriers seen more commonly in adult hospice, including fear of addiction to pain medication, fear of hastening death through use of opioids, and concerns about legal action. There are also unique barriers to referral of children to home-based palliative care and hospice, which can be roughly divided into two groups: those that are associated with constraints within medical culture and those that are related to clinical practice.

Constraints on PPC within our medical culture include limited financial resources for specialized PPC, limited access specifically in underresourced areas, lack of research, lack of evidence-based guidelines and quality metrics, and lack of provider training and expertise. All of these barriers have been best addressed at the levels of resource allocation, policy, local and governmental advocacy, and curriculum development.[64] As a result, specialty PPC programs have increased at specialty children's hospitals,[65,66] pediatric hospice and palliative medicine fellowship programs have grown in number,[67] and guidelines and quality metrics are being developed.[60] Despite these changes, the growth of pediatric home-based palliative care and hospice program lags behind hospital-based programs,[65,66] leaving opportunities for growth to better meet patient and family needs.

From the provider standpoint, the barriers to home-based palliative care and hospice are the same as barriers to palliative care in general: uncertainty of prognosis, the perception that families are not ready to acknowledge that their child is going to die as a result of their illness, language barriers, time constraints, and families' preferences for life-sustaining care.[68] Specific to hospice, referrals have traditionally been reserved for children whose doctors were willing to predict that they had 6 months or less to live and whose families were willing to forgo curative treatment. The somewhat-arbitrary prognostic threshold of 6 months and the dichotomization of palliative and cure-oriented therapies often leads to introducing hospice care late in the child's illness, thus preventing children and their families from receiving beneficial support, symptom management, and home-based care at or toward the end of life and may perpetuate the myth that hospice care is synonymous with "giving up." Providers themselves may have emotional reactions to referring their patients to hospice, especially providers who managed cure-oriented treatment that was unsuccessful.

Logistical barriers exist for home-based palliative care and hospice services in the form of reimbursement and insurance coverage. In the United States, Medicare legislation passed in 1982 opted to cover either disease-directed therapy or hospice-based services, mandating that patients having primary insurance through Medicare must opt for these now-competing forms of care. In 2010, the Affordable Care Act included Concurrent Care for Children, which states that patients younger than age 21 years are legally eligible to receive hospice services while still undergoing curative or life-extending therapy.[69] Importantly this provision only applies to children covered by federal insurance (Medicaid or the state Children's Health Insurance Program) and applies only to hospice services (not palliative care services). (Further specifics are discussed in Chapter 4, "Settings of Care.") The example of hospice insurance policy in the United States highlights how systems in place can lead to confusion, misconceptions, and logistical hurdles that create a barrier for referral to home-based palliative care and hospice services.

Uncertainty of prognosis is much more common in pediatric patients than in adults. In most PPC programs, cancer represents less than half of all diagnostic groups.[65] Children with chronic and complex life-limiting conditions have a wide variety of illnesses, including those caused by prematurity, congenital disorders of every organ system, neurodegenerative abnormalities, and malignancies. All of these disorders are relatively rare and often do not lend themselves to accurate predictions about either the response to treatment or the likelihood of survival.

In light of this uncertainty, counseling on timing of hospice referral can be difficult and often varies from provider to provider. Many providers often delay referring patients to home-based palliative care and hospice until death is inevitable or expected in the immediate future, despite a large body of evidence that suggests physicians are poor predictors of life expectancy in the setting of serious illness.[70]

Families may also share the misconception that hospice is equivalent with "giving up" and may decline these services as a result.[71] Families often remain hopeful for their child to be cured or greatly outlive their prognosis even as the end of life approaches. The uncertainty of prognosis means that some experience unexpected improvements, idiosyncratic responses to therapy, and plateaus of relative stability that inspire families' hope for a positive resolution of the child's illness. Hopes for recovery are also fueled by the promises of innovative treatments, new technologies, medications or gene therapies, and by accounts of miraculous recoveries in the media and social media and in the marketing of children's hospitals. Families also often worry about the effect of end-of-life care in the home on siblings.

Transitions of care to hospice often involve a change in the care setting, intensity, and providers, which can create additional barriers. Patients and their families often have formed strong relationships with their long-time providers. Providers may also form very strong attachments to their patients and have intimate knowledge of families' needs and strengths.[72] An abrupt transfer to a new team, regardless of the skills of its members and the best intentions of all those involved, has a profound and usually negative effect on the continuity of care that the child and the family need.[73] Introducing new providers and asking families to take on more responsibility for the child's care during the most challenging times can discourage families from accepting hospice services and, at its worst, can take on the quality of abandonment.

OVERCOMING BARRIERS TO HOME-BASED PALLIATIVE CARE AND HOSPICE REFERRALS

Similar to advance care planning, conversations about hospice can be held as an extension of goals-of-care conversations, specifically as end of life approaches. As such, home-based palliative care and hospice should be considered in terms of the patient's and family's needs along a continuum, rather than signifying a change in philosophy of care or signaling a certain location on or the inevitability of a disease trajectory. For the children and families cared for by palliative care providers, the barriers are worth overcoming and can be overcome by deliberately designed systems and transitions of care and thoughtful communication. When palliative care and hospice are introduced as services that seek to prevent, relieve, reduce, or mitigate symptoms and improve or maintain the quality of life for seriously ill children and their families, they can be integrated with curative or life-extending care.

As with discussions of goals of care or advance care planning, discussions about home-based palliative care and hospice are best initiated with an accurate discussion of diagnosis and prognosis. Considering the prognosis, goals can be reviewed and reframed where necessary in order to identify the needs of the child and family. Once needs are identified, providers can discuss how home-based palliative care and hospice can help meet these stated goals and needs. Examples of needs toward the end of life may include medications and comfort in the home, managing the logistics of a death in the home, providing medical equipment in the home, and additional supportive services from social workers, chaplains, expressive therapists, child life specialists, and bereavement or grief counselors. Throughout this conversation, it is important to reinforce that all providers are committed to collaborating across the continuum of care to support the child and family. As mentioned earlier, children and their families may have misunderstandings (often negative) about the word "hospice" itself, even though they may benefit from the services provided. One strategy for introducing home-based palliative care and hospice is to first introduce the services provided, emphasizing how they align with the identified goals and needs, and only then refer to hospice by name. This approach enables the provider to define what hospice means for the child and family, rather than allow that definition to be determined by previously held beliefs. Box 14.2 offers communication strategies for discussing hospice.

This approach allows home-based palliative care and hospice services to be framed as coincident treatment. Many home-based palliative care programs that provide community-based care without the strict eligibility requirement for hospice allow patients to transition into hospice when it is appropriate. This approach helps to establish palliative care providers earlier, address child and family needs earlier, and ease transitions toward end of life, and it may shift focus away from dying, thus mitigating the effects of uncertainty and the dichotomization between curative therapies and hospice care.[74] As palliative care and hospice become more recognized as early interventions for children with serious illness, palliative care providers can help to create an environment in which starting home-based palliative care and hospice is less abrupt, more readily accepted by families, and associated with better quality-of-life outcomes at the end of life.[74] Programs of this nature do exist, but further development and advocacy are needed to better match the needs of all children and their families who could benefit from home-based palliative care and hospice.

Compassion and continuity are two key components to support hope during times of transition to hospice care. Compassionate relationships impart hope, regardless of the trajectory of illness.[23] Children and their families benefit from maintaining the relationship with those providers who have cared for them throughout their illness. Even after most of the disease-directed therapy has concluded, continuity of care can continue to support and nurture hope. Parents' hopes are supported by continuing efforts that maintain the integrity of the parent–child relationship and by continuing to integrate their spiritual beliefs into their lives throughout the course of the illness.[75] Transitions of care often require care coordination, and hope can be supported by relieving some of these burdens.

Hope extends into bereavement by affirming a lifelong bond with the child that continues after death. In bereavement, parents strive to find ways of sustaining that lifelong bond and attempt to make meaning of their forever-changed life.[76] Home-based palliative care and hospice programs that include bereavement, sibling programs, and ongoing support groups can assist families as they find hope in their search for meaning in their child's death and grow in the relationship with their child after death.[77]

BOX 14.2 COMMUNICATION STRATEGIES FOR DISCUSSING HOSPICE

"In order to best support your goals of receiving care in the home setting and working to ensure your child's best quality of life for as many days as possible, we would recommend home-based care from a multidisciplinary team of care providers. This team would provide support in the home setting to help with pain and symptoms and to support the needs of your child and family. The type of care I am describing is provided by a team of providers called *hospice*. This may not be what you thought about hospice, but I want to assure you this is how we work with these teams with our patients and families."

Vignette Reflection

Advance Care Planning for End-of-Life and Legacy

James was diagnosed with metastatic alveolar rhabdomyosarcoma at age 12. He started chemotherapy but relapsed several months later. Over the next 12 months, James continued to receive various chemotherapies, including investigational therapies. These treatments provided some, albeit minimal, reduction in disease burden. During that year, he had recurrent admissions for complications related to his cancer and therapies including anemia, infection, pain, and malignant pleural effusions. Subspecialty palliative care was consulted and joined an extensive team of medical and psychosocial providers caring for James. During initial encounters for pain management, the palliative care team began to develop rapport and learn about James's interests and hobbies. With time, advance care planning was gently introduced as a way to help James and his parents think about the future. Initial conversations included James and his mother. Later, his parents encouraged him to have conversations with the palliative care team alone, to offer him individual support. Voicing My CHOiCE was introduced and, while not formally completed, guided conversations between James and various members of the palliative care team. James shared his understanding that he was going to die from his cancer. With further exploration, he shared his worries about his parents and younger siblings, wanting to know that they would be okay without him and that they would remember him. As a result of these discussions, James wrote letters to his family members for after his death and worked with art therapy to complete a large mural project that celebrated his time and relationships with his family. James also shared his desire to enjoy life and have as much time as possible out of the hospital. To achieve this goal, he underwent draining catheter placement for his pleural effusions. He was able to attend professional sporting events and completed a cross-country trip to the ocean to swim with dolphins. Earlier in his illness, James had a short ICU stay requiring intubation for pneumonia. Reflecting on that experience, James voiced a preference to pursue intensive care if it might lead to recovery or improvements that would allow him to enjoy his life. He was clear that if providers were not certain about his ability to recover, he wanted to be given a time-limited trial to do so. He voiced his preference for his parents to make these decisions for him when the time came, even if he was able to participate in discussions. Several months later he had worsening respiratory distress related to his malignant pleural effusions and tumor progression. His parents agreed to an ICU admission and intubation based on his stated wishes. Without improvements in his respiratory status, and radiographic evidence of worsening lung involvement of his cancer, life-sustaining medical treatments were discontinued, and he died comfortably, shortly thereafter in the ICU, surrounded by his family.

CARE DURING AND AFTER THE DEATH

Advance care planning may also include arranging spiritual or religious ceremonies for after the child has died, planning organ donation, and making autopsy decisions. These topics may be emotionally challenging for children and their families as they often require them to imagine a time after the child has died. Additionally, discussions about organ donation and autopsy have issue-specific nuances with which clinicians frequently dealing with end-of-life care need be familiar.

SPIRITUAL AND RELIGIOUS CONSIDERATIONS

Discussions about spiritual or religious ceremonies and events at and after death may facilitate preparation, coping, legacy work, and meaning-making for children and their families. Many advance care planning documents (Five Wishes, Voicing My Choices) include prompts dedicated to spiritual and religious customs and preferences for care after the child's death. Families have varying prior experience with the logistics of postmortem care. Explicitly stating what does or does not need to be in place before a child's death can relieve anxiety and a sense of unpreparedness. Some families may find comfort in planning ahead and being prepared. Supporting these discussions in an individualized and family-centered manner is paramount for this delicate topic. Collaboration with chaplains and members or leaders of the family's spiritual community can help address family concerns as well as inform providers about their beliefs and customs. (Further discussion of religious and spiritual considerations can be found in Chapters 18 and 27.)

ORGAN DONATION

Organ transplantation is a potentially life-saving treatment option for those with end-stage organ failure. In the United States, the Uniform Anatomical Gift Act, passed in 1968, authorized individuals to donate all or a part of their or a family member's body after death for education, research, therapy, or transplantation. The Act was revised in 1987 and then again in 2006, to emphasize an individual's choice in donation, including language prohibiting others from overruling a person's decision regarding organ donation after their death.[78]

In the United States in 1984, the National Organ Transplant Act was approved, establishing the Organ Procurement and Transplantation Network (OPTN). The OPTN is responsible for the nationwide, equitable distribution of organs for transplantation using specific allocation policies, which are managed regionally by Organ Procurement Organizations (OPOs).[79] From 1998 to 2020, there have been more than 790,000 transplantations in the United States: 79% from deceased donors and 21% from living donors. Patients younger than 18 years old comprise 7% of all transplant recipients and 14% of deceased donors.[79] The demand for organs continues to exceed the supply: as of January 2020, approximately 112,000 people were awaiting transplantation, of which 2,000 were younger than 18 years.[79] For more information on the lived experience of awaiting transplantation, see Chapter 32. Palliative care providers may find themselves caring for children who may be donors and for children who may be recipients. As such, providers need to be aware of systems and factors influencing organ donation; child, family, and provider perspectives about organ donation; ethical considerations; and best practices in discussing organ donation with families.

DEFINITIONS

Organ donation, by law, occurs after an individual has died. In the United States, death has been defined, legally, as the irreversible cessation of function of either circulatory or respiratory functions, or all functions of the entire brain, including brainstem.[80] Practically, organ donation can occur in distinct ways after either a circulatory and respiratory death or after death by neurologic criteria (often referred to as "brain death"). If an individual has died by neurologic criteria, the body's functional status is maintained with cardiorespiratory support, and organs are subsequently procured. When an individual is critically ill, dependent on cardiorespiratory support, and the family or surrogate has decided to forgo life-sustaining medical treatment, organ donation may be able to occur after circulatory death. (Commonly referred to as donation after circulatory death [DCD]). In this setting, the individual is taken to an operating room, life-sustaining medical treatment is discontinued, and the individual receives standard end-of-life care. Once pulselessness occurs, a predetermined waiting period (commonly 5 minutes) elapses, after which time the organ procurement team enters the room, and the organs are procured. If the individual has not died within a predetermined amount of time (commonly 1 hour), then the organ donation is cancelled.[80]

A wide array of tissues can be donated in the postmortem period, including heart valves, musculoskeletal tissue (ligaments/tendons and bone), nerves, reproductive tissue, skin, and vascular tissue (veins/arteries).[81] Tissue donation does not have the same immediate time-sensitive considerations as organ donation. For both organ and tissue donation, patient characteristics and comorbidities determine what can be donated. Collaboration with OPOs is essential in determining what options may exist.

ETHICAL CONSIDERATIONS

Organ donation and criteria used to define death are ethically complicated and nuanced entities.[80,82] Examples of ethical challenges include caring for patients for whom the legal definition of death by neurologic criteria is not accepted as death from a personal, religious, spiritual, or cultural standpoint; how long to wait between pulselessness and organ procurement in DCD; and ensuring that patients who die in the operating room after discontinuation of life-sustaining medical treatments receive the same quality end-of-life care, including symptom management and desired presence of family members, if possible.[80]

Additionally, given the imbalance between potential recipients and available organs, laws and regulations have been put in place to optimize organ donation. At their best, policies that focus on process can minimize the implication that not consenting to organ donation is negative[83] and allow many children and their families who want to donate organs to be able to do so.[84]

Most applicable to palliative care providers is an awareness of real or perceived conflict of interest. Palliative care providers care for children who are both organ donors and organ recipients, often concomitantly. To mitigate potential conflict of interest, best practices are to use available organ-donation–specific resources (through OPOs or otherwise), to ensure that providers discussing organ donation are appropriately trained, to not serve in roles that may call into question conflict of interest, and to separate conversations about organ donation from those about prognosis and end-of-life. Specifically, in situations where DCD is being considered, discussions of discontinuing life-sustaining medical treatment should occur prior to discussions of organ donation, and a clear boundary should exist between palliative care providers and organ procurement representatives.[80] Specifics of communication around organ donation requests are discussed later in this chapter.

FACTORS INFLUENCING DONATION

Multiple studies have evaluated factors influencing a person's willingness to donate their own or a family member's organs.[83,85–90] Specific patient and family characteristics, beliefs, attitudes, and experiences have been correlated with both consenting to and declining organ donation (Box 14.1).[85–87,90,91] Families deciding about organ donation on behalf of their children have a higher consent rate than do families deciding on behalf of adult relatives.[92] As with any complex, multifactorial decision, the many variables determining a person's willingness to donate organs are likely to be weighed differently for each individual. Awareness of these factors can allow providers a better starting point to understanding what factors may help determine decisions about organ donation. However, previously correlated factors are not a substitute for open-minded and judgment-free discussions to help understand a patient's and family's perspective on organ donation, when applicable.

RELIGION

Most major religions recognize organ donation as an act of compassion and altruism and thus support organ donation, leaving decisions up to individuals in the religious community.[91,93,94] A significant number of people cite their religious beliefs as a reason not to donate.[86,91,93,95] In particular, persons who are concerned about maintaining the body's integrity after death and/or believe that organ transplantation is against God's will have less favorable attitudes toward organ donation.[91,93,95] The role of religious beliefs on the organ-donation process has been explored, with many conflicting conclusions.[86,91,93,95,96] This may be due to an incomplete understanding of the complex interactions among religion, societal norms, family dynamics, and personal organ-donation beliefs.[93] Religion is a part of many peoples' lives and may influence perspectives on organ donation in ways that may not be predictable at population or community levels. It is essential for the medical team to understand and respect the religious beliefs of patients and families if the team is to provide unconditional support during the decision-making process. Chaplains and members or leaders of the child and family's spiritual or religious community may be helpful in supporting the religious or spiritual needs of children and their families faced with decisions about organ donation.

RACE AND ETHNICITY

Organ donation does not occur in a vacuum of social and cultural context of healthcare and society. The same challenges that exist for healthcare delivery based on race and ethnicity also exist in organ donation. In the United States, individuals from minority racial and ethnic groups tend to have less trust in the healthcare system and are less likely to donate organs, discuss organ donation with family members, or carry an organ donor card,[86,91,97–99] and are more likely to believe that doctors will not try as hard to save a person's life or pronounce death correctly if doctors know that the person is willing to be an organ donor.[95,97] Healthcare providers and systems may also be contributing to differences in consent to organ donation. For example, one study of factors associated with willingness to donate found that black families were less likely to have spoken with a chaplain or OPO representative and received counseling on fewer organ-donation topics than did white families.[97] In pluralistic societies, providers should be aware of beliefs and experiences of individuals from minority racial or ethnic groups. Policies and systems that standardize processes may allow for a more just approach to discussions about organ donation.

CHILD AND PARENT PERSPECTIVES

In 2019, children younger than 18 years made up 8% of the donor pool, and nearly half were aged 11 to 17 years.[79] As with other aspects of advance care planning, the views and preferences of both child and family should be incorporated in the organ donation planning process.

Many students recognize the benefit of organ donation and transplantation to help others and would be willing to donate their organs.[100–104] Opposition to or discomfort with organ donation includes lack of trust, lack of information, uneasiness with a body being cut up, fear of being disrespectful to the dead, discomfort with having one's organ in another's body, and fear of not being dead.[102,103] In one study, one-fourth of students with driver's licenses or learner's permits had designated themselves as organ donors, with increased knowledge and previous discussions with friends and family serving as positive predictors of willingness to donate. However, of those intended donors, only slightly more than half shared this with their family, despite survey data showing that adolescents are willing to discuss organ donation with their parents.[101,103] Families' knowledge of patient preference increases the likelihood of consent to organ donation, highlighting the importance of helping to facilitate conversations between children and their families.

Several factors influence parents' willingness to consent to organ donation on behalf of their children[105–107] (Box 14.2). Most notably, parents valued rapport with the person making the request, especially when members of the child's healthcare team first mention organ donation.[106] Bereaved parents who were not approached about organ donation believe they would have been open and welcomed the conversation. Interestingly, these parents made assumptions about why they were not asked, specifically centered on the health or value of the child's organs.[107] Consenting to organ donation has a positive effect on parental bereavement.[108,109] Very few surrogate decision-makers for adults (6–14%) regretted the decision to consent to organ donation, but as many as 38% of individuals who did not consent to donation regretted their decision.[110] In pediatrics, no parent regretted their decision to donate, and several expressed regret that they had not consented to donate more organs or tissue.[109]

PROVIDER ROLES AND PERSPECTIVES

Organ donation involves an interdisciplinary team, including members from organ procurement organizations and other institutions who have various backgrounds, training, and perspectives. Understanding the roles and perspectives of the many providers involved in organ donation is essential to ensure collaboration and provide consistent and compassionate care to children and their families.

PASTORAL CARE

Chaplains are especially skilled in communication and providing support to bereaved families, and they are sensitive to ethnic, cultural, and religious values; thus, they are a valuable resource during the organ donation process.[111] Chaplains' participation in the organ donation process varies with surveys showing that one-third to one-half of hospital-based chaplains are involved in the organ donation process.[111,112] Most chaplains view organ donation as consistent with their religious values.[113] As with any diverse group of providers, individual chaplain's views may vary.[114] As a group, chaplains highly value respect for the donor, not viewing the donor as a means to an end, and the importance of families being free from coercion and having the right to decline organ donation on religious grounds.[113] Overwhelmingly, chaplains believe they can be an extremely valuable source of support during the organ donation process because of their training in grief and crisis counseling.[113]

SOCIAL WORK

Social workers may be involved with families for whom organ donation is a consideration, often meeting families at the time of accident or other traumatic injury that may lead to a situation in which organ donation is being considered. Social workers may also provide support around decision-making and grief that surrounds end-of-life care[115] and support other providers in navigating the organ donation process in the setting of a dying child and grieving families.[116] These providers' role in hospitals helping families navigate postmortem care may put them in communication with families during the organ donation process.[117]

NURSING

Nurses spend a large amount of time at the bedside providing direct patient care and are in a strong position to support families considering organ donation.[88,118] Nurses focus on respect and dignity of a child and their family during the organ donation process and view protecting the child and family as a major responsibility.[119] Barriers to high-quality nursing care during organ donation include a lack of education, experience, and involvement in decision-making process.[120] Most pediatric critical care nurses see the benefit of organ donation to both the child's family and society. Specific to DCD, they report feeling less knowledgeable or comfortable answering questions from families.[121] Strategies to assist nurses in this role include educational programs related to organ donation, programs to improve communication skills, and ensuring a work environment that promotes excellent end-of-life care. Intensive care unit leadership must promote a culture that recognizes nurses as valued members of the team. As such, the bedside nurse should be present at family conferences, nurse performance evaluations should include end-of-life care skills, patient assignments must promote continuity of care, and unit policies and guidelines regarding the care of potential organ donors must be readily accessible.[118]

PHYSICIAN

Initiating the request for organ donation has typically been the attending physician's responsibility. In 1998, changes in federal regulations concerning organ and tissue donation stipulated that individuals initiating the organ donation request process must be properly trained.[122] This was misinterpreted by some to mean that only OPO staff members could approach families, thus excluding physicians from the process.[83] However, a donation request is now recognized as a collaborative process between OPOs and the medical team. The physician's relationship with the family is invaluable, as are the training and skill of the OPO representatives. An important physician responsibility is to incorporate OPO staff members into the medical team and coordinate efforts in the organ request process.[83]

ORGAN PROCUREMENT ORGANIZATIONS

There are 58 OPOs in the United States and Puerto Rico.[123] These organizations serve specific geographic areas and coordinate organ procurement efforts. OPOs evaluate potential organ donors, discuss donation with families, facilitate surgical removal and preservation of donated organs, and coordinate these organs' distribution according to national organ-sharing policies.[123] Factors that are important for the success of OPOs include experienced leadership, adequate staffing, allocation of responsibilities, strong relationships with donor hospitals and transplant centers, and support of donor families. Highly efficient and successful OPOs have a management team that is focused on the donation process, systems for monitoring activity and tracking outcomes, and efficient mechanisms for resolving conflict with hospitals and within the organization itself.[124]

The US Healthcare Financing Administration changed the federal Conditions of Participation for tissue and organ donation such that hospitals must notify their OPO of any patients who are potential donors. The intention was to increase OPO referral rates so that all families would have the option of tissue and/or organ donation. Furthermore, the person making the donation request must be adequately trained to do so. This stipulation was based on evidence suggesting that healthcare providers lack sufficient knowledge and training to effectively approach families about organ donation.[83] Involvement of the local OPO is imperative to the process, and families have reported that discussing organ donation with an OPO representative is crucial to their decision-making process. In fact, talking with an OPO staff member prior to the request for organ donation and spending more time with an OPO representative are positively correlated with the decision to donate.[85]

DISCUSSING ORGAN DONATION

Palliative care providers may find themselves engaging in discussions about organ donation as a part of advance care planning or in the setting of a dying or dead child. Palliative care providers need to be familiar with logistical, ethical, and societal beliefs and practices surrounding organ donation to meet the needs of the child and family.

ORGAN DONATION AS ADVANCED CARE PLANNING

In the United States, most people are in favor of organ donation and would donate organs themselves, but only a minority are registered organ donors.[125,126] Organ donation advocates encourage individuals to have conversations with loved ones about organ donation.[126] Primary care providers have been encouraged to talk to their patients about organ donation to provide education and dispel misconceptions.[125] One study included discussion of organ and tissue donation as a part of advance care planning for adults, and found that this was more likely to be completed by younger patients.[127] Most organ donation occurs from individuals after determination of death by neurologic criteria,[128] which is unlikely to be the cause of death for pediatric patients with serious illness, for whom advance care planning typically occurs. Often, organ and tissue donation discussions are initiated by children and their families who, in the face of the death of a child, may ask about organ or tissue donation as an altruistic act to help another individual or contribute to scientific research. Palliative care providers may have the opportunity to answer basic questions about organ donation and refer children and their families to OPOs for further information. In some instances, children and their families receiving palliative care services have been able to donate tissue to tissue banks and research institutions even after a death in the home hospice setting. This requires logistical coordination with hospice, the OPO, and the research institution. Discussions about organ donation as part of advance care planning may allow children and their families to have the opportunity to participate in organ donation and have preparations in place prior to end of life. This can often be done without greatly altering end-of-life care.

APPROACHING FAMILIES ABOUT ORGAN DONATION

In the end-of-life or near-end-of-life setting, any provider on the healthcare team may be approached by a child's family about organ donation, and providers must be able to provide support and resources when this occurs.[129] The standard approach for adults is that requests are initiated by OPO staff who have specific training. In pediatric populations, consent to donation increases when a trusted person from the healthcare team and a trained member of the OPO initiate the discussion.[106]

Best practices in pediatric organ donation include a collaborative approach with providers and members of the OPO and supporting the decision of the family or surrogate decision-maker.[129,130] Special attention should be paid to the child's preference when known[131] and to cultural differences and language barriers. Collaboration with interpreter services, social work, and chaplaincy can provide culturally competent communication and offer providers insight into family and cultural dynamics.[130] Higher consent rates occur when the approaching provider is of the same racial, cultural, or ethnic background of the family, with some hospitals being deliberate about these characteristics of the approaching team.[130] Together, these best practices enable continuation of the individualized, clear, consistent, and compassionate communication that families should be receiving during these challenging times.

Several communication frameworks have been put forth for when families are approached. These include the standard approach, the presumptive approach, and dual advocacy.[132–134] The *standard approach* may be described as value-neutral, unbiased, and balanced. The goal is to help the family reach the choice that is best for them.[132,134] However, the goal of the *presumptive approach* is to increase the number of organs available for transplantation. Requestors view themselves as advocates for both donors and recipients. There is a shift from value-neutral language to value-positive language, and the discussion is biased toward supporting organ donation.[132,134] *Dual advocacy* considers the interests of both donors and recipients and promotes the family's right to make a decision based on complete information, including the positive impact that organ donation can have. Dual advocacy recognizes that requestors must also consider the needs of the family.[133] Currently, there is controversy concerning the best way to approach families.[132–134] The ideal approach would allow for maximum consent to organ donation for those families for whom donation aligns with patient and family preferences while respecting the rights of the child and family. Fully transparent, fair, and even-handed discussions prioritize the rights of children and their families,[134] which is most consistent with the standard approach.[132]

Several programs piloted around organ donation place providers (chaplains or social workers) in roles where they can provide support and coordination for families for whom organ donation discussions are likely to occur.[111,135] These programs have led to improved communication during organ donation discussions, improved relationships with OPOs, and increased support of staff, thus highlighting the importance of interdisciplinary care in the setting of organ donation. Box 14.3 offers communication strategies for introducing organ donation. Boxes 14.4 and 14.5 offer additional considerations regarding organ donation.

BOX 14.3 COMMUNICATION STRATEGIES FOR INTRODUCING ORGAN DONATION

When faced with the death of a child, many families wonder about organ donation. Is this something you have thought about?

As we plan ahead about end-of-life care, sometimes the details change if a child or a family is considering the possibility of organ donation. Would you like to hear more information?

Please note and comply with any local laws and policies regarding the introduction of organ donation to families.

AUTOPSY

Autopsy (synonymous with *postmortem examination*) has been practiced in some form since the third century BCE, became standardized in the mid-19th century,[131] and remains a gold standard for diagnosis of disease.[136] Autopsy may occur when consent is obtained from family or surrogate to better understand the cause of death or when legally mandated as part of a forensic investigation into death. PPC providers need

BOX 14.4 ORGAN DONATION DECISIONS

FACTORS ASSOCIATED WITH CONSENT TO ORGAN DONATION

- Sense of altruism
- Perceived good quality of patient care
- Understanding the concept of brain death
- Families given enough information and time to make an informed decision
- Separation in the timing of discussions relating to brain death and organ donation
- High level of interpersonal skill of the person making the donation request
- High level of trust in the physician and healthcare system
- Communication with others about organ donation preferences
- Young adult
- Private location to hold organ donation discussions
- Families being informed of the potential to help others
- Death resulting from trauma
- Increased knowledge about organ donation and transplantation

FACTORS ASSOCIATED WITH DECLINING ORGAN DONATION

- Poor communication between healthcare providers and family members
- Emotional exhaustion
- Religious beliefs
- Family's belief that a patient would not have wanted to be an organ donor
- Family's perception of uncaring healthcare providers
- Feeling pressured to make a decision
- Families being told that healthcare providers are required to ask about donation
- Potential for disfigurement
- Poor timing of the request

BOX 14.5 ORGAN DONATION CONSENT ON BEHALF OF CHILDREN

FACTORS ASSOCIATED WITH FAMILIES CONSENTING TO ORGAN DONATION ON BEHALF OF THEIR CHILDREN

- Parents being registered organ donors
- Parents holding favorable beliefs about organ donation
- Parents receiving organ donation information prior to the child's death
- Organ donation first mentioned by a member of the child's healthcare team
- Parents perceiving the requester as sensitive to the family's needs
- Family feeling that they had sufficient time to discuss donation
- Family members agreeing about donation

FACTORS ASSOCIATED WITH FAMILIES DECLINING ORGAN DONATION ON BEHALF OF THEIR CHILDREN

- Just knowing organ donation was not something they wanted for their child
- Perception that child has been through enough
- Potential to interfere with other end-of-life choices (e.g., holding child, taking child home)
- Fears of disfiguring of child's body
- Overwhelming grief

to be versed in the basics of autopsy, legal considerations, and its potential impact on families and providers to help provide optimal care at the end of life and into bereavement.

DESCRIPTION

In addition to its understood meaning of anatomical dissection, autopsy may include photography, medical imaging (X-rays, magnetic resonance imaging [MRI], and computed tomography), and chemistry, microbiological, toxicological, cytogenetic, and molecular evaluation.[137] An autopsy's extent can vary depending on family preference and on the information being sought. Limited autopsy can include external examination only, imaging only, organ-specific autopsy, or specific tissue sampling (e.g., skin biopsy to isolate fibroblasts for genetic analysis, or body fluid aspiration to evaluate microbiological causes of death).[138] Collaboration with pathologists and other medical providers can help better meet the needs of a family for whom autopsy remains a conflicted decision.

For a standard autopsy, two incisions are typically made: a Y-shaped incision from the anterior axillary line at the level of clavicle, to the xiphoid process, and then to the opposite anterior axillary line, and extended down to the pubic bone; and an incision from behind one ear, over the top of the head, to behind the opposite ear.[137] Additionally, organs are removed and examined; those not undergoing additional testing may be returned to the body.[137] Providers should be familiar with specifics of autopsy at their place of practice if they are to be able to best guide patients and families. Autopsy may be more extensive when performed by a coroner for forensic purposes than when performed in the hospital setting.[137]

LOGISTICS

Autopsy requests for children who die in the home or hospice setting require an additional degree of logistical support. Collaboration with funeral homes is necessary to assist with transportation of the body, as is collaboration with the hospital and hospital staff to ensure that questions about cost, timing, and consent for autopsy are all in place prior to the child's death. Timing of autopsy may be of significant importance when metabolic disorders are suspected, as many of the tests should be performed as close to time of death as possible.[138] In many cases, some financial costs associated with the transportation of the child's body and autopsy may not be covered by the insurance plan or by the hospital where the autopsy takes place, which may present a barrier to autopsy and merits discussion with families before the autopsy is arranged.

Autopsy (for both medical and forensic evaluation) can also be compatible with organ and tissue donation,[139] which requires knowledge of local practices for both and coordination among teams.

BENEFITS AND YIELD OF PEDIATRIC AUTOPSY

Multiple studies, prospective and retrospective, have reported autopsy findings in different contexts of pediatric care, including general pediatrics, neonatology, cardiology, hematology-oncology, critical care, and emergency medicine.[140–148] Autopsy has consistently discovered new major diagnoses in 20–50% of cases.[140–148] Limited autopsy can also have a high yield in pediatric postmortem evaluation. Postmortem MRI, along with noninvasive evaluation of both fetuses and children was shown to have a greater than 90% concordance rate with conventional full autopsy in a prospective validation study. This concordance was greatest in fetuses (95%), newborns (81%), and infants (85%) and less so for children ages 1–16 (54%).[149]

Autopsy can also generate stored tissue samples, which may allow for future genetic or molecular testing.[150] Additional testing may be of high yield for sudden unexplained deaths, including sudden infant death syndrome (SIDS). One meta-analysis showed cases of sudden infant death that remained unexplained after standard autopsy and clinical review were likely to resolved when more genes were tested.[151] One program has expanded the clinicopathologic testing often used in undiagnosed disease programs for living patients to the postmortem evaluation of children less than 3 years old who died unexpectedly, with success in providing new information to families about the death of their child.[152] Genetic evaluation leading to novel information can inform the future reproductive decisions of the deceased child's parents and siblings. As novel tools in genomics, transcriptomics, proteomics, and metabolomics continue to be developed, there is likely to be increased knowledge of dysregulated pathophysiological pathways that can shed light on causes of unexplained death.[153] Palliative care providers should collaborate with subspecialist colleagues to determine the implication of postmortem testing on the details of the autopsy, including timing. For example, metabolic autopsy often requires significant advance planning and time-sensitive testing. Palliative care providers should also be aware of the evolving landscape of postmortem evaluation and collaborate with pathologists and other specialists so that families are aware of potential benefits of autopsy.

LEGAL CONSIDERATIONS AND CONSENT

Informed consent for autopsy should follow the same principles as for any procedure.[154] Although autopsy may be discussed beforehand, the formal consent to autopsy is typically signed after death, except in states or regions that permit signing the consent before death. The individual who is legally allowed to give autopsy consent is generally the person assuming custody of the child's body for burial. Next of kin and the person authorized to consent to autopsy are dictated by the law in the jurisdiction where the child died. In the absence of any of those individuals, the consent to autopsy may need to be obtained from a representative of governmental agencies charged by law with the responsibility for burial. The consent to autopsy may differ from initial discussions and information sharing about autopsy and should be obtained by a healthcare provider who is knowledgeable about autopsy process and can adequately address the questions and concerns raised by families. Children may receive specialized care far from home, and consent for autopsy may need to be obtained over the phone. Laws within the jurisdiction where the child died dictate whether telephone consent is permissible and what specifically is required for telephone consent.

Legal requirements for autopsy consent vary among countries, regions, and states; therefore, providers should know existing laws both where the death occurs and where the autopsy takes place. Some countries, for example, allow autopsies to be done without consent for medical, scientific, or educational reasons.[155] The form used to obtain autopsy consent needs to provide details about the type of autopsy to be done, such as complete or limited, whether tissue retention is requested, and whether tissue or other samples will be kept for any purpose. The examiner can be liable for failure to obtain consent to autopsy or failure to comply with the scope of the consent to autopsy.[156] In the United States, organ retention is regulated under state, not federal, law.[157] No uniform national legislation has been instituted to regulate organ retention after autopsy, and the judicial authorities in the different states have not reached a consensus about this issue. With few exceptions, state statutes do not address the retention of body remains whether the autopsy is performed after consent from next of kin or if it is mandated by the state.[157] Organ retention in the United States is regulated under the common law, which typically considers that the survivors of the deceased have no property rights over the human body or its parts. Therefore, the courts have generally not imposed liability over unauthorized tissue and/or organ retention after autopsy in the United States except in cases where no consent to a general autopsy was given.

The United States has no national standards for the practice of medicolegal death investigation in children[158]; however, most jurisdictions authorize autopsies when the death of someone younger than 18 years is traumatic, unexpected, obscure, suspicious, or otherwise unexplained. This is consistent with the AAP recommendations to perform a complete autopsy in such cases, including suspected SIDS and unexplained deaths in children with chronic conditions.[158] Clinicians should be familiar with the local laws, as some states allow exceptions for autopsies in unexplained deaths if the procedure is contrary to the religious beliefs of the decedent.[156]

FACTORS CONTRIBUTING TO AUTOPSY DECISION

When a child's death occurs and an autopsy is not legally required for forensic purposes, the child's family or surrogate may consider autopsy. A decision about autopsy is multifactorial and is more likely when cause of death is unknown, after a short hospital stay, when autopsy is discussed by a trusted provider, and when discussions occur after families and providers agree that the child will die from the underlying illness.[147,159-161] Despite the potential benefits of autopsy, autopsies are declined by parents for many reasons[162] (Box 14.3). Timing of autopsy and bodily integrity may be of specific importance to certain spiritual or religious groups because these factors may interfere with practices or contradict beliefs about postmortem care of the body. Some religions have fairly permissive attitudes toward autopsies; others limit autopsy because of the need to bury all body parts within a short interval.[155] Open and honest discussions with families and collaboration with chaplaincy and members or leaders of the family's spiritual or religious community can help families navigate decisions around autopsy when such concerns arise. Cultural influences on autopsy decisions are presumed to exist but have not been well researched.

Decision about autopsy is also influenced by which provider initiates the discussion. Autopsies are more likely when the discussion is led by a provider who was directly involved in the care of the deceased child and/or acquainted with the family.[161] Additionally, more experienced clinicians have more positive and accepting views of the procedure than do junior colleagues, which may affect how the conversation around autopsy is framed.[163,164] Involving the pathologist who will perform the autopsy may benefit bereaved parents if more information about the specifics of the autopsy is needed.[165]

PARENT PERSPECTIVES

Compared to families of deceased adults, families of deceased children who consented to autopsy report more comfort in knowing the cause of death.[166] Data on parental perception of autopsy include many surveys of bereaved parents whose children died in different contexts, specifically after intrauterine fetal loss and SIDS. In these studies, parental consent is largely impacted by the desire to obtain answers about cause of death and to obtain information that would impact future pregnancies.[166–168] Parents in these surveys declined autopsy out of the desire to protect their child, including concerns of body disfiguration, when there was an absence of questions to be answered or when they felt their child had already suffered too much.[161,166,167,169,170] Parents whose infant or child died report similar reasons for pursuing autopsy, with an additional emphasis on contributing to medical knowledge and research, all with the intent to help other children and their families.[161,170–172] Parents also express the desire to respect the wishes of their children.[173]

Several studies have shown no or low (<10% of surveyed families) regret about the decision to pursue an autopsy.[161,166,167,170] One study of 53 parents whose infant or child died showed that 8% regretted the decision of autopsy, 42% felt that the autopsy decision added to their grief, and 35% felt that the autopsy left the question of why their child died unanswered.[171] Very little data exist on the perspectives of bereaved parents of children and infants who were not offered autopsy. One study of bereaved parents who lost a child to cancer showed that nearly two-thirds of parents did not recall a discussion about autopsy, though 90% of them would have considered autopsy had it been discussed.[172]

Data from parents suggest that families benefit from an individualized approach as they decide about autopsy. Providers should disclose the risk that autopsy may not contribute to a better understanding of the child's death and explain that although autopsy offers many benefits and regret is rare, parents may have mixed emotional responses.[170,171]

PROVIDER PERSPECTIVES

Limited data exist on the attitudes or beliefs of healthcare providers about pediatric autopsy. Ninety-eight percent of practicing physicians surveyed about autopsy believe that autopsy provided valuable information. They were less likely to pursue consent for autopsy if they felt that the family would be concerned about bodily disfiguration, if they thought little information would be obtained, or if they were concerned that discussions would upset the family.[164] Two studies have shown that pediatric residents lacked knowledge about autopsy and that training was variable and often inadequate for pediatric residents to feel confident in their ability to talk to families about autopsy.[174,175] As technology has allowed for autopsies to be performed less invasively, healthcare professionals across multiple disciplines feel that these minimally invasive autopsies will allow for more choices for parents, and discussing autopsy with families will be easier.[176,177]

DISCUSSING AUTOPSY WITH FAMILIES

The discussion of autopsy typically occurs after the child's death, which is in line with most families' preferences. However, it is not uncommon for an autopsy to be discussed before death along with other end-of-life issues in children with chronic conditions or when death is expected. Providers may have the opportunity to engage with the child and family and incorporate discussions about autopsy into advance care planning. Providers' knowledge of laws and policies where they practice can allow them to serve as a guide for families, particularly in situations with complicated logistics, such as death in the home setting, when organ donation is being considered, or any specific limitations or unique tests to be performed at the time of the autopsy. Basic knowledge of the autopsy procedure can allow palliative care providers to address concerns or questions about body integrity or disfiguration that may arise when autopsy is discussed.

When discussions of autopsy occur after the child's death, best practices involve collaboration, as members of the treating team can be joined by relevant specialists. Some have even called for specific providers to be trained in discussing autopsy and partner with primary providers for the consent process.[160] Specifics of autopsy, including extent of autopsy, what may be tested, and the potential yields and limitations of postmortem testing should be discussed. Concerns about bodily disfiguration and timing of autopsy as it relates to funeral or other ceremonial plans deserve special attention.

Inevitably, providers will find themselves in the situation where autopsy is legally mandated and consent is not necessary. In such cases, an individualized approach to gauge the family's information preferences about specifics about autopsy can precede further discussion about autopsy details. This gives the family a modicum of control in a painful situation in which autopsy is required against family wishes.

AUTOPSY REVIEW

The consent process for autopsy should include a discussion of when results are expected and how they will be reviewed. Timing of the return of results depends on the extent of testing being performed. Providers should collaborate with pathologists performing the autopsy to obtain best estimates to provide families. In our experience, many families expect autopsy results sooner than they are available, which can take weeks.[178]

The AAP and the Society of Critical Care Medicine recommend physician–parent meetings to discuss the death and review autopsy results.[179,180] Often called an "autopsy review," this meeting can help families to receive this information in a timely, clear, and compassionate manner. One study of bereaved parents whose children died in the PICU found that most parents wanted to meet with their child's physician to discuss details (including but not limited to autopsy) about the child's death, although these meetings rarely occurred.[181] The preferred location and timing of a meeting were variable.[181] Providers should consider discussing specifics about autopsy review at the time of consent.

Written reports of the results may be difficult for families to interpret because they are often written in medical language/terminology and may be devoid of context or, more specifically, meaning. An autopsy review offers the option for families to meet with subspecialists and clinicians who can provide bereavement support, including palliative care teams. Palliative care providers can use the review to help ensure that families are getting information that matches their preferences and can provide guidance about grief and bereavement. The

BOX 14.6 REASONS BEREAVED PARENTS DECLINE AUTOPSY

Dislike of invasiveness
Practical considerations (transfer or cost)
Organ retention
Ambivalent feelings
Poor communication about the procedure
Quality and length of the consent form
Religious or cultural concerns

autopsy report can also be summarized in a letter to the family written in nonmedical terminology, emphasizing what was learned or not learned. Autopsy results should be shared with other healthcare providers who cared for the child, including the primary care provider. Box 14.6 reviews specific reasons parents decline autopsy and Box 14.7 offers communication strategies for introducing autopsy.

BOX 14.7 COMMUNICATION STRATEGIES FOR INTRODUCING AUTOPSY

I'd like to talk with you about autopsy. Is this something you've heard about?

Sometimes autopsy can provide additional information to families, and to providers. Details are different for each child. Would you like to hear more about an autopsy specific to your child?

An autopsy occurs after death and is an internal and external examination using surgical techniques. It is performed by medical professionals who treat your child's body with respect and dignity. We partner with families to provide information and decide about which parts of autopsy match your preferences and what we might be able to learn.

Used with permission from Zehm A, Rosenberg LB, Daubman BR. Discussing autopsy with bereaved families #400. *J Palliat Med.* 2020;23(10):1400–1402.[182]

Team Reflection

Autopsy After End-of-Life Care with Home Hospice

Amanda was a 16-year-old girl diagnosed early in life with a rare genetic mutation that resulted in progressive worsening neurological impairment and dysfunction. When palliative care was consulted at age 12, she had profound developmental delay and was completely dependent on her parents for routine care. She had epilepsy requiring multiple antiepileptic medications and received nutrition and fluids via gastrostomy tube. Her worsening ability to handle secretions resulted in frequent hospitalizations for respiratory distress and aspiration pneumonia often requiring prolonged ICU stays. The interdisciplinary palliative care team saw her during these admissions, which increased over time in both frequency and length. Her parents increasingly recognized that her underlying condition was progressing and that she was approaching the end of her life. After one lengthy and complicated ICU stay, her parents decided to forgo further hospitalizations, electing to enroll her in hospice, and a POLST form was completed limiting cardiac resuscitation, intubation and noninvasive respiratory support. Amanda lived for 9 months on hospice and would often receive enteral antibiotics for respiratory infections, per her parents' request. Prior to her death her parents expressed their desire to have Amanda undergo a complete autopsy and to have her brain tissue donated to a research lab, located more than 1,500 miles away, that studied her specific genetic mutation. Collaboration between palliative care, her primary care provider, the community-based hospice, the funeral home, the hospital pathology department, and the research lab allowed for a time-sensitive postmortem plan to be put in place preemptively. Amanda had worsening respiratory distress from an aspiration pneumonia, received careful opioid titration to manage her dyspnea and died peacefully at home. Per prearranged plan, her body was transported from her home to the hospital by the funeral home, who offered this service free of charge. A signed autopsy consent had been previously obtained. The pathologist completed the autopsy in a timely manner, and her brain tissue was preserved according to the research lab's specification. Her body was returned to the funeral home where a religious ceremony was held. Several months later, on the family's request, an autopsy review was conducted at the children's hospital where Amanda had received her care. In attendance were Amanda's mother and older sister, an intensivist with a long-standing relationship with Amanda and her family, Amanda's neurologist, and members of the interdisciplinary palliative care team. The team reviewed her autopsy results, including inflammation and scarring of her lungs. Her family felt the autopsy results validated their assessment that her underlying disease and respiratory complications had been progressing and supported their decision-making to enroll Amanda in hospice. They were grateful for the coordination that allowed her brain tissue to be donated to research, which brought them a tremendous amount of meaning. Last, Amanda's family appreciated coming back to the hospital, seeing her providers, and being able to donate dozens of fleece blankets for other hospitalized children.

CONCLUSION

The AAP Policy Statement on Pediatric Palliative Care and Hospice Care Commitments, Guidelines, and Recommendations emphasizes the importance of the process of advance care planning over time, stating that "at a minimum, goals of care and treatment choices should be revisited whenever requested by the patient or family, with every hospitalization or with any significant change in treatment course or prognosis, and at least annually for children with complex chronic conditions."[5] As we have discussed here, advance care planning discussions are best thought of as an extension of goals-of-care conversations that address future-oriented topics and imagine the child in a worse state of health, along an expected or possible trajectory, including at end of life. These conversations provide opportunities for patient and family education about resuscitative measures, medical technology, hospice, and other end-of-life considerations, as well as organ donation and autopsy. These conversations should aim to be relationship-based and occur frequently throughout the illness trajectory. Advance care planning should involve the patient in the manner they desire and should work to ensure that a patient- and family-centered approach to communication and decision-making is supported. This is best done through utilization of an interdisciplinary team taking a holistic approach to advance care planning. When advance care planning is integrated effectively into the ongoing trajectory of care, our patients and families receive compassionate and thoughtful goal-concordant care.

REFERENCES

1. Singer PA, Robertson G, Roy DJ. Bioethics for clinicians: 6. Advance care planning. *CMAJ*. 1996;155(12):1689–1692.
2. Sudore R, Lum H, You J, et al. Defining advance care planning for adults: A consensus definition from a multidisciplinary Delphi Panel (S740). *J Pain Symptom Manage*. 2017;53(2):431–432.
3. Lotz JD, Jox RJ, Borasio GD, Fuhrer M. Pediatric advance care planning: A systematic review. *Pediatrics*. 2013;131(3).
4. Katz AL, Webb SA, Committee on Bioethics. Informed consent in decision-making in pediatric practice. *Pediatrics*. 2016;138(2):e20161485.
5. American Academy of Pediatrics. Pediatric palliative care and hospice care commitments, guidelines, and recommendations. *Pediatrics*. 2013;132(5):966–972.
6. Curtis JR, Patrick DL, Engelberg RA, Norris K, Asp C, Byock I. A measure of the quality of dying and death. *J Pain Symptom Manage*. 2002;24(1):17–31.
7. Mack JW, Weeks JC, Wright AA, Block SD, Prigerson HG. End-of-life discussions, goal attainment, and distress at the end of life: Predictors and outcomes of receipt of care consistent with preferences. *J Clin Oncol*. 2010;28(7):1203–1208.
8. Decourcey DD, Silverman M, Oladunjoye A, Wolfe J. Advance care planning and parent-reported end-of-life outcomes in children, adolescents, and young adults with complex chronic conditions. *Crit Care Med*. 2019;47(1):101–108.
9. Wharton RH, Levine KR, Buka S, Emanuel L. Advance care planning for children with special health care needs: A survey of parental attitudes. *Pediatrics*. 1996;97(5):682–687
10. Lyon ME, Wang J. Longitudinal randomized controlled trial of advance care planning for teens: Religiousness and end of life treatment preferences. *J Adolesc Health*. 2016;58(2):S84.
11. Durall A, Zurakowski D, Wolfe J. Barriers to conducting advance care discussions for children with life-threatening conditions. *Pediatrics*. 2012;129:e975.
12. Liberman DB, Pham PK, Nager AL. Pediatric advance directives: Parents' knowledge, experience, and preferences. *Pediatrics*. 2014;134(2).
13. Heckford E, Beringer AJ. Advance care planning: Challenges and approaches for pediatricians. *J Palliat Med*. 2014;17(9):1049–1053.
14. Kon AA, Morrison W. Shared decision-making in pediatric practice: A broad view. *Pediatrics*. 2018;142(Supplement 3):S129–S132.
15. Opel DJ. A 4-step framework for shared decision-making in pediatrics. *Pediatrics*. 2018;142(Supplement 3):S149–S156.
16. Jacobsen J, Brenner K, Greer JA, et al. When a patient is reluctant to talk about it: A dual framework to focus on living well and tolerate the possibility of dying. *J Palliat Med*. 2018;21(3):322–327.
17. Back AL, Arnold RM, Baile WF, Tulsky JA, Fryer-Edwards K. Approaching difficult communication tasks in oncology. *CA Cancer J Clin*. 2005;55(3):164–177.
18. Miyaji NT. The power of compassion: Truth-telling among American doctors in the care of dying patients. *Soc Sci Med*. 1993;36(3):249–264.
19. Tobias JS, Souhami RL. Fully informed consent can be needlessly cruel. *BMJ*. 1993;307(6913):1199–1201
20. Lamont EB, Christakis NA. Prognostic disclosure to patients with cancer near the end of life. *Ann Intern Med*. 2001;134(12):1096–1105.
21. Wolfe J, Klar N, Grier HE, et al. Understanding of prognosis among parents of children who died of cancer: Impact on treatment goals and integration of palliative care. *JAMA*. 2000;284(19):2469–2475.
22. Mack JW, Wolfe J, Grier HE, Cleary PD, Weeks JC. Communication about prognosis between parents and physicians of children with cancer: Parent preferences and the impact of prognostic information. *J Clin Oncol*. 2006;24(33):5265–5670.
23. Mack JW, Wolfe J, Cook EF, Grier HE, Cleary PD, Weeks JC. Hope and prognostic disclosure. *J Clin Oncol*. 2007;25(35):5636–5642.
24. Wright AA, Zhang B, Ray A, et al. Associations between end-of-life discussions, patient mental health, medical care near death, and caregiver bereavement adjustment. *JAMA*. 2008;300(14):1665–1673.
25. Mack JW, Wolfe J, Cook EF, Grier HE, Cleary PD, Weeks JC. Peace of mind and sense of purpose as core existential issues among parents of children with cancer. *Arch Pediatr Adolesc Med*. 2009;163(6):519–524.
26. van Vliet LM, van der Wall E, Plum NM, Bensing JM. Explicit prognostic information and reassurance about nonabandonment when entering palliative breast cancer care: Findings from a scripted video-vignette study. *J Clin Oncol*. 2013;31(26):3242–3249.
27. Feudtner C. The breadth of hope. *N Engl J Med*. 2009;361(24):2306–2307.
28. Quill TE, Arnold RM, Platt F. "I wish things were different": Expressing wishes in response to loss, futility, and unrealistic hopes. *Ann Intern Med*. 2001;135(7):551.
29. Klick JC, Hauer J. Pediatric palliative care. *Curr Probl Pediatr Adolesc Health Care*. 2010;40(6):120–151.
30. Siden H, Chavoshi N. Shifting focus in pediatric advance care planning: From advance directives to family engagement. *J Pain Symptom Manage*. 2016;52(3):e1–3.
31. Hinds PS, Oakes L, Furman W, et al. End-of-life decision making by adolescents, parents, and healthcare providers in pediatric oncology. *Cancer Nurs*. 2001;24(2):122–134.
32. Mchaffie HE, Lyon AJ, Hume R. Deciding on treatment limitation for neonates: The parents' perspective. *Eur J Pediatr*. 2001;160(6):339–344.
33. Hinds PS, Oakes LL, Hicks J, et al. "Trying to be a good parent" as defined by interviews with parents who made phase I, terminal care, and resuscitation decisions for their children. *J Clin Oncol*. 2009;27(35):5979–5985.
34. Hauer JM. Caring for Children Who Have Severe Neurological Impairment: A Life with Grace. The Johns Hopkins University Press; 2013.
35. Renjilian CB, Womer JW, Carroll KW, Kang TI, Feudtner C. Parental explicit heuristics in decision-making for children with life-threatening illnesses. *Pediatrics*. 2013;131(2):e566–572.
36. Feudtner C. Collaborative communication in pediatric palliative care: A foundation for problem-solving and decision-making. *Pediatr Clin North Am*. 2007;54(5):583–607.
37. Morrison W, Berkowitz I. Do not attempt resuscitation orders in pediatrics. *Pediatr Clin North Am*. 2007;54(5):757–771.
38. Jones BL, Parker-Raley J, Higgerson R, Christie LM, Legett S, Greathouse J. Finding the right words: Using the terms allow natural death (and) and do not resuscitate (DNR) in pediatric palliative care. *J Healthc Qual*. 2008;30(5):55–63.

39. Hinds PS, Oakes L, Furman W, et al. Decision making by parents and healthcare professionals when considering continued care for pediatric patients with cancer. *Oncol Nurs Forum.* 1997;24(9):1523–1528.
40. Burns JP, Edwards J, Johnson J, Cassem NH, Truog RD. Do-not-resuscitate order after 25 years. *Crit Care Med.* 2003;31(5):1543–1550.
41. Smith CB, Oneill LB. Do not resuscitate does not mean do not treat: How palliative care and other modalities can help facilitate communication about goals of care in advanced illness. *Mt Sinai J Med.* 2008;75(5):460–465.
42. Hickman SE, Nelson CA, Moss AH, et al. Use of physician orders for life-sustaining treatment (POLST) paradigm program in the hospice setting. *J Palliat Med.* 2009;12(2):133–141.
43. Boss RD, Hutton N, Griffin PL, Wieczorek BH, Donohue PK. Novel legislation for pediatric advance directives: Surveys and focus groups capture parent and clinician perspectives. *Palliat Med.* 2015;29(4):346–353.
44. Committee on School Health and Committee on Bioethics. Do not resuscitate orders in schools. *Pediatrics.* 2000;105(4):878–879.
45. Diekema DS, Botkin JR. Forgoing medically provided nutrition and hydration in children. *Pediatrics.* 2009;124(2):813–822.
46. Dussel V, Kreicbergs U, Hilden JM, et al. Looking beyond where children die: Determinants and effects of planning a childs location of death. *J Pain Symptom Manage.* 2009;37(1):33–43.
47. Foster TL, Gilmer MJ, Davies B, et al. Bereaved parents' and siblings' reports of legacies created by children with cancer. *J Pediatr Oncol Nurs.* 2009;26(6):369–376.
48. Foster TL, Dietrich MS, Friedman DL, Gordon JE, Gilmer MJ. National survey of childrens hospitals on legacy-making activities. *J Palliat Med.* 2012;15(5):573–578.
49. Wiener L, Zadeh S, Battles H, et al. Allowing adolescents and young adults to plan their end-of-life care. *Pediatrics.* 2012;130(5):897–905.
50. Fletcher S, Hughes R, Pickstock S, Auret K. Advance care planning discussions with adolescent and young adult cancer patients admitted to a community palliative care service: A retrospective case-note audit. *Journal of Adolescent and Young Adult Oncology.* 2018;7(1):112–119.
51. Lyon M, Mccabe M, Patel K, D'angelo L. What do adolescents want? An exploratory study regarding end-of-life decision-making. *J Adolesc Health.* 2004;35(6):529.e1–6.
52. Lyon ME, Garvie PA, Mccarter R, Briggs L, He J, Dangelo LJ. Who will speak for me? Improving end-of-life decision-making for adolescents with HIV and their families. *Pediatrics.* 2009;123(2):e199–206.
53. Wiener L, Ballard E, Brennan T, Battles H, Martinez P, Pao M. How I wish to be remembered: The use of an advance care planning document in adolescent and young adult populations. *J Palliat Med.* 2008;11(10):1309–1313.
54. Hinds PS, Drew D, Oakes LL, et al. End-of-life care preferences of pediatric patients with cancer. *J Clin Oncol.* 2005;23(36):9146–9154.
55. Weir RF, Peters C. Affirming the decisions adolescents make about life and death. *Hastings Cent Rep.* 1997;27(6):29.
56. Zadeh S, Pao M, Wiener L. Opening end-of-life discussions: How to introduce Voicing My CHOiCES™, an advance care planning guide for adolescents and young adults. *Palliat Support Care.* 2014;13(3):591–599.
57. Lyon ME, Jacobs S, Briggs L, Cheng YI, Wang J. Family-centered advance care planning for teens with cancer. *JAMA Pediatr.* 2013;167(5):460.
58. Davies B, Sehring SA, Partridge JC, et al. Barriers to palliative care for children: Perceptions of pediatric health care providers. *Pediatrics.* 2008;121(2):282–288.
59. Feudtner C, Feinstein JA, Satchell M, Zhao H, Kang TI. Shifting place of death among children with complex chronic conditions in the United States, 1989-2003. *JAMA.* 2007;297(24):2725.
60. Chirico J, Donnelly JP, Gupton A, et al. Costs of care and location of death in community-based pediatric palliative care. *J Palliat Med.* 2019;22(5):517–521.
61. Friedrichsdorf SJ, Postier A, Dreyfus J, Osenga K, Sencer S, Wolfe J. Improved quality of life at end of life related to home-based palliative care in children with cancer. *J Palliat Med.* 2015;18(2):143–150.
62. Niswander LM, Cromwell P, Chirico J, Gupton A, Korones DN. End-of-life care for children enrolled in a community-based pediatric palliative care program. *J Palliat Med.* 2014;17(5):589–591.
63. Kassam A, Skiadaresis J, Alexander S, Wolfe J. Parent and clinician preferences for location of end-of-life care: Home, hospital or freestanding hospice? *Pediatr Blood Cancer.* 2013;61(5):859–864.
64. Himelstein BP, Hilden JM, Boldt AM, Weissman D. Pediatric palliative care. *N Engl J Med.* 2004;350(17):1752–1762.
65. Feudtner C, Womer J, Augustin R, et al. Pediatric palliative care programs in childrens hospitals: A cross-sectional national survey. *Pediatrics.* 2013;132(6):1063–1070.
66. Weaver MS, Rosenberg AR, Tager J, Wichman CS, Wiener L. A summary of pediatric palliative care team structure and services as reported by centers caring for children with cancer. *J Palliat Med.* 2018;21(4):452–462.
67. Klick JC, Friebert S, Hutton N, et al. Developing competencies for pediatric hospice and palliative medicine. *Pediatrics.* 2014;134(6):e1670–e1677.
68. Johnston EE, Rosenberg AR, Kamal AH. Pediatric-specific end-of-life care quality measures: An unmet need of a vulnerable population. *J Oncol Pract.* 2017;13(10):e874–e880.
69. Kang TI, Munson D, Hwang J, Feudtner C. Integration of palliative care into the care of Community. *Pediatr Rev.* 2014;35:318–326.
70. Glare P, Virik K, Jones M, et al. A systematic review of physicians' survival predictions in terminally ill cancer patients. *BMJ.* 2003;327(7408):195–190.
71. Jünger S, Pastrana T, Pestinger M, Kern M, Zernikow B, Radbruch L. Barriers and needs in paediatric palliative home care in Germany: A qualitative interview study with professional experts. *BMC Palliat Care.* 2010;9(1):10.
72. Docherty SL, Miles MS, Brandon DH. Searching for "the dying point": Providers' experiences with palliative care in pediatric acute care. *Pediatr Nurs.* 2007;33:335–341.
73. Back AL, Young JP, Mccown E, et al. Abandonment at the end of life from patient, caregiver, nurse, and physician perspectives. *Arch Intern Med.* 2009;169(5):474–479.
74. Hays RM, Valentine J, Haynes G, et al. The Seattle Pediatric Palliative Care Project: Effects on family satisfaction and health-related quality of life. *J Palliat Med.* 2006;9(3):716–728.
75. Meyer EC, Ritholz MD, Burns JP, Truog RD. Improving the quality of end-of-life care in the pediatric intensive care unit: Parents' priorities and recommendations. *Pediatrics.* 2006;117(3):649–657.
76. Finkbeiner AK. *After the Death of a Child: Living with Loss through the Years.* Johns Hopkins University Press; 1998.
77. Murphy SA, Johnson LC, Lohan J. Finding meaning in a child's violent death: A five-year prospective analysis of parents' personal narratives and empirical data. *Death Stud.* 2003;27(5):381–404.
78. National Conference of Commissioners on Uniform State Laws. The Uniform Determination of Death Act 1981.
79. Organ Procurement and Transplantation Network. http://optn.transplant.hrsa.gov/
80. Macauley RC. *Ethics in Palliative Care: A Complete Guide.* Oxford University Press; 2018.
81. The American Association of Tissue Banks. 2020. http://www.aatb.org/
82. Truog RD. Defining death: Getting it wrong for all the right reasons. *Texas Law Review.* 2015;93(7):1885–1914.
83. Williams MA, Lipsett PA, Rushton CH, et al. The physician's role in discussing organ donation with families. *Crit Care Med.* 2003;31(5):1568–1573.
84. Brierley J, Larcher V. Organ donation from children: Time for legal, ethical and cultural change. *Acta Paediatrica.* 2011;100(9):1175–1179.
85. Siminoff LA, Gordon N, Hewlett J, Arnold RM. Factors influencing families consent for donation of solid organs for transplantation. *JAMA.* 2001;286(1):71–77.
86. Thornton JD, Wong KA, Cardenas V, Curtis JR, Spigner C, Allen MD. Ethnic and gender differences in willingness among high school students to donate organs. *J Adolesc Health.* 2006;39(2):266–274.

87. Jeffres L, Carroll J, Rubenking B, Amschlinger J. Communication as a predictor of willingness to donate one's organs: An addition to the theory of reasoned action. *Prog Transplant.* 2008;18(4):257–262.
88. Thomas SL, Milnes S, Komesaroff PA. Understanding organ donation in the collaborative era: A qualitative study of staff and family experiences. *Intern Med J.* 2008;39(9):588–594.
89. Siminoff L, Marshall H, Dumenci L, Bowen G, Swaminathan A, Gordon N. Communicating effectively about donation: An educational intervention to increase consent to donation. *Prog Transplant.* 2009;19(1):35–43.
90. Simpkin AL, Robertson LC, Barber VS, Young JD. Modifiable factors influencing relatives' decision to offer organ donation: Systematic review. *BMJ.* 2009;338:b991.
91. Alden DL, Cheung AHS. Organ donation and culture: A comparison of Asian American and European American beliefs, attitudes, and behaviors. *J Appl Soc Psychol.* 2000;30(2):293–314.
92. Siminoff LA, Molisani AJ, Traino HM. A comparison of the request process and outcomes in adult and pediatric organ donation. *Pediatrics.* 2015;136(1):e108–114.
93. Stephenson MT, Morgan SE, Roberts-Perez SD, Harrison T, Afifi W, Long SD. The role of religiosity, religious norms, subjective norms, and bodily integrity in signing an organ donor card. *Health Communication.* 2008;23(5):436–447.
94. Al-Mousawi M, Hamed T, Al-Matouk H. Views of Muslim scholars on organ donation and brain death. *Transplant Proc.* 1997;29(8):3217.
95. Alvaro EM, Jones SP, Robles AS, Siegel J. Hispanic organ donation: Impact of a Spanish-language organ donation campaign. *J Natl Med Assoc.* 2006;98(1):28–35.
96. Morse CR, Afifi WA, Morgan SE, et al. Religiosity, anxiety, and discussions about organ donation: Understanding a complex system of associations. *Health Communication.* 2009;24(2):156–164.
97. Siminoff LA, Burant CJ, Ibrahim SA. Racial disparities in preferences and perceptions regarding organ donation. *J Gen Intern Med.* 2006;21(9):995–1000.
98. Manninen DL, Evans RW. Public attitudes and behavior regarding organ donation. *JAMA.* 1985;253(21):3111–3115.
99. Lietz C, Mayes T, Naclerio A, Taylor R. Pediatric organ transplantation and the Hispanic population: Approaching families and obtaining their consent. *Transplant Proc.* 2004;36(5):1237–1240.
100. Afri T, Tellis V. Attitudes of high school students regarding organ donation. *Transplant Proc.* 2001;33(1-2):968–969.
101. López-Navidad A, Vilardell J, Aguayo M, et al. Introducing an informative program on donation and transplantation into secondary education. *Transplant Proc.* 2002;34(1):25–28.
102. Sanner MA. A Swedish survey of young peoples' views on organ donation and transplantation. *Transpl Int.* 2002;15(12):641–648.
103. Pierini L, Valdez P, Pennone P, et al. Teenager donation: Investigation of 848 high school students. *Transplant Proc.* 2009;41(8):3457–3459.
104. Siebelink MJ, Geerts EAHM, Albers MJIJ, Roodbol PF, Van De Wiel HBM. Childrens' opinions about organ donation: A first step to assent? *Eur J Public Health.* 2011;22(4):529–533.
105. Weiss A, Fortinsky R, Laughlin J, et al. Parental consent for pediatric cadaveric organ donation. *Transplant Proc.* 1997;29(3):1896–1901.
106. Rodrigue JR, Cornell DL, Howard RJ. Pediatric organ donation: What factors most influence parents' donation decisions?. *Pediatr Crit Care Med.* 2008;9(2):180–185.
107. Darlington AS, Long-Sutehall T, Randall D, Wakefield C, Robinson V, Brierley J. Parents' experiences of requests for organ and tissue donation: The value of asking. *Arch Dis Child.* 2019;104(9):837–843.
108. Bellali T, Papadatou D. Parental grief following the brain death of a child: Does consent or refusal to organ donation affect their grief? *Death Stud.* 2006;30(10):883–917.
109. Hoover SM, Bratton SL, Roach E, Olson LM. Parental experiences and recommendations in donation after circulatory determination of death. *Pediatr Crit Care Med.* 2014;15(2):105–111.
110. Rodrigue JR, Cornell DL, Howard RJ. The instability of organ donation decisions by next-of-kin and factors that predict it. *Am J Transplant.* 2008;8(12):2661–2667.
111. Tartaglia A, Linyear AS. Organ donation: A pastoral care model. *J Pastoral Care.* 2000;54(3):277–286.
112. Carey LB, Robinson P, Cohen J. Organ procurement and health care chaplaincy in Australia. *J Relig Health.* 2009;50(3): 743–759.
113. Delong WR. Organ donation and hospital chaplains: Attitudes, beliefs, and concerns. *Transplantation.* 1990;50(1):25–28.
114. Bradby H, Kenten C, Deedat S, Morgan M. 'Having a different conversation around death': Diverse hospital chaplains' views on end-of-life care. *Ethn Health.* 2013;18(6):530–543.
115. Geva J, Weinman ML. Social work perspectives in organ procurement. *Health & Social Work.* 1995;20(4):287–293.
116. Truog RD, Christ G, Browning DM, Meyer EC. Sudden traumatic death in children: "We did everything, but your child didn't survive." *JAMA.* 2006;295(22):2646–2654.
117. Sefansky S. Involved in the business of death: The social work role in postmortem care. *Health Social Work.* 2016;42(1):e8–e14.
118. Daly BJ. End-of-life decision making, organ donation, and critical care nurses. *Crit Care Nurse.* 2006;26(2):78–86.
119. Meyer K, Bjørk IT. Change of focus: From intensive care towards organ donation. *Transpl Int.* 200;21(2):133–139.
120. Jawoniyi OO, Gormley K. How critical care nurses' roles and education affect organ donation. *Br J Nurs.* 2015;24(13):698–700.
121. Mathur M, Taylor S, Tiras K, Wilson M, Abd-Allah S. Pediatric critical care nurses' perceptions, knowledge, and attitudes regarding organ donation after cardiac death. *Pediatr Crit Care Med.* 2008;9(3):261–269.
122. Medicare and Medicaid programs; hospital conditions of participation; identification of potential organ, tissue, and eye donors and transplant hospitals' provision of transplant-related data—HCFA. Final rule. *Fed Regist.* 1998;63(119):33856–33875.
123. Association of Organ Procurement Organizations. http://www.aopo.org/
124. Bollinger RR, Heinrichs DR, Seem DL, Rosendale JD, Johnson KS, Metzger RA. Organ procurement organization (OPO), best practices. *Clin Transplant.* 2001;15(s6):16–21
125. Ladin K, Hanto DW. Family physicians role in discussing organ donation with patients and the public. *AMA J Ethics.* 2012;14(3):194–200.
126. Sadler BL, Sadler NR. Having conversations about organ donation. *Hastings Center Rep.* 2015;45(5):inside back cover.
127. Kelly CM, Masters JL, Deviney S. End-of-life planning activities: An integrated process. *Death Stud.* 2013;37(6):529–551.
128. Kotloff RM, Blosser S, Fulda GJ, et al. Management of the potential organ donor in the ICU: Society of Critical Care Medicine/ American College of Chest Physicians/Association of Organ Procurement Organizations consensus statement. *Crit Care Med.* 2015;43(6):1291–1325.
129. Martin DE, Nakagawa TA, Siebelink MJ, et al. Pediatric deceased donation—a report of the Transplantation Society meeting in Geneva. *Transplantation.* 2015;99(7):1403–1409.
130. Bratton SL, Kolovos NS, Roach ES, Mcbride V, Geiger JL, Meyers RL. Pediatric organ transplantation need: Organ donation best practices. *Arch Pediatr Adolesc Med.* 2006;160(5):468.
131. King LS, Meehan MC. A history of the autopsy: A review. *Am J Pathol.* 1973;73(2):514–544.
132. Zink S, Wertlieb S. A study of the presumptive approach to consent for organ donation: A new solution to an old problem. *Crit Care Nurse.* 2006;26(2):129–136.
133. Luskin RS, Glazier AK, Delmonico FL. Organ donation and dual advocacy. *N Engl J Med.* 2008;358(12):1297–1298.
134. Truog RD. Consent for organ donation—balancing conflicting ethical obligations. *N Engl J Med.* 2008;358(12):1209–1211.
135. Thall C, Jensen G, Wright C, Baker S, Meade R. The role of hospital-based family support teams in improving the quality of the organ donation process. *Transplant Proc.* 1997;29(8):3252–3253.
136. Friberg N, Ljungberg O, Berglund E, et al. Cause of death and significant disease found at autopsy. *Virchows Archiv.* 2019;475(6):781–788.

137. Conran RM, Stocker TJ. The Pediatric Autopsy. In Collins KA, Byard RW. Forensic Pathology of Infancy and Childhood. Springer Science + Business Media New York. 2014:59–80.
138. Olpin SE. The metabolic investigation of sudden infant death. *Ann Clin Biochem*. 2004;41(4):282–293.
139. Twamley H, Haigh A, Williment C, Hudson C, Whitney J, Neuberger J. Prospective audit to evaluate the potential of the coronial system to increase solid organ donation. *BMJ Open*. 2016;6(7):e010231.
140. Goldstein B, Metlay L, Cox C, Rubenstein JS. Association of pre mortem diagnosis and autopsy findings in pediatric intensive care unit versus emergency department versus ward patients. *Crit Care Med*. 1996;24(4):683–686.
141. Kumar P, Taxy J, Angst DB, Mangurten H. Autopsies in children: Are they still useful? *Pediatr Res*. 1996;39:135–135.
142. Berge JT, Gast-Bakker D-AHD, Plötz FB. Circumstances surrounding dying in the paediatric intensive care unit. *BMC Pediatrics*. 2006;6(1):22
143. Buckner T, Blatt J, Smith SV. The autopsy in pediatrics and pediatric oncology: A single-institution experience. *Pediatr Dev Pathol*. 2006;9(5):374–380.
144. Cardoso MP, Bourguignon DC, Gomes MM, Saldiva PH, Pereira CR, Troster EJ. Comparison between clinical diagnoses and autopsy findings in a pediatric intensive care unit in Sao Paulo, Brazil. *Pediatr Crit Care Med*. 2006;7(5):423–427.
145. Feinstein JA, Ernst LM, Ganesh J, Feudtner C. What new information pediatric autopsies can provide. *Arch Pediatr Adolesc Med*. 2007;161(12):1190–1196.
146. Narayanan A, Thorburn K, Baines P. Autopsies in children continue to reveal unanticipated discrepancies between autopsy findings and antemortem clinical diagnoses. *Arch Dis Child*. 2009;94(8):645–645.
147. von Dessauer B, Velozo L, Benavente C, Bobenrieth F, Bongain J, Irazuzta J. Postmortem studies in the contemporary pediatric intensive care unit. *Pediatr Crit Care Med*. 2011;12(6):617–621.
148. Widmann R, Caduff R, Giudici L, et al. Value of postmortem studies in deceased neonatal and pediatric intensive care unit patients. *Virchows Archiv*. 2016;470(2):217–223.
149. Thayyil S, Sebire NJ, Chitty LS, et al. Post-mortem MRI versus conventional autopsy in fetuses and children: A prospective validation study. *Lancet*. 2013;382(9888):223–233.
150. Scheimberg I. The genetic autopsy. *Curr Opin Pediatr*. 2013;25(6):659–665.
151. Heathfield L, Martin L, Ramesar R. A systematic review of molecular autopsy studies in sudden infant death cases. *J Pediatr Genet*. 2018;07(04):143–149.
152. Goldstein RD, Nields HM, Kinney HC. A new approach to the investigation of sudden unexpected death. *Pediatrics*. 2017;140(2):e20170024.
153. Hutchinson JC, Arthurs OJ, Sebire NJ. Postmortem research: Innovations and future directions for the perinatal and paediatric autopsy. *Arch Dis Child Educ Pract Ed*. 2015;101(1):54–56.
154. Griffiths BT, Sebire NJ, Brierley J. Learning from investigation after death. *Pediatr Crit Care Med*. 2018;19(8S):S72–S78.
155. Burton JL, Underwood J. Clinical, educational, and epidemiological value of autopsy. *Lancet*. 2007;369(9571):1471–1480.
156. Bierig, JR. A potpourri of legal issues relating to the autopsy. *Arch Path Lab Med*. 1996;120(8):759–762.
157. Klaiman MH. Whose brain is it anyway? *J Leg Med*. 2005;26(4):475–490.
158. Mitchell RA, Diangelo C, Morgan D. Medicolegal death investigation of sudden unexpected infant deaths. *Pediatric Annals*. 2017;46(8):e297–e302.
159. Committee on Child Abuse and Neglect and Committee on Community Health Services. Investigation and review of unexpected infant and child deaths. *Pediatrics*. 1999;104(5):1158–1160.
160. Henry J, Nicholas N. Dead in the water: Are we killing the hospital autopsy with poor consent practices? *J Roy Soc Med*. 2012;105(7):288–295.
161. Wiener L, Sweeney C, Baird K, et al. What do parents want to know when considering autopsy for their child with cancer? *J Pediatr Hematol/Oncol*. 2014;36(6):464–470.
162. Lewis C, Hill M, Arthurs O, Hutchinson C, Chitty L, Sebire N. Factors affecting uptake of postmortem examination in the prenatal, perinatal and paediatric setting. *BJOG*. 2017;125(2):172–181.
163. Vanmarter LJ, Taylor F, Epstein MF. Parental and physician-related determinants of consent for neonatal autopsy. *Arch Pediatr Adolesc Med*. 1987;141(2):149–153.
164. Stolman CJ, Castello F, Yorio M, Mautone S. Attitudes of pediatricians and pediatric residents toward obtaining permission for autopsy. *Arch Pediatr Adolesc Med*. 1994;148(8):843–847
165. Mcdermott MB. Obtaining consent for autopsy. *BMJ*. 2003;327(7418):804–806.
166. Mchaffie HE, Fowlie P, Hume R, Laing I, Lloyd D, Lyon A. Consent to autopsy for neonates. *Arch Dis Child Fetal Neonatal Ed*. 2001;85(1):F4–F7.
167. Vennemann MMT, Rentsch C, Bajanowski T, Zimmer G. Are autopsies of help to the parents of SIDS victims? A follow-up on SIDS families. *Int J Legal Med*. 2006;120(6):352–354.
168. Human M, Goldstein RD, Groenewald C, Kinney HC, Odendaal H. Bereaved mothers' attitudes regarding autopsy of their stillborn baby. *S Afr J Obstet Gynaecol*. 2017;23(3):93–96.
169. Meaney S, Gallagher S, Lutomski JE, Odonoghue K. Parental decision making around perinatal autopsy: A qualitative investigation. *Health Expect*. 2014;18(6):3160–3171.
170. Rankin J, Wright C, Lind T. Cross sectional survey of parents' experience and views of the postmortem examination. *BMJ*. 2002;324(7341):816–818.
171. Sullivan J, Monagle P. Bereaved parents perceptions of the autopsy examination of their child. *Pediatrics*. 2011;127(4):e1013–e1020.
172. Alabran JL, Hooper JE, Hill M, et al. Overcoming autopsy barriers in pediatric cancer research. *Pediatr Blood Cancer*. 2012;60(2):204–209.
173. Baker JN, Windham JA, Hinds PS, et al. Bereaved parents intentions and suggestions about research autopsies in children with lethal brain tumors. *J Pediatr*. 2013;163(2):581–586.
174. Rosenbaum GE, Burns J, Johnson J, Mitchell C, Robinson M, Truog RD. Autopsy consent practice at US teaching hospitals. *Arch Intern Med*. 2000;160(3):374–380.
175. Mccabe ME, Hunt EA, Serwint JR. Pediatric residents clinical and educational experiences with end-of-life care. *Pediatrics*. 2008;121(4):e731–737.
176. Ben-Sasi K, Chitty LS, Franck LS, et al. Acceptability of a minimally invasive perinatal/paediatric autopsy: Healthcare professionals' views and implications for practice. *Prenat Diagn*. 2013;33(4):307–312.
177. Lewis C, Hill M, Arthurs OJ, Hutchinson JC, Chitty LS, Sebire N. Health professionals' and coroners' views on less invasive perinatal and paediatric autopsy: A qualitative study. *Arch Dis Child*. 2018;103(6):572–578.
178. Putman MA. Perinatal perimortem and postmortem examination. *Adv Neonat Care*. 2007;7(6):281–288.
179. Committee on Bioethics and Committee on Hospice Care. Palliative care for children. *Pediatrics*. 2000;106:351–357.
180. Truog RD, Campbell ML, Curtis JR, et al. Recommendations for end-of-life care in the intensive care unit: A consensus statement by the American College of Critical Care Medicine. *Crit Care Med*. 2008;36(3):953–963.
181. Meert KL, Eggly S, Pollack M, et al. Parents' perspectives regarding a physician-parent conference after their child's death in the pediatric intensive care unit. *J Pediatr*. 2007;151(1)50–55.
182. Zehm A, Rosenberg LB, Daubman BR. Discussing autopsy with bereaved families #400. *J Palliat Med*. 2020;23(10):1400–1402.

15 | ANTICIPATORY GRIEF AND BEREAVEMENT

JENNIFER M. SNAMAN, TERRAH FOSTER AKARD, SUE E. MORRIS, AND LORI WIENER

I often say I have a hole in my heart and I can hear the wind blow through it. Some days I actually hear that wind whistle through my heart. If I don't feel that way, I think there's something wrong

BEREAVED PARENT

Anticipatory grief and bereavement—the before, during, and after of a death—comprise many different physical, psychological, spiritual, social, and cultural facets. The grief following the death of a child is never-ending and ebbs and flows over the lifetime of those who experience the loss.[1–4] At the core of pediatric grief and bereavement is the child, surrounded by concentric circles of family, friends, members of the interdisciplinary care team, and the wider community (Figure 15.1).

Over the past two decades of research, the perspectives of bereaved parents have proved to be invaluable in the development and expansion of the field of pediatric palliative care (PPC).[5–8] This burgeoning research area has explored the care provided to the child and family throughout the illness trajectory, at the end of life, and into bereavement, rather than exclusively focusing on the death itself.[9–16] Approaching bereaved families (including parents and siblings) for research purposes had previously been questioned given concerns about inflicting psychological harm or distress in this vulnerable population.[17] Yet multiple studies have shown that parents find participation to be a positive and therapeutic experience—often even more so than nonbereaved parents.[18,19]

This chapter addresses the interplay between the universality of the grief experience and the uniqueness of the individual's and family's response. The phenomenon of anticipatory grief is described, followed by a discussion of bereavement. Emphasis is on the role of ongoing assessment in bereaved families and the implications for intervention, including cultural and spiritual dimensions of care and support. The roles that various interdisciplinary members of the primary and specialty palliative care teams play in supporting families throughout the illness and following the child's death are outlined in Table 15.1.

Quotations from bereaved families are woven throughout the chapter to highlight important themes. The grief of clinicians is also addressed, including interventions designed to support interdisciplinary team members who care for children with serious illnesses and their families.

THE CHILD, FAMILY, AND COMMUNITY

THE FAMILY UNIT

The definition of "family" has expanded over time to encompass many diverse constellations. From the outset, a family's own definition of their family unit and the role of each member within that unit should be elicited. Without such information, clinicians' assumptions of inclusion or exclusion may be faulty. This may result in overlooking members who are themselves valuable sources of support or those who are in need of additional support. The nuclear family of child,

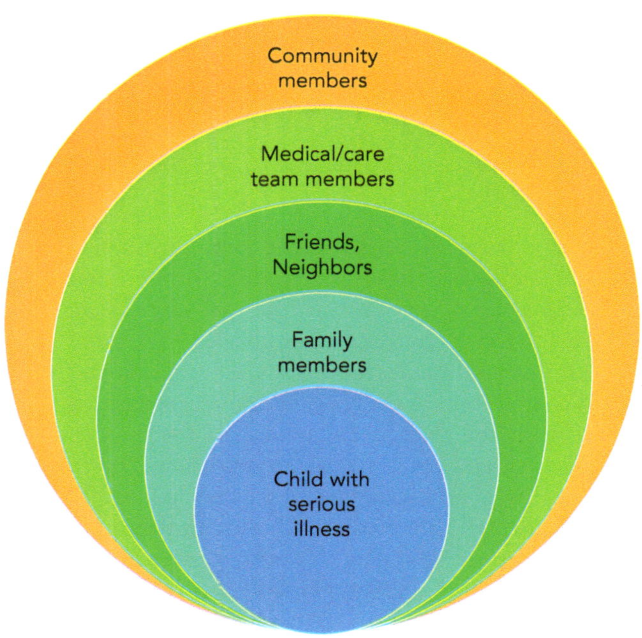

Figure 15.1 The cascading effect of grief.

TABLE 15.1 Interdisciplinary team members and roles. Interdisciplinary team members play various roles in supporting children with serious illness and their families throughout the disease course, at the end of life, and following the child's death.

TEAM MEMBER/ROLE	ROLE DURING DISEASE COURSE AND AT END OF LIFE	ROLE IN BEREAVEMENT (FOLLOWING CHILD'S DEATH)
Child life specialist (Includes art and/or music therapists)	Support for child and siblings Communicating with child and siblings around treatment and end of life issues Memory making and legacy activities	Individual support Group support for siblings as part of a siblings' bereavement program
Resource specialist	Help with financial assistance with housing, meals and parking	Financial assistance for funerals, other bills
Physician/NP (primary medical team)	Medical care, communication around treatment, prognosis,	Condolence call following death Personalized sympathy card Invitation to meet as a team to discuss lingering issues or answer questions
Interdisciplinary team, including bedside nurses	Psychosocial support, empathetic listening and reassurance Role-specific care	Team sympathy card to parents and family Attending wake or funeral if desired/appropriate Provision and participation in hospital-wide memorial services
Palliative care physician/NP	Pain and symptom management Advanced care planning Anticipatory guidance around end of life Coordination with home care/hospice	Condolence call following death Personalized sympathy card Invitation to meet as a team to discuss lingering issues or answer questions
Psychiatrist	Consultation and liaison	Consultation and Liaison as needed for distressing symptoms Providing team support and facilitation of team debriefs
Social worker	Psychosocial support for parents, child, siblings, parents, and extended family, including funeral planning	Condolence call following death Personalized sympathy card Bereavement outreach to family Facilitation of bereavement support groups Facilitation of bereavement rounds for teams (ideally with Chaplaincy) Providing team support and facilitation of team debriefs
Psychologist	Emotional support for parents and child Management of behavioral health problems	Condolence call following death Personalized sympathy card Bereavement outreach to family Facilitation of bereavement support groups Facilitation of bereavement rounds for teams (ideally with Chaplaincy) Providing team support and facilitation of team debriefs
Chaplain	Spiritual support for parents, child and family	Condolence call Sympathy card Bereavement outreach to family Officiating at funeral or memorial services for child Facilitation of bereavement rounds for teams (with social work and/or psychology)

siblings, and parents is usually at the core, surrounded by the extended family. For families of children with serious illness, grandparents may play a major role and serve as informal caregivers to the ill child as well as siblings.[20,21] Close friends may be indistinguishable from family, especially during acute clinical changes and as the child or adolescent nears the end of life. With the changing structure of the family, teams must be open and accepting of nontraditional, alternative, and complicated arrangements. These may include divorced and reconstituted (blended) families, with their inherently conflicted histories and new alliances; single or lone-parent families; children of lesbian, gay, bisexual, transgender, and queer or questioning (LGBTQ) parents; and children raised by grandparents. The composition of the family likely frames other factors, including developmental level, psychological history (including coping with past losses and trauma), sources of support, and cultural and spiritual beliefs.

A universal phenomenon in the bereavement process is that individuals in the same family grieve in different ways and on different schedules.[1,2,22,23] Despite mourning the same child, family members are often out of sync with one another in their experience and expressions of grief. Misunderstanding, guilt, anger, resentment, and a profound loneliness often arise when this phenomenon is not understood.[1,2] Additionally, the death of a child can send parents reeling into uncertainty about their identity.[24] This may be especially true for parents who have lost an only child or for those who have lost more than one child: Are they still parents? Are they still a family?

As for siblings of children who die, their modes of expressing grief may differ substantially from that of their parents or other adults. Thus, their grief's meaning and depth may be underestimated or even missed completely.[25] All too often siblings become disenfranchised grievers,[25] whereby their loss is minimized compared to that of their parents'. Bereaved siblings have also been described as "forgotten mourners" as they adjust to the loss of the sibling relationship and the resultant change in family dynamics and roles.[26]

CULTURE AND BACKGROUND, COMMUNITY, AND PEERS

There is a growing diversity of familial, cultural, and community influences throughout the world. It is crucial to recognize the impact of background, culture, and language on the family's experience of the child's illness and treatment, how they make decisions along the illness trajectory and at the end of life, and on the grief process.[27] Cultural perceptions may challenge the use of language. For instance, in English, the word "compassion" connotes a deep caring. In some Spanish traditions, however, the word is primarily connoted with care for the dying. Thus, the use of this term in the wrong context may communicate an unintended message to the family.

Many issues at the end of life and after a child's death vary by culture, including the meaning of pain and suffering, illness, and death; the role of religion and spirituality; the role of family; and practices or preferences. There may be cultural differences in the expectations of the medical team, the expected role of family members and the community, and beliefs about the inclusion of children in discussions. Information regarding customs and rituals for specific cultures or ethnic groups is available and can provide a broad framework for beginning to explore a family's beliefs. However, team members must be aware that significant differences can exist in these practices within the same ethnic groups (or even within the same family). Therefore, rather than make assumptions about preferences based on their race, religion, or culture, clinicians should incorporate a deep sense of humility and curiosity in developing a partnership with families.[28] Awareness of these nuances and differences may also enable bereavement care to be better individualized.[29]

ANTICIPATORY GRIEF

> It might sound a little bit strange, but I guess I would have to say that the grieving process started with the diagnosis.
>
> Bereaved parent

Anticipatory grief is a universal process among families of children with serious illness.[30,31] It begins at time of diagnosis, wends its way along the illness trajectory, and—for children with incurable disease—continues until the moment of death. Anticipatory grief often resembles the grief that immediately follows a death: emotions are alternately raw and numb and very much evident.[32] The classic definition of anticipatory grief is "grief expressed in advance when the loss is perceived as inevitable."[33] Experientially, the process reflects the emotional response to the pain of separation before the actuality of loss.[32] The ill child may grieve multiple losses: the loss of his or her healthy self, of function and role, of separation from loved ones. Parents and other family members also experience anticipatory grief, grieving the loss of "normalcy," of a healthy child and a typical future for that child. Throughout the illness course, parents move from the conceptualization that "our child may not survive" to "our child is going to die" to an even more anguished dawning that "we are going to lose our child." It is at this juncture that the recognition of an inevitable separation has begun.[32] The ebb and flow of anticipatory grief is unique for each person and family, depending on the nature and length of the illness trajectory, as well as psychological and cultural factors.[34]

The child and family may feel overwhelmed by their intense emotions, not understanding the source. Often, they do not recognize that below the sadness lies the deeper and more complex phenomenon of anticipatory grief. Articulating this distinction and explicitly naming this phenomenon can be a powerful therapeutic intervention for both children and parents. It is important to explain that grief arises not only around the finality of death, but also for the cumulative losses that occur over the course of an illness.

> A mother berated herself: "I can't understand why I cry all the time. My daughter is doing reasonably well right now. It makes me feel guilty when I cry like this—I feel as if I am burying her before she actually dies." Once the psychologist explained the concept of anticipatory grief, she experienced enormous relief at being able to attribute a meaning to her tears.

The grief of seriously ill children has its own immediacy.[35–37] Being in the hospital for extended periods of time separates them from their family and friends—at home, school, and in other activities, in the neighborhood and their faith community. They often express longing for these relationships, so disrupted by the illness. Children facing death may become fearful and express anxiety about being separated from their families. It is crucial that parents reassure children that they will always be loved and will never be forgotten. Children may feel isolated or fearful if they are not given permission to talk openly about their illness and impending death.[38] For parents who feel that such conversations could be in the best interest of their child and family, age- and developmentally appropriate tools to facilitate these discussions may be provided. However, parents should not be pressured or forced to initiate them.

Siblings of children with serious illness also experience anticipatory grief, which may be manifested in behavioral changes, school difficulties, or symptoms of acute and posttraumatic stress.[39] Awareness of these needs and provision of support to siblings during treatment and into bereavement is essential.[40] Child life specialists and mental health professionals can engage these children in discussions around their experience of the sibling's illness and assist parents in talking with them to ensure that their unique needs are being met.

Grief following the death of a fellow patient can be intense, especially when the children have similar diseases or clinical courses. On one level, the child and family grieve the loss of their acquaintance or friend. On a deeper level, they are struck with the awareness that: "This could have been me/our child . . . and will I/our child be next?"[32] A recent study indicated that for adolescents and early young adults with cancer, the death of a peer resulted in grief that was slow to ease[41] and was associated with increased risk of adverse psychological outcomes. This close sense of identification provides an opening for the patient and family to address their own sadness and fear. It may also be an ideal time for medical and psychosocial clinicians to help them explore these fears and provide additional support as needed.

The exhaustion that accompanies the long course of a serious illness, with its many ups and downs, is inordinate. The family may find it difficult to know whether to prepare for loss or for life—and how to apportion their emotional energy. Discomfort may occur when a patient's life extends beyond its prognostic expectancy. The family may at first feel jubilant to have more time with the child, while at the same time they may wonder how they will continue to manage under the ongoing threat of death and permanent loss.

A certain degree of disengagement from the child on the part of family members, or from one another, may be part of the anticipatory grief process. In a self-protective move against loss and further pain, the family may seem "to leave before being left."[32] Such disengagement may be seen in a general emotional withdrawal from the child, or it may take specific forms, including parents beginning to take a less active role in caring for the dying child. These phenomena are neither inevitable nor, when they occur, irreversible. However, they do signify a family's difficulty in negotiating the anticipatory grief process. It is crucial that the family not feel chastised by the team. Furthermore, a timely referral to a mental health clinician for individual, marital, or family therapy[32] may be considered.

Because there are no social rituals to mark anticipatory grief, as there are in bereavement, even close family and friends may be unaware of or confused by what the family is experiencing or how to help. Family members frequently describe a profound sense of loneliness and separateness from others. One of the most therapeutic interventions that clinicians can introduce at this time is to facilitate support among families going through the same experience (Box 15.1).

> Right now, we are living in a different world. . . . Our friends in the "outside world" care about us, but they can't really understand what we are living through. Our closest people right now are the other families at the hospital and our team.

INTERVENTIONS AS DEATH APPROACHES

The trajectories of life-threatening illnesses in children are variable and may include cycles of relapse and remission, steady or stepwise deterioration, or acute declines due to illness, injury, or accident. With the approach of the child's death, everyone confronts the full intensity of anticipatory grief. The child faces the ultimate leave-taking from everyone and everything[32]; the family stands at the brink of their new life ahead, facing the specter of life without the child. During this period, there may be the need for planning and critical decision-making interwoven with legacy- or memory-making activities with the child.[42,43]

Decisions may include setting of end-of-life care and death (home-based or hospital), specific needs, advance care planning (ACP) and/or advance directives, autopsy, and funeral arrangements. Many families must consider (or reconsider) decisions to continue or discontinue interventions based on the balance between increased time versus increased suffering.

Children with cancer have reported their preference for honesty and parental involvement in communication about their illness.[44] Almost all children surveyed (aged 3–17) wanted to be told if they were dying.[45] Involvement in discussions and decisions, if they so choose, can help them to maintain a sense of autonomy.[46] How and when to include them is often a collaborative decision among the child, family, and primary team, along with guidance from the palliative care team.

Children near the end of life may confide wishes to loved ones and prepare for death.[47] Younger children may communicate their awareness via their actions and the implications of their words rather than through explicit discussions. Family communication tools (e.g., Hello, Hear My Voice, ShopTalk) and ACP guides that provide age-appropriate methods of voicing preferences (e.g., My Wishes, Voicing My Choices) provide a way for children and adolescents to express their opinions about their care and how they wish to be remembered in the future.[48,49]

Many adolescents and young adults have an opinion about what they would want to happen to their body after death (including autopsy, burial, or cremation) and funeral planning. Research has shown that they would like the option of donating their body or tissues for research into their disease,[48] yet this conversation rarely occurs. Parents who agreed to an autopsy for research purposes found it to be feasible[50] and satisfying,[51] with no parents regretting the decision.[52] Interestingly, most parents who had not discussed autopsy would have considered it for the advancement of science and better understanding of their child's condition.[53,54]

Hospitals may offer *legacy-building activities* (e.g., shared artwork, making a memory box or book, storytelling, videos and portraits, tracing family members' hands, making prints and molds of the child's hands and feet) to assist seriously ill children and their families in documenting the child's legacy. These are provided primarily by child life specialists, social workers, chaplains, and bedside nurses. Although the

BOX 15.1 ANTICIPATORY GRIEF AND BEREAVEMENT: KEY CONCEPTS

Anticipatory grief and bereavement—the before, during, and after loss—begin at the time of the child's diagnosis and extend years after the child's death

ANTICIPATORY GRIEF

- Grief expressed in advance when a loss is perceived to be threatening or inevitable.
- The child may grieve for others and lost things in his or her life.
- The family faces multiple and cumulative losses leading up to the child's death. The multiple losses may continue throughout bereavement.
- The child and family may feel overwhelmed by the intensity of their emotions, not recognizing that underlying their sadness is the even deeper phenomenon of anticipatory grief. Clarifying this distinction and naming the phenomenon can provide patients and families with relief and comfort.
- The death of another patient engenders powerful grief—and anticipatory grief—for children with serious illness, their families, and the wider community.

BEREAVEMENT

- An experience that ebbs and flows over a lifetime. There is no absolute time frame for, or expectation of, its resolution.
- Families often express a sense of multiple losses: the death of their child as an individual and a member of the family and community; the loss of their professional family, the team who cared for the child, often over months and years; the loss of their role as a parent, caregiver, and protector of their child
- Bereavement follow-up is an integral part of comprehensive PPC and may assuage the family's sense of abandonment.
- Bereavement assessment, and reassessment over time, is both prevention and intervention, particularly for those families determined to be at high risk for mental- and health-related complications from grief.
- Despite mourning the same child, individuals in the family grieve in different ways and on different schedules. Being out of sync with one another is a normal phenomenon.
- Siblings grieve deeply for their brother or sister. However, because children's ways of expressing grief may differ substantially from that of their grieving parents, their mourning may be underestimated or missed entirely.

activities are typically not empirically based, some have demonstrated improved psychosocial outcomes and comfort in bereavement.[42,43,47,55,56] Legacy research in pediatric oncology has shown that children desire that others remember their personal characteristics, things they like to do, and connectedness with others.[57] It is important to offer a variety of activities to find those that appeal to ill children and their family members while also respecting a decision for them to decline.[58] Those who decline can be reassured that children have already created a legacy by simply being who they are.

Parents have specific beliefs about their role in being a "good parent" to their seriously ill child.[59] Attributes include the recognition of their role in instilling hope within themselves and in their child as they strive to maintain the optimal quality of life possible for the child. As death approaches, families often need assurance that they have done all they could for their child. The team's availability is crucial and usually appreciated, even by those families who appear to be coping well on their own. Mental health and spiritual care professionals can be of enormous importance for some families during this time.

Another dimension of the anticipatory grief process involves spirituality. The illness experience may challenge the beliefs and search for meaning of many children and parents, at times leading to significant spiritual suffering.[60] The task of spiritual care in PPC is to offer support to persons of many faiths, cultures, and practices.[61] In most spiritual practices, prayer is a demonstration of faithfulness. In some traditions, the belief is that prayers are answered if they are asked properly and with faith. When prayers go unanswered and children become sicker, the notions of doubt and punishment may loom large.

> A 16-year-old boy explained that he no longer prayed because God did not listen to him, but if the chaplain prayed for him, God might hear his prayers.

When the practices that comfort a child differ from what brings solace to the family, the chaplain and palliative care team search for ways to reconcile them.

> Tommy, a 15-year-old teenager, was devastated when his disease recurred for the third time. His parents, devout Catholics, invited the priest to visit Tommy to provide support through prayer and sacraments. However, over the previous year, Tommy had been reading about Buddhist beliefs and had participated in a meditation workshop that brought him great comfort. The hospital chaplain arranged for Tommy to speak with a monk about his fears and search for peace as he continued to provide spiritual support for the parents. At Tommy's request, after his death, his parents invited several monks to chant mantras. Knowing that they had honored their son's spiritual preferences provided them with a sense of peace.

When families lose access to their primary spiritual and religious community (often because of geographical distance), making new connections is another of many adjustments. Interdisciplinary team members can help to facilitate access to the needed spiritual support.[60]

> A Muslim boy had end-stage kidney disease. His mother was a "match" for transplant and said that she would do anything not to lose her son. His father expressed fear of

losing both his son and his wife. They requested to talk with an Islamic chaplain. Although the hospital chaplain was not Islamic, the social worker encouraged the family to meet with her nonetheless. They accepted the suggestion and found her to be deeply understanding. The father requested that she pray for the family. The fact that she represented "faith" was enough for the family to accept her.

For deeply spiritual or religious families, the chaplain's accompaniment through the process of anticipatory grief and into bereavement can be of inestimable importance.

BEREAVEMENT

THE GRIEF EXPERIENCE

Parenting is a permanent change in the individual: a person never gets over being a parent. Parental bereavement is also a permanent condition. The bereaved parent, after a time, will cease showing the symptoms of grief, but the parent does not "get over" the death of a child.[62(p. 178)]

The death of a child is described as one of the worst and most stressful life events.[63] The resultant intense and prolonged grief [2,64,65] may be compounded when parents have witnessed their child's protracted physical and emotional suffering throughout the course of the illness.[5,10,65,66] Bereaved parents are at increased risk of short- and long-term psychosocial and physical morbidities.[67–75] Likely related to the impact of grief on psychological health, there have also been documented deleterious effects on marriage quality, occupational status, and finances.[72,76] The significant morbidities and intensity and extent of the grief response are thought to be due to the disruption of the natural order of life[77] (a child dying before the parent), a sense of guilt and/or feelings of failure in protecting their child from harm,[78,79] and the profound disruption of family structure and roles following the child's death.[80] Despite experiencing such a shattering event, the vast majority of parents are able to integrate their loss into their life over time. Although their grief is never-ending, it ebbs and flows, changes, and may abate in intensity over time with ongoing support.

CURRENT RESEARCH ON PARENTAL GRIEF AND BEREAVEMENT

Early research in the field of parental grief and bereavement was primarily descriptive or conceptual in nature. These studies provided a rich context within which the characteristics of an individual family may be viewed and have led to an expansion of data in larger populations of bereaved parents. Importantly, previously used frameworks for understanding the concept of grief as a whole may not accurately reflect the grief experience of parents.[81] Popular and commonly understood concepts of the trajectory of "normal" grief, such as the Kubler-Ross model, suggested stages of coping leading to acceptance.[82,83] However, newer models of grief focus on finding meaning in the loss and living with it as opposed to recovering from grief.[15,84–86] Additionally, multidomain models of parental grief highlight the importance of ongoing relationships with others and continuing supportive bonds with their deceased child.[72,87–89]

Much of the bereavement literature has focused on aspects of the child's diagnosis, treatment, and end-of-life care to ascertain characteristics of the experience that are associated with poor outcomes in parents. Some of these factors may be fixed, whereas others can be modified in the healthcare setting. It is important to note that many of the correlations cited are from small, retrospective qualitative studies or those that include parents many years out from their child's death; few are prospective quantitative studies examining the parental grief experience over time. Despite these limitations, there is much to learn from the available literature and innovative ways to support parents and families in their grief during treatment, at the end of life, and following the child's death into bereavement.

Although "long-term" consequences often refer to sequelae 1 or 2 years following a loss, a time frame for parental bereavement has not been established in the literature. Qualitative data indicate that acute grief reactions in the first 2 years may be different from descriptions of parental grief at later points.[4] Additionally, bereaved parent's psychological and social needs may change over time. For examples, within cohorts of bereaved parents, parents closer to the death of their child (average of 4–6 years vs. 7–9 years from child's death) had worse psychological well-being and poorer quality of life.[10]

Compared to nonbereaved parents, parents who experienced the death of a child have higher rates of hospitalization for psychological morbidity and physical health issues, including an increased risk for development of cancer, cardiac disease, and diabetes.[8–11] Additionally, an elevated incidence of both natural and unnatural death has been reported.[90] Bereaved parents are at increased risk of significant psychosocial morbidities,[67] including higher rates of psychiatric hospitalization, suicide, and substance misuse.[68–69] *Unresolved grief* emerges as a specific risk factor for the psychological and physical health of both mothers and fathers in the long term.[68] Bereaved fathers with unresolved grief are seven times more likely to report sleep disturbances, with ensuing impact on their capacity for work and overall well-being.[68]

Importantly, bereaved parents can experience positive and negative changes in both personal and relational domains.[91] A common and damaging misconception is that the incidence of separation or divorce is elevated in couples whose child has died. Yet a study on long-term marital status shows the opposite: bereaved parents actually are less likely to divorce or separate than are nonbereaved.[92] Another study indicated bereaved parents were more satisfied with their relationship if they perceive that their partner has a similar level of grief intensity,[93] thus highlighting the importance of inclusion of both parents (or other caregivers) in supportive interventions.

PARENTAL GRIEF: IMPACT OF PARENTAL DEMOGRAPHICS AND CHILD'S DIAGNOSIS AND TREATMENT

Parental demographics, a family's history of previous losses, premorbid conditions, and financial problems likely affect the grief experience and bereavement outcomes. Although most of these factors are fixed, they are important because they have been found to influence parental outcomes. There are documented differences in grief experience by gender, both in coping strategies as well as in psychological and physical outcomes.[72,94] For example, fathers who were able to say farewell to their deceased child in the way they wanted and mothers who were able to talk about their feelings with family and trusted that the care team had made every effort to cure their child reported lower levels of prolonged grief symptoms.[11] Differences between genders may also be related to the parental role during the child's illness; the secondary parent-caregiver may spend less time at the bedside given the need to work and maintain family income and health insurance. *In general*, fathers' coping tends to be more work-focused and task-oriented in their grieving.[72] The differing needs of mothers and fathers have implications for the types of interventions provided during the child's illness, immediately after the death, and for family bereavement support. However, it is important to note that the literature on parental bereavement may not reflect the actual experience of all parents and may propagate certain stereotypes.

The child's age at the time of death has been associated with parental outcomes of distress[95] and prolonged grief.[96] Aspects of the child's illness and type of treatment have also been associated with long-term parental outcomes.[3,97] Finally, previous loss experiences have been associated with poorer adjustment in bereavement.[3] This may be especially true in parents who have experienced the death of more than one child.

QUALITY OF CARE, COMMUNICATION, AND CARE AT THE END-OF-LIFE

Many modifiable factors relating to parental grief are related to the quality of care (perceived and actual) during treatment and at the child's end of life. Open and honest communication is essential throughout the disease course and the child's end of life.[14,16,98,99] Moreover, positive parental perception of doctor–patient communication has been directly correlated with perceptions of high-quality physician care at the end of life.[100,101] Parents who reported receiving high-quality prognostic information were less likely to experience decisional regret, and higher parental ratings of communication have been associated with lower levels of long-term parental grief.[102]

Parents desire support and information about how to prepare practically and emotionally for the death of their child. Although most parents want to be fully informed of their child's status, many clinicians avoid this type of communication. Parents who have been informed that their child's death is imminent are more likely to be prepared.[103,104] Furthermore, these parents are more likely to talk about death with their child, even more so when they perceive the child also to be aware, an approach that has been shown to reduce the risk of psychological morbidity in bereavement.[105]

Location of the child's death is another factor in bereaved parents' bereavement: one study indicated that fathers reported high levels of depression, anxiety, and stress when the child died in the hospital rather than at home. The chance of a child dying at home was greater when the parents received information that the child's illness was incurable and were more cognizant of his or her imminent death.[106] It remains to be determined whether the significant factor is the actual location of the child's death or the ability of parents (and patients) to discuss and plan the location of death.[107]

The severity of symptoms and perceived suffering at the end of life have been associated with higher levels of long-term parental grief.[102] Most parents who reported that their child experienced pain that could not be relieved or a "difficult moment of death" were still affected by this experience many years later.[9] Knowing the many factors that have been associated with parental outcomes in bereavement, interdisciplinary team members can work together to facilitate high-quality communication, including issues related to dying and death, and address and manage distressing symptoms throughout the illness and at the end of life.

POST-DEATH FACTORS ASSOCIATED WITH PARENTAL GRIEF OUTCOMES

Understanding the parental perception of the child's death is crucial to understanding the family's response to the loss. Did they feel their child died peacefully? Was there disappointment in the care their child received at the time of death? Did they feel their child suffered or had poor symptom management? Was the timing of the death unanticipated? Did they perceive a sense of abandonment from their child's medical team or close friends as death neared or following death?

There are other factors that are associated with parental grief outcomes. Parents who were not able to be physically and/or emotionally present at the time of their child's death may have long-lasting regrets or feelings of guilt and inadequacy about their caregiving. Parental perception of the oncologist's care, the child's quality of life during the last month, preparedness for the child's death, and economic hardship have been found to predict grief and depression outcomes.[108] Resilience has also been associated with healthier outcomes for bereaved parents, including factors such as perception of self, social resources, and family cohesion.[11,109] Family cohesion remains critically important. In studies conducted over the decades, communication within the family (being able to talk about feelings freely and comfortably) has been associated with more positive grief outcomes.

Many bereaved parents express a strong desire for something positive to come from their child's death. For example, parents and siblings have reported choosing special activities to honor the deceased child,[55] such as a ritual or gathering on the child's birthday or anniversary of the death or walking to raise money for a significant cause. Importantly, many aspects of the care the child received at the end of life and at the time of death appeared to be fixed or not modifiable, such as end-of-life course, location of death, and symptoms at the end of life. However, these details may change and shift over time as parents retell their stories and restructure the narrative of their child's life. This process of making sense of and attempting to find some meaning in the illness and death (a desire expressed by some, not all, families) can be facilitated by mental health professionals.

> A 15-year-old girl with multiply relapsed leukemia shared with her therapist that she did not want any more disease-directed treatment—but was worried because her mother was searching hard for new therapies. The therapist first worked with the mother, helping her to communicate with her daughter about their respective wishes. This was followed by joint sessions in which mother and daughter were able to share their concerns and fears. Together they made the decision to go home and not pursue more treatment. After her daughter's death, the mother's letter to the therapist exemplifies the meaning offered by such open communication: "Thank you for the enlightened guidance that opened us up to talk about so many vital things that have really given me the peace of mind I cling to. Nothing was left unsaid and so many pitfalls avoided because all of her wishes were spelled out for me to follow."

THE GRIEF EXPERIENCE OF SIBLINGS AND CURRENT RESEARCH

> Three healthy siblings complained to the psychologist: "Every holiday our parents say: 'Let's make this holiday perfect for your brother, since it may be his last.' Meanwhile, he has lived for four years. How long are we supposed to keep this up?[32(p. 73)]

Bereaved siblings face many challenges that may continue for years. With the death of the patient, they suffer multiple losses: not just of their brother or sister but also of the roles that were inherent in the relationship.[110–112] Siblings must negotiate this permanent loss while feeling the psychological distance of their parents who are immersed in their own grief. Siblings struggle with overwhelming sadness and other intense feelings that are strikingly similar to those faced by bereaved adults. Children often report previous losses; thus a "loss history" is crucial in understanding their strengths and vulnerabilities. Young children's prior experience with death, if any, is typically the loss of a grandparent or a pet. They may also talk about objects that they have lost, especially if they are associated with their brother or sister. Children often report traumatic memories as well as express fears for the future. Frightening images tend to focus on the illness itself, such as how the person looked, visible symptoms, medical technology, or on the viewing, funeral, or burial. Children may express several worries, including the possibility of other losses, possible harm to themselves, loss of a specific aspect of the sibling relationship, religious concerns, and/or contagion and familial risk of illness. Adolescents often express sadness about the future (e.g., my brother or sister will never know my children). Anger at the injustice of the loss, as well as at the pain that they must now suffer, takes on many forms including verbal outbursts, physical aggression or other forms of acting out, sleep and somatic disorders, and school difficulties. Somewhat paradoxically, some children may withdraw from others, especially their family, as a part of their grief experience.

One of the most common—and most painful—aspects of sibling bereavement is a child's sense of guilt. The guilt may focus on an act, word, or thought that was committed or omitted, real or imagined, rational or irrational. Whatever the source, its existence may sharply exacerbate the loss and complicate grief.

> A 17-year-old girl who had served as a stem cell donor for her sister created the drawing in (Figure 15.2), 2 years after her sister's death. (She also wrote the "Sibling Reflection," later in this chapter.)

The frequent and inset intrusion of traumatic thoughts or an unrelenting sense of guilt often signals the need for psychological treatment. Children may also grapple with the fact that their loss reverberates throughout the social environment, often bearing a combination of both positive and negative consequences, such as the outpouring of support versus stigmatization.

Although limited, research on bereaved siblings is growing and new scales and instruments are being developed to better understand the sibling grief experience and how this may change over time.[113,114] Siblings are often referred to as being invisible because of the parents' intense involvement in

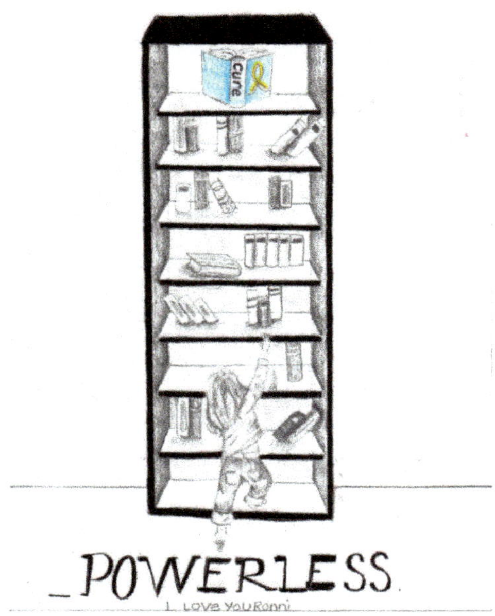

Figure 15.2 Powerless.

the care of their ill child.[115] During the illness, the siblings desire open and honest communication within the family, adequate information from clinicians, involvement in the care of the sick child, and support to continue their own interests and activities.[115–118] In fact, bereaved siblings who reported dissatisfaction with communication, poor preparation for death, missed opportunities to say goodbye, and perceived negative impact of the cancer experience had higher levels of distress and lower social support scores.[119] Parents often try to protect siblings from involvement in the child's illness, particularly end-of-life care, thinking that it will shelter them from trauma. Yet this well-intentioned approach may instead lead siblings to feel abandoned and potentially excluded from the family tragedy,[112,120] with long-term impact caused by these feelings.[119]

Like parental grief, the bereavement experience of siblings is slow to improve and long-lasting. In a survey-based study including siblings 2–9 years after the death of a sibling, the majority of siblings noted that they had not "worked through" their grief.[121] Following the child's death, bereaved siblings may experience both a positive and negative change to their lives.[122] For example, bereaved siblings have reported that family relationships may become closer in some families, but more distant for others. Some bereaved siblings have improvements in school performance after the death, whereas others have experienced greater difficulties post-death. Siblings may experience changes in personality, schoolwork, goals and life perspective, activities/interests, and relationships with family members and peers; these changes have been found to continue for years following the death.[122,123]

Siblings may be at increased risk of psychological sequalae [124] Compared to nonbereaved individuals, bereaved siblings are at increased risk of low self-esteem, low levels of maturity and difficulty falling asleep.[125] During the first year after a sibling's death, rates of anxiety, depression, and illicit substance use increased before returning to baseline.[119] All bereaved siblings indicated that their loss still affected them an average of 12 years later.[119] A population-based study in Denmark showed bereavement in childhood due to sibling death was associated with an increased risk of both short- and long-term mortality.[126] There has been no significant change in self-reported peer relationships in siblings of children who died from cancer.[127]

There is some evidence that certain groups may be particularly vulnerable to negative effects following a sibling's death. One study indicated that younger (elementary school aged) and male siblings may have more social difficulties in bereavement, including more isolation, less acceptance, and fewer friends.[128] Additionally, children who serve as a donor of hematopoietic stem cells for their sibling may require special consideration. Studies have found sibling donors from transplants that resulted in the recipient's death reported anger, guilt, and blame.[129] Negative emotions were reported by siblings who felt inadequately informed of possible complications from the procedure and/or the cause of the recipient's death, perceived a lack of support from family and doctors after the sibling's death, and internalized their feelings.[129,130] Further investigation into understanding the unique needs of these bereaved siblings is needed to advance specific support for this population.[131] The following reflection is by a bereaved sibling, in which she shares her experience during her sister's treatment and following her death. She also is the artist of Figure 15.2: *Powerless.*

Family Reflection

Sibling Reflection

When my big sister Ronni was diagnosed with stage 4 Ewings Sarcoma, I remember thinking that she will get better, and everything will go back to normal. I never thought she would die. Almost immediately after diagnosis I saw her go through so much treatment and pain. We were constantly surrounded by people trying to help her. Doctors, nurses, surgeons, counselors, my parents, and so many more. Then there was me. How could I be so much a part of this but unable to do anything. I felt helpless. I remember giving Ronni a list of remedies to help cure cancer, things I found online. She seemed as into it as I was at the time, but I also remember getting upset when she didn't follow them. It's hard to see everything and be able to do nothing. Sometimes I couldn't even get her to smile, let alone cure her cancer. At some point it was brought up to our parents about Ronni receiving a stem cell donor. I was tested to determine if I was a good match. I remember the day my parents came into our TV room and told me I was a perfect match for Ronni. This was everything. I thought this was my chance to finally help her like everyone else. I was so proud to do this. My mom and dad were so proud of me and seeing how happy Ronni was, is still one of the best moments I've ever experienced. When Ronni passed away, it was a lot of disbelief. I put a lot of blame on myself. Why didn't my stem cells help her? At the time I felt like I let my parents down, like I let Ronni down. Almost 11 years later, although I understand so much more about the process and I'm so happy that I did it, I still can't help but sometimes feel this way. I just wish she was here.

BEREAVEMENT ASSESSMENT

Under ideal circumstances, a mental health clinician carries out a comprehensive family bereavement assessment. When a mental health clinician is not available for direct clinical involvement, another palliative care team member may carry out the evaluation and then seek consultation about the family's status, risk, and supportive needs.

A bereavement assessment is often performed over several sessions, usually beginning shortly after the child's death, with follow-up over the subsequent weeks and months.[132] The clinician must carefully monitor the pace of the assessments, both within meetings and in scheduling subsequent times, always based on the family's cues. Moving quickly through an interview for the sake of completing the assessment frequently results in distress and the loss of important information. Fundamental concepts of a bereavement assessment are described in Box 15.2.

BOX 15.2 FUNDAMENTALS OF BEREAVEMENT ASSESSMENT

- Allow for time, without interruption, to speak with the family in a manner that conveys your complete attention.
- Provide a comfortable and confidential physical setting, with items such as facial tissues and water available. If children are included, set out toys, books, and drawing or writing materials.
- Welcome the family, express your condolences, and acknowledge the enormity of their loss.
- Refer to the deceased child by name. Be open to looking at photographs or videos of the child if the family offers them. Use clinical judgment about initiating a request to see pictures.
- Approach the family in an open and nonjudgmental manner to facilitate trust and reduce any sense of intimidation.
- Pose questions in a way that reflects the family's cognitive, developmental, and educational levels and cultural background.
- Always ask, never assume.
- Before focusing on the child's illness and death, allow time for the family to describe and reminisce about the child.
- Invite families to tell the story of their child in their own way and at their own pace. It is common for bereaved individuals to repeat details of the illness and death numerous times as they move through the grief experience.
- Pace the assessment. Avoid overwhelming the family; use clinical judgment as to whether it is time to take a break or end the session. Moving quickly through an interview for the sake of completing the assessment often results in unnecessary distress and the risk of missing important information.
- Let the family express their feelings and opinions regardless of if you agree. Refrain from interrupting or trying to fill silences.
- Verify your impressions with the family. When necessary, ask explicitly if your understanding is accurate. If you make a mistake or misunderstand something, apologize and continue. Families tend to be very forgiving.
- If red flags emerge in the assessment, consult with a mental health clinician.
- Bereavement interviews elicit the expression of intense emotions. Closely monitor your own reactions during and after the session. Just as all families are different, each clinician brings his or her background and vulnerabilities to the setting.

Although only the word "family" is used in the box, these points apply to individual grief/bereavement assessments as well.

In the immediate aftermath of the child's death, it is important to assess each family member's response and determine what is needed to carry the family through the crisis, including referrals for medical or mental health issues. Initial discussions often include family member's wishes for a funeral and/or memorial service and burial and, in some instances, the clarification of logistical issues around transporting the body. If the family has not made advance arrangements, they often need assistance in these aspects of planning. This initial assessment also may include sensitive inquiry into the family's financial resources and identification of people who can aid them in the days and weeks ahead. Questions about the course of the child's illness and death, or unresolved issues with the medical team, can usually wait until after the service and other arrangements have taken place. Other major areas of bereavement assessment include developmental level of the sibling(s) of the parent(s) and sibling(s) and the family; family composition, relationships, and background; significant medical issues; psychological history, particularly coping with past losses or trauma; ethnicity, culture, and spiritual beliefs; available support within the family and community; and access to professional services. A "loss history" encompasses loss in its broadest sense;[32] for example, loss of individuals through illness and death, trauma, change in relationships (e.g., divorce); loss of employment and/or financial security; and/or geographical moves. A critical dimension of the loss history includes the experience of immigrant or refugee families. In addition to the loss of their home country, many of these individuals have suffered unspeakable trauma in their past. Given the extreme sensitivity of these issues, which may include fear of legal repercussions if disclosed, utmost care must be exercised in any inquiry.

The heart of the bereavement assessment is the family's experience of the child's illness and death. In broaching this segment of the interview, the family should be invited first to describe and reminisce about their child. Hearing the family's story as they choose to recount it is essential, both for its content and for how it is told. Other issues, including both the facts and the accompanying emotions, are important to listen for or elicit as the family relates their experience; these are outlined in Box 15.3.

"Red flags" in the family that may indicate a predisposition to a particularly complicated bereavement period include a history of multiple losses or trauma, psychiatric disturbance (especially suicidal ideas or behavior), and misuse of drugs or alcohol.[133] Family relationships that were already fragile or stressed before the child's death are at risk for further deterioration. If the individual or family has an existing relationship with a mental health clinician, the team may seek permission to contact that individual to ensure timely follow-up. For others, it is crucial to have an emergency plan, including access to immediate psychiatric assessment at the time of the child's death. The importance of helping a family to create a "safety net" of extended family and friends before the child's death cannot be overestimated.

Exploring a family's ethnic and cultural background—and degree of acculturation in immigrant families—is

BOX 15.3 BEREAVEMENT ASSESSMENT ITEMS FOCUSED ON THE CHILD'S ILLNESS AND END-OF-LIFE EXPERIENCE

- How was information about your child's illness (diagnosis, prognosis, end of life) communicated?
- How did you and the staff share information with your child? What did he or she know or understand?
- Did you and your child participate in decisions about treatment and end-of-life care?
- Did you and your child communicate about nearing the end of life and death? Did your child express any preferences around the end of their life (preferred location of death, rituals, etc.) or after their death (involvement in legacy items, planning funeral, concern for you or other family members, etc.)?
- Was there any staff member with whom you felt especially comfortable or uncomfortable?
- When and how did you realize, or when and how were you told, that your child was going to die?
- Were you given information about home and hospice care for your child?
- Were you prepared for what to expect at the time of death (medically, including physical changes, as well as emotionally)?
- Did your child seem to be suffering before he or she died? If so, how?
- Was your family with your child before his or her death and/or at the time of death? Was everyone there that you wanted to be present? Did you have the support you needed from staff?

essential for assessment and formulation of an optimal bereavement care plan. Family members may vary considerably in their attachments to beliefs and customs from their home country; consequently, individual beliefs and needs can be quite different. Through sensitive and thorough inquiry, important information can be gleaned to frame the family's psychological responses within the context of their own cultural background. The clinician's effort to understand these factors promotes respect and candor within the therapeutic relationship.

A key underlying premise of the assessment process is "always ask, never assume." Assumptions about behavior based on gender, ethnic or cultural background, age or even the type of loss suffered must be evaluated against the information provided by the individual. Furthermore, while the assessment marks a starting point for working with a bereaved family, the process of evaluation continues. Periodic check-ins with the family provide ongoing supportive contact as well as a lens through which to monitor for changes in emotion or behavior that might otherwise be missed. For example, a parent may go through periods of seeming "almost normal," only to be followed by incapacitating grief when he or she is unable to leave the house or even get out of bed. Another example may be a sibling who appears to be functioning well who is suddenly stricken with nightmares, becomes inconsolable and fearful, and withdraws from friends and activities.

Families may experience increased financial strain following the death of a child, with the high cost of medical treatment and funeral/burial costs.[76] Significant household financial effects of a child's death may be compounded further by work disruptions or job loss due to ongoing parental grief. A comprehensive assessment of finances is essential, and interdisciplinary team members, including social workers and resource specialists, can develop a plan to ease this distress.

BEREAVEMENT INTERVENTIONS

Ongoing bereavement assessments of individuals and families helps to guide the clinician in what type of intervention would be most valuable at a given time. The best "fit" for bereavement support must be based on astute clinical judgment in combination with the unique needs and wishes of the individual or family. These needs may fluctuate over time, and thus a variety of support and treatment modalities may be accessed concurrently or sequentially in the bereavement process. Some parents choose to cope on their own, with or without support from family or friends. Many families find tremendous strength and support in their local community and/or spiritual organization. Others turn to self-help bereavement groups at local agencies that rely on volunteers and trained peer or online support groups.

The most common supportive interventions for bereaved parents are support groups, counseling, psychotherapy, and crisis intervention. Several studies have shown that both professional and social support are beneficial for parents' grief outcomes, although not all parents find these resources to be helpful. Some people choose more intensive or personalized intervention in the form of individual, marital, or family psychotherapy to examine the enduring impact of the child's illness and death on their lives. A critical topic for future research is the identification of parents at risk for complicated or prolonged grief reactions[134,135] and the design of optimal intervention for these individuals. Emerging from existing research are recommendations in caring for bereaved parents, outlined in Box 15.4.

COMMUNITY SUPPORT FOR BEREAVED PARENTS AND FAMILY MEMBERS

Over the long term, the social network, including connections with other bereaved families, has proved to be particularly valuable for many bereaved parents and siblings.[103,136] Research indicates that fathers talk mainly with their spouse, while mothers often confide in family, friends, and other bereaved parents. Both types of sharing have a beneficial impact on grief.[10] Community-based support for bereaved family members includes hospice-based bereavement programs, nonprofit agencies, faith-based programs, and private practitioners. Accessing community resources helps bereaved families meet other local families and can lessen

BOX 15.4 EVIDENCE-BASED RECOMMENDATIONS TO SUPPORT BEREAVED PARENTS AND FAMILIES

- Seek out the preferred methods of support unique to each family to best facilitate open communication.
- Attempt to reduce the child's suffering throughout the illness and at the end of life through optimal symptom management.
- Communicate openly and honestly with parents, include children when possible.
- Communicate with families after the death of a child, both in the moments and days as well as the weeks, months, and years after the death.
- Inform parents about the demonstrated value of open communication with and support from family and friends.
- Recommend that parents seek professional psychological support during the child's illness and following the death, particularly when there are risk factors in the family. Normalize the need for this support and aid families in finding support in their local community.

Adapted with permission from Snaman JM, Kaye EC, Torres C, Gibson DV, Baker JN. Helping parents live with the hole in their heart: The role of health care providers and institutions in the bereaved parents' grief journeys. *Cancer.* 2016 Sep 1;122(17):2757–2765.

their sense of isolation. Often support organizations have "chapters" in different communities (e.g., the Compassionate Friends). Importantly, hospice-based bereavement programs are available for families even if the patient was not enrolled for care. Most states or regions have a hospice locator to identify locations and services offered.

ONLINE GRIEF AND BEREAVEMENT SUPPORT AND SHARED MATERIALS

There is a great deal of information and support online for grieving individuals, including Facebook groups, podcasts, and online forums or posts. The challenge, especially for the newly bereaved, is finding support that promotes connection while decreasing their sense of isolation. A suggested starting point is to search national or state organizations for online groups that focus on a similar loss or ask psychosocial team members or the bereavement coordinator for recommendations. In any online forum, individuals risk opening up to others who might not be supportive. Should this occur, it is important to encourage the bereaved to leave and explore other sites or alternative resources.

INDIVIDUAL SUPPORT FOR BEREAVED PARENTS AND FAMILY MEMBERS

Psychotherapy can be critical for those individuals or families who have preexisting or current vulnerabilities in addition to or inextricable with the child's death. While there is much debate about the precise characterization of *pathological grief*, current research supports the concept of *prolonged grief disorder* (PGD), which is characterized by an intense, unabating longing or yearning for the deceased and unremitting, debilitating grief symptoms and depressive symptoms.[137] PGD includes challenges to one's sense of identity and feeling that life is empty or meaningless following the loss. It is important that assessments look for extremes of emotion that persist over time (e.g., consuming rage that envelops the individual and alienates the family or the total suppression of any sign of feeling). Such symptoms, particularly those of PGD, appear particularly prominent among bereaved parents, who may struggle with their sense of identity and purpose, the meaning of their child's life, and making sense of their untimely loss. Psychotherapy facilitates the unfolding of the grief process within a well-contained and safe context. It can play a pivotal role in rebuilding, strengthening, and sustaining the individual's and family's resources as they move forward into the future. An adaptation of the evidence-based meaning-centered psychotherapy,[138,139] a brief intervention originally developed for advanced cancer patients that incorporates the principles of Viktor Frankl's logotherapy[140] has shown early efficacy for parents who have lost a child to cancer.[141,142]

The exigencies of bereavement demand that mental health clinicians have a solid base in normative grief responses, psychopathology, evaluation, and different forms of psychotherapy. In addition, for those who work with bereaved siblings, knowledge of child development and psychotherapy is critical. Without a broad foundation, clinicians lack a context in which to place the intense issues of bereavement, and their ability to intervene effectively may be severely compromised.

INVENTIONS FOR SIBLINGS

> When we first went to the psychologist, my little brother thought she was a checkup doctor. But I explained to him, "You know how we lost our older sister? This doctor tries to get the sadness out of your heart."
>
> 7-year-old child

Findings suggest that, after the death, siblings perceive their life to change, not only within the family but also in relationships outside the family.[122,123] Whenever possible, clinicians should communicate directly with siblings and educate parents about the importance of addressing their unique needs. Importantly, psychological outcomes for siblings have been linked to maternal mental health symptoms, including posttraumatic stress disorder, depression, and PGD,[143] highlighting the need for increased support for all members of the family. Support groups and/or camps or other group activities can provide bereaved siblings a chance to meet other children who have experienced the death of a loved one and may serve to normalize the feelings that the child may be experiencing. Individual or family-based psychotherapy may also be helpful for certain individuals. The death of a child will be experienced by the wider community, including by the child's peers, neighbors, schoolmates, and other families.

Recent evidence indicated that school-based support, particularly support from friends, peers, and teachers, facilitates adjustment in bereaved siblings.[144] There are available resources for clinicians and school staff to help support individuals who may be grieving.[145,146] Interdisciplinary clinicians, where possible, should outreach to schools and community members to find ways to support siblings as well as their class- or schoolmates, neighbors, and community members as they process and grieve the death of a child.

SUPPORT FOR BEREAVED PARENTS PROVIDED BY THE CARE TEAM

Bereavement follow-up by primary care, specialty palliative care, and bereavement teams is considered an intrinsic component of comprehensive pediatric care. The vast majority of pediatric oncologists believe that bereavement support is a part of good clinical care,[147] and bereavement care is now an evidence-based standard in pediatric oncology (Box 15.5).[148]

Despite this validation, comprehensive longitudinal support for families following a child's death is sporadic.[149] Given ongoing clinical responsibilities, members of the primary care team may not be able to provide intensive follow-up for all bereaved families. Many families express anguish that the clinicians who cared for their child—their "professional family"—usually do not follow them into bereavement (referred to as a "double loss").[8,13,14,103,150] However, a skilled "hand-off" to a bereavement support counselor or team, including pertinent information about the family and deceased child as well as risk factors for severe grief reactions, can provide some continuity for families.

Whether or not the family chooses to meet with the bereavement team, contact with a primary team member may assuage the family's sense of abandonment or thoughts that the child was unimportant and will not be missed.[151] Clinicians may consider attending the viewing or funeral, meeting with the family to review medical/end-of-life care issues or autopsy results, or making a home visit.[152,153] Events such as an annual hospital memorial service provide valuable opportunities for connection. The families who attend are eager to talk with the staff who knew their child and often spontaneously describe their life since the child's death. These touch points are opportunities to assess the family's functioning and may serve a crucial preventive role by identifying those at risk for serious physical, psychological, and social sequelae.

In many circumstances, the opportunity for ongoing face-to-face assessment and follow-up does not exist. The condolence letter, card, or phone call is one of the simplest gestures that can be made by a clinician, and it is typically highly valued by family members.[133,154] This letter has two goals: to express a tribute to the deceased child and to be a source of comfort or support to the survivors. Many clinicians worry about finding the "right words" to express their condolences or worry that a note or phone call may remind parents of their loss or cause additional distress. Typical themes to include in the letter or phone call and example language are provided in Table 15.2.[133]

Clinicians should avoid attempting to understand the loss or compare it to other losses ("I know how you feel, my dog recently died") or impose religious or other personal beliefs on others ("At least she is in a better place now"). Finally, providers should be alert to risk factors for adverse mental health outcomes in bereaved parents or other family members that may be identified during condolence calls or other contact. These include isolation or poor social support, history of mental health illness, substance use issues, existential distress, hopelessness, and other concurrent stressors.[152] If risk factors are identified, clinicians should contact psychosocial and/or mental health providers to help identify next steps and additional supports for bereaved family members and plan for close follow-up.

BOX 15.5 EVIDENCE-BASED STANDARDS FOR EARLY INTEGRATION OF PPC AND BEREAVEMENT INTO ROUTINE ONCOLOGY CARE

- Children, adolescents, and young adults with cancer and their families should be introduced to palliative care concepts to reduce suffering throughout the disease process regardless of disease status.
- When necessary, youth and families should receive developmentally appropriate end-of-life care (which includes bereavement care after the child's death).
- A member of the healthcare team should contact the family after a child's death to assess family needs, identify those at risk for negative psychosocial sequelae, continue care, and provide resources for bereavement support.

Adapted with permission from Lichtenthal WG, Corner GW, Sweeney CR, et al. Mental health services for parents who lost a child to cancer: if we build them, will they come? *J Clin Oncol.* 2015;33(20):2246–2253.

148

HOSPITAL-BASED BEREAVEMENT PROGRAMS

Bereavement care for parents and other family members is considered an essential component of quality care. The development of bereavement services, however, appears to have fallen behind that of other essential elements of palliative care.[155] Bereavement support for families is often haphazard, varying greatly by hospitals, teams, and available resources.[149] Research findings, as outlined earlier, indicate that bereaved parents are at heightened risk of poor bereavement outcomes.[65,156] As such, hospital-based pediatric bereavement programs should be implemented as a standard of care to ensure that *all* bereaved families receive support after the death of a child, not just those patients who received support from a specialty palliative care team or had certain medical diagnoses. Clinical and administrative staff must recognize the importance of a hospital-wide response to the death of all patients, as well as the more personalized bereavement follow-up that teams and clinicians typically provide. In a study that explored hospital-based bereavement services following the

TABLE 15.2 Themes or topics to consider including in condolence letters and calls and example phrases.

Offer condolence	"I was so saddened to hear about [child's] death" or "I am so sorry for the loss of your sweet daughter [child's name]."
A personal memory of the patient and family	"I will always remember his big eyes and his belly laughs."
Specific references to qualities of the child, such as courage, humor, kindness, can bring life to the letter	"He was always so kind and caring."
An acknowledgment of all the family did for the child	"You were always at her bedside holding her hand. She was incredibly fortunate to have you as a father."
A statement that it was a privilege to have participated in the child's care	"It was a privilege to get the chance to care for [child's name]."
Offer opportunities to return to the hospital or contact the medical team	"Please reach out to our team if you would like to come back to the hospital to visit with the staff. We would love to see you and your family again."
Commit to an ongoing relationship with the parents and other family members, including ways to reach out for additional support	"If you find you need some additional support for you or for [child's name]'s sister(s)/brother(s), please call us and we can provide you with some additional resources."
Conclude with a statement that the child and family will be remembered	"I will always remember [child's name]. Please know [child's name] and your family and will remain in my thoughts."

Adapted with permission from Weaver MS, Lichtenthal WG, Larson K, Wiener L. How I approach expressing condolences and longitudinal remembering to a family after the death of a child. *Pediatr Blood Cancer.* 2019;66(2):e27489.[152]

death of a child, parents who received bereavement support materials described feeling cared for and supported by staff, a reduction in sense of isolation and improved coping and personal growth.[157] Importantly, the provision of services seems to be most effective for parents experiencing more complex mourning.[157] Coordinated bereavement programs not only help bereaved families navigate the many changes brought about by the death of a child but also facilitate the identification of those individuals who might be at risk for prolonged grief or negative psychosocial outcomes, thus permitting early intervention and ongoing support.[158]

The development of hospital-based pediatric bereavement programs is also consistent with recommendations for best practice guidelines for hospital-based bereavement care.[157] Within the framework of prevention, the primary goal of bereavement programs is to help bereaved parents and families adapt to the permanent absence of their child.[158] An "education, guidance and support model"[159] lends itself to a building-block approach where different components can be added as funding and resources become available. The essential components of a pediatric-focused institution-based bereavement program is outlined in Box 15.6.[158]

There are many challenges to developing a bereavement program. New or growing programs need to identify champions who can promote and sustain the program. Securing regular funding for a bereavement coordinator position and required materials may also be difficult. Other challenges include identifying deceased patients and tracking family contact information, accessing the hospital-based supports (especially if families live some distance away), dealing with the emotional difficulty some families have upon returning to the hospital, addressing expected and unexpected death, and determining the timing and frequency of contact and the format of the program. Bereaved parents may be key stakeholders in creating and expanding a bereavement program as well as in developing supportive materials for other families that experienced the death of a child.[160] It is recommended that pediatric programs maintain flexibility in terms of range, timing, location, and types of services offered, including services for fathers, siblings, and grandparents.[157] If it is not feasible to offer support groups or individual counseling within the hospital, someone from the interdisciplinary team should work to identify local community-based organizations that provide these services. Making a referral is especially important given that many parents simply may not have the energy to make contact themselves in the initial weeks and months following the death of their child. Having a clinician from the organization call the family facilitates outreach. If a family member declines a referral, pass along the contact/or connection information for local community-based organizations that provide these services so that the family may access these at a later date.

SUPPORT FOR THE CARE TEAM

THE EXPERIENCE OF GRIEF AND LOSS FOR THE CARE TEAM

Working with families through death and bereavement can be treacherous ground for clinicians from all disciplines, especially for those who are inexperienced or poorly supported. Although witnessing suffering may be unavoidable when caring for seriously ill children, exposure to suffering can have a profound effect on clinicians and is often referred to as the "cost of caring."[161] Caring for seriously ill children frequently evokes painful reactions of inadequacy, helplessness, and even guilt and can contribute to burnout in clinicians[162] (see Chapter 12).

Healthcare providers, particularly physicians, have historically found it difficult to discuss their feelings with colleagues, close friends, or even spouses and instead discuss technical difficulties in treatment.[163,164] The ability to handle the stresses associated with caring for patients and avoid resorting to maladaptive defenses is important as the patient

BOX 15.6 ESSENTIAL COMPONENTS OF A HOSPITAL-BASED BEREAVEMENT PROGRAM

1. Acknowledgment of the death of the patient by the hospital, including a formal hospital letter of condolence and individual or group sympathy cards from members of the care team who knew the child and family.
2. Psychoeducational information about the experience of grief, including written materials, web-based information, and seminars for families about coping with grief and loss.
3. Support services, including the invitation to meet with the team, individual support, group programs, and meeting with peer mentors; information about community-based resources (individual counseling, support groups, camps etc.), and memorial services.
4. Staff support and education about the nature of grief, offering condolences, and self-care strategies for clinicians, including debriefing opportunities after a difficult death.

Adapted with permission from Morris SE, Dole OR, Joselow M, Duncan J, Renaud K, Branowicki P. The development of a hospital-wide bereavement program: ensuring bereavement care for all families of pediatric patients. *J Pediatr Health Care.* 2017;31(1):88–95.158

can rarely be helped without meaningful relationships that entail emotional involvement on the part of the medical provider.[165] It is therefore critical that clinicians closely monitor their own reactions and expressed beliefs and withhold judgment about the way a family grieves. Consultation with a colleague from a mental health discipline can be valuable in maintaining perspective when working with families in crisis.[166] Furthermore, while many families feel honored and moved at witnessing professionals' grief for their child, this compassion must be demonstrated without taking over and superseding the family's own intensity. Clinicians can judge the appropriateness of their involvement in response to the question: "Whose needs are being served?" The answer is unequivocally, "The family's."[32] This balanced perspective is an absolute of effective bereavement intervention.

SUPPORTIVE INTERVENTIONS FOR STAFF

Processing the death of patients is important to prevent burnout and compassion fatigue. Clinicians must develop coping strategies to help them deal with distressing emotions that inevitably arise when caring for seriously ill and dying children and their families. With repeated and cumulative exposure to suffering and death, self-care is the foundation for being able to sustain oneself, grow personally, and care for others (see also Chapter 12).

Adopting a prevention framework, clinicians from all disciplines should receive ongoing training to address the importance of self-care as a core competency and learn how to incorporate these strategies into their daily lives, both at work and at home. Taking appropriate breaks or vacations, spending time in mindful meditation, completing self-help interventions,[167] sharing personal/professional struggles with colleagues, and seeking necessary medical and mental health treatment should be viewed as a marker of professionalism, not a sign of weakness.[168] Fortunately, hospital programs are beginning to implement interventions in an attempt to combat burnout and improve well-being. Peer support has begun to gain traction as a mechanism for improving well-being in medicine.[169] At the same time, institutions must also examine workplace practices and provide opportunities for clinicians to reduce tasks that are inefficient and draining while focusing on clinical practice that is effective and rewarding.[166]

Supportive interventions for staff fall into three categories: institutional strategies, team-based strategies, and individual strategies. Institutional strategies include the provision of employee assistance programs and opportunities for staff to attend continuing education courses about serious illness, end-of-life care, and bereavement. Other strategies include discipline-specific education sessions or debriefings or interdisciplinary case forums such as Schwartz Center Rounds[170,171] (https://www.theschwartzcenter.org/programs/schwartz-rounds). Memorial services to commemorate the children who have died are also a tribute to the staff members who cared for them. These events can be a time for both grieving and for the renewal of professional commitment.

> It is my pleasure to help out and to meet these families again. The spirit of this gathering is so beautiful, and I love to feel shaken by emotions and let the emotions overwhelm me, instead of restraining them as we need to when working in the hospital. (Social worker)

Team-based strategies are tailored to meet the specific needs of the team and may vary depending on the cause of death and the length of the relationship between the team and the patient and family. They include informal and formal debriefing opportunities, memorial services for staff and families, and bereavement rounds. These events are times in which patients are remembered, and clinicians are encouraged to discuss how their deaths impacted them personally and professionally while also identifying those family members potentially at risk of a difficult bereavement outcome.[172]

Finally, individual strategies ideally include practices at both work and home. Supportive work practices may include speaking to a psychosocial provider or chaplain during a patient's end-of-life period or debriefing with a peer or supervisor after a difficult situation. A role exists, therefore, for mental health clinicians and chaplains in supporting team members throughout the child's illness and following their death.

> I've had Jewish and Hindu doctors, Catholic and Muslim nurses, Protestant and secular social workers, Christian and non-believing child life specialists, Buddhist and Bahai respiratory therapists (and almost every other combination of belief and profession within the interdisciplinary team!) seek spiritual

support for themselves—not only for the children and families they care for. (Hospital chaplain)

Other strategies include creating a pause during the day to spend time away from the workplace or following a patient's death and offering condolences by either making bereavement calls or writing condolence cards.[133] At home, strategies for healthcare professions include limiting access to email and reaching out for professional help if feeling overwhelmed. Each of these strategies can reduce stress and decrease the risk for burnout while also fostering personal growth and well-being. For each person, different types of situations, cases, or deaths will trigger deep emotional reactions or distress. Some self-care strategies are listed in Box 15.7.

CONCLUSION AND FUTURE DIRECTIONS

Bereavement is a process of converting presence into absence, actuality into memory. Families must construct a narrative of the child's life and a framework for memories of the child that can endure over a lifetime. There remain many unanswered questions about how best to support parents, siblings, and other individuals affected by the death of a child. Opportunities abound for future research and development of interventions to improve both short- and long-term outcomes in bereaved parents. What is clear is that most individuals, adults and children alike, demonstrate remarkable resilience in their emergence from the child's death. They derive strength from the deep commitment of the clinicians who care for them.

BOX 15.7 SELF-CARE STRATEGIES TO MAINTAIN A HEALTHY WORK-LIFE "BALANCE"

- Let go of overinvolvement: Set personal limits, create personal boundaries, pick and choose.
- Create a "feel good" email folder.
- Find and nurture real friendships—engage with social events.
- Patch minor differences as they occur.
- Ask for help—we are generally not very good at this.
- Work toward a balanced life—fill up, empty out, fill up, empty out.
- Embrace spirituality—it can be watching the waves come in, observing the sunrise or sunset, listening to birds migrate.
- Be mindful—be 100% present in what you are doing.
- Ask yourself when the last time was when you had fun. What can you do to have fun "now"?
- Sit down for breakfast.
- Pack a healthy snack.
- Clear your desk before you leave, if you can; create a tomorrow "to-do" list.
- Make your transition to home peaceful and restorative.
- Schedule at least one "down time" event during the week.
- Read for pleasure.
- Play music that relaxes you while working.
- Walk outside whenever you can—even around the block between patients.
- Take "mini" vacations.
- Send a sweet note to someone you know is hurting.

ACKNOWLEDGMENTS

Portions of this chapter are reprinted from B. Sourkes (1982), *The Deepening Shade: Psychological Aspects of Life-Threatening Illness*, with permission from the University of Pittsburgh Press. We would like to acknowledge the patients, their family members and staff who so courageously shared their inner lives with us.

REFERENCES

1. Raphael B. *The Anatomy of Bereavement*. Basic Books; 1994.
2. Rando T, ed. *Parental Loss of a Child*. Research Press; 1986.
3. Rando TA. An investigation of grief and adaptation in parents whose children have died from cancer. *J Pediatr Psychol*. 1983;8(1):3–20.
4. Snaman JM, Kaye EC, Torres C, Gibson D, Baker JN. Parental grief following the death of a child from cancer: The ongoing odyssey. *Pediatr Blood Cancer*. 2016;63(9):1594–1602.
5. Wolfe J, Grier HE, Klar N, et al. Symptoms and suffering at the end of life in children with cancer. *N Engl J Med*. 2000;342(5):326–333.
6. Contro N, Larson J, Scofield S, Sourkes B, Cohen H. Family perspectives on the quality of pediatric palliative care. *Arch Pediatr Adolesc Med*. 2002;156(1):14–19.
7. Kreicbergs U, Valdimarsdóttir U, Steineck G, Henter J-I. A population-based nationwide study of parents' perceptions of a questionnaire on their child's death due to cancer. *Lancet*. 2004;364(9436):787–789.
8. Field M, Behrman, RE. *When Children Die: Improving Palliative and End-of-Life Care for Children and Their Families*. National Academies Press; 2003.
9. Kreicbergs U, Valdimarsdottir U, Onelov E, Bjork O, Steineck G, Henter JI. Care-related distress: A nationwide study of parents who lost their child to cancer. *J Clin Oncol*. 2005;23(36):9162–9171.
10. Kreicbergs UC, Lannen P, Onelov E, Wolfe J. Parental grief after losing a child to cancer: Impact of professional and social support on long-term outcomes. *J Clin Oncol*. 2007;25(22):3307–3312.
11. Pohlkamp L, Kreicbergs U, Sveen J. Factors during a child's illness are associated with levels of prolonged grief symptoms in bereaved mothers and fathers. *J Clin Oncol*. 2020;38(2):137–144.
12. Pohlkamp L, Kreicbergs U, Sveen J. Bereaved mothers and fathers' prolonged grief and psychological health 1 to 5 years after loss-a nationwide study. *Psychooncology*. 2019;28(7):1530–1536.
13. D'Agostino NM, Berlin-Romalis D, Jovcevska V, Barrera M. Bereaved parents' perspectives on their needs. *Palliat Support Care*. 2008;6(1):33–41.
14. Snaman JM, Kaye EC, Torres C, Gibson DV, Baker JN. Helping parents live with the hole in their heart: The role of health care providers and institutions in the bereaved parents' grief journeys. *Cancer*. 2016;122(17):2757–2765.
15. Snaman J, Morris SE, Rosenberg AR, Holder R, Baker J, Wolfe J. Reconsidering early parental grief following the death of a child from cancer: A new framework for future research and bereavement support. *Support Care Cancer*. 2019.
16. Wiener L, Tager J, Mack J, Battles H, Bedoya SZ, Gerhardt CA. Helping parents prepare for their child's end of life: A

retrospective survey of cancer-bereaved parents. *Pediatr Blood Cancer.* 2020;67(2):e27993.
17. Hynson JL, Aroni R, Bauld C, Sawyer SM. Research with bereaved parents: A question of how not why. *Palliat Med.* 2006;20(8):805–811.
18. Weaver MS, Mooney-Doyle K, Kelly KP, et al. The benefits and burdens of pediatric palliative care and end-of-life research: A systematic review. *J Palliat Med.* 2019;22(8):915–926.
19. Jager J, Battles H, Bedoya SZ, Gerhardt CA, Young-Saleme T, Wiener L. Participation in online research examining end-of-life experiences: Is it beneficial, burdensome, or both for parents bereaved by childhood cancer? *J Pediatr Oncol Nurs.* 2019;36(3):170–177.
20. Moules NJ, Laing CM, McCaffrey G, Tapp DM, Strother D. Grandparents' experiences of childhood cancer, part 1: Doubled and silenced. *J Pediatr Oncol Nurs.* 2012;29(3):119–132.
21. Moules NJ, McCaffrey G, Laing CM, Tapp DM, Strother D. Grandparents' experiences of childhood cancer, part 2: The need for support. *J Pediatr Oncol Nurs.* 2012;29(3):133–140.
22. Rosen EJ. *Families Facing Death.* Revised ed. Jossey-Bass; 1998.
23. Rosof BD. *The Worst Loss.* Henry Holt; 1994.
24. O'Connor K, Barrera M. Changes in parental self-identity following the death of a child to cancer. *Death Stud.* 2014;38(6–10):404–411.
25. Doka A, Tucci, A. *Living with Grief: Children and Adolescents.* Hospice Foundation of America; 2008.
26. Buckle J, Fleming, SJ. *Parenting After the Death of a Child: A Practioner's Guide.* Routledge; 2011.
27. Crawley LM. Racial, cultural, and ethnic factors influencing end-of-life care. *J Palliat Med.* 2005;8(Suppl 1):S58–69.
28. Tervalon M, Murray-Garcia J. Cultural humility versus cultural competence: A critical distinction in defining physician training outcomes in multicultural education. *J Health Care Poor Underserved.* 1998;9(2):117–125.
29. Wiener L, McConnell DG, Latella L, Ludi E. Cultural and religious considerations in pediatric palliative care. *Palliat Support Care.* 2013;11(1):47–67.
30. Al-Gamal E. Quality of life and anticipatory grieving among parents living with a child with cerebral palsy. *Int J Nurs Pract.* 2013;19(3):288–294.
31. Al-Gamal E, Long T. Anticipatory grieving among parents living with a child with cancer. *J Adv Nurs.* 2010;66(9):1980–1990.
32. Sourkes B. *The Deepening Shade: Psychological Aspects of Life-Threatening Illness.* Pittsburgh University of Pittsburgh Press; 1982.
33. Aldrich CE. Some dynamics of anticipatory grief. In Schoenberg B, Carr, A., Kutscher, A., eds. *Anticipatory Grief.* Columbia University Press; 1974.
34. Rando TA. *Clinical Dimensions of Anticipatory Mourning: Theory and Practice in Working with the Dying, Their Loved Ones, and Their Caregivers.* Research Press Company; 2000.
35. Huntley T. *Helping Children Grieve: When Someone They Love Dies.* Augsburg; 2002.
36. Kemp DM. *Children Are . . . Images of Grace: A Pediatrician's Trilogy of Faith, Hope and Love.* MI Zonderman Publishing; 1996.
37. Grossoehme D. *The Pastoral Care of Children.* Haworthe Pastoral Press; 1999.
38. Holden JM, Watterson J, Chrastek J. Tell the children [In Process Citation]. *J Clin Oncol.* 2000;18(17):3193–3195.
39. Long KA, Lehmann V, Gerhardt CA, Carpenter AL, Marsland AL, Alderfer MA. Psychosocial functioning and risk factors among siblings of children with cancer: An updated systematic review. *Psycho-oncology.* 2018;27(6):1467–1479.
40. Alderfer MA, Hodges JA. Supporting siblings of children with cancer: A need for family-school partnerships. *School Ment Health.* 2010;2(2):72–81.
41. Johnson LM, Torres C, Sykes A, Gibson DV, Baker JN. The bereavement experience of adolescents and early young adults with cancer: Peer and parental loss due to death is associated with increased risk of adverse psychological outcomes. *PloS One.* 2017;12(8):e0181024.
42. Akard TF, Dietrich MS, Friedman DL, et al. Digital storytelling: An innovative legacy-making intervention for children with cancer. *Pediatr Blood Cancer.* 2015;62(4):658–665.
43. Akard TF, Wray S, Friedman DL, et al. Transforming a Face-to-Face Legacy Intervention to a Web-Based Legacy Intervention for Children With Advanced Cancer. *J Hosp Palliat Nurs.* 2020;22(1):49–60.
44. Smith LE, Maybach AM, Feldman A, Darling A, Akard TF, Gilmer MJ. Parent and Child Preferences and Styles of Communication About Cancer Diagnoses and Treatment. *J Pediatr Oncol Nurs.* 2019;36(6):390–401.
45. Ellis R, Leventhal B. Information needs and decision-making preferences of children with cancer. *Psycho-oncology.* 1993;2:277–284.
46. Wicks L, Mitchell A. The adolescent cancer experience: Loss of control and benefit finding. *Eur J Cancer Care.* 2010;19(6):778–785.
47. Foster TL, Gilmer MJ, Davies B, et al. Bereaved parents' and siblings' reports of legacies created by children with cancer. *J Pediatr Oncol Nurs.* 2009;26(6) 369–376.
48. Wiener L, Zadeh S, Battles H, et al. Allowing adolescents and young adults to plan their end-of-life care. *Pediatrics.* 2012;130(5):897–905.
49. Zadeh S, Pao M, Wiener L. Opening end-of-life discussions: How to introduce Voicing My CHOiCES, an advance care planning guide for adolescents and young adults. *Palliat Support Care.* 2015;13(3):591–599.
50. Broniscer A, Baker JN, Baker SJ, et al. Prospective collection of tissue samples at autopsy in children with diffuse intrinsic pontine glioma. *Cancer.* 2010;116(19):4632–4637.
51. Caretti V, Jansen MH, van Vuurden DG, et al. Implementation of a multi-institutional diffuse intrinsic pontine glioma autopsy protocol and characterization of a primary cell culture. *Neuropathol Applied Neurobiol.* 2013;39(4):426–436.
52. Angelini P, Hawkins C, Laperriere N, Bouffet E, Bartels U. Post mortem examinations in diffuse intrinsic pontine glioma: Challenges and chances. *J Neuro-Oncol.* 2011;101(1):75–81.
53. Wiener L, Sweeney C, Baird K, et al. What do parents want to know when considering autopsy for their child with cancer? *J Pediatr Hematol Oncol.* 2014;36(6):464–470.
54. Baker JN, Windham JA, Hinds PS, et al. Bereaved parents' intentions and suggestions about research autopsies in children with lethal brain tumors. *J Pediatr.* 2013;163(2):581–586.
55. Foster TL, Gilmer MJ, Davies B, et al. Comparison of continuing bonds reported by parents and siblings after a child's death from cancer. *Death Stud.* 2011;35(5):420–440.
56. Foster TL, Dietrich MS, Friedman DL, Gordon JE, Gilmer MJ. National survey of children's hospitals on legacy-making activities. *J Palliat Med.* 2012;15(5):573–578.
57. Akard TF, Gilmer MJ, Friedman DL, Given B, Hendricks-Ferguson VL, Hinds PS. From qualitative work to intervention development in pediatric oncology palliative care research. *J Pediatr Oncol Nurs.* 2013;30(3):153–160.
58. Rosenberg A, Jones, B, Wolfe, J. Palliative care for children with cancer and their families. In Abrams AN, Muriel, AC, Wiener L, eds. *Textbook for Multidisciplinary Care.* Springer International Publishing; 2016:243–264.
59. Hinds PS, Oakes LL, Hicks J, et al. "Trying to be a good parent" as defined by interviews with parents who made phase I, terminal care, and resuscitation decisions for their children. *J Clin Oncol.* 2009;27(35):5979–5985.
60. Foster TL, Bell CJ, Gilmer MJ. Symptom management of spiritual suffering in pediatric palliative care. *J Hosp Palliat Nurs.* 2012;14(2):116–117.
61. Mitchell K, Anderson, H. *All Our Losses, All Our Griefs: Resources for Pastoral Care.* Westminster Press; 1983.
62. Klass D. *Parental Grief: Solace and Resolution.* Springer; 1988.
63. Wheeler I. Parental bereavement: The crisis of meaning. *Death Stud.* 2001;25(1):51–66.
64. Middleton W, Raphael B, Burnett P, Martinek N. A longitudinal study comparing bereavement phenomena in recently bereaved

spouses, adult children and parents. *Aust N Z J Psychiatry.* 1998;32(2):235–241.

65. Morris S, Fletcher K, Goldstein R. The Grief of Parents After the Death of a Young Child. *J Clin Psychol Med Settings.* 2019;26(3):321–338.
66. Jalmsell L, Kreicbergs U, Onelov E, Steineck G, Henter JI. Symptoms affecting children with malignancies during the last month of life: A nationwide follow-up. *Pediatrics.* 2006;117(4):1314–1320.
67. Hendrickson KC. Morbidity, mortality, and parental grief: A review of the literature on the relationship between the death of a child and the subsequent health of parents. *Palliat Support Care.* 2009;7(1):109–119.
68. Lannen PK, Wolfe J, Prigerson HG, Onelov E, Kreicbergs UC. Unresolved grief in a national sample of bereaved parents: Impaired mental and physical health 4 to 9 years later. *J Clin Oncol.* 2008;26(36):5870–5876.
69. Youngblut JM, Brooten D, Cantwell GP, del Moral T, Totapally B. Parent health and functioning 13 months after infant or child NICU/PICU death. *Pediatrics.* 2013;132(5):e1295–1301.
70. Brooten D, Youngblut JM, Caicedo C, Del Moral T, Cantwell GP, Totapally B. Parents' Acute Illnesses, Hospitalizations, and Medication Changes During the Difficult First Year After Infant or Child NICU/PICU Death. *Am J Hospice Palliat Care.* 2018;35(1):75–82.
71. Goodenough B, Drew D, Higgins S, Trethewie S. Bereavement outcomes for parents who lose a child to cancer: Are place of death and sex of parent associated with differences in psychological functioning? Psychooncology. 2004;13(11):779–791.
72. Alam R, Barrera M, D'Agostino N, Nicholas DB, Schneiderman G. Bereavement experiences of mothers and fathers over time after the death of a child due to cancer. *Death Stud.* 2012;36(1):1–22.
73. Li J, Hansen D, Mortensen PB, Olsen J. Myocardial infarction in parents who lost a child: A nationwide prospective cohort study in Denmark. *Circulation.* 2002;106(13):1634–1639.
74. Li J, Johansen C, Hansen D, Olsen J. Cancer incidence in parents who lost a child: A nationwide study in Denmark. *Cancer.* 2002;95(10):2237–2242.
75. Li J, Johnsen SP, Olsen J. Stroke in parents who lost a child: A nationwide follow-up study in Denmark. *Neuroepidemiology.* 2003;22(3):211–216.
76. Dussel V, Bona K, Heath JA, Hilden JM, Weeks JC, Wolfe J. Unmeasured costs of a child's death: Perceived financial burden, work disruptions, and economic coping strategies used by American and Australian families who lost children to cancer. *J Clin Oncol.* 2011;29(8):1007–1013.
77. Davies R. New understandings of parental grief: Literature review. *J Adv Nurs.* 2004;46(5):506–513.
78. Fletcher PN. Experiences in family bereavement. *Fam Community Health.* 2002;25(1):57–70.
79. Bjork M, Sundler AJ, Hallstrom I, Hammarlund K. Like being covered in a wet and dark blanket - parents' lived experiences of losing a child to cancer. *Eur J Oncol Nurs.* 2016;25:40–45.
80. Lang A, Goulet C, Amsel R. Explanatory model of health in bereaved parents post-fetal/infant death. *Int J Nurs Stud.* 2004;41(8):869–880.
81. Rosenberg AR, Baker KS, Syrjala K, Wolfe J. Systematic review of psychosocial morbidities among bereaved parents of children with cancer. *Pediatr Blood Cancer.* 2012;58(4):503–512.
82. Kubler-Ross E. *On Death and Dying.* Macmillan; 1969.
83. Kessler D, Kubler-Ross E. *On Grief and Grieving: Finding the Meaning of Grief Through the Five Stages of Loss.* Scribner; 2005.
84. Stroebe M, Schut H. The dual process model of coping with bereavement: Rationale and description. *Death Stud.* 1999;23(3):197–224.
85. Field NP, Gao B, Paderna L. Continuing bonds in bereavement: An attachment theory-based perspective. *Death Stud.* 2005;29(4):277–299.
86. Stroebe M, Schut H, Boerner K. Continuing bonds in adaptation to bereavement: Toward theoretical integration. *Clin Psychol Rev.* 2010;30(2):259–268.
87. Barrera M, O'Connor K, D'Agostino NM, et al. Early parental adjustment and bereavement after childhood cancer death. *Death Stud.* 2009;33(6):497–520.
88. Klass D. Solace and immortality: Bereaved parents' continuing bonds with their children. *Death Stud.* 1993;17(4):343–368.
89. Foster TL, Gilmer MJ. Continuing bonds: A human response within paediatric palliative care. *Int J Palliat Nurs.* 2008;14(2):85–91.
90. Li J, Precht DH, Mortensen PB, Olsen J. Mortality in parents after death of a child in Denmark: A nationwide follow-up study. *Lancet.* 2003;361(9355):363–367.
91. Gilmer MJ, Foster TL, Vannatta K, et al. Changes in parents after the death of a child from cancer. *J Pain Sympt Manage.* 2012;44(4):572–582.
92. Eilegard A, Kreicbergs U. Risk of parental dissolution of partnership following the loss of a child to cancer: A population-based long-term follow-up. *Arch Pediatr Adolesc Med.* 2010;164(1):100–101.
93. Buyukcan-Tetik A, Finkenauer C, Schut H, Stroebe M, Stroebe W. The impact of bereaved parents' perceived grief similarity on relationship satisfaction. *J Fam Psychol.* 2017;31(4):409–419.
94. Barrera M, D'Agostino NM, Schneiderman G, Tallett S, Spencer L, Jovcevska V. Patterns of parental bereavement following the loss of a child and related factors. *Omega (Westport).* 2007;55(2):145–167.
95. Kreicbergs U, Valdimarsdottir U, Onelov E, Henter JI, Steineck G. Anxiety and depression in parents 4–9 years after the loss of a child owing to a malignancy: A population-based follow-up. *Psychol Med.* 2004;34(8):1431–1441.
96. Pohlkamp L, Kreicbergs U, Prigerson HG, Sveen J. Psychometric properties of the Prolonged Grief Disorder-13 (PG-13) in bereaved Swedish parents. *Psychiatry Res.* 2018;267:560–565.
97. Michon B, Balkou S, Hivon R, Cyr C. Death of a child: Parental perception of grief intensity—end-of-life and bereavement care. *Paediatr Child Health.* 2003;8(6):363–366.
98. Snaman JM, Torres C, Duffy B, Levine DR, Gibson DV, Baker JN. Parental perspectives of communication at the end of life at a pediatric oncology institution. *J Palliat Med.* 2016;19(3):326–332.
99. Mack JW, Joffe S. Communicating about prognosis: Ethical responsibilities of pediatricians and parents. *Pediatrics.* 2014;133(Suppl 1):S24–30.
100. Mack JW, Hilden JM, Watterson J, et al. Parent and physician perspectives on quality of care at the end of life in children with cancer. *J Clin Oncol.* 2005;23(36):9155–9161.
101. Mack JW, Cronin AM, Kang TI. Decisional regret among parents of children with cancer. *J Clin Oncol.* 2016;34(33):4023–4029.
102. van der Geest IM, Darlington AS, Streng IC, Michiels EM, Pieters R, van den Heuvel-Eibrink MM. Parents' experiences of pediatric palliative care and the impact on long-term parental grief. *J Pain Sympt Manage.* 2014;47(6):1043–1053.
103. deCinque N, Monterosso L, Dadd G, Sidhu R, Lucas R. Bereavement support for families following the death of a child from cancer: Practice characteristics of Australian and New Zealand paediatric oncology units. *J Paediatr Child Health.* 2004;40(3):131–135.
104. Valdimarsdottir U, Kreicbergs U, Hauksdottir A, et al. Parents' intellectual and emotional awareness of their child's impending death to cancer: A population-based long-term follow-up study. *Lancet Oncol.* 2007;8(8):706–714.
105. Kreicbergs U, Valdimarsdottir U, Onelov E, Henter JI, Steineck G. Talking about death with children who have severe malignant disease. *N Engl J Med.* 2004;351(12):1175–1186.
106. Surkan PJ, Dickman PW, Steineck G, Onelov E, Kreicbergs U. Home care of a child dying of a malignancy and parental awareness of a child's impending death. *Palliat Med.* 2006;20(3):161–169
107. Dussel V, Kreicbergs U, Hilden JM, et al. Looking beyond where children die: Determinants and effects of planning a child's location of death. *J Pain Symptom Manage.* 2009;37(1):33–43.
108. McCarthy MC, Clarke NE, Ting CL, Conroy R, Anderson VA, Heath JA. Prevalence and predictors of parental grief and depression after the death of a child from cancer. *J Palliat Med.* 2010;13(11):1321–1326.
109. Vegsund HK, Reinfjell T, Moksnes UK, Wallin AE, Hjemdal O, Eilertsen MB. Resilience as a predictive factor towards a healthy adjustment to grief after the loss of a child to cancer. *PloS One.* 2019;14(3):e0214138.

110. Rosen H. *Unspoken Grief: Coping with Sibling Loss.* Lexington Books; 1986.
111. Davies B. *Shadows in the Sun: The Experiences of Sibling Bereavement in Childhood.* Brunner/Maze; 1999.
112. DeVita-Raeburn E. *The Empty Room: Understanding Sibling Loss.* Scribner; 2004.
113. Patterson P, McDonald FEJ, Costa DSJ, Tindle R, Allison KR, Morris SE. Initial validation of a needs instrument for young people bereaved by familial cancer. *Support Care Cancer.* 2019;28(8):3637–3648.
114. Hogan NS, Schmidt LA, Howard Sharp KM, et al. Development and testing of the Hogan Inventory of Bereavement short form for children and adolescents. *Death Stud.* 2021;45(4):313–321. Epub July 5, 2019.
115. Wilkins KL, Woodgate RL. A review of qualitative research on the childhood cancer experience from the perspective of siblings: A need to give them a voice. *J Pediatr Oncol Nurs.* 2005;22(6):305–319.
116. Nolbris M, Hellstrom AL. Siblings' needs and issues when a brother or sister dies of cancer. *J Pediatr Oncol Nurs.* 2005;22(4):227–233.
117. Alderfer MA, Long KA, Lown EA, et al. Psychosocial adjustment of siblings of children with cancer: A systematic review. *Psychooncology.* 2010;19(8):789–805.
118. Steele AC, Kaal J, Thompson AL, et al. Bereaved parents and siblings offer advice to health care providers and researchers. *J Pediatr Hematol Oncol.* 2013;35(4):253–259.
119. Rosenberg AR, Postier A, Osenga K, et al. Long-term psychosocial outcomes among bereaved siblings of children with cancer. *J Pain Sympt Manage.* 2015;49(1):55–65.
120. Ballard KL. Meeting the needs of siblings of children with cancer. *Pediatr Nurs.* 2004;30(5):394–401.
121. Sveen J, Eilegard A, Steineck G, Kreicbergs U. They still grieve-a nationwide follow-up of young adults 2-9 years after losing a sibling to cancer. *Psychooncology.* 2014;23(6):658–664.
122. Foster TL, Gilmer MJ, Vannatta K, et al. Changes in siblings after the death of a child from cancer. *Cancer Nurs.* 2012;35(5):347–354.
123. Alkard TF, Skeens MA, Fortney CA, et al. Changes in siblings over time after the death of a brother or sister from cancer. *Cancer Nurs.* 2018.
124. Bolton JM, Spiwak R, Sareen J. Consequences of sibling death: Problematic, potentially predictable, and poorly managed. *JAMA Pediatr.* 2017;171(6):519–520.
125. Eilegard A, Steineck G, Nyberg T, Kreicbergs U. Psychological health in siblings who lost a brother or sister to cancer 2 to 9 years earlier. *Psychooncology.* 2013;22(3):683–691.
126. Yu Y, Liew Z, Cnattingius S, et al. Association of mortality with the death of a sibling in childhood. *JAMA Pediatr.* 2017;171(6):538–545.
127. Alderfer MA, Stanley C, Conroy R, et al. The social functioning of siblings of children with cancer: A multi-informant investigation. *J Pediatr Psychol.* 2015;40(3):309–319.
128. Gerhardt CA, Fairclough DL, Grossenbacher JC, et al. Peer relationships of bereaved siblings and comparison classmates after a child's death from cancer. *J Pediatr Psychol.* 2012;37(2):209–219.
129. MacLeod KD, Whitsett SF, Mash EJ, Pelletier W. Pediatric sibling donors of successful and unsuccessful hematopoietic stem cell transplants (HSCT): A qualitative study of their psychosocial experience. *J Pediatr Psychol.* 2003;28(4):223–230.
130. Wiener LS, Steffen-Smith E, Fry T, Wayne AS. Hematopoietic stem cell donation in children: A review of the sibling donor experience. *J Psychosoc Oncol.* 2007;25(1):45–66.
131. Weaver MS, Diekema DS, Carr A, Triplett B. Matched marrow, sibling shadow: The epidemiology, experience, and ethics of sibling donors of stem cells. *J Adolesc Young Adult Oncol.* 2015;4(3):100–104.
132. Contro N, Scofield, S. The power of their voices: Child and family assessment in pediatric palliative care. In Goldman A, Haines, R, Liben, S, eds. *Oxford Textbook of Pediatric Palliative Care.* Oxford University Press; 2006:143–153.
133. Weaver MS, Lichtenthal WG, Larson K, Wiener L. How I approach expressing condolences and longitudinal remembering to a family after the death of a child. *Pediatr Blood Cancer.* 2019;66(2):e27489.
134. Endo K, Yonemoto N, Yamada M. Interventions for bereaved parents following a child's death: A systematic review. *Palliat Med.* 2015;29(7):590–604.
135. Lichtenthal WG, Corner GW, Sweeney CR, et al. Mental health services for parents who lost a child to cancer: If we build them, will they come? *J Clin Oncol.* 2015;33(20):2246–2253.
136. Snaman J, Kaye, EC, Torres, C, Gibson, DV, Baker, JN. Helping parents live with the hole in their heart: The role of health care providers and institutions in bereaved parents' grief journeys. *Cancer.* 2016;122(17):2757–2765.
137. Prigerson HG, Horowitz MJ, Jacobs SC, et al. Prolonged grief disorder: Psychometric validation of criteria proposed for DSM-V and ICD-11. *PLoS Med.* 2009;6(8):e1000121.
138. Breitbart W, Pessin H, Rosenfeld B, et al. Individual meaning-centered psychotherapy for the treatment of psychological and existential distress: A randomized controlled trial in patients with advanced cancer. *Cancer.* 2018;124(15):3231–3239.
139. Breitbart W, Poppito, SR. *Individual Meaning-Centered Psychotherapy for Patients with Advanced Cancer: A Treatment Manual.* Oxford University Press; 2014.
140. Frankl V. *Man's Search for Meaning: An Introduction to Logotherapy.* 4th ed. Beacon Press; 1992.
141. Lichtenthal WG, Breitbart W. The central role of meaning in adjustment to the loss of a child to cancer: Implications for the development of meaning-centered grief therapy. *Curr Opin Support Palliat Care.* 2015;9(1):46–51.
142. Lichtenthal WG, Catarozoli C, Masterson M, et al. An open trial of meaning-centered grief therapy: Rationale and preliminary evaluation. *Palliat Support Care.* 2019;17(1):2–12.
143. Morris AT, Gabert-Quillen C, Friebert S, Carst N, Delahanty DL. The indirect effect of positive parenting on the relationship between parent and sibling bereavement outcomes after the death of a child. *J Pain Sympt Manage.* 2016;51(1):60–70.
144. Howard Sharp KM, Russell C, Keim M, et al. Grief and growth in bereaved siblings: Interactions between different sources of social support. *School Psychology Quarterly.* 2018;33(3):363–371.
145. Schonfeld DJ, Demaria T, Committee on Psychosocial Aspects of Child and Family Health, Disaster Preparedness Advisory Council. Supporting the grieving child and family. *Pediatrics.* 2016;138(3):e20162147.
146. Schonfeld DJ, Quakenbush, M. *After a Loved One Dies—How Children Grieve and How Parents and Other Adults Can Support Them.* New York Life Foundation; 2014.
147. Jensen J, Weng C, Spraker-Perlman HL. A provider-based survey to assess bereavement care knowledge, attitudes, and practices in pediatric oncologists. *J Palliat Med.* 2017;20(3):266–272.
148. Lichtenthal WG, Sweeney CR, Roberts KE, et al. Bereavement follow-up after the death of a child as a standard of care in pediatric oncology. *Pediatr Blood Cancer.* 2015;62(Suppl 5):S834–869.
149. Wiener L, Rosenberg AR, Lichtenthal WG, Tager J, Weaver MS. Personalized and yet standardized: An informed approach to the integration of bereavement care in pediatric oncology settings. *Palliat Support Care.* 2018;16(6):706–711.
150. Contro NA, Larson J, Scofield S, Sourkes B, Cohen HJ. Hospital staff and family perspectives regarding quality of pediatric palliative care. *Pediatrics.* 2004;114(5):1248–1252.
151. Ives T. Just tell me: A bereaved parent's thoughts on expressing condolences and longitudinal remembering to a family after the death of their child. *Pediatr Blood Cancer.* 2019;66(2):e27521.
152. Weaver MS, Lichtenthal WG, Larson K, Wiener L. How I approach expressing condolences and longitudinal remembering to a family after the death of a child. *Pediatr Blood Cancer.* 2018;66(2):e27489.
153. October T, Dryden-Palmer K, Copnell B, Meert KL. Caring for parents after the death of a child. *Pediatr Crit Care Med.* 2018;19(8S Suppl 2):S61–S68.

154. Bedell SE, Cadenhead K, Graboys TB. The doctor's letter of condolence. *N Engl J Med.* 2001;344(15):1162–1164.
155. Agnew A, Manktelow R, Taylor B, Jones L. Bereavement needs assessment in specialist palliative care: A review of the literature. *Palliat Med.* 2010;24(1):46–59.
156. Friebert S, Huff, S. *Standards of Practice for Pediatric Palliative Care: Professional Development and Resource Series.* National Hospice and Palliative Care Organization; 2009.
157. Donovan LA, Wakefield CE, Russell V, Cohn RJ. Hospital-based bereavement services following the death of a child: A mixed study review. *Palliat Med.* 2015;29(3):193–210.
158. Morris SE, Dole OR, Joselow M, Duncan J, Renaud K, Branowicki P. The development of a hospital-wide bereavement program: Ensuring bereavement care for all families of pediatric patients. *J Pediatr Health Care.* 2017;31(1):88–95.
159. Morris SE, Block SD. Adding value to palliative care services: The development of an institutional bereavement program. *J Palliat Med.* 2015;18(11):915–922.
160. Snaman JM, Kaye EC, Levine DR, et al. Empowering bereaved parents through the development of a comprehensive bereavement program. *J Pain Sympt Manage.* 2017;53(4):767–775.
161. Costa DK, Moss M. The cost of caring: Emotion, burnout, and psychological distress in critical care clinicians. *Ann Am Thorac Soc.* 2018;15(7):787–790.
162. Maslach C, Leiter MP. Understanding the burnout experience: Recent research and its implications for psychiatry. *World Psychiatry.* 2016;15(2):103–111.
163. Mermann AC. Coping strategies of selected physicians. *Perspect Biol Med.* 1990;33(2):268–279.
164. Fanos JH. "Coming through the fog, coming over the moors": The impact on pediatric oncologists of caring for seriously ill children. *J Cancer Educ.* 2007;22(2):119–123.
165. Marten G, Mauer AM. Interaction of health-care professionals with critically ill children and their parents. *Clinical Pediatrics.* 1982;21:540–544.
166. Muriel AC, Tarquini S, Morris SE. The "liaison" in consultation-liaison psychiatry: Helping medical staff cope with pediatric death. *Child Adolesc Psychiatr Clin N Am.* 2018;27(4):591–598.
167. Shanafelt TD, Kaups KL, Nelson H, et al. An interactive individualized intervention to promote behavioral change to increase personal well-being in US surgeons. *Ann Surg.* 2014;259(1):82–88.
168. Merlo LJ. A piece of my mind: Healing physicians. *JAMA.* 2016;316(23):2489–2490.
169. Shapiro J, Galowitz P. Peer support for clinicians: A programmatic approach. *Acad Med.* 2016;91(9):1200–1204.
170. Lintz KC, Penson RT, Chabner BA, Lynch TJ. Schwartz Center rounds. A staff dialogue on caring for an intensely spiritual patient: Psychosocial issues faced by patients, their families, and caregivers. *Oncologist.* 1998;3(6):439–445.
171. Schwartz Center Rounds can make staff effective. *Nurs Manag (Harrow).* 2017;24(2):7.
172. Morris SE, Kearns JP, Moment A, Lee KA, deLima Thomas J. "Remembrance": A self-care tool for clinicians. *J Palliat Med.* 2019;22(3):316–318.
173. Contro N, Sourkes B. Opportunities for quality improvement in bereavement care at a children's hospital: Assessment of interdisciplinary staff perspectives. *J Palliat Care.* 2012;28(1):28–35.

16 | RESOLVING CONFLICTS IN PEDIATRIC PALLIATIVE CARE

ROBERT MACAULEY, JODY CHRASTEK, AMIE BRANDTJEN, HARVEY COHEN, AND THADDEUS M. POPE

Conflict is inevitable but combat is optional.

MAX LUCADO[1]

Conflict at one level or another is a common occurrence in personal and professional relationships, and the field of interdisciplinary pediatric palliative care (IPPC) is no exception. These conflicts may be structural—involving unequal power, authority, control, and time constraints—as well as relational, in which stereotyping, misinformation, and negative behavior can provoke intense reactions.[2] In general, people are averse to the high emotions that often arise in the face of disagreements. However, when conflict is ignored, trust is compromised, and a minor disagreement can devolve into a fracturing of relationships and a breakdown in communications. Conversely, when appropriately addressed, conflicts can lead to deeper team understanding and cohesion. In these instances, what may initially be viewed as a failure may in fact become an opportunity.

This chapter examines clinical scenarios in which conflict could potentially jeopardize desired outcomes for patients and families. It also identifies practical approaches to identify and work through conflict with the goal of arriving at meaningful patient- and family-centered care plans. This chapter specifically addresses conflicts between families and teams, conflicts between pediatric patients and their parents, and conflicts within teams.

CONFLICTS BETWEEN FAMILIES AND TEAMS

Clinical Vignette

Eric was a 14-year-old boy with Hunter syndrome (mucopolysaccharidosis Type II) who experienced cardiac failure requiring endotracheal intubation and two pressors in the pediatric intensive care unit (PICU). Given the progressive nature of his condition, the critical care and specialty palliative care teams recommended focusing on comfort. Despite being apprised on several occasions of the seriousness of his condition—as well as his poor prognosis—his parents were unwilling to consider any limitation of treatment, including a do-not-attempt-resuscitation (DNAR) order.

As a result, the team experienced moral distress, feeling as if they were causing Eric to needlessly suffer. Discussions with the parents became increasingly heated, to the point where the parents declined offers of future care conferences.

"We know what's best for our son," they told the palliative care consultant, "and we've said all we're going to say."

Cases like Eric's—in which parents request treatment that seems excessively burdensome, especially when a child is dying—are among the most challenging in pediatric palliative care. They often prompt ethics (or even legal) consultation in order to clarify the scope of parental rights. These consultations will likely explore the role of the best interest standard in the care of children who lack decision-making capacity, the increased latitude afforded parents compared to other surrogates, and the threshold for state intervention.[3] (The latter, however, is more often applied to the reverse situation: where the parents refuse treatment that the medical team recommends.) Some hospitals and health systems have formalized protocols for responding to such requests[4] based on professional consensus statements.[5]

Yet, no matter how thoughtful the analysis of ethical obligations and legal recourse, it may be unlikely to sway parents' opinions or meaningfully impact practical outcomes. The reason is that the primary issue here is not one of dueling moralities. Everyone involved in Eric's care—both his parents as well as the members of the medical team—share the same motivation and goal: to do what is best for Eric. The problem is that they have different opinions about what, precisely, that entails.

In that respect, it may feel as if the parents and the clinicians are speaking different languages. Clinicians in particular may respond in the same way that people often do when attempting to communicate with someone who doesn't speak their language by saying the same thing again, louder each time. Rising volume, however, does not produce proportional increase in comprehension. Quite the contrary: it usually leads to entrenchment and heightened conflict.

Navigating such conflict requires what some have called "crucial conversations," referring to discussions in which the stakes are high, opinions vary, and emotions run strong.[6] (By that definition, one might argue that most palliative care conversations are "crucial.") In preparing for such conversations, it is often helpful to "work on oneself first." In other words, rather than trying to change the other person (in this case, Eric's parents), it is incumbent on the palliative care professionals to explore and "own" their personal views and how these might be influencing the conversation. Since one of the primary mandates of palliative care is to ameliorate suffering, the team might understandably be frustrated that they are not able to achieve this goal for Eric. Frustration might then be directed at the perceived obstacle to accomplishing that goal (i.e., his parents), including labeling and judging them. But "judgments of others are alienated expressions of our own unmet needs,"[7] and the best way to avoid making such judgments is to change oneself, not others.

One way that team members can identify their own needs and preconceptions is through thoughtful reflection. This can take many forms, including quiet introspection, writing down one's thoughts about the dilemma, discussion with a close colleague, consultation from a mentor, psychotherapy, and team debriefing. A specific modality that has been used in palliative care is the *Balint group*, named for a British psychoanalyst who recognized that unconscious emotions and misunderstandings produce "secondary effects" on the physician–patient relationship.[8] These groups are composed of several clinicians and a facilitator who meet regularly to discuss an actual case that involves challenging clinician–patient relational dynamics. Whoever has presented the case is required to remain silent during the ensuing discussion, offering the opportunity for additional insight and reflection to previously unrecognized dynamics within the clinical encounter. Studies have shown that the process increases clinicians' coping ability, psychological mindedness, and patient-centeredness.[9] This process can be particularly effective in the training context.[10]

One particularly dangerous assumption—especially in situations where a child may be enduring what is perceived to be burdensome treatment—is thinking on the part of clinicians that, "I would never do that, if he were my child." Such a bias is important to identify because not only is it unhelpful, it may not even be true. For example, nearly 90% of physicians say they would want to forgo resuscitation if they were terminally ill.[11] However, in one study more than one-quarter of physicians who ultimately died were admitted to the ICU.[12]

Thus, there is no way to be sure what we as professionals would do in a certain situation, since we're not actually in that situation. Given professionals' focus on maximizing quality of life—and the recognition of the low likelihood of benefit of certain burdensome treatments—if Eric were our child and that treatment was the only chance he had at survival, we might well make the same decision as his parents.

Furthermore, even if we somehow could be certain that we wouldn't make the same decision, the fact remains that Eric is not our child. Each family comes with its own cultural background, values, beliefs and loss history—all of which affect their decision-making about what is right for their child. Professionals have an obligation to honor the decisions that parents make, within reasonable limits. Only in rare cases will the courts override parental requests for potentially beneficial treatment, although these outliers often gain significant attention due to their unusual nature and often extreme circumstances.[13] In the majority of cases that never go to court, professionals are left either to make peace with a decision that runs contrary to their values or to deepen the conversation with the parents in the hopes of reaching mutual understanding.

In attempting the latter, it might be tempting to provide additional factual information in the belief that if the other person truly understood, then they would agree with the team's recommendations. Such an intellectual approach, however, can often be perceived as criticism or even badgering.[7] Palliative care professionals are well aware that emotional responses often override intellectual analysis, so the first step should be to address the parents' emotional needs.

Eric's parents' refusal to attend future care conferences is a sign that they don't feel safe having such conversations, which in turn has led to their withdrawal from further conversation. Other manifestations of feeling unsafe include masking true feelings through sarcasm and avoiding sensitive topics in conversation. Lack of safety can also lead to violence, usually not in the physical sense—although this has been known to occur—but in the form of controlling or verbally attacking.

To feel safe in a conversation, people need two things: mutual purpose and mutual respect. Both of these are threatened in the interactions with Eric's parents. They might believe the medical team's purpose is to prevent him from continuing to receive life-sustaining treatment—rather than to spare him additional suffering—and do not feel that their viewpoint is respected. "Contrasting statements" may be helpful here, by acknowledging the parents' concern that their beliefs are not being respected and proceeding to confirm that the team does, in fact, deeply value those beliefs and perspectives.[5]

To restore safety, the team can explicitly state what their purpose is: minimizing suffering while continuing to support Eric in ways that might provide benefit. Rather than assuming that his parents share that goal—let alone the means of achieving it—the team can then engage in "humble inquiry." In contrast to the focused (and sometimes leading) questions that medical professionals often ask parents, humble inquiry is "the fine art of drawing someone out, of asking questions to which you do not already know the answer, of building a relationship based on curiosity and interest in the other person."[14] By maximizing curiosity and interest in the other person and their views, the risk of bias and preconceptions is minimized.

This approach also evens the playing field in the conversation. Power dynamics are endemic in the practice of medicine, and conflict often occurs when parents feel that their authority to make decisions for their child is threatened. By inquiring about the parents' values and opinions, palliative care professionals render themselves "temporarily dependent and vulnerable. It is precisely [that] temporary subordination that creates psychological safety for [the parents] and, therefore, increases the chances that [they] will tell [us] what [we] need to know."[15]

What we need to know, in short, is what Eric's parents need. According to the methodology known as *nonviolent communication* (NVC)—with that term used in the Gandhian sense, referring to "our natural state of compassion when violence has subsided from our heart"[7]—feelings stem from unmet needs. In the case of Eric's parents these might include needing to believe they are making the right decisions for Eric, to view themselves as "good parents,"[16] and to minimize the possibility of decisional regret over not having done enough for him.

A starting point is to name the emotion that the parents seem to be expressing and then inquire about what unmet need might be prompting it. One might therefore say, "It seems as if you're upset and frustrated. Can you tell me a little about what is making you feel that way?" There is no judgment in that question, nor any attempt to persuade the parents to change their position. Instead, it is purely an attempt to receive the parents' needs with empathy, a foundational value in palliative care. Such an approach reflects one of the core principles of NVC: "Listen to what people are needing rather than what they are thinking."[7]

If the palliative care professional has not guessed correctly, there is the opportunity for further inquiries about other possible explanations for the parents' response. The primary stimulus may ultimately turn out to be something the palliative care team never considered but that the parents eventually share when they feel respected and honored by the open discussion. The mere process of humble inquiry can, therefore, begin to restore damaged trust. This is a deferential, empathy-based approach, not a technique that guarantees a particular outcome.

Parents themselves may not be aware of what need is unmet, especially if there is an unrecognized trauma or loss history. But once the unmet need is identified, the palliative care team can explore what concrete actions the parent would like taken in order to meet that need. In some instances of profound trauma, extreme care must be exercised in eliciting the issues and may belong in the hands of mental health professionals.

Such openness requires us to accept the possibility that—even after the parents' needs are identified and hopefully met—they may remain steadfast in requesting maximal treatment. In all but the most extreme cases (where state intervention may be considered), this may appear to leave the medical team exactly where it started: watching a child suffer needlessly.

Upon closer analysis, though, the situation has markedly improved in several ways. First, the team is more attuned to their own opinions and preconceptions—including any judgment that had been directed toward the parents—which might have influenced how they were approaching the case. Second, there is deeper trust in the relationship with the parents, thus reopening the lines of communication and allowing for deeper and more candid sharing going forward. Third, this improved communication may allow for exploration of some middle ground that might satisfy the needs of both the team and the parents, such as by continuing intensive treatment while also maximizing symptom management.

Entrenched conflict leads to a black-and-white view of the world, whereas trust-based communication shifts away from "either/or"—referred to in the NVC literature as a "sucker's choice"—toward solutions that satisfy the needs of all parties. An example of this might be a do-not-escalate-treatment (DNET) order, which preserves the parents' hope of recovery while also preventing increased suffering as well as addressing the staff's moral distress. Such a middle ground may address parental concerns for decisional regret by "absolving" them of ultimate responsibility. Thus, when Eric dies, it will be due to his body failing rather than the discontinuation of a treatment he was dependent on.[17] Such an order may make it easier for the parents to consider subsequent further limitations, which in some studies occurs in the majority of cases of DNET orders.[18]

Family Reflection

A mother recounted a disagreement with a physician about placing a DNR order for her son. She vividly explained the implications of that interchange for parents who are faced with making life-and-death decisions for their children. Her son, James, is an 18-year-old with lissencephaly. This conflict occurred when he was about 7 years old and hospitalized. His G-tube was very painful and had been leaking constantly.

"What we put James through sometimes. . . ," I said to his doctor.

"This is a perfect time to be talking about this," he replied.

"No. This is *not* the time to be talking about it. The time to talk about it is when it's *not* something critical happening and I can process things. When something like this happens, your emotions take over and you just want your child treated."

I left and completely disregarded the conversation that had just occurred. The following morning James started hemorrhaging.

"Why isn't anything happening?" I asked his nurse. "Why isn't he being taken to the PICU?"

"Well," the nurse replied, "it's probably because of the DNR."

"What DNR? We talked about it yesterday but . . . I didn't . . . tell me where I consented to it."

"It was an order from the doctor," the nurse explained, showing it to me in the chart.

I told the nurse that I wanted it removed, but he said only a doctor could do that. On my insistence, they did take James to the PICU where he received transfusions and platelets. And the doctor took the DNR order off, but he was not happy about it.

In the conversation the day before, there had been no conclusion. I had no idea that the DNR order was there. Just because we talked about the importance of James's quality of life.... But this decision is something you definitely want to feel you are a part of deciding.

The DNR issue is brought up almost every time we are admitted. How it is brought up depends entirely on the person—whether or not they can empathize and have experienced what it is like to lose a part of yourself. Other than that one time, I have never felt coerced. And with you guys [the pediatric palliative care team] I almost feel as if we are holding hands walking—making decisions together.

What reason could ever be satisfying to me about putting a DNR on a child without my consent? We want our child to be treated the same way the doctor would want his child to be treated. Maybe sometimes we parents do wait longer than would be the perfect thing.... But there can't be any regret—that's one thing you cannot have doubts about. You can't question: "Did I kill my child? Did I not do enough?" It's your child's life and that's more important than your own life.

You don't place the order unless you know for sure that's what you both agreed to. Not that you think that's where you were, not that you suggested... hinted... that maybe.... It has to be 100%. This is *final*. You can't change that. You can't fix *dead*. You can't.

James's mother

CONFLICTS BETWEEN CHILDREN OR ADOLESCENTS AND THEIR PARENTS

Clinical Vignette

Anne was a 16-year-old girl with cystic fibrosis and end-stage lung disease. Over the past few years, she and her family had argued often about her nonadherence with prescribed medications and doing her pulmonary treatments. Her family desperately wanted her to be considered for a lung transplant. Anne, when informed about the process and what it would entail, felt strongly that she did not want to pursue this treatment and wanted to spend the rest of her time at home with her family and friends. However, she also felt that she could not disobey her parents. Based on her wishes and the probability of the transplant not being successful, the medical team recommended to her parents that she be allowed to transition to comfort care at home with hospice services. Her father reluctantly agreed with this recommendation, but her mother, a deeply religious person, felt that with God's help and with a transplant, Anne could be cured and that she needed to stay in the hospital to receive care until a transplant was performed. When Anne understood that this was what her mother wanted, she stopped asking about going home and became less communicative with the staff and her family. Despite continued intensive therapy, Anne died a few weeks later, having never discussed her own desires again.

The specialty palliative care team may be called upon when there is conflict between the child or adolescent and their parent. This may occur when the medical team is offering disease-related therapies and the child does not want to pursue them, or when the medical team feels that the child or adolescent should have a voice in decision-making and the parents do not agree. These are often very frustrating phenomena for the entire team. The issues are complex and involve individual psychological and familial factors. Social workers and psychology/psychiatry personnel may have particular insight into the nature of these dynamics. In addition, community, religious, ethnic, historical, and other parameters may play a significant role. Given such complexity, it is incumbent on the palliative care team to listen carefully to both the patient and the parents, as well as to the treating team.

There are three situations in which minors are legally permitted to make their own medical decisions: meeting the criteria for emancipation, being deemed "mature" in the eyes of the law (in some states), or suffering from a condition that permits consent for specific treatment under the minor treatment statutes of that state (typically including sexually transmitted infection or addiction to drugs or alcohol).[19] Yet even when none of these apply, the American Academy of Pediatrics (AAP) believes that "children should be involved in discussions about their healthcare." Even when a child is incapable of giving true informed consent or refusal, their assent should still be sought. Such involvement has three core elements: "1) helping the child achieve a developmentally appropriate awareness of the condition, 2) telling the child what should be expected with tests and treatment, 3) assessing the child's understanding and factors that influence their response."[20]

A fourth element —"soliciting an expression of the child's willingness to accept the proposed care"—is only relevant if the intent is to give the child's opinion serious consideration.[20] As Leikin observes, "If assent is to be honored, then dissent should be binding. If not, a promise has been broken, showing disrespect for the minor, which leads to mistrust of the physician or parents or both."[21]

Thus, prior to speaking with the child, it is important for the specialty palliative care team to first clarify, in conversations with the parents and treating team, whether or not the willingness of the child to accept the proposed therapy will be considered before a decision is made. If not, the treatment plan should still be explained to the child in developmentally appropriate terms. However, the child would not be asked for assent. Unfortunately, this discussion with the family and team does not always happen.

Yet even when a child may be able to give assent to a certain intervention, parents may not want these decisions discussed with their children, regardless of their age. It is important to realize that the role of the individual, including a child—which is such a critical part of our culture—is not shared by many other cultures. In some cultures, the expectation is that medical and other decisions are made by the parents or other authority figures, whatever the age of the patient. Attempting to impose our cultural values on these families will not only be ineffectual, but will diminish our ability to help families, including the children, navigate their way through the disease process. Thus, while the team may not have felt that it was "right" to follow the mother's rather than Anne's wishes, it was judged to be necessary in order to maintain the therapeutic relationship at this critical phase of the illness.

Clinical Vignette

Edward was a 16-year-old son of immigrant Mexican parents who had multiply relapsed acute lymphocytic leukemia. His physicians recommended to the family that additional chemotherapy was unlikely to help him and would only make him suffer more. His parents insisted that he receive more disease-oriented treatment and further insisted that he not be told that his disease was no longer curable. The specialty palliative care team was consulted and held long discussions with Edward and his parents, both separately and together. Eventually the family agreed that while the team would not initiate discussion about prognosis with Edward, they could respond honestly if he asked. When Edward did ask and was informed that his disease was no longer curable, he expressed a strong desire to return home to be with his friends and family. Initially, his parents could not accept that decision, but with guidance from both the oncology and the palliative care teams and the realization of the thoughtfulness that went into Edward's decision, they agreed.

Despite the long-standing stance of the AAP that older children and adolescents should be involved in the medical decision-making and consent process, there still has not been widespread understanding and endorsement among practitioners of the concept of pediatric assent or refusal.[22–24]

While it would often be helpful to obtain the assent of most children to the treatment being given, the issues of disagreements almost always pertain to older children and adolescents. Although age is an important variable, it is equally (if not more) important to consider the developmental maturity of the child and be sensitive to the culture and history of the family regarding decision-making. The Midwest Bioethics Center (now called the Center for Practical Bioethics) rightly notes that "there is a morally relevant distinction among three categories of minors: those lacking any decision-making capacity, those with developing capacity, and those having decision-making capacity."[25]

In pediatrics, the physician's duties to protect and promote health-related interests of the child and adolescent are grounded in the fiduciary relationship between the physician and patient. However, these duties may conflict with the patient's or parents' wishes and create tensions within the family. Most commentators believe that parents have an ethically parallel fiduciary obligation to protect and promote both the health-related and the non–health-related interests of their child or adolescent, with the pediatrician and the parents acting as "co-fiduciaries" for health matters.[26]

This parental responsibility for medical decision-making in caring for their child or young adult is not an absolute right, however, because the state also has a societal interest in protecting the child or young adult from harm and can challenge parental authority in situations in which the child or young adult is put at risk (the doctrine of *parens patriae*).[26] Note that one should not solicit a child's assent if the treatment or intervention is determined to be necessary by the physician and family; the patient should be told that fact and should not be deceived. Unless one of the three exceptions just noted applies, the child is not the final decision-maker; the parent or surrogate is, although a child's lack of assent may be a factor in determining whether the parent is acting in the child's best interest.

Parents represent the interests of the family as a whole as well as their own interests. They have responsibility for the care and custody of the children and for their personal and physical development. As long as a decision resides within the zone of parental discretion—with the balance of benefits and burdens not extremely disproportionate in either direction—we should not interfere with this authority. If the likely benefits of treatment in conditions with a good prognosis outweigh the burdens, parents may choose a treatment plan over the objections or dissent of the child. In situations with a poor prognosis and interventions associated with a heavy patient burden—as in this vignette—more consideration should be given to the adolescent's opportunity to provide assent or refusal.[27]

Clinical Vignette

Joe was a 17-year-old with Hodgkin disease. He presented at the age of 15 with Stage IV disease and was treated with 6 months of intensive chemotherapy. Although his disease responded to the therapy, Joe suffered many side effects that greatly affected his life. He had been very popular and had several girlfriends. The chemotherapy resulted in a dramatic change in his appearance, and, most painful of all, his friends abandoned him. Joe also was very symptomatic during the course of his therapy and would only come to the hospital reluctantly. After completing therapy, he regained his physical appearance and his social life. Unfortunately, one year later, he was found to have recurrent disease. He and his family were advised that although his chances of survival were not as good as they had been, with additional chemotherapy and a stem cell transplant he had a reasonable chance to be cured. However, without this therapy, he would die of his disease. His parents favored further chemotherapy leading to transplant, but Joe was very reluctant to embark on more treatment that would again severely impact his personal life. His parents asked that his physicians convince him to undergo the planned treatment. Despite multiple efforts by many members of the team, he ultimately refused to come to the hospital for his treatment.

It is important to realize that many children and adolescents want to be invited into the decision-making process;[28] however, they also want choice over their actual degree of involvement. When the adolescent does wish to participate, though, some structural barriers may yet exist. For example, the Center for Practical Bioethics recommends that "minors with decisional capacity should have the right to make advance directives [including] the right to name a surrogate decision maker other than their parents."[29] But advance directives executed by nonemancipated minors are not legal in any state. At present, the most that can be said of such a document is that it carries "moral weight."[29]

Furthermore, it is one thing to say that "minors with decisional capacity should be allowed to make treatment decisions,"[25] but whether that extends to refusing treatments for which the benefits clearly outweigh the burdens remains unclear. Furthermore, once one acknowledges exceptions to the rule, an attempt to validate the right of minors to make their own decisions may slide down the slippery slope to a place where only decisions that adults agree with qualify.

Ross offers a contrary view on the subject as to whether to allow adolescents who are not emancipated to counter what their parents have decided. In describing her approach of "constrained parental autonomy," she provides two arguments to justify overriding the decisions of a mature minor.[30] The first argument is that the adolescent's current autonomy can be overridden to promote their long-term autonomy. She recognizes that this is quite different from how adults are treated but concludes that there are moral reasons for treating the decision-making capacity of adults and adolescents differently. These include that adolescents need the opportunity to develop habits such as self-control that can advance their lifetime autonomy and that this may not occur if they make certain decisions regarding important therapeutic choices. Second, parental interest in raising their child according to their own vision of the good life does not abruptly terminate when the adolescent has achieved some degree of decisional capacity.[31]

The mature minor doctrine fails to acknowledge the limitations of judgment seen in many adolescents and the right and responsibility of parents to promote their adolescent's long-term autonomy. Adolescent maturity is necessary, but not sufficient, to justify sole decision-making authority in cases where effective life-saving therapies exist. Parents should retain ultimate authority to consent to potentially effective life-saving treatment over their adolescent's refusal. As Ross writes, "Parents should have a presumptive right to noninterference, a right that is restricted only if they fail to provide for their child's basic needs."[30]

This view is reflected in the prevailing US Supreme Court opinion on this topic: "Most children, even in adolescence, simply are not able to make sound judgments concerning many decisions, including their need for medical care or treatment. Parents can and must make those judgments."[32] Admittedly, since that 1979 decision there has been a significant movement toward empowering adolescents to make their own decisions. More recently, however, a combination of neurocognitive evidence (recognizing the "dual process" of adolescent brain development whereby the locus of emotional decision-making matures faster than the cognitive[33]) and the recognition of unintended legal consequences has highlighted the ways in which an adolescent's decision-making is not equivalent to an adult's, especially in high-stakes situations. Thus, for example, if minors are mature enough to make their own medical decisions, they are also mature enough to be held responsible for other decisions, even to the point of life imprisonment or, worse, being convicted of murder. Indeed, the Supreme Court has more recently reaffirmed "the fundamental right of parents to make decisions concerning the care, custody, and control of their children."[34]

Yet, for all the theories that underlie ethical analysis, the final decision must be able to be implemented. Thus, the preceding vignette demonstrates that even though both the parents and the medical team agreed that further disease-directed treatment was the most beneficial course for Joe, there was no way to force him to undertake the therapy. Even assuming compulsory treatment could be logistically feasible, the burden on Joe—in the form of restricted freedom at the very least and potentially including sedation or restraint—would be extreme, tilting the balance of benefits and burdens far toward the latter. It is thus clear that while ethical principles and legal rules are important, they cannot always determine how clinicians deal with patient–family disagreements. Practical options may also be limited when therapeutic decisions require the cooperation of the whole family.

All the vignettes in this section demonstrate the difficulties involved in dealing with life-and-death situations in which children and parents disagree. Even when the treating, specialty palliative care, and ethics teams intervene there is no guarantee that they will be successful. While the palliative care team can often help to clarify the issues and give voice to the patient, family, and treating team, myriad complex factors often determine the process of decision-making and the eventual course of action.

CONFLICT WITHIN THE TEAM

IPPC teams are at heightened risk of conflict for several reasons, starting with the intense nature of the work, which requires focus and compassion not only for the patient and families but also among the team members. (In addition to intrateam conflict, the possibility of interteam conflict between the IPPC and the primary team also exists, often manifested in terms of disparate opinions and role overlap.) The nature of a team fluctuates over time, as a function of changes in staffing, life circumstances, and relationships. The interdisciplinarity of the team, while a source of strength in providing whole-person care to seriously ill children and their families, may simultaneously heighten the risk of intrateam conflict. For example, as the physician and nurse focus on the patient's comfort through effective symptom management, the social worker is providing emotional support and guidance for the family as well as assisting with instrumental needs. While the overall goals of the physician, nurse, and social worker are certainly connected, their difference in focus has the potential to lead to misunderstandings (Table 16.1).

Many times, when past and present, external and internal pressures build up, small conflicts can intensify significantly. As Radford observes, "Differences themselves are not necessarily the cause of conflict. They become a source of conflict when people believe they are not respected, valued, or understood."[2]

Clinical Vignette

An IPPC team was stressed and overstretched. They had recently cared for two children whose deaths had not gone as hoped, and both situations had consumed a great deal of time and energy.

At their interdisciplinary team (IDT) rounds the week following these deaths, they discussed Tara, a 4-year-old girl with a degenerative neurological condition. Bryan, the social worker, opened the discussion with the observation that Tara's overall condition seemed to be worsening, with fewer "good days" and increased feeding intolerance. He wondered whether it was time to stop her enteral feeds. Although he knew that artificial nutrition and hydration (ANH) can be a controversial subject, he felt that Tara might be suffering and he wanted the team's input.

Tara's primary nurse, Sonia, arrived at the meeting late, emotionally spent from having just been present at the death of a 6-month-old baby. When she heard Bryan's assessment of Tara's condition, Sonia was annoyed. She had been Tara's nurse for 2 years and felt that she knew her medical needs best, and she was not sure if it was time to stop the ANH. The chaplain, Don, doubted that reducing or stopping artificial nutrition and hydration would even be an option for her parents, as he knew that it might conflict with their faith, which was paramount in their lives. Bryan wondered aloud why parents' religious beliefs should cause a child to suffer. Al, the medical director, did not notice the rising tension among the nurse, social worker, and chaplain, because he and the pharmacist were discussing which medications could be used to relieve some of Tara's symptoms. Furthermore, with many patients to see, Al was in a hurry to finish IDT rounds. Jill, the nurse manager, saw what was going on but did not intervene at that time as she too was pressed for time.

In the past, the psychosocial clinicians had felt that their input was not valued, while others on the team felt there was too much "story telling" and not enough focus on medical issues. The discussion about Tara brought up those feelings again for many of the team members. Everyone began to talk at once, as many felt they had important information that was not being acknowledged. Then several members spoke up and said that sort of discord was why they hated to come to team meetings.

Just then, Al was paged to meet with an upset family, and asked Bryan to join him. The IDT discussion was wrapped up quickly, leaving many team members fuming inside. The team psychologist, Yasmine, knew that something had to be done to rebuild the trust and cohesiveness so important to a team's functioning.

TABLE 16.1 The interdisciplinary pediatric palliative care (IPPC): Roles in conflict resolution based on discipline expertise

DISCIPLINE	ROLE LEADERSHIP	CONFLICT MANAGEMENT
Physician	Symptom management and treatment option expert	Guides discussions with clear explanation of options for patient, identifying strengths and weakness of varying recommendations. Supports families through complex decision-making.
RN–NP case manager	Offers support through direct care of the child, education with family caregivers, demonstration and assistance with use of equipment and supplies. Often assists in the development of care action plans for family to refer to in a medical crisis.	Facilitates communication among team members regarding family wishes and preferences. Supports complex decision making with clear information. Explores treatment options through collaboration with practice subspecialties.
Social worker	Offers support to patient and family through the lens of the bio-psycho-social model of social work, adhering to a discipline-specific code of ethics. Offers counseling, enhanced medical literacy.	May be seen as the broker of communication based on education and training. Specializes in support for complex decision making while attending to social, cultural, and religious or spiritual considerations. Attends to needs with a 'person in environment' perspective.
Chaplain/Spiritual care	Offers support for emotional, spiritual and faith-based concerns. Specializes in attention to the patient and family's faith background and seeks to honor faith traditions.	May offer critical support for emotional needs of parents when decision making is complicated by religious or spiritual beliefs. Supports the team with information that would enhance their understanding of the patient/family position.

TABLE 16.2 Radford's steps toward resolving conflict

Recognition	Admit that conflict exists, rather than engaging in denial or falling prey to "emotional hijack" (e.g., by raising your voice or engaging in unproductive nonverbal communication, such as sitting with arms crossed).
Responsibility	Take responsibility for your own actions, while acknowledging the role of other's actions as well as that of random unpredictable factors.
Restoration	Take active steps to resolve the conflict, including seeking other people's perspectives and expressing remorse.

As described in the preceding vignette, intrateam conflicts are often pushed aside and deemed "low priority" in the face of emotionally laden work with seriously ill children and their families. People may try to avoid conflict by not dealing with it, but eventually such unresolved conflicts can weaken the very infrastructure of the team. As Radford writes, "The most common way to 'avoid conflict' is to talk about people, instead of to them. Little issues become big ones. Minor grievances chafe and resentment eats away at contentment."[2]

In every conflict there is also an opportunity for healing and restoration of trust. How intrateam conflict is handled is specific to the situation and to each team's individual and group history, as well as to the cultural backgrounds of the team members. Some cultures may emphasize nonverbal communication, for instance, deeming what some view as candor more as confrontation.

If the conflict involves only a few individuals, the conflict may best be addressed privately among them, together with a neutral professional. Conflicts that involve the entire team, as in the preceding scenario, often require a facilitated discussion—or series of discussions—with everyone present.

A wide variety of methods have been proposed for resolving conflict, including principled negotiation[1] and conflict transformation.[35] Radford proposes specific steps in resolving conflict within a team: Recognition, Responsibility, and Restoration (Table 16.2).[2] These steps can be tailored to each specific situation and team.

RECOGNITION

The first step in resolving conflict is to recognize that conflict exists and that it has the potential to negatively impact the functioning of the team. Absent such an acknowledgment, team members may write off the tension as "someone else's problem" or grow to accept the suboptimal communication and unsafe atmosphere as "the best that can be hoped for." Ideally, each member of the team will both perceive and admit that a conflict exists. If not, "inviting" individuals into this recognition—rather than simply declaring it—is more likely to foster active participation in ultimately resolving the conflict.

Recognition of conflict can be an opportunity to model good communication, flexible leadership, and mutual respect when facing the challenges of an emotionally complex clinical practice. Once the conflict has been acknowledged by the team, identifying an optimal context for addressing it is crucial. This involves creating a "safe space" where individuals are able to share candidly and without fear of repercussions, within specific ground rules (such as using "I statements" to avoid being accusatory). In establishing clear expectations for the group, it may be helpful to enlist an impartial mediator to help move the discussion forward. It can also be helpful to proactively reassure team members that conflict is a normal, albeit difficult part of the healthy growth of a team. By identifying conflict and labeling the issues without blame, team members have the opportunity to explore how they each felt impacted within the scope of their role.

Team Reflection

Sensing that unresolved conflict was harming the team, Yasmine sent an email to the team leaders, Al and Jill, requesting to meet with everyone as soon as possible. At first, Al said the team was too busy. Sonia groaned inside wondering how there would be time for yet another meeting. Bryan was afraid of not feeling listened to, while Don wondered what might be different this time.

But as Yasmine met individually with each team member to better understand their perspective, it became clear to everyone that a team meeting was necessary. If individuals could not get back to trusting each other, the intense and important work of the team would suffer. Al and Jill agreed that it made sense to let Yasmine take the lead in the meeting.

A meeting time was set up and coverage provided for the team so that urgent matters would not call people away. It was important that the meeting place was private and comfortable, and an unused family lounge worked well for this purpose. Yasmine began by stressing the importance of trust within the team, setting the expectation of mutual respect and a safe environment. She acknowledged that team members had told her that, due to the underlying tensions, it was hard to be at work now, when it used to be enjoyable. She reviewed the issue of ANH and acknowledged that it is often a difficult topic to discuss but can be done in a trusting environment such as a well functioning team. The quiet presence of Al and Jill showed their support for the work the team was doing.

RESPONSIBILITY

The next step is responsibility, understanding how one's actions can affect situations and other people. It means developing emotional intelligence to consider how words or actions may be perceived, regardless of intention. When a word or action inadvertently causes hurt and conflict, one must accept accountability and work to ease the situation.

Rarely does someone intend to injure or disrespect another team member, although that may have been the impact of that person's words or actions. In assuming good intent on the part of the other, it is wise to avoid using words like "blame" and "fault." These can evoke strong emotions and trigger a "fight/flight/freeze response."[2] It is more constructive to invite participants to accept responsibility for their own contribution to the conflict, rather than to attribute that responsibility to others. Conflict may influence how a person acts, both consciously in their words and also unconsciously in their body language. Such stress may also impair a person's ability to view the situation objectively and even cause physical symptoms (e.g., tension headaches).

It is also important to establish realistic expectations for the conflict resolution process, with an emphasis on the term "process." A single team meeting is often insufficient to "solve" a conflict, and thus it is more realistic to establish an expectation that concrete, action-oriented next steps will be identified. As Stephen Covey observes, "You cannot talk your way out of things you behaved your way into. You've just got to behave your way out."

Team Reflection

Yasmine handed out sheets of paper and asked everyone to privately write five short sentences about their feelings regarding the recent team conflict situation and five different ways they could have reacted to help de-escalate the conflict. This was a challenge for some but was helpful for self-reflection.

After a few minutes, Yasmine asked if anyone was willing to share their thoughts on what they could have done differently. She started by acknowledging how she could have been more proactive when the conflict started by speaking up more quickly. Some team members mentioned being more careful before making assumptions or taking things too personally, while others acknowledged that they had not considered the consequences of their actions. As Yasmine had anticipated, not everyone was willing to share their feelings, so she planned to follow up individually with those who were silent.

Yasmine then asked each team member to respectfully offer their perspective on the conflict while the others listened. Not surprisingly, the interpretation of the meaning of actions and situation varied among the members of the team. The team then had the opportunity both to offer feedback on what they'd heard and suggest possible solutions. Sonia was able to tell Bryan that she felt, at times, he was questioning her ability as a nurse when he brought up medical issues, while Bryan was able to express how he felt his opinions were often disregarded as not being "clinical enough." Don shared his concern that the team devalued spiritual concerns, often viewing them as a crutch that parents shouldn't be leaning on. All of these perceptions contributed to the conflict over whether to continue ANH for Tara.

Yasmine deftly shifted the conversation from feeling wronged by others to what responsibility each person had in contributing the conflict. Bryan expressed his appreciation for Sonia's commitment to their patients, admitting that he sometimes felt jealous of her critical acumen. For her part, Sonia confessed to similar jealousy of the emotional connection Bryan and Don made with patients, while Don granted that he might have overreacted to Bryan's suggestion because he wished he'd been consulted before the question of stopping ANH was raised.

RESTORATION

Restoration is necessary when trust on a team has been broken. With the recognition of the misstep, understanding what went wrong and acknowledgment of individual responsibility, the next step is to offer an apology (Table 16.3).[2] A true apology acknowledges another person's hurt feelings and one's own actions that contributed to them. It is also inquisitive, seeking to understand the other person's response and thinking through what could be done in the future to prevent such an event from recurring.

Team Reflection

As the team members listened to one another and began to understand the differing feeling and perceptions, the group began to come to a consensus of how to move forward. Al admitted that he was somewhat conflict-averse and expressed his intention to pay greater attention to team dynamics. Sonia acknowledged that she had not been devoting enough attention to her own self-care, leading to her increased stress level which then impacted her team relationships. Bryan recognized that he could preface statements on medical management with more inquisitiveness and less conclusion. Don promised to work harder at "assuming good intent" on the part of his teammates if they didn't happen to recognize the role religion played in a particular family's life.

The team decided to develop a plan to address conflicts promptly in the future and continue to rebuild the trust that had been lost. Each member took responsibility to ensure better team communication and personal accountability and to be respectful of one another as professionals.

TABLE 16.3 ABC when trust is broken

A	Acknowledge that something is wrong. Admit your part. Apologize for any action that hurt the other. Ask for what you can do to put things right. Accept that the other may not be ready to heal or forgive. Act as though you can be trusted.
B	Believe the other acted from an unsatisfied need. Behave as though you want to repair the relationship. Build on common values.
C	Care for the other. Be consistent. Clarify your intentions. Have compassion for yourself and the other involved. Choose your path wisely.

Used with permission from Radford N. *Conflict First Aid: How to Stop Personality Clashes from Damaging You or Your Organization.* Business Expert Press; 2018.

Broken trust and hurt within a team can linger. These are situations in which leadership must consider how the team can move forward and prioritize what is most important. These decisions and vision must be shared openly and honestly with the team, asking if everyone is ready to accept and support them. Those individuals whose vision does not align with the leaders' may face a decision to leave.

By the nature of the work and the teamwork necessary to accomplish it, all teams will experience conflict. If the work environment becomes toxic, the team suffers, and, in turn, the vulnerable children and families in their care are adversely affected. Effective resolution within an IPPC team is, therefore, of crucial importance.

CONCLUSION

Conflict is not a sign of failure. Rather, it is a sign that the stakes are high and members of an IPPC team have strong beliefs about what patients and their families need and how to best provide that to them. So, rather than denying that conflict exists—or avoiding it when it becomes too obvious to ignore—it is preferable to address the conflict in a constructive and collaborative fashion. Different contexts may demand distinct responses, depending on whether the conflict is between the family and the team, between the child or adolescent and the family, or within the team itself. Effective resolution of conflict leads to improved patient care, as well as to greater candor and depth of the relationship among children, families, and clinicians.

REFERENCES

1. Lucado M. *When God Whispers Your Name*. Thomas Nelson; 2011.
2. Radford N. *Conflict First Aid: How to Stop Personality Clashes from Damaging You or Your Organization*. New York, NY: Business Expert Press; 2018.
3. Diekema DS. Parental refusals of medical treatment: The harm principle as threshold for state intervention. *Theor Med Bioeth*. 2004; 25(4):243–264.
4. Children's Hospital (Boston) Ethics Advisory Committee. Resolving conflicts over possibly inappropriate or harmful life-sustaining therapies. https://www.childrenshospital.org/~/media/BE0A0DA60589 43D79F7AF2551E72C52A.ashx
5. Bosslet GT, Pope TM, Rubenfeld GD, et al. An official ATS/AACN/ACCP/ESICM/SCCM policy statement: Responding to requests for potentially inappropriate treatments in intensive care units. *Am J Respir Crit Care Med.* 2015; 191:1318–1330.
6. Patterson K, Grenny J, McMillan R, Switzler A. *Crucial Conversations: Tools for Talking When Stakes Are High*. McGraw Hill; 2002.
7. Rosenberg MB. *Nonviolent Communication: A Language of Life.* PuddleDancer Press; 2015.
8. Pedraz-Petrozzi B. Balint groups and palliative care. *Hospice Palliat Med Int J.* 2018;2:149–151.
9. Kjeldmand D, Holmström I. Balint groups as a means to increase job satisfaction and prevent burnout among general practitioners. *Ann Fam Med.* 2008;6(2):138–145.
10. Arnold R. The challenges of integrating palliative care into postgraduate training. *J Pall Med.* 2003;6:801–817.
11. Periyakoil VJ, Neri E, Fong A, Kraemer H. Do unto others: Doctors' personal end-of-life resuscitation preferences and their attitudes toward advance directives. *PLOS One*. 2014. https://doi.org/10.1371/journal.pone.0098246
12. Weissman JS et al. End-of-life care intensity for physicians, lawyers, and the general population. *JAMA*. 2016;315(3):303–305.
13. Wilkinson D, Savulescu J. *Ethics, Conflict and Medical Treatment for Children: From Disagreement to Dissensus.* Elsevier. 2018. Chapter 1, The Charlie Gard case. https://www.ncbi.nlm.nih.gov/books/NBK537990/
14. Schein EH. *Helping: How to Give, Offer, and Receive Help*. Berrett-Koehler Publishers; 2011.
15. Schein EH. *Humble Inquiry: The Gentle Art of Asking Instead of Telling*. Berrett-Koehler Publishers; 2013.
16. Feudtner C, Walter JK, Faerber JA, et al. Good-parent belief of parents of seriously ill children. *JAMA Pediatr*. 2015;169(1):39–47.
17. Seymour JE. Negotiating natural death in intensive care. *Soc Sci Med.* 2000;51(8);1241–1252.
18. Morgan, CK, Varas, GM, Pedroza C, Almoosa, KF. Defining the practice of "no escalation of care" in the ICU. *Crit Care Med.* 2014;42(2):357–361.
19. Coleman DL, Rosoff PM. The legal authority of mature minors to consent to general medical treatment. *Pediatrics*. 2013;131:786–793.
20. Mercurio MR, Adam MB, Forman EN, Ladd RE, Ross LF, Silber TJ. American Academy of Pediatrics Policy Statements on Bioethics. *Pediatr Rev*. 2008;29:e1–8.
21. Leikin SL. Minors' assent or dissent to medical treatment. *J Peds.* 1983;102:169–176.
22. Lee KJ, Havens PL, Sato TT, Hoffman GM, Leuthner SR. Assent for treatment: Clinician knowledge, attitudes, and practice. *Pediatrics.* 2006;118(2):723–730.
23. Talati ED, Lang CW, Ross LF. Reactions of pediatricians to refusals of medical treatment for minors. *J Adolesc Health*. 2010;47(2):126–132.
24. Duncan RE, Sawyer SM. Respecting adolescents' autonomy (as long as they make the right choice). *J Adolesc Health*. 2010;47(2):113–114.
25. Midwest Bioethics Center Task Force. Health care decision-making treatment guidelines for minors. Center for Practical Bioethics. 1991. https://practicalbioethics.org/files/ethics-consortium-guidelines/Minors-Decision-Making-Guidelines.pdf
26. McCullough LB. Contributions of ethical theory to pediatric ethics: Pediatricians and parents as co-fiduciaries of pediatric patients. In Miller G, ed. *Pediatric Bioethics*. Cambridge University Press; 2010:11–21.
27. American Academy of Pediatrics. Informed consent in decision-making in pediatric practice. *Pediatrics.* 2016;138:e1–e16.
28. Kelly K, Mowbray C, Pyke-Grimm K, Hinds PS. Identifying a conceptual shift in child and adolescent-reported treatment decision-making: "Having a say, as I need at this time." *Pediatr Blood Cancer.* 2017;64:e26262–e26294.
29. Weir RF, Peters C. Affirming the decisions adolescents make about life and death. *The Hastings Center Report.* 1997;27(6):29–40.
30. Ross LF. *Children, Families and Healthcare Decision-Making*. Oxford University Press; 1998.
31. Strong C. Respecting health care decision-making capacity of minors. *Bioethics Forum.* 1995;11:7–12.
32. *Parham v. J.R.* 1979. 442 U.S. 584.
33. Giedd JN. The teen brain: Insights from neuroimaging. *J Adolesc Health*. 2008;42(4):335–343.
34. *Troxel v. Granville*. 2000. 530 U.S. 57.
35. Kriesberg L. The state of the art in conflict transformation. Available at https://berghof-foundation.org/library/the-state-of-the-art-in-conflict-transformation

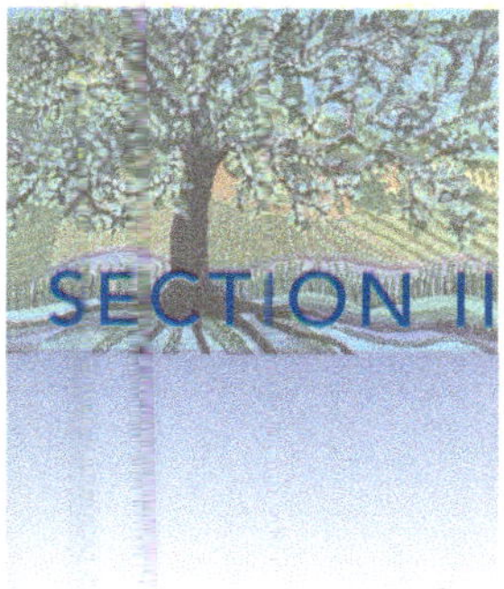

SECTION III | EASING SUFFERING

Pain has an element of blank;
It cannot recollect
When it began, or if there were
A day when it was not.
It has no future but itself,
Its infinite realms contain
Its past, enlightened to perceive
New periods of pain.

EMILY DICKINSON

Pain is the symptom most commonly associated with suffering, and studies from across the globe suggest that suffering from pain remains highly prevalent in seriously ill children. The chapters in this section show that seriously ill children face a myriad of symptoms including pain, and they experience suffering throughout their illness trajectory.

According to Dr. Eric Cassell, suffering is a specific state of distress that occurs when the intactness or integrity of the person is threatened or disrupted. It lasts until the threat is gone or integrity is restored.[1] The meanings and fears related to suffering are personal and individual, so that even if two patients have the same symptoms, their suffering is different. This far-reaching definition of suffering can be applied to the seriously ill child and family. Importantly, when the integrity of a child is threatened and disrupted, so, too, is the integrity of the entire family; when there is child suffering, there is family suffering. The "threats" as described by Cassell can be *visible*, such as the underlying illness and observable symptoms, and they can be *invisible*, such as disruptions to everyday life, social needs, and psychological and existential concerns.

It is the primary responsibility of the interdisciplinary pediatric palliative care team to ease suffering of the child and family with the goal of rebuilding child and family integrity. Though the family's pre-illness integrity can never be fully restored, a reintegration can be achieved that incorporates the experience of the family living with an ill child. Strategies to reestablish family integrity include *global approaches* such as teamwork, and *targeted strategies* such as symptom management. The preceding section and chapters focused on broad approaches to ease suffering in seriously children and their families through relationships and communication. The chapters that follow focus primarily on specific symptom experiences of the child and comprehensive strategies to evaluate and treat such symptoms. We chose to order these chapters from broad symptoms experiences to more specific, closing the section with distress in the child and family when death is near. And, as is the case throughout this textbook, the interdisciplinary team emerges as the common thread to achieve comfort for the child and family.

REFERENCE

1. EJ Cassell. *The nature of suffering and the goals of medicine* (2nd ed.) New York: Oxford University Press; 2004.

17 | PSYCHOLOGICAL SYMPTOMS

CHASE SAMSEL, KATHLEEN PERKO, LORI WIENER, AND MARYLAND PAO

As I stand in the night the fear approaches
I stand strong and face it with all I have
It tears and beats down on me
I stand my ground and face whatever it comes at me with
It reaches to the darkest part of my soul
It flows through me and never seems to go away
It comes right back
But I stand my ground
For the hopes of the end and of something better
I stand strong for the things that help me fight it
In the end it does not end but I still stand strong
Into the night I stand bold till the end
But then there is another journey ahead
Another challenge to face
I will face sadness, humiliation, opinion, pain, disgrace, and choice as they tear me apart.
The medicine from friendship, family, love, and life experiences heal me.

DERICK MOUNT, *diagnosed with osteosarcoma at age 12 (December 3,1986–August 17, 2005)*

When a child faces a chronic or life-threatening illness, families inherit myriad challenges. First and foremost, the family is thrust into living with uncertainty. Concerns about the child's health status—the diagnosis, prognosis, and rigors of the treatment regimen—are accompanied by additional stresses, including parental ability to maintain employment with associated financial implications, the child's ability to negotiate school and maintain relationships, and the ongoing challenges of difficult events or traumas that occur in everyday life. Worry and sadness are natural psychological reactions in this context. When should clinicians be concerned that these responses, secondary to the illness or treatment, are becoming pathologic in and of themselves? When do worry and sadness become clinically relevant anxiety and depression?

Symptoms such as anxiety and depressed mood are evaluated on a continuum (Figure 17.1).

In general, increasing frequency of a symptom, lasting longer than two continuous weeks, and the presence of significant impairment in functioning or quality of life, or the expressed desire for death should alert clinicians to pursue an in-depth mental health assessment to explore the need for specific psychological intervention. Such assessments must consider the cultural background of the family because psychological symptoms may be either minimized or emphasized in certain cultural contexts.[1]

There are junctures in the illness where strong psychological reactions may be expected. The diagnosis of a life-threatening illness such as cancer and the subsequent intensive treatment may be disruptive, frightening, and potentially traumatic for children and their families. Anxiety or depression may emerge at multiple stages of illness: during and immediately after diagnosis and treatment from the uncertainty of outcome, as well as during survivorship, treatment for relapses, and end-of-life care and when worries emerge about how death might affect the family. Hospitalization may create more anxiety in children under the age of 5 years or in those who already had difficulty separating from caregivers. Just

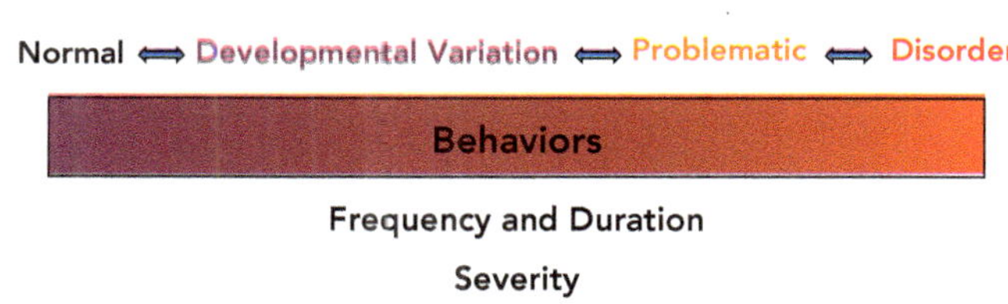

Figure 17.1 Spectrum of clinical concerns.

thinking about chemotherapy or hospital smells may trigger feelings of anxiety. Youth, particularly adolescents, are concerned about the effects the illness and treatment may have on their appearance. Additionally, the further a child gets from a normal routine, the more anxiety-inducing it may be to try to reenter his or her previous life with school, family, and friends. Anxiety, depression, posttraumatic stress, disordered sleep, and adequate pain control must all be addressed for optimal care to be provided.

ANXIETY IN PEDIATRIC PATIENTS

Anxiety emerges in response to perceived or real threats to our physical integrity or our sense of self (i.e. our identity or self-regard). It is a universal but subjective experience often based on a person's knowledge, judgment, expectations, and previous experiences. Anxiety can range from transient mild discomfort or uneasiness to pervasive and paralyzing fear. It is accompanied by psychological, cognitive, and behavioral symptoms. Psychological symptoms of anxiety include dread and anticipation of negative outcomes, an inability to turn off one's thoughts, and feelings of helplessness. Physical symptoms include feeling tense, palpitations, chest tightness or shortness of breath, nausea, stool urgency, tremors, crying spells, and difficulty sleeping. Behaviorally, children may become jumpy, irritable, avoidant, talk too fast, and have trouble concentrating.

Anxiety is considered to be problematic when its intensity and duration begin to affect functioning and quality of life, especially in the context of childhood cancer or other life-threatening illness. It can develop as a primary disorder, as a psychological reaction to illness, as a secondary disorder (e.g., due to medication side effects, neurotransmitter-secreting tumors, neurologic injury) or may be comorbid with other psychiatric disorders such as depression. Anxiety may be acute or chronic. It is important to identify any underlying treatable medical etiologies for new-onset anxiety (Table 17.1). For example, akathisia, a common side effect of medications, may be misdiagnosed as anxiety in children and young adults.

Anxiety disorders are common in the general population in the United States, with the prevalence of any lifetime anxiety disorder estimated to be 31.9% among adolescents.[2] Anxiety is common in children, with a lifetime prevalence of any anxiety disorder at 15–20%, representing all levels of severity.[3] In children with chronic illness, an estimated 20–35% have an anxiety disorder. In a study assessing anxiety in pediatric oncology patients, 14.3% of 63 children met diagnostic criteria for an anxiety disorder.[4] The prevalence of anxiety in other disorders, such as asthma, ranges from 9%[5] to 37%,[6] while in diabetes anxiety symptoms range from 0.8% to almost 20%.[7] One study found anxiety symptoms persisting 10 years after diagnosis of diabetes.[8] High rates of anxiety, up to 63%, have been reported in children with epilepsy.[9] Among adolescent patients with cystic fibrosis, researchers found a 22% prevalence rate of anxiety.[10] Clearly, age at onset, sample selection, method, and timing of appraisal of anxiety disorders need to be considered when interpreting the literature on anxiety disorders in chronically ill children.

Recognition of severe anxiety is important because it may affect symptom management, treatment adherence, and/or the ability of the patient to cope with the illness. Severe anxiety may even exacerbate preexisting physical conditions such as nausea, pain, and irritable bowel syndrome. Procedural anxiety related to the anticipation or performance of specific medical procedures could interfere with treatment. Anxiety is also common in parents and can exacerbate the

TABLE 17.1 Anxiety disorders seen in medically ill children

DIAGNOSIS	KEY SYMPTOMS AND/OR CONSIDERATIONS
Generalized anxiety disorder	Excessive worry with associated restlessness, fatigue, difficulty concentrating, irritability, muscle tension, sleep disturbance
Obsessive-compulsive disorder	Obsessive preoccupation or fears about physical illness; time-consuming repetitive compulsive behaviors (e.g., handwashing)
Acute stress/ posttraumatic stress disorder	Numbness, avoidance, intrusiveness and hyperarousal; can occur as a reaction to hearing diagnosis, aspects of medical treatment, or memories of treatment; common in chronic physical illness
Separation anxiety disorder	Inappropriate and/or excessive worry about separation from home and/or the family; common in children younger than age 6, resurgence around age 12
Phobias	Specific fear of blood and/or needle, claustrophobia, agoraphobia, white coat syndrome; may lead to difficulty with MRI scans, confinement in isolation, treatment compliance, etc.
Panic disorder	Severe palpitations, diaphoresis, and nausea; feeling of impending doom; resulting panic attacks lasting at least several minutes
Anxiety disorder caused by general medical condition	Direct pathophysiologic consequence of a general medical condition (e.g., panic attacks from sympathetic storms). Should be considered if history is not consistent with symptoms of primary anxiety disorder and physical symptoms such as shortness of breath, tachycardia, or tremor are pronounced

Adapted from the *Diagnostic and Statistical Manual of Mental Disorders*, Text Revision, Fifth Edition (DSM-5).[12]

child's anxiety. It is critical to document if there is a family history of anxiety and monitor the parents' anxiety when discussing treatment options and decisions, communicating with them throughout the course of treatment, and coordinating posttreatment care.

Posttraumatic stress has emerged as a possible model for understanding cancer-related distress across family members during the illness and beyond.[11] Pediatric medical traumatic stress is a set of psychological and physiological responses of children and their families to pain, injury, serious illness, medical procedures, and invasive or frightening treatment experiences. Traumatic stress responses include symptoms of arousal, reexperiencing, and avoidance or a constellation of these symptoms consistent with posttraumatic stress disorder (PTSD) or acute stress disorder.[12] Traumatic stress responses are more related to one's subjective experience of the medical event than its objective severity and are seen in children as well as in parents across the course of treatment and into survivorship.[13] Anticipatory anxiety can develop initially or during the course of treatment, and clinicians need to monitor vigilantly for increased irritability, resistance, and outright refusal to cooperate with procedures. Many clinicians have found that providing anticipatory guidance about normative psychological symptoms (including anxiety about tests, procedures, and hospitalizations) to children and their parents is helpful in decreasing the stress of uncertainty.

EVALUATION OF ANXIETY IN A PEDIATRIC SETTING

Assessment by a palliative care team member for anxiety begins with a careful medical history, including the current subjective symptoms to rule out possible medical conditions precipitating anxiety in the child, such as the use of drugs or alcohol (Box 17.1).

It is critical to evaluate for pain because pain can affect mood and anxiety (see Chapter 23). It is also imperative to ask if the child has a history of anxiety disorders, current or previous use of anxiolytic medications, and any family psychiatric history, especially anxiety or mood disorders. It is important to learn about previous anxiety and coping around the initial diagnosis in child and caregivers, anxiety surrounding hospitalizations, fear of needles and/or procedures, anticipatory anxiety, or the physical effects of illness and any treatments or medications. Be specific as to whether there are rooms, people, sights, times during the day, days of the week, sounds, or smells that the child finds aversive to better understand how to modify these factors. The clinician should be alert to previous difficulties with separation from home and/or other familiar settings or people. Worries about death or dying need to be explicitly questioned, using developmentally appropriate language. Assessment of sources of anxiety such as academic and social impact and financial burden of illness may add important information as well as family understanding of anxiety in the system. Screening and assessment tools for anxiety include the State-Trait Anxiety Inventory for

BOX 17.1 POSSIBLE MEDICAL CONDITIONS PRECIPITATING ANXIETY IN MEDICALLY ILL PATIENTS

METABOLIC

- Electrolyte disturbances
- Uremia
- Vitamin B_{12} and/or folate deficiency

PULMONARY

- Hypoxia
- Pneumothorax
- Pulmonary edema and/or embolism
- Asthma
- Anaphylaxis

NEUROLOGIC

- Encephalopathy/Delirium
- Encephalitis
- Mass/lesion
- Post stroke
- Post concussion
- Seizure
- Vertigo

ENDOCRINOLOGIC

- Cushing syndrome
- Adrenal insufficiency
- Hypopituitarism
- Pheochromocytoma and other neurosecretory tumors
- Thyroid dysfunction

CARDIOVASCULAR

- Ischemic heart disease
- Arrhythmias
- Congestive heart failure
- Hematologic, such as anemia

NEOPLASMS

- Brain tumors
- Insulinoma
- Lymphoma
- Small cell carcinoma
- Pancreatic cancer
- Leukemia

OTHER

- Transplantation
- Pain (uncontrolled)
- Caffeine
- Substance abuse or withdrawal

Adapted with permission from the Clinical Manual of Pediatric Psychosomatic Medicine.

American Psychiatric Association

Children (STAI-C), the Multidimensional Anxiety Scale for Children (MASC), and the Generalized Anxiety Disorder Scale (GAD-7) including others.[14]

A thorough assessment for an anxiety disorder may include a review of

- Heart rate, respiratory rate, and temperature
- Complete blood count
- Glucose
- Electrolytes
- Blood urea nitrogen
- Creatinine
- Liver enzymes
- Thyroid function tests
- Urinalysis with toxicology screening
- Arterial blood gas and/or oxygen saturation measurements to rule out respiratory causes
- Central nervous system scans

DEPRESSION IN PEDIATRIC PATIENTS

Depression describes transient sad feelings in combination with a sustained low mood leading to impairment in overall functioning; it may present with both psychological and physical symptoms. In general, the most prominent symptoms of depression are sadness, dysphoria, and anhedonia (inability to experience pleasure). Depression may exist as a primary disorder, as a psychological reaction to illness, or as a secondary disorder to an organic etiology, or it may be comorbid with other psychiatric disorders such as anxiety. Even if patients do not meet full diagnostic criteria for a depressive disorder, they should still receive appropriate clinical follow-up and continued monitoring. (Table 17.2)

Childhood depression does not look identical to adult depression and may be more difficult to diagnose, particularly with a concurrent medical illness. Children are more likely than adults to present with irritability, guilt, and somatic complaints. Physical symptoms include joint, limb back, and abdominal pain; headaches; gastrointestinal problems; fatigue; weakness; and changes in appetite. Depression may be expressed in apathetic mood, nonadherence, and changes in behavior, including regression. Depression affects school

TABLE 17.2 Depressive disorders seen in medically ill children

DIAGNOSIS	KEY SYMPTOMS AND/OR CONSIDERATIONS
Major depressive episode	Primary mood disorder most often associated with previous psychiatric history. Must exhibit at least 5 symptoms persisting most of the time for at least 2 weeks of: persistent depressed mood, anhedonia, irritability, change of weight, change of appetite, sleep disturbance, fatigue, feelings of worthlessness and/or guilt, diminished ability to concentrate, recurrent thoughts of death.
Persistent depressive disorder/Dysthymia	Chronically depressed or irritable mood for at least 1 year that is less disabling than MDD. At least 2 symptoms of: sleep disturbance, fatigue, diminished ability to concentrate, feelings of hopelessness.
Adjustment disorder (adjustment to diagnosis, course, and treatment of illness)	Depressed mood in reaction to medical illness; the most common mood disorder in cancer patients. Symptoms of depression do not meet criteria for major depression but are associated with mildly impaired functioning or shorter duration.
Mood disorder caused by general medical condition	Depressed mood, elevated mood, or irritability pathophysiologically caused by underlying medical condition (e.g., to any central nervous system (CNS) lesions in frontal, limbic, and temporal lobes); may be one of first symptoms of medical illness. Relationship to significant physical examination and study findings
Substance-induced mood / affective disorder	Depression induced by medication, drugs, or alcohol. Usually resolves within 2 weeks of abstinence. Important to note the course of depression in initiation and/or dosage of a medicine (e.g., high-dose α interferon).
Primary or secondary mania	Manic symptoms as a primary bipolar disorder, secondary to medical condition, induced by medication (e.g., corticosteroids) or toxicity. Symptoms include abnormally elevated, expansive, or irritable mood, rapid speech, decreased sleep needs. Patients with brain atrophy or sleep deprivation are more prone.
Behavioral considerations	
Regression	When stress of illness leads to behavioral regression and manifests as clinginess, social withdrawal, tearfulness, depressed mood. Very common in children and adolescents. Generally resolves after illness and/or hospitalization.
Bereavement	Feelings of emptiness and loss with fleeting thoughts of sadness or suicide that are part of normal mourning process. Complicated bereavement may signify a major depressive episode if it includes prolonged sadness and inability to experience any happiness or pleasure.

Adapted from the *Diagnostic and Statistical Manual of Mental Disorders*, Text Revision, Fifth Edition (DSM-5).[12]

performance and peer relationships and can be associated with substance use and suicidal thoughts and behaviors. When diagnosing depression in a child with a medical illness, consideration must be given to the fact that the medical symptoms and/or side effects of serious illness can be confused with, or coexist with, symptoms of depression. Depressive responses may be a normal response to the diagnosis and treatment of cancer and to medical events that occur during treatment. Physicians and nurses are less accurate at assessment of depression than of physical distress and can sometimes over- or underestimate psychological distress because of strong personal feelings toward patients, their own burnout, and/or lack of background training in behavioral health. However, persistent depressed mood or irritability associated with anhedonia and withdrawn behavior that lasts for more than half the time during a continuous period of 2 or more weeks should signal the need for additional monitoring and intervention.

The lifetime prevalence of a major depressive disorder in the general US population is 16.6%. Approximately 2% of school-age children[15] and 11% of adolescents[2] meet criteria for major depressive disorder (MDD), with gender differences becoming more apparent with age (females greater than males).[2,15] A recent updated meta-analysis described a 22% higher prevalence of depression in chronically ill children compared to their non–physically ill peers.[16] Generally, studies using clinical interview methodologies rather than self-report tend to report higher levels of depression. Some large samples have shown no difference in the prevalence of depression in children with other conditions such as asthma,[6] while others[17] found that 16.3% of youths with asthma compared with 8.6% of youths without asthma met criteria from the *Diagnostic and Statistical Manual of Mental Disorders* (DSM) for one or more anxiety or depressive disorders. The prevalence of depression in youth with diabetes is believed to be two to three times greater than in those without diabetes.[18] A study[8] found that in the 10 years of post-diabetes diagnosis, 27% of the children and adolescents developed depression. Children with complex partial seizures and absence epilepsy are five times more likely to have a mood or anxiety disorder than are healthy children.[9] Depression, although common, is often unrecognized and untreated in children and adolescents with epilepsy[19] and cystic fibrosis.[10] These data, taken across chronic illnesses, suggest that screening at regular intervals for depression and anxiety should be considered in chronically ill children, but rates may vary with the particular disease group.

Depression affects quality of life and psychological well-being. In the medically ill, depression may affect symptom management, treatment adherence, and thus medical outcomes. Depression is associated with higher morbidity, increased hospital length of stay, and increased complaints of somatic symptoms, and it is a risk factor for nonadherence with medical care. As with anxiety, patients may feel depressed at multiple points throughout the illness. The diagnosis and subsequent arduous treatment for many serious conditions may trigger feelings of overwhelming helplessness and depression and lead to delays in seeking or receiving care.

At terminal stages of an illness, clinicians can help the child and family work through feelings of loss and should recognize symptoms of depression as part of the grieving process. Whenever possible, it is important to find ways to help children communicate their worries to family or the clinical team so that the diagnosis of depression or anxiety can be properly made or ruled out. For example, emotional withdrawal should not be confused with depression. Emotional distancing provides the opportunity to conserve energy to focus on a few significant relationships rather than dealing with multiple painful separations.[20] In addition, chronic and severe pain is exhausting, and, once under control, the child's distress may improve. Therefore, it is essential that the palliative care team assess for the role that pain and withdrawal might have in depressive symptoms. Yet, as psychiatric symptoms can be reactive to the stresses and disruptions being experienced, a good history that includes knowledge of these conditions can help the palliative care team anticipate problems and provide them with the time to engage additional resources as needed.

One of the most frequent reasons for a psychiatric consult in a pediatric hospital setting is depression, especially within 1 year of a cancer diagnosis. Pediatric oncologists in the United States commonly prescribe antidepressants despite the lack of robust randomized controlled trials of antidepressants in youth with cancer. A survey of 40 pediatric oncologists found that half had prescribed a selective serotonin reuptake inhibitor (SSRI),[21] while a review of a single children's hospital reported that 10% of pediatric oncology patients received an antidepressant medication within 1 year of diagnosis.[22] On admission to the National Institutes of Health (NIH) Clinical Center, 14% of pediatric oncology patients had been prescribed a psychotropic medication.[23] These prescribing clinicians appear to be responding to significant distress associated with medical illness and its treatments.

EVALUATION OF DEPRESSION IN A PEDIATRIC SETTING

A detailed patient history is needed to determine the etiology of psychological and physical symptoms consistent with depression. Symptoms of depression can be difficult for clinicians to differentiate from medical and treatment side effects of cancer, which often include vegetative symptoms such as fatigue, decreased appetite, and sleep disturbances. Careful attention is needed to discern whether physical symptoms can be attributed to the illness process and/or treatment, or to a depressive disorder. Often, the diagnosis of depression in pediatric cancer patients is based on psychological symptoms such as anhedonia, feelings of worthlessness, guilt, feeling like a burden to others, and/or suicidal thoughts and actions.

Determining whether depressive symptoms are related to an expected course of grief and demoralization or to a clinical depressive episode is an important consideration, particularly in patients at the end of life. Consideration must be given to the patient's and family's psychiatric history, which may reveal genetic vulnerability for mood disorders. Evaluation for depression includes the assessment of symptom severity, duration, and impact on functioning and quality of life. Both the patient and primary caregivers should be interviewed to obtain information most comprehensively.

Assessment for depression in a child begins with a careful medical history including the current subjective symptoms to rule out possible medical conditions precipitating depression, such as use of drugs or alcohol (Box 17.2; see also Box 17.1). It is critical to evaluate for pain, as significant pain can affect mood and anxiety (see Chapter 23). It is also imperative to ask if the child has a history of mood disorders, previous suicide attempts, current or previous use of prescribed medications, or a family history of psychiatric disorders, especially suicidal behavior. It is extremely important to elicit a history of prior losses, including serious illness and/or death of family members, parental divorce, loss of pets, disappointments in school or social relationships, bullying (including cyberbullying), and how the child has, until this point, coped with his or her illness. Screening and assessment tools with high reliability and validity often require extensive time and expertise for use (e.g., Child Behavioral Checklist [CBCL], Behavioral Assessment Scale for Children [BASC]) whereas briefer tools are less reliable and valid (e.g., Patient Health Questionnaire for Adolescents [PHQ-A], Childhood Depression Inventory [CDI][14]).

A thorough assessment for major depression may include

- A review of vital signs and laboratory tests and/or procedures including heart rate respiratory rate and temperature
- Complete blood count
- Glucose
- Electrolytes
- Blood urea nitrogen
- Creatinine
- Liver enzymes
- Thyroid function tests
- Urinalysis with toxicology screening
- Central nervous system scans
- Possibly an electroencephalogram (EEG)

ASSESSMENT AND MANAGEMENT OF SUICIDE RISK IN CHILDREN AND ADOLESCENTS

Completed suicide is rare in children. The prevalence is unknown in children with chronic illness because few healthcare professionals assess for suicide risk in pediatric patients presenting with medical complaints.[24] Suicide risk increases with age in the general population. Increased rates of suicidal ideation are found in pediatric epilepsy,[9] adult survivors of childhood cancer,[25] and in adults with medical diagnoses that are also common in childhood such as asthma[26] and pulmonary disease.[27] Given that many previous studies indicate that chronic physical illness is a risk factor for suicide in adults[28,29] and adolescents[30] with variability by individual underlying medical diagnoses, a case has been made for universal suicide risk screening in medical settings.[31] There are now pediatric and adult suicide risk screening tools that have been validated on general medical populations.[32] While many children who attempt suicide or die by suicide are depressed, studies have that shown up to 20–60% of youth did not have clinically significant depression at the time of their attempt.[33] Therefore, assessing risk specific to suicide in addition to depression is critical. To provide a comprehensive evaluation, clinicians should inquire about suicidal ideation and history of previous suicide attempts and/or ideation, along with the stated intent and belief of lethality of attempt of suicide with or without

BOX 17.2 ADDITIONAL CONSIDERATIONS FOR MEDICAL CONDITIONS PRECIPITATING DEPRESSION IN MEDICALLY ILL PATIENTS

MEDICATIONS

- Corticosteroids (may cause depressive or mania symptoms)
- Opioid analgesics
- Benzodiazepines
- Barbiturates
- Narcotics
- Interferon-α
- Interleukin-2
- Retinoic acid variants
- Immunotherapeutics and immunomodulators
- Calcineurin Inhibitors (e.g., cyclosporine, tacrolimus)
- Chemotherapy agent (e.g., prednisone, vincristine, vinblastine, procarbazine, l-asparaginase)

METABOLIC ABNORMALITIES

- Electrolytes
- Calcium
- B_{12}
- Folic acid
- Parathyroid function
- Thyroid function

TUMOR

- Primary brain tumors
- Central nervous system lymphomas or metastases
- Carcinoma of pancreas

PAIN

- Severe, uncontrolled pain
- Fear of unrelieved pain

Adapted with permission from Abraham J, Gulley JL, Allegra CJ, editors: The Bethesda Handbook of Clinical Oncology, Lippincott, Williams and Wilkins, Philadelphia, 2005.

a plan. Other risk factors include comorbid psychiatric disorders; symptoms of helplessness, hopelessness, impulsivity; social isolation; uncontrolled pain; advanced disease; male or nonconforming gender; history of abuse or violence; and family history of suicidal behavior or psychopathology.[34]

Ongoing assessment of suicide risk begins with the first report of suicidal ideation, including passive thoughts such as being tired of fighting or feeling it would be okay not to wake up from sleep. Other specific times for assessment should occur with any change in mental status, during worsening of illness-related symptoms and pain, and at times of management transition such as a change of healthcare provider. A clinical pathway for management of a positive screens for suicide risk in pediatric hospitals assists clinicians in determining the range of possible interventions.[35] For example, if a patient is found to have acute current suicidal ideation (which is actually rare in a medical setting), immediate interventions should include environmental restrictions, particularly removal of any firearms and other lethal means from the home, appropriate support, observation, and monitoring at home or in the hospital if actively suicidal, with available care providers to be contacted in an emergency. More commonly identified are passive suicidal thoughts or a history of past behaviors which should be taken seriously for the distress and possible depression they indicate; this positive screen may not always require immediate one-to-one monitoring. Specific mental health consultation is essential to further assess suicidal comments even in the medically ill. Treatment must simultaneously address underlying psychopathology, disease-related factors, and pain, and may include psychopharmacology and/or psychotherapy.[36]

INTERVENTIONS FOR ANXIETY AND DEPRESSION

PSYCHOTHERAPEUTIC INTERVENTIONS

One of the challenges in evaluating anxiety or depression in children is the differentiation of symptoms that are secondary to the physical illness or treatment. Somatic symptoms of depression, such as difficulty sleeping or fatigue, are also common symptoms of both depression and physical illness. It is also important to differentiate symptoms that might be interpreted as depression because they may more accurately be an expression of grief or demoralization. Such symptoms, regardless of whether they are normal rather than pathological, warrant intervention. Therapeutic interventions are designed to reduce distress and help the child integrate the facets of his or her illness and life into expression.[37]

Psychotherapy is an established and effective treatment modality within adult oncology.[38] In pediatrics, the role of psychotherapy continues to evolve. Psychotherapy provides an opportunity for the child to reintegrate shattered facets of their life[39] and a place to develop positive emotional responses and learn coping skills to address changes in their day-to-day life, health status, and relationships. As each child is unique, the approach to the particular type of psychotherapy needs to consider a therapeutic method that is individualized, flexible, multidisciplinary, and inclusive so that it includes all members of the child's social system who may be impacted by the illness.[40]

Considering that parents are an integral part of the child's social system and may contribute to the onset and maintenance of anxiety and depression, parallel parental or family intervention should be offered.[41,42] Familial and cultural beliefs such as protecting the child from being included in medical treatment discussions may need to be further explored, as these often-unspoken attitudes may interfere with communication between the team and the patient. A thorough assessment of the characteristics of the child, psychosocial concerns and/or psychiatric history, background of illness, and the therapy being considered must precede deciding on a specific therapeutic modality. The depth and accuracy of the assessment and how these factors impact on each other often drives the choices of therapy and therapist, allowing for optimal conditions for a successful therapeutic relationship and outcome. Several types of psychotherapy have been very effective with seriously ill children.

For some, psychotherapy—through words, play and art—can provide a vehicle for communication of profound grief. For others, different forms of coping skill-work and/or self-expression are equally powerful and effective, including behavioral and cognitive techniques, play, bibliotherapy, storytelling, writing, art, music, and animal-assisted therapy. Most often, a combination of these specialized treatments is used.

Behavioral and cognitive behavioral approaches for reducing procedural distress are well-established.[43] These should be tailored developmentally and include distraction, guided imagery, self-hypnosis, biofeedback, and relaxation.[44] Parents and staff members can be trained in the use of these approaches. Other treatments for anxiety and depression include family therapy and psychodynamic psychotherapy to reduce anxiety and provide patients and families with adaptive strategies, identify underlying causes of dysfunction and distress, and focus on meaningfulness.

Effective treatment of a depressive disorder is best accomplished in collaboration with a mental health professional. Clinical social workers, child psychologists and psychiatrists, and marriage and family therapists familiar with children with serious illness should be consulted in this process. There are few reports of interventions for depression that are specific and exclusive to pediatric cancer or other life-threatening illnesses. Fortunately, literature in this area is growing and the results of more general literatures are relevant. For example, individual psychotherapy for depression, especially cognitive-behavioral therapy (CBT), is effective for youth in general, both alone and in combination with medication.[45] Emerging adult meaningfulness and psychodynamic-based psychotherapies such as CALM and Dignity Therapy have also shown significant benefits and could be appropriate for some adolescents and young adults with advanced illness and/or facing end-of-life care.[46]

While most adults use words to express emotions as well as to address conflicts, play is the language and vehicle for a child's expression and the mechanism for therapists to promote healing. There are a variety of play therapy approaches to reduce the anxiety and depression that critically ill children may experience at the end of life. To create a therapeutic relationship based on trust, safety, and acceptance, a nondirective or child-centered approach during the first few sessions with the child is useful.[47] The therapist provides several games, objects, and therapeutic toys the child can choose from. These may be medical play materials such as oxygen masks, alcohol pads, syringes, blood pressure cuffs, or stethoscopes. Objects that the child can control and can be used to facilitate mastery include modeling clay, bubbles, finger paints, and sand. Board games created to allow the child to share end-of-life worries, concerns, and fears in a nonthreatening and dynamic way can also be informative and effective in identifying major stressors.[48] Because an important goal is to create open communication and closeness between the child and parents, it may be useful to have the parents join the child in playing such games. For the child who may be too ill or weak to play, vicarious enjoyment and expression may be accomplished by playing for the child. Creating an environment of safety and trust that fosters freedom and acceptance is particularly significant for children who often experience a loss of control, privacy, and freedom of choice.

Bibliotherapy is an interactive therapeutic intervention that uses literature and storytelling as a means to reduce anxiety, gain insight into behavioral or psychological symptoms, enhance self-understanding, and promote coping skills and personal growth.[49] Stories can shape one's response to later events, make connections between seemingly random events, address unfair suffering, and provide meaning. After an assessment and the identification of clear therapy goals, the basic technique begins with a therapist choosing a story to read to a child that includes characters the child may relate to and whose struggles and triumphs the child can identify with. The therapist reads the story, followed by a discussion of the themes by the child and the therapist.[50,51] The child may be asked to suggest additions or changes in the story, or they may share stories that are similar but have different outcomes. Together, the child and therapist might write a book or story that exemplifies the individual child's struggles and strengths and gives meaning to his or her life. By externalizing a problem and recreating the ending, children can begin to experience a sense of mastery over their circumstances.

Bibliotherapy is effective in groups as well as in individual sessions. For children able to address end-of-life concerns, reading books allows group participants to talk about their personal thoughts about death, transitions, spiritual concerns, the afterlife or even to make together a book that has a different ending.[52] Viewing films can also be used to impart therapeutic messages and help the child obtain greater insight into his or her own life circumstances.[53,54] The goal of each of these techniques is to foster emotional expressiveness, which in turn reduces psychic distress.

Writing is another useful medium for working with medically ill children. Anxiety about the unknown is common and therefore, at the end of each session, providing validation of one's existence and a sense of continuity from one session to the next is useful. It can be helpful to complete a page of a personalized workbook for children living with a life-threatening illness[55] or a list of feelings or statements written by both the therapist and child about what activities and feelings were evident that day. A narrative therapy approach of letter writing, postal or e-mail, between sessions can also be used to maintain open communication. Computer-assisted art therapy[56] can enable online interactive communication between the child and the therapist in real time.

Children often fear that they will be forgotten after death. The workbook and letters written during sessions may be material that the children wish their parents to keep and cherish following their death. "My Mock Will," a page in the workbook, *This Is My World,* created by and available through the National Cancer Institute, has been especially instructive for parents who were not able to communicate with their child about their last wishes or who the child would like to have some of their most meaningful belongings. As death approaches, feelings of loneliness and the need for expression often intensify. Adolescents particularly appreciate the opportunity to use writing techniques to counteract their anxiety, sadness, and grief. This can take the form of a personal narrative, song, poem, or combination of these. Many find that addressing issues such as funeral arrangements, giving away belongings, and a discussion of how they wish to be remembered[57] are less threatening through writing than verbal communication. Offering children the opportunity to use creative writing to document what they would want to happen after they are gone and to leave something of themselves behind can often lessen anxiety—despite family and team fears of the opposite—because it affirms that an important part of their existence is still under their control.

Art therapy is another creative technique to enable children to express their conscious and unconscious concerns and externalize their fears and anxieties. Art media can be used as memory-making or legacy-building activities for the child to do alone or with family members. Treasure boxes, pillowcases, outlining and then painting of a parent and child's hands touching, and family quilts, especially those that includes photographs, can also be a potent form of self-expression and healing. Structured art therapy consists of asking children to draw consistent themes, once or repeatedly. Examples include the "change in family" drawing and the "scariest" drawing.[39,59] Another impactful art exercise is the mandala.[39,58] Instead of asking children to fill in a blank circle to express how they are feeling at this particular moment, Sourkes created a structured intervention that includes defining a topic that is central to the child.[39] This is followed by a guided visualization of that topic, and then an active approach in which the child draws the identified feelings within the circle, representing their importance through chosen colors and proportions. This technique allows the therapist to ask highly focused questions and interpret the drawings within the context of the individual child's reality.[39]

Photography can be used as a powerful avenue to reduce distress, increase a sense of control, and promote family interactions and communication. Following instructions pertaining to confidentiality, providing a child with a camera and asking them to take pictures (e.g., daily pictures for a specified number of days) that will show others what it is like to be sick can provide the family and providers insight into the child's perspective. Self-portraits are perhaps the most powerful and valuable photographs to work with therapeutically. Asking the child to choose where they would like their portrait taken or what they would like to be doing or wearing when their portrait is created allows others to bear witness to what is most important to that child. Using phototherapy techniques, children can connect the past with the present,[59] critical steps in integrating their life experience.

Animal-assisted therapy has regained popularity. Animal-facilitated therapy (AFT) or "pet therapy," has had an increased presence in the literature with a surge of recent research methodologies exploring this complementary alternative medicine (CAM) intervention.[60] Some hospitals and long-term care facilities have also reported placing an animal on a unit, with patients and staff sharing responsibilities for the animal's care. Dogs are most commonly involved, although therapeutic activities with cats, fish, guinea pigs, dolphins, and horses have also been described. Interaction between the patient and animal may simply be an informal, unstructured visit that includes play, petting, and talking with the animal and its owner. The presence of an animal seems to lessen the threat of the hospital setting, reminding many children and families of their own pet. Time with the animal may also be integrated into the goals of a therapeutic intervention. For example, a child who is resistant to leaving the hospital room or having social interaction may be willing to take a dog for a walk around the unit. Similarly, for a child who is feeling alone, snuggling with an assist animal can provide a sense of unconditional love, acceptance, and a connection to the world outside of the hospital environment.

The contact comfort of tactile stimulation and the gentle presence of the animal has both physical and psychosocial effects on children.[61] Animal-assisted therapy tends to reduce heart rate, blood pressure, and respiration rate, thus inducing a physiologic relaxation response. Reduction in anxiety and improvement in confidence, self-image, and self-esteem has been reported.[62] Children participating in animal-assisted therapy may also experience a significant reduction in pain, perhaps due to the release of endorphins that occurs during interaction with a friendly animal.[63] Additionally, the animal provides a distraction from pain and the hospital experience as well as direct enjoyment. According to a review of articles addressing the healing power of the human–animal connection, the affection shared between the child and animal promotes healing and provides energy and activation. Patients also enjoy having a sense of control and a sense of calm when they are able to help care for the animal.[61]

The need for intervention may continue after the end of treatment or throughout critical periods of development in a child with a chronic illness. For adolescent survivors of childhood cancer and their families, participation in a combined CBT and family therapy intervention reduced symptoms of traumatic stress in all members of the family.[74,75] Resources for interdisciplinary members of pediatric oncology teams to promote trauma-informed practice are found in the Medical Traumatic Stress Toolkit[76] produced by the National Child Traumatic Stress Network and available by download at www.nctsnet.org/nccts/nav.do?pid=typ_mt_ptlkt.

Team Reflection

Sandra was a 16-year-old high school sophomore when she was diagnosed with osteosarcoma. As a cross-country runner and an avid dancer, she was devastated not only by the diagnosis itself but also by the recommendation that she undergo an above the knee amputation. For weeks, she refused to listen to any discussion by her oncologists of surgery. She was referred to a psychosocial clinician for counseling. During the first session, Sandra tearfully reflected on all the losses she had already experienced and anticipated experiencing in her life. She was concerned about how poorly her mother was handling the thought of her daughter losing her leg, not being able to run with her cross-country team or dance in competitions, as well as how much more difficult it would be to fulfill her dream of becoming a doctor. Taking risks was something Sandra had always avoided, and the surgery represented such an enormous "unknown" that just the thought of it initiated mild panic attacks. During the following 2 weeks, Sandra met with the psychosocial clinician several times a week and explored the range of intense emotions associated with her diagnosis and future surgery. The team social worker also worked closely with the family on how best to support and prepare Sandra for surgery and on how to help her to maintain healthy self-esteem afterward. In addition, the whole psychosocial team identified several goals with Sandra that were mutually agreed upon and carried out.

1. Sandra identified two activities that previously had frightened her. Together with the recreational therapist, she participated in both of these activities.
2. Sandra loved to sing. Together with a music therapist, they searched for and recorded songs that best described the anxiety that she was experiencing and how she would like to ultimately conquer her fears.
3. Sandra read short stories by peers who had also lost a limb and learned how they had adapted to their life since the amputation. A librarian worked closely with Sandra to help identify these stories.
4. Sandra was introduced by her nurse practitioner to another teenager who recently had an amputation. It took a little time before she was ready to look at the stump.
5. Sandra wrote a letter to her leg during an individual psychotherapy session.
6. Sandra met with a psychologist, and together they identified soothing images. A relaxation CD was created that included a guided imagery of all that Sandra could and would do with one leg.

7. Sandra met with a child psychiatrist who agreed with the multimodal therapies and recommended in addition the limited use of short-acting benzodiazepines for acute procedures such as scans but did not recommend additional psychotropic medication during this time.
8. Sandra met with a chaplain to discuss her spiritual concerns.
9. Sandra met with the surgeon and expressed her thoughts, wishes, questions, and fears about the amputation.

The interventions listed here took place over the course of a month. At the meeting with the surgeon, Sandra said she had two remaining questions to ask. The first question was whether she would be able to obtain a prosthetic leg that would allow her to wear high heels. The second was whether he would keep the leg, so that when she became a doctor, she could study the tumor and "eradicate this disease once and for all."

Sandra and her family coped well with her surgery. No one provider could have helped Sandra grieve, prepare for her surgery, or prepare for her life without a limb. Each specialist brought an approach that complemented the others and allowed her physical, psychological, social, and spiritual concerns to be integrated into her care. Each discipline also provided a web of support to Sandra and her family. With each person, Sandra developed a strong relationship—each of which brought unique meaning to her experience.

Within a year of Sandra's surgery, she joined a Special Olympics cross-country team. As a result of significant neurotoxicity, she was not able to pursue a medical degree. A vocational therapist helped Sandra identify other skills and areas of strength. She currently works with children and hopes to run her own daycare center one day.

PHARMACOLOGIC INTERVENTIONS

When anxiety or depression is so severe that the child cannot participate or make use of the psychotherapeutic techniques offered, pharmacologic interventions may need to be considered (Table 17.3). Combining pharmacological and psychological interventions is often effective. Before prescribing anxiolytic or antidepressant agents, considerations include knowing body weight, renal and hepatic impairments, and clinical status. Drug-drug interactions should also be factored into medication and dose selection.

When prescribing psychoactive medications in a seriously physically ill patient, it is critical to consider the increased risks of medications in this population in addition to the potential benefits. Two medication classes with great potential to improve or worsen quality of life are benzodiazepines and antihistamine/anticholinergics. Benzodiazepines may be helpful as premedication for procedures such as bone marrow biopsies or magnetic resonance imaging (MRIs) that may precipitate an acute anxiety reaction. Often used for anxiety when SSRI use is medically contraindicated or due to drug-drug interactions, benzodiazepines can cause sedation, delirium/confusion, and behavioral disinhibition, especially in young children and children with autism and/or neurodevelopmental disorders. Abrupt discontinuation, particularly of short-acting benzodiazepines, can lead to withdrawal symptoms, irritability, and rebound anxiety. Chronic use of benzodiazepines can lead to tolerance and dependence even in youth, and best practices urge clinicians to prescribe benzodiazepines thoughtfully in a time-limited manner. Antihistamines/anticholinergics such as diphenhydramine are sometimes utilized for sleep or anxiety. However, they are not helpful for persistent anxiety, paradoxical reactions as seen in benzodiazepine use can also occur, and they can precipitate or worsen delirium as well.

For pharmacologic treatment of depression, both citalopram and fluvoxamine have been shown to be well-tolerated in empirical trials in pediatric oncology patients.[63,64] Case reports for use of tricyclic antidepressants,[65,66] low-dose atypical antipsychotics (e.g., risperidone),[67,68] and low-dose stimulants[69] in medically ill children are covered in the literature. Similarly, there is evidence for family interventions in childhood disorders, including depression.[70] Many families may be reluctant to try psychotropic medications for a variety of cultural and personal beliefs. However, they are often more willing to consider them when it is explained, for example, how the symptoms of cancer and cancer treatment may be due to a shared biologic mechanism of cytokine-induced mood changes.[71,72] Given the complexity of prescribing psychotropic medications in this population, primary teams may consider consultation with a child and adolescent consultation-liaison psychiatrist or palliative care specialist.

Anxiety and depression can sometimes be the direct result of some disease processes and/or the necessary medical treatments for pediatric diseases (i.e., substance-induced affective disorder/medication-induced affective disorders). Corticosteroids are a common treatment for many children with serious physical illness and are well-documented to cause irritability, anxiety, depression, and sometimes even mania or psychosis that warrant consideration of psychotropic management.[73] Some studies are showing promise for psychotropic interventions for pediatric patients with corticosteroid-induced affective disorders.[70] Many existing and emerging immunotherapeutics also have potential to cause neurobehavioral side effects (Box 17.2).

Very young children, children with neurocognitive insults, and children with developmental delays and/or autism spectrum disorders are particularly vulnerable to the neurobehavioral side effects of medications. Sometimes the best psychotropic intervention is adjusting or altering existing offending medications to improve mood and anxiety symptoms in children (e.g., switching very anticholinergic diphenhydramine for less anticholinergic hydroxyzine for pruritis).

TABLE 17.3 Preparations and dosages of anxiolytics and antidepressants in children

MEDICATION	DOSAGE[b]	CLINICAL INDICATIONS	SIDE EFFECTS/NOTES
Benzodiazepines			
Clonazepam	0.01 mg/kg/24 hour divided every 8 hour PO	Longer coverage of persistent, pervasive anxiety, may decrease anxiety rebound symptoms	Drowsiness, sedation, may lead to behavioral disinhibition
Diazepam	0.04–0.2 mg/kg/dose IV 0.12–0.8 mg/kg/24 hour divided every 6–8 hour PO	Long coverage of persistent, pervasive anxiety, may decrease anxiety rebound symptoms.	Drowsiness, sedation, may lead to behavioral disinhibition Long-half-life may interfere with other medications.
Lorazepam	0.05 mg/kg/dose every 4–8 hours PO/IV, max 2 mg/dose	Quick onset, useful for acute anxiety and procedures.	Drowsiness, sedation, may lead to behavioral disinhibition. Should be tapered
Midazolam	0.025–0.05 mg/kg IV Max 0.4 mg/kg 0.25–1.0 mg/kg PO Max 20 mg	Quick onset, useful for acute anxiety and procedures. Continuous infusion at end of life	Drowsiness, sedation, may lead to behavioral disinhibition. Amnestic effects Should be tapered
Selective Serotonin Reuptake Inhibitors (SSRI)			Black box warning for suicidal ideation in children under 18 years. Risk of serotonin syndrome with toxicity
Citalopram	10 mg/day once by mouth; children >12 start at 20 mg/day. Increase by 5–10 mg every 2 weeks as clinically indicated. Maximum dose 40 mg/day	Anxiety and depression Has fewest drug-drug interactions	Dry mouth, somnolence, insomnia, nausea, vomiting
Escitalopram[a]	5 mg/day once by mouth; children >12 start at 10 mg/day. Increase by 5–10 mg every 2 weeks as clinically indicated. Maximum dose 20 mg/day	Anxiety and [a]depression Has few drug-drug interactions	Dry mouth, somnolence, insomnia, nausea, vomiting
Fluoxetine[a]	5–20 mg/day once by mouth based on weight. Increase after 2 weeks as clinically indicated. Maximum dose 60 mg/day	Anxiety, depression[a], and OCD[a] Has many drug-drug interactions and more serotonergic side-effects than other SSRIs	Dry mouth, headache, somnolence, insomnia, nausea, vomiting Long half life
Sertraline[a]	12.5 mg/day once by mouth; >12 start at 25 mg. Increase by 12.5–25 mg after at least 1 week as clinically indicated. Maximum dose 200 mg/day	Anxiety[a], depression, and OCD[a]	Dry mouth, somnolence, insomnia, nausea, vomiting
Serotonin norepinephrine reuptake Inhibitors (SNRIs)			Black box warning for suicidal ideation in children under 18 years.
Venlafaxine	37.5 mg/day once by mouth; Increase by 37.5 mg every 4–7 days as clinically indicated. Maximum dose 225 mg/day	Anxiety, depression, and OCD May provide neuropathic pain benefits	Dry mouth, somnolence, insomnia, nausea, vomiting
Duloxetine[a]	30 mg/day once by mouth; increase by 30 mg after 2 weeks as clinically indicated Maximum dose 120 mg/day	Anxiety[a], depression, and OCD May provide neuropathic pain benefits	Dry mouth, somnolence, insomnia, nausea, vomiting
Tricyclic Antidepressants (TCA)			Black box warning for suicidal ideation in children under 18 years. Generally very sedating and anticholinergic at the doses needed to achieve antidepressant and anxiolytic effects (e.g. higher than for neuropathic pain and migraines)
Amitriptyline[a]	1 mg/kg/day divided three times a day; increase by 0.5 mg/kg/day every 2–3 days as clinically indicated Maximum dose 200 mg/day	Anxiety, depression, and OCD	Dry mouth, constipation, weight gain, hypotension. Increased sedation than with other TCA

(continued)

TABLE 17.3 Continued

MEDICATION	DOSAGE[b]	CLINICAL INDICATIONS	SIDE EFFECTS/NOTES
Benzodiazepines			
Desipramine	10 mg/day once by mouth Increase as clinically indicated. Maximum dose 150 mg/day	Anxiety, depression, and OCD Not recommended as first-line medication.	Sedation, dry mouth, constipation, weight gain, hypotension
Nortriptyline	30 mg/day once or divided three times a day by mouth. Increase as clinically indicated. Maximum dose 150 mg/day	Anxiety, depression, and OCD Not recommended as first-line medication	Sedation, dry mouth, constipation, weight gain, hypotension. TCA blood levels easily monitored
Other antidepressants			
Bupropion	37.5 mg/day divided twice a day by mouth; increase dose as clinically indicated every three days. Maximum dose 300 mg/day	Depression Fewer sexual side effects	Activation, agitation, anxiety, headaches, GI symptoms. Increased risk of seizures
Alternative anxiolytics			
Buspirone	15 mg/day divided twice a day; increase as clinically indicated. Maximum dose 60 mg/day	Anxiety	Tachycardia, headache, GI symptoms, dizziness, insomnia
Stimulants			
Methylphenidate[a]	2.5 mg by mouth twice a day, increase as clinically indicated Maximum dose 40 mg/day	ADHD[a] Useful for fatigue, depressed, sedated person at end-of-life, rapid on and off.	Insomnia, appetite suppression
Amphetamine/ dextroamphetamine[a]	2.5 mg by mouth twice a day, increase as clinically indicated Maximum dose 40 mg/day	ADHD[a] Useful for fatigue, depressed, sedated person at end-of-life, rapid on and off.	Insomnia, appetite suppression
Antipsychotics			
Haloperidol[a]	3–12 years: 0.025–0.05 mg/kg/day divided 2/three times; increase every 5–7 days as clinically indicated >12 years: 1–2 mg by mouth twice a day; increase as clinically indicated. Maximum dose 100 mg/day	Psychosis/schizophrenia[a], bipolar mania[a], irritability in autism spectrum disorder, tics/Tourette's syndrome[a] Can help with nausea	Can decrease WBC count; consider discontinuing if ANC<1000 More prone to extrapyramidal symptoms
Atypical Antipsychotics			
Risperidone[a]	0.5 mg/day PO divided qd–bid x4 days, then increase to target 1 mg/day Maximum dose 3 mg/day	Self-injurious behavior in autism spectrum disorders[a], schizophrenia[a], bipolar mania[a] Can help with nausea	Can decrease WBC count; consider discontinuing if ANC<1000 Hyperprolactinemia
Olanzapine[a]	2.5 mg/day PO divided qd–bid × 4 days, then increase to target 5–10 mg/day Maximum dose 10 mg/day	Self-injurious behavior in autism spectrum disorders, schizophrenia[a], bipolar mania[a] Can help with nausea with specific studies in nausea from highly emetogenic chemotherapy	Can decrease WBC count; consider discontinuing if ANC<1000 Very anticholinergic
Quetiapine[a]	50 mg/day PO divided qd–tid × 4 days, then increase to target 100 mg/day Maximum dose 150 mg/day	Self-injurious behavior in autism spectrum disorders, schizophrenia[a], bipolar mania[a]	Can decrease WBC count; consider discontinuing if ANC<1000 Fairly anticholinergic

[a] Has a US Food and Drug Administration (FDA) indication in children or adolescents.

[b] Children <12 years old warrant lower dosing.

Prescribing information adapted from Johns Hopkins Hospital, Custer, Rau, and Lee (eds.), *The Harriet Lane handbook*, 18th ed. Mosby, 2008; and Taketomo, C., Hoddomg, J., Kraus, D., *Pediatric and neonatal dosage handbook*, 24th ed., Lexicomp, 2018.

mg, milligram; kg, kilogram; hr, hour; PO, per os or by mouth; IV, intravenous; Max, maximum dose/day; GI, gastrointestinal.

CONCLUSION

Anxiety and depression are common symptoms in the seriously medically ill child. This chapter has reviewed clinical presentations of anxiety and depression along with means for assessing and treating these symptoms. As the child's well-being is intrinsically linked to parents' overall functioning,[77] the establishment and maintenance of a developmentally appropriate therapeutic relationship that involves the family in a meaningful way is of utmost importance, regardless of the specific intervention. Most children and families are eager for help and support. By understanding their worries, concerns, symptoms, and grief, we can build on their strengths and utilize specialized treatments throughout the course of the illness to achieve symptom reduction, psychological growth, and resilience.

REFERENCES

1. Field MJ, Behrman RE, eds. *When Children Die: Improving Palliative and End-of-Life Care for Children and Their Families.* National Academies Press; 2003.
2. Merikangas KR, He JP, Burstein M, et al. Lifetime prevalence of mental disorders in U.S. adolescents: Results from the National Comorbidity Survey Replication–Adolescent Supplement (NCS-A). *J Am Acad Child Adolesc Psychiatry.* 2010;49(10):980–989. https://doi.org/10.1016/j.jaac.2010.05.017
3. Beesdo K, Knappe S, Pine D. Anxiety and anxiety disorders in children and adolescents: Developmental issues and implications for DSM-V. *Psychiatr Clin North Am.* 2009;32(3):483–524. https://doi.org/10.1016/j.psc.2009.06.002
4. Gothelf D, Rubinstein M, Shemesh E, et al. Pilot study: Fluvoxamine treatment for depression and anxiety disorders in children and adolescents with cancer. *J Am Acad Child Adolesc Psychiatry.* 2005;44(12):1258–1262. https://doi.org/10.1097/01.chi.0000181042.29208.eb
5. Richardson L, Lozano P, Russo J, McCauley E, Bush T, Katon W. Asthma symptom burden: Relationship to asthma severity and anxiety and depression symptoms. *Pediatrics (Evanston).* 2006;118(3):1042–1051. https://doi.org/10.1542/peds.2006-0249
6. Ortega A, Huertas S, Canino G, Ramirez R, Rubio-Stipec M. Childhood asthma, chronic illness, and psychiatric disorders. *J Nerv Mental Dis.* 2002;190(5):275–281. https://doi.org/10.1097/00005053-200205000-00001
7. Chavira D, Garland A, Daley S, Hough R. The impact of medical comorbidity on mental health and functional health outcomes among children with anxiety disorders. *J Dev Behav Pediatr.* 2008;29(5):394–402. https://doi.org/10.1097/dbp.0b013e3181836a5b
8. Kovacs M, Goldston D, Obrosky D, Bonar L. Psychiatric disorders in youths with IDDM: Rates and risk factors. *Diabetes Care.* 1997;20(1) 36–44. https://doi.org/10.2337/diacare.20.1.36
9. Caplan R, Siddarth P, Gurbani S, Hanson R, Sankar R, Shields W. Depression and anxiety disorders in pediatric epilepsy. *Epilepsia.* 2005;46(5):720–730. https://doi.org/10.1111/j.1528-1167.2005.43604.x
10. Quittner A, Goldbeck L, Abbott J, et al. Prevalence of depression and anxiety in patients with cystic fibrosis and parent caregivers: Results of the International Depression Epidemiological Study across nine countries. *Thorax.* 2014;69(12):1090–1097. https://doi.org/10.1136/thoraxjnl-2014-205983
11. Kazak A, Simms S, Barakat L, et al. Surviving cancer competently intervention program (SCCIP): A cognitive-behavioral and family therapy intervention for adolescent survivors of childhood cancer and their families. *Family Process.* 1999;38(2):175–191.
12. American Psychiatric Association. *Diagnostic and Statistical Manual of Mental Disorders: DSM-5.* 5th ed. American Psychiatric Association; (2013).
13. Stuber M, Shemesh E. Post-traumatic stress response to life-threatening illnesses in children and their parents. *Child Adolesc Psychiatr Clin North Am.* 2006;15(3):597–609. https://doi.org/10.1016/j.chc.2006.02.006
14. American Academy of Pediatrics. Mental health screening and assessment tools for primary care. *Am Acad Pediatr.* 2010;125(Supplement 3):S173–S192. https://doi.org/10.1542/peds.2010-0788R
15. Kessler R, Berglund P, Demler O, Jin R, Merikangas K, Walters E. Lifetime prevalence and age-of-onset distributions of DSM-IV disorders in the national comorbidity survey replication. *Arch Gen Psychiatry.* 2005;62(6):593–602. https://doi.org/10.1001/archpsyc.62.6.593
16. Pinquart M, Shen Y. Depressive symptoms in children and adolescents with chronic physical illness: An updated meta-analysis. *J Pediatr Psychol.* 2011;36(4):375–384. https://doi.org/10.1093/jpepsy/jsq104
17. Katon W, Lozano P, Russo J, McCauley E, Richardson L, Bush T. The prevalence of DSM-IV anxiety and depressive disorders in youth with asthma compared with controls. *J Adolesc Health.* 2007;41(5):455–463. https://doi.org/10.1016/j.jadohealth.2007.05.023
18. Kokkonen J, Taabuka A, Kokkonen ER, et al. Diabetes in adolescence: The effect of family and psychologic factors on metabolic control. *Nordic J Psychiatry.* 1997;51(3):165–172. https://doi.org/10.3109/08039489709109091
19. Plioplys S, Dunn D, Caplan R. 10-year research update review: Psychiatric problems in children with epilepsy. *J Am Acad Child Adolesc Psychiatry.* 2007;46(11):1389–1402. https://doi.org/10.1097/chi.0b013e31815597fc
20. Kübler-Ross E. *On Death and Dying.* The Macmillan Company; 1969.
21. Kersun L, Kazak A. Prescribing practices of selective serotonin reuptake inhibitors (SSRIs) among pediatric oncologists: A single institution experience. *Pediatr Blood Cancer.* 2006;47(3):339–342. https://doi.org/10.1002/pbc.20484
22. Portteus A, Ahmad N, Tobey D, Leavey P. The prevalence and use of antidepressant medication in pediatric cancer patients. *J Child Adolesc Psychopharmacol.* 2006;16(4):467–473. https://doi.org/10.1089/cap.2006.16.467
23. Pao M, Ballard E, Rosenstein D, Wiener L, Wayne A. Psychotropic medication use in pediatric patients with cancer. *Arch Pediatr Adolesc Med.* 2006;160(8):818–822. https://doi.org/10.1001/archpedi.160.8.818
24. Habis A, Tall L, Smith J, Guenther E. Pediatric emergency medicine physicians' current practices and beliefs regarding mental health screening. *Pediatr Emerg Care.* 2007;23(6):387–393. https://doi.org/10.1097/01.pec.0000278401.37697.79
25. Recklitis CJ, Lockwood RA, Rothwell MA, Diller LR. Suicidal ideation and attempts in adult survivors of childhood cancer. *J Clin Oncol.* 2006;24(24):3852–3857. https://doi.org/10.1200/JCO.2006.06.5409
26. Goodwin R, Eaton W. Asthma, suicidal ideation, and suicide attempts: Findings from the Baltimore epidemiologic catchment area follow-up. *Am J Public Health.* 2005;95(4):717–722. https://doi.org/10.2105/AJPH.2003.019109
27. Goodwin R, Kroenke K, Hoven C, Spitzer R. Major depression, physical illness, and suicidal ideation in primary care. *Psychosom Med.* 2003;65(4):501–505. https://doi.org/10.1097/01.psy.0000041544.14277.ec
28. Ratcliffe G, Enns M, Belik S, Sareen J. Chronic pain conditions and suicidal ideation and suicide attempts: An epidemiologic perspective. *Clin J Pain.* 2008;24(3):204–210. https://doi.org/10.1097/ajp.0b013e31815ca2a3
29. Hughes D, Kleespies P. Suicide in the medically ill. *Suicide Life-Threat Behav.* 2001;31(Supp):48–59. https://doi.org/10.1521/suli.31.1.5.48.24226
30. Blumenthal SJ. Youth suicide: Risk factors, assessment, and treatment of adolescent and young adult suicidal patients. *Psychiatr Clin North Am.* 1990;13(3):511–556.
31. Horowitz L, Roaten K, Pao M, Bridge J. Suicide prevention in medical settings: The case for universal screening. *Gen Hosp Psychiatry.* 2020;63:7–8. https://doi.org/10.1016/j.genhosppsych.2018.11.009
32. Thom R, Hogan C, Hazen E. Suicide risk screening in the hospital setting: A review of brief validated tools. *Psychosomatics.* 2020;61(1):1–7. https://doi.org/10.1016/j.psym.2019.08.009
33. Cash S, Bridge J. Epidemiology of youth suicide and suicidal behavior. *Curr Opin Pediatr.* 2009;21(5):613–619. https://doi.org/10.1097/mop.0b013e32833063e1
34. Simon RI, Hales RE. *The American Psychiatric Publishing Textbook of Suicide Assessment and Management.* American Psychiatric Press; 2006.

35. Brahmbhatt K, Kurtz B, Afzal K, et al. Suicide risk screening in pediatric hospitals: Clinical pathways to address a global health crisis. *Psychosomatics*. 2019;60(1):1–9. https://doi.org/10.1016/j.psym.2018.09.003
36. Berman A, Jobes D, Silverman M. *Adolescent Suicide: Assessment and Intervention*. American Psychological Association; 2006.
37. Sourkes B, Frankel L, Brown M, et al. Food, toys, and love: Pediatric palliative care. *Curr Probl Pediatr Adolesc Health Care*. 2005;35(9):350–386. https://doi.org/10.1016/j.cppeds.2005.09.002
38. Chong Guan N, Mohamed S, Kian Tiah L, Kar Mun T, Sulaiman AH, Zainal NZ. Psychotherapy for cancer patients. *Int J Psychiatry Med*. 2016;51(5):414–430. https://doi.org/10.1177/0091217416680197
39. Sourkes B. *Armfuls of Time: The Psychological Experience of the Child with a Life-Threatening Illness*. University of Pittsburgh Press; 1995.
40. Kearney J, Bartell A. Psychotherapy with paediatric and adolescent cancer patients. In Watson M., Kissane C, eds. *Handbook of Psychotherapy in Cancer Care*. Wiley; 2011:213–223.
41. Weisz J, Kazdin A, eds. *Evidence-Based Psychotherapies for Children and Adolescents*. 3rd ed. Guilford Press; 2017.
42. Lewinsohn PM, Rohde P, Hops H, Clarke G. *Leader's Manual for Parent Groups: Adolescent Coping with Depression Course*. Castalia Publishing; 1991.
43. Spirito A, Kazak AE. *Effective and Emerging Treatments in Pediatric Psychology*. Oxford University Press; 2006.
44. Powers S. Empirically supported treatments in pediatric psychology: Procedure- related pain. *J Pediatr Psychol*. 1999;24(2):131–145. https://doi.org/10.1093/jpepsy/24.2.131
45. TADS Team. The Treatment for Adolescents with Depression Study (TADS). *Arch Gen Psychiatry*. 2007;64:1132–1144.
46. Rodin G, Lo C, Rydall A, et al. Managing Cancer and Living Meaningfully (CALM): A randomized controlled trial of a psychological intervention for patients with advanced cancer. *J Clin Oncol*. 2018;36(23):2422–2432. https://doi.org/10.1200/jco.2017.77.1097
47. Landreth, GL. *Innovations in Play Therapy: Issues, Process, and Special Populations*. Brunner-Routledge; 2001.
48. Wiener L. Shop talk: A new therapeutic game for youth living with cancer and other life-threatening illnesses. *Psychooncology*. 2009;18(Suppl 2):S240S241.
49. Arruda-Colli M, Weaver M, Wiener L. Communication about dying, death, and bereavement: A systematic review of children's literature. *Journal of Palliative Medicine*. 2017;20(5):548–559. https://doi.org/10.1089/jpm.2016.0494
50. Kreitler S, Oppenheim D, Segev-Shoham E. Fantasy, art therapies, and other expressive and creative psychosocial interventions. In Kreitler S, ed. *Psychosocial Aspects of Pediatric Oncology*. Wiley; 2012: 351–388.
51. Rokke K. Bibliotherapy: A place for childrens' literature in dealing with cancer. *J Pediatr Oncol Nurs*. 1993;10(2):57. https://doi.org/10.1177/104345429301000219
52. Brown CD. Therapeutic play and creative arts. In Armstrong-Daily A, ed. *Hospice Care for Children*. Oxford University Press; 2009:305–338.
53. Kalm MA. *The Healing Movie Book—Precious Images: The Healing Use of Cinema in Psychotherapy*. Lulu Press; 2004.
54. Wolz B. *E-motion Picture Magic: A Movie Lover's Guide to Healing and Transformation*. Glenbridge; 2005.
55. Wiener L. *This is My World*. CWLA Press; 1998.
56. Malchiodi CA. *Art Therapy and Computer Technology: A Virtual Studio of Possibilities*. Jessica Kingsley; 2000.
57. Wiener L, Ballard E, Brennan T, Battles H, Martinez P, Pao M. How I wish to be remembered: The use of an advance care planning document in adolescent and young adult populations. *J Palliat Med*. 2008;11(10):1309–1313. https://doi.org/10.1089/jpm.2008.0126
58. Wiener LS, Battles H. Mandalas as a therapeutic technique for HIV-infected children and adolescents: What do they reveal? *J HIV AIDS Soc Serv*. 2002:1(3):27–39. https://doi.org/10.1300/J187v01n03_04
59. Weiser J. Phototherapy techniques: Using clients' personal snapshots and family photos as counseling and therapy tools; in memory of Arnold Gassan photographer, poet and phototherapy pioneer—feature. 2009. http://findarticles.com/p/articles/mi_m2479/is_3_29/ai_80757504/
60. Urbanski B, Lazenby M. Distress among hospitalized pediatric cancer patients modified by pet-therapy intervention to improve quality of life. *J Pediatr Oncol Nurs*. 2012;29(5):272–282. https://doi.org/10.1177/1043454212455697
61. Halm M. The healing power of the human-animal connection. *Am J Crit Care*. 2008;17(4):373–376. https://doi.org/10.4037/ajcc2008.17.4.373
62. Willis D. Animal therapy. *Rehabil Nurs*. 1997;22(2):78–81. https://doi.org/10.1002/j.2048-7940.1997.tb01738.x
63. Braun C, Stangler T, Narveson J, Pettingell S. Animal-assisted therapy as a pain relief intervention for children. *Complement Ther Clin Pract*. 2009;15(2):105–109. https://doi.org/10.1016/j.ctcp.2009.02.008
64. DeJong M, Fombonne E. Citalopram to treat depression in pediatric oncology. *J Child Adolesc Psychopharmacol*. 2007;17(3):371–377. https://doi.org/10.1089/cap.2006.0076
65. Maisami M, Sohmer B, Coyle J. Combined use of tricyclic antidepressants and neuroleptics in the management of terminally ill children: A report on three cases. *J Am Acad Child Psychiatry*. 1985;24(4):487–489.
66. Pfefferbaum-Levine B, Kumor K, Cangir A, Choroszy M, Roseberry E. Tricyclic antidepressants for children with cancer. *Am J Psychiatry*. 1983;140(8):1074–1076. https://doi.org/10.1176/ajp.140.8.1074
67. Bealke J, Meighen K. Risperidone treatment of three seriously medically ill children with secondary mood disorders. *Psychosomatics*. 2005;46(3):254–258. https://doi.org/10.1176/appi.psy.46.3.254
68. Samsel C, Muriel A. Risk factors and treatment for steroid-related mood and behavior symptoms in preschool children with leukemia: A case series. *Pediatr Blood Cancer*. 2017;64(2):343–345. https://doi.org/10.1002/pbc.26220
69. Walling V, Pfefferbaum B. The use of methylphenidate in a depressed adolescent with AIDS. *J Dev Behav Pediatr*. 1990;11(4):195–197. https://doi.org/10.1097/00004703-199008000-00007
70. Diamond G, Josephson A. Family-based treatment research: A 10-year update. *J Am Acad Child Adolesc Psychiatry*. 2005;44(9): 872–887. https://doi.org/10.1097/01.chi.0000169010.96783.4e
71. Cleeland C, Bennett G, Dantzer R, et al. Are the symptoms of cancer and cancer treatment due to a shared biologic mechanism? A cytokine-immunologic model of cancer symptoms. *Cancer*. 2003;97(11):2919–2925. https://doi.org/10.1002/cncr.11382
72. Miller A, Maletic V, Raison C. Inflammation and its discontents: The role of cytokines in the pathophysiology of major depression. *Biol Psychiatry*. 2009;65(9):732–741. https://doi.org/10.1016/j.biopsych.2008.11.029
73. Warris L, van den Heuvel-Eibrink M, Aarsen F, et al. Hydrocortisone as an intervention for dexamethasone-induced adverse effects in pediatric patients with acute lymphoblastic leukemia: Results of a double-blind, randomized controlled trial. *J Clin Oncol*. 2016;34(19):2287–2293. https://doi.org/10.1200/jco.2015.66.0761
74. Kazak A, Alderfer M, Streisand R, et al. Treatment of posttraumatic stress symptoms in adolescent survivors of childhood cancer and their families: A randomized clinical trial. *J Fam Psychol*. 2004;18(3): 493–504. https://doi.org/10.1037/0893-3200.18.3.493
75. Stuber M, Shemesh E. Post-traumatic stress response to life-threatening illnesses in children and their parents. *Child Adolesc Psychiatr Clin North Am*. 2006;15(3):597–609. https://doi.org/10.1016/j.chc.2006.02.006
76. Stuber ML, Schneider S, Kassam-Adams N, Kazak AE, Saxe G. The medical traumatic stress toolkit. *CNS Spectrums*. 2006;11(2): 137–142. https://doi.org/10.1017/s1092852900010671
77. Schor EL, American Academy of Pediatrics. Family pediatrics: Report of the task force on the family. *Pediatrics*. 2003;111:1541–1571

18 | EXISTENTIAL SUFFERING AND DISTRESS

ELISHA WALDMAN AND MARK BARTEL

The way care is given can reach the most hidden places.

Dame Cicely Saunders[1]

Suffering—its identification, prevention, and alleviation—lies at the heart of the work of palliative care. Suffering may take any number of forms, ranging from the physical to the psychological to the social and the spiritual. This chapter deals with the particular yet difficult to define domain of existential suffering. The first part of the chapter explores how we define and identify existential suffering. The second part explores where, in the context of the practice of pediatric palliative care (PPC), clinicians might encounter existential suffering. The third part explores ways in which interdisciplinary teams might address existential suffering.

Family Vignette

The teenaged patient was known as "the angry one" on the unit. Everyone experienced her dismissal and struggled to connect with her. She wanted to throw everyone out of her room and withdrew even from her parents. The curtains were left closed, the television was off, and she refused to eat more than a minimal amount each day. All attempts to help offered by her doctors, nurses, social workers, chaplains, and child life specialists were rejected. The existential suffering she experienced was worsening her condition, distressing her family, and overwhelming the medical team. Several ideas for the sources of her existential suffering were circulating, but it was the child life specialist who pinpointed the issue: her parents did not want to speak to her about her terminal condition. After a long discussion with the child life specialist and the chaplain, the parents were able to reflect on the importance of honesty and decided to speak with their daughter.

After the patient died, the mother shared the outcome of their discussion with us. Opening up this topic began an existential healing and gave both mother and daughter the priceless gift of communication. During a late-night conversation, as they lay in bed together, the daughter brought up one of the losses she faced: she asked her mother what it is like to have a baby, something this girl knew she would never experience.

IDENTIFYING EXISTENTIAL SUFFERING

The experience of existential suffering in humans extends back to the earliest emergence of a self-aware *Homo sapiens*. Among the earliest recorded evidence of such suffering is a clay tablet from the Near East that dates to about 3,000 years ago. It is inscribed with what is known as the Babylonian theodicy, a poem describing two friends debating the meaning of suffering: "You are kind, my friend; behold my grief. / Help me; look on my distress; know it. / I, though humble, wise, and a suppliant, / Have not seen help or succour for one moment."[2] The Biblical Book of Job, likely more familiar to the modern reader, is believed to have its origins in that poem.[3] In Job we read of the protagonist, suffering one tragedy after another, saying, "When I looked for good, evil came, and when I waited for light, darkness came. My inward parts are in turmoil and are never still; days of affliction come to meet me. I go about in sunless gloom; I stand up in the assembly and cry for help" (30:26–28).[4] This cry resonates across the ages and is surely recognizable to the modern reader as an expression of existential distress; this could very easily have been written just today.

Numerous examples from art and literature over the past two millennia attest to human interest in and recognition of the importance of suffering, ranging from the passions of Bach and Verdi, to the painting and sculpture of Michelangelo and Picasso, to the writings of Dostoevsky and Dickens. Interest in the topic of existential suffering as reflected specifically in the medical literature has grown in recent years. This may reflect relatively recent and continually improving developments in interventions which may not "cure" a condition but can prolong life. While such interventions are introduced with the hope of simultaneously improving quality of life, all too often this is not the case. Instead, they may result in tradeoffs involving more time lived but with diminished quality, during which time existential issues might arise. Regardless, it is clear that over the past three decades there has been increased acceptance of the idea of whole-person care and the importance of addressing nonphysical symptoms along with physical symptoms and root causes of illness. This includes the idea of existential distress.

DEFINING EXISTENTIAL SUFFERING

Clinicians often use the term "existential suffering" or "existential distress," yet what is meant by this term and how to address it remain poorly understood. As one review paper states: "The most prevalent finding in this review has been a lack of consistency in the way existential suffering is defined and understood."[5] It also often seems that the terms "existential suffering" and "existential distress" are used interchangeably. The difference, if any, between the two terms may not be meaningful, but some have ventured that "suffering" is more indicative of an ongoing and critical process, whereas "distress" may represent a broader range of states, encompassing everything from what might be considered "normal" worries and sadness through disabling anxiety and panic.[6] That understanding should not indicate that distress about an issue is any less deserving of attention than had it been labeled "suffering." Rather, the label may indicate a degree of depth and gravity, with distress encompassing a potentially milder range. There may also be a difference in degree of temporality implied by the two terms, with the idea of suffering indicating an experience that is more sustained. Ultimately, the difference may be academic and less critical when it comes to the bedside. For the purposes of this chapter, we will primarily use the term "existential suffering" but acknowledge that many may use that term and "existential distress" interchangeably without making a distinction.

A review of the literature suggests that there may be upward of 50 different definitions of existential suffering, which speaks to the lack of a common language around the issue.[5] Despite the lack of consensus, attempts have been made to create classification systems as a way of defining types, or root causes, of existential suffering.[7] It is then possible to extract a number of themes that appear to be consistent across definitions. Existential suffering often touches on or overlaps with spirituality, psychological distress, social distress, and physical symptoms. It is important to recognize that these other forms of suffering may be at once distinct from yet linked to existential suffering; for example, the experience of ongoing physical suffering may well exacerbate the experience of existential suffering. Identifying and addressing these potential contributing issues is a vital part of addressing existential suffering. The often-multifaceted nature of existential suffering also speaks to the importance of an interdisciplinary approach.

Existential suffering is often discussed in the context of spiritual distress, at times even interchangeably; certainly there is much shared language in discussing existential issues and spiritual issues. Spiritual distress is not limited just to those who identify with a faith community or specific set of religious beliefs.[7] Taken in its broadest form, the idea of spiritual distress is so closely aligned with, and even encompassed by, the idea of existential suffering that they are practically indistinguishable. Because of this, much of the literature that addresses existential suffering is also literature that addresses spiritual distress, and vice-versa. In addition (and as will be discussed later in this chapter) addressing existential suffering demands a broad interdisciplinary approach in which chaplaincy plays a specific and significant role.

There is limited research on the identification and management of existential suffering; most of the literature focuses on adult patients and is grounded in the psychiatric literature. An increasingly robust body of literature is exploring spiritual needs and distress in different populations, and this research contributes to the discussion of existential suffering. Often it seems that by "existential suffering" clinicians mean some sort of ineffable level of soul-deep suffering that is distinct from all other forms of more corporeal suffering[8] and is difficult to plumb and engage. In fact, the phrase "existential suffering" often seems as if it is appended to perceived suffering that is beyond our comprehension or skills to manage as clinicians, as though clinicians are acknowledging that "this is just the way it is." What makes existential suffering seem so elusive? Eric Cassel, a physician and one of the great modern writers on suffering in medicine wrote, "Suffering occurs when an impending destruction of the person is perceived; it continues until the threat of disintegration has passed or until the integrity of the person can be restored in some other manner."[9]

Classification systems as ways of defining types, or root causes of, existential suffering, are important to explore.[5] Although none of the proposed systems may be completely satisfactory, they can provide a framework for understanding what people mean by "existential suffering." The typologies presented in Table 18.1 may also be instructive when thinking about how to elicit and address concerns around such suffering.

An additional proposed classification scheme, drawing on the work of Yalom, has direct relevance for the world of palliative care. It proposes four domains through which existential suffering can exist.[10] The first domain is that of *mortality*, meaning a recognition of one's own mortality and an accompanying anxiety around death itself. Second is the domain of *freedom*, wherein an individual may experience regret about past choices and unresolved conflicts. Third is a struggle

TABLE 18.1 One typology of Existential Suffering, Or: Categories of Existential Suffering

Meaninglessness, purposelessness	Hopelessness, futility	Loneliness, isolation, abandonment
Life legacy	Crisis of faith	Loss of autonomy
Life review	Where is God?	Loss of social role
Unfinished business	Fear of dying	Grief over imminent separation/loss of relationships
Disappointment	Worry about life after death	Worry about becoming a burden to others
Guilt	Disruption of personal identity	Dependency
Remorse	Lack of peace	

TABLE 18.2 Domains of existential distress

EXISTENTIAL DOMAIN	CLINICAL EXAMPLE
Mortality	Expressing anxiety about dying or the afterlife. Worries about separating from loved ones
Freedom	Feelings of regret about past choices or unresolved conflict with one's self or others
Meaninglessness	Feelings of loss of purpose and meaning. Questioning the meaning of illness, suffering, or faith
Isolation	Feelings of abandonment by or disconnectedness from one's family, community, or God.

Used with permission from Grech T, Marks A. Fast facts and concepts #319: Existential suffering Part 1: Definition and diagnosis. *J Palliat Med.* 2017;20(1):93–94.[11]

around *meaning*, which may entail concerns around purpose and meaning of one's life, one's illness, and one's legacy. Finally is the domain of *isolation*, in which an individual may feel lost and abandoned by family, community, or God. Although the domains as described in Table 18.2 may not apply directly to all children and their families, they are nonetheless useful across a range of settings in which clinicians encounter existential suffering.

The idea of existential suffering is often met by staff with a sense of despair, perhaps frustration, and at times even a bit of a distancing, as though identifying an area of concern that is "other" (i.e., not the clinician's area of expertise and therefore something to be acknowledged from a distance but not directly engaged). Why is this? In part it may be that we lack the language to fully describe what this entity, existential suffering, really is. The concept gets at something fundamentally human, yet without an easily identifiable locus (as opposed to, e.g., pain caused by a tumor which can be localized and addressed). Even psychological concerns somehow seem easier to describe, as they can be identified as coming from the mind and/or brain and linked to how a person is processing emotions, feelings, and perceptions. Existential suffering, on the other hand, is harder to pin down. As Eric Cassell wrote, "Suffering is ultimately a personal matter. Patients sometimes report suffering when one does not expect it, or do not report suffering when one does expect it. Furthermore, a person can suffer enormously at the distress of another, especially a loved one."[9]

Existential suffering is also daunting because, unlike many other forms of suffering clinicians encounter, in addition to challenges around definitions, it may not be amenable to "treatment" the way most medical issues are treated. For medical professionals, so often focused on "fixing" things, this inability to solve an issue may feel very disconcerting and dissatisfying. Often, rather than "fix" existential suffering, what is asked of clinicians is simply to be present (as reflected in the palliative care teaching, "don't just do something, sit there!"). Being fully present in the face of human suffering can be terribly challenging and places great demands on the clinician who may feel uncomfortable and inadequately trained for such an "intervention."

An additional complexity for the clinician may stem from the fact that existential suffering may actually arise not just contemporaneously with—but possibly even as a result of—attempts at treating an underlying condition or illness. For example, feelings of existential suffering could easily be exacerbated by the experience of side effects of chemotherapy or organ transplantation such as pain or chronic negative impacts on quality of life. This can lead to feelings of clinician guilt and self-doubt (as in the case of a patient who experiences serious permanent organ damage or even death in the course of stem cell transplantation). Yet medical professionals and healers are obliged to try to relieve suffering. How does one even begin to engage in this daunting undertaking? At times, compassionate presence may be the only possible response to existential suffering.

ENCOUNTERING EXISTENTIAL SUFFERING IN CHILDREN

At the center of every story in PPC is a child. Many studies, in particular from the pediatric oncology literature, suggest that, certainly by adolescence, many children want to be involved in discussions about prognosis and treatment.[12] Alternately, a recent paradigm of "Having a Say" has also been proposed as an approach that focuses more on child and adolescent communication preferences and that recognizes that those preferences may change through the course of an illness.[13] Unfortunately, even when clinicians do engage children in direct discussions, existential suffering may often be underappreciated. This may be due to parental concerns about clinicians exploring such issues with children, as well as to clinician discomfort with delving into these domains. In addition, simply recognizing signs of existential suffering, as well as the language used by children to express it, may fall outside the knowledge base and comfort zone of some providers. And yet existential suffering in children is a very real entity and, in fact, is one that can involve devastating psychological and emotional distress. Trauma and illness can impact children's sense of identity and grounding, affecting their faith, worldview, and sense of security. It is important to recognize that adult-based constructs around suffering and existential issues are not always directly transferrable to children.

Part of the challenge stems from variability in developmental maturity as "children" grow from a legal age of minority to one of adulthood. In addition, the idea of existential suffering is linked with personal concepts of meaning, spirituality, and place in the world that mature with time, developing along with one's experience of the surrounding world. How distress is experienced and expressed by a child depends on developmental stage and neurologic status and may change over time. Fowler's proposed stages of spiritual development provide one model of how an individual's understanding and expression of spirituality may develop through the life cycle.[14,15] This model is fluid and individuals may move through different stages of spiritual development in nonlinear fashion depending on life events.

It has also been well established, in the work of Robert Coles and others, that even from a very young age children may experience rich spiritual lives.[16] These experiences may be expressed nonverbally, for example through artwork. Table 18.3 presents one model of how children's spiritual development may track with developing concepts of illness and death, along with potentially helpful interventions at each stage.[17]

How young can a child be and still experience existential suffering? It is important to note here that we are talking about not just suffering in the general sense (e.g., exploring the question of who decides if a neurologically compromised child is suffering), but rather specifically *existential suffering*, which implies some distress around one's sense of self, one's security, and one's place in the world. Many clinicians who work with neonates attest to a definite sense that even newborns can experience distress that is distinct from pain, hunger, or discomfort and which may be more related to a sense of disruption of "normal" neonatal attachment: a loss of parental presence, parental comfort and contact. In short, a form of existential suffering.

> The newborn's condition was declining, and her mother was brought from the recovery room. It was hoped that there would time for her to say goodbye. When the mother arrived, she spoke to her baby and touched her gently. The baby then stabilized.

Human beings, from the moment of first contact with the outside world, are capable of experiencing some form of existential suffering. To be sure, the means of expressing that distress, the nonverbal cues or language and constructs used to describe it, change with time, experience, and developmental maturity. But the capacity to experience existential suffering is a fundamental aspect of humanity, and the burden is on clinicians and caretakers to be sensitive to those expressions and adapt language and sensibilities to the needs of our patients.

As is accepted practice in pediatrics, clinicians should attempt, when possible, to speak directly with patients in an age- and developmentally appropriate way. Studies suggest, for example, that adolescents are largely willing to engage in discussions about spirituality, but that the language and framing they use may be different from what we expect of adults.[18] For example, adolescents may not speak explicitly about religion or religious practices and may even express a lack of interest in those ideas, but instead may speak more broadly about "energies," karma, meaning, or hopes for the future. Entering into discussions with an awareness

TABLE 18.3 Children's spiritual development and concepts of death

AGE RANGE	CHILDREN'S SPIRITUAL DEVELOPMENT	CHILDREN'S DEVELOPMENTAL UNDERSTANDING OF THE DEATH	SUPPORTIVE INTERVENTIONS FOR EXPRESSION OF CHILDREN'S FEELINGS AND WORRIES
1–4	The child models spirituality based on their loved ones' beliefs. Religious symbols bring forth feelings of love and companionship or terror and guilt	The child has a very limited understanding of the concrete aspects of death. They view death as temporary and reversible	Play activities assist children in expressing their emotional or spiritual concerns. Medical toys such as puppets, coloring books, encourage expression of concerns
5–10	The child's development of spiritual beliefs arises through fantasy and stories of good and evil	They can think concretely and have imaginative belief systems. However, they lack the ability to understand the intricacies of death. Children may be afraid of going to sleep and not waking. They fear that they may have done something wrong to cause their illness and feel guilt for bringing suffering to the family	The incorporation of drama, play therapy, and drawings helps children express their worries about their illness. Discussions about symbols in their play create opportunities for children to discuss their fears and guilt
10–13	They begin to understand the larger meanings of punishment and rewards. They may question God about their illness and wonder why they must suffer	They can grasp the permanence of death. They fear the specifics of what will happen as the approach death and after they die	Discussions with youth about their worries may help in the processing of emotions and release of existential and spirtual distress. They may wish to talk with family and friends about dying, their fears, and to gather comfort knowing family will eventually heal after their death. Games and time with friends foster therapeutic distractions for children
14–18	The adolescent ponders	Adolescents typically have a clear understanding of their illness and grasp the realities of their life-threatening condition. However, they may lack the emotional maturity to cope with the enormity of their situation	Support groups, teen play rooms, and flexible visitation rules help to promote socialization and adolescent development. Allowing adolescents to participate in their medical decisions enhances their sense of control and self-efficacy

Reproduced with permission from Currin-McCulloch J, Proserpio T, Podda M, Clerici C. Easing existential distress in pediatric cancer care. In Wolfe J et al., eds. Palliative Care in Pediatric Oncology. Springer International; 2018. P189-201.[17]

of and curiosity about these possible differences is critical. Clinicians must also be thoughtful about soliciting parental permission and partnering with parents before exploring serious topics with a child. This may be especially challenging when it comes to exploring potential existential suffering, as parents desperate to protect their child may feel defensive about allowing any provider to delve into such profound and intimate subjects. Tools such as Voicing My Choices may provide some language and a mechanism to open up these discussions with parents and children alike.[19] Providers should also remain alert to the possibility of cultural differences, especially when dealing with patients and families from a different background, as they may have different perspectives on disclosure and acceptability of involving children in discussions.[20,21]

> The adolescent was clearly declining and knew she was going to die, but her parents refused to let staff speak openly with her. At one point she was asked by a child life specialist if there was a song she'd like to hear on her tablet, and she replied with the name of a song about heaven. She was trying to signal to her mother that she had questions about her future and wanted to talk, but it was not until later, the day she died, that the parents openly acknowledged her impending death.

ENCOUNTERING EXISTENTIAL SUFFERING IN FAMILIES

Adding to the complexity of identifying existential suffering is that, in pediatrics in particular, clinical teams engage with the family as a unit, with that unit's collective sense of values and identity. Simultaneously, clinicians engage with the members of that family unit as individuals—parents, children, extended family—and each individual's sense of identity both acts upon and is acted on by the identities of the others in the group. Clinicians must therefore be attuned to the values and needs of all family members involved in the care of a patient, both because each of those family members may themselves be at risk for existential suffering and because what each member is experiencing will potentially have an impact on others.

PARENTS

Much of the existing literature on existential suffering is, perhaps unsurprisingly, focused on the adult experience, and, in fact, much of the work done by PPC teams may be parent-focused. In addition, given that PPC often requires us to interface more with adults than with the children themselves (e.g., in situations where the children are unable to communicate or are simply too young), clinicians are often more likely to pick up on existential suffering in parents.

For parents, having a child facing potentially life-limiting illness may impact the parental role, limiting or even destroying their sense of control, their sense that they are able to protect their child.[22] This experience may also undermine parents' faith and worldview, destroying their sense of identity, structure, and grounding. Essentially everything that in the past may have given a parent meaning in life is disrupted and called into question.

> The Trauma Center team had done its best but the boy did not survive his injuries. When his mother was told, she became distraught and ran from the hospital out into the adjacent highway's busy traffic. She was successfully rescued from harm and brought back inside, later explaining that she was trying to be hit by a car because she had nothing to live for without her beloved son.

Conversely, many parents may find spirituality and faith communities to be a source of support and a place that provides them with strength and meaning.[23,24] This appears to be true not just after a child has died, but throughout the stages of a child's illness, regardless of outcome.[24,25] Some tools for screening for spiritual needs have been developed; perhaps the best known of these is the Faith, Importance, Community, Address (FICA) in care tool, designed to help facilitate discussions about spirituality between clinicians and adult patients.[26]

SIBLINGS

Clinicians should also consider the possibility of existential suffering in other family members. This may include grandparents or other extended family members, but siblings in particular are at risk of being forgotten, often suffering from the changing dynamics in the nuclear family brought on by the demands of caring for a sick child.[27] Siblings may experience anxiety around their own well-being as well as that of their affected sibling.[28,29] Mental health professionals such as child psychologists, child psychiatrists, and social workers, as well as child life specialists and chaplains, may prove helpful in both evaluating and addressing needs.[30,31] In addition, hospital or community-based support groups may be helpful in providing support.

> As the infant's condition continued to decline, his 10-year-old sister became more and more anxious. She was unable to complete school tasks that were previously easy for her, and she spent more time alone at home. Her parents finally understood more fully when she was able to explain her self-assigned existential role to them: "I am his second Mommy—I need to fix this!" After the tears slowed, she and her parents were able to talk through the feelings of helplessness and love that they were all sharing.

ENCOUNTERING EXISTENTIAL SUFFERING IN PROVIDERS

Finally, it should not be overlooked that clinicians themselves may experience existential suffering. Those in fields such as PPC, intensive care, and oncology are at risk for existential suffering through ongoing exposure to intense, often emotional situations.[32] Though many clinicians are taught as part of their training to separate the personal from their professional lives and exercise good self-care, it can be extremely challenging when working in the midst of great suffering. It may not be possible or even desirable to attempt to so divide ourselves.

> The Emergency Department nurse shared her worries about coping: "If I maintain a 'cast iron' heart in order to protect myself here at work, I might take that home, becoming cold to those I love."

There is an inevitable spillover between the spheres of our lives. Acknowledging both, and their influences on the other, is an honest start to managing our own existential suffering. More research in this area would be welcome, for it is not surprising that some clinicians find themselves grappling with questions of faith and meaning, struggling with their own roles in the dramas they face daily. It is always important for clinicians to remember that they are not alone: speaking with trusted colleagues allows expression and reflection on these deep feelings. Utilizing an interdisciplinary approach, the palliative care team may play a crucial role in providing support for fellow clinicians and trainees.

ADDRESSING EXISTENTIAL SUFFERING

How to approach existential suffering in patients and families? The first step is, of course, to remain alert to the possibility of its presence. Unfortunately, this may be also the easiest step to miss. It is far easier to focus on the concrete and mechanistic aspects of care: the next step in a treatment plan, the next medication to be tried. But to recognize, explore, and address existential suffering, clinicians must be willing to identify those vulnerable moments, even seek them out, and explore them with patients and families.

A number of formalized interventions have been proposed in addressing existential suffering in adults; it should also be noted that most are grounded in psychiatric and psychoanalytic approaches. Some of these interventions provide valuable guidance for all clinicians in addressing existential issues in parents, siblings, patients, and staff alike. An example of one such proposed intervention is "dignity therapy," a type of focused psychotherapy designed by Chochinov, the aim of which is to bring a sense of meaning to individuals facing life-limiting illness.[33–35] Other approaches, for example, include group and individual meaning-centered psychotherapy (based on the teachings of Viktor Frankl) and hypnosis-facilitated therapy. Clearly not all of these approaches will be feasible when addressing existential suffering in children; furthermore, these approaches require the expertise of specialty-trained mental health professionals. Yet incorporating some of the basic tenets into care, such as careful use of language and monitoring our own behavior, may prove useful in opening the door for patients and families to discuss existential concerns. Through these discussions, many of these concerns may be alleviated. Chochinov described four components of dignity-conserving therapy: attitudes, behavior, compassion, and dialogue.[34] Box 18.1 includes some helpful suggestions based on these categories that may be useful for clinicians from any discipline.

With awareness of the possibility of existential distress clinicians can cultivate an inner courage to engage, be fully present, and be willing to listen and enter into a relationship. At that point we clinicians can let the child and family teach us what they are experiencing and understand how we may best walk alongside them. Each child approaches the end of life differently, with unique strengths and stressors. If clinicians can become trustworthy companions in their eyes, they will feel more open about sharing their fears, hopes, and feelings. With this isolation aspect of existential suffering alleviated, the child can then express specific ways that teams may further serve them at end of life.

BOX 18.1 EXAMPLES OF APPROACHES TO DIGNITY-CONSERVING CARE

Attitudes and assumptions can affect practice.

Be aware of how your own and other clinicians' past experiences, attitudes, and assumptions may affect provision of care.

Teach learners to be mindful of how their attitudes and assumptions may shape behaviors.

Behaviors should always enhance patient dignity.

Use nonverbal techniques to convey caring and attentiveness.

Don't rush; sit down and make eye contact.

Turn off digital devices and avoid jargon when talking with patients and their families.

Acknowledge personhood beyond the illness.

Elicit personal stories; encourage sharing of reflections and memories.

Acknowledge the effect of sickness on a patient and family's broader life experience.

Recognize and acknowledge suffering.

Explore patient and family values.

Explore whether to involve extended family or community supports.

Adapted with permission from 40. Cook D, Rocker G. Dying with dignity in the intensive care unit. *N Engl J Med.* 2014;370:2506–2514.

CHAPLAINCY AND OTHER INTERDISCIPLINARY TEAM MEMBERS

Given the significant overlap between existential issues and spirituality, it is essential to emphasize the role that chaplaincy plays in addressing existential suffering. Some PPC teams have successfully integrated a dedicated chaplain as part of the core team, while others may rely on chaplains available through their institutions.[36] Regardless of team structure, having a close working relationship with a chaplain allows for integration of a critical skill set into palliative care interventions. In addressing existential suffering, chaplains function to complement and enhance work being done by palliative care providers, as well as add yet another layer to the support provided by the PPC team. Box 18.2 outlines aspects of the role of chaplaincy in providing palliative care.

BOX 18.2 FIVE ASPECTS OF CHAPLAINCY'S ROLE ON THE PALLIATIVE CARE TEAM

Spiritual concerns heard

- Assessing patient/family spiritual concerns and needs
- Listening in witness to distress and existential suffering
- Interpreting these concerns to the team (including hopes, fears, denial, miracle language, misunderstandings of medical issues)

Spiritual support provided

- Addressing expressed patient/family spiritual concerns and needs
- Including life review and difficult ethical and end-of-life decision-making
- Including assisting the team in providing spiritual care to their level of expertise and comfort

Creating sacred space and providing rituals for end of life

- Rituals from patient/family's own spiritual, cultural and/or worldview traditions
- Rituals devised with patient/family for their specific needs

Establishing partnership with patient/family religious leaders

- Interpreting medical messages for community-based religious leaders and way-finding in the medical setting
- Supplementing spiritual care when community-based religious leaders cannot be present or when patient/family have no religious preference
- Serving as alternate spiritual listener when patient or family wishes to explore other possibilities or emotions

Assisting in team resilience

- Offering opportunities including reflection, "defusing," debriefings, memorial gatherings, and education as the palliative care team shares in emotionally laden end-of-life relationships
- Offering the same for the rest of the medical staff who may struggle with strong emotions and moral distress while working with the patient and the palliative care team

Figure 18.1 illustrates a model of how spiritual providers, in partnership with other clinicians, may bring these skills to bear across the course of a child's illness in order to provide comprehensive spiritual support. This model can also illustrate how other psychosocial clinicians such as psychologists, social workers, and child life specialists can collaborate with other clinicians to provide whole-person care. Chaplains, with their specific focus on spirituality, play a central role in identifying and addressing existential suffering. Psychologists, social workers, child life specialists, and expressive arts therapists address it as well. Given the complex and often multifaceted nature of existential suffering and its root causes, such collaborative models and partnerships are essential in the care of any individual, whether it be a be a child, family member, or staff clinician experiencing existential suffering. Additionally, this model applies to care delivery across a spectrum of settings, not just the inpatient setting, reflecting the importance of exploring needs in an ongoing fashion throughout the course of an illness.

Just as palliative care specialists differentiate between primary palliative care (basic skills for all clinicians to master) and specialty palliative care (those skills acquired through advanced training), it is important for all providers to have some degree of comfort in exploring existential issues with seriously ill patients. By approaching patients and their families with curiosity and an openness to the possibility of existential suffering, clinicians can begin to identify how overlapping issues might be addressed (e.g., depression, social support issues, spiritual distress). If no other issues are identified, the focus is on exploring the nuances of the experience of existential suffering. Cross-training (i.e., improving primary spiritual, psychological, and psychosocial skill sets) should be an essential part of training for all clinicians, regardless of discipline, who care for children with serious illness. Opportunities for further training are emerging, such as the Interprofessional Spiritual Care Educational Curriculum (ISPEC, now being adapted into the pediatric-specific ISPEC-Peds) at the George Washington Institute for Spirituality and Health. Such courses are much-needed steps toward improving primary skills in exploring existential suffering.[38,39] This sort of cross-training, combined with close partnering between disciplines (whether part of an interdisciplinary palliative care team or not), results in a team whose sum is truly greater than its parts.

FUTURE DIRECTIONS

While it is gratifying to see how far the idea of whole-person care and spiritual care has come in recent years, much work remains. Understanding the spiritual and existential needs of children across developmental stages, as well as those of parents and clinicians, is critical to knowing how to best address them. In addition to research to improve the evidence base, conferences and publications where experiences are

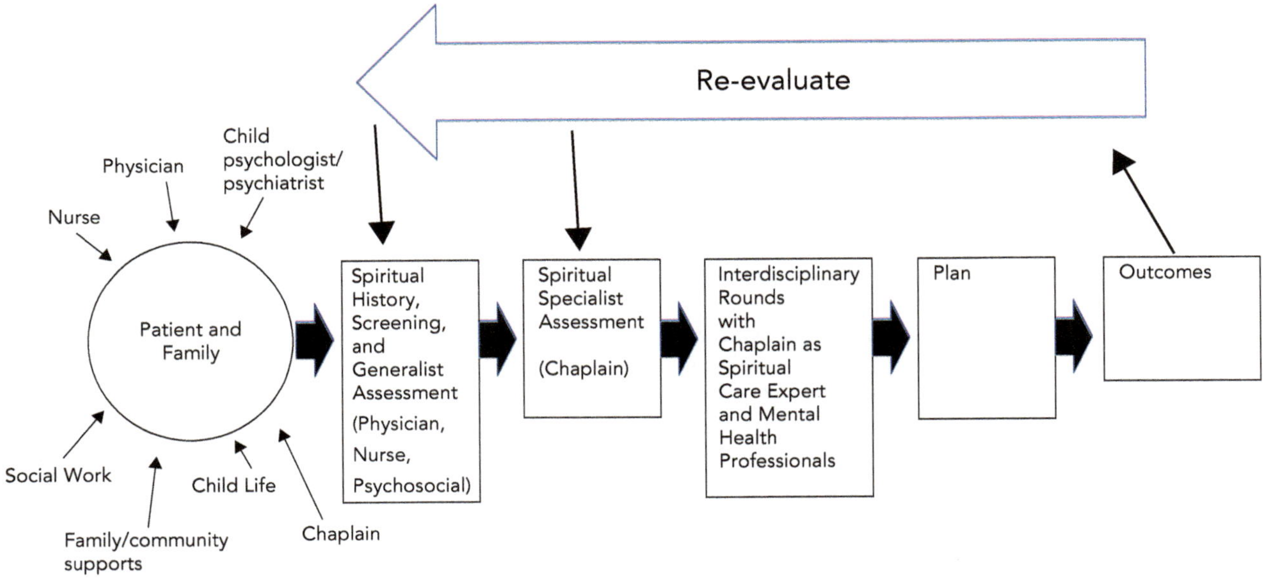

Figure 18.1 Inpatient spiritual care implementation model.[37]

Used with permission from Puchalski C, Ferrell B, Virani R, et al. Improving the quality of spiritual care as a dimension of palliative care: The report of the Consensus Conference. *J Palliat Med.* 2009;12(10):885–904.

shared are critical. Especially given the varying composition of palliative care teams at different centers, as well as the variable availability of other specialists such as chaplains, models for how teams explore existential distress will likely need to be adjusted to meet specific needs: there is not likely to be just one answer. The more information and experiences are shared, the stronger and more agile the palliative care community will be in responding to these needs.

Clinicians also must continue to advocate with healthcare systems at the local, state, and federal levels for funding to support interdisciplinary teams, without which care cannot be truly holistic. As noted earlier, educational opportunities are emerging, and continued growth of these opportunities, plus exploration of novel educational methods (such as online learning) should be developed to help improve accessibility to all providers. Finally, clinicians must continue to look inward with courage, into their own hearts as clinicians and healers, and acknowledge their own strengths, fears, and weaknesses. They must recognize and accept that not everything can be "fixed." Sometimes even just the act of opening up to exploring existential issues, or of simply listening and being present, can provide just enough space for patients and families to unburden themselves and find comfort and meaning, even if the ultimate questions remain unanswered.

"Oh that I had one to hear me!" Job 31:35

Family Reflection: Existential Suffering Across the Family Unit

Our daughter, Nora, was 16 when she was diagnosed with cancer in her liver and lungs. Her older brother was home from college when she started treatment, so our full family of four leapt into caregiving mode. Close to a year later, Nora passed away.

Everyone in our family experienced existential suffering. There are painful memories of Nora in bed, almost inconsolable, questioning why this was happening; her brother trying to summon the courage to be by her side in her final hours; and, as parents, confronting the absolute worst thing that could happen to a parent.

Some specifics: Nora found the persistent nausea even worse than the pain. We tried so many different combinations of medicines, never quite sure what was actually working and in what combination. If I could go back in time, I would have kept a medicine diary that would register what she was taking and the positive or negative effect.

Although it was rare, there were a few caregivers with poor bedside manner. Those interactions were always extremely upsetting to Nora. The opposite was also true: the vast majority of our nurses, palliative care team, doctors were excellent and warm communicators—the impact they had on Nora was profound. When she felt seen, she felt taken care of; her anxiety was reduced and she was able to joke and enjoy things.

In retrospect, I wish we had a better sense of how we could also tend to Nora's brother during this time. We were so focused on Nora—necessarily so—but he was and still is suffering. I know that there were sibling groups available to him, but he's not a joiner in that way. I don't think Nora felt his pain, but as parents we could see it.

As a parent, you have to fight from operating with a scarcity mindset and lapsing into catastrophic thinking. Like Nora, when we were not "seen" by our caregivers, we suffered. There was a time in the summer when they turned over the whole staff of doctors, and that was a very rough period for all of us. Even though we had our main oncologist, nurse practitioners, and palliative group the resident team managed our hourly care and we faced some real struggles when the new team came on board and included some folks who were very poor communicators. The good news was that our core team was so connected with us that they were able to right the ship pretty quickly.

We never had to contend with what I know would have been the absolute worst part of this journey—telling Nora she wasn't going to live. By the time we knew this as fact she was moving into liver and kidney failure and was too medicated to discuss her condition.

Her death and the days, weeks, and months after, were the most difficult and dark days of our lives. The fact that our caregiving team and the hospital stayed in touch with us—through notes and messages—was a key part in treating our true existential despair. If we hadn't had that I worry that we would have had a much harder time making it out of the depth of our sadness. We were reminded that Nora mattered and that we mattered. We were all continuing to be seen.

REFERENCES

1. Doyle D, Hanks GWC, MacDonald N, eds. Foreword. *The Oxford Textbook of Palliative Medicine*. 2nd ed. Oxford University Press; 1998: ix.
2. Lambert WG, trans. Translation from Electronic Tools and Near East Archives (etana.org), *Babylonian Theodicy*. Lines 287–290.
3. Clarke B. Misery loves company: A comparative analysis of Theodicy Literature in ancient Mesopotamia and Israel. *Intermount West J Relig Stud*. 2010;2:78–92.
4. Biblical quotes. *The Harper Collins Study Bible* (New Revised Standard Version). Harper Collins; 1993.
5. Boston P, Bruce A, Schreiber R. Existential suffering in the palliative care setting: An integrated literature review. *J Pain Symp Manag*. 2011;41(3):604–618.
6. National Comprehensive Cancer Network. *NCCN Clinical Practice Guidelines in Oncology: Distress Management*. NCCN; 2010. Version 1, 2011.
7. Cai S, Guo Q, Luo Y, et al. Spiritual needs and communicating about death in nonreligious theistic families in pediatric palliative care: A qualitative study. *Palliat Med*. 2020;34(4):533–540.
8. Bruce A, Schreiber R, Petrovskaya O, Boston P. Longing for ground in a ground(less) world: A qualitative inquiry of existential suffering. *BMC Nursing*. 2011;10(2)p 1-9.
9. Cassel EJ. The nature of suffering and the goals of medicine. *N Engl J Med*. 1982;306(11):639–645.
10. Yalom ID. Existential Psychotherapy. Basic Books; 1980.
11. Green T, Marks A. Fast facts and concepts #319: Existential suffering Part 1: Definition and diagnosis. *J Palliat Med*. 2017;20(1):93–94.
12. Sisk BA, Fasciano K, Block SD, Mack JW. Longitudinal prognostic communication needs of adolescents and young adults with cancer. *Cancer*. 2020;126(2):400–407.
13. Kelly K, Mowbray C, Pyke-Grimm K, Hinds P. Identifying a conceptual shift in child and adolescent-reported treatment decision making: "Having a say, as I need at this time." *Pediatr Blood Cancer*. 2017;64(4) p1-8.
14. Fowler JW, Dell ML, Fowler JW, et al. Stages of faith and identity: Birth to teens. *Child Adolesc Psychiatr Clin N Am*. 2004;13(1): 17–33.
15. Neuman ME Addressing children's beliefs through Fowler's stages of faith. *J Pediatr Nurs*. 2011;26(1):44–50.
16. Coles R. *The Spiritual Life of Children*. Houghton Mifflin; 1990.
17. Currin-McCulloch J, Proserpio T, Podda M, Clerici C. Easing existential distress in pediatric cancer care. In Wolfe J et al., eds. Palliative Care in Pediatric Oncology. Springer International; 2018. P189-201.
18. Barton KS, Tate T, Lau N, et al. "I'm not a spiritual person." How hope might facilitate conversations about spirituality among teens and young adults with cancer. *J Pain Symptom Manage*. 2018;55(6):1599–1608.
19. Weiner L, Zadeh S, Battles H, et al. Allowing adolescents and young adults to plan their end-of-life care. *Pediatrics*. Nov;130(5):897–905.
20. Wiener L, McConnell DG, Latella L, et al. Cultural and religious considerations in pediatric palliative care. *Palliat Support Care*. 2013 Feb;11(1):47–67.
21. Rosenberg AR, Bona K, Coker T, et al. Pediatric palliative care in the multicultural context: Findings from a workshop conference. *J Pain Symptom Manage*. 2019;57(4):846–855.
22. Bluebond-Langner M. *The Private Worlds of Dying Children*. Princeton University Press; 1978.
23. Scneider MA, Mannell RC. Beacon in the storm: An exploration of the spirituality and faith of parents whose children have cancer. *Issues Compr Pediatr Nurs*. 2006;29(1):3–24.
24. Hexem KR, Moller CJ, Carroll K, et al. How parents of children receiving pediatric palliative care use religion, spirituality, or life philosophy in tough times. *J Palliat Med*. 2011;14(1):39–44.
25. Robinson MR, Thiel MM, Backus MM, et al. Matters of spirituality at the end of life in the pediatric intensive care unit. *Pediatrics*. 2006;118(3):e719–e729.
26. Puchalski C, Romer AL. Taking a spiritual history allows clinicians to understand patients more fully. *J Palliat Med*. 2000;3(1):129–137.
27. Sloper P. Experiences and support needs of siblings of children with cancer. *Health Social Care Community* 2000;8(5):298–306.
28. Nolbris M, Enskar k, Hellstrom A. Experience of siblings of children treated for cancer. *Eur J Oncol Nurs*. 2007;11(2):106–112.
29. Bluebond-Langner M. *In the Shadow of Illness: Parents and Siblings of the Chronically Ill Child*. Princeton University Press; 2000.
30. Murray JS. A qualitative exploration of psychosocial support for siblings of children with cancer. *J Pediatr Nurs*. 2002;17(5):327–337.
31. Steele AC, Kaal J, Thompson AL, et al. Bereaved parents and siblings offer advice to healthcare providers and researchers. *J Pediatr Hematol Oncol*. 2013;35(4):253–259.
32. Pessin H, Fenn N, Hendriksen E, et al. Existential distress among caregivers or professionals taking care of dying patients. *Curr Opin Support Palliat Care*. 2015;9(1):77–86.
33. Chochinov HM. *Dignity Therapy: Final Words for Final Days*. Oxford University Press; 2012.
34. Chochinov HM. Dignity and the essence of medicine: The A, B, C, and D of dignity-conserving care. *BMJ*. 2007;335(18):184–187.
35. Martinez M, Arantzamendi M, Belar A, et al. "Dignity therapy," a promising intervention in palliative care: A comprehensive systematic literature review. *Palliat Med*. 2017;31(6):492–509.
36. Fitchett G, Lyndes KA, Cadge W, et al. The role of professional chaplains on pediatric palliative care teams: Perspectives from physicians and chaplains. *J Palliat Med*. 2011;14(6):704–707.
37. Puchalski C, Ferrell B, Virani R, et al. Improving the quality of spiritual care as a dimension of palliative care: The report of the Consensus Conference. *J Palliat Med*. 2009;12(10):885–904.
38. Puchalski C, Jafari N, Buller H, et al. Interprofessional spiritual care education curriculum: A milestone toward the provision of spiritual care. *J Palliat Med*. 2019.
39. Robinson M, Thiel MM, Shirkey K, et al. Efficacy of training interprofessional spiritual care generalists. *J Palliat Med*. 2016;19(8):814–821.
40. Cook D, Rocker G. Dying with dignity in the intensive care unit. *N Engl J Med*. 2014;370:2506–2514.

19 | NEUROLOGICAL SYMPTOMS

SHIH-NING LIAW, JENNA E. FREITAS, AND JULIE HAUER

We could not foresee what we might meet upon our road. Torment in the dark was the danger that I feared, and it did not hold me back. But I would not have come, had I known the danger of light and joy.

GIMLI, *in the Lord of the Rings by J. R. R. Tolkien*

Children with neurological conditions comprise one of the largest populations of individuals who receive pediatric palliative care (PPC). In a multicenter demographic study of hospital-based PPC programs in North America, nearly half of all children enrolled in palliative care were identified as having cognitive impairment, with the most common categories of principal diagnoses being genetic/congenital and neuromuscular conditions.[1] Other serious illnesses, such as primary brain tumors and malignancies with metastatic brain disease (discussed in Chapter 33), place children at risk for neurological symptoms. PPC clinicians should be familiar with management strategies of common neurological symptoms, which can be a major source of distress for these patients and their families.

This chapter addresses symptoms that arise due to impairment of the central nervous system (CNS). These symptoms may manifest from a variety of conditions that cause dysfunction of the CNS, including congenital anomalies, genetic/metabolic conditions that cause degenerative CNS disease, and brain lesions or injury acquired after birth. Neurological symptoms present particular difficulties for PPC clinicians for multiple reasons. Regardless of etiology, these symptoms are often difficult to treat, are sometimes intractable, and may evolve over time. Furthermore, children with severe neurological impairment (SNI) are at risk for more than one CNS etiology for observed symptoms. For example, a child with SNI who experiences dystonia is also at risk for central neuropathic pain, which can trigger and worsen dystonic features. The evidence base is limited for symptom interventions among children with SNI, and the complex clinical presentation of neurological symptoms makes assessment and management an inexact science that may require trials of pharmacological treatment for multifactorial causes. This chapter presents a general treatment approach for all neurological symptoms, followed by management strategies for specific symptoms, such as seizures, spasticity, dystonia, chorea, myoclonus, autonomic dysfunction, and central neuropathic pain.

GENERAL APPROACH TO CARE

The most important principle in providing palliative care for children with SNI is an effective partnership among the caregivers and members of the healthcare team. Families caring for children with SNI often rely on multiple pediatric providers, including primary care clinicians and pediatric subspecialists, to identify, evaluate, and manage chronic neurological symptoms. Neurologists, physiatrists, and palliative care clinicians have complementary yet distinct skill sets to promote comfort and optimize management of distressing neurological symptoms. Subspecialists in gastroenterology, orthopedics, pulmonology, complex care, and pain medicine may serve crucial roles in addressing comorbidities that contribute to increased symptomatology. Comprehensive care of children with neurological conditions also includes an array of clinicians in the home and community setting, and an interdisciplinary approach will provide the most holistic support for a child with SNI (Table 19.1).

Open communication is an essential element of effective palliative care for children with SNI. Family members and caregivers have an intimate knowledge of their child's likes, dislikes, behavioral patterns, and rhythms of daily life and are the most reliable reporters of any symptoms that deviate from their child's norm. Healthcare providers attending to concerns raised by families must consider the broader impact of these symptoms on the child's relational and emotional well-being within the context of the family's psychosocial health.

An important dimension of open communication with a trusted clinician is anticipatory guidance about what to expect in the future. Many families report greater peace of mind and increased hopefulness when provided honest prognostic information, even if the news is difficult to hear.[2,3] In any discussion about prognostication, clinicians must acknowledge the inherent uncertainty that exists as they provide guidance about potential outcomes, complications, and decisions that may arise in the future. For families who find advance care planning helpful, clinicians can offer the approach of "hoping

TABLE 19.1 Interdisciplinary approaches to management of neurological symptoms

Physicians and advanced practice providers (nurse practitioners, physician assistants)	Physicians and advanced practice providers play an integral role in caring for children with SNI. Given the complex nature of neurological symptoms, many subspecialties are often involved in management, including neurology, physiatry, orthopedics, gastroenterology, pulmonology, complex care, pain medicine, and palliative care. Providers work together to manage seizures, spasticity, dystonia, autonomic dysfunction, neuro-irritability, and pain
Nurses	Nurses play a crucial role in caring for children with SNI across healthcare settings (e.g., home, clinics, schools, hospitals, long-term care). Nurses are often the first-line providers who can assess a child's symptomatology and offer immediate, hands-on support through nonpharmacologic and pharmacologic interventions. Nurses can work with a child and family to recognize pain behaviors and identify the appropriate pain assessment tool that can be implemented across settings to identify and treat discomfort.
Social workers	Social workers support children with SNI and their families in a variety of ways. Social workers can help to identify psychosocial factors that may contribute to symptomatology. They can also assess the impact of challenging symptoms on the psychosocial functioning of the family, assisting with caregiver coping and anticipatory grief.
Psychologists	Psychologists perform focused assessments that allow families and teams to understand a child's neurocognitive abilities. This sets the stage for the multidisciplinary team to best support a child's development considering the level of neurologic impairment. An evaluation by a psychologist is often required for a child with SNI to receive appropriate community services. Psychologists may also assist with the assessment and management of behavioral issues and delirium.
Child life specialists	Child life specialists (CLS) are trained to support a child coping with illness. CLS are usually available in inpatient pediatric settings and are commonly members of home-based palliative care services. CLS implement developmentally appropriate, nonpharmacologic interventions to improve comfort and enhance quality of life for children with SNI.
Other: Chaplains, music therapists, integrative therapy providers, bereavement counselors	Various other specialists play important roles in supporting the physical, psychosocial, and spiritual needs of children with SNI and their families.

for the best while preparing for the worst" to aid in developing plans for potential clinical scenarios.[4]

Effective collaboration and open communication empower families of children with SNI and their healthcare teams to develop a proactive approach to managing neurological symptoms. This entails having a shared understanding about anticipated symptoms and the goals of treatment for each of these symptoms. In most situations, a reasonable goal for treatment is to achieve an acceptable level of symptom control with a tolerable level of medication side effects. For every neurological symptom, a comprehensive management plan should include nonpharmacological and pharmacological interventions that address both maintenance of symptom control and treatment of breakthrough symptoms. This often requires a scheduled medication regimen to decrease the frequency and severity of symptom episodes and a plan to treat breakthrough symptoms (Box 19.1).[5]

Acute changes in symptomatology should prompt consideration of a new nociceptive trigger. Neurological symptoms are often exacerbated by any cause of discomfort, including acute illness, pain, constipation, poor sleep, and medication toxicity. Given the nonspecific clinical presentation and the broad range of possible triggers, a thoughtful evaluation that incorporates a detailed history of new symptoms, a careful consideration of previous exacerbation patterns, and a thorough physical examination is imperative to establishing a reasonable evaluation and treatment plan that effectively addresses safety concerns without overly burdensome diagnostic testing. Clinicians can also engage families in other helpful strategies, such as maintaining a symptom diary, recording videos of symptom episodes, and reviewing medication side effects, to better characterize the symptoms.[6]

Children who receive nutrition and fluids by feeding tubes are at high risk for overfeeding when there is a gradual decline in health and function, as there is no easy way to measure this gradual decline in metabolic expenditure.[7] Palliative care teams should remain vigilant to the risk of symptoms arising

BOX 19.1 EXAMPLE OF A NEUROLOGICAL SYMPTOM MANAGEMENT PLAN

Interventions for persistent crying and increased tone above baseline:

1. Utilize nonpharmacological strategies:
   a. Swaddle tightly with legs flexed toward abdomen
   b. Apply vibratory mat, 15 minutes on followed by 15 minutes off
   c. Apply weighted blanket, 30 minutes on followed by 30 minutes off
2. If pain is suspected, administer as-needed dose of acetaminophen or ibuprofen via gastrostomy tube
3. If no benefit from the above, administer as-needed dose of diazepam via gastrostomy tube
4. Continue nonpharmacological strategies, and, if no relief after 30 minutes, notify provider

from overfeeding, such as pain, emesis, retching, and respiratory symptoms. Children with SNI may exhibit an increase in neurological symptoms, including spasticity and dystonic movements. Palliative care teams can guide families in the reduction of feeds while attending to worries about such plans, as illustrated in the Family Vignette. A 25–30% reduction of enteral feeds and fluids may be suggested as a trial to assess for symptom improvement.[7]

Family Reflection

We were told of Grace's medical issues when she was 5 months old. We will never forget hearing, "Kids like Grace typically don't live to their first birthday, and we never see them live past their second birthday." Given the numerous health issues Grace would endure due to an undiagnosed disorder of her brain, our goal became one of living the best life possible in the short one we were going to have with her. This is why palliative care became so important to us! This was the team that helped not only to manage Grace's symptoms and comfort, but also to support our whole family emotionally. We were blessed to make it past both those 1- and 2-year marks relatively smoothly. With the exception of a couple of short hospital stays for illness and surgeries to aid in her care, such as G-tube placement and orthopedic surgery, Grace was doing well! It was in Grace's fourth year that things really started to change. We noticed her respiratory needs changing, resulting in more interventions to help maintain health and treat acute illness. Her irritability really increased with what we believed to be nerve pain. After some long stays in the hospital trying to understand the cause, we decided it was time to take her home and do what we could to make her comfortable. Palliative care worked with us to adjust and add to her medications so that Grace could be comfortable at home over the next year. Due to this support, we were also able to do things our family loved, like travel and spend time at the lake, valuing every precious moment. The following spring, we noticed another change; Grace's body was becoming puffier, and she was having vomiting spells. Again, palliative care helped make adjustments to medications, and we decreased her feedings. Grace was showing us signs that her body was no longer able to process what she was given. The palliative care team was amazing at helping us understand what this all meant. Soon we were having more discussions as decreasing the formula seemed to play a big part in improving her comfort. While this was easy to identify, it was also heartbreaking to see and accept as a parent. Eventually, stopping feeds entirely was the best way to ensure her comfort. Two days later, our Gracie passed away in our arms surrounded by all her favorite people. To this day, we attribute her ability to enjoy those 5 and a half years of living, with an impaired nervous system, to the care and support we were provided through palliative care and all those people we will always affectionately refer to as "Team Grace."

Optimizing overall comfort through nonpharmacological interventions is important in maintaining a holistic approach to symptom management. Just as adjuvant medications are used synergistically with opioids to treat pain, nonpharmacologic strategies and integrative therapies work together with pharmacologic management to address distressing symptoms.[8] Nonpharmacological options that may provide benefit for children with SNI include comfort strategies, positional support, sensory interventions, and integrative therapies (Table 19.2). Simple strategies such as repositioning, rocking, swaddling, and light massage can be easily utilized by parents, caregivers, and bedside nurses. While there is a paucity of published data regarding the use and efficacy of integrative therapy in children with SNI, families often report benefits from these types of interventions. When thinking about which strategies to try, considerations should include sources of discomfort, developmental level of the child, potential physical limitations, and replicability of the intervention.[9]

Unfortunately, each of the neurological symptoms discussed in this chapter has the potential to become persistent and intractable despite best attempts to address contributing factors, enhance comfort, and treat with multiple medications. Children with intractable symptoms are at risk for experiencing undesirable adverse effects from polypharmacy, and these situations should prompt families and healthcare teams to weigh the anticipated benefits and burdens of escalation of pharmacological treatment. Open communication within a trusted therapeutic relationship allows for exploration of values that are most important to the family and shared decision-making about goals of treatment. For example, if a family is worried that their child who is receiving multiple medications for treatment of intractable seizures is too sedated to interact and participate in activities, clinicians can partner with the family to develop a shared understanding about the desired functional goals of treatment (e.g., ability to engage with therapies), the potential tradeoffs (e.g., increased risk of breakthrough seizures), and the changes needed in the management plan to achieve these goals.

TABLE 19.2 Nonpharmacological strategies to promote comfort in children with severe neurological impairment (SNI)

Comfort strategies	Cuddling, rocking, massage, warm baths, music Adjusting enteral feed rate, venting gastrostomy tube
Positional support	Repositioning, supportive seating systems, supportive bedding/mattresses
Sensory interventions	Weighted blankets, vibratory mats and pillows
Integrative therapies	Essential oils, aromatherapy, Reiki, craniosacral therapy, acupuncture/acupressure

MANAGEMENT OF NEUROLOGICAL SYMPTOMS AT THE END OF LIFE

Children with neurological conditions may experience intensification of neurological symptoms as they near the end of life. This may be particularly marked in children with progressive neurological conditions, such as a neurodegenerative disorder or brain malignancy. Determination of whether symptomatic changes represent irreversible progression of the underlying disease requires careful consideration of the trajectory of a child's condition and compassionate communication with the family. Escalation of medications may be necessary to treat distressing neurological symptoms at the end of life, and ongoing conversations with the family are important to establish shared prognostic understanding and modified treatment goals. In these situations, the family and healthcare team may agree that prioritizing comfort allows for intensifying pharmacological treatment with the expectation of increased somnolence. Because this plan of care may also diminish respiratory function and the effectiveness of respiratory clearance, clinicians must engage the family in considering the potential role and impact of advanced respiratory technologies, hospitalizations, intensive care, and resuscitative efforts in the care of their child. In addition to managing distressing symptoms, interdisciplinary palliative care clinicians serve a crucial role in supporting the family through difficult decisions, attending to anticipatory grief, and providing bereavement care.

NEUROLOGICAL SYMPTOMS

The following sections describe management strategies for specific symptoms, such as seizures, spasticity, dystonia, chorea, myoclonus, autonomic dysfunction, central neuropathic pain, visceral hyperalgesia, and neuro-pain (neuro-irritability). For a summary of doses and indications of medications in this chapter, see Table 19.3.

TABLE 19.3 Medications for neurological symptoms (maximum weight of 50 kg for dosing)

MEDICATIONS	MECHANISMS OF ACTION	INITIAL STARTING DOSE (MAXIMUM STARTING DOSE)
Autonomic Dysfunction/Dysautonomia		
Clonidine	Centrally acting alpha-2-adrenergic receptor agonist, reducing sympathetic outflow	Days 1–4: 0.002 mg/kg PO TID Days 5–8: 0.004 mg/kg PO TID Option to start with once a day dose to minimize sedation, then increase to BID, then TID Option to increase further: 0.02 mg/kg per day was the average dose identified for spasticity[5] Autonomic storm: 0.003–0.006 mg/kg q4h prn Sleep: 0.003–0.006 mg/kg nightly
Gabapentin	Inhibit excitation by binding to alpha-2-delta protein of the voltage-gated calcium channels in the CNS	Day 1–3: 2 mg/kg (100 mg), PO TID Day 4–5: 4 mg/kg PO TID Increase every 2–4 days by 5–6 mg/kg/day until: Effective analgesia reached (may be noted at 30–45 mg/kg/day) Side effects experienced (nystagmus, sedation, tremor, ataxia, swelling) Maximum total dose of 50–72 mg/kg/day reached (2,400–3,600 mg/day) Younger children (<5 years) may require a 30% higher dose, such as a total dose of 45–60 mg/kg/day Half of the total daily dose may be given as the evening dose if symptoms occur more in the evening Titrate more rapidly for severe pain or as tolerated, titrate more gradually if sedation noted
Morphine	CNS opioid receptors	Autonomic storm: 0.2–0.3 mg/kg (10–15 mg) PO q4h prn
Propranolol	Beta-1 adrenergic receptor antagonist	0.2–0.4 mg/kg PO q8h (20 mg), increase every 3–4 days up to 1.6 mg/kg q8h (80 mg)
Bromocriptine	D2 receptor agonist	0.025 mg/kg (1.25 mg) PO q12h
Central Neuropathic Pain/Visceral Hyperalgesia		
Gabapentin	See above	See above
Pregabalin	See gabapentin	Day 1–3: 1 mg/kg (50mg) PO nightly Day 4–5: 1 mg/kg PO BID Increase every 2–4 days up to 3 mg/kg/dose PO given BID or TID (maximum 6 mg/kg/dose)
Nortriptyline Amitriptyline	Presynaptic reuptake inhibition in the CNS of norepinephrine and serotonin	Day 1–4: 0.2 mg/kg (10 mg) PO nightly Day 5–8: 0.4 mg/kg PO nightly Increase every 4–5 days by 0.2 mg/kg/day until: Effective analgesia, side effects (constipation, dry mouth, urinary retention, sedation), or dosing reaches 1–1.5 mg/kg/day (50–75 mg/day maximum) Obtain ECG before further dose escalation up to 1.5–2 mg/kg/day (100 mg/day maximum); higher rate of side effects with higher doses including anticholinergic Consider plasma level if concerns with GI tract absorption Option of twice-daily dosing, giving 25–30% in the morning and 70–75% in the evening

(continued)

TABLE 19.3 Continued

MEDICATIONS	MECHANISMS OF ACTION	INITIAL STARTING DOSE (MAXIMUM STARTING DOSE)
Methadone	NMDA receptor antagonist, mu-opioid receptor agonist	0.1 mg/kg (5 mg) PO q8h; titrate slowly due to long biphasic half-life, monitor for cumulative effects in first 3–7 days
Spasticity		
Baclofen	Modulates GABA-B receptors	2.5–5 mg PO TID; increase every 3 days by 5–15 mg/day up to a maximum of 60–80 mg/day
Tizanidine	See clonidine above	0.04–0.08 mg/kg (2–4 mg) PO nightly, increase up to 0.16 mg/kg q8h (max 8–12 mg q8h)
Clonidine	See clonidine above	See dysautonomia above
Diazepam	Increases affinity of GABA for GABA-A receptor	0.03–0.05 mg/kg (2 mg) PO/IV q6–8 hr, titrate to effect (max 10 mg)
Dystonia		
Trihexylphenidyl	Anticholinergic	1 mg/day PO, increase every 3–5 days up to 4–5 mg TID; some children will benefit from and tolerate up to 60–100 mg/day (side effects may be managed with pyridostigmine)
Tetrabenazine	Dopamine depletion	12.5 mg/day PO, increase weekly up to 25 mg q12h
Clonidine	See clonidine above	Status dystonicus: 0.003–0.006 mg/kg q3–4h prn[17]
Myoclonus		
Clonazepam	See diazepam above	0.005–0.01 mg/kg PO q8–12h (0.25–0.5 mg)
Seizures (acute therapy for prolonged seizure)		
Lorazepam	See diazepam above	0.1 mg/kg (4–6 mg) PO/SL/PR/IV every 15 min × 2
Midazolam	See diazepam above	0.2 mg/kg SL, intranasal, or IV (10 mg)
Diazepam rectal gel	See diazepam above	2–5 years: 0.5 mg/kg every 15 min × 3 6–11 years: 0.3 mg/kg every 15 min × 3 >12 years: 0.2 mg/kg every 15 min × 3 Round dose to 2.5, 5, 10, 15, or 20 mg/dose
Fosphenytoin Phenytoin	Sodium-channel modulator	15–20 mg/kg IV loading dose followed by maintenance dose of 4–10 mg/kg/day (age-dependent dosing)
Seizures at end of life		
Phenobarbital	Enhances inhibition at GABA-A receptor	15–20 mg/kg IV/SC/PO/PR loading dose for seizures, followed by maintenance dose 4–6 mg/kg/day IV/SC/PO/PR
Clonazepam	See diazepam above	0.005–0.01 mg/kg PO q8–12h (0.25–0.5 mg), increase up to 0.05–0.1 mg/kg PO q8–12h
Midazolam infusion	See diazepam above	Loading dose of 0.03–0.04 mg/kg (maximum 2 mg) followed by 0.03–0.1 mg/kg/hour IV or SC infusion titrated to effect

5HT, serotonin; ACh, acetylcholine; CNS, central nervous system; D2, dopamine; H, histamine; hr, hours; IV, intravenous; min, minutes; NMDA, N-methyl-D-aspartate; PO, by mouth (also enteral by feeding tube); PR, per rectum; PRN, as needed; q, every; SC, subcutaneous; SL, sublingual.

SEIZURES

All children with SNI and oncology patients with tumors of the CNS are at risk of experiencing seizures. Comprehensive epilepsy management is best done under the expert guidance of a neurologist and requires a careful treatment approach that optimizes seizure control, monitors for medication toxicities, and minimizes adverse effects. Many children with SNI are on antiepileptic drug (AED) therapy for maintenance seizure control. However, some medications used in palliative care may lower the seizure threshold, including baclofen, neuroleptics, and stimulants. Though the initial goal is to be seizure-free, children with SNI are at high risk for intractable seizures. For these children, palliative care teams can facilitate review of treatment goals by engaging families, neurologists, and interdisciplinary team members to assess factors that impact health and quality of life.

Palliative care teams may be asked about novel or unconventional therapies to treat seizures, including the use of cannabidiol and medical marijuana. In 2018, the US Food and Drug Administration approved the first pharmaceutical-grade, cannabidiol-based medication to treat seizures associated with Lennox-Gastaut and Dravet syndromes.[10] Emerging evidence supports the efficacy of cannabidiol products to treat drug-resistant epilepsy in these genetic seizure syndromes. However, children with SNI without genetically defined seizure syndromes may not experience similar benefits in seizure control and quality of life outcomes.[11,12] Neurologists should engage families in determining the role of cannabidiol products in the treatment plan, and palliative care teams can facilitate communication and support parental preferences.

In addition to seizure maintenance, a comprehensive palliative care plan should include an action plan for management of prolonged breakthrough seizures. This plan should be readily accessible and identify what is normal for the child, when a seizure has become prolonged and requires medication, and to what level further help should be sought if seizure activity continues. During a seizure, caregivers should implement environmental measures to support safety and comfort, and, if the seizure becomes prolonged, a rapid-acting benzodiazepine can be administered as first-line therapy. Options include diazepam rectal gel, which can be repeated after 10 minutes if the seizure has not subsided. Sublingual or buccal administration of lorazepam or midazolam may also be considered, as there is evidence that these options are not inferior to rectal diazepam and may be more cost-effective.[13] If further medical attention is required, other parenteral agents, such as lorazepam (intravenous/intramuscular) or midazolam (intranasal/intravenous/intramuscular), may be administered.[14]

An important role of the palliative care clinician is to provide reassurance that seizures are more unpleasant and frightening for those observing them than they are for the child who experiences them. If seizures do not appear to distress the child, then vigorous attempts to abolish them may result in undesirable adverse effects, such as oversedation or respiratory compromise. These situations provide opportunities for clinicians and families to refine the goals of treatment and engage in advance care planning.

Palliative care teams can work with neurologists to revisit care plans for breakthrough seizures when goals shift to prioritizing comfort, minimizing hospitalizations, and avoiding repeated use of intravenous treatment. One approach may be to modify the medication plan for persistent seizures to include repeated administration of buccal, intranasal, or enteral medications to allow for care in the home setting. Plans can also include the use of loading doses of rectal or enteral AEDs in the context of adjusted goals and expectations of treatment. At end of life, phenobarbital remains an excellent choice for treating seizures due to its efficacy for a broad range of seizure types, pharmacokinetics, and low cost.[15] Its onset of action is fast enough to be utilized as adjunctive therapy for status epilepticus, and its long half-life enhances maintenance control of seizures. It promotes comfort through its sedative and anxiolytic effects. It comes in a variety of formulations that can be given through enteral and parenteral routes, making it a highly versatile AED in palliative care.

In rare instances, management of status epilepticus may benefit from a continuous infusion to provide optimal comfort. Midazolam is the most commonly used agent, while barbiturates are also used for this indication. In pediatrics, these infusions are typically initiated in an intensive care setting, and, depending on the goals of care, home care and hospice agencies may be able to support continuation of these therapies in the community. If venous access is not available, subcutaneous administration of intravenous medications provides therapeutic equivalence and allows for management and titration under hospice supervision.

SYMPTOMS OF MUSCLE TONE AND MOVEMENT

Children with neurological conditions experience alterations to their muscle tone and involuntary movements. Because of underlying injury to the CNS, most children with SNI exhibit upper motor neuron signs on physical examination, such as hypertonia, spasticity, exaggerated deep tendon reflexes, and clonus. Children with SNI may also experience movement disorders, such as dystonia, chorea, and myoclonus. The extent to which these symptoms cause discomfort or distress varies from child to child. Goals for pharmacological treatment of these symptoms are to improve comfort, enhance ease of care, decrease risk of musculoskeletal deformities, and improve function. Complete cessation of these symptoms may not be possible, and treatment should be aimed at finding an acceptable balance between desired improvements and adverse effects of medications. At times, repetitive abnormal movements may mimic seizures, and families should work closely with their child's neurologist to determine whether to pursue diagnostic testing with electroencephalogram (EEG) or to initiate an empiric trial of therapy.

HYPERTONIA AND SPASTICITY

Hypertonia is the increased resistance of muscle to passive movement that is not dependent on the velocity of the movement. Spasticity is a specific type of hypertonia in which muscle tone increases with increasing velocity of passive movement.[16] Hypertonia itself is not painful, though children with severe hypertonia are often unable to tolerate long periods of time in certain positions. Children with hypertonia are also at risk for painful, acute muscle spasm, in which a muscle suddenly contracts involuntarily. In children with SNI, acute pain from other sources often triggers increases in tone and acute muscle spasm, which unfortunately sets up a feedback loop that propagates pain behaviors. In the context of an acute increase in tone, diazepam is recommended as the first-line agent for short-term treatment of spasticity.[17] It is important to remember that diazepam functions as a muscle relaxant but is not an analgesic. Concurrent use of analgesic agents, such as acetaminophen, nonsteroidal anti-inflammatory drugs, or opioids, may be necessary to adequately treat pain.

Chronic management of spasticity involves a multidisciplinary approach that includes physical therapy and some combination of locally injected medications, systemic enteral medications, and an implanted intrathecal pump. Targeting specific muscle groups with botulinum toxin and/or phenol injections may be effective at reducing localized spasticity with a duration of effect that can last for 3–4 months.[17] For generalized spasticity, systemic agents, such as baclofen and diazepam, are commonly used, but the utility of systemic therapy may be limited by impairment of truncal tone and inability to maintain posture.[18] Other enteral medications that may help with tone management include tizanidine, clonidine, dantrolene, and gabapentin.[18] All of these medications cause sedation, and treatment should always aim to balance desired outcomes with adverse effects.

Intrathecal baclofen (ITB) is a modality to consider for children with severe spasticity of the lower extremities who experience significant side effects from systemic pharmacological treatment. A pump that is implanted in the abdominal wall delivers a continuous infusion of baclofen into the intrathecal space of the spinal cord. The direct exposure of nerve roots allows for the dose of baclofen to be one-thousandth of its systemic dose, thereby offering the intended benefits of reducing muscle tone and minimizing side effects. The goals of ITB include reducing functional limitations, improving mobility, enhancing comfort, facilitating ease of care, and optimizing overall quality of life.[19] The ITB pump is refilled every 3 months and replaced every 4–7 years. Serious complications of ITB include soft tissue infection, meningitis, and pump malfunction.

DYSTONIA

Dystonia is a movement disorder in which involuntary muscle contractions, which can be intermittent or sustained, lead to twisting, repetitive movements and/or abnormal postures. Dystonia can be a prominent feature in individuals with injury to the basal ganglia. Primary dystonia syndromes, in which dystonia is the most prominent symptom and no other neurological impairments are identified, are rare. When dystonia is identified in children with SNI, it is typically characterized as a secondary dystonia caused by the underlying condition.[20] Like spasticity, dystonia can be triggered or exacerbated by acute illness or pain. Prolonged dystonia is referred to as *status dystonicus* and carries the risk of rhabdomyolysis.[21]

When a child experiences acute dystonia, triggers to consider include acute illness, pain, and potentially inciting medications. Any dopamine receptor antagonist, including metoclopramide, haloperidol, risperidone, and olanzapine, can cause dystonia. Because these are common medications used to treat other symptoms, including nausea, delirium, behavioral dysregulation, and sleep disturbance, palliative care clinicians must maintain a high index of suspicion for drug-induced dystonia. The treatment of acute dystonic reactions should include consideration of therapeutic alternatives to the inciting medication, as well as administration of an anticholinergic agent, such as diphenhydramine.[21]

Temporizing management of status dystonicus involves management of triggers and use of medications, including clonidine and at times the addition of an intravenous midazolam infusion.[21] Long-term management of dystonia is difficult and requires multidisciplinary expertise. In addition to physical therapy, treatment options include botulinum injections for focal dystonias, systemic medications, and surgical interventions, such as ITB or deep brain stimulation of the globus pallidus. Pharmacological strategies for dystonia include the use of muscle relaxants (benzodiazepines, baclofen), gabapentin, anticholinergics (diphenhydramine, trihexyphenidyl, benztropine), and dopamine mediators (levodopa, tetrabenazine).[21,22]

CHOREA

Chorea is a movement disorder characterized by abrupt, irregular, involuntary movements that range from fidgeting to larger dance-like movements that flow limb to limb. It is associated with injury to the basal ganglia and is seen more frequently in neurodegenerative conditions. As with other disorders of tone and movement, chorea is typically exacerbated by acute illness or pain. Many medications, including metoclopramide, haloperidol, phenothiazines, and phenytoin, may induce chorea. The approach to managing acute worsening of chorea should include evaluation for painful stimuli, acute illness, and medication side effects.[23]

Chorea does not cause pain but may be distressing to experience and to watch. The mainstay of management is to incorporate nonpharmacological strategies to enhance comfort, improve function, and decrease the risk of injury. Positioning, soft splinting, and proprioceptive feedback may help to reduce and control the movements and enable a child to function or rest. For example, a therapist may improve the repetitive, writhing movements of an upper limb by placing a firm, but not restrictive, hand on the shoulder of the child and applying firm, but gentle, pressure diagonally over the child's chest toward the opposite hip with the therapist's forearm. Movement is not restricted, and the proprioceptive feedback provided around the shoulder and across the core of the trunk may normalize the fluctuating tone and reduce distal involuntary movement. If effective, this technique can be taught to the family and caregivers as part of the treatment plan. The ability to soothe through touch benefits not only the child but also the family by empowering them to employ a therapeutic intervention.

MYOCLONUS

Myoclonus describes brief, involuntary, jerking movements that are due to sudden contraction and relaxation of a muscle or muscle group. It can be a chronic symptom experienced by children with SNI. Because of its involuntary, repetitive nature, myoclonus may be hard to distinguish from seizure activity, and diagnostic correlation with EEG and/or electromyography to determine treatment options may be beneficial.[24] As with other neurological symptoms, myoclonic movements may be triggered by physiological stressors, such as acute illness and pain. Myoclonus has been associated with renal failure, liver failure, hypoglycemia, and hyponatremia. In addition, many classes of medications, including fluoroquinolones, AEDs, tricyclic antidepressants (TCAs), selective serotonin reuptake inhibitors, cannabinoids, and opioids, have been implicated as potential triggers.[25]

When an acute exacerbation of myoclonus develops, the palliative care clinician serves an important role to troubleshoot for inciting physiological triggers and critically consider the potential of polypharmacy. In particular, for a child undergoing titration of opioids for pain, opioid-induced myoclonus must be considered and treated effectively to optimize comfort. Myoclonus is one of several neuroexcitatory signs of opioid toxicity and may precede the onset of opioid-induced hyperalgesia, delirium, and seizures. These symptoms are thought to be due to the accumulation of neurotoxic metabolites of opioids, often in the clinical setting of rapid dose escalation or impaired renal clearance.[26]

Treatment of opioid-induced myoclonus should include administration of benzodiazepines for short-term symptom relief and modification of opioid therapy to reduce the risk of recurrence. If pain is adequately controlled, opioid dose reduction may suffice to mitigate the risk of myoclonus. However, if the patient requires continued high-dose opioid therapy, opioid rotation with a 25–50% decrease in the equianalgesic dose may be effective in decreasing myoclonus while allowing for continued titration. In patients with renal impairment, the hepatically cleared opioids, fentanyl and methadone, carry less risk of opioid neurotoxicity.[26]

AUTONOMIC DYSFUNCTION

Children with SNI are at risk for autonomic dysfunction due to alterations in the areas of the nervous system that control autonomic function, including the hypothalamus. Other terms used include *dysautonomia*, *autonomic storm*, *sympathetic storm*, *thalamic storm*, and *paroxysmal autonomic instability with dystonia*. Features of autonomic dysfunction include tachycardia, hyperthermia, flushing and redness of the face and body, retching, vomiting, bowel dysmotility, abdominal pain, urinary retention, diaphoresis, increased salivation, and discomfort.[5,27–30]

The study of treatment is limited to case reports, predominantly in adults with hypoxic and traumatic brain injury. Benefit has been reported with gabapentinoids, clonidine, and opioids.[5,28] Children with SNI assessed to have autonomic dysfunction are at risk for other comorbid problems due to the altered nervous system, with presenting clinical features similar to central neuropathic pain and visceral hyperalgesia. Dysautonomia can be a source of discomfort, and pain can trigger the features that occur with dysautonomia.

CENTRAL NEUROPATHIC PAIN

Neuropathic pain is caused by a lesion or disease of the somatosensory nervous system. This includes central neuropathic pain due to impairment of the spinothalamic tract or thalamus. Neuropathic pain has characteristics described as burning, shock-like, shooting, or needle-like pain. Symptoms with central neuropathic pain can be constant, involve sudden bursts of intense pain with no known trigger, and include visceral pain associated with normal to mild distention of the gastrointestinal (GI) tract and bladder. Neuropathic pain can result in pain from a stimulus that does not normally result in pain (allodynia) or an increased pain response to a painful stimulus (hyperalgesia). Neuropathic pain is suggested in children with SNI by higher baseline pain ratings and the significant intensity and duration of symptoms that were attributed to routine problems.[5]

Central neuropathic pain is best studied in adults with multiple sclerosis or following a cerebral vascular accident. Thalamic magnetic resonance imaging findings have been reported with various pediatric conditions, including numerous metabolic and genetic disorders, infections of the CNS, osmotic demyelination syndrome, and hypoxic-ischemic injury.[5] This information suggests risk for central neuropathic pain in children with SNI but does not indicate which child may develop pain due to this problem.

The goals of treatment are pain control, not cure, given the inability to correct the cause of pain. Medications for neuropathic pain include gabapentinoids, clonidine, TCAs, and opioids (see Table 19.3 for dosing guidelines). Benefit from neuropathic agents, such as gabapentin and TCAs, in children with SNI who exhibit persistent pain behaviors provides indirect evidence of neuropathic pain as a chronic pain source.[31–34] A proposed pharmacological strategy entails a step-wise approach to treatment, with gabapentinoids as first-line medications, clonidine and TCAs as second-line agents, and methadone as a third-line option.[5]

VISCERAL HYPERALGESIA

Visceral hyperalgesia occurs when pain is generated in response to a stimulus in the GI tract. It is attributed to sensitization of visceral afferents and central sensitization in the CNS. Symptoms caused by visceral hyperalgesia overlap with autonomic dysfunction and central neuropathic pain. Nonpharmacological treatment strategies focus on decreasing gut distention, and families can be advised to induce a bowel movement, vent a feeding tube, and decrease the rate and volume of enteral feedings.[7] Pharmacological strategies utilize medications to treat neuropathic pain, utilizing the step-wise approach described for central neuropathic pain.

NEURO-PAIN (NEURO-IRRITABILITY)

Children with SNI are at high risk for both chronic and acute pain. Differences are noted in Table 19.4. Multiple pain sources can coexist and occur intermittently. Acute on chronic pain can be due to "routine" sources of discomfort, which families commonly manage each day (e.g., need for personal care or to be repositioned), a new cause of nociceptive pain (e.g., urinary tract infection), and breakthrough symptoms from the chronic pain source.

"Neuro-pain" is a term proposed to indicate chronic pain generated by the impaired nervous system.[35] Neuro-pain

TABLE 19.4 Acute versus chronic pain

	ACUTE	CHRONIC
Cause	Tissue inflammation and injury (nociceptive pain)	Musculoskeletal, visceral, postsurgical, and neuropathic
Duration	Hours to days	> 3 months, persists
Identification	Sources typically identified by diagnostic tests	No established diagnostic tests or criteria
Goals	Resolution after treatment of cause and healing of tissue injury	Pain control

is defined as chronic pain in children with SNI without diagnostic tests or distinct features to differentiate one from another (i.e., central neuropathic pain, autonomic dysfunction, visceral hyperalgesia, chronic postsurgical pain).[35] Pain behaviors often present with other neurological problems with overlapping features, such as spasticity, dystonia, and seizures.[35] A screening tool has been developed to aid in the assessment of chronic neuro-pain and serve as a guide to the initiation of medication trials.[35]

When a child with SNI exhibits pain behaviors, the first step is a comprehensive assessment for acute nociceptive pain sources. When episodes with pain behaviors are noted to recur, treatment of chronic pain sources should be considered. Box 19.2 provides a framework to guide assessment of acute and chronic pain sources.[35]

BOX 19.2 SCREENING CHILDREN WITH SNI FOR RISK OF NEURO-PAIN

1. Does your child have any of the following for more than 3 months?
   - Frequently not calm: intermittently agitated, irritable, cranky, uncomfortable, without a consistent explanation
   - Problems include any of the following and symptoms may recur after treatment:
     - o Autonomic dysfunction and storms
     - o Spasticity or dystonia
     - o Gastrointestinal reflux disease (GERD) and vomiting
     - o Constipation with discomfort
     - o Pain with feeds, not tolerating tube feeds
     - o Chronic poor sleep
     - o Symptoms continue for more than 2–3 months after surgery without an explanation
2. Review prior testing for sources of nociceptive pain to determine need for further testing*
3. Review for testable chronic pain sources, such as:
   - Dental, hip subluxation, chronic dry eyes, renal stones
   - Note: Some findings can be incidental and not the reason for symptoms
4. Screen for risk of chronic pain due to CNS sources without diagnostic tests
   - Assess with Neuro-Pain Risk Assessment Tool (N-PRAT)
   - Use score to guide decision to initiate medication trial
   - Causes, history, and exam pg e6-e7 of AAP clinical report [5]
   - Minimum assessment in the prior 3 months:
     - o Specific findings from history and exam (e.g., imaging of shunt, X-ray if fracture suspected, place longer G-tube if tight against abdomen due to weight gain, ophthalmology assessment if persistent erythema of eyes)
     - o Blood (CMP, CBC, lipase); Urine (analysis and culture)
   - Other assessments to consider: abdominal ultrasound, dental exam if no recent exam

*Nociceptive assessment guidelines

Team Reflection

The palliative care team is consulted to assist with symptom treatment and decision-making for a 2-year-old boy with severe motor and intellectual disability, microcephaly, intractable seizures, spasticity, and dystonia. He lives with his parents, who are expecting their second child. His medical problems result in frequent and prolonged hospitalizations, often due to concerns for prolonged seizures, and continuous EEG studies identify no epileptiform correlates for the events. His medication regimen includes scheduled baclofen, clonazepam, and three AEDs, and the family administers lorazepam as needed for breakthrough symptoms. He is also on a proton pump inhibitor and a bowel regimen for constipation. Clinical features during breakthrough events include facial grimacing, flushing, tears, and severe back arching. His heart rate and blood pressure are elevated during these episodes. His parents worry that he is experiencing pain and express, "They keep explaining it is his brain but we think they are missing something." The palliative care team recommends initiating gabapentin, and, over several weeks, the dose is titrated to approximately 50 mg/kg/day. The parents are noticeably more relieved as they describe his comfort as "over 75% better," noting that this is "the first time he has smiled and been able to lay on his back in a long time." There is a decrease in symptom benefit 3 months later, and clonidine is added, both scheduled (0.028 mg/kg/day) for maintenance and as needed (0.007 mg/kg every 4 hours as needed) for breakthrough symptoms. This regimen results in symptom benefit that has been sustained for more than 3 years. The parents are grateful for how much better their child's life has been since the addition of medications for symptom treatment.

Chronic symptom management requires a multimodal approach.[5,35] In addition to nonpharmacological interventions to enhance comfort, pharmacological intervention to treat neuro-pain requires several considerations. Consider initiating a scheduled medication for recurrent episodes that do not respond to typical comfort strategies and are of significant severity, duration, and frequency. As described for central neuropathic pain, medication trials should follow a step-wise approach. Gabapentinoids are the first-line agents given their safety and efficacy for several neurological symptoms (central neuropathic pain, visceral hyperalgesia, autonomic dysfunction). Clonidine and TCAs can be used as second-line therapies, and methadone can be considered if other agents have not controlled the pain. For most children with neuro-pain, scheduled medications can help to decrease the severity and frequency of pain episodes, but breakthrough symptoms can still occur. A treatment plan for breakthrough symptoms should include nonpharmacological and pharmacological interventions (see Box 19.1). Consider strategies to lessen the distention of the GI tract and assess for excessive caloric intake.[7]

CONCLUSION

There are many opportunities to better understand how palliative care teams can best support the management of neurological problems in seriously ill children. Further research is needed to describe the extent of distress caused by neurological symptoms, understand the efficacy of different treatment options, and explore the impact of palliative care interventions on quality of life outcomes for seriously ill children and their families.

REFERENCES

1. Feudtner C, Kang TI, Hexem KR, et al. Pediatric palliative care patients: A prospective multicenter cohort study. *Pediatrics.* 2011;127(6):1094–1101.
2. Mack JW, Wolfe J, Cook EF, et al. Hope and prognostic disclosure. *J Clin Oncol.* 2007;25(35):5636–5642.
3. Mack JW, Wolfe J, Cook EF, et al. Peace of mind and sense of purpose as core existential issues among parents of children with cancer. *Arch Pediatr Adolesc Med.* 2009;163(6):519–524.
4. Lotz JD, Daxer M, Jox RJ, et al. "Hope for the best, prepare for the worst": A qualitative interview study on parents' needs and fears in pediatric advance care planning. *Palliat Med.* 2017;31(8):764–771.
5. Hauer J, Houtrow AJ, AAP Section on Hospice and Palliative Medicine, Council on Children with Disabilities. Pain assessment and treatment in children with significant impairment of the central nervous system. *Pediatrics.* 2017;139(6):e20171002.
6. Rasmussen LA, Grégoire M. Challenging neurological symptoms in paediatric palliative care: An approach to symptom evaluation and management in children with neurological impairment. *Paediatr Child Health.* 2015;20(3):159–165.
7. Hauer J. Feeding intolerance in children with severe impairment of the central nervous system: Strategies for treatment and prevention. *Children (Basel).* 2018;5(1):1.
8. Culbert TP, Olness K. *Integrative Pediatrics.* Oxford University Press; 2010.
9. Shafto K, Gouda S, Catrine K, Brown ML. Integrative approaches in pediatric palliative care. *Children (Basel).* 2018;5(6):75.
10. Food and Drug Administration. FDA approves first drug comprised of an active ingredient derived from marijuana to treat rare, severe forms of epilepsy. Updated March 27, 2020. https://www.fda.gov/news-events/press-announcements/fda-approves-first-drug-comprised-active-ingredient-derived-marijuana-treat-rare-severe-forms
11. Elliott J, DeJean D, Clifford T, et al. Cannabis-based products for pediatric epilepsy: An updated systematic review. *Seizure.* 2020;75:18–22.
12. Devinsky O, Cross HJ, Laux L, et al. Trial of cannabidiol for drug-resistant seizures in the Dravet syndrome. *N Engl J Med.* 2017;376(21):2011–2020.
13. Nickels KC. Less effective and more expensive: Is it time to move on from rectal diazepam? *Epilepsy Curr.* 2018;18(1):27–28.
14. Arya R, Kothari H, Zhang Z, Han B, Horn PS, Glauser TA. Efficacy of nonvenous medications for acute convulsive seizures. *Neurology.* 2015;85(21):1859–1868.
15. Pal DK. Phenobarbital for childhood epilepsy: Systematic review. *Paediatr Perinat Drug Ther.* 2006;7(1):31–42.
16. Sanger TD, Delgado MR, Gaebler-Spira D, Hallett M, Mink JW. Classification and definition of disorders causing hypertonia in childhood. *Pediatrics.* 2003;111(1):e89–97.
17. Quality Standards Subcommittee of the American Academy of Neurology and the Practice Committee of the Child Neurology Society; Delgado MR, Hirtz D, et al. Practice parameter: Pharmacologic treatment of spasticity in children and adolescents with cerebral palsy (an evidence-based review): Report of the Quality Standards Subcommittee of the American Academy of Neurology and the Practice Committee of the Child Neurology Society. *Neurology.* 2010;74(4):336–343.
18. Chang E, Ghosh N, Yanni D, Lee S, Alexandru D, Mozaffar T. A review of spasticity treatments: Pharmacological and interventional approaches. *Crit Rev Phys Rehabil Med.* 2013;25(1–2):11–22.
19. Hasnat MJ, Rice JE. Intrathecal baclofen for treating spasticity in children with cerebral palsy. *Cochrane Database Syst Rev.* 2015;11:CD004552.
20. Fernández-Alvarez E, Nardocci N. Update on pediatric dystonias: Etiology, epidemiology, and management. *Degener Neurol Neuromuscul Dis.* 2012;2:29–41.
21. Allen NM, Lin JP, Lynch T, King MD. Status dystonicus: A practice guide. *Dev Med Child Neurol.* 2014;56(2):105–12.
22. National Institute of Neurological Disorders and Stroke. Dystonias fact sheet. Updated March 13, 2020. https://www.ninds.nih.gov/Disorders/Patient-Caregiver-Education/Fact-Sheets/Dystonias-Fact-Sheet
23. Sanger TD, Chen D, Fehlings DL, et al. Definition and classification of hyperkinetic movements in childhood. *Mov Disord.* 2010;25(11):1538–1549.
24. Caviness JN. Treatment of myoclonus. *Neurotherapeutics.* 2014;11(1):188–200.
25. Levy A, Chen R. Myoclonus: Pathophysiology and treatment options. *Curr Treat Options Neurol.* 2016;18(5):21.
26. Wilson RK, Weissman DE. Neuroexcitatory effects of opioids: Treatment. Fast Facts and Concepts. May 2015; 58. https://www.mypcnow.org.
27. Park ES, Park CI, Cho SR, et al. Assessment of autonomic nervous system with analysis of heart rate variability in children with spastic cerebral palsy. *Yonwei Med J.* 2002;43(1):65–72.
28. Axelrod FB, Berlin D. Pregabalin: A new approach to treatment of the dysautonomic crisis. *Pediatrics.* 2009;124(2):743–746.
29. Chelimsky G, Chelimsky T. Familial association of autonomic and gastrointestinal symptoms. *Clin Auton Res.* 2001;11(6):383–386.
30. Chelimsky G, Hupertz VF, Chelimsky TC. Abdominal pain as the presenting symptom of autonomic dysfunction in a child. *Clin Pediatr (Phila).* 1999;38(12):725–729.
31. Hauer JM, Solodiuk JC. Gabapentin for management of recurrent pain in 22 nonverbal children with severe neurological impairment: A retrospective analysis. *J Palliat Med.* 2015;18(5):453–456.
32. Hauer J, Wical B, Charnas L. Gabapentin successfully manages chronic unexplained irritability in children with severe neurologic impairment. *Pediatrics.* 2007;119(2):e519–e522.
33. Siden HB, Carleton BC, Oberlander TF. Physician variability in treating pain and irritability of unknown origin in children with severe neurological impairment. *Pain Res Manag.* 2013;18(5):243–248.
34. Haney AL, Garner SS, Cox TH. Gabapentin therapy for pain and irritability in a neurologically impaired infant. *Pharmacotherapy.* 2009;29(8):997–1001.
35. Hauer JM. Chronic pain in children with severe impairment of the central nervous system: A framework for assessment and initial management. *Complex Care Journal.* 2020;1(1). http://complexcarejournal.org/2020/03/24/chronic-pain-in-children-with-severe-impairment-of-the-central-nervous-system/.

20 | PEDIATRIC DELIRIUM IN THE PALLIATIVE CARE SETTING

PAULA TRAN, JEFFREY MOSS, EUNICE KOH, KATHERINE ORT, RICHARD J. SHAW, AND MICHELLE GOLDSMITH

The English word delirium arises from an agricultural metaphor to break away from the ploughed straightness of the furrow, *līra* in Latin. The related Latin verb, *dēlīrāre*, reveals the meaning of our chosen topic, "to be deranged, to be crazy out of one's wits."
So there beyond the furrow lies the madness and wisdom of the mind's vagaries.

Michelle Goldsmith

INTRODUCTION

Pediatric delirium, an often underrecognized and reversible complication of illness, is a clinical emergency demanding immediate management.[1] New research on the clinical presentation of pediatric delirium and age-appropriate assessment tools for prompt identification highlight some of the phenomenological differences between adults and children.[2–6] In the context of palliative care, delirium requires an immediate response and a collaboratively developed plan of care similar to that for pain, anxiety, nausea, and dyspnea.[7] In the adult palliative care setting, delirium has been carefully studied and identified commonly in the elderly, medically ill, and toward the end of life.[8,9] Delirium is the most common neuropsychiatric disorder, with prevalence estimated as high as 85% among those who are terminally ill.[10] In a palliative care setting, researchers[11] identified 42% of the patients with a diagnosis of delirium at the time of hospital admission and an additional 45% who developed delirium during their hospital stay. These data suggest that delirium occurs in the majority of adult patients nearing the end of life and that improved methods of diagnosis and management are warranted for this highly distressing and often reversible condition.

Between children and adults, much overlap exists in the presentation of delirium such as waxing and waning sensorium and disorientation; however, several pertinent symptoms emerge in our younger patients which distinguish them from adults. Changes in affect with increased irritability, inconsolability, decreased eye contact with close care givers, and the loss of previously achieved developmental milestones should raise suspicion that a child is experiencing delirium.[12,13] Frequently parents will say things such as "this is not my child," or "I don't know how to help her." While hallucinations and delusions remain a *sine qua non* in established criteria for adult delirium, the absence of psychotic features among children does not rule out the phenomenon. Therefore, in all critically ill patients of every age, mental status, and relatability to loved ones should be carefully evaluated in addition to the conventional monitoring of pulse, temperature, respiratory rate, blood pressure, and pain.[14]

The study of delirium is at the confluence of several clinical disciplines including anesthesiology, critical care medicine, pediatrics, geriatrics, oncology, pain medicine, palliative medicine, neurology, psychiatry, psychology, nursing, pharmacy, and bioethics. Across these domains, there has been a recent groundswell of interest in delirium,[15] and specifically pediatric delirium, after a long period of neglect between 1980 and 2003.[2,3] Advances in medical care that prolong life place critically ill patients at greater risk for delirium. In addition, awareness of potential cognitive and psychological sequelae of delirium has led to efforts directed at early recognition and treatment. Goals of palliative and general clinical care target delirium as a symptom that necessitates immediate attention.[16]

This chapter offers an overview of pediatric delirium, its clinical relevance, and its emotional impact in seriously ill children, families, and clinical providers. An additional goal includes underscoring the interdisciplinary nature of delirium. Any clinician or caregiver, including respiratory therapist, nurse, doctor, intensive care unit (ICU) pharmacist, and parent, can screen patients for delirium. Delirium stems from many causes, occurs in both simple and complex clinical situations, and should be suspected in all circumstances when mental status is altered. One long-term study involving adult inpatients has shown that nurse-directed delirium prevention and management programs involving multidisciplinary education and collaboration have led to a decrease in delirium and clinician workload.[17] Every member of the treatment team serves as a resource in the prevention, recognition, and management of delirium.

Topics addressed in this chapter include definitions, clinical presentation, prevalence and epidemiology, etiology and risk factors, pathogenesis, assessment, and treatment. Finally, there is a review of the relationship between delirium and posttraumatic stress symptoms, including its effects on caregivers.

DEFINITION

According to the *Diagnostic and Statistical Manual* (DSM),[13] the core features of delirium include a disturbance of consciousness, change in cognition, and perceptual disturbance that develops over a short period, usually hours to days, and fluctuates over time (see Box 20.1). Delirium has been associated with rates of morbidity and mortality that surpass those of all other psychiatric diagnoses.[19] Across clinical disciplines and countries, many ambiguities prevail in the terminology used to describe delirium.[20] Such terms as "acute brain failure," "encephalopathy," "acute confusional state," and "ICU psychosis" have been widely employed, and the critical care literature now conforms to the recommendations of the American Psychiatric Association and other experts that the term "delirium" be used uniformly to describe this syndrome of brain dysfunction.[21] The need for shared terminology reflects the challenges clinicians face in diagnosing delirium across clinical settings and age groups.

BOX 20.1 DSM-5 DIAGNOSTIC CRITERIA FOR DELIRIUM

Change in consciousness

- Reduced clarity in awareness of the environment, that is a reduced ability to focus, sustain, or shift attention

Change in cognition

- Memory deficit, disorientation, language disturbance, or development of a perceptual disturbance not better accounted for by a preexisting cognitive disorder

Temporal character

- Develops over a short period, usually hours to days, and fluctuates during the course of the day

Etiology

- There is evidence from the history, physical examination, or laboratory findings of a general medical condition, including possible substance intoxication or substance withdrawal, that is deemed etiologically related to the disturbance
- Changes in consciousness and cognition are not due to neurocognitive disorder or state of decreased alertness

Adapted with permission from the American Psychiatric Association, *Diagnostic and Statistical Manual of Mental Disorders*, 5th edition revised (DSM-V). American Psychiatric Association; 2013).

CLINICAL PRESENTATION

Although the clinical presentation of delirium in children and adolescents is similar to that of adults, there are observed differences in the type and frequency of symptoms across various age groups.[4–6] Clinician-observed features of pediatric delirium vary across several studies. Pediatric patients are described as having more frequent fluctuation in symptoms, greater affective lability, impaired attention, and disturbances in their sleep–wake cycle.[4] By contrast,[6] a study described pediatric patients as having lower rates of sleep disturbance, fewer cognitive deficits, and lower levels of symptom fluctuation.

With regard to psychotic symptoms, authors have described both lower and higher prevalence of perceptual disturbances and delusions among children compared to adults.[4,6] Some have suggested that delusions and hallucinations may not be core symptoms of pediatric delirium.[4] Alternatively, a study of pediatric patients emerging from anesthesia reported that younger children had higher rates of hallucinations and other perceptual disturbances when compared with older children.[22] These differences may reflect variations in brain function across the age span, developmental immaturity in children, functional decline in old age, and differences in the expression of distress during hospitalization.[23] The variance in observed clinical features is wide and may result from the fluctuating nature of the illness, the subjective nature of clinical assessment, limitations of age-appropriate screening tools, and the various causes of delirium.

SUBTYPES

The adult literature well-describes three motoric subtypes of delirium: hypoactive, hyperactive, and mixed.[24] Delirium is also categorized on the basis of symptom severity, with terms such as "pre-delirium," "subsyndromal," "veiled," and "full-blown," all of which designate differences in presentation.[25] These additional terms reflect increasing research into the phenomenology of delirium. Although few studies have focused on categorizing delirium temporally or by severity, the practical finding from this work is that delirium may be detectable earlier in its course with vigilant screening. In this chapter, a discussion of motoric subtypes is reviewed with vignettes.

The term "hyperactive" refers to patients who present with symptoms of confusion, psychosis, disorientation, agitation, hypervigilance, hyper-alertness, fast or loud speech, combativeness, and behavioral problems such as pulling out catheters and lines. These patients quickly come to the attention of the medical staff and are less likely to be overlooked.

TABLE 20.1 Characteristics of delirium subtypes

SUBTYPE	HYPERACTIVE	HYPOACTIVE	MIXED
Clinical features	Psychomotor agitation Increased verbal fluency and volume Restlessness Hyperarousal Hallucinations	Psychomotor retardation Diminished speech production and volume Apathy Withdrawal	Presence of hyperactive and hypoactive symptoms
Notes	More easily identified May demand a higher level of care May need restraint for safety of self and others Often more distressing to family, staff, and patient	Often overlooked Often misdiagnosed as depression or oversedation from medication	Diagnosis confounded by mixed clinical picture
Likely etiologies	Drug withdrawal Anticholinergic-induced	Hepatic Metabolic encephalopathies Acute sedative or analgesic intoxication Hypoxia	Multiple etiologies
Common electroencephalogram (EEG) findings and pathophysiology	EEG: fast or normal Increased cerebral metabolism Reduced activity in the GABA system	EEG: diffuse slowing Decreased cerebral metabolism Increased activity in the GABA system	Multiple pathways
Treatment options	Haloperidol	Second-generation antipsychotic	Second-generation antipsychotic

Clinical Vignette: Hyperactive Delirium

Anna is a 14-year-old previously healthy girl who presented with the sudden onset of dizziness, shortness of breath, lethargy, and chest pain. Chest x-ray showed signs of cardiomegaly which prompted cardiology consultation. Following a cardiology workup, including an echocardiogram, Anna was diagnosed with idiopathic dilated cardiomyopathy, and hospitalized in the ICU. By hospital Day 4, Anna's cardiac function had declined rapidly, and she was placed on the cardiac transplant waiting list. Despite intensive pharmacologic treatment, her worsening cardiac status necessitated Anna being placed on a ventricular assist device. Anna's course was further complicated by a small cerebral vascular accident on hospital Day 17. The night following her stroke, Anna was unable to sleep, became acutely agitated, and needed soft physical restraints to prevent her from pulling out her lines and catheters. She was clearly confused and disoriented, and unable to reason with the medical staff. By the following morning, Anna said she was hearing the voice of her deceased grandfather and believed that he had visited her the previous night. She also reported seeing blood coming out of the faucet in her room and the feeling of spiders walking over her face.

Following psychiatric consultation, Anna was diagnosed with hyperactive delirium and a score of 22/32 on the Delirium Rating Scale-Revised-98 (DRS-R-98). Recommendations were made for treatment with intravenous (IV) haloperidol 0.5 mg every 6 hours, pending review of her electrocardiogram (ECG). Although Anna's ECG showed evidence of a prolonged QTc interval (410 ms), it was considered safe to prescribe the haloperidol with close cardiac monitoring. In addition, blinds were opened during the day to maintain a circadian rhythm, and an effort was made to minimize ambient noise in the room, including television and multiple conversations. This was very helpful in reducing her level of agitation and reestablishing her normal sleep–wake cycle. By hospital Day 20, Anna's symptoms of delirium had resolved, and her DRS-R-98 score was 5/32. The following day, an organ became available, and Anna underwent cardiac transplant surgery.

By contrast, patients with *hypoactive* or *silent delirium* present with somnolence, decreased activity, slow or decreased speech, psychomotor slowing, withdrawal, apathy, and confusion. These patients may also be perceived as calm and somnolent by the medical and nursing staff. Patients with this latter presentation who demand less care do not as frequently raise concern for delirium or may be misdiagnosed with depression. In these cases, parental opinion comparing current presentation and baseline functioning can be very useful. Often parental observations, such as "this is not my child" alerts clinicians to reassess mental status more carefully and frequently.

Clinical Vignette: Hypoactive Delirium

Barry is a 16-year-old male with a history of acute lymphoblastic leukemia with CNS involvement. Although he initially responded well to chemotherapy, his treatment was complicated by both herpes simplex virus as well as hemorrhagic stroke requiring intensive rehabilitation. Although Barry made a good recovery, residual damage to his frontal lobes was evident on magnetic resonance imaging (MRI) scan. After 3 years in remission, Barry relapsed and was restarted on a reinduction regimen of methotrexate, vincristine, daunorubicin, and asparaginase. After his second dose of chemotherapy, Barry developed fever and signs of neutropenia, and he was admitted for IV antibiotics. By hospital Day 3, although Barry's fever had resolved and his white blood count was recovering, he was noted to be increasingly withdrawn, spending much of the day in silence, avoiding eye contact, and appearing internally distracted. He started to refuse food, was sleeping excessively during the day, and became almost mute. On hospital Day 5, Barry was referred for psychiatric consultation due to concerns about possible depression related to his relapse. Barry was quite uncommunicative during the assessment and either unable or unwilling to cooperate with simple tests of attention and cognition. However, he did appear quite profoundly impaired even with respect to simple questions about orientation and memory.

Due to concerns about a possible hypoactive delirium, recommendations were made for a comprehensive medical workup, including an MRI scan, as well as a trial of treatment with risperidone at a dose of 0.5 mg twice daily. By the following day, although still slowed motorically, Barry improved remarkably. He was more talkative, affectively expressive, and able to answer questions. On mental status exam, he continued to have difficulty with orientation, attention and memory, and visual-spatial abilities. He also hesitantly endorsed a strongly held belief that "men in black were outside his room, waiting for him to die." His score on the DRS-R-98 was 18/32, and he was thought to meet criteria for hypoactive delirium. Barry was continued on risperidone for another 5 days. His medical workup was unremarkable, and no etiology identified to explain his symptoms. His psychotic symptoms resolved by hospital Day 9, and he was fully oriented, with a score of 3/32 on the DRS-R-98. One week after discharge Barry was titrated down to risperidone 0.5 mg at night, and, after 5 days, the medication was discontinued. Both he and his mother reported that his mood and affect remained appropriate, and he did not exhibit any further symptoms of delirium.

Mixed delirium describes patients who fluctuate between hyperactive and hypoactive states.[23,27] These critically ill patients present with an array of symptoms in the context of possible pain, anxiety, and nausea, thus making it difficult to recognize delirium and identify the cause.

Clinical Vignette: Mixed Delirium

Jackie is a 9-year-old girl with a glioblastoma who, during hospitalization for chemotherapy, developed pressured speech, periods of confusion, and occasional disorientation. She was noticed to be sleeping as little as 4 hours a night. Her level of activity was also increased, and nursing staff reported that she would spend significant periods of time cleaning and ordering items in her hospital room. She expressed less interest in toys and games or participating in care. She had a score of 18/32 on the DRS-98 and was diagnosed with acute delirium. Jackie was initially treated with risperidone 0.5 mg nightly. She seemed to improve on this regimen, with better sleep and less pressured activity, but continued to have episodes of increased confusion, disorientation, apathy, and talking to herself during the day. Her risperidone was increased to 0.5 mg twice daily, with the addition of zolpidem 5 mg for insomnia. Her mother was encouraged to walk her around the unit three times per day to promote mobility and purposeful activity. She showed improvement on this regimen and gradually returned to her baseline over several days, at which time she had a score of 4/32 on the DRS-R-98.

PREVALENCE AND EPIDEMIOLOGY

One of the largest retrospective pediatric studies on delirium[3] reported a 9% prevalence of delirium in a sample of 1,027 patients referred for psychiatric consultation. Another study[5] reported a lower prevalence of 4.6% in a pediatric sample of 877 critical care patients. By comparison, among adult studies, delirium has been reported in 15% to 18% of patients on acute medical and surgical wards, with higher rates in specific populations.[19]

Regarding age, a study of 1,027 patients[3] identified 84 patients with delirium ages 6 months to 18 years, and there was no significant difference in mean and median age based on the cause of delirium. The study did not assess whether age itself was a risk factor for delirium. According to the study[5] that presented data stratified by age, the greatest incidence of delirium occurred among the oldest children (15–18 years), but these data were not analyzed for statistical significance. Conversely, another study[28] found a negative correlation between age and delirium among post-anesthesia patients suffering with emergence delirium.

Although studies to assess the prevalence of delirium in children receiving end-of-life care have not yet been undertaken, data from adult studies suggest potentially much higher rates in this population. For example, immediately before death, delirium rates of 68–88% have been reported in adult oncology patients.[11,29] More specifically, according to a review,[8] hypoactive delirium, which is easily overlooked, has been reported as being as high as 40–78% in adult palliative care patients.[11,30,31]

Attempts to quantify the prevalence of delirium by subtype among adults have resulted in a range of findings. For example, a study[32] reported hypoactive delirium (43.5%) occurring considerably more often than "purely" hyperactive delirium (1.6%), and mixed delirium was the most frequently observed subtype (54.1%). The low number of cases with hyperactive delirium in this cohort is unusual when compared with other studies that report rates of hyperactive delirium ranging from 15% to 80%.[24,33] On the other hand, the high number of cases in the cohort[32] of 375 elderly diagnosed with hypoactive delirium suggests that careful screening may accurately identify more subtle presentations of delirium. The only comparison[4] of prevalence of delirium subtype between adults to children found that, across three adult studies, there was an average of 59% hypoactive delirium, similar to a pediatric prevalence of 69%. Agitation was noted in the adult studies at a combined rate of 44%, which was significantly lower than the pediatric rate of hyperactive delirium of 68%.

Figures for the prevalence of delirium by subtype in the pediatric palliative care setting are not known. In adult palliative care literature, the rates of hypoactive delirium are as high as 86%, with a mean prevalence 48% in one meta-analysis, while rates of hyperactive delirium vary between 13% and 46% of patients.[31,34]

Despite the varied estimates on prevalence, numerous studies suggest that the motoric subtypes of delirium differ beyond the degree of psychomotor activity. Studies show variation between hypoactive, hyperactive, and mixed delirium with regard to other nonmotoric features of delirium,[35] etiology and pathophysiology,[36] ease of detection and assessment, response to treatment,[26] and outcome.[37] Notably, clinician observations of patient psychomotor disturbance were less reliable when compared with data from electronic motion detectors.[38] Because recognition of delirium continues to be challenging and machine-assisted assessment is helpful, there is the potential that future technological innovations may enhance clinician assessment. For example, similar to the use of heart monitors in the ICU, motion detection may be used to help alert clinicians to the presence of delirium among high-risk groups.

ETIOLOGY AND RISK FACTORS

Causes and risk factors for delirium are often multifaceted and include vascular, infectious, neoplastic, degenerative, organ failure, toxic, deficiencies including vitamin, congenital, CNS pathologic, traumatic, endocrinological, metabolic, dehydration, heavy metal, and anoxic phenomena.[19] Medication-related etiologies, as a result of toxic effects or withdrawal reactions, are also common. As with adults, certain classes of medications, such as steroids, opiates, benzodiazepines, and anticholinergic agents, are frequent precipitants.

Clinical Vignette

Tristan, a 16-year-old boy with chronic myelogenous leukemia (CML), was scheduled to receive a blood transfusion. He was pretreated with IV diphenhydramine to prevent allergic reactions. He had previously received three doses of diphenhydramine in the prior 36-hour period for itching and insomnia. After transfusion he complained of blurry vision, appeared flushed, and became agitated. He also reported that there were cameras in his room and snakes coming out of his arm. On examination, he had dilated pupils, dry mucous membranes, and flushed skin. He was assessed as having classic signs of an anticholinergic delirium related to his treatment with diphenhydramine.

At end of life, delirium often results from intensive treatment of pain and suffering, which can lead to drug-induced change in mental status.[9] A study of 40 critically ill children[5] found that the most frequent causes of delirium in decreasing order included a change in analgosedative medication, infections, and neurological and respiratory disorders. Often there were multiple causes for delirium. Infection was twice as often the precipitating factor compared with drug induced-delirium in one report.[4] A thorough diagnostic workup to identify the cause is the standard of care[39]; however, in the palliative care setting where the goal of care is to decrease pain and suffering, this approach is often modified

PATHOGENESIS

Delirium as a neuropsychiatric disorder involves global encephalopathic dysfunction caused by multiple impaired neural pathways and physiologic compromises. The neurotransmitters implicated in the pathophysiology of delirium include acetylcholine, dopamine, glutamine, gamma-aminobutyric acid (GABA), and serotonin.[36] Dopamine modulates mood and cognitive function, and in excess can lead to psychotic disorders. Similarly, acute alterations in dopamine levels may contribute to the characteristic symptoms of delirium. Antipsychotic medications that inhibit the dopamine pathway effectively treat delirium.[40] Alteration of GABA, an inhibitory neurotransmitter, may also cause changes in cerebral functioning, possibly by affecting sleep patterns. In the critical and palliative care setting, benzodiazepines and propofol, which directly affect GABA receptors, are frequently administered, and contribute to the development of delirium.[41] Likewise, the use of anticholinergic drugs precipitate and worsen symptoms of delirium.[42] These neurotransmitter perturbations are thought to cause neuronal membrane hyperpolarization, thus spreading neuronal depression, which is seen on electroencephalogram (EEG) as a diffuse slowing.[43]

Other insults to cerebral functioning such as inflammation, hypoxia, metabolic encephalopathies, and drugs or toxins, compound the development of delirium. Inflammation, caused by infection, surgery, or other tissue injury, heightens blood–brain barrier permeability leading to translocation of inflammatory mediators, such as cytokines and chemokines, into the CNS, causing encephalopathy dysfunction.[44] Cytokines such as interleukin (IL)-1, IL-2, interferon (IFN), and tumor necrosis factor (TNF) can affect neuronal pathways by inhibiting acetylcholine, leading to agitation, perceptual disturbances, seizures, and delirium.[45] There are reports of chemokine elevations in patients with delirium, and one study found IL-6 increases in children with influenza who developed delirium.[46] Inability to meet oxygen needs, either because of increased demand or decreased delivery, contributes to development of delirium because of disruption of ionic gradients, neurotransmitter homeostasis, and neurotoxic byproduct elimination. The compromise of oxygen metabolism can be due to hypoglycemia, hyper- or hypothermia, and vitamin or amino acid deficiencies. Impaired oxygen metabolism leads to reduced neurotransmitter synthesis, causing a deregulation of sleep–wake cycle, behavior, and mood, and psychomotor activity, all of which are clinical manifestations of delirium.[40,47]

ASSESSMENT

The diagnosis of pediatric delirium is primarily made on clinical examination, which should always include an interview with parents and primary caregivers. Suspicion of delirium also necessitates a review of the medical chart, including laboratory and imaging test results. Nursing staff and parents' observations are particularly important to evaluate fluctuations in levels of consciousness and sleep disturbance. The Nursing Staff Delirium Screening Scale (NDSS) provides a quick and consistent measure for those clinicians who have the most frequent clinical contact with patients.[43] Although not generally standard of care, EEG findings may offer diagnostic support of delirium and perhaps subtype.[43] Additionally, family members serve as a valuable clinical resource regarding the patient's state of arousal, activity, and orientation, especially in the pediatric population. In palliative care, the education of patients and family members in recognizing signs of delirium can aid in assessment and early intervention, minimize distress to the patient and family, and support clinical decision-making in end-of-life care.

STRUCTURED DELIRIUM ASSESSMENT INSTRUMENTS

To supplement and help guide the direct clinical evaluation, there are several structured assessments and rating scales to diagnose and track symptoms related to delirium. These tools include assessment for cognitive impairment, such as Mini Mental Status Exam[49]; screening for delirium using DSM-IV-TR diagnostic criteria including the Confusion Assessment Measure[50,51]; and delirium-specific numeric scales to rate severity, including the Delirium Rating Scale-Revised-98 (DRS-R-98).[50]

DELIRIUM RATING SCALE-REVISED-98

The DRS-R-98 is widely used to assess delirium in adults using a 16-item scale with items that include disturbances of cognition, perception, thought, language, sleep, affect, and psychomotor function. Items are rated based on direct observation, data from the medical record, and accounts from caregivers. The DRS-R-98 has been proved reliable for both the diagnosis and serial assessment of delirium and has been used and validated for pediatric patients. The scale was validated for children based on retrospective chart review identifying 84 individuals ages 6 months to 19 years. All of these highly medically compromised patients experienced lengthy hospital stays with an average hospitalization of 43 days.[52,53]

PEDIATRIC ANESTHESIA EMERGENCE DELIRIUM SCALE

The Pediatric Anesthesia Emergence Delirium Scale (PAEDS) is a measure designed to rate postsurgical emergence delirium and has been validated for use in children.[26] Unlike other scales, the PAEDS is a clinician report of observed behaviors and responses to stimuli, which differentiate it from the DRS-R-98.

PEDIATRIC CONFUSION ASSESSMENT MEASURE

The Pediatric Confusion Assessment Measure (p-CAM) is a two-part assessment tool that screens for overall cognitive impairment using the Richmond Agitation Sedation Scale (RASS) and then distinguishes delirium from other causes of cognitive impairment.[54,55] Unlike the DRS-R-98, the p-CAM is designed to diagnose delirium rather than to rate symptom severity. The Pre-School Confusion Assessment Method (ps-CAM) is designed to assess for delirium in critically ill infants and preschool-aged children.[56]

CORNELL ASSESSMENT OF PEDIATRIC DELIRIUM

The Cornell Assessment of Pediatric Delirium (CAP-D) is a screening tool adapted from the PAED to improve identification of hypoactive and hyperactive delirium by using a behavioral scale. It has been validated for use in children of all ages and provides developmental anchor points to help guide clinicians' assessment of CAP-D symptoms based on a developmental understanding of the presentation of delirium.[57]

PEDIATRIC INDEX OF MORTALITY AND PEDIATRIC RISK OF MORTALITY

The Pediatric Index of Mortality (PIM)[58] and the Pediatric Risk of Mortality (PRISM II)[59] are scales used in the pediatric intensive care setting to predict outcome. Using PIM and PRISM, one study[60] found the positive predictive value was low mostly due to few identified cases of delirium (40 out of 877 patients), but the negative predictive value was very high at 99%, suggesting that these scales can be used to rule out nonoccurrence of delirium.[60] A 2009 study suggested an algorithm for diagnosing and managing pediatric delirium using the RASS and PAEDS.[25] As the authors point out, further research is required to validate any proposed methods. Likewise, the overview (see Figure 20.1) included in this chapter highlights important aspects of identifying and

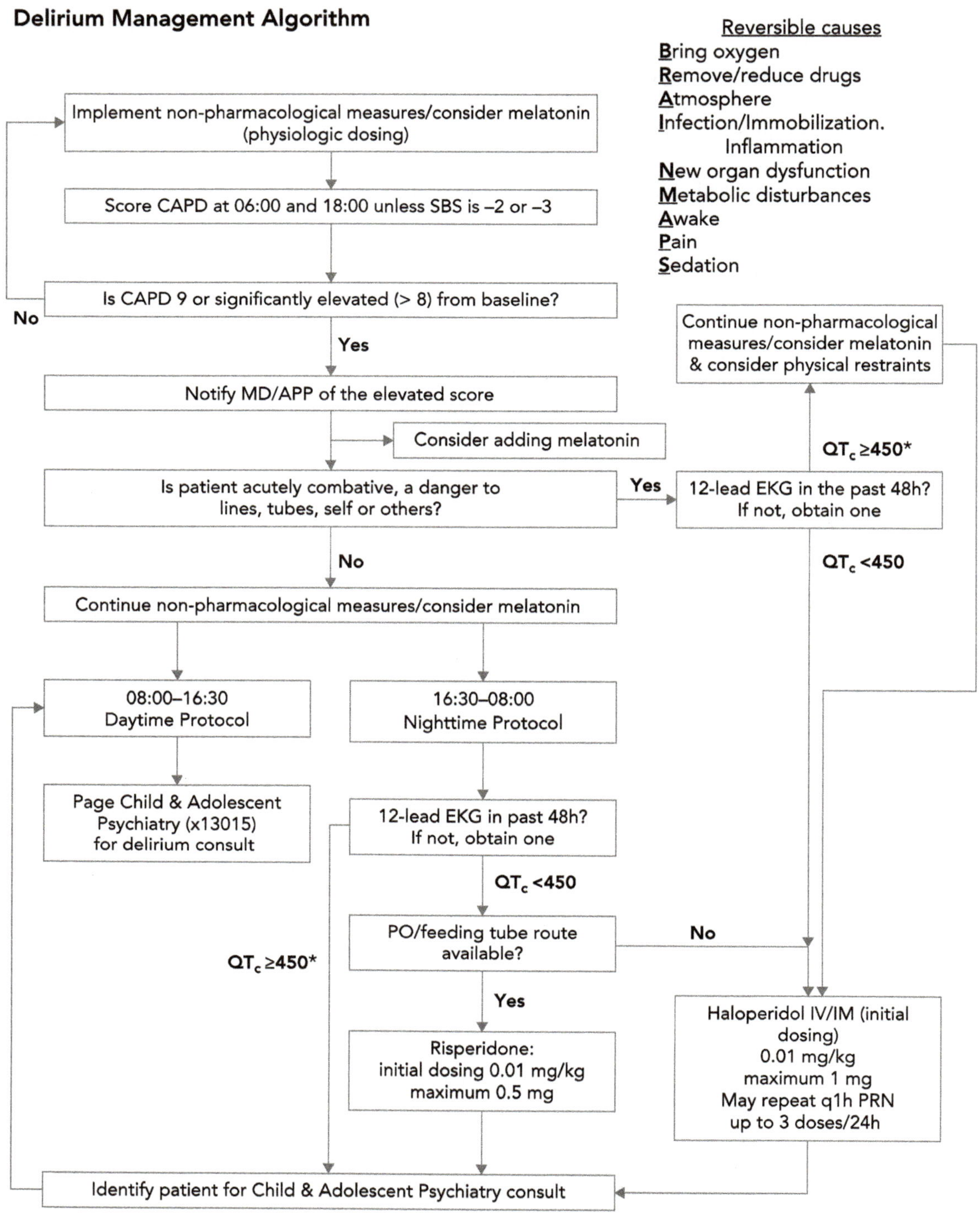

*if QTc 450–500 may consider a single dose of haloperidol based on clinical scenario

Figure 20.1 *Delirium management algorithm.*

treating pediatric delirium. Further research will be needed to establish best evidenced-based practices.

CATATONIA

Delirium always includes a change in mental status and may be accompanied by other alterations in sensorium such as catatonia. Distinguishing these clinical phenomena remains difficult, even among adults, as each syndrome can present with both agitated and negativistic features. Careful and repeated assessment by experienced clinicians remains necessary because treatment approaches for each entity are quite different. Like delirium, catatonia can present with changes in behavior, motor activity, affect, and responsiveness to the surrounding environment. Catatonia though may also include autonomic instability, fever, and leukocytosis, and it possesses less of a waxing and waning quality. Both diagnoses may be related to underlying medical conditions. However, neuroleptic medications, the first-line pharmacologic treatment for delirium, can worsen catatonia; benzodiazepines, helpful for catatonia, can exacerbate delirium.

BUSH FRANCIS CATATONIA RATING SCALE

The DSM-5 defines catatonia as the presence of at least 3 of the following 12 symptoms: catalepsy, waxy flexibility, stupor, agitation, mutism, negativism, posturing, mannerisms, stereotypies, grimacing, echolalia, and echopraxia.[18] The Bush Francis Catatonia Rating Scale (BFCRS) is a clinical tool that captures these symptoms as well as their severity. Although the DSM-5 characterizes catatonia related to a medical cause as being diagnostically possible only in the absence of a delirium diagnosis, studies have shown that the two conditions can coexist. In one study of more than 200 adult hospital patients diagnosed with delirium, 12.7–30.2% also met criteria for catatonia.[61] In another prospective study involving more than 130 adult intensive care patients, delirium and catatonia were both present in 31% of the cohort.[62]

Catatonia has been studied in pediatric patients, including in those with neurodevelopmental disorders such as autism.[63] Identifying and addressing catatonia in pediatric cases resembles the process in adult medical care.[64] Experts in the diagnosis and treatment of catatonia have argued that the condition is often underrecognized[65] and have reasoned for routine screening in the pediatric population. Esseveld and colleagues have proposed that catatonia be considered in critically ill pediatric patients exhibiting changes in behavior or affect.[66] Differentiation of delirium from catatonia prevents healthcare teams from proceeding down the wrong treatment path and delaying appropriate medical intervention.

STRUCTURED ASSESSMENTS

Despite the availability of validated tools to rapidly and accurately detect delirium, few ICUs, worldwide, are routinely evaluating patients for delirium using a validated screening tool.[67–72] In an international online survey of PICUs, 71% of respondents reported they did not practice delirium screening, and only 2% reported screening every patient at least once per 12-hour shift.[73–74]

Although there is no evidence that the use of a structured assessment tool results in improved outcomes,[75] the use of such tools has been shown to lead to an understanding of risk factors, associated morbidities, and strategies to prevent and treat delirium in adults.[76–82] In adults, without the use of a structured screening tool, delirium goes undetected in up to 60–75% of patients.[75,83,84]

In 2013, the Society of Critical Care Medicine's clinical practice guidelines for the management of pain, agitation, and delirium (PAD) in adult patients in the ICU recommended routine monitoring of delirium.[77] The 2018 guidelines updated and expanded the 2013 PAD guidelines with the addition of immobility and sleep disruption (PADIS) and issued a good practice statement that critically ill adults should be regularly assessed for delirium using a valid tool because early detection may lead to prompt identification of cause, guide treatment, and determine effectiveness of treatment.[85]

TREATMENT

PREVENTION AND NONPHARMACOLOGIC INTERVENTIONS

The recognition and treatment of delirium in the hospital setting requires a team effort. This includes observational input from and implementation of treatment recommendations by nursing staff and caretakers at the bedside. Ancillary staff involved with the delirious patient's care, including physical therapists, occupational therapists, and art therapists, also play important roles in communicating clinical information to the rest of the hospital team as they may observe changes in a patient's behaviors and alertness when parents, nursing staff, and physicians are not in the room. Thus, it is important that psychoeducation on the prevention, identification, and treatment of delirium be provided to all those involved in the patient's care. Silver and colleagues have outlined a clinical pathway with suggestions regarding delirium prevention measures.[86]

RISK FACTORS FOR DELIRIUM

Knowledge of the risk factors for delirium allows for their mitigation, when possible. The risk factors for pediatric delirium are like those seen in adult delirium and can be categorized as (1) predisposing, (2) precipitating, and (3) environmental (see Table 20.2). A documented predisposing risk factor for pediatric delirium is younger age, described as younger than 5 years old in one prospective study involving almost 100 critically ill patients ranging from infant age to 21 years old[87] and identified as less than 2 years of age in a separate multisite study involving 25 critical care centers throughout the world.[88] Though predisposing risk factors are often unchangeable, many precipitating and environmental risk factors are either reversible or reducible. For example,

TABLE 20.2 Risk factors for delirium

PREDISPOSING	PRECIPITATING	ENVIRONMENTAL
Age	Electrolyte imbalance	Immobility, including physical restraints
Genetic predisposition	Hypoxia, fever or hypotension	Bothersome light and noise
Neurological disease	Acidosis	Reduced social interactions
Psychiatric illness	Hypoalbuminemia	Pain
Visual or hearing impairment	Infection including sepsis	Lines and catheters
Surgery	Deliriogenic medications	
	Sleep disturbance	

an electrolyte imbalance caused by an acute illness would be considered a precipitating risk factor that can be corrected. Likewise, a precipitating infection can be treated. Loud noise and limited social interactions are examples of environmental risk factors that may be addressed in a timely fashion. The use of physical restraints, known to independently increase risk of delirium fourfold,[88] is another environmental risk factor that can be directly modified.

PREVENTION

Especially in high-risk populations where multiple risk factors for developing delirium are present, close observation, monitoring, and optimization of the patient's surroundings by the entire treatment team is critical to minimize the risk of developing delirium. Promotion of the sleep–wake cycle, constant reorientation with calendars and clocks, providing reassurance with familiar objects from home, keeping a calm environment by minimizing bright lights and loud activity, adequate treatment of pain, and encouraging mobility are additional recommended environmental interventions. Nighttime interruptions can be reduced by clustering clinical care and administration of scheduled medications at the same time.

Given the potential of medications to cause and/or worsen delirium, checking medication lists for drug-drug interactions, minimizing use of known deliriogenic medications such as anticholinergics,[89,90] benzodiazepines,[91,92] corticosteroids,[93] and sedating medications,[94] as well as ensuring appropriate tapering of medications such as opiates and benzodiazepines to prevent withdrawal symptoms, are all critical steps to minimize delirium risk. Management guidelines for pediatric delirium that do not involve introducing an antipsychotic medication are provided in Table 20.3.

In an effort to reduce the frequency and magnitude of adverse outcomes associated with ICU delirium and weakness, the Society of Critical Care Medicine implemented a quality improvement initiative called the Intensive Care Unit Liberation Collaborative which is designed to facilitate implementation of the PAD guidelines using the integrated, interdisciplinary, evidence-based strategies of the ABCDEF bundle[77,85]:

Assess, prevent, and manage pain

Both spontaneous awakening trials (SAT) and spontaneous breathing trials (SBT)

Choice of analgesia and sedation

Delirium: assess, prevent, and manage

Early mobility and exercise

Family engagement and empowerment[95,96]

This bundled approach to care has shown a reduction in the time critically ill adults have been delirious, with as much as 50% reduction risk in delirium compared to patients who did not receive the bundle.[97–99] Implementation of a bundle has been shown to decrease incidence of delirium in the pediatric ICU (PICU).[100] It has also been shown to reduce the monthly prevalence of delirium in adults and children and is associated with improved patient outcomes, ICU and hospital length of stay, and mortality.[73,83]

TABLE 20.3 Management guideline for pediatric delirium to be used with or without neuroleptics

INTERVENTION TYPE (BY WHOM?)	POTENTIAL ACTIONS/ACTIVITIES
Reversing medical causes (Medical team)	Correcting lab abnormalities Correcting abnormal vital signs Treating underlying infections
Sensory and environmental modification (Nursing staff, parents at bedside, ancillary staff)	Favorite or soothing music Gentle touch and massage Minimize immobilizing lines, catheters, and restraints Minimize noise Calming and clear speech Lighting Familiar objects in the room and with patient when leaving the room
Caregiver measures (Nursing staff, parents, medical providers)	Proper body alignment • Assist with passive range of motion • Avoid immobility Time and place reorientation • Boards to communicate with pictures or words • Clocks • Photos • Daily schedules to promote sleep–wake cycles Sleep protocols Play favorite movies and/or shows Parental participation in care Parental and significant other presence Parents holding child in bed or chair Scheduling medications and treatments to accommodate child's routine and minimize intrusion

Melatonin has been investigated as a potential intervention for preventing delirium in critically ill patients. A naturally occurring hormone, melatonin has roles in circadian rhythms and sleep. Two studies have shown that nightly, low-dose melatonin administration was associated with decreased incidence of delirium in elderly and critically ill adults, respectively.[101,102] Data surrounding the use of melatonin in critically ill children are lacking. Preoperative melatonin in children undergoing surgery was associated with a dose-dependent reduction in emergence reactions compared to preoperative oral midazolam.[103] Melatonin has been used for pediatric sleep disturbance and has a favorable side-effect profile.[104] Despite lack of data in hospitalized pediatric patients, it is regularly prescribed in PICUs for regulating sleep disturbances.[105]

PHARMACOLOGIC STRATEGIES TO REDUCE THE INCIDENCE OF DELIRIUM

While a diagnostic workup of potential causes is being conducted, pharmacologic interventions may still be required to manage symptoms in patients with delirium (Table 20.4).

TABLE 20.4 Pharmacologic management guidelines for pediatric delirium

MEDICATION	COMMERCIALLY AVAILABLE FORMULATIONS	SUGGESTED DOSING STRATEGY[a]	NOTABLE ADVERSE EFFECTS/MONITORING	COMMENTS
Haloperidol	Tablet Solution IM injection (IV-off label)	0.01 mg/kg IM/IV (max 1 mg) at bedtime or twice daily and/or every 1 hour as needed for up to 3 doses in 24-hour period	Extrapyramidal symptoms (dystonia) QT prolongation (significant)	Acute agitation Patient unable to tolerate enteral medication Useful in hyperactive delirium
Risperidone	Solution Tablets ODT	0.01 mg/kg (max 0.5 mg) at bedtime or twice daily, titrate to max 0.08 mg/kg/day (max 4 mg) in 2–4 doses	Extrapyramidal symptoms (dystonia) Orthostatic hypotension QT prolongation	Useful in mixed/ hypoactive delirium
Quetiapine	Tablets	0.5 mg/kg, rounded to nearest 6.25 mg increment (max 50 mg, at bedtime or twice daily, titrated to max	Sedation Orthostatic hypotension QT prolongation	
Olanzapine	Tablet ODT IM injection	7–10 years: 1.25 mg at bedtime, titrated to max 10 mg in 1–2 doses >10 years: 2.5–5 mg at bedtime, titrated to max 20 mg in 1–2 doses	Sedation Metabolic changes (weight gain, hyperglycemia) QT Prolongation	
Aripiprazole	Solution Tablets	6–10 years: 2 mg daily 7–10 years: 2.5–5 mg daily, titrated to 10 mg daily	Extrapyramidal symptoms (akathesia) Orthostatic hypotension	Useful in hypoactive delirium

[a]Dosages may need to be adjusted for evidence of hepatic and/or renal dysfunction.

ODT, oral disintegrating tablet.

Antipsychotic and sedative agents can be used to diminish levels of agitation, correct disturbances in the sleep cycle, and minimize perceptual disturbances. Second-generation antipsychotics and haloperidol have all been used in the treatment of delirium, with varying degrees of success. The side-effect profile of each agent should be considered and individualized to each patient. Moreover, treatments should always be accompanied by adequate pain management and monitoring of potential medication withdrawal reactions.

FIRST-GENERATION ANTIPSYCHOTIC AGENTS

Haloperidol, one of the first-generation antipsychotics, has been a commonly used agent for the management of delirium.[106] While haloperidol is commonly used for patients who require IV administration for acute agitation, or who are unable to tolerate enteral medications; it is, however, neither approved by the US Food and Drug Administration (FDA) for the treatment of delirium at any age nor approved for IV use. However, the IV route results in more reliable absorption and decreased incidence of extrapyramidal reactions as compared to enteral administration, with minimal effects on blood pressure, respiration, and heart rate.[107,108] Of note, the intravenous dose (e.g., 5 mg) is twice as potent as oral administration (2.5 mg). This high-potency agent may be preferred to low-potency antipsychotics because of the decreased likelihood of hypotensive and anticholinergic effects, and it has been found to be safe and effective in managing cases of pediatric delirium.[109] At end of life, subcutaneous administration is also a convenient option. The primary mechanism of haloperidol's action is inhibition of dopaminergic pathways that may be overstimulated in states of hyperactive delirium, thus helping restore normal thought patterns and sensorium. The cautious use of haloperidol is recommended in patients with hypoactive delirium who may already have dopaminergic suppression and consequently its use may exacerbate symptoms of delirium.[43] A double-blinded, randomized control trial comparing haloperidol, chlorpromazine, and lorazepam for the treatment of delirium reported both haloperidol and chlorpromazine as effective in improving symptoms of delirium and cognitive function, while lorazepam was not only ineffective but also worsened symptoms in some patients.[110]

All antipsychotics have side effects, and patients must be closely monitored. Serious adverse reactions requiring immediate medical attention include malignant hyperthermia; extrapyramidal movement disorders, including laryngeal spasm; hypotension; glucose and lipid dysregulation; anticholinergic effects, such as constipation, urinary retention, and dry mouth; and cardiac effects such as QTc prolongation and torsades de pointes, need to be monitored. ECG monitoring is strongly recommended for those on IV haloperidol. Significant complications such as dystonia, hypotension, and hyperpyrexia were reported in more than 20% of pediatric burn patients treated with haloperidol.[111]

SECOND-GENERATION ANTIPSYCHOTIC AGENTS

Atypical antipsychotic agents, including risperidone, quetiapine, and olanzapine, are increasingly being used instead of haloperidol for the management of delirium in the ICU.[105,112] Case reports and single-center retrospective case series have described the utility of second-generation antipsychotics for management of delirium.[113–115] Data supporting the safety of quetiapine and olanzapine have been established in pediatric delirium.[115,116] Although there have been few efficacy studies directly comparing the second-generation antipsychotic agents and haloperidol, there may be some benefits in terms of the second-generation antipsychotic side-effect profile.[117,118] A review on the topic concluded that second-generation antipsychotics are effective in treating delirium and have fewer side effects compared with high-dose haloperidol. Most second-generation antipsychotics act on both dopaminergic and serotonergic receptors. In the case of hypoactive or mixed delirium, second-generation antipsychotics may be indicated because their mechanisms of action extend beyond dopamine blockade and affect other pathways likely implicated in the pathophysiology of delirium.[26] Disadvantages of second-generation antipsychotic agents include the lack of IV formulations. Although most of these agents must be given orally, some, such as risperidone and olanzapine, have sublingual formulations (see Table 20.4).

Controlled studies for delirium in the pediatric population, comparing both classes of antipsychotics for efficacy and safety, have yet to be undertaken. Of note, all of the antipsychotics are employed off-label when used to treat delirium. The second-generation antipsychotics have been tested in children, with approval, for other indications. For example, risperidone has been approved for use in children ages 5–16 for management of aggressive behavior related to autism. Olanzapine is indicated for the treatment of schizophrenia and manic or mixed episodes of bipolar disorder in 13- to 17-year-olds. These medications can be safely used at low doses in young children with appropriate monitoring when treating delirium.[119]

DEXMEDETOMIDINE

Dexmedetomidine, a centrally acting alpha-2 adrenergic agonist, has shown some promise in preventing and managing delirium in the ICU, particularly when sedation is indicated for facilitating care such as mechanical ventilation. Studies in adult patients have shown a reduction in the incidence of delirium in patients receiving dexmedetomidine versus benzodiazepines.[120] Nocturnal dexmedetomidine may also contribute to reduction in incidence of delirium.[121] It is difficult to determine whether the benefits associated with dexmedetomidine are direct or due to avoidance or minimization of other sedative agents. Last, dexmedetomidine has also been compared to haloperidol or used in cases of haloperidol-refractory delirium.[122,123] There is a paucity of data in the pediatric critical care population directly comparing rates of delirium with dexmedetomidine versus alternative sedative agents.

BENZODIAZEPINES

Benzodiazepines, such as lorazepam and diazepam, are GABA agonists that treat distress related to anxiety and sleep–wake cycle disturbance in delirious patients. They have amnesic properties and consequently can worsen cognitive impairment. There are also reports of paradoxical effects, such as aggression, violence, and irritability in pediatric patients.[124] In general, there appears to be some consensus that benzodiazepines should not be used as first-line agents in the treatment of pediatric delirium. In addition, a longer duration of benzodiazepines and opioid use in critically ill children was associated with increased reports of delusional memory, which is associated with greater risk for post-traumatic stress disorder (PTSD).[125] Benzodiazepines have been linked as an independent risk factor for development and duration of delirium in a dose-dependent manner.[126,127] In some cases when a benzodiazepine is required, lorazepam combined with haloperidol for severe agitation in older adolescent and adult patients has been beneficial.[117]

Figure 20.1 describes an algorithm that depicts the key factors and decision points salient to education, assessment, and treatment of delirium in the pediatric palliative care setting. Although this algorithm is not an evidenced-based protocol, it does suggest a paradigm for understanding delirium and its management.

PHARMACOLOGIC TREATMENT CHALLENGES

Treatment of a delirious pediatric patient with antipsychotic medications presents with some challenges. If catatonia is missed, introduction of an antipsychotic medication may worsen or complicate the clinical picture by contributing to neuroleptic malignant syndrome (NMS).[62] If there is the acute onset of pyrexia, autonomic dysfunction, muscle rigidity, an alteration in mental status, and/or other signs and symptoms consistent with NMS after introduction of an antipsychotic medication, the antipsychotic agent should be immediately discontinued and supportive measures should be implemented.

First- and second-generation antipsychotics share risks that require close monitoring. Possible side effects of all antipsychotic medications include prolongation of the QTc interval and increasing the risk of torsades de pointes and ventricular fibrillation; extrapyramidal side effects (EPS) of akathisia, dystonia, and tardive dyskinesia, the latter of which is irreversible; hypotension; metabolic side effects; and anticholinergic side effects including dry mouth, confusion, blurry vision, urinary retention, and constipation. The relative risks of each antipsychotic medication depend on receptor activity. For example, haloperidol, which has more significant D_2 receptor activity compared with olanzapine, bears a higher risk of EPS. Generally, as a group, the second-generation antipsychotics have less risk of EPS but increased risk of metabolic side effects. Haloperidol has been the most studied neuroleptic medication in the treatment of delirium. However, there is literature supporting the safety and efficacy of second-generation antipsychotics.[128] Furthermore, second-generation antipsychotics may be more effective than first-generation antipsychotics at targeting symptoms of hypoactive delirium, given their activity beyond the D_2 receptor and the involvement of serotonergic, cholinergic, and dopaminergic dysfunction in this specific subtype of delirium.[129]

Some antipsychotic medications are available in various formulations: liquid, sublingual or orally disintegrating, intramuscular (rarely indicated), or IV. In selecting which antipsychotic medication to select for delirium, knowledge of the limitations of each medication as well as the restrictions of the patient (e.g., if the patient is able to tolerate oral medication) can guide decision-making. End-of-life considerations should also factor into antipsychotic choice.

Parents may voice concerns over the short-term use of antipsychotic agents. They may express worry about adding on an additional medication to the polypharmacy in a critically ill pediatric patient. They may also question starting a medication with potential drug-drug interactions or serious side effects. Psychoeducation regarding when and why to treat delirium often requires an in-depth and compassionate discussion regarding goals of care, including risks of not treating, benefits of medication, possible side effects of treatment, and each aspect of informed consent.

Close monitoring of the QTc interval with an ECG, checking for motor abnormalities with a physical examination, documenting abnormal involuntary movements, screening for hypotension with vital sign checks, and monitoring for other possible side effects through close communication with nursing staff and caretakers further ensures safety and tolerability of antipsychotic medications in the setting of delirium. For patients who cannot safely tolerate antipsychotics due to concerns about their cardiac status, valproic acid has been shown in adult patients to be safe and efficacious although with not quite the same effect as antipsychotics.[130]

SEQUELAE OF DELIRIUM

Leonard and colleagues[8] have reviewed the many psychological and cognitive sequelae of delirium for inpatients, families, and caregivers of critically ill adults in the palliative care setting. Delirium has been associated with longer lengths of hospital stays, increased rates of morbidity and mortality, and other negative outcomes post-recovery.[131,132] It is now widely recognized that PTSD may follow episodes of delirium in adults in the hospital setting.[133–135] In pediatric patients, delirium has also been linked with increased lengths of stay and hospital costs and higher rates of morbidity and mortality, as well as cognitive impairment and psychological distress in both patients and caregivers.

LENGTH OF STAY

Several studies have demonstrated increased lengths of hospital stay in pediatric patients with delirium.[3,136,137] Pediatric patients with delirium have been shown to have a more than two times lengthier PICU admission and overall hospitalization outside of the ICU, even after controlling for confounding variables.[137,138] Given that longer lengths of ICU stay are a significant risk factor for traumatic responses in patients and their caregivers, measures to prevent delirium are essential to improve medical outcomes.[139,140]

ECONOMIC COSTS

The economic burden of pediatric delirium extends beyond the increased medical costs related to extended lengths of hospital stays. In adults, data show that yearly critical care spending surpasses $80 billion in the United States.[141] Annually, approximately more than $4 billion of healthcare costs are related to delirium.[142] Pediatric delirium has been linked to more serious underlying medical conditions, mechanical intervention, and longer hospitalizations, considerably adding to hospital expenses. In one particular study, a delirium diagnosis in a PICU correlated with a hospitalization cost surge of 85%.[143] Early detection of delirium not only facilitates timely intervention, but also is likely to shorten the duration of delirium, and result in cost savings.

MEDICAL OUTCOMES

Delirium in the critically ill pediatric population anticipates unfavorable medical results, similar to delirium in their adult counterparts.[138] Research has now demonstrated a convincing positive correlation between a history of delirium and in-hospital mortality for pediatric patients. Mirroring adult data, mortality rates of 20–26% have been found in cases of pediatric delirium.[138,144] This association may help identify patients who have a poor prognosis. Data on the neurocognitive impact of delirium on children are also emerging. Research has shown children who are critically ill to have visual and spatial memory disturbances and deficits in both executive function and attention in contrast to generally medically hospitalized pediatric patients.[145–147]

POSTTRAUMATIC STRESS DISORDER

The recognition of PTSD symptoms in medically ill patients, including those receiving treatment in ICUs, is now well-recognized. These symptoms include flashbacks, nightmares, avoidance, anger, and hypervigilance.[7] In children, 5–28% of patients discharged from a PICU meet criteria for PTSD 3 months after discharge, and up to 62% of patients had PTSD symptoms without experiencing full PTSD criteria.[146,148] Furthermore, research has found that up to 84% of parents of children in the PICU develop PTSD symptoms.[139]

More recently, studies examining the relationship between PTSD and the experience of delirium have emerged. These qualitative inquiries provide evidence that a great number of patients with mild to moderate delirium (43% of those with hypoactive delirium and 66% of patients with hyperactive features) recall their experience.[133] In sum, these studies suggest the importance of recognizing the potential negative effects of pediatric delirium on psychosocial functioning and mental health outcomes in both patients and their caregivers.[144] The following vignette describes the traumatic experience of delirium and its impact.

Clinical Vignette

Cassie, a 14-year-old girl with a history of asthma, was admitted for treatment of acute respiratory distress syndrome. After initial continuous nebulized albuterol treatments, she went into respiratory failure and was intubated and transferred to the ICU. She remained on the ventilator for 3 days before being extubated. Although Cassie improved medically, she became increasingly anxious, particularly when approached by nursing staff. She also had increased difficulty sleeping at night. At one point, she became combative and hit her nurse while she was attempting to administer an IV medication with a syringe.

Cassie received a psychiatry consultation and was noted to be confused and disoriented during her evaluation. Careful questioning elicited the history that Cassie believed that her nurse was attempting to kill her by injecting poison into her IV line. She also reported being afraid to fall asleep at night, believing that someone might come into her room at night to turn off her oxygen supply. Cassie was diagnosed with acute delirium and started on risperidone 0.5 mg b.i.d. She made a rapid recovery and was soon transferred to a general pediatric unit and then home.

Cassie was seen in follow-up a month after her discharge. A psychiatric consultation was requested again after her mother reported that Cassie was still having difficulties sleeping at night and had missed 13 of her last 17 regular school days. Cassie reported persistent distressing dreams as well as intrusive memories of her hospitalization, prompted by events such as watching television episodes of *ER* or visiting the hospital. She described conscious efforts to avoid things that reminded her of her experience. She tried to be outside as much as possible because being indoors gave her a boxed-in feeling that reminded her of the ICU. She was also reluctant to take her asthma medications and stated that she worried that they might be contaminated, even though she knew this to be impossible. In addition, she described a feeling of a foreshortened future and fear that she was likely to die at an early age because of asthma. Cassie was assessed as having symptoms of PTSD related to the traumatic medical experience during her inpatient hospitalization. Her symptoms persisted despite vigorous attempts by her parents to reassure her and were clearly interfering with her ability to function at school. She was referred to the local university child psychiatry clinic for further evaluation and treatment.

Adult and pediatric studies exploring the association between delirium and PTSD in intensive care patients have found that those with delusional memories have increased risk of developing PTSD symptoms compared with those with factual memories.[125,149] Because alterations in memory and perception are common presentations of delirium, children with delirium may be at greater risk of developing PTSD. Such sequelae should not be taken lightly because it can cause significant social impairment and can negatively impact academic performance.[150]

In cases of pediatric delirium, caregivers and clinicians should ask what they remember after the resolution of their symptoms. Some children do not recall the experience or report positive associations.[125] The specifics of delusions should not be overinterpreted (e.g., IV lines being perceived as snakes); rather, themes of fear, anxiety, loss, and mortality can be considered and explored. Further psychological support is recommended both for the patient and the family, if delirium has been distressing whether for themselves or for anyone else, including caregivers and staff.

Little research is available for clinical interventions for treating PTSD in palliative care patients; however, research on treatment of pediatric PTSD in other settings can be extrapolated. Interventions based on principles of trauma-focused cognitive-behavioral therapy (CBT) and, in specific cases, selective serotonin reuptake inhibitors have been found to be helpful for medically ill children PTSD symptoms.[1[illegible]]

IMPACT ON CAREGIVERS

Delirium affects not only patients but also family members and medical staff. For adult cancer patients, mean distress levels regarding delirium on a 4.0 scale were highest among their spouses (3.75), nurses (3.09), and then patients (3.02).[135] For families, hyperactive delirium and severe physical debilitation were the strongest predictors of distress in contrast to nurses who rated the severity of the delirium and perceptual disturbances more highly.[135] Interviews conducted with bereaved family members who witnessed delirium revealed they were often troubled by feelings of guilt and helplessness, struggled with making proxy decisions, and worried about the burden of care.[151] Families often equate signs of delirium with pain or discomfort, going crazy, and death anxiety.[15[illegible]] In addition, family members of patients with delirium reported both concerns about inadequate medical care as well as a desire for more information about the condition.[152]

These accounts by families likely reflect the challenge that medical staff face when caring for patients with delirium. Nurses commonly reported stress from increased workload, safety concerns for themselves and their patients, and difficulty finding a balance between connecting with the patient and being on guard.[153] Parents who have children hospitalized in intensive care are at increased risk of developing PTSD.[154] All caregivers, including parents, siblings, nurses, doctors, other clinicians, social workers, and clergy are at risk of psychological sequelae from traumatic experiences with critically ill patients.

Understanding traumatic stress in the medically ill population is an important intervention for both providers and families. There is broad consensus that treatment should be "trauma-informed." It is important for providers to understand traumatic stress and responses and incorporate this knowledge into their care practices when treating patients with delirium at the end of life. The toolkit created by the National Child Traumatic Stress Network (NCTSN), with support from the Substance Abuse and Mental Health Services Administration of the National Institute of Mental Health, can be useful to providers, patients, and parents in managing traumatic stress in the hospital setting. The toolkit includes an introduction to traumatic stress as it relates to children facing illness, injury, other medical events; practical tips and tools for healthcare providers; and handouts that can be given to parents that present evidence-based tips for helping their child cope. These materials are available free of charge from the NCTSN website, www.nctsnet.org.

FAMILY EXPERIENCES WITH DELIRIUM

As described earlier, delirium is often a stressful experience for families and caregivers. Schmitt et al.[155] identified three major themes that relate to a family's experience of delirium. *Symptom burden* refers to the caregiver's experience of distressing symptoms in their child, for example, disorientation or not recognizing a caregiver. *Emotional burden* refers to the impact delirium can have on a caregiver's emotional state. For a child at the end of their life, this can result in caregivers feeling that they have already lost their child ahead of their imminent death. Last, *situational burden* refers to concerns about the environment, for example, the patient engaging in self-harm behaviors or interfering with medical equipment and procedures.

We include a couple's perspective of delirium during their child's stay in the pediatric ICU (the name has been changed for privacy):

Clinical Vignette

Our 5-year-old son, Darren, went into septic shock from a viral infection which resulted in intubation for 2 weeks. He was heavily sedated to prevent him from moving. When he was finally extubated, we were excited to see him wake up. Unfortunately, when they woke him up and he was extubated, he had a frightening combination of opioid and benzodiazepine withdrawal resulting in delirium. We were seriously concerned that he had suffered some brain damage from his illness. He was awake but appeared to be hallucinating and had to be restrained as he was pulling at IVs. Normally Darren has an extensive vocabulary and is very chatty, but he was barely saying one or two words a day. He would seem to come in and out of awareness, sometimes recognizing familiar videos and shows on his iPad and watching them, but other times just looking off at the ceiling and moaning or screaming. It was devastating and scary to watch a 5-year-old in this state. We didn't know if he was in pain, or whether he was scared . . . we had no idea what was going on inside his head.

Unfortunately, he remained in this state for about 2 weeks. Each day he was slowly weaned off different drugs, and he would have slightly longer periods of attentiveness and give us the odd smile before wandering back off into space. We would leave the lights on during the day and tried to recreate his regular night-time routine. He started coming back to us and showing moments of his old self; he was still far from where he had been before he got sick. Each day we would wonder "Is this the new Darren? Is he still feeling sick? Did the virus damage his brain?"

Once at home, playing with other kids seemed to be his cure. Even though he was still on some of the opioids (he had a long wean schedule), within just a few more days Darren was right back to his old self again!

Partnering with families in the management of delirium can be therapeutic for both patients and families. If parents are distressed, this can heighten the stress in a child's environment and can cause delirium to intensify.[156] It is helpful for parents to help provide a consistent presence at bedside. Parents should be encouraged to talk to the patient and calmly reorient them without challenging delusions. They can be encouraged to ask simple questions. Familiar toys or comfort items at bedside can soothe the child. Parents should be encouraged to be with their child as much as possible. It is also important to recognize the impact of delirium on parents, which can lead to caregiver burnout. This added stress may affect the relationship between the parent and medical team as well as the parent's relationship with other members of the family. Parents should be educated about all aspects of delirium so they may be better able to manage their own expectations and in turn support their child.

CONCLUSION

Pediatric patients experiencing delirium constitute a high-risk population because of developmental vulnerabilities associated with their neurophysiology, challenges in assessment, and advancements in life-prolonging medical therapies. Delirium is associated with a number of indices of medical morbidity that include increased length of hospital stay and elevated rates of both morbidity and mortality.[157,158] In addition, research has shown associations with poor functional outcome, cognitive decline, and patient and family emotional distress in patients with delirium.[135,151,159] Research in adult intensive care patients has shown a threefold increase in mortality in patients diagnosed with delirium independent of other risk factors.[160] Similarly, studies in pediatric patients have reported mortality rates as high as 20%.[3] Because pediatric delirium is an often underdiagnosed and reversible complication of serious illness with significant negative impact, further research has the potential to improve patient care and outcome across all disciplines.

Many challenges await additional study. The diagnosis of delirium in children is based on DSM-5 criteria described for adult patients and may not be applicable to the pediatric population. Efforts to improve the prospective assessment of pediatric delirium may benefit from incorporating advancements in medical technology, including motion detectors, as well as expanded knowledge of motoric subtypes. Valid and reliable assessment tools that are age-appropriate and based on interdisciplinary agreed-upon diagnostic criteria are few. There are no evidence-based treatment guidelines existing for the management of pediatric delirium or for pediatric delirium in the palliative care setting. In addition, variations in the treatment of delirium based on differences in genetic predisposition, etiology, and pathophysiological disturbance demand further exploration. Finally, educational materials for clinicians and families about the risk factors and signs of delirium, as well as the potential for cognitive impairment and PTSD, are limited. Delirium should be recognized as a medical complication that spans many clinical domains and all age groups. In managing delirium, clinicians can capitalize on interdisciplinary collaboration and research with the goal of enhancing patient care, family support, and clinical outcomes.

REFERENCES

1. Smith HA, Fuchs DC, Pandharipande PP, Barr FE, Ely EW. Delirium: An emerging frontier in the management of critically ill children. *Crit Care Clin.* 2009;25(3):593–614.
2. Prugh DG, Wagonfeld S, Metcalf D, Jordan K. A clinical study of delirium in children and adolescents. *Psychosom Med.* 1980;42(1 Suppl):177–195.
3. Turkel SB, Tavaré CJ. Delirium in children and adolescents. *J Neuropsychiatry Clin Neurosci.* 2003;15(4):431–435.
4. Turkel SB, Trzepacz PT, Tavaré CJ. Comparing symptoms of delirium in adults and children. *Psychosomatics.* 2006;47(4):320–324.
5. Schieveld JN, Leroy PL, van Os J, Nicolai J, Vos GD, Leentjens AF. Pediatric delirium in critical illness: Phenomenology, clinical correlates and treatment response in 40 cases in the pediatric intensive care unit. *Intensive Care Med.* 2007;33(6):1033–1040.
6. Leentjens AF, Schieveld JN, Leonard M, Lousberg R, Verhey FR, Meagher DJ. A comparison of the phenomenology of pediatric, adult, and geriatric delirium. *J Psychosom Res.* 2008;64(2):219–223.
7. Nauck F, Alt-Epping B. Crises in palliative care: A comprehensive approach. *Lancet Oncol.* 2008 Nov;9(11):1086–1091.
8. Leonard M, Agar M, Mason C, Lawlor P. Delirium issues in palliative care settings. *J Psychosom Res.* 2008;65(3):289–298.
9. Breitbart W, Lawlor P. Delirium in the terminally ill. In Chochinov M, ed. *Oxford Handbook of Psychiatry in Palliative Care Medicine.* 2nd ed. Oxford University Press; 2012: 81–100.
10. Massie MJ, Holland J, Glass E. Delirium in terminally ill cancer patients. *Am J Psychiatry.* 1983;140(8):1048–1050.
11. Lawlor PG, Gagnon B, Mancini IL, et al. Occurrence, causes, and outcome of delirium in patients with advanced cancer: A prospective study. *Arch Intern Med.* 2000;160(6):786–794.
12. Schieveld JN, Janssen NJ. Delirium in the pediatric patient: On the growing awareness of its clinical interdisciplinary importance. *JAMA Pediatr.* 2014;168(7):595–596.
13. Hatherill S, Flisher AJ. Delirium in children and adolescents: A systematic review of the literature. *J Psychosom Res.* 2010;68(4):337–344.
14. Flaherty JH, Rudolph J, Shay K, et al. Delirium is a serious and underrecognized problem: Why assessment of mental status should be the sixth vital sign. *J Am Med Dir Assoc.* 2007;8(5):273–275.
15. Leentjens AF, Maclullich AM, Meagher DJ. Delirium, Cinderella no more. . . ? *J Psychosom Res.* 2008;65(3):205.
16. Institute of Medicine (US) Committee on Palliative and End-of-Life Care for Children and Their Families; Field MJ, Behrman RE, eds. *When Children Die: Improving Palliative and End-of-Life Care for Children and Their Families.* National Academies Press (US); 2003
17. Pretto M, Spirig R, Milisen K, Degeest S, Regazzoni P, Hasemann W. Effects of an interdisciplinary nurse-led Delirium Prevention and Management Program (DPMP) on nursing workload: A pilot study. *Int J Nurs Stud.* 2009;46(6):804–812.
18. American Psychiatric Association. *Diagnostic and Statistical Manual of Mental Disorders.* 5th ed. American Psychiatric Publishing 2013.
19. Wise MG, Trzepacz PT. Delirium (confusional states). In Rundell JR, Wise MG, eds. *Textbook of Consultation-Liaison Psychiatry.* American Psychiatric Press; 1996: 258–275.
20. Morandi A, Pandharipande P, Trabucchi M, et al. Understanding international differences in terminology for delirium and other types of acute brain dysfunction in critically ill patients. *Intensive Care Med.* 2008;34(10):1907–1915.
21. Girard TD, Pandharipande PP, Ely EW. Delirium in the intensive care unit. *Crit Care.* 2008;12 Suppl 3(Suppl 3):S3.
22. Przybylo HJ, Martini DR, Mazurek AJ, Bracey E, Johnsen L, Coté CJ. Assessing behaviour in children emerging from anaesthesia: Can we apply psychiatric diagnostic techniques? *Paediatr Anaesth.* 2003;13(7):609–616.
23. Gupta N, de Jonghe J, Schieveld J, Leonard M, Meagher D. Delirium phenomenology: What can we learn from the symptoms of delirium? *J Psychosom Res.* 2008;65(3):215–222.
24. Liptzin B, Levkoff SE. An empirical study of delirium subtypes. *Br J Psychiatry.* 1992;161:843–845.
25. Schieveld JN, van der Valk JA, Smeets I, et al. Diagnostic considerations regarding pediatric delirium: A review and a proposal for an algorithm for pediatric intensive care units. *Intensive Care Med.* 2009;35(11):1843–1849.
26. Karnik NS, Joshi SV, Paterno C, Shaw RJ. Subtypes of pediatric delirium: A treatment algorithm. *Psychosomatics.* 2007;48(3):253–257.
27. Gupta AK, Saravay SM, Trzepacz PT, Chiray P. Delirium motoric subtypes. *Psychosomatics.* 2005;46:158.
28. Sikich N, Lerman J. Development and psychometric evaluation of the pediatric anesthesia emergence delirium scale. *Anesthesiology.* 2004;100(5):1138–1145.
29. Morita T, Tei Y, Tsunoda J, Inoue S, Chihara S. Underlying pathologies and their associations with clinical features in terminal delirium of cancer patients. *J Pain Symptom Manage.* 2001;22(6):997–1006.
30. Lam PT, Tse CY, Lee CH. Delirium in a palliative care unit. *Prog Palliat Care.* 2003;11:126–133.
31. Spiller JA, Keen JC. Hypoactive delirium: Assessing the extent of the problem for inpatient specialist palliative care. *Palliat Med.* 2006;20(1):17–23.
32. Peterson JF, Pun BT, Dittus RS, et al. Delirium and its motoric subtypes: A study of 614 critically ill patients. *J Am Geriatr Soc.* 2006;54(3):479–484.
33. Kobayashi K, Takeuchi O, Suzuki M, Yamaguchi N. A retrospective study on delirium type. *Jpn J Psychiatry Neurol.* 1992;46(4):911–917.
34. Ross CA, Peyser CE, Shapiro I, Folstein MF. Delirium: Phenomenologic and etiologic subtypes. *Int Psychogeriatr.* 1991;3(2):135–147.
35. Meagher DJ, O'Hanlon D, O'Mahony E, Casey PR, Trzepacz PT. Relationship between symptoms and motoric subtype of delirium. *J Neuropsychiatry Clin Neurosci.* 2000;12(1):51–56.
36. Maldonado JR. Pathoetiological model of delirium: A comprehensive understanding of the neurobiology of delirium and an evidence-based approach to prevention and treatment. *Crit Care Clin.* 2008 Oct;24(4):789–856,ix.

37. O'Malley G, Leonard M, Meagher D, O'Keeffe ST. The delirium experience: A review. *J Psychosom Res.* 2008;65(3):223–228.
38. Godfrey A, Conway R, Leonard M, Meagher D, Olaighin G. A classification system for delirium subtyping with the use of a commercial mobility monitor. *Gait Posture.* 2009;30(2):245–252.
39. Practice guideline for the treatment of patients with delirium. American Psychiatric Association. *Am J Psychiatry.* 1999;156(5 Suppl):1–20.
40. van der Mast RC. Pathophysiology of delirium. *J Geriatr Psychiatry Neurol.* 1998;11(3):138–158.
41. Maldonado JR. Delirium in the acute care setting: Characteristics, diagnosis and treatment. *Crit Care Clin.* 2008;24(4):657–vii.
42. Rummans TA, Evans JM, Krahn LE, Fleming KC. Delirium in elderly patients: Evaluation and management. *Mayo Clin Proc.* 1995;70(10):989–998.
43. Jacobson S, Jerrier H. EEG in delirium. *Semin Clin Neuropsychiatry.* 2000;5(2):86–92.
44. Rudolph JL, Ramlawi B, Kuchel GA, et al. Chemokines are associated with delirium after cardiac surgery. *J Gerontol A Biol Sci Med Sci.* 2008;63(2):184–189.
45. Dunlop RJ, Campbell CW. Cytokines and advanced cancer. *J Pain Symptom Manage.* 2000;20(3):214–232.
46. Fukumoto Y, Okumura A, Hayakawa F, et al. Serum levels of cytokines and EEG findings in children with influenza associated with mild neurological complications. *Brain Dev.* 2007;29(7):425–430.
47. Eikelenboom P, Hoogendijk WJ, Jonker C, van Tilburg W. Immunological mechanisms and the spectrum of psychiatric syndromes in Alzheimer's disease. *J Psychiatr Res.* 2002;36(5):269–280.
48. Gaudreau JD, Gagnon P, Harel F, Tremblay A, Roy MA. Fast, systematic, and continuous delirium assessment in hospitalized patients: The nursing delirium screening scale. *J Pain Symptom Manage.* 2005;29(4):368–375.
49. Folstein MF, Folstein SE, McHugh PR. "Mini-mental state". A practical method for grading the cognitive state of patients for the clinician. *J Psychiatr Res.* 1975;12(3):189–198.
50. Inouye SK, van Dyck CH, Alessi CA, Balkin S, Siegal AP Horwitz RI. Clarifying confusion: The confusion assessment method. A new method for detection of delirium. *Ann Intern Med.* 1990;113(12):941–948.
51. Ely EW, Margolin R, Francis J, et al. Evaluation of delirium in critically ill patients: Validation of the Confusion Assessment Method for the Intensive Care Unit (CAM-ICU). *Crit Care Med.* 2001;29(7):1370–1379.
52. Trzepacz PT, Mittal D, Torres R, Kanary K, Norton J, Jimerson N. Validation of the Delirium Rating Scale-revised-98: Comparison with the delirium rating scale and the cognitive test for delirium [published correction appears in J Neuropsychiatry Clin Neurosci 2001 Summer;13(3):433]. *J Neuropsychiatry Clin Neurosci.* 2001;13(2):229–242.
53. Turkel SB, Braslow K, Tavaré CJ, Trzepacz PT. The delirium rating scale in children and adolescents. *Psychosomatics.* 2003;44(2):126–129.
54. Smith HA, Boyd J, Fuchs DC, et al. Diagnosing delirium in critically ill children: Validity and reliability of the Pediatric Confusion Assessment Method for the intensive care unit. *Crit Care Med.* 2011;39(1):150–157.
55. Sessler CN, Gosnell MS, Grap MJ, et al. The Richmond Agitation-Sedation Scale: Validity and reliability in adult intensive care unit patients. *Am J Respir Crit Care Med.* 2002;166(10):1338–1344.
56. Smith HA, Gangopadhyay M, Goben CM, et al. The Preschool Confusion Assessment Method for the ICU: Valid and reliable delirium monitoring for critically ill infants and children. *Crit Care Med* 2016;44(3):592–600.
57. Silver G, Kearney J, Traube C, Hertzig M. Delirium screening anchored in child development: The Cornell Assessment for Pediatric Delirium. *Palliat Support Care.* 2015;13(4):1005–1011.
58. Shann F, Pearson G, Slater A, Wilkinson K. Paediatric index of mortality (PIM): A mortality prediction model for children in intensive care. *Intensive Care Med.* 1997;23(2):201–207.
59. Pollack MM, Ruttimann UE, Getson PR. Pediatric risk of mortality (PRISM) score. *Crit Care Med.* 1988;16(11):1110–1116.
60. Schieveld JN, Leusberg R, Berghmans E, et al. Pediatric illness severity measures predict delirium in a pediatric intensive care unit. *Crit Care Med.* 2008;36(6):1933–1936.
61. Grover S, Ghosh A, Ghormode D. Do patients of delirium have catatonic features? An exploratory study. *Psychiatry Clin Neurosci.* 2014;68(8):644–651.
62. Wilson JE, Carlson R, Duggan MC, et al. Delirium and catatonia in critically ill patients: The delirium and catatonia prospective cohort investigation. *Crit Care Med.* 2017;45(11):1837–1844.
63. Wing L, Shah A. Catatonia in autistic spectrum disorders. *Br J Psychiatry.* 2000;176:357–362.
64. Dhossche DM, Wachtel LE. Catatonia is hidden in plain sight among different pediatric disorders: A review article. *Pediatr Neurol.* 2010;43(5):307–315.
65. van der Heijden FM, Tuinier S, Arts NJM, Hoogendoorn MLC, Kahn RS, Verhoeven WMA. Catatonia: Disappeared or under-diagnosed? *Psychopathology.* 2005;38:3–8
66. Esseveld MM, Leroy PLMN, Leue C. et al. *Intensive Care Med.* 2013;39:528.
67. Shehabi Y, Botha JA, Boyle MS, et al. Sedation and delirium in the intensive care unit: An Australian and New Zealand perspective. *Anaesth Intens Care* 2008;36(4):570–578.
68. Van Eijk MM, Kesecioglu J, Slooter AJ: Intensive care delirium monitoring and standardised treatment: A complete survey of Dutch intensive care units. *Intensive and Critical Care Nursing.* 2008;24(4):218–221.
69. Mac Sweeney R, Barber V, Page V, et al. A national survey of the management of delirium in UK intensive care units. *QJM.* 2010;103(4):243–251.
70. Patel RP, Gambrell M, Speroff T, et al. Delirium and sedation in the intensive care unit: Survey of behaviors and attitudes of 1384 healthcare professionals. *Crit Care Med.* 2009;37(3):825–832.
71. Mistarz R, Eliott S, Whitfield A, Ernest D. Bedside nurse-patient interactions do not reliably detect delirium: An observational study. *Aust Crit Care.* 2011;24(2):126–132.
72. Kudchadkar SR, Yaster M, Punjabi NM. Sedation, sleep promotion, and delirium screening practices in the care of mechanically ventilated children: A wake-up call for the pediatric critical care community. *Crit Care Med.* 2014;42(7):1592–1600.
73. Simone S, Edwards S, Lardieri A, et al. Implementation of an ICU bundle: An interprofessional quality improvement project to enhance delirium management and monitor delirium prevalence in a single PICU. *Pediatr Crit Care Med.* 2017;18(6):531–540.
74. Traube C, Silver G, Kearney J, et al. Cornell Assessment of Pediatric Delirium: A valid, rapid, observational tool for screening delirium in the PICU. *Crit Care Med.* 2014;42(3):656–663.
75. van den Boogaard M, Pickkers P, van der Hoeven H, Roodbol G, van Achterberg T, Schoonhoven L. Implementation of a delirium assessment tool in the ICU can influence haloperidol use. *Crit Care.* 2009;13(4):R131.
76. Alvarez RV, Palmer C, Czaja AS, et al. Delirium is a common and early finding in patients in the pediatric cardiac intensive care unit. *J Pediatr.* 2018;195:206–212.
77. Barr J, Fraser GL, Puntillo K, et al. Clinical practice guidelines for the management of pain, agitation, and delirium in adult patients in the intensive care unit. *Crit Care Med.* 2013;41(1):263–306.
78. Ely EW, Pandharipande PP. The evolving approach to brain dysfunction in critically ill patients. *JAMA.* 2016;315(14):1455–1456.
79. Ely EW, Inouye SK, Bernard GR, et al. Delirium in mechanically ventilated patients: Validity and reliability of the confusion assessment method for the intensive care unit (CAM-ICU). *JAMA.* 2001;286(21):2703–2710.

80. Ely EW, Margolin R, Francis J, et al. Evaluation of delirium in critically ill patients: Validation of the Confusion Assessment Method for the Intensive Care Unit (CAM-ICU). *Crit Care Med.* 2001;29(7):1370–1379.
81. Ely EW, Siegel MD, Inouye SK. Delirium in the intensive care unit: An under-recognized syndrome of organ dysfunction. *Semin Respir Crit Care Med.* 2001;22(2):115–126.
82. Ely EW, Shintani A, Truman B, et al. Delirium as a predictor of mortality in mechanically ventilated patients in the intensive care unit. *JAMA.* 2004;291(14):1753–1762.
83. Brummel NE, Vasilevskis EE, Han JH, Boehm L, Pun BT, Ely EW. Implementing delirium screening in the ICU: Secrets to success. *Crit Care Med.* 2013;41(9):2196–2208.
84. Immers HE, Schuurmans MJ, van de Bijl JJ. Recognition of delirium in ICU patients: A diagnostic study of the NEECHAM confusion scale in ICU patients. *BMC Nurs.* 2005;4:7.
85. Devlin JW, Skrobik Y, Gélinas C, et al. Clinical practice guidelines for the prevention and management of pain, agitation/sedation, delirium, immobility, and sleep disruption in adult patients in the ICU. *Crit Care Med.* 2018;46(9):e825–e873.
86. Silver GH, Kearney JA, Bora S, et al. A clinical pathway to standardize care of children with delirium in pediatric inpatient settings. *Hosp Pediatr.* 2019;9(11):909–916.
87. Silver G, Traube C, Gerber LM, Sun X, Kearney J, Patel A, Greenwald B. Pediatric delirium and associated risk factors: A single-center prospective observational study. *Pediatr Crit Care Med.* 2015;16(4):303–309.
88. Traube C, Silver G, Reeder RW, et al. Delirium in critically ill children: An international point prevalence study. *Crit Care Med.* 2017;45(4):584–590.
89. Naja M, Zmudka J, Hannat S, et al. In geriatric patients, delirium symptoms are related to the anticholinergic burden. *Geriatr Gerontol Int.* 2016;16:424–431.
90. Madden K, Hussain K, Tasker RC. Anticholinergic medication burden in pediatric prolonged critical illness: A potentially modifiable risk factor for delirium. *Pediatr Crit Care Med.* 2018;19(10):917–924.
91. Pandharipande P, Shintani A, Peterson J, Pun BT, Wilkinson GR, Dittus RS, Bernard GR, Ely EW Lorazepam is an independent risk factor for transitioning to delirium in intensive care unit patients. *Anesthesiology.* 2006;104:21–26.
92. Smith HAB, Gangopadhyay M, Goben CM, et al. Delirium and benzodiazepines associated with prolonged ICU stay in critically ill infants and young children. *Crit Care Med.* 2017;45:1427–1435.
93. Schreiber MP, Colantuoni E, Bienvenu OJ, et al. Corticosteroids and transition to delirium in patients with acute lung injury. *Crit Care Med.* 2014;42(6):1480–1486.
94. van den Boogaard M, Pickkers P, Slooter AJ, et al. Development and validation of PRE-DELIRIC (PREdiction of DELIRium in ICu patients) delirium prediction model for intensive care patients: Observational multicentre study. *BMJ.* 2012;344:e420.
95. Marra A, Ely EW, Pandharipande PP, Patel MB. The ABCDEF bundle in critical care. *Crit Care Clin.* 2017;33(2):225–243.
96. Ely EW. The ABCDEF bundle: Science and philosophy of how ICU liberation serves patients and families. *Crit Care Med.* 2017;45(2): 321–330.
97. Balas MC, Vasilevskis EE, Burke WJ, et al. Critical care nurses' role in implementing the "ABCDE bundle" into practice. *Crit Care Nurse.* 2012;32(2):35–48.
98. Balas MC, Vasilevskis EE, Olsen KM, et al. Effectiveness and safety of the awakening and breathing coordination, delirium monitoring/management, and early exercise/mobility bundle. *Crit Care Med.* 2014;42(5):1024–1036.
99. Frimpong K, Stollings JL, Carlo ME, Ely EW. ICU delirium viewed through the lens of the PAD guidelines and the ABCDEF implementation bundle. In Balas M, Clemmer T, Hargett K, eds. *ICU Liberation: The Power of Pain Control, Minimal Sedation, and Early Mobility.* Society of Critical Care Medicine; 2015.
100. Simone S, Edwards S, Lardieri A, et al. Implementation of an ICU bundle. *Pediatric Critical Care Medicine.* 2017;18(6):531–540.
101. Al-Aama T, Brymer C, Gutmanis I, Woolmore-Goodwin SM, Esbaugh J, Dasgupta M. Melatonin decreases delirium in elderly patients: A randomized, placebo-controlled trial. *Int J Geriatr Psychiatry.* 2010;26(7):687–694.
102. Baumgartner L, Lam K, Lai J, et al. Effectiveness of melatonin for the prevention of intensive care unit delirium. *Pharmacotherapy.* 2019;39(3):280–287.
103. Bain ZN, MacLaren JE, Herrmann L, Mayes L, Rosenbaum A. Preoperative melatonin and its effects on induction and emergence in children undergoing anesthesia and surgery. *Surv Anesthesiol.* 2010;54(3):126–127.
104. Esposito S, Laino D, D'Alonzo R, et al. Pediatric sleep disturbances and treatment with melatonin. *J Translat Med.* 2019;17(1):77.
105. Staveski SL, Pickler RH, Lin L, et al. Management of pediatric delirium in pediatric cardiac intensive care patients. *Pediatr Criti Care Med.* 2018;19(6):538–543.
106. Ely EW, Stephens RK, Jackson JC, et al. Current opinions regarding the importance, diagnosis, and management of delirium in the intensive care unit: A survey of 912 healthcare professionals. *Crit Care Med.* 2004;32(1):106–112.
107. Beliles KE. Alternative routes of administration of psychotropic medications. In Stoudemire A, ed. *Psychiatric Care of the Medical Patient.* 2nd ed. Oxford University Press; 2000: 395–405.
108. Menza MA, Murray GB, Holmes VF, Rafuls WA. Decreased extrapyramidal symptoms with intravenous haloperidol. *J Clin Psychiatry.* 1987;48(7):278–280.
109. Brown RL, Henke A, Greenhalgh DG, Warden GD. The use of haloperidol in the agitated, critically ill pediatric patient with burns. *J Burn Care Rehabil.* 1996;17(1):34–38.
110. Breitbart W, Marotta R, Platt MM, et al. A double-blind trial of haloperidol, chlorpromazine, and lorazepam in the treatment of delirium in hospitalized AIDS patients. *Am J Psychiatry.* 1996;153(2):231–237.
111. Ratcliff SL, Meyer WJ 3rd, Cuervo LJ, Villarreal C, Thomas CR, Herndon DN. The use of haloperidol and associated complications in the agitated, acutely ill pediatric burn patient. *J Burn Care Rehabil.* 2004;25(6):472–478.
112. Turkel SB, Hanft A. The pharmacologic management of delirium in children and adolescents. *Pediatric Drugs.* 2014;16(4):267–274.
113. Schieveld JNM, Leroy PLJM, Os JV, Nicolai J, Vos GD, Leentjens AFG. Pediatric delirium in critical illness: Phenomenology, clinical correlates and treatment response in 40 cases in the pediatric intensive care unit. *Intensive Care Med.* 2007;33(6):1033–1040.
114. Brahmbhatt K, Whitgob E. Diagnosis and management of delirium in critically ill infants: Case report and review. *Pediatrics.* 2016;137(3). doi:10.1542/peds.2015-1940.
115. Khan SS, Mican LM. A naturalistic evaluation of intramuscular ziprasidone versus intramuscular olanzapine for the management of acute agitation and aggression in children and adolescents. *J Child Adolesc Psychopharmacol.* 2006;16(6):671–677.
116. Joyce C, Witcher R, Herrup E, et al. Evaluation of the safety of quetiapine in treating delirium in critically ill children: A retrospective review. *J Child Adolesc Psychopharmacol.* 2015;25(9): 666–670.
117. Breitbart W, Alici Y. Agitation and delirium at the end of life: "We couldn't manage him." *JAMA.* 2008;300(24):2898–E1.
118. Liu CY, Juang YY, Liang HY, Lin NC, Yeh EK. Efficacy of risperidone in treating the hyperactive symptoms of delirium. *Int Clin Psychopharmacol.* 2004;19(3):165–168.
119. Turkel SB. Delirium. In Shaw RJ, DeMaso DR, eds. *Textbook of Pediatric Psychosomatic Medicine.* American Psychiatric Publishing; 2010: 63–75.
120. Pandharipande PP, Pun BT, Herr DL, et al. Effect of sedation with dexmedetomidine vs lorazepam on acute brain dysfunction in mechanically ventilated patients: The MENDS randomized controlled trial. *JAMA.* 2007;298(22):2644–2653.

121. Skrobik Y, Duprey MS, Hill NS, Devlin JW. Low-dose nocturnal dexmedetomidine prevents ICU delirium: A randomized, placebo-controlled trial. *Am J Respir Crit Care Med.* 2018;197(9):1147–1156.
122. Reade MC, Eastwood GM, Bellomo R, et al. Effect of dexmedetomidine added to standard care on ventilator-free time in patients with agitated delirium: A randomized clinical trial [published correction appears in JAMA. 2016;316(7):775]. *JAMA.* 2016;315(14):1460–1468.
123. Carrasco G, Baeza N, Cabré L, et al. Dexmedetomidine for the treatment of hyperactive delirium refractory to haloperidol in nonintubated ICU patients. *Crit Care Med.* 2016;44(7):1295–1306. doi:10.1097/ccm.0000000000001622.
124. Saïas T, Gallarda T. Paradoxical aggressive reactions to benzodiazepine use: A review. *Encephale.* 2008;34(4):330–336.
125. Colville G, Kerry S, Pierce C. Children's factual and delusional memories of intensive care. *Am J Respir Crit Care Med.* 2008;177(9):976–982.
126. Mody K, Kaur S, Mauer EA, et al. Benzodiazepines and Development of Delirium in Critically Ill Children. *Crit Care Med.* 2018;46(9):1486–1491.
127. Smith HAB, Gangopadhyay M, Goben CM, et al. Delirium and benzodiazepines associated with prolonged ICU stay in critically ill infants and young children. *Crit Care Med.* 2017;45(9):1427–1435.
128. Turkel SB, Jacobson J, Munzig E, Tavare CJ. Atypical antipsychotic medications to control symptoms of delirium in children and adolescents. *J Child Adolesc Psychopharmacol.* 2012;22(2):126–130.
129. Karnik NS, Joshi SV, Paterno C, Shaw R: Subtypes of pediatric delirium: A treatment algorithm. *Psychosomatics.* 2007;48(3):253–257.
130. Crowley KE, Urben L, Hacobian G, Geiger KL. Valproic acid for the management of agitation and delirium in the intensive care setting: A retrospective analysis. *Clin Ther.* 2020;42(4):e65–e73.
131. Levkoff SE, Evans DA, Liptzin B, et al. Delirium: The occurrence and persistence of symptoms among elderly hospitalized patients. *Arch Intern Med.* 1992;152(2):334–340.
132. Newman MF, Grocott HP, Mathew JP, et al. Report of the substudy assessing the impact of neurocognitive function on quality of life 5 years after cardiac surgery. *Stroke.* 2001;32(12):2874–2881.
133. DiMartini A, Dew MA, Kormos R, McCurry K, Fontes P. Posttraumatic stress disorder caused by hallucinations and delusions experienced in delirium. *Psychosomatics.* 2007;48(5):436–439.
134. Dew MA, Kormos RL, DiMartini AF, et al. Prevalence and risk of depression and anxiety-related disorders during the first three years after heart transplantation. *Psychosomatics.* 2001;42(4):300–313.
135. Breitbart W, Gibson C, Tremblay A. The delirium experience: Delirium recall and delirium-related distress in hospitalized patients with cancer, their spouses/caregivers, and their nurses. *Psychosomatics.* 2002;43(3):183–194.
136. Thom RP. Pediatric delirium. *Am J Psychiatry Resid J.* 2017:6–8.
137. Smeets IA, Tan EY, Vossen HG, et al. Prolonged stay at the paediatric intensive care unit associated with paediatric delirium. *Eur Child Adolesc Psychiatry.* 2010;19(4):389–393.
138. Traube C, Silver G, Gerber LM, et al. Delirium and mortality in critically ill children: Epidemiology and outcomes of pediatric delirium. *Crit Care Med.* 2017;45(5):891–898.
139. Nelson LP, Gold JI. Posttraumatic stress disorder in children and their parents following admission to the pediatric intensive care unit: A review. *Pediatr Crit Care Med.* 2012;13(3):338–347.
140. Stuber ML, Shemesh E. Post-traumatic stress response to life-threatening illnesses in children and their parents. *Child Adolesc Psychiatr Clin N Am.* 2006;15(3):597–609.
141. Chang B, Lorenzo J, Macario A. Examining health care costs: Opportunities to provide value in the intensive care unit. *Anesthesiol Clin.* 2015;33(4):753–770.
142. Barr J, Fraser GL, Puntillo K, et al. Clinical practice guidelines for the management of pain, agitation, and delirium in adult patients in the intensive care unit. *Crit Care Med.* 2013;41(1):263–306.
143. Traube C, Mauer EA, Gerber LM, et al. Cost associated with pediatric delirium in the ICU. *Crit Care Med.* 2016;44(12):e1175–e1179.
144. Malas N, Brahmbhatt K, McDermott C, Smith A, Ortiz-Aguayo R, Turkel S. Pediatric delirium: Evaluation, management, and special considerations. *Curr Psychiatry Rep.* 2017;19(9):65.
145. Jones SM, Fiser DH, Livingston RL. Behavioral changes in pediatric intensive care units. *Am J Dis Child.* 1992;146(3):375–379.
146. Turkel SB. Pediatric delirium: Recognition, management, and outcome. *Curr Psychiatry Rep.* 2017;19(12):101.
147. Als LC, Nadel S, Cooper M, Pierce CM, Sahakian BJ, Garralda ME. Neuropsychologic function three to six months following admission to the PICU with meningoencephalitis, sepsis, and other disorders: A prospective study of school-aged children. *Crit Care Med.* 2013;41(4):1094–1103.
148. van den Boogaard M, Schoonhoven L, Evers AW, van der Hoeven JG, van Achterberg T, Pickkers P. Delirium in critically ill patients: Impact on long-term health-related quality of life and cognitive functioning. *Crit Care Med.* 2012;40(1):112–118.
149. Jones C, Griffiths RD, Humphris G, Skirrow PM. Memory, delusions, and the development of acute posttraumatic stress disorder-related symptoms after intensive care. *Crit Care Med.* 2001;29(3):573–580.
150. Yasik AE, Saigh PA, Oberfield RA, Halamandaris PV. Posttraumatic stress disorder: Memory and learning performance in children and adolescents. *Biol Psychiatry.* 2007;61(3):382–388.
151. Morita T, Akechi T, Ikenaga M, et al. Terminal delirium: Recommendations from bereaved families' experiences. *J Pain Symptom Manage.* 2007;34(6):579–589.
152. Namba M, Morita T, Imura C, Kiyohara E, Ishikawa S, Hirai K. Terminal delirium: Families' experience. *Palliat Med.* 2007;21(7):587–594.
153. Lou MF, Dai YT. Nurses' experience of caring for delirious patients. *J Nurs Res.* 2002;10(4):279–290.
154. Balluffi A, Kassam-Adams N, Kazak A, Tucker M, Dominguez T, Helfaer M. Traumatic stress in parents of children admitted to the pediatric intensive care unit. *Pediatr Crit Care Med.* 2004;5(6):547–553.
155. Schmitt EM, Gallagher J, Albuquerque A, et al. Perspectives on the delirium experience and its burden: Common themes among older patients, their family caregivers, and nurses. *Gerontologist.* 2019;59(2):327–337.
156. Schieveld JNM, Ista E, Knoester H, Molag ML. Pediatric delirium: A practical approach. In Rey JM, ed. *IACAPAP e-Textbook of Child and Adolescent Mental Health.* International Association for Child and Adolescent Psychiatry and Allied Professions; 2015: 1–17.
157. Inouye SK, Rushing JT, Foreman MD, Palmer RM, Pompei P. Does delirium contribute to poor hospital outcomes? A three-site epidemiologic study. *J Gen Intern Med.* 1998;13(4):234–242.
158. McCusker J, Cole M, Abrahamowicz M, Primeau F, Belzile E. Delirium predicts 12-month mortality. *Arch Intern Med.* 2002;162(4):457–463.
159. Trzepacz PT, Meagher DJ. In Levenson JL, ed. *Textbook of Psychosomatic Medicine.* American Psychiatric Publishing; 2005: 91–130.
160. Ely EW, Shintani A, Truman B, et al. Delirium as a predictor of mortality in mechanically ventilated patients in the intensive care unit. *JAMA.* 2004;291(14):1753–1762.

ADDITIONAL READING

Kishk OA, Simone S, Lardieri AB, Graciano AL, Tumulty J, Edwards S. Antipsychotic treatment of delirium in critically ill children: A retrospective matched cohort study. *J Pediatr Pharmacol Therap.* 2019;24(3):204–213. doi:10.5863/1551-6776-24.3.204.

21 | FATIGUE

CHRISTINA ULLRICH, SHANA JACOBS, AND PAMELA S. HINDS

An 11-year-old boy with osteosarcoma defined fatigue as "being tired, not being able to do much, feeling sleepy, and feeling mentally tired but you can't go to sleep."

A 10-year-old girl with Burkitt lymphoma defined fatigue as "feeling so tired that you can't even keep your head up."

A 14-year-old girl with rhabdomyosarcoma said fatigue is when "you sleep a lot but still feel tired, heavy eyelids."

When asked to describe how her body feels, a 12-year-old girl with acute lymphocytic leukemia said, "my body feels tired and sometimes sad and sometimes in a bad mood like I don't want to get up sometimes."

Vignette

Dave is a 19-year-old man with a rare immunodeficiency that was diagnosed when he was 2 years old. As an adolescent, he developed chronic hepatitis as well as pulmonary complications, for which he received a liver transplant. At the age of 18, he underwent a bone marrow transplant with the goal of curing his immunodeficiency. He has been working to recover from his bone marrow transplant and is currently working part-time. He hopes to attend college in the near future.

David began to experience bothersome fatigue prior to his liver transplant. He continues to contend with it, even as he approaches the 2-year mark after his bone marrow transplant. He described his fatigue as follows:

> Fatigue is very hard to describe and it's not easy, it's not necessarily a feeling that you can control nor can you expect. It's kind of like having your engine running on low fuel, you feel sluggish tired and irritated.
>
> There's really nothing but time that can help fatigue. It's not something that just goes away when you want it to. But trying to actually move around and get some fresh air or going for a walk in the sun or just doing an activity that you might enjoy can help.
>
> Advice I would give to someone with serious illness and fatigue. . . . It'll pass, you won't realize it but you're gonna get better with time and you'll eventually forget about it and start moving on with your life. It'll take a while but you'll realize that there are so many things we take for granted. Once you start doing those things again you'll appreciate not being too tired to do 'em.

INTRODUCTION

Children with life-threatening illness commonly experience fatigue, a unique experience that is complex in its origins and multidimensional in its presentation. The National Comprehensive Cancer Network defines cancer-related fatigue as "a distressing, persistent, subjective sense of physical, emotional and/or cognitive tiredness or exhaustion related to cancer or cancer treatment that is not proportional to recent activity and interferes with usual functioning."[1] Distinct from the "everyday fatigue" experienced by health individuals, fatigue experienced by children with serious illness is generally more severe; it is also persistent and can be unrelated to an energy imbalance (i.e., lack of rest). Other distinguishing features are its interference with function and distressing nature. For children with life-threatening illness, fatigue results in physical, social, and psychological consequences. It can exacerbate other symptoms, impair well-being and quality of life, and impede participation in meaningful activities, detracting from a child's hope, sense of self, and connection to others. Child fatigue may also be detrimental to the well-being of parents. In the adult realm, *patient* fatigue is also associated with fewer caregiver work and social activities and greater caregiver strain.[2]

For these reasons, palliative care and other clinicians should routinely monitor for the presence of fatigue and intervene when needed. By monitoring routinely, clinicians legitimate the existence of what can be a baffling symptom to the affected child and the ill child's parents. While there is a belief that little can be done for this distressing symptom, evidence supporting interventions to mitigate fatigue is emerging. Often, just preparing patients and families for the experience of fatigue and validating the experience can provide benefit.

During the final stages of life, a child's body slows, and the child may withdraw from family and friends. These changes may provide a form of protection, a shield from suffering when the child's death is imminent. As such, educating family and caregivers to anticipate such changes is important, and interventions at this time to increase the child's energy and awareness may be detrimental to the child's state. Though these changes at this point in care may be referred to as fatigue, they can differ from fatigue occurring upstream in the illness trajectory. The types of fatigue and their chief characteristics, causative factors, probable mechanisms of action, measures of fatigue in ill children, analytic strategies for fatigue scores, and interprofessional interventions to prevent or diminish fatigue are the subjects of this chapter.

DEFINING FATIGUE IN ILL CHILDREN AND ADOLESCENTS

Fatigue is characterized as a distressing, pervasive symptom with physical, mental, social, and emotional components characterized by a lack of energy that is both perceived internally by the ill child and observed by others around the child.[2] Children are able to use expressive descriptors of physical fatigue such as "not being able to run or play with friends" or looking in a mirror and seeing themselves as a "dull face." They also describe aspects of emotional fatigue in terms of withdrawing from others, being irritable and feeling "mad" or "sad." Researchers exploring fatigue in seriously ill children confirm that perceptions of fatigue differ by developmental age 6–8 years. Younger children tend to emphasize the physical sensation of fatigue ("I am too tired to lift my head up from this table") somewhat more than emotional and cognitive aspects. Relatedly, they can describe how fatigue has altered their usual activities from playing and running to watching television or reading. Adolescents tend to report the impact of fatigue on their thinking, their physical sensations and limitations, and their social interactions and feelings. They also highlight mental tiredness that alternates and at times merges with the physical sensation of fatigue.[3–5] Adolescents report being aware of friends and relatives being in their hospital room to visit with them but being "too tired to open my eyes" or "too tired to talk or answer questions." Their reports of fatigue may also include their interpretation of this symptom being linked to a more serious illness or other contributory condition. In a qualitative study of children receiving treatment for cancer, researchers generated a detailed description of fatigue that reflected loss of or diminished energy and a typology of three types of fatigue: typical tiredness, treatment fatigue, and shutdown fatigue.[6] Although the majority of descriptors are from studies involving children in treatment for cancer, including those with advanced cancers,[7] the descriptors are similar from other groups of ill children as well.[8] However, not yet documented is whether or to what extent these descriptions offered by seriously ill children differ from descriptions by children with non–life-threatening illnesses or how the descriptions vary or not in seriously ill children over the course of their illness.

FATIGUE IN VARIOUS CONDITIONS AND POPULATIONS

Fatigue is prevalent among children with a range of chronic or serious conditions. For example, children with rheumatologic conditions such as juvenile rheumatoid (idiopathic) arthritis commonly report fatigue.[9,10] Fatigue is also encountered in children with multiple sclerosis,[11] with a prevalence as high as 79%, and it has a well-established association with impaired quality of life.[12] Almost two-thirds (59%) of children with mild to moderate physical disabilities (Gillette Functional Assessment Questionnaire levels 7–10) experience fatigue greater than that experienced by healthy children.[13] Children with epilepsy also experience more fatigue than do their healthy counterparts, with higher seizure frequency being associated with greater fatigue.[14] Sleep impairment and depression also aggravate fatigue in this population.[15] Among patients aged 8–47 with cystic fibrosis at end of life, the majority (96%) experienced fatigue that their caregivers described as distressing, second only in prevalence to dyspnea. Similarly, 77% of parents of children older than 2 years who died of advanced heart disease reported that their child suffered from a high degree of fatigue, and fatigue was the most commonly reported symptom in the child's last month of life.[16]

In pediatric cancer, cancer-related fatigue is known to be common and highly burdensome. In one study of 58 children with cancer, the most commonly reported symptom was fatigue (52%).[17] In one large, cross-sectional study of 502 children, 414 (82.5%) reported some degree of bothersome fatigue,[18] while in a longitudinal study of 104 children with advanced cancer followed over 9 months, 87% reported fatigue at least once. Of these children, 97% reported highly distressing fatigue.[19,20]

Like fatigue occurring earlier in the illness trajectory, fatigue occurring in advanced illness is also common and may be bothersome. Within the oncology population, a study of symptoms and suffering during the last month of life found that 96% of 141 parents surveyed reported that their child had experienced fatigue.[21] Such fatigue is also associated with impaired child well-being. In a Swedish nationwide survey of 449 parents of children with cancer, 86% reported physical fatigue as the most frequently reported symptom that had moderate or high impact on their child's well-being during the last month of life.[22] Indeed, at least in some instances, parents of children with advanced cancer view it as a source of significant suffering for their children at end of life and find it highly concerning.[23–27]

In looking even further along the illness trajectory, interviews with 30 parents whose children had received pediatric home hospice services for any diagnosis, fatigue was one of the most frequently identified symptoms during the last week of their child's life.[28] In an integrative overview of selected physical and psychosocial symptoms experienced by children approaching end of life, fatigue was described as an independent symptom, rather than a symptom taken as a "given" of the effects of illness or activity. Additionally, fatigue was described as an intrinsic part of a child dying and that its presence may actually bring relief to the dying child.[8] For children in the last moments of life, it may be helpful to describe this type of fatigue as an expected part of the process at the close of their child's life. In some instances, framing it as protective for the child may also be helpful.

Among children who survive cancer, the experience of fatigue is somewhat variable. Among adolescents and young adults who have recently completed cancer treatment (median 18 months), fatigue was the most prevalent symptom, experienced by 85%, and was ranked as more severe than any other symptom. Interestingly, those greater than 1 year out from treatment reported worse fatigue than those closer to treatment.[29,30] Other studies also support the finding of unmitigated fatigue even more than three decades after treatment. In contrast, a study of 286 childhood cancer survivors, aged 12–49 years, did not report higher rates of fatigue (14%) compared with healthy populations. However, the few who did report bothersome fatigue were more likely to have multiple chronic conditions, report depressive symptoms, and have lower quality of life scores. Fatigue as a late effect may be related to the original cancer diagnosis, as well as to other late effects. Long-term childhood acute lymphoblastic leukemia survivors with fatigue concurrently experienced poor neurocognitive function, such as executive function, task efficiency, and emotional regulation.[31,32]

CHILD IMPACT

A key characteristic of fatigue in pediatric life-threatening illness is its profound impact on the child's experience. For instance, a qualitative study exploring factors that influenced quality of life in 49 children and adolescents with epilepsy found excessive fatigue as a barrier to academic and social pursuits. Participants described how intermittent or continuous fatigue made it difficult to think clearly and fully participate in classroom learning.[33] For children with cerebral palsy, fatigue is negatively associated with duration of physical activity and motivations to participate in social activities.[34] Children with leukemia describe fatigue, both disease- and treatment-related, as having the greatest impact on their quality of life by altering participation in school, sports, and family activities.[35]

Multiple studies have documented cancer-related fatigue to be a debilitating symptom with physical, cognitive, social, and emotional components that are detrimental to health-related quality of life (HRQL).[36–40] For example, interviews with 6- to 19-year-olds unveiled multiple terms that children use to refer to their fatigue. The negative effects of the fatigue on daily functioning and mood and their need for rest were also revealed. Perceived alleviators varied by the ill child's age and included distractions, rest, nutrition, and exercise. Through impairment of a child's function and ability to participate in meaningful activities, fatigue may lead to loss of control in a situation that likely already feels out of control and a sense of loneliness and isolation. It is no wonder that, for many, fatigue is one of the most distressing symptoms that children may experience.[41–43]

Beyond the child's day-to-day experience, fatigue may also be relevant in terms of its relationship with indicators of worsening health or health complications and worse prognosis (i.e., survival). Adults with cancer who experience fatigue are most likely to require unplanned clinic visits and emergency room visits.[44,45] Several studies of adults with both early-stage and advanced cancer have demonstrated that fatigue independently predicts worse prognosis.[46–49] While it seems logical that similar relationships between fatigue and prognosis and healthcare utilization would exist in pediatrics, they have yet to be examined.

FATIGUE IN CAREGIVERS

Note should also be taken of the significant fatigue that parents (and other caregivers) are likely to experience throughout a child's illness. Caregiving for the ill child (e.g., obtaining and coordinating services, medical and therapy appointments, providing hands-on care, being "on-call" 24/7), parenting siblings, household and/or employment responsibilities, and emotional factors (e.g., depression, anxiety, coping with the experience) may all contribute to parent fatigue. Experiencing such fatigue of their own may influence how a parent perceives fatigue in their ill child. The inpatient setting can also contribute to parent fatigue through sleep disturbance.

Parents/caregivers of children undergoing hematopoietic stem cell transplant, who often actively care for and remain with their child throughout the hospitalization, experience profound sleep disruption. In one sample of parents/caregivers, 71% demonstrated significant sleep disturbance, and the same proportion rated sleep quality as poor. Parents/caregivers attributed their sleep disturbance to cardiac monitor alarms (76%), infusion pump alarms (82%), staff assessments (82%), and door openings (71%).[50]

Parents of children with progressive neurodegenerative conditions also report fatigue to be a common problem for themselves. It can impact them in multiple ways, including their relationships, ability to work outside the home, injuries, and exacerbation of their own medical conditions.[51] Interventions such as those supporting coping skills may be helpful to caregivers and can improve caregiver distress and burden and reduce fatigue.[52]

CLINICIAN RECOGNITION AND TREATMENT OF FATIGUE

As depicted in Table 21.1, multiple challenges exist in clinician recognition and response to fatigue, as well as in patient–clinician and family–clinician communication about the ill child's fatigue. The greatest challenge may be to effectively inquire about a child's fatigue, as several studies demonstrate

TABLE 21.1 Considerations and challenges in initial response to the ill child's fatigue

CHALLENGES IN CLINICIAN DETECTION AND RESPONSE TO FATIGUE	STRATEGIES TO ADDRESS CHALLENGES	CHALLENGES IN PATIENT–CLINICIAN COMMUNICATION ABOUT FATIGUE	STRATEGIES TO ADDRESS CHALLENGES
Prevalence (and impact) under-appreciated. For example, fatigue may be overshadowed by more visible symptoms	Clinician education	Not wanting to "bother" the clinician	Anticipatory guidance and education (see text) Routine inquiry about child's fatigue, including the question: "How tired have you been in the past 7 days?" (see text)
Multidimensional presentation of fatigue	More investigation into the presentation and patient descriptions of fatigue Further incorporation of fatigue assessments into practice Clinician education regarding assessment queries to ask of the ill child	Fear of appearing to be a "complainer"	Anticipatory guidance and education (see text) Routine inquiry about child's fatigue (see text)
Belief that fatigue is "to be expected"	Clinician education	Belief that fatigue is "to be expected"	Anticipatory guidance and education (see text) Routine inquiry about child's fatigue (see text)
Belief that fatigue is unavoidable/effective interventions do not exist	Clinician education Further research into current and novel interventions	Belief that fatigue is unavoidable/effective interventions do not exist	Anticipatory guidance and education (see text) Routine inquiry about child's fatigue (see text)
Focus on disease-directed treatment	Clinician education	Worry that fatigue indicates disease progression or will result in de-intensification of treatment	Anticipatory guidance and education (see text)
Systems issues (e.g., time, documentation practices)	Systems changes that allow routine assessment and that facilitate documentation and clinician attention to fatigue Adoption of single item fatigue measure[119]	Need for standardized clinical query regarding fatigue to facilitate communication and accurate assessment	Development and adoption of measures, such as the PROMNIS single-item fatigue measure[119]
Lack of established risk factors for fatigue (particularly ones that are modifiable)	Research elucidating (modifiable) risk factors for fatigue		
Need for pediatric-specific guidelines and evidence-based interventions	Further research in both existing and novel interventions		

underrecognition of fatigue by clinicians.[53,54] Complicating the challenges of assessment is the changeability of fatigue in terms of its presence, intensity, and interference in a child's life. Because of these challenges, clinicians should routinely inquire about fatigue. By doing so, clinicians convey their recognition that it is reasonable and acceptable for a child or parent to raise concerns about fatigue, if it occurs. If fatigue is not a problem for the child, education and anticipatory guidance that fatigue is common, is manifest in many ways, and need not be simply endured will open the door to future conversations, if the need arises.

These challenges to recognizing and labeling fatigue in ill children account in part for the undertreatment of fatigue which has been documented.[21,25] In one study of children with advanced cancer and fatigue, only 13% received fatigue-directed treatment.[21] Undertreatment of recognized fatigue may stem from a variety of factors, including a need for more education regarding fatigue interventions and their effectiveness.[55,56] When guidance or treatment is provided, clinicians usually recommend rest, which is not an intervention well-supported by evidence.[57,58] Among the children with advanced cancer and fatigue described earlier, treatment was successful in only 25%, suggesting that education and evidence from rigorous studies to guide clinicians and provide them with effective interventions for fatigue are likely both essential.

FATIGUE ASSESSMENT AND MEASUREMENT

Fatigue assessment clinically receives guidance from the Guidelines from the National Comprehensive Cancer Network (NCCN) that recommend routine screening for fatigue as the sixth vital sign.[1] According to the NCCN guidelines, children older than 12 years of age should be screened using a simple numeric rating scale such as 0, "no fatigue," to 10, "worst fatigue you can imagine." For children 7–12 years of age, a 5-point scale is recommended with the word anchors being "not tired" to "worst." For children aged 5 and 6 years, the words "tired" or "not tired" are recommended for use to assess the presence of fatigue. If the screening confirms the presence of fatigue, the clinical assessment moves to a deeper level with an assessment of eight treatable contributing factors to fatigue: anemia, pain, sleep disturbance or poor sleep hygiene, nutritional deficits, changes in functional status, emotional distress, medications or side effects and drug interactions, and presence of comorbidities. The healthcare team should assess for the onset and type of fatigue, aggravating or alleviating factors, and degree of interference with the child's functioning.[1] This assessment should be done at standardized points in care and at times of change in the ill child's condition.

Quantitative measurement of fatigue by the ill child, caregiver (parent or other proxy), and clinician occurs in two forms: disease-specific or general measures. Caregiver and clinician reports have a longer history of use than do child reports. Because ill children, their caregivers, and their clinicians define fatigue differently and identify different causative factors,[59,60] soliciting reports from all three may be essential to the clinical management of fatigue. Another principle in fatigue measurement is timing. Because fatigue has features such as persistence and intensity, it is important to solicit the reports of the ill child, caregiver, and clinician over time. This would include scheduled, standardized times as well as at unexpected changes in the ill child's health status.

Examples and descriptions of disease-specific and general pediatric fatigue and multisymptom measures that include items about fatigue follow. Completed reviews of pediatric measures being used to index fatigue indicate that all three types of fatigue measures have been assessed for key characteristics including their psychometric properties. Fatigue measures declared ready for incorporation into clinical research by one or both of the fatigue instrument reviews include the Fatigue Scale-Child, Fatigue Scale-Adolescent (FS-A), the PedsQL Multidimensional Fatigue Scale, and the PROMIS Pediatric Fatigue measure.[5,61–66] Original studies have reported on these established measures and support their psychometric properties, including responsiveness to change over time.

The Childhood Fatigue Scale (CFS) is a 10-item (4-point Likert scale) questionnaire that asks children (7–12 years) about their tiredness during the previous week. The three subscales are lack of energy, inability to function, and altered mood. The Parent Fatigue Scale (PFS) is a 17-item inventory of parents' perception of their child's fatigue in the previous week. In addition to the three subscales on the children's version, it also includes a scale of altered sleep. The FS-A is a 13-item questionnaire that asks adolescents (13–18 years) to evaluate their fatigue experience during the previous week. The child and parent scales are available in English and Spanish; the adolescent form in English only. The CFS, PFS, and FS-A are validated research instruments, easy to administer, and require limited time to complete in the clinical setting.

The PedsQL Multidimensional Fatigue Scale is an 18-item research instrument (ages 2–18) with three subscales of six items each: general fatigue, sleep-rest fatigue, and cognitive fatigue. The scale is self-administered for 8- to 18-year-olds, interview-administered in 5- to 7-year-olds, and done by parent proxy for the youngest children. The 5-point Likert response option format solicits ratings to the prompt: "How much of a problem has this been for you in the past month?" The measure has strong reliability and construct validity coefficients in its testing in children with cancer, sickle cell disease, and other health conditions. It is available in 22 languages.[62,67,68] The Pediatric Functional Assessment of Chronic Illness Therapy-Fatigue (Peds FACIT-F) is an 11-item scale for children with cancer that measures fatigue in the past 7 days.[69] The Peds FACIT-F has very acceptable internal consistency coefficients and concurrent validity. It is available in English and Spanish.[69]

The PROMIS Pediatric Measures, including the PROMIS Pediatric Fatigue measures were developed using item response theory (IRT) and created to document child and adolescent reports of their symptom, function, and quality-of-life experience with illness and treatment. The measures were developed first from qualitative methods with children 8 years and older for item development, identification of extant questionnaire items for an item pool, item review, and revision by experts.[70,71] Very acceptable item and scale reliability, as well as diverse forms of validity have been reported for the measures and specifically for the PROMIS Pediatric Fatigue measure, including responsiveness to change over time. Items are scored from 0 ("never") to 4 ("almost always") for symptom (fatigue) interference. Items are considered equivalent psychometrically and therefore can be selected from the item bank to be used for the same measurement purpose. Generally, 6–8 items are recommended to achieve acceptable to strong internal consistency coefficients. The time period is "in the past 7 days."

The PROMIS Pediatric Fatigue measure has been tested in diverse pediatric groups such as children with advanced disease receiving palliative care and children receiving treatment for cancer, sickle cell disease, and nephrotic syndrome.[62,72–77] Additionally, the PROMIS Pediatric Fatigue measure has been evaluated for clinically important change over time using the scale-judgment method to establish the minimally important difference (MID); the MID is a 3-point difference in scores over time.[77]

More recently validated multisymptom measures that include fatigue items validated in pediatric samples include the Symptom Screening in Pediatrics Tool (SSPedi) (https://www.sungresearch.com/sspedi), the Pediatric PRO-CTCAE measurement system, and the Pediatric Quality of Life and Evaluation of Symptoms Technology (PediQUEST). The SSPedi is a 15-item, 5-point Likert measure for children aged 8–18 years to report their symptoms "since yesterday" during cancer treatment and stem cell transplantation. The tool is viewed as a screening measure and has a matching proxy version. Reliability, different forms of validity, and responsiveness to change have been positively assessed. A mini-SSPedi for children 4–7 years of age has been derived from the older age group version and is in testing now.

The Pediatric PRO CTCAE measurement system, begun from qualitative work with pediatric oncology experts and followed by cognitive interviewing involving children and their caregivers, includes 62 subjective cancer treatment toxicities and 1–3 questions per toxicity in terms of frequency, intensity, and interference. The recall period is "the past 7 days," and child- or proxy-reported scores can be mapped onto the National Cancer Institute's Common Toxicity Criteria Adverse Events (CTCAE) grades.[78] The items have been validated in 7- to 18-year-olds in treatment for cancer (i.e., content validity, construct validity), including for responsiveness to change over time. In addition, the items have been mapped to clinician-reporting of treatment toxicities.[78] A matching proxy measure is also available and has been validated in 7- to 18-year-olds in treatment for cancer.[76,79–83]

PediQUEST is a computer-based child or parent report of multiple symptoms including the child's fatigue as well as the child's quality of life and includes an adapted version of the MSAS.[19,20] The age of eligible children is 2–18 years, with parents typically completing the items on behalf of their child younger than 7 years. Response options use a 4- or a 5-point Likert format for the 24 physical or psychological symptoms in three age-specific versions: 2–6 years (proxy), 7–12 years, and 13–18 years. The symptom presence, frequency, severity, and bother in the preceding week are solicited. Psychometric characteristics including responsiveness to change have not yet been reported.

In summary, multiple validated measures exist of fatigue or inclusive of fatigue items in ill children. The measures have been most commonly validated in children with cancer, including advanced stages and at end of life. Several of the preceding measures and fatigue items have the documented ability of capturing responsiveness to change over time, and it is these measures that would be most well-suited for longitudinal and clinical trial studies. This includes children with incurable cancer. The multiplicity of validated fatigue measures, including in pediatrics, is considered to be a research challenge and was addressed by one working group in oncology convened by the National Cancer Institute. After weighing the features of multiple fatigue measures, the working group recommended the use of the PROMIS Fatigue measures in cancer research (adult or pediatric) whenever possible.[84] Certainly, the selection of a measure is based on multiple factors including preference of the study team, match with study purpose, and target participants but having the same measure used across studies has the advantage of allowing for direct comparison of findings from different patient groups.

ASSESSMENT OF FATIGUE AS A DOSE-LIMITING TOXICITY

Clinicians have reported that fatigue can be a dose-limiting toxicity in pediatric oncology for some patients enrolled on a Phase I study.[85,86] Importantly, children enrolled on Phase I/II trials for incurable cancers have willingly completed self-report fatigue measures (e.g., PROMIS Pediatric Fatigue) at more than one time point, among other symptom and function measures, with a minimal amount of missing data, indicating that the measures are not perceived by these children as burdensome or troublesome.[87] Being able to collect subjective treatment toxicity information, such as fatigue, from the ill child at this point in their cancer treatment would enhance the completeness and accuracy of the impact of the Phase I agent on the child.

FATIGUE MECHANISMS

As depicted in Figure 21.1, fatigue in children with serious illness is a complex process. Across illness conditions, research aimed at defining fatigue mechanisms has been limited. It is likely that significant differences between populations of children (e.g., differences in disease pathophysiology, disease-directed treatments, and in child characteristics such as age and gender) result in fatigue stemming from different mechanisms. However, such varying mechanisms have yet to be described and delineated.

At the same time, there may be factors associated with fatigue that are common to many populations. Disease activity may be one such factor; children with worse asthma control, on active cancer treatment, worse chronic kidney disease, sickle cell disease, and rheumatic disease all report greater fatigue.[73] Child factors not directly linked to their illness, such as (older) age and (female) sex, also seem to be associated with fatigue.[18,39,88] For example, among children with physical disabilities (Gillette Functional Assessment Questionnaire levels 7–10), fatigue was associated with being female,[13] among other factors. This pattern has been observed in children with cancer, as well. Age is another factor that may influence the experience of fatigue, with older adolescents in treatment for cancer typically reporting higher fatigue than younger patients.[89,90] Little is known about whether child characteristics, some of which may predate the child's illness, influence the child's experience of fatigue and, if they do, whether or not the level of influence is constant or varies over time and situations.

Factors potentially contributing to child fatigue are most thoroughly characterized in the cancer population. Physical factors, such as type of cancer and cancer treatment, are associated with fatigue.[18,39,88] Such treatments include dexamethasone (disrupts sleep)[91] and tyrosine kinase inhibitors (which may cause hypothyroidism or adrenal insufficiency). Fatigue caused by these endocrinologic perturbations improves after correction.[92]

Sleep disturbance, a common occurrence when children are hospitalized, also plays a role in fatigue. Hospitalized children experience multiple nocturnal awakenings, which are associated with increased fatigue; those who experienced 20 or more awakenings had significantly higher fatigue scores than those with fewer awakenings.[93] Some studies have also found that anemia is associated with fatigue.[20,88,94] While one

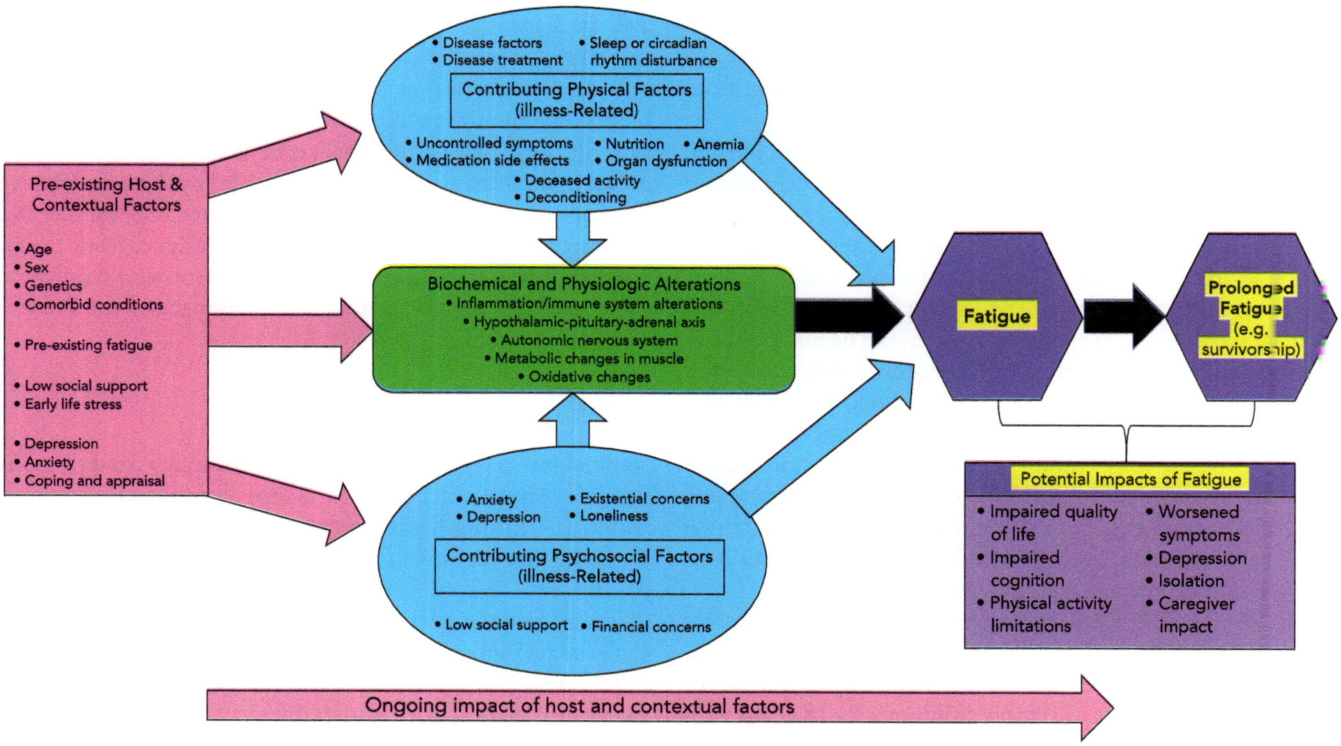

Figure 21.1 *Diagram representing predisposing host and contextual factors that may exacerbate or mitigate fatigue; physical and psychosocial (illness-related) factors, as well as biochemical and physiologic alterations contributing to fatigue and prolonged fatigue. The potential impact of fatigue and prolonged fatigue are also displayed.*

of these studies (focused on children with advanced cancer) found that lower hemoglobin is associated with child report of fatigue, it was not associated with child reports of *bothersome* fatigue.[20] In this sample, only other distressing symptoms, but not other factors, such as anemia or cancer treatment factors, were associated with bothersome fatigue. This suggests that suffering from other symptom(s) may reduce a child's threshold for experiencing fatigue distress or that the treatment of other troubling symptoms may help to relieve the fatigue experience. And, for children with advanced cancer, symptom distress may figure more prominently in the experience of fatigue than other factors such as cancer-directed therapy or anemia. This also reminds us that factors underlying fatigue are unlikely to be static and may well change across the trajectory of illness.

Given the impact of fatigue on function and quality of life as described earlier, an association with emotional distress would not be a surprise. While these studies describe simultaneous emotional distress and fatigue, few have documented it in a quantitative fashion. In the previously described study of children with advanced cancer, sadness and worry were associated with fatigue.[20] A study of adolescents and young adults with cancer revealed that greater psychological distress correlated with greater fatigue severity.[39] The association between fatigue and worse psychological well-being is well-documented in adults across multiple diagnoses,[95–99] including cancer, end-stage kidney disease, multiple sclerosis, and chronic obstructive pulmonary disease (COPD). In adults, factors such as childhood adversity, coping, and appraisal (e.g., catastrophizing) may influence response to fatigue, regulation of that response, and how it is experienced and expressed.[100] In children, whether and how psychological distress leads to fatigue in serious illness, or vice versa, is not as well studied. A recent study used the Pediatric PRO CTCAE measurement system (including fatigue) to identify groups of children and adolescents in treatment for cancer, distinguished by their pattern of toxicity suffering (high adverse-event suffering, moderate and low adverse-event suffering). The findings indicated the presence of all three groups and that group membership was able to predict the distal outcome of psychological stress. That being said, it is quite possible that the relationship is bidirectional.

Much of how these child and clinical factors result in pathophysiologic changes giving rise to fatigue is yet to be elucidated. However, there has been a rapid expansion in research focusing on the biological pathways and genetic factors contributing to the genesis and persistence of fatigue. Alterations in biochemistry and physiology hypothesized to cause fatigue are often divided into peripheral and central mechanisms. Peripheral mechanisms include the muscles and related tissues; central mechanisms (e.g., immune, neuroendocrine) occur in the central nervous system, resulting in impairment of motor neuron impulses.

Existing studies of nonmalignant conditions, when taken together, suggest that alterations in the hypothalamic-pituitary-adrenal (HPA) axis and autonomic nervous system and/or inflammation play a role in nonmalignant conditions such as heart failure, chronic kidney disease, COPD, and multiple sclerosis.[101] The degree to which these conditions have common fatigue pathway alterations is unknown. It seems likely that they share some mechanisms giving rise to fatigue, with disease-specific mechanisms also at play.

As with other aspects of fatigue, most research has focused on its occurrence in the setting of cancer. Proinflammatory cytokines such as interleukin (IL)-1-beta, IL-6, and tumor necrosis factor (TNF)-alpha, which can signal the central nervous system to generate fatigue symptoms, have been the subject of great interest. Both cancer and its treatment are associated with increases in cytokines, and the tumor microenvironment has been demonstrated to include the listed cytokines. Persistent fatigue in breast cancer survivors is also associated with cytokine dysregulation.

Neuroendocrine derangements have also been implicated in fatigue in cancer. Initial studies of sympathetic and parasympathetic activity in breast cancer survivors suggest that the autonomic nervous system, which also plays a role in inflammation, may contribute to fatigue.[102] The HPA axis controls release of cortisol by the adrenal cortex, usually in response to stress, and it also plays an important role in cytokine regulation and modulation of inflammation. Several studies suggest that dysregulation of this axis may also contribute to fatigue. As an example, abnormal patterns of cortisol levels in breast cancer survivors are associated with fatigue.[103]

A variety of other biochemical and physiologic perturbations have been implicated in fatigue, circadian rhythm disruption, serotonin dysregulation, and peripheral mechanisms, such as skeletal muscular and mitochondrial dysfunction. While there is a great paucity of research on this topic in children, one small study found an association between fatigue and low carnitine levels in children receiving chemotherapy, suggesting that an abnormality in adenosine triphosphate synthesis may contribute to fatigue.[104] Research demonstrating differential gene expression lends additional support to the hypotheses that immune function/inflammation, neurotransmission, neurotransmission, energy metabolism, and circadian rhythms play a role in fatigue.[105]

There are other theories regarding the potential mechanisms of action related to fatigue. Some ideas related to the cause of fatigue are disease- or treatment-specific. For example, one theorized mechanism of action is a phenotypic biochemical mechanism that has been studied in children in treatment for acute lymphocytic leukemia (ALL).[106] Failure of the antioxidant body defense system is viewed as secondary to genetic variation. In this theory, nitrosative stress during the treatment for ALL increases in the cerebral spinal fluid as measured by certain biomarkers, chief among those being protein 3-nitrotyrosine (3NT). This biomarker is associated with high fatigue at different points in treatment and suggests that cell damage results when antioxidant defenses are low and contributes to fatigue. Ongoing work to elucidate the biological mechanisms of fatigue will inform the development of targeted interventions mitigating fatigue and ultimately improve quality of life and other outcomes for children impacted by fatigue and serious illness.

Treatment of Fatigue

EDUCATION AND COUNSELING

One of the most important aspects of helping children and families deal with the distressing symptom of fatigue is preparing them for it and educating them about it.[1] Many families may be very worried when their children become fatigued, while it may be a common symptom of either the disease or the treatment. Providers should give anticipatory guidance about the likelihood of experiencing fatigue and that experiencing fatigue is not necessarily an indicator of disease progression. Children and families can be advised on setting realistic expectations about what activities children may be able to participate in and how to choose the most meaningful activities when energy is limited. Additionally, parents can be counseled in some general strategies to help minimize fatigue, including

- Limit naps to not interfere with nighttime sleep
- Maintain a structured daily routine
- Incorporate relaxation strategies for sleep[107]

NONPHARMACOLOGIC INTERVENTIONS

Most of the trials investigating interventions for reducing fatigue in children have been in children with cancer. Nonpharmacologic interventions include physical activity (exercises such as walking, swimming, light weight, yoga, physical therapy) and mind-body interventions (massage; energy therapies like healing touch, acupressure, mindfulness/relaxation). In adults with cancer, physical activity has been found to significantly decrease the severity of fatigue.[108] Aerobic, neuromotor, resistance, and combination exercises were all effective in a meta-analysis in reducing fatigue (although smaller effects were observed with resistance). Additionally, this meta-analysis found that the effect of physical activity did not differ based on presence of fatigue at the time of the intervention or whether the intervention was supervised or conducted in a group or its duration measured in weeks or minutes per week.[108]

In pediatric patients, the evidence for fatigue and nonpharmacologic interventions is more limited but still promising.[109,110] Exercise interventions in children have been used even in very sick patients, such as those undergoing bone marrow transplant,[111,112] as well as with patients in the home setting.[113] Challenges with exercise interventions include getting children to stick with the prescribed program and finding programs applicable to children of different ages and underlying medical conditions.[114] Additionally, exercise interventions may require a prolonged period of time to see effect and may require a lot of encouragement to continue.[113] While the evidence in pediatrics is limited, it was sufficient for a recent clinical practice guideline to make a strong recommendation of physical activity "based on the consistent benefit across patient and intervention characteristics in adults, universal availability, very low risk of harm, low costs, and likelihood of other associated health benefits."[115]

Several studies of mind-body interventions have been performed in children with cancer to decrease fatigue, and there have been several reviews and meta-analyses published in recent years. Most of these found inconclusive evidence for the role of any nonpharmacologic intervention for management of fatigue, citing problems with diverse age groups and diagnoses and the short duration of studies making it difficult to conclude if the interventions were helpful, as well as lack of blinding and insufficiently sensitive fatigue measures in children.[110,116] Duong et al. performed a systematic review in pediatric and adult studies aiming to determine whether nonphysical activity in mind and body practices reduce the severity of fatigue in patients with cancer or hematopoietic stem cell transplant (HSCT) recipients compared to control interventions: 55 studies were included. When combined, all interventions significantly reduced the severity of fatigue when compared to all control groups (SMD −0.51, 95% confidence interval [CI] −0.73 to −0.29) and when compared to usual care or waitlist control, but not when compared to sham alone. When compared to all controls, only mindfulness (SMD −0.50, P = 0.005) and relaxation techniques (SMD −0.94, P = 0.006) significantly reduced the severity of fatigue.[117] Based on this evidence, a recent clinical practice guideline made a strong recommendation to use "relaxation or mindfulness or both for children with cancer or undergoing stem cell transplant on the basis of the consistent benefit across patient and intervention characteristics in adults, very low risk of harm, and low costs. Furthermore, we noted that, once learned, these interventions could be used without assistance."[115]

TREATMENT OF UNDERLYING CAUSES

While it is important to educate families that some degree of fatigue is to be expected, it is important to always rule out any treatable causes and to offer treatment if that is in line with the family's goals and the clinical condition. These include treatment of anemia, weaning of pain and other sedating medications as tolerated, or alternatively adequately treating pain and depression and optimizing nutrition as able.

PHARMACOLOGIC

More evidence for pharmacologic interventions is documented in the pediatric cancer population, though again there is better evidence in the adult cancer population that has been extrapolated to children. Tomlinson et al. performed a meta-analysis of pharmacological interventions in cancer and stem cell transplant patients of all ages (though in the end they were all adult studies as there were no pediatric studies to include). Based on 117 studies the authors evaluated

- erythropoietins (EPO) ($n = 31$, 26.5%)
- stimulants ($n = 19$, 16.2%)
- l-carnitine ($n = 6$, 5.1%)
- corticosteroids ($n = 5$, 4.3%)
- antidepressants ($n = 5$, 4.3%)
- appetite stimulants ($n = 3$, 2.6%)
- others ($n = 48$, 41.0%)

The comparison groups were placebo ($n = 75$, 64.1%), usual care ($n = 26$, 22.2%), and other pharmacologic interventions ($n = 16$, 13.7%). Of the studies analyzed, EPO and stimulants (notably methylphenidate) were helpful in improving fatigue, though neither made a meaningful improvement.[118] Based on this evidence, a recent clinical practice guideline includes a strong recommendation against using pharmacological interventions to treat fatigue in children.[115] It is possible that such studies are limited by instrumentation, our limited understanding of the different potential mechanisms underlying fatigue, and the challenge of conducting symptom intervention studies in the pediatric population. Given this, and the fact that none of the studies on which this recommendation was made is based on pediatric studies, it is reasonable to consider a trial of a pharmacologic intervention such as a stimulant for specific children.

CONCLUSION

Children with serious illness frequently experience fatigue that is complex, multifaceted, and multifactorial in nature. This fatigue may significantly impact them and their caregivers with respect to their quality of life, function, and other developmental and disease outcomes. We have learned a great deal about fatigue from the concurrent study of fatigue in ill adults. In recent years, pediatric-focused studies have also taught us a great deal about the nature and impact of fatigue on ill children. Much of our deepened knowledge about fatigue in seriously ill children has emanated from the specialty of oncology.

For some time, the lack of rigorously developed assessment instruments was a significant impediment to the study and treatment of fatigue in seriously ill children. However, impressive advances have recently been made in defining, assessing, and measuring fatigue in this population. We are now well-positioned to focus on mechanisms of action that cause or contribute to fatigue. This knowledge will, in turn, inform interventions to treat seriously ill children experiencing distressing fatigue, or even prevent it in those who are most vulnerable to it. Although certain interventions may be narrowly targeted in nature, more likely effective interventions will take a more global approach, such as supporting coping or adaptation and scheduling physical, cognitive, and other activities to take place during higher energy time periods for each affected child. Because fatigue is an issue for both ill children and their families, impactful interventions will likely need to be directed at both.

REFERENCES

1. National Comprehensive Cancer Network. NCCN clinical practice guidelines in oncology: Cancer-related fatigue. version 1.2021. www.nccn.org
2. Passik SD, Kirsh KL. A pilot examination of the impact of cancer patients' fatigue on their spousal caregivers. *Palliat Support Care.* 2005;3(4):273–279.
3. Hockenberry-Eaton M, Hinds PS, Alcoser P, et al. Fatigue in children and adolescents with cancer. *J Pediatr Oncol Nurs.* 1998;15(3): 172–182.
4. Ullrich CK, Mayer OH. Assessment and management of fatigue and dyspnea in pediatric palliative care. *Pediatr Clin North Am.* 2007;54(5):735–756, xi.
5. Hockenberry MJ, Hinds PS, Barrera P, et al. Three instruments to assess fatigue in children with cancer: The child, parent, and staff perspectives. *J Pain Symptom Manage.* 2003;25(4):319–328.
6. Davies B, Whitsett SF, Bruce A, McCarthy P. A typology of fatigue in children with cancer. *J Pediatr Oncol Nurs.* 2002;19(1):12–21.
7. Tomlinson D, Zupanec S, Jones H, O'Sullivan C, Hesser T, Sung L. The lived experience of fatigue in children and adolescents with cancer: A systematic review. *Support Care Cancer.* 2016;24(8):3623–3631.
8. Scurkes BM. Children's experience of symptoms: Narratives through words and images. *Children (Basel).* 2018;5(4):53.
9. Ward TM, Brandt P, Archbold K, et al. Polysomnography and self-reported sleep, pain, fatigue, and anxiety in children with active and inactive juvenile rheumatoid arthritis. *J Pediatr Psychol.* 2008;33(3):232–241.
10. Sallfors C, Hallberg LR, Fasth A. Well-being in children with juvenile chronic arthritis. *Clin Exp Rheumatol.* 2004;22(1):125–130.
11. Carroll S, Chalder T, Hemingway C, Heyman I, Moss-Morris R. Understanding fatigue in paediatric multiple sclerosis: A systematic review of clinical and psychosocial factors. *Dev Med Child Neurol.* 2016;58(3):229–239.
12. Storm Van's Gravesande K, Blaschek A, Calabrese P, et al. Fatigue and depression predict health-related quality of life in patients with pediatric-onset multiple sclerosis. *Mult Scler Relat Disord.* 2019;36:101368.
13. Maher C, Crettenden A, Evans K, et al. Fatigue is a major issue for children and adolescents with physical disabilities. *Dev Med Child Neurol.* 2015;57(8):742–747.
14. Kanemura H, Sano F, Ohyama T, Sugita K, Aihara M. Association between seizure frequency and fatigue levels in children with epilepsy. *J Paediatr Child Health.* 2018;54(12):1336–1340.
15. Kwon OY, Park SP. Interictal fatigue and its predictors in epilepsy patients: A case-control study. *Seizure.* 2016;34:48–53.
16. Balkin EM, Wolfe J, Ziniel SI, et al. Physician and parent perceptions of prognosis and end-of-life experience in children with advanced heart disease. *J Palliat Med.* 2015;18(4):318–323.
17. Torres V, Nunes MDR, Silva-Rodrigues FM, et al. Frequency, severity, and distress associated with physical and psychosocial symptoms at home in children and adolescents with cancer. *J Pediatr Health Care.* 2019;33(4):404–414.
18. Tomlinson D, Baggott C, Dix D, et al. Severely bothersome fatigue in children and adolescents with cancer and hematopoietic stem cell transplant recipients. *Support Care Cancer.* 2019;27(7):2665–2671.
19. Wolfe J, Orellana L, Ullrich C, et al. Symptoms and distress in children with advanced cancer: Prospective patient-reported outcomes from the PediQUEST study. *J Clin Oncol.* 2015;33(17):1928–1935.
20. Ullrich CK, Dussel V, Orellana L, et al. Self-reported fatigue in children with advanced cancer: Results of the PediQUEST study. *Cancer.* 2018;124(18):3776–3783.
21. Ullrich CK, Dussel V, Hilden JM, et al. Fatigue in children with cancer at the end of life. *J Pain Symptom Manage.* 2010;40(4):483–494.
22. Jalmsell L, Kreicbergs U, Onelov E, Steineck G, Henter JI. Symptoms affecting children with malignancies during the last month of life: A nationwide follow-up. *Pediatrics.* 2006;117(4):1314–1320.
23. von Lutzau P, Otto M, Hechler T, Metzing S, Wolfe J, Zernikow B. Children dying from cancer: Parents' perspectives on symptoms, quality of life, characteristics of death, and end-of-life decisions. *J Palliat Care.* 2012;28(4):274–281.
24. Wolfe J, Hammel JF, Edwards KE, et al. Easing of suffering in children with cancer at the end of life: Is care changing? *J Clin Oncol.* 2008;26(10):1717–1723.
25. Hechler T, Blankenburg M, Friedrichsdorf SJ, et al. Parents' perspective on symptoms, quality of life, characteristics of death and end-of-life decisions for children dying from cancer. *Klin Padiatr.* 2008;220(3):166–174.
26. Heath JA, Clarke NE, Donath SM, McCarthy M, Anderson VA, Wolfe J. Symptoms and suffering at the end of life in children with cancer: An Australian perspective. *Med J Aust.* 2010;192(2):71–75.
27. Pritchard M, Burghen E, Srivastava DK, et al. Cancer-related symptoms most concerning to parents during the last week and last day of their child's life. *Pediatrics.* 2008;121(5):e1301–1309.
28. Hendricks-Ferguson V. Physical symptoms of children receiving pediatric hospice care at home during the last week of life. *Oncol Nurs Forum.* 2008;35(6):E108–115.
29. Spathis A, Hatcher H, Booth S, et al. Cancer-related fatigue in adolescents and young adults after cancer treatment: Persistent and poorly managed. *J Adolesc Young Adult Oncol.* 2017;6(3):489–493.
30. Hicks J, Bartholomew J, Ward-Smith P, Hutto CJ. Quality of life among childhood leukemia patients. *J Pediatr Oncol Nurs.* 2003;20(4):192–200.
31. Clanton NR, Klosky JL, Li C, et al. Fatigue, vitality, sleep, and neurocognitive functioning in adult survivors of childhood cancer: A report from the Childhood Cancer Survivor study. *Cancer.* 2011;117(11):2559–2568.
32. Cheung YT, Brinkman TM, Mulrooney DA, et al. Impact of sleep, fatigue, and systemic inflammation on neurocognitive and behavioral outcomes in long-term survivors of childhood acute lymphoblastic leukemia. *Cancer.* 2017;123(17):3410–3419.
33. Elliott IM, Lach L, Smith ML. I just want to be normal: A qualitative study exploring how children and adolescents view the impact of intractable epilepsy on their quality of life. *Epilepsy Behav.* 2005;7(4):664–678.
34. Brunton LK. Descriptive report of the impact of fatigue and current management strategies in cerebral palsy. *Pediatr Phys Ther.* 2018;30(2):135–141.
35. Gedaly-Duff V, Lee KA, Nail L, Nicholson HS, Johnson KP. Pain, sleep disturbance, and fatigue in children with leukemia and their parents: A pilot study. *Oncol Nurs Forum.* 2006;33(3):641–646.
36. Gibson F, Mulhall AB, Richardson A, Edwards JL, Ream E, Sepion BJ. A phenomenologic study of fatigue in adolescents receiving treatment for cancer. *Oncol Nurs Forum.* 2005;32(3):651–660.
37. Ream E, Gibson F, Edwards J, Seption B, Mulhall A, Richardson A. Experience of fatigue in adolescents living with cancer. *Cancer Nurs.* 2006;29(4):317–326.
38. Erickson JM, Beck SL, Christian B, et al. Patterns of fatigue in adolescents receiving chemotherapy. *Oncol Nurs Forum.* 2010;37(4): 444–455.
39. Poort H, Kaal SEJ, Knoop H, et al. Prevalence and impact of severe fatigue in adolescent and young adult cancer patients in comparison with population-based controls. *Support Care Cancer.* 2017;25(9):2911–2918.
40. Anderson LM, Allen TM, Thornburg CD, Bonner MJ. Fatigue in children with sickle cell disease: Association with neurocognitive and social-emotional functioning and quality of life. *J Pediatr Hematol Oncol.* 2015;37(8):584–589.
41. Moody K, Meyer M, Mancuso CA, Charlson M, Robbins L. Exploring concerns of children with cancer. *Support Care Cancer.* 2006;14(9):960–966.
42. Walker AJ, Gedaly-Duff V, Miaskowski C, Nail L. Differences in symptom occurrence, frequency, intensity, and distress in adolescents prior to and one week after the administration of chemotherapy. *J Pediatr Oncol Nurs.* 2010;27(5):259–265.

43. Hedstrom M, Ljungman G, von Essen L. Perceptions of distress among adolescents recently diagnosed with cancer. *J Pediatr Hematol Oncol.* 2005;27(1):15–22.
44. Aprile G, Pisa FE, Follador A, et al. Unplanned presentations of cancer outpatients: A retrospective cohort study. *Support Care Cancer.* 2013;21(2):397–404.
45. Barbera L, Atzema C, Sutradhar R, et al. Do patient-reported symptoms predict emergency department visits in cancer patients? A population-based analysis. *Ann Emerg Med.* 2013;61(4):427–437 e425.
46. Paiva CE, Paiva BS. Prevalence, predictors, and prognostic impact of fatigue among Brazilian outpatients with advanced cancers. *Support Care Cancer.* 2013;21(4):1053–1060.
47. Stauder MC, Romero Y, Kabat B, et al. Overall survival and self-reported fatigue in patients with esophageal cancer. *Support Care Cancer.* 2013;21(2):511–519.
48. Trajkovic-Vidakovic M, de Graeff A, Voest EE, Teunissen SC. Symptoms tell it all: A systematic review of the value of symptom assessment to predict survival in advanced cancer patients. *Crit Rev Oncol Hematol.* 2012;84(1):130–148.
49. Lacourt TE, Kavelaars A, Ohanian M, et al. Patient-reported fatigue prior to treatment is prognostic of survival in patients with acute myeloid leukemia. *Oncotarget.* 2018;9(58):31244–31252.
50. Coleman K, Flesch L, Petiniot L, et al. Sleep disruption in caregivers of pediatric stem cell recipients. *Pediatr Blood Cancer.* 2018;65(5):e26965.
51. Steele R, Davies B. Impact on parents when a child has a progressive, life-threatening illness. *Int J Palliat Nurs.* 2006;12(12):576–585.
52. Mosher CE, Secinti E, Johns SA, et al. Examining the effect of peer helping in a coping skills intervention: A randomized controlled trial for advanced gastrointestinal cancer patients and their family caregivers. *Qual Life Res.* 2018;27(2):515–528.
53. Madden K, Magno Charone M, Mills S, et al. Systematic symptom reporting by pediatric palliative care patients with cancer: A preliminary report. *J Palliat Med.* 2019;22(8):894–901.
54. Chidambaram S, DeShields T, Potter P, Olsen S, Chen L. Patient and provider concordance on symptoms during the oncology outpatient clinic visit. *J Community Support Oncol.* 2014;12(10):370–377.
55. Pearson EJ, Morris ME, McKinstry CE. Cancer-related fatigue: A survey of health practitioner knowledge and practice. *Support Care Cancer.* 2015;23(12):3521–3529.
56. Yilmaz HB, Tas F, Muslu GK, Basbakkal Z, Kantar M. Health professionals' estimation of cancer-related fatigue in children. *J Pediatr Oncol Nurs.* 2010;27(6):330–337.
57. Stone P, Ream E, Richardson A, et al. Cancer-related fatigue--a difference of opinion? Results of a multicentre survey of healthcare professionals, patients and caregivers. *Eur J Cancer Care (Engl).* 2003;12(1):20–27.
58. Gibson F, Garnett M, Richardson A, Edwards J, Sepion B. Heavy to carry: A survey of parents' and healthcare professionals' perceptions of cancer-related fatigue in children and young people. *Cancer Nurs.* 2005;28(1):27–35.
59. Hinds PS, Hockenberry-Eaton M, Quargnenti A, et al. Fatigue in 7- to 12-year-old patients with cancer from the staff perspective: An exploratory study. *Oncol Nurs Forum.* 1999;26(1):37–45.
60. Ullrich CK, Rodday AM, Bingen KM, et al. Three sides to a story: Child, parent, and nurse perspectives on the child's experience during hematopoietic stem cell transplantation. *Cancer.* 2017;123(16):3159–3166.
61. Pinheiro LC, McFatrich M, Lucas N, et al. Child and adolescent self-report symptom measurement in pediatric oncology research: A systematic literature review. *Qual Life Res.* 2018;27(2):291–319.
62. Tomlinson D, Hinds PS, Ethier MC, Ness KK, Zupanec S, Sung L. Psychometric properties of instruments used to measure fatigue in children and adolescents with cancer: A systematic review. *J Pain Symptom Manage.* 2013;45(1):83–91.
63. Hinds PS, Yang J, Gattuso JS, et al. Psychometric and clinical assessment of the 10-item reduced version of the Fatigue Scale-Child instrument. *J Pain Symptom Manage.* 2010;39(3):572–578.
64. Mandrell BN, Yang J, Hooke MC, et al. Psychometric and clinical assessment of the 13-item reduced version of the fatigue scale-adolescent instrument. *J Pediatr Oncol Nurs.* 2011;28(5):287–294.
65. Macpherson CF, Wang J, DeWalt DA, Stern ED, Jacobs S, Hinds PS. Comparison of legacy fatigue measures with the PROMIS Pediatric Fatigue Short Form. *Oncol Nurs Forum.* 2018;45(1):106–114.
66. Rogers VE, Zhu S, Ancoli-Israel S, Liu L, Mandrell BN, Hinds PS. A pilot randomized controlled trial to improve sleep and fatigue in children with central nervous system tumors hospitalized for high-dose chemotherapy. *Pediatr Blood Cancer.* 2019;66(8):e27814.
67. Varni JW, Burwinkle TM, Szer IS. The PedsQL Multidimensional Fatigue Scale in pediatric rheumatology: Reliability and validity. *J Rheumatol.* 2004;31(12):2494–2500.
68. Varni JW, Burwinkle TM, Katz ER, Meeske K, Dickinson P. The PedsQL in pediatric cancer: Reliability and validity of the Pediatric Quality of Life Inventory Generic Core Scales, Multidimensional Fatigue Scale, and Cancer Module. *Cancer.* 2002;94(7):2090–2106.
69. Lai JS, Cella D, Kupst MJ, et al. Measuring fatigue for children with cancer: Development and validation of the pediatric Functional Assessment of Chronic Illness Therapy-Fatigue (pedsFACIT-F). *J Pediatr Hematol Oncol.* 2007;29(7):471–479.
70. Irwin DE, Gross HE, Stucky BD, et al. Development of six PROMIS pediatrics proxy-report item banks. *Health Qual Life Outcomes.* 2012;10:22.
71. Irwin DE, Varni JW, Yeatts K, DeWalt DA. Cognitive interviewing methodology in the development of a pediatric item bank: A patient reported outcomes measurement information system (PROMIS) study. *Health Qual Life Outcomes.* 2009;7:3.
72. Hinds PS, Nuss SL, Ruccione KS, et al. PROMIS pediatric measures in pediatric oncology: Valid and clinically feasible indicators of patient-reported outcomes. *Pediatr Blood Cancer.* 2013;60(3):402–408.
73. DeWalt DA, Gross HE, Gipson DS, et al. PROMIS((R)) pediatric self-report scales distinguish subgroups of children within and across six common pediatric chronic health conditions. *Qual Life Res.* 2015;24(9):2195–2208.
74. Menard JC, Hinds PS, Jacobs SS, et al. Feasibility and acceptability of the patient-reported outcomes measurement information system measures in children and adolescents in active cancer treatment and survivorship. *Cancer Nurs.* 2014;37(1):66–74.
75. Reeve BB, Edwards LJ, Jaeger BC, et al. Assessing responsiveness over time of the PROMIS pediatric symptom and function measures in cancer, nephrotic syndrome, and sickle cell disease. *Qual Life Res.* 2018;27(1):249–257.
76. Reeve BB, McFatrich M, Mack JW, et al. Expanding construct validity of established and new PROMIS pediatric measures for children and adolescents receiving cancer treatment. *Pediatr Blood Cancer.* 2020:e28160.
77. Thissen D, Liu Y, Magnus B, et al. Estimating minimally important difference (MID) in PROMIS pediatric measures using the scale-judgment method. *Qual Life Res.* 2016;25(1):13–23.
78. McFatrich M, Brondon J, Lucas NR, et al. Mapping child and adolescent self-reported symptom data to clinician-reported adverse event grading to improve pediatric oncology care and research. *Cancer.* 2020;126(1):140–147.
79. Reeve BB, Withycombe JS, Baker JN, et al. The first step to integrating the child's voice in adverse event reporting in oncology trials: A content validation study among pediatric oncology clinicians. *Pediatr Blood Cancer.* 2013;60(7):1231–1236.
80. Reeve BB, McFatrich M, Pinheiro LC, et al. Eliciting the child's voice in adverse event reporting in oncology trials: Cognitive interview findings from the Pediatric Patient-Reported Outcomes version of the Common Terminology Criteria for Adverse Events initiative. *Pediatr Blood Cancer.* 2017;64(3).
81. Reeve BB, McFatrich M, Pinheiro LC, et al. Cognitive interview-based validation of the patient-reported outcomes version of the common terminology criteria for adverse events in adolescents with cancer. *J Pain Symptom Manage.* 2017;53(4):759–766.

82. Reeve BB, McFatrich M, Mack JW, et al. Validity and reliability of the pediatric patient-reported outcomes—common terminology criteria for adverse events. *J Natl Cancer Inst.* 2020;112(11):1143–1152.
83. Reeve BB, McFatrich M, Lin L, et al. Validation of the caregiver pediatric patient-reported outcomes version of the common terminology criteria for adverse events measure. *Cancer.* 2020;127(9):1483–1494.
84. Barsevick AM, Irwin MR, Hinds P, et al. Recommendations for high-priority research on cancer-related fatigue in children and adults. *J Natl Cancer Inst.* 2013;105(19):1432–1440.
85. Becher OJ, Millard NE, Modak S, et al. A phase I study of single-agent perifosine for recurrent or refractory pediatric CNS and solid tumors. *PLoS One.* 2017;12(6):e0178593.
86. Chuk MK, Widemann BC, Minard CG, et al. A phase 1 study of cabozantinib in children and adolescents with recurrent or refractory solid tumors, including CNS tumors: Trial ADVL1211, a report from the Children's Oncology Group. *Pediatr Blood Cancer.* 2018;65(8):e27077.
87. Hinds PS, Wang J, Stern ED, et al. Voices of children and adolescents on phase 1 or phase 2 cancer trials: A new trial endpoint? *Cancer.* 2017;123(19):3799–3806.
88. Hinds PS, Hockenberry M, Tong X, et al. Validity and reliability of a new instrument to measure cancer-related fatigue in adolescents. *J Pain Symptom Manage.* 2007;34(6):607–618.
89. Nagarajan R, Gerbing R, Alonzo T, et al. Quality of life in pediatric acute myeloid leukemia: Report from the Children's Oncology Group. *Cancer Med.* 2019;8(9):4454–4464.
90. Zhukovsky DS, Rozmus CL, Robert RS, et al. Symptom profiles in children with advanced cancer: Patient, family caregiver, and oncologist ratings. *Cancer.* 2015;121(22):4080–4087.
91. Vallance K, Liu W, Mandrell BN, et al. Mechanisms of dexamethasone-induced disturbed sleep and fatigue in paediatric patients receiving treatment for ALL. *Eur J Cancer.* 2010;46(10):1848–1855.
92. Colombo C, De Leo S, Di Stefano M, Vannucchi G, Persani L, Fugazzola L. Primary adrenal insufficiency during lenvatinib or vandetanib and improvement of fatigue after cortisone acetate therapy. *J Clin Endocrinol Metab.* 2019;104(3):779–784.
93. Hinds PS, Hockenberry M, Rai SN, et al. Nocturnal awakenings, sleep environment interruptions, and fatigue in hospitalized children with cancer. *Oncol Nurs Forum.* 2007;34(2):393–402.
94. Yeh CH, Chiang YC, Lin L, et al. Clinical factors associated with fatigue over time in paediatric oncology patients receiving chemotherapy. *Br J Cancer.* 2008;99(1):23–29.
95. Zordan R, Manitta V, Nandurkar H, Cole-Sinclair M, Philip J. Prevalence and predictors of fatigue in haemo-oncological patients. *Intern Med J.* 2014;44(10):1013–1017.
96. Hwang SS, Chang VT, Rue M, Kasimis B. Multidimensional independent predictors of cancer-related fatigue. *J Pain Symptom Manage.* 2003;26(1):604–614.
97. Bossola ADH, Lenaert B, Van Heugten CM, Gambaro G, Bossola M. Exploring the diurnal course of fatigue in patients on hemodialysis treatment and its relation with depressive symptoms and classical conditioning. *J Pain Symptom Manage.* 2019;57(5):890–898 e894.
98. Greeke EE, Chua AS, Healy BC, Rintell DJ, Chitnis T, Glanz BI. Depression and fatigue in patients with multiple sclerosis. *J Neurol Sci.* 2017;380:236–241.
99. Lewko A, Bidgood PL, Garrod R. Evaluation of psychological and physiological predictors of fatigue in patients with COPD. *BMC Pulm Med.* 2009;9:47.
100. Bower JE. The role of neuro-immune interactions in cancer-related fatigue: Biobehavioral risk factors and mechanisms. *Cancer.* 2019;125(3):353–364.
101. Maura LA, Malone S, Jaime-Lara R, Riegel B. A systematic review of biological mechanisms of fatigue in chronic illness. *Biol Res Nurs.* 2018;20(4):410–421.
102. Fagundes CP, Murray DM, Hwang BS, et al. Sympathetic and parasympathetic activity in cancer-related fatigue: More evidence for a physiological substrate in cancer survivors. *Psychoneuroendocrinology.* 2011;36(8):1137–1147.
103. Bower JE, Ganz PA, Aziz N. Altered cortisol response to psychologic stress in breast cancer survivors with persistent fatigue. *Psychosom Med.* 2005;67(2):277–280.
104. Hockenberry MJ, Hooke MC, Gregurich M, McCarthy K. Carnitine plasma levels and fatigue in children/adolescents receiving cisplatin, ifosfamide, or doxorubicin. *J Pediatr Hematol Oncol.* 2009;31(9):664–669.
105. Flowers E, Miaskowski C, Conley Y, et al. Differential expression of genes and differentially perturbed pathways associated with very high evening fatigue in oncology patients receiving chemotherapy. *Support Care Cancer.* 2018;26(3):739–750.
106. Hockenberry MJ, Moore IMK, Scheurer ME, et al. Influence of Nitrosative Stress on Fatigue During Childhood Leukemia Treatment. *Biol Res Nurs.* 2018;20(4):403–409.
107. Zupanec S, Jones H, McRae L, Papaconstantinou E, Weston J, Stremler R. A sleep hygiene and relaxation intervention for children with acute lymphoblastic leukemia: A pilot randomized controlled trial. *Cancer Nurs.* 2017;40(6):488–496.
108. Oberoi S, Robinson PD, Cataudella D, et al. Physical activity reduces fatigue in patients with cancer and hematopoietic stem cell transplant recipients: A systematic review and meta-analysis of randomized trials. *Crit Rev Oncol Hematol.* 2018;122:52–59.
109. Chang CW, Mu PF, Jou ST, Wong TT, Chen YC. The effectiveness of non-pharmacological interventions on fatigue in children and adolescents with cancer: A systematic review. *JBI Libr Syst Rev.* 2012;10(10):574–614.
110. Nunes MDR, Bomfim E, Olson K, et al. Interventions minimizing fatigue in children/adolescents with cancer: An integrative review. *J Child Health Care.* 2018;22(2):186–204.
111. Bogg TF, Broderick C, Shaw P, Cohn R, Naumann FL. Feasibility of an inpatient exercise intervention for children undergoing hematopoietic stem cell transplant. *Pediatr Transplant.* 2015;19(8):925–931.
112. Diorio C, Celis Ekstrand A, Hesser T, et al. Development of an individualized yoga intervention to address fatigue in hospitalized children undergoing intensive chemotherapy. *Integr Cancer Ther.* 2016;15(3):279–284.
113. Lam KKW, Li WHC, Chung OK, et al. An integrated experiential training programme with coaching to promote physical activity, and reduce fatigue among children with cancer: A randomised controlled trial. *Patient Educ Couns.* 2018;101(11):1947–1956.
114. Lopes-Junior LC, Bomfim EO, Nascimento LC, Nunes MD, Pereira-da-Silva G, Lima RA. Non-pharmacological interventions to manage fatigue and psychological stress in children and adolescents with cancer: An integrative review. *Eur J Cancer Care (Engl).* 2016;25(6):921–935.
115. Robinson PD, Oberoi S, Tomlinson D, et al. Management of fatigue in children and adolescents with cancer and in paediatric recipients of haemopoietic stem-cell transplants: A clinical practice guideline. *Lancet Child Adolesc Health.* 2018;2(5):371–378.
116. Bhardwaj T, Koffman J. Non-pharmacological interventions for management of fatigue among children with cancer: Systematic review of existing practices and their effectiveness. *BMJ Support Palliat Care.* 2017;7(4):404–414.
117. Duong N, Davis H, Robinson PD, et al. Mind and body practices for fatigue reduction in patients with cancer and hematopoietic stem cell transplant recipients: A systematic review and meta-analysis. *Crit Rev Oncol Hematol.* 2017;120:210–216.
118. Tomlinson D, Robinson PD, Oberoi S, et al. Pharmacologic interventions for fatigue in cancer and transplantation: A meta-analysis. *Curr Oncol.* 2018;25(2):e152–e167.
119. Wang J, Jacobs S, Dewalt DA, Stern E, Gross H, Hinds PS. A longitudinal study of PROMIS pediatric symptom clusters in children undergoing chemotherapy. *J Pain Symptom Manage.* 2018;55(2):359–367.

22 | SLEEP AND CIRCADIAN RHYTHMS

TOLUWALASE A. AJAYI, ERIC S. ZHOU, AND VALERIE E. ROGERS

Golden slumbers kiss your eyes,
Smiles awake you when you rise;
Sleep, pretty wantons, do not cry,
And I will sing a lullaby,
Rock them, rock them, lullaby.
Care is heavy, therefore sleep you,
You are care, and care must keep you;
Sleep, pretty wantons, do not cry,
And I will sing a lullaby,
Rock them, rock them, lullaby.

"Cradle Song," by Thomas Dekker

INTRODUCTION

Sleep is a biological necessity, a time of healing, mending, and restoration. Lack of restful sleep can affect daytime functioning, increase pain, promote mood disturbances, alter immune function, negatively impact developmental outcomes in children, and contribute to cardiovascular and metabolic disease.[1–3] Healthy, or robust, circadian rhythms, likewise, are increasingly recognized as important to good health.[4]

Sleep and circadian rhythm disturbances are common among children and adolescents, particularly among those with life-threatening illnesses. This chapter reviews normal sleep and circadian rhythms, and common sleep and circadian disturbances in children. It further discusses current evidence for sleep and circadian disturbances in children with common life-threatening illnesses. Finally, assessment and interdisciplinary management strategies for sleep and circadian rhythm disorders are discussed.

SLEEP AND CIRCADIAN RHYTHM PROBLEMS IN CHILDREN

Sleep is regulated by two independent processes. The first is the homeostatic sleep drive, wherein the longer one is awake, the stronger the drive to sleep becomes. Sleep needs vary by developmental age group, and daily sleep recommendations have been established (Table 22.1).[5] The second is the circadian timing system, which regulates the timing of diurnal physiological processes such as core body temperature, blood pressure, and hormone levels. Circadian rhythms are generated by clock genes controlled by the central circadian pacemaker in the hypothalamus. In contrast to the homeostatic sleep drive, the circadian timing system operates independently of time spent awake but can be modified by environmental cues (*zeitgebers*) such as light and noise exposure, physical and social activities, and food intake, with light being the most important.[6]

TABLE 22.1 Sleep recommendations by age group

AGE GROUP	RECOMMENDED 24-HOUR SLEEP DURATION
Newborns (0–3 months)	14–17 hours
Infants (4–11 months)	12–15 hours
Toddlers (1–2 years)	11–14 hours
Preschoolers (3–5 years)	10–13 hours
School-aged children (8–13 years)	9–11 hours
Teenagers (14–17 years)	8–10 hours
Young adults (18–25 years)	7–9 hours

Used with permission from Hirshkowitz M, Whiton K, Albert SM, et al. National Sleep Foundation's sleep time duration recommendations: Methodology and results summary. *Sleep Health.* 2015;1(1):40–43.

Sleep problems are common, reported in 20–50% of healthy children.[7] The most common pediatric sleep disorder is *insomnia*, affecting nearly one-third of children. It is characterized by persistent problems with sleep initiation, maintenance, or quality despite age-appropriate opportunity for sleep and that result in daytime impairment.[8] Behavioral insomnias are most common in children. They result from inadequate sleep training or caregiver difficulties with setting limits around sleep in younger children or from poor sleep hygiene habits such as excessive caffeine intake and use of electronic devices near bedtime in older children.[9] Insomnia can also co-occur with medical or psychiatric disorders due to sleep-disrupting symptoms such as pain, mood disorders or depression, or sleep-related breathing disorders (SRBDs).[10–12]

Parasomnias are undesirable events that occur when falling asleep or awakening from sleep (disorders of arousal) or during sleep. They involve bizarre sleep-related movements, behaviors and emotions.[8] Parasomnias affect about 13% of children and are typically outgrown by adolescence.[13] Although generally benign, they can result in injuries and further disrupted sleep, and their symptoms overlap those of nocturnal frontal lobe epilepsy.[13] Disorders of arousal are the most common parasomnias and include confusional arousals, sleep walking, and sleep terrors. Sleep terrors, the most striking of these, are characterized by sudden onset of screaming, intense fear, and autonomic activation (e.g., increased heart and respiratory rates). They are distinguished from nightmares in that they occur earlier in the sleep cycle, and these children exhibit significant motor activity, are difficult to awaken during the terror, and have little memory of it.[14]

SRBDs range from primary snoring (snoring without significant upper airway obstruction), to obstructive sleep apnea (OSA) or central sleep apnea. OSA involves intermittent partial (hypopneas) or complete (apneas) cessation of airflow during sleep despite continued respiratory effort due to collapse of the upper airway on inspiration. An obstructive apnea-hypopnea index (AHI) of 1 or more per hour is diagnostic of pediatric OSA.[8] Central nervous system (CNS)-mediated intermittent apneas without accompanying respiratory effort reflect central apneas and are diagnostic of central sleep apnea when the central AHI is 5 or more per hour.[8] Snoring occurs in about 12% of children[15] and OSA and central sleep apnea in about 5% each.[16,17] Both types of sleep apnea result in intermittent oxygen desaturations and sleep fragmentation.

Restless legs syndrome (RLS), or Willis-Ekbom disease, occurs in 2–4% of children. It is characterized by a strong urge to move affected limbs, accompanied by uncomfortable sensations in the limbs. Symptoms start or worsen during rest, are relieved with movement, and occur predominantly in the evening or at night.[8] In children, sleep disruption is commonly the presenting complaint.[18] Symptoms can occur in association with low iron stores, but are also seen in children with neurologically based disorders such as attention deficit-hyperactivity disorder and depression. The presence of periodic limb movements in sleep (PLMS)—episodes of repetitive, stereotyped movements of the limbs—are supportive of an RLS diagnosis but require polysomnography with limb electromyography for diagnosis.

Narcolepsy is a rare disorder characterized by an irresistible need to sleep or lapses into sleep during the day. Narcolepsy results from genetic and environmental factors,[19] but tumors, surgery, or radiation of the brain can also play a role. Narcolepsy is the most common cause of excessive daytime sleepiness (EDS), but other symptoms may be present such as disturbed sleep, hypnagogic hallucinations (vivid dreams occurring during sleep–wake transitions), and sleep paralysis (temporary inability to move at sleep–wake transitions). The presence of *cataplexy* (brief, sudden loss of muscle tone while maintaining consciousness) is the key feature distinguishing type 1 from type 2 narcolepsy.[8]

The most common circadian rhythm disorder in pediatrics is *delayed sleep–wake phase disorder*, with a prevalence of 3% in adolescents.[20] Hormonal changes and physiological lengthening of the circadian period during adolescence, as well as external factors such as academic and social demands, can delay bedtime and contribute to its development. Adolescents are typically unable to fall asleep before midnight and have difficulty waking in the morning to meet school and social obligations.[15] Delayed sleep–wake phase disorder is often confused with sleep onset insomnia. Importantly, it is highly associated with depression.[21]

SLEEP AND CIRCADIAN RHYTHM PROBLEMS IN CHILDREN WITH LIFE-THREATENING ILLNESSES

Sleep disturbances are among the most commonly reported symptoms in pediatric palliative care (PPC) patients. However, the complex clinical presentations of many of these children, and the frequency of life-threatening symptoms may be so overwhelming to providers that problematic sleep may easily be dismissed as less important[22] or may not be recognized.[23] Current evidence for sleep and circadian disorders in children with several life-threatening illnesses is presented. Table 22.2 presents definitions for sleep terms and normal values.

CANCER

Cancer, its treatment, and its late effects all impact the regulation of sleep and circadian rhythms. Children experience a high level of sleep fragmentation, demonstrated by frequent nighttime awakenings and daytime naps, and catch-up sleep on weekends in response to chronic sleep loss on school days (referred to as *social jet lag*).[24,25] Problems initiating and maintaining sleep have been described,[26] with insomnia reported by 24% of a sample of children with mixed tumors and 39% of those with leukemia.[27] Studies exploring symptoms of children during the last week or month of life, or children with advanced cancer, found that changes in sleep patterns or insomnia were among the most commonly reported problems.[28,29] Even still, medical teams referring children for

TABLE 22.2 Definition of sleep terms

SLEEP TERMS	DEFINITION
Actigraph	Wrist-worn device that records movement and estimates sleep and wake variables via algorithms using activity counts downloaded from the actigraph.
Awakenings	Number of episodes of wake during sleep. By actigraphy, duration of an awakening is usually ≥5 minutes; fewer than 4 per night indicates good quality sleep.
Sleep efficiency (SE)	Percent of time a person actually slept versus how long they tried to sleep; 85% or more indicates good quality sleep.
Sleep onset latency (SOL)	Time from bedtime to sleep onset; less than 30 minutes indicates good quality sleep.
Sleep quality	Reflects the soundness of sleep. Frequent awakenings or low SE result in sleep fragmentation and decreased sleep quality.
Total sleep time (TST)	Amount of sleep achieved between nighttime sleep onset and final morning awakening.
Wake after sleep onset (WASO)	Time spent awake between sleep onset and final awakening; 20 minutes or less indicates good quality sleep.

Parameters for good quality sleep from Ohayon M, Wickwire EM, Hirschkowitz M, et al. National Sleep Foundation's sleep quality recommendations: first report. *Sleep Health*. 2017;3(1):6–19.

palliative care consults significantly underdiagnose less clinically evident symptoms, including sleep disturbances.[23]

Among the most frequent sleep-related problems are EDS and hypersomnolence.[27] Children with CNS tumors report significantly higher somnolence than children with other types of cancer,[26,30] and childhood brain tumor survivors have a prevalence of hypersomnia/narcolepsy up to 80 times higher than the general population.[31] Among children and young adults with advanced cancer receiving palliative care, EDS was one of the most common and distressing symptoms, reported by 59%, with few differences by gender, age, ethnicity, or tumor type.[28,29,32]

SRBDs have gained recognition as sleep disorders in children with cancer. One study reported that 40% of a sample of children with mixed tumor types had symptoms of SRBDs, which increased to 46% in children with tumors of the hypothalamus, thalamus, or brainstem, areas of the brain responsible for sleep and respiratory control.[27]

Circadian rhythm disturbances have been little studied in children with cancer, unlike in the adult cancer population. In a sample of children with mixed tumor types, 4% had a circadian rhythm disorder,[27] while circadian activity rhythms measured by actigraphy became dysregulated during dexamethasone therapy in children with acute lymphoblastic leukemia.[33]

SICKLE CELL DISEASE

Children with sickle cell disease (SCD) and parents reporting on their children have reported frequent nighttime awakenings and poor quality sleep by questionnaire or sleep diary.[34,35] More than one-third of adolescents have reported moderate or severe sleep disturbances, and 18% required a sleeping medication at least three times per week.[36] Symptoms of insomnia are also common, with 29–50% reporting difficult or delayed sleep onset.[34–36] Studies using objective measures have also identified suboptimal sleep quality and duration in children with SCD.[37,38]

Parasomnias are common, with a prevalence of 16% reported for night terrors, 27% for sleep talking, and 25% for nightmares,[34] and an overall prevalence of parasomnias of 26%.[39] Symptoms of RLS are also common, although underrecognized.[34,40,41] EDS with accompanying daytime dysfunction has been reported by 60% of children with SCD and 70% of parents reporting on their child.[42]

Children with SCD have a high prevalence of SRBDs, with snoring reported in up to 54%.[34,43] OSA is also common, ranging from 11% in children with sickle cell anemia[44] to 41% in children with SCD recruited without regard to SRDB status.[43]

NEUROMUSCULAR DISORDERS

Disease-related respiratory muscle weakness and decreased ventilatory responses common in neuromuscular disorders and associated obesity, scoliosis, and chest wall and upper airway abnormalities predispose to the development of SRBDs (OSA, central sleep apnea, nocturnal hypoxemia, and hypoventilation).[22,45] Their prevalence exceeds 40%.[46] Children with neuromuscular disorders who also have untreated SRBDs are at higher risk of developing complications of SRBDs compared to the general population. These include neurocognitive deficits, cardiac and metabolic dysfunction, and pulmonary hypertension.[47] SRBDs in Duchenne muscular dystrophy has a bimodal presentation, with OSA most common during the first decade of life and hypoventilation more common in the second decade. Among children and adolescents, 65% reported sleep-related symptoms (snoring, sleep disturbance) and 24% reported daytime symptoms[48] including EDS, fatigue, and headaches.[45]

Prader-Willi syndrome is characterized by increased fat mass, hypotonia, appetite dysregulation, behavioral difficulties, and endocrinopathies, all of which predispose to sleep disorders. Compared to age- and sex-matched controls, these children demonstrate shorter sleep onset latency (SOL), higher wake after sleep onset (WASO), and higher EDS.[49] SRBDs include nocturnal hypoxemia, hypoventilation, central sleep apnea, and OSA, which has a prevalence in these children of 80%.[50] Respiratory failure during illness is the most common cause of death, with sleep apnea considered the likely cause of most deaths.[51]

HUMAN IMMUNODEFICIENCY VIRUS

Human immunodeficiency virus (HIV)-related sleep disturbances have been well studied in adults but are less well described in children. HIV-infected children experience significantly less total sleep time (TST), more WASO, lower sleep efficiency (SE), and more frequent awakenings during sleep than noninfected children,[52] as well as significantly more EDS.[53] A high prevalence of insomnia (20%) was identified in HIV-infected adolescents and was significantly associated with age, fatigue, depression, and anxiety.[54] Adolescents also reported significantly higher scores on a SRBDs questionnaire compared to noninfected peers,[53] while 4 of 11 HIV-infected adolescents who underwent polysomnography had an AHI of 1 per hour or greater.[55]

CYSTIC FIBROSIS

While the prevalence of sleep disturbances in children with cystic fibrosis is unknown, they are common due to disease-related factors such as nocturnal hypoxemia, cough, SRBDs, medications, and pain.[56–58] On average, children with cystic fibrosis experience more frequent and longer nighttime awakenings, lower SE, longer SOL, and more WASO.[57–61] Symptoms of insomnia are common, with 43% of children reporting problems with sleep onset and 39% reporting sleep maintenance problems,[60] while insomnia was reported by 38% of adolescents.[62] EDS has been reported at a prevalence of 48–74%.[60,63]

Children have a high prevalence of SRBDs, including snoring in 30–58% and witnessed apneas in 88%.[59,60] Shorter TST, lower SE, higher WASO, and more frequent awakenings during the night were associated with more severe lung disease,[57,60] while lower nocturnal oxygen saturation (SpO_2) was associated with poorer lung function and structural lung changes.[64] This is important, as progressive decline in lung function and recurrent lung infections lead to respiratory failure, the most common cause of death.

HEART DISEASE

Among children and adolescents with heart disease, only half achieve at least 8 hours of sleep per night, and adolescents report significant social jet lag, with only 18% reporting 8 hours or more of sleep on school nights versus 79% on weekends. TST did not differ by presence or absence of heart failure or by illness severity.[65] Adolescents and young adults with an implanted cardiodefibrillator report more trouble falling asleep, restless/disturbed sleep, and early morning awakenings compared to a normative sample.[66]

Most studies of children with heart disease have focused on respiratory-related sleep disorders, reporting lower mean and nadir SpO_2 and greater sleep time with SpO_2 of less than 90% in children with congenital heart diseases compared to healthy children.[67,68] In a study of infants with congenital heart disease, three-quarters were found to have an AHI of 1 per hour or more,[67] while among children with clinically stable primary cardiomyopathy aged 1 month to 18 years, 9 out of 10 had an obstructive AHI of 1 per hour or more. A central AHI of 5 per hour or more on polysomnography was found in 5 of 10 children, and central sleep apnea was associated with severity of cardiac dysfunction.[69]

CHRONIC KIDNEY DISEASE

Sleep disturbances in chronic kidney disease (CKD) are caused by a variety of disease-related factors including stress, pain, malnutrition, anemia, reduced airway muscle tone, and upper airway edema.[70] Among nondialyzed children with CKD, 39% of whom were post-renal transplant with a stable graft, 10% reported insomnia and 37% had a sleep disorder.[71] One-quarter of children and adolescents on either peritoneal dialysis or hemodialysis slept less than 7 hours per night, and 86% endorsed sleep disturbing symptoms,[72] with greater sleep disturbance associated with lower quality of life.[73] Children on hemodialysis for end-stage renal failure reported significantly more nighttime awakenings and difficult morning arousals, and a greater need for sleeping medications than age- and sex-matched controls; they also achieved significantly less deep sleep and more arousals on polysomnography.[74]

One of the most common sleep disorders in children with CKD is RLS. Prevalence of RLS symptoms vary from 10% in children recruited regardless of dialysis or transplant status, to 30% in children on either peritoneal dialysis or hemodialysis, and 35% in children most of whom had mild CKD.[71–73] Importantly, only one-quarter of children with CKD and RLS had reported their symptoms to their healthcare provider.[75] EDS was reported by parents of 12% of children with CKD who were not dialysis-dependent,[71] while 46% of children studied without regard to their dialysis or transplant status reported EDS or presence of daytime napping.[73]

Studies of SRBDs in children with CKD are limited. Snoring has been reported in 46% of children on dialysis,[72] while SRBDs were identified in 6% of nondialysis-dependent children with CKD[71] and in 23% of children with CKD regardless of dialysis or transplant status.[73]

ENVIRONMENTAL AND PSYCHOSOCIAL FACTORS RELATED TO SLEEP PROBLEMS

Identifying factors that influence sleep must move beyond individual-based models and examine sleep within a larger environmental context. Environments that promote a sense of safety and security also promote longer and higher quality sleep (Figure 22.1). Mental health, home and family dynamics, electronic media use, nutrition/diet, and hospital setting are discussed separately here, yet each of these factors is interrelated.

MENTAL HEALTH

Fear, anxiety, depression, or anger at bedtime make it difficult for a child to transition to sleep at bedtime and at subsequent awakenings throughout the night. Children may

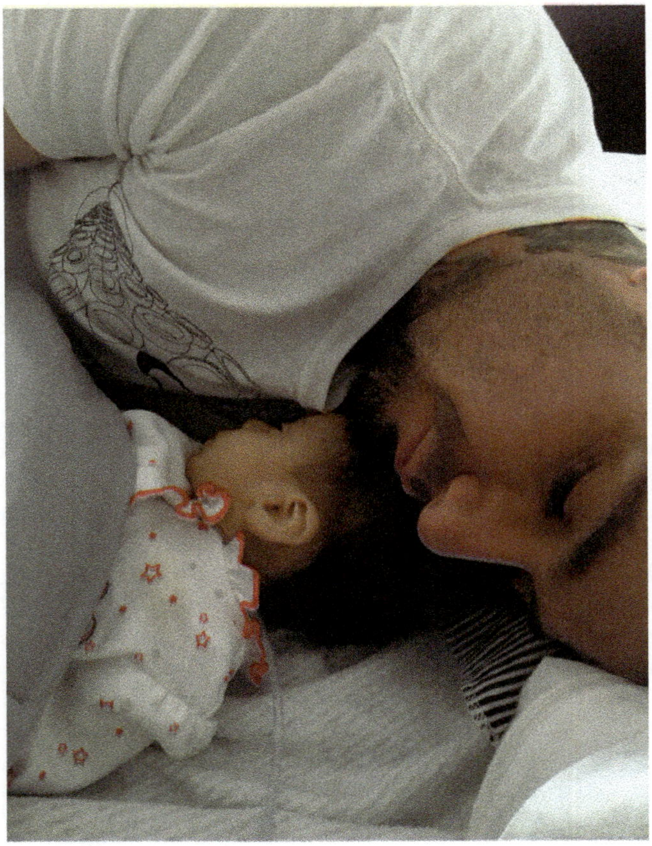

Figure 22.1 *Patient finding peace and security in the arms of her family as she sleeps.* Used with family permission.

worry about their health, their situation, and fears of the dark compounded by legitimate fears of death. For the transition to sleep to be smooth, a child must feel safe. Adolescents with a life-threatening illness also have concerns about growing up and planning for the future, combined with a grief relating to multiple losses including friendships, physical appearance, and modification of future aspirations. Supportive communication with their parents may be lacking, and, as a consequence, adolescents may remain awake in bed trying to deal with poorly understood anxieties.[76]

Research and clinical experience support a relationship between childhood sleep problems and anxiety or other alterations in mood. Even modest sleep restriction results in difficulties regulating emotions and subsequent elevations in anxiety and depression. As many as 83% of anxious children experience significant sleep disturbance.[77] Difficulty falling asleep, refusing to sleep alone, and nightmares are common in children with anxiety, along with reduced TST on school nights, frequent nighttime awakening, and decreased deep sleep.[76] Children who require a high level of parental involvement at bedtime are more likely to have problems with nighttime awakenings and vice versa.[78] Thus, the interaction between anxiety, sleep problems, and parent–child bedtime interactions may be particularly complex in the palliative care context.

Sleep disturbances are reported in up to 90% of adolescents with major depression.[79] Among young people, depression is associated with symptoms of insomnia, with polysomnography studies identifying reduced TST, longer SOL, and shorter latency to rapid eye movement (REM) sleep.[80] Poor sleep quality and EDS are also frequently reported. Increasingly, there is evidence of a bidirectional relationship between sleep and emotional and behavioral functioning.

HOME AND FAMILY DYNAMICS

Multiple aspects of family functioning in families of children with serious illness have been linked with child sleep problems. Taking care of a seriously or chronically ill child is one of the most difficult tasks a parent can endure, leading to extreme physical and emotional stress. Stress can lead to disturbed sleep of the primary caregiver, which can then affect the sleep of the child.[81] The reciprocal nature of the child–parent sleep relationship has been well-studied, such that children's sleep problems predict parent mental well-being, and parent sleep problems predict children's behavior and functioning.[82,83]

Family chaos can also impact the seriously ill child's sleep. Family chaos is defined as family disorganization and environments that are unstructured, pressured for time, noisy, and unpredictable—themes commonly experienced when a child is diagnosed with a serious illness. Depending on illness severity and chronicity, there can also be significant employment and financial consequences[84] contributing to the sense of instability and leading to sustained family disorganization. Stressful family environments, lack of parental rules, and family conflict are all associated with sleep problems in children and adolescents.[85] High levels of family disorganization debilitate children from developing stable sleep onset and good quality sleep.[85,86]

ELECTRONIC MEDIA

Children and adolescents are growing up in a technological age, with 75% of children having electronic screen-based devices in their bedrooms and 60% of adolescents interacting with screens in the hour before bedtime.[87,88] Research is emerging on how blue light emitted by electronic devices contributes to hyperarousal and decreased sleepiness at bedtime.[89] Presence of a television and or computer/electronic gaming console in a child's or adolescent's bedroom has been related to delayed bedtimes, shorter time in bed and TST, increased bedtime resistance, sleep anxiety, parasomnias, more SRBDs and higher overall sleep disturbance.[90] This is particularly relevant in children receiving home-based hospice or palliative care, where the living room may become their bedroom to provide space to accommodate medical equipment.

NUTRITION/DIET

Malnutrition and poor nutrition are common complications in infants and children with serious illnesses including heart disease, metabolic disorders, and cancer. Concerns of poor caloric or protein delivery and loss of ability to orally feed tend to center around growth, neurodevelopment, and family distress, but nutrition is also a significant factor in sleep. Research is emerging on how dietary patterns and specific foods impact sleep. Some studies, for example, highlight a potential effect of macronutrients on sleep, particularly alterations in slow wave sleep (deep sleep) and REM sleep with changes in carbohydrate and fat intakes.[91]

Caffeine, alcohol, and tobacco can also lead to sleep disturbances. Higher caffeine intake, occurring as early as 12 years of age, is associated with shorter TST, and increased SOL, WASO, and EDS.[92] Alcohol, tobacco, and cannabis use are not uncommon in adolescents living with serious illness, and their use is well-documented in adolescent cancer survivors and those with active disease.[93,94] Large quantities of alcohol before falling asleep leads to decreased SOL early in the night when blood alcohol levels are high, with subsequent disrupted, poor-quality sleep later in the night as blood alcohol levels fall.[95]

HOSPITAL SETTING

Reasons for disturbed sleep in the hospital are multifactorial. A systematic review of sleep in hospitalized pediatric cancer patients found that noise, light levels, and staff interruptions were associated with decreased TST and increased nighttime awakenings.[96] Additionally, as the complexity of a child's illness increases, their sleep becomes increasingly fragmented, with increased awakenings.[97] Parents report sleep disruptions by nighttime nursing care such as vital signs, intravenous medications and procedures, and by sequelae of treatment such as nausea and vomiting, diarrhea, fever, and trips to the bathroom (Figure 22.2).[98] Children admitted to intensive care lost up to 50% of their usual sleep time.[99] In children with CNS tumors hospitalized for high-dose chemotherapy, only half achieved the recommended TST for age, and the longest continuous sleep period averaged 88 minutes,[98] about the length of a single sleep cycle. Changes in sleep in young children persisted for up to 7 weeks after discharge from intensive care.[100] Circadian rhythms can also become severely dysregulated during hospitalization.[101]

Persistent/recurrent pain is also common among children with serious illnesses, and poor sleep is a common comorbidity, with a bidirectional relationship between the two.[102,103] Approximately half of pediatric patients with pain reported disturbed sleep, with pain frequently associated with

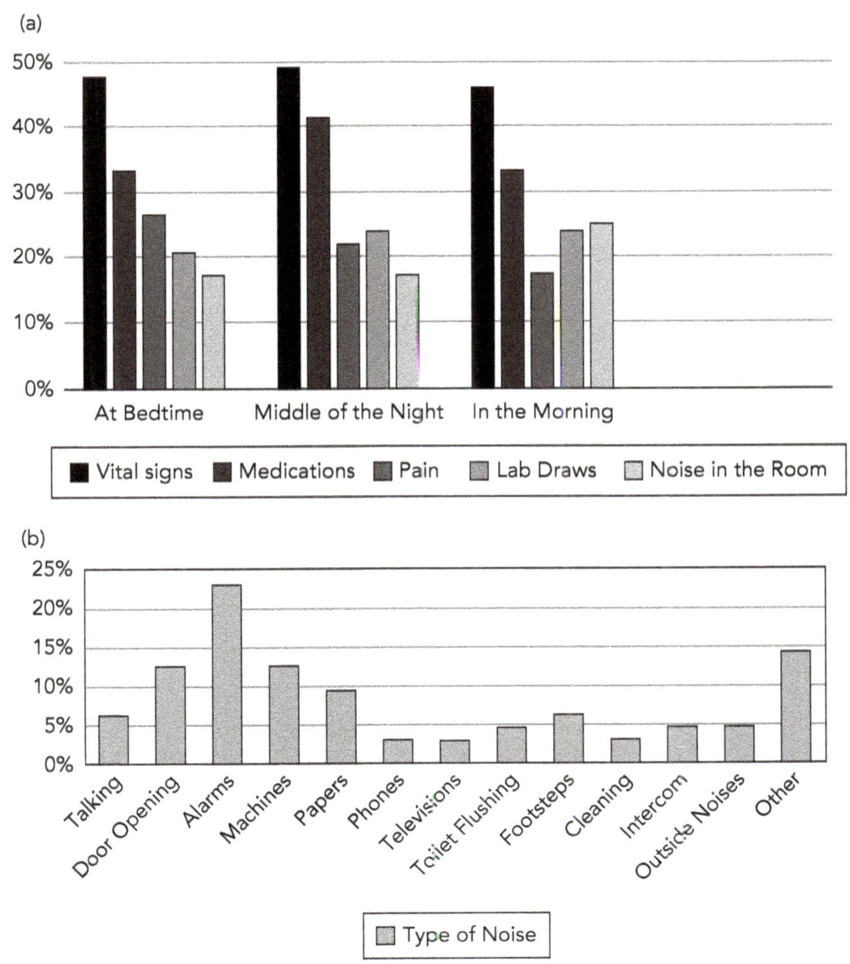

Figure 22.2 Timing of hospital staff activities that wake children or keep them awake (panel A) and types of noises that disturb their sleep (panel B). Reproduced with permission from Crawford S., et al. Quality of sleep in a pediatric hospital. *J Nurs Adm.* 2019;49(5):273–279.

sleep-onset and sleep maintenance difficulties, increased cognitive and somatic arousal at bedtime, difficulty awakening in the morning, higher EDS, and poorer sleep quality compared to healthy peers.[104] Parents able to stay with their children during hospitalization have identified poor sleep as a significant additional burden to their child's hospital admission.[99]

ASSESSMENT

Assessment of sleep and circadian health in children requires consideration of a patient's physical, psychological, social, economic, and environmental health. Because of the medical complexities of a child with a serious illness and increased risk for developing sleep problems, all children in the palliative care setting should be screened for sleep and circadian disturbances initially and at regular intervals, asking open-ended questions rather than specifying sleep concerns presumed to be present. The following domains are important to include.

The chief sleep/circadian complaint(s) should be elicited from the patient and family early in the interview. The typical sleep–wake patterns of the child and differences between week days and weekends should be identified, including usual bedtimes/wake times, SOL, frequency and length of nighttime awakenings, need for an alarm clock to awaken, and timing/length of naps, if taken. Sleep opportunity is also important. Patients engaged in ongoing medical care while attending school and engaging in extracurricular activities may not have sufficient sleep opportunity. Daytime consequences of sleep/circadian disruptions can include child-, caregiver-, or teacher-reported difficulty concentrating, EDS, fatigue, or mood disturbances.

Environmental factors may also exacerbate poor sleep. Inquire about the age and comfort of the child's mattress and bedding, and noise and light levels at bedtime and over the course of the night. Explore events leading up to bedtime (e.g., RLS symptoms) or during the night (e.g., SRBDs, parasomnias) that might disrupt sleep. Electronic devices in the bedroom can distract from sleep, and blue light emitted from screens can disrupt melatonin production.

Medical and psychiatric comorbidities and their treatments should be explored to assess their impact on sleep, including a thorough review of medications (prescribed, over the counter, and herbal supplements). Among children who are hospitalized, 3–6% are prescribed medication for sleep.[105] Use of these medications may persist after discharge, without clear instructions for discontinuation. Finally, sleep disorders such as insomnia are potentially heritable,[106] therefore inquiries should include sleep disorders among family members and the interventions used by them that are deemed most effective.

If time constraints preclude a thorough sleep evaluation, use of screening instruments, such as the BEARS, can be helpful.[107] BEARS stands for Bedtime issues, Excessive daytime sleepiness, night Awakenings, Regularity and duration of sleep, and Snoring. Age-appropriate questions are presented in each domain. This tool was shown to increase the amount of sleep information gathered and the likelihood of identifying sleep problems in the pediatric primary care setting. Other questionnaires are available although not all have undergone adequate psychometric evaluation.[108]

Sleep diaries can be a useful assessment tool. Diaries should include bedtime, SOL, frequency/duration of nighttime awakenings, morning wake time, and length and timing of daytime naps.[109] They are most helpful for screening for sleep disorders such as insomnia, which are based on subjective perception rather than objective assessments. Actigraphy is useful in assessing sleep–wake patterns over time, although disagreement with sleep diaries in pediatric populations is not unusual.[110] Polysomnography is typically recommended to evaluate SRBDs and certain parasomnias (e.g., to rule out nocturnal seizures).[111]

Finally, it is worth noting that caregivers of children who are seriously ill often struggle with sleep, too. It is important to help them understand how their poor sleep can influence their ability to provide care and how they, too, may benefit from intervention.

MANAGEMENT

NONPHARMACOLOGIC

Nonpharmacologic management of sleep disturbances should be informed by a comprehensive assessment of the child's sleep and daytime functioning, their family's response to this sleep, and ongoing or previous treatments (e.g., behavioral strategies, medications). Several evidence-based intervention strategies can be used to improve sleep onset, continuity, and quality. *Extinction* is principled in reducing reinforcement, in the form of parental attention, of a child's inappropriate bedtime behaviors (e.g., repeatedly getting out of bed). Unmodified or graded extinction techniques can be used.[112] This approach is typically not recommended for children who are under 6 months of age, are ill or need close monitoring. Another technique involves establishing a *consistent bedtime routine* (e.g., bath, pajamas, read story, say prayers, get tucked in). Consistent routines immediately preceding bedtime have been shown to improve a range of sleep outcomes in children.[113] A third technique, establishing *consistent sleep/wake times*, can improve sleep consistency. Extending sleep on weekends or after a poor night of sleep can further delay bedtime. Total sleep opportunity should be appropriate for age.[5]

Cognitive-behavioral therapy for insomnia is the gold standard treatment for insomnia in adults, with limited trials in pediatric populations.[114] Multiple components are implemented simultaneously. Among these are *sleep restriction*, or restricting the sleep period to increase sleep drive; *stimulus control*, or controlling stimuli that prevent sleep onset (e.g., associating the bedroom with activities other than sleep); *cognitive restructuring*, or therapy to restructure dysfunctional beliefs that maintain insomnia (e.g., catastrophizing the consequences of insomnia); *sleep hygiene* measures (e.g., regular bedtimes/wake times, limited napping, avoiding caffeine late in the day); and *relaxation techniques* (e.g., meditation, yoga, massage, psychotherapy, etc.).

Adolescents who present with circadian rhythm disturbances such as delayed sleep–wake phase disorder can benefit from approaches that reset their circadian timing. These include morning bright light therapy[115] using a commercial light box with or without evening melatonin supplementation, or gradual advancement of sleep and wake times.

The evidence base for integrative and complementary therapies for symptom management is limited in PPC,[116,117] and even fewer studies examine sleep as an outcome.[117–119] Integrative and complementary therapies are, nevertheless, used by families of children with serious illnesses, including 31–84% of children with cancer.[120] Several, including massage,[113] yoga,[121] acupuncture,[122] and mindfulness-based stress reduction[123] have been helpful for symptom management, which could in turn improve sleep.

As mentioned, hospitalized children face medical and environmental challenges disruptive to sleep. Considering ways in which the hospital team can work together with families to reduce their impact on a child's sleep is essential element to a comprehensive intervention strategy.[124] Measures could be implemented during hospitalization to protect sleep and promote healthy circadian rhythms such as continuing home bedtime routines, limiting evening noise and light exposure, establishing protected sleep periods, providing adequate medical management of sleep-disrupting symptoms, and promoting daytime light exposure and social activities to the extent children are able.[98] See Table 22.3 for other interdisciplinary strategies.

PHARMACOLOGIC

Clinical trials for pharmacological management of most sleep disorders in children are lacking, thus recommendations

TABLE 22.3 Interdisciplinary contributions to improving children's sleep

DISCIPLINE	DISCIPLINE SPECIFIC CONTRIBUTION	OVERLAPPING CONTRIBUTIONS
Medicine	Assess for underlying medical conditions. Collaborate with/referral to other providers, such as a sleep specialist. Collaborate with family physician(s) for management of sleep problems of parents or siblings. Prescribe medications to assist sleep and manage symptoms. Advanced practice nurses assume some roles.	Monitor poor sleep as a symptom and provide empathetic support during ongoing assessment. Avoid prescription of medications at nighttime that disrupt sleep, where possible. Avoid painful and fearful procedures around bedtime and in the room in which the child sleeps where possible. Ensure required observations (e.g., vital signs) maximize comfort and sleep, minimize light and noise at night. Provide emotional and spiritual support, including active listening and focusing on the patient, and maximize family's strengths. Provide information and brochures on the importance of sleep and how it can be improved. Provide practical assistance and equipment, such as a suitable hospital bed, blankets, pillows. Wake patients at night only when essential, and incorporate protected sleep periods with no interruptions. Referral to community agencies and supports. Flexibility to allow different sleeping arrangements (e.g., co-sleeping), particularly during end-of-life care. Collaborative effort to promote continuation of home bedtime routines in the hospital as closely as possible.
Nursing	Work collaboratively with other team members to implement and evaluate treatment in home, hospice or hospital settings. Provide care in a hospital or hospice setting or at home including after-hours support by telephone. Administer prescribed sleep-related medications as needed, and in conjunction with behavioral sleep measures and protected sleep time. Offer the patient measures designed to assist sleep: • Environment: lighting, temperature • Diet: healthy snacks, avoidance of caffeine • Quiet activities: relaxation, music, reading a story.	
Psychosocial	Supportive counseling for patient and family. Evidence-based management of pain, anxiety, depression resulting from/comorbid with the illness. Adjustment to physical deterioration and psychological distress associated with end-of-life phase of illness. Bereavement care to the family and siblings, including anticipatory care before death of the child.	
Behavioral sleep medicine	Comprehensive sleep evaluation. Psycho-education about sleep. Cognitive-behavioral therapy for insomnia.	
Child life	Connect patients and families with expressive therapies (such as music, art, play). Provide access to developmentally appropriate media for expression of emotions such as fear and anxiety (such as use of a worry doll).	
Allied health	Physiotherapy: assist with mobility and activity, including exercise. Occupational therapy: Equipment, relaxation or mindfulness-based techniques, therapeutic play. Speech pathology: Communication.	
Integrative care	Implement interventions such as massage, yoga, acupuncture, mindfulness techniques or other.	

TABLE 22.4 Pharmacological management of sleep problems

MEDICATION (CLASS)	USES	RECOMMENDED DOSE	ADDITIONAL NOTES
Clonazepam (benzodiazepine)	Insomnia PLMS RLS	0.1–0.75 mg; maximum 0.2 mg/kg/ dose or 1 mg total dose	Increases TST, REM latency, slow-wave (deep) sleep; decreases awakenings, PLMS. Associated with daytime sleepiness, rebound insomnia. Requires dose taper. Most commonly used in adolescents, or in children with neurodevelopmental disorders with RLS/PLMS.
Clonidine (alpha-2 agonist)	Insomnia	25–50 mcg at bedtime; maximum dose 10 mcg/kg/day or weight-based maximum dose	Decreases SOL, REM sleep; increases slow wave sleep. Tolerance can develop. Requires dose taper to prevent hypertensive rebound.
Diphenhydramine (antihistamine)	Insomnia	0.5 mg/kg; maximum dose 25 mg	Small decrease in SOL, TST. Paradoxical arousals can occur. Tolerance can develop. Evidence for efficacy conflicting.
Gabapentin (anticonvulsant)	Insomnia PLMS RLS	3–7.5 mg/kg, 30–45 min before bedtime; maximum dose 15 mg/kg	Increases slow wave sleep and SE, decreases WASO, awakenings. At higher doses, difficulty falling asleep, agitated nighttime awakenings.
Melatonin (hormone, chronobiotic)	Insomnia Circadian disorders	Sedation: 1–3 mg, 30–60 min before bedtime; typical maximum dose 10 mg Chronobiotic: 0.3–0.5 mg 5–6 hours before bedtime	Used as sedative, decreases SOL, TST, WASO. Most effective in children with autism/ neurodevelopmental disorders. Used as chronobiotic, can advance sleep–wake cycle. Tolerance can develop. Not regulated by FDA; concentrations may differ from label.
Ramelteon (synthetic selective melatonin agonist)	Insomnia Circadian disorders	2–8 mg	Reliable melatonin concentration. Case reports only: decreases SOL, awakenings.
Trazodone (atypical antidepressant)	Insomnia	1 mg/kg; up to 25 mg in children ≥3 years and 50 mg in adolescents	Most commonly prescribed in children with comorbid mood/anxiety disorders. Increases TST, decreases awakenings. Effectiveness appears unrelated to dose, low doses may be effective. Risk for QT prolongation.

FDA, US Food and Drug Administration; kg, kilogram; mcg, microgram; mg, milligram; PLMS, periodic limb movements in sleep; RLS, restless legs syndrome; SE, sleep efficiency; SOL, sleep onset latency; TST, total sleep time; WASO, wake after sleep onset.

Information compiled from reviews of pharmacological management of pediatric sleep disorders discussed in this chapter. Consultation with a clinical pharmacist for patient-specific dosing is recommended.

discussed here and in Table 22.4 are based on expert opinion.[9,125–127]

No sleep medication is approved by the US Food and Drug Administration (FDA) for treatment of insomnia in children. Therefore, a stepwise approach to treatment should be used that includes good nutrition and sleep hygiene measures, behavioral interventions to improve sleep, appropriate management of sleep disruptors such as pain and anxiety, and sleep medications used as an adjunct to nonpharmacological measures for acute sleep disturbances or when those measures alone fail to improve sleep. Medications should be used at the lowest effective dose for the shortest possible duration. The most common medications and supplements used to promote sleep in children are discussed here.

Melatonin is considered the first-line agent. Its safety and efficacy in improving SOL, TST, and WASO have been demonstrated in children.[127–129] It is also useful for advancing the circadian phase in adolescents with delayed sleep phase disorder.[130] Side effects are generally mild (e.g., morning drowsiness, headache) and resolve within a few days. Melatonin can potentially decrease blood pressure and serum glucose levels, so children concurrently taking medications that affect these levels should be monitored.[131] Newer prescription melatonin receptor agonists such as ramelteon provide reliable dosing. Studies of use of ramelteon in children are currently limited to case series, but outcomes are encouraging, with only mild side effects.[127]

First-generation antihistamines, particularly diphenhydramine, are the most prescribed medications for pediatric insomnia,[132,133] due to their sedating effect, familiarity to pediatric prescribers, and over-the-counter availability. However, side effects are common, including impaired consciousness and paradoxical arousal, and studies have not consistently demonstrated their effectiveness.[127,128] Therefore, antihistamines are not recommended as first-line therapy.

Benzodiazepines are commonly used to treat insomnia in adults and have been used in clinical practice to treat pediatric insomnia, particularly in adolescents. Clonazepam is the most commonly prescribed medication in this class for children.[132,133] Small studies in children have shown improvement in nighttime awakenings and daytime behavior. However, the muscle relaxing properties of benzodiazepines can limit their use in seriously ill children. Use of clonazepam may be appropriate in children with movement arousal sleep disorders (e.g., RLS or PLMS), but side effects such as EDS and withdrawal symptoms can be significant.

Other prescription medications for pediatric insomnia that have demonstrated preliminary safety and efficacy in pediatric case series are clonidine, trazodone, and gabapentin.[127] Non-benzodiazepine sedative-hypnotics, such as zolpidem, have not shown efficacy in pediatric clinical trials and have a high side effect profile (e.g., parasomnias, daytime sedation) so their use is discouraged.[127] Chloral hydrate is contraindicated in children due to its side effect of respiratory depression and increased risk of sleep apnea.

As a disorder of iron metabolism, RLS symptoms are common in PPC populations. Children may be sensitive to low iron or ferritin levels and become symptomatic with levels in the low normal range. Oral iron repletion has been used as an effective treatment for RLS/PLMS symptoms[134] and may also improve sleep.[135] In adults with RLS, dopamine agonists are effective treatment, although limited clinical data exist for children. Gabapentin, likewise, has been used clinically to treat RLS in children.[136] These medications may be considered when distressing symptoms are not managed with iron therapy and nonpharmacological interventions such as good sleep hygiene, exercise, and avoidance of caffeine and nicotine.

Several life-threatening illnesses place children at high risk for SRBDs. Adenotonsillectomy is the gold standard treatment for pediatric OSA. Continuous positive airway pressure therapy (CPAP) is second-line therapy where adenotonsillectomy is ineffective or inappropriate, as in children on hospice care, but compliance is poor. Some evidence suggests that nasal steroids may reduce the AHI.[137,138] Montelukast, alone or as adjunct to nasal steroids, reduces adenoid size and AHI with limited side effects.[138] These options can be beneficial for short-term pharmacological management of mild OSA, although are unlikely to adequately treat more severe OSA.

Critical in managing sleep disturbances in children with serious illnesses are ongoing conversations between the healthcare team and families to establish goals of care.[139] As exemplified in Box 22.1, caregivers (or children themselves) may have goals for sleep that differ from that of team members. Important in helping patients and families establish appropriate goals is presenting the realm of possibilities for improving sleep in lay language, tailoring interventions to the needs of the child, and avoiding overwhelming families with information or increasing their burden with therapies inappropriate for the child's stage of illness.

BOX 22.1 FAMILY PERSPECTIVES ON SLEEP

Jayden is our son whose childhood has been complicated with hypoxic-ischemic encephalopathy/intracranial hemorrhage that led to non-shunted hydrocephalus. Sleep was never "normal" for Jayden. At first we tried giving him medications at the request of his medical team to "normalize" his sleep, but none of it worked. So we decided to let Jayden sleep when Jayden wants to sleep, and it has worked well. In the hospital, sleep for us, his parents, didn't really happen. In the pediatric intensive care unit (PICU), there was no space for us to sleep together. We took turns, and even though we could have stayed at Ronald McDonald House, it was important that we stay together. So, in the hospital all those days, sleep just didn't happen. There were interruptions every 2 hours for medications, alarms going off, his team needing to see him. It was just hard.

When we went home on hospice, we continued to let Jayden sleep how he wanted, and he is doing well. Our sleep—well—we are together as a family and can sleep in our bed, so that is better. We are also grateful for our home care nurses, who we have throughout the day and night. When Jayden is doing well, we sleep better. When he is sicker and needs oxygen or something else, even when the nurses are there, we are on high alert. He still has his feeding tube, tracheostomy, and is ventilator dependent. But he is here with us, and we are together as a family at home. That is what matters to us.

Retold by Jaden's mother. Used with permission.

Clinical vignette

Joey, an 8-year-old female, was diagnosed with relapsed rhabdomyosacroma involving her lungs and sacrum. She developed back and abdominal pain on the fourth day post-bone marrow transplant, and patient-controlled analgesia with fentanyl was commenced. Subsequently she developed bright and vivid dreams, which were distressing. Her analgesia was changed to hydromorphone, and she concurrently received diazepam for 3 nights to assist with sleep. Although her dreams settled down, her sleep continued to be disturbed.

A sleep specialist conducted a thorough evaluation of Joey's sleep and circadian health. During their discussion, a number of factors were discovered that could influence Joey's sleep. With the aid of the sleep specialist, Joey and her family put these factors into groups and explored ways to improve them. Environmental factors included Joey's father noticing that lighting in the hospital room was constantly dim, even during the daytime when it was sunny. This resulted in Joey feeling sleepy and taking naps throughout the day, which reduced her drive to sleep at night. The family had also been leaving the television on in the room all evening as "background noise." This was not something Joey was used to, and it bothered her. Hospital factors included Joey acknowledging that she was "annoyed" by frequent interruptions when she slept. This included nurses performing overnight vital sign checks and cleaning staff emptying the wastebasket. Individual factors included that Joey had struggled previously with vivid dreams and had started to become anxious about bedtime.

An interdisciplinary effort was undertaken to assist Joey. Her family worked at turning on lights during the day and reducing light exposure in the evening, including turning off the television. They arranged with the nurse manager to delay one of her nighttime vitals checks by 1 hour to allow Joey to wake naturally in the morning. Next, they arranged for cleaning staff to come every other day to empty the wastebasket as the timing of their cleaning shift could not be altered. Finally, Joey began to keep a sleep diary and recognized that she was napping too much during the daytime. As a result, she limited her nap duration and didn't nap late in the day. The efforts that Joey and her family made to understand and correct sleep-disturbing factors was rewarded by a team effort that ultimately resulted in better sleep.

CONCLUSION

Sleep-related problems are common among children with life-threatening conditions, exceeding prevalence rates in the general pediatric population. The etiology of sleep impairment can be multifaceted and include the child's medical condition, physical health impairments, mental health disorders, psychosocial factors, and environmental disturbances. There are well-established associations between sleep-related disturbances and poorer physical and psychological health outcomes in children, as well as in their families. Clinicians working with this population would be wise to evaluate sleep health concerns at routine intervals and refer families for appropriate treatment when issues are identified.

Comprehensive assessment and treatment is best achieved by a sleep specialist. It is also important to consult with the full interdisciplinary team to understand the myriad factors impacting a child's sleep and how the team can work to improve sleep outcomes. Nonpharmacological approaches to management should be considered first (with the exception of SRBDs), before introducing psychopharmacological agents. Staff should be educated on techniques that could be implemented to improve sleep in the hospital or hospice environment. To date, most research on sleep and circadian disturbances has been carried out in children with specific illnesses, those with stable disease, and among limited developmental age groups. Thus these recommendations are based on populations that may differ from those seen in the reader's clinic. Future research should expand to studying sleep in children in a wide variety of illnesses and age groups, and interventions to improve sleep in palliative care populations should be tested in clinical trials, as these children may have needs that are different from those of otherwise healthy children with sleep disorders.

REFERENCES

1. Asif N, Iqbal R, Nazir CF. Human immune system during sleep. *Am J Clin Exp Immunol.* 2017;6(6):92–96.
2. Medic G, Wille M, Hemels MEH. Short- and long-term health consequences of sleep disruption. *Nat Sci Sleep.* 2017;9:151–161.
3. Astill RG, Van der Heijden KB, Van Ijzendoorn MH, Van Someren EJ. Sleep, cognition, and behavioral problems in school-age children: A century of research meta-analyzed. *Psychol Bull.* 2012;138(6):1109–1138.
4. Masri S, Sassone-Corsi P. The emerging link between cancer, metabolism, and circadian rhythms. *Nat Med.* 2018;24(12):1795–1803.
5. Hirshkowitz M, Whiton K, Albert SM, et al. National Sleep Foundation's sleep time duration recommendations: Methodology and results summary. *Sleep Health.* 2015;1(1):40–43.
6. Roenneberg T, Merrow M. The circadian clock and human health. *Curr Biol.* 2016;26(10):R432–443.
7. Mindell JA, Owens JA. *A Clinical Guide to Pediatric Sleep: Diagnosis and Management of Sleep Problems.* 2nd ed. Lippincott Williams & Wilkins; 2010.
8. American Academy of Sleep Medicine. *International Classification of Sleep Disorders.* 3rd ed. American Academy of Sleep Medicine; 2014.
9. Brown KM, Malow BA. Pediatric insomnia. *Chest.* 2016;149(5):1332–1339.
10. Primhak R, Kingshott R. Sleep physiology and sleep-disordered breathing: The essentials. *Arch Dis Child.* 2012;1(1):54–58.
11. Baglioni C, Battagliese G, Feige B, et al. Insomnia as a predictor of depression: A meta-analytic evaluation of longitudinal epidemiological studies. *J Affect Disord.* 2011;135(1-3):10–19.
12. Finan PH, Goodin BR, Smith MT. The association of sleep and pain: An update and a path forward. *J Pain.* 2013;14(12):1539–1552.
13. Ekambaram V, Maski K. Non-rapid eye movement arousal parasomnias in children. *Pediatr Ann.* 2017;46(9):e327–e331.
14. Mason TBA, 2nd, Pack AI. Pediatric parasomnias. *Sleep.* 2007;30(2):141–151.
15. Ali NJ, Pitson D, Stradling JR. Natural history of snoring and related behaviour problems between the ages of 4 and 7 years. *Arch Dis Child.* 1994;71(1):74–76.
16. Marcus CL, Brooks LJ, Draper KA, et al. Diagnosis and management of childhood obstructive sleep apnea syndrome. *Pediatrics.* 2012;130(3):e714–755.
17. Kritzinger FE, Al-Saleh S, Narang I. Descriptive analysis of central sleep apnea in childhood at a single center. *Pediatr Pulmonol.* 2011;46(10):1023–1030.
18. Picchietti DL, Bruni O, de Weerd A, et al. Pediatric restless legs syndrome diagnostic criteria: An update by the International Restless Legs Syndrome study group. *Sleep Med.* 2013;14(12):1253–1259.
19. Nallu S, Guerrero GY, Lewis-Croswell J, Wittine LM. Review of narcolepsy and other common sleep disorders in children. *Adv Pediatr.* 2019;66:147–159.
20. Sivertsen B, Pallesen S, Stormark KM, Boe T, Lundervold AJ, Hysing M. Delayed sleep phase syndrome in adolescents: Prevalence and correlates in a large population-based study. *BMC Public Health.* 2013;13:1163.
21. Regestein QR, Monk TH. Delayed sleep phase syndrome: A review of its clinical aspects. *Am J Psychiatry.* 1995;152(4):602–608.
22. Gadoth N, Oksenberg A. Sleep and sleep disorders in rare hereditary diseases: A reminder for the pediatrician, pediatric and adult neurologist, general practitioner, and sleep specialist. *Front Neurol.* 2014;5:133.
23. Madden K, Magno Charone M, Mills S, et al. Systematic symptom reporting by pediatric palliative care patients with cancer: A preliminary report. *J Palliat Med.* 2019;22(8):894–901.
24. Brimeyer C, Adams L, Zhu L, et al. Sleep complaints in survivors of pediatric brain tumors. *Support Care Cancer.* 2016;24(1):23–31
25. Orsey AD, Wakefield DB, Cloutier MM. Physical activity (PA) and sleep among children and adolescents with cancer. *Pediatr Blood Cancer.* 2013;60(11):1908–1913.
26. Verberne LM, Maurice-Stam H, Grootenhuis MA, Van Santen HM, Schouten-Van Meeteren AY. Sleep disorders in children after treatment for a CNS tumour. *J Sleep Res.* 2012;21(4):461–469.
27. Rosen G, Brand SR. Sleep in children with cancer: Case review of 70 children evaluated in a comprehensive pediatric sleep center. *Support Care Cancer.* 2011;19(7):985–994.

28. Theunissen JM, Hoogerbrugge PM, van Achterberg T, Prins JB, Vernooij-Dassen MJ, van den Ende CH. Symptoms in the palliative phase of children with cancer. *Pediatr Blood Cancer.* 2007;49(2):160–165.
29. Van Cleve L, Munoz CE, Savedra M, et al. Symptoms in children with advanced cancer: Child and nurse reports. *Cancer Nurs.* 2012;35(2):115–125.
30. Jacola LM, Conklin HM, Scoggins MA, et al. Investigating the role of hypothalamic tumor involvement in sleep and cognitive outcomes among children treated for craniopharyngioma. *J Pediatr Psychol.* 2016;41(6):610–622.
31. Khan RB, Merchant TE, Sadighi ZS, et al. Prevalence, risk factors, and response to treatment for hypersomnia of central origin in survivors of childhood brain tumors. *J Neurooncol.* 2018;136(2):379–384.
32. Jalmsell L, Kreicbergs U, Onelov E, Steineck G, Henter JI. Symptoms affecting children with malignancies during the last month of life: A nationwide follow-up. *Pediatrics.* 2006;117(4):1314–1320.
33. Rogers VE, Zhu S, Ancoli-Israel S, Hinds PS. Impairment in circadian activity rhythms occurs during dexamethasone therapy in children with leukemia. *Pediatr Blood Cancer.* 2014;61(11):1986–1991.
34. Hankins JS, Verevkina NI, Smeltzer MP, Wu S, Aygun B, Clarke DF. Assessment of sleep-related disorders in children with sickle cell disease. *Hemoglobin.* 2014;38(4):244–251.
35. Valrie CR, Trout KL, Bond KE, et al. Sleep problem risk for adolescents with sickle cell disease: Sociodemographic, physical, and disease-related correlates. *J Pediatr Hematol Oncol.* 2018;40(2):116–121.
36. Graves JK, Jacob E. Pain, coping, and sleep in children and adolescents with sickle cell disease. *J Child Adolesc Psychiatr Nurs.* 2014;27:109–120.
37. Souza LC, Viegas CA. Quality of sleep and pulmonary function in clinically stable adolescents with sickle cell anemia. *J Bras Pneumol.* 2007;33(3):275–281.
38. Rogers VE, Lance EI. Sleep, fatigue and neurodevelopmental outcomes in pediatric sickle cell disease. *Austin Pediatrics.* 2017;4(2):1056–1058.
39. Mascarenhas MI, Loureiro HC, Ferreira T, Dias A. Sleep pathology characterization in sickle cell disease: Case-control study. *Pediatr Pulmonol.* 2015;50(4):396–401.
40. Downes M, de Haan M, Kirkham FJ, Telfer PT. Parent reported sleep problems in preschool children with sickle cell anemia and controls in East London. *Pediatr Blood Cancer.* 2017;64(6):5.
41. Rogers VE, Marcus CL, Jawad AF, et al. Periodic limb movements and disrupted sleep in children with sickle cell disease. *Sleep.* 2011;34(7):899–908.
42. Valrie CR, Gil KM, Redding-Lallinger R, Daeschner C. The influence of pain and stress on sleep in children with sickle cell disease. *Children's Health Care.* 2007;36(4):335–353.
43. Rosen CL, Debaun MR, Strunk RC, et al. Obstructive sleep apnea and sickle cell anemia. *Pediatrics.* 2014;134(2):273–281.
44. Salles C, Ramos RTT, Daltro C, Barral A, Marinho JM, Matos MA. Prevalence of obstructive sleep apnea in children and adolescents with sickle cell anemia. *J Bras Pneumol.* 2009;35(11):1075–1083.
45. Arens R, Muzumdar H. Sleep, sleep disordered breathing, and nocturnal hypoventilation in children with neuromuscular diseases. *Paediatr Respir Rev.* 2010;1(1):24–30.
46. Katz SL. Assessment of sleep-disordered breathing in pediatric neuromuscular diseases. *Pediatrics.* 2009;123(Suppl 4):S222–225.
47. Alves RS, Resende MB, Skomro RP, Souza FJ, Reed UC. Sleep and neuromuscular disorders in children. *Sleep Med Rev.* 2009;1(2):133–148.
48. Suresh S, Wales P, Dakin C, Harris MA, Cooper DG. Sleep-related breathing disorder in Duchenne muscular dystrophy: Disease spectrum in the paediatric population. *J Paediatr Child Health.* 2005;41(9-10):500–503.
49. Miller J, Wagner M. Prader-Willi syndrome and sleep-disordered breathing. *Pediatr Annals.* 2013;42(10):200–204.
50. Sedky K, Bennett DS, Pumariega A. Prader Willi syndrome and obstructive sleep apnea: Co-occurrence in the pediatric population. *J Clin Sleep Med.* 2014;10(4):403–409.
51. Miller A, Enright PL. PFT interpretive strategies: American Thoracic Society/ European Respiratory Society 2005 guideline gaps. *Respir Care.* 2012;57(1):127–133.
52. Franck LS, Johnson LM, Lee K, et al. Sleep disturbances in children with human immunodeficiency virus infection. *Pediatrics.* 1999;104(5):e62.
53. Gazini CC, Reimão RNAA, Rossini SRG, et al. Quality of sleep and quality of life in adolescents infected with human immunodeficiency virus. *Arq Neuropsiquiatr.* 2012;70(6):422–427.
54. Coetzee BJ, Loades ME, Du Toit S, Kagee A. Correlates of fatigue among South African adolescents living with HIV and receiving antiretroviral therapy. *Aids Behav.* 2019;23(3):602–608.
55. Kier C, Manta D, Ahmad KS, Dixon D, Malea JM. Polysomnogram findings of obstructive sleep apnea for children with HIV. *Chest.* 2009;136(4):38S.
56. Shakkottai A, O'Brien LM, Nasr SZ, Chervin RD. Sleep disturbances and their impact in pediatric cystic fibrosis. *Sleep Med Rev.* 2018;42:100–110.
57. Amin R, Bean J, Burklow K, Jeffries J. The relationship between sleep disturbance and pulmonary function in stable pediatric cystic fibrosis patients. *Chest.* 2005;128(3):1357–1363.
58. Vandeleur M, Walter LM, Armstrong DS, Robinson P, Nixon GM, Horne RSC. How well do children with cystic fibrosis sleep? An actigraphic and questionnaire-based study. *J Pediatr.* 2017;182:170–176.
59. Silva AM, Descalco A, Salgueiro M, et al. Respiratory sleep disturbance in children and adolescents with cystic fibrosis. *Rev Port Pneumol (Barc).* 2016;22(4):202–208.
60. Naqvi SK, Sotelo C, Murry L, Simakajornboon N. Sleep architecture in children and adolescents with cystic fibrosis and the association with severity of lung disease. *Sleep Breath.* 2008;12(1):77–83.
61. Fauroux B, Pepin JL, Boelle PY, et al. Sleep quality and nocturnal hypoxaemia and hypercapnia in children and young adults with cystic fibrosis. *Arch Dis Child.* 2012;97(11):960–966.
62. Tomaszek L, Cepuch G, Pawlik L. Evaluation of selected insomnia predictors in adolescents and young adults with cystic fibrosis. *Biomed Pap Med Fac Univ Palacky Olomouc Czech Repub.* 2018;162(3):212–218.
63. Vandeleur M, Walter LM, Armstrong DS, Robinson P, Nixon GM, Horne RSC. What keeps children with cystic fibrosis awake at night? *J Cyst Fibros.* 2017;16(6):719–726.
64. van der Giessen L, Bakker M, Joosten K, Hop W, Tiddens H. Nocturnal oxygen saturation in children with stable cystic fibrosis. *Pediatr Pulmonol.* 2012;47(11):1123–1130.
65. Brubaker JA. *Sleep and Health Related Quality of Life in Children with Cardiac Disease* [dissertation]. ProQuest: Nursing, Case Western Reserve University School of Graduate Studies; 2011.
66. Koopman HM, Vrijmoet-Wiersma CMJ, Langius JND, et al. Psychological functioning and disease-related quality of life in pediatric patients with an implantable cardioverter defibrillator. *Pediatr Cardiol.* 2012;33(4):569–575.
67. Ykeda DS, Lorenzi-Filho G, Lopes AA, Alves RS. Sleep in infants with congenital heart disease. *Clinics (Sao Paulo).* 2009;64(12):1205–1210.
68. Hiatt PW, Mahony L, Tepper RS. Oxygen desaturation during sleep in infants and young children with congenital heart disease. *J Pediatr.* 1992;121(2):226–232.
69. Al-Saleh S, Kantor PF, Chadha NK, Tirado Y, James AL, Narang I. Sleep-disordered breathing in children with cardiomyopathy. *Ann Am Thorac Soc.* 2014;11(5):770–776.
70. Maung SC, El Sara A, Chapman C, Cohen D, Cukor D. Sleep disorders and chronic kidney disease. *World J Nephrol.* 2016;5(3):224–232.
71. Sinha R, Davis ID, Matsuda-Abedini M. Sleep disturbances in children and adolescents with non-dialysis-dependent chronic kidney disease. *Arch Pediatr Adolesc Med.* 2009;163(9):850–855.
72. Davis ID, Baron J, O'Riordan M A, Rosen CL. Sleep disturbances in pediatric dialysis patients. *Pediatr Nephrol.* 2005;20(1):69–75.

73. Davis ID, Greenbaum LA, Gipson DS, et al. Prevalence of sleep disturbances in children and adolescents with chronic kidney disease. *Pediatr Nephrol.* 2012;27(3):451–459.
74. El-Refaey AM, Elsayed RM, Sarhan A, et al. Sleep quality assessment using polysomnography in children on regular hemodialysis. *Saudi J Kidney Dis Transpl.* 2013;24(4):714–718.
75. Riar SK, Leu RM, Turner-Green TC, et al. Restless legs syndrome in children with chronic kidney disease. *Pediatr Nephrol.* 2013;28(5):773–795.
76. Brown WJ, Wilkerson AK, Boyd SJ, Dewey D, Mesa F, Bunnell BE. A review of sleep disturbance in children and adolescents with anxiety. *J Sleep Res.* 2018;27(3):e12635.
77. Alfano CA, Beidel DC, Turner SM, Lewin DS. Preliminary evidence for sleep complaints among children referred for anxiety. *Sleep Med.* 2006;7(6):467–473.
78. Adair R, Bauchner H, Philipp B, Levenson S, Zuckerman B. Night waking during infancy: Role of parental presence at bedtime. *Pediatrics.* 1991;87(4):500–504.
79. Meltzer LJ, Mindell JA. Nonpharmacologic treatments for pediatric sleeplessness. *Pediatr Clin North Am.* 2004;51(1):135–151.
80. Benca RM, Obermeyer WH, Thisted RA, Gillin JC. Sleep and psychiatric disorders. a meta-analysis. *Arch Gen Psychiatry.* 1992;49(8):651–668.
81. Meltzer LJ, Mindell JA. Relationship between child sleep disturbances and maternal sleep, mood, and parenting stress: A pilot study. *J Fam Psychol.* 2007;21(1):67–73.
82. Kouros CD, El-Sheikh M. Within-family relations in objective sleep duration, quality, and schedule. *Child Dev.* 2017;88(6):1983–2000.
83. Bajoghli H, Alipouri A, Holsboer-Trachsler E, Brand S. Sleep patterns and psychological functioning in families in northeastern Iran: Evidence for similarities between adolescent children and their parents. *J Adolesc.* 2013;36(6):1103–1113.
84. Nicholas DB, Beaune L, Barrera M, Blumberg J, Belletrutti M. Examining the experiences of fathers of children with a life-limiting illness. *J Soc Work End Life Palliat Care.* 2016;12(1-2):126–144.
85. Koopman-Verhoeff ME, Serdarevic F, Kocevska D, et al. Preschool family irregularity and the development of sleep problems in childhood: A longitudinal study. *J Child Psychol Psychiatry.* 2019;60(8): 857–865.
86. Billows M, Gradisar M, Dohnt H, Johnston A, McCappin S, Hudson J. Family disorganization, sleep hygiene, and adolescent sleep disturbance. *J Clin Child Adolesc Psychol.* 2009;38(5):745–752.
87. Buxton OM, Chang AM, Spilsbury JC, Bos T, Emsellem H, Knutson KL. Sleep in the modern family: Protective family routines for child and adolescent sleep. *Sleep Health.* 2015;1(1):15–27.
88. Hysing M, Pallesen S, Stormark KM, Jakobsen R, Lundervold AJ, Sivertsen B. Sleep and use of electronic devices in adolescence: Results from a large population-based study. *BMJ Open.* 2015;5(1):e006748.
89. Chang AM, Aeschbach D, Duffy JF, Czeisler CA. Evening use of light-emitting eReaders negatively affects sleep, circadian timing, and next-morning alertness. *Proc Natl Acad Sci USA.* 2015;112(4): 1232–1237.
90. Cain N, Gradisar M. Electronic media use and sleep in school-aged children and adolescents: A review. *Sleep Med.* 2010;11(8):735–742.
91. St-Onge MP, Mikic A, Pietrolungo CE. Effects of diet on sleep quality. *Adv Nutr.* 2016;7(5):938–949.
92. Orbeta RL, Overpeck MD, Ramcharran D, Kogan MD, Ledsky R. High caffeine intake in adolescents: Associations with difficulty sleeping and feeling tired in the morning. *J Adolesc Health.* 2006;38(4):451–453.
93. Rosenberg AR, Bona K, Ketterl T, Wharton CM, Wolfe J, Baker KS. Intimacy, substance use, and communication needs during cancer therapy: A report from the Resilience in Adolescents and Young Adults study. *J Adolesc Health.* 2017;60(1):93–99.
94. Phillips-Salimi CR, Lommel K, Andrykowski MA. Physical and mental health status and health behaviors of childhood cancer survivors: Findings from the 2009 BRFSS survey. *Pediatr Blood Cancer.* 2012;58(6):964–970.
95. Colrain IM, Nicholas CL, Baker FC. Alcohol and the sleeping brain. *Handb Clin Neurol.* 2014;125:415–431.
96. Lee S, Narendran G, Tomfohr-Madsen L, Schulte F. A systematic review of sleep in hospitalized pediatric cancer patients. *Psychooncology.* 2017;26(8):1059–1069.
97. Hinds PS, Hockenberry M, Rai SN, et al. Nocturnal awakenings, sleep environment interruptions, and fatigue in hospitalized children with cancer. *Oncol Nurs Forum.* 2007;34(2):393–402.
98. Rogers VE, Zhu S, Ancoli-Israel S, Liu L, Mandrell BN, Hinds PS. A pilot randomized controlled trial to improve sleep and fatigue in children with CNS tumors hospitalized for high dose chemotherapy. *Pediatr Blood Cancer.* 2019;61:1986–1991.
99. Stickland A, Clayton E, Sankey R, Hill CM. A qualitative study of sleep quality in children and their resident parents when in hospital. *Arch Dis Child.* 2016;101(6):546–551.
100. Corser NC. Sleep of 1- and 2-year-old children in intensive care. *Issues Compr Pediatr Nurs.* 1996;19(1):17–31.
101. Rogers VE, Zhu S, Ancoli-Israel S, Liu L, Mandrell BN, Hinds PS. Relationship between circadian activity rhythms and fatigue in hospitalized children with CNS cancers receiving high dose chemotherapy. *Support Care Cancer.* 2020:28(3):1459–1467.
102. Valrie CR, Gil KM, Redding-Lallinger R, Daeschner C. Sleep in children with sickle cell disease: An analysis of daily diaries utilizing multilevel models. *J Pediatr Psychol.* 2007;32(7):857–861.
103. Fisher K, Laikin AM, Sharp KMH, Criddle CA, Palermo TM, Karlson CW. Temporal relationship between daily pain and actigraphy sleep patterns in pediatric sickle cell disease. *J Behav Med.* 2018;41(3):416–422.
104. Allen JM, Graef DM, Ehrentraut JH, Tynes BL, Crabtree VM. Sleep and pain in pediatric illness: A conceptual review. *CNS Neurosci Ther.* 2016;22(11):880–893.
105. Meltzer LJ, Mindell JA, Owens JA, Byars KC. Use of sleep medications in hospitalized pediatric patients. *Pediatrics.* 2007;119(6):1047–1055.
106. Beaulieu-Bonneau S, LeBlanc M, Merette C, Dauvilliers Y, Morin CM. Family history of insomnia in a population-based sample. *Sleep.* 2007;30(12):1739–1745.
107. Owens JA, Dalzell V. Use of the 'BEARS' sleep screening tool in a pediatric residents' continuity clinic: A pilot study. *Sleep Med.* 2005;6(1):63–69.
108. Spruyt K, Gozal D. Pediatric sleep questionnaires as diagnostic or epidemiological tools: A review of currently available instruments. *Sleep Med Rev.* 2011;15(1):19–32.
109. Carney CE, Buysse DJ, Ancoli-Israel S, et al. The consensus sleep diary: Standardizing prospective sleep self-monitoring. *Sleep.* 2012;35(2):287–302.
110. Short MA, Gradisar M, Lack LC, Wright H, Carskadon MA. The discrepancy between actigraphic and sleep diary measures of sleep in adolescents. *Sleep Med.* 2012;13(4):378–384.
111. Beck SE, Marcus CL. Pediatric polysomnography. *Sleep Med Clin.* 2009;4(3):393–406.
112. Didden R, Sigafoos J, Lancioni GE. Unmodified extinction for childhood sleep disturbance. In Perlis M, Aloia MS, Kuhn BR, eds. *Behavioral Treatments for Sleep Disorders.* Academic Press; 2011: 257–263.
113. Mindell JA, Li AM, Sadeh A, Kwon R, Goh DYT. Bedtime routines for young children: A dose-dependent association with sleep outcomes. *Sleep.* 2015;38(5):717–722.
114. Zhou ES, Owens J. Behavioral treatments for pediatric insomnia. *Curr Sleep Med Rep.* 2016;2(3):127–135.
115. Gradisar M, Dohnt H, Gardner G, et al. A randomized controlled trial of cognitive-behavior therapy plus bright light therapy for adolescent delayed sleep phase disorder. *Sleep.* 2011;34(12):1671–1680.
116. Jacobs SS. Integrative therapy use for management of side effects and toxicities experienced by pediatric oncology patients. *Children (Basel).* 2014;1(3):424–440.
117. Zhou ES, Gardiner P, Bertisch SM. Integrative medicine for insomnia. *Med Clin North Am.* 2017;101(5):865–879.

118. Jacobs S, Mowbray C, Cates LM, et al. Pilot study of massage to improve sleep and fatigue in hospitalized adolescents with cancer. *Pediatr Blood Cancer.* 2016;63(5):880–886.
119. Hinds PS, Hockenberry M, Rai SN, et al. Clinical field testing of an enhanced-activity intervention in hospitalized children with cancer. *J Pain Symptom Manage.* 2007;33(6):686–697.
120. Ladas EJ. Integrative medicine in childhood cancer. *J Altern Complement Med.* 2018;24(9-10):910–915.
121. Hooke MC, Gilchrist L, Foster L, Langevin M, Lee J. Yoga for children and adolescents after completing cancer treatment. *J Pediatr Oncol Nurs.* 2016;33(1):64–73.
122. Yeh CH, Chien LC, Chiang YC, Lin SW, Huang CK, Ren D. Reduction in nausea and vomiting in children undergoing cancer chemotherapy by either appropriate or sham auricular acupuncture points with standard care. *J Altern Complement Med.* 2012;18(4):334–340.
123. Kimes D, Levine E, Timmins S, Weiss SR, Bollinger ME, Blaisdell C. Temporal dynamics of emergency department and hospital admissions of pediatric asthmatics. *Environ Res.* 2004;94(1):7–17.
124. Alonso PB, Hickey V, Flesch L, et al. Quality improvement I initiative to improve sleep in pediatric HSCT patients and caregivers. *Biol Blood Marrow Transplant.* 2019;25(3):S68.
125. Troester MM, Pelayo R. Pediatric sleep pharmacology: A primer. *Semin Pediatr Neurol.* 2015;22(2):135–147.
126. Bruni O, Angriman M, Calisti F, et al. Practitioner review: Treatment of chronic insomnia in children and adolescents with neurodevelopmental disabilities. *J Child Psychol Psychiatry.* 2018;59(5):489–508.
127. Blackmer AB, Feinstein JA. Management of sleep disorders in children with neurodevelopmental disorders: A review. *Pharmacotherapy.* 2016;36(1):84–98.
128. McDonagh MS, Holmes R, Hsu F. Pharmacological treatment for sleep disorders in children: A systematic review. *J Child Neurol.* 2019;34(5):237–247.
129. Goldman SE, Adkins KW, Calcutt MW, et al. Melatonin in children with autism spectrum disorders: Endogenous and pharmacokinetic profiles in relation to sleep. *J Autism Dev Disord.* 2014;44(10):2525–2535.
130. Szeinberg A, Borodkin K, Dagan Y. Melatonin treatment in adolescents with delayed sleep phase syndrome. *Clin Pediatr (Phila).* 2006;45(9):809–818.
131. Esposito S, Laino D, D'Alonzo R, et al. Pediatric sleep disturbances and treatment with melatonin. *J Transl Med.* 2019;17(1):77.
132. Bock DE, Roach-Fox E, Seabrook JA, Rieder MJ, Matsui D. Sleep-promoting medications in children: Physician prescribing habits in Southwest Ontario, Canada. *Sleep Med.* 2016;17:52–56.
133. Stojanovski SD, Rasu RS, Balkrishnan R, Nahata MC. Trends in medication prescribing for pediatric sleep difficulties in US outpatient settings. *Sleep.* 2007;30(8):1013–1017.
134. Picchietti MA, Picchietti DL. Advances in pediatric restless legs syndrome: Iron, genetics, diagnosis and treatment. *Sleep Med.* 2010;11(7):643–651.
135. Dosman CF, Brian JA, Drmic IE, Senthilselvan A, Harford MM, Smith RW, et al. Children with autism: Effect of iron supplementation on sleep and ferritin. *Pediatr Neurol.* 2007;36(3):152–158.
136. Frenette E. Restless legs syndrome in children: A review and update on pharmacological options. *Curr Pharm Des.* 2011;17(15):1436–1442.
137. Kuhle S, Hoffmann, DU, Mitra S, Urschitz MS. Anti-inflammatory medications for obstructive sleep apnoea in children. *Cochrane Database Sys Rev.* 2020;1(1):CD007074.
138. Liming BJ, Ryan M, Mack D, Ahmad I, Camacho M. Montelukast and nasal corticosteroids to treat pediatric obstructive sleep apnea: A systematic review and meta-analysis. *Otolaryngol Head Neck Surg.* 2019;160(4):594–602.
139. Edmonds KP, Ajayi TA, Cain J, Yeung HN, Thornberry K. Establishing goals of care at any stage of illness: The PERSON mnemonic. *J Palliat Med.* 2014;17(10):1087.

23 | PREVENTION AND TREATMENT OF PAIN IN CHILDREN WITH SERIOUS ILLNESS

STEFAN J. FRIEDRICHSDORF, LAUREN HEATHCOTE, MICHAEL SANGSTER, DONNA EULL, AND AMBER BORUCKI

"There were little computers. And there were little people. And you could tell them if you want the pain to go down. Or the nausea to go down."

11-year-old girl with advanced cancer during her end-of-life period, who while practicing hypnosis followed the suggestion to imagine going inside her own brain and successfully turned down pain and nausea.

FAMILY REFLECTION

Our two daughters suffer from an extremely rare genetic disorder, RTD-2/BVVLS, which presents itself differently depending on the mutation. They have multiple organ systems affected by this disease including autonomic dysautonomia, respiratory failure, deafness/blindness, chronic pain, and neuromuscular/nervous system disfunction. Over the years we have learned so much from our palliative care team. They have been vital to our daughters' health management. They taught us about pain management—the different levels and types of pain. This was so critical for us to keep them comfortable which allowed them to thrive. Our daughters would not be alive or have had the quality of life if it wasn't for Dr. Friedrichsdorf and his palliative team.

When our oldest first met the team, she was screaming in pain which contributed to her already multiple apneic episodes because of her compromised respiratory drive. She was not able to tolerate any feedings, neither gastric nor jejunum feedings—she was failing to thrive. She couldn't even lift up her arms. It was only until the palliative care program managed and prescribed her a regiment of pain medication, specifically Tramadol that she stopped having feeding intolerance and began to develop. Many doctors were concerned about pain control and use of opioids for respiratory-compromised children, but with the proper pain management and the attentiveness of the palliative program we never had an issue with any of those medications. The palliative care program became part of our medical team and worked with our other specialist in managing their complex medical care.

Not only did the palliative team care for our daughters' medical needs, but they also reached out to our whole family and made sure that our well-being was being addressed as well. This compassionate outreach, especially during the multiple intensive care hospital visits and crisis situations was extremely valuable to us. They made sure that our two older boys were coping and helped them understand what was happening to their sisters. Providing for and ensuring caregivers are doing OK is so important and unique to this program.

We have a very close relationship with the team as we have to contact them to make adjustments and make new plans as our daughters' conditions change. Thinking out of the box is important with children with rare diseases, especially with children like our daughters who are nonverbal and not able to express what is wrong.

Not only did the palliative care program provide us with an array of pain control methods, but they also included holistic therapies like massage, aroma therapy, distraction techniques, music therapy, and sensory interventions. These methods were successful and helpful when used in conjunction with their pain medications.

Our experience with our palliative program has had a great impact not only on our daughters, but on our whole family. We believe what makes the program successful and important for all chronically ill children is their philosophy to treat the whole child and not just their pain with medication. They focus on the child's well-being and ensure they have the best quality of life.

Deborah and Grant Toma

INTRODUCTION

PAIN IN CHILDREN WITH SERIOUS ILLNESS

Pain is among the most distressing and most prevalent symptoms children with serious illness experience in their disease trajectory and especially during their end-of-life period.[1] Most published data stem from children with cancer and show a significant symptom burden in this population.[2–5] Self-reports from children with malignancies show high distress from pain in 39% of pediatric patients with advanced cancer, which increased to 58% at end of life.[5] Children who were enrolled into North American pediatric palliative care (PPC) programs experienced on average eight additional distressing symptoms other than pain.[1] In these patients with advanced serious illness, the majority of distressing symptoms, such as unrelieved pain, were not treated during the end-of-life period, and, when treated, the therapy was commonly ineffective.[2–7]

MULTIMODAL ANALGESIA

Advanced pain treatment and prevention for children with serious illness usually requires multimodal analgesia, which means, based on the individual patient, combining multiple analgesic agents (such as basic analgesia, opioids, adjuvant analgesia), regional anesthesia, rehabilitation, and psychological and integrative (previously called "nonpharmacological") therapies which act synergistically for more effective pain control with fewer side effects than a single analgesic or modality.[8–10]

Analgesic medications, especially opioids, remain the foundation of advanced pain treatment in children with serious illness. However, the past few years, and promoted by PPC curricula,[11] have brought a paradigm shift away from "medications-only" toward offering "multimodal analgesia," as a large number of children with complex pain do *not* achieve adequate analgesia solely with pharmacology.

Figure 23.1 shows the components of multimodal analgesia, with the implication that an individual child may require one, several, or all of the components listed in each circle to achieve excellent analgesia. Each of these therapeutic options is described later in more detail.

PAIN IN NONVERBAL CHILDREN WITH IMPAIRMENT OF THE CENTRAL NERVOUS SYSTEM

While nearly all published PPC data come from children with malignancies, the majority of children with serious illness in high-income countries do not have cancer, but metabolic, genetic, or neurologic diseases with impairment of the central nervous system (CNS), which usually leaves them nonverbal.[1,7] Assessing pain may be complicated in these children by possible altered pain processing,[12] and validated multidimensional observational tools are available.[13] Frequently used tools in this population include the revised Face, Legs, Activity, Cry, Consolability (r-FLACC),[14] Pediatric Pain

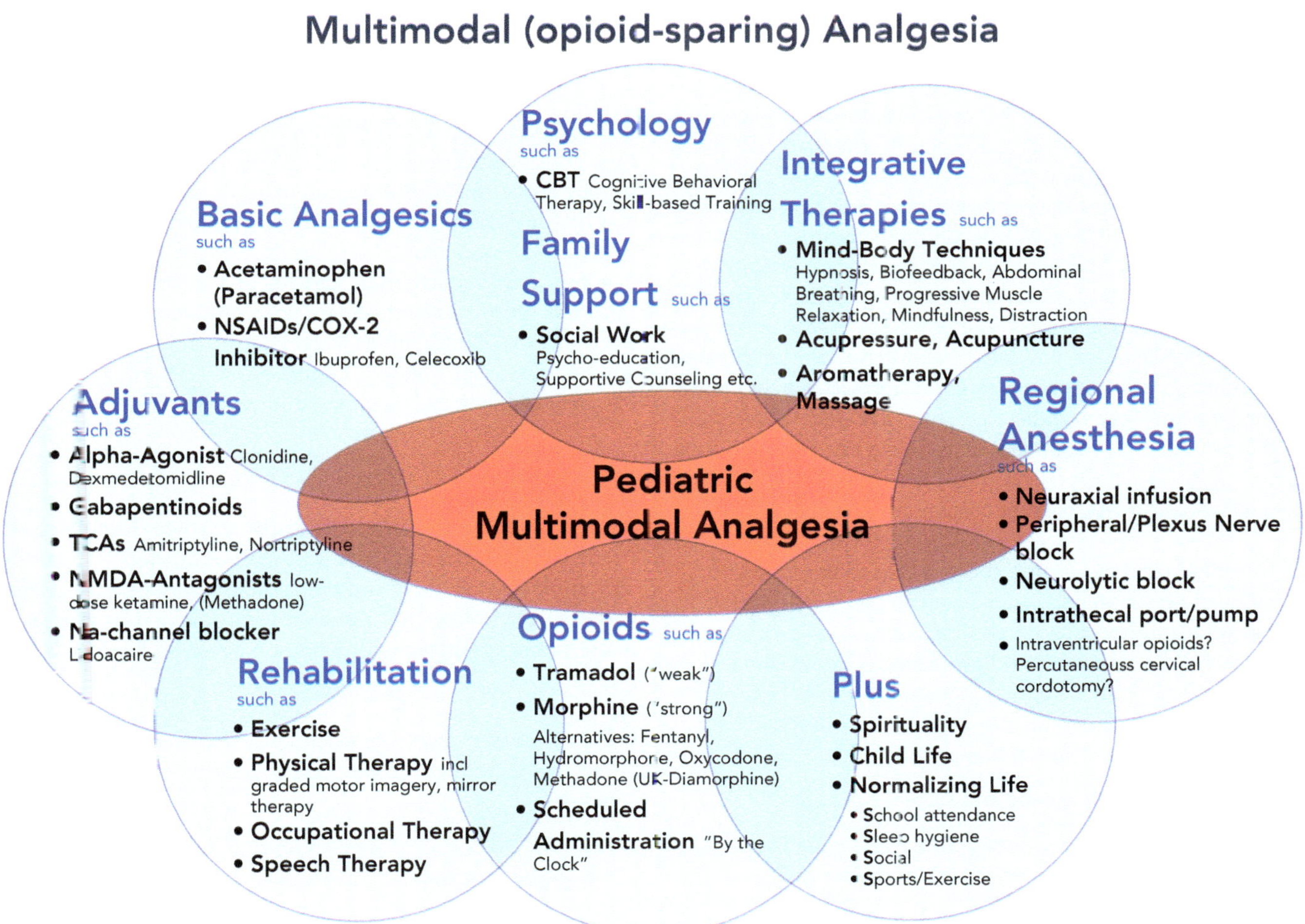

Figure 23.1 *Multimodal analgesia.* Used with permission from Stefan Friedrichsdorf, Benioff Children's Hospitals in Oakland and San Francisco, University of California at San Francisco (UCSF).

Profile (PPP),[15,16] or Noncommunicating Children's Pain Checklist-revised (NCCPC-R).[17]

Pinpointing the correct underlying pathology causing pain in nonverbal pediatric patients with impairment of the CNS remains a challenge for clinicians and caregivers alike. The pain experience may be driven by the underlying disease, comorbidities, and/or painful procedures and interventions. In addition to the pain pathophysiologies discussed here (acute, chronic, total, neuropathic, and/or visceral pain) many children receiving artificial hydration and nutrition via feeding tubes may also develop feeding intolerance and visceral hyperalgesia, and their clinical course may be further complicated by spasticity/contracture, reflux, medication withdrawal, hypoactive or hyperactive delirium, dysautonomia, and/or nausea. Of note, autonomic stress responses, including, changes in blood pressure, heart rate, temperature, respiratory rate, and epinephrine/norepinephrine serum levels, do not usually correlate with severity of pain.[18]

PREVENTION AND TREATMENT OF PAIN AND ANXIETY CAUSED BY NEEDLES

A majority of children and their families report needle pain as the worst pain experienced in the hospital setting.[19,20] Children with complex illness and PPC needs are at high risk for frequent exposure to needle procedures in the course of diagnosis and treatment. To prevent emotional trauma and other long-term effects of poorly managed pain in this vulnerable population, it is essential for all healthcare providers to make every effort to prevent and treat needle pain effectively. Untreated needle pain caused by procedures such as blood draws, injections, and venous cannulation can have long-term consequences including needle phobia, preprocedural anxiety, hyperalgesia, and avoidance of healthcare, resulting in increased morbidity and mortality.[8] Current evidence strongly supports the consistent use of four bundled modalities for elective needle procedures to reduce or eliminate pain experienced by children.[8,21] Although use in clinical practice may present challenges, the four bundle elements have been successfully implemented as the standard of care for needle procedures system-wide in children's hospitals and pediatricians' offices on several continents.[8,21] Bundle elements include

- Topical anesthesia "Numb the skin" for term infants 36 weeks of gestation and older, for example, 4% lidocaine cream (administered at least 30 minutes prior procedure), EMLA (lidocaine 2.5% and prilocaine 2.5%) cream (60 minutes prior), amethocaine [tetracaine] 4% gel (30–60 minutes prior) or needle-free lidocaine application via a sterile, single-use, disposable injector (J-tip).[22–24]
- *Sucrose or breastfeeding* for infants 0–12 months.[25–27]
- *Comfort positioning* provides a choice and encourages parents to hold children on their laps or be nearby.
    - For infants, facilitate skin-to-skin, warmth, swaddling, or facilitated tucking.[28–35]
    - For children 6 months and older, *upright is best.*
    - *Children should never be held down* as restraining children for procedures is never supportive, creates a negative experience, and increases resistance, anxiety, and pain.[36]
- *Distraction* appropriate for age and developmental level, such as toys, stories, books, music, bubbles or pinwheels, stress balls, and apps, videos, or games on electronic devices.[37–39]

These four simple modalities (or three to children older than 12 months) and not just some of them should be offered for all needle procedures for all children.[20,21]

Plan B. For children who have already had suboptimal needle procedure experiences and anxiety and fear preclude them from being successful with the listed four strategies, consider referrals to psychology or child life for a coping plan and/or the use of minimal sedation, such as nitrous gas, to help them be successful and avoid retraumatization.[40–42]

Note that all procedures, including needle procedures, should be carefully considered for children in PPC, especially at end of life, to evaluate the potential benefits and burdens, importance to the overall treatment plan, and the alignment with the established goals of care.

CONSIDERATIONS FOR TREATING PAIN IN CHILDREN WITH SERIOUS ILLNESS

This chapter suggests a 12-step approach for advanced analgesia consideration in neonates, children, and adolescents with serious illness, based on the Education in Palliative and End-of-Life Care (EPEC)-Pediatrics curriculum.[11] The appropriate treatment choices depend on the clinical scenario and the context of the individual child and his or her family (including cancer vs. nonmalignant disease, infant vs. older child, verbal vs. nonverbal child, underlying pain pathophysiology, and goals of care). See Figure 23.2 for step-by-step considerations for advanced pain treatment in children with serious illness.

STEP 1: EVALUATION

As of July 2020, the internationally accepted International Association for the Study Pain (IASP) definition[43] of pain is "An unpleasant sensory and emotional experience associated with, or resembling that associated with, actual or potential tissue damage" and is expanded upon by the following six key points:

- Pain is always a personal experience that is influenced to varying degrees by biological, psychological, and social factors.
- Pain and nociception are different phenomena. Pain cannot be inferred solely from activity in sensory neurons.
- Through their life experiences, individuals learn the concept of pain.

Consideration for Pain Treatment in Children with Serious Illness

(1) Evaluation
- Talking history & perform clinical exam (medical tests only as required)

(2) Treat underlying causes
- If within goals of Care. (Palliative CNS emergency....? Radiation, Glucocorticosteroids, Surgery?)

(3) Integrative Therapies
- e.g. Active mind-body techniques; acupuncture/acupressure; music/art/pet therapy, massage, aromatherapy, apps

(4) Social Work, Rehabilitation, Psychology, Spirituality, Child Life
- Family Support, psycho-education, supportive counseling, parent guidance. Respite needed?
- Manage Comorbidities e.g. anxiety, depression, sleep disturbances, poor exercise tolerance/deconditioned, school absenteeism etc.

(5) Basic Analgesia and Opioids
- Acetaminophen (Paracetamol) and NSAIDs/COX-2 Inhibitor
- Opioids for new-onset neuropathic pain, tissue injury (not for chronic pain/primary pain disorders). Tramadol? Methadone?

(6) Gabapentinoids and/or Tricyclic Antidepressants
- Gabapentin (or pregabaline); amitriptyline (or nortriptyline)

(7) Alpha-2-adrenergic agonists
- Clonidine or dexmedetomidine

(8) NMDA-receptor-channel blocker
- Low-dose ketamine (and/or methadone?)

(9) Sodium-channel Blockers
- Lidocaine (transdermal patch? Intravenous?)

(10) Regional Anesthesia
- e.g. Neuraxial infusion (epidural: tunneled catheter); peripheral/plexus nerve block; neurolytic block; intrathecal port/pump

(11) Other Adjuvants
- Botox A? Low-dose propofol? Benzodiazepines? Capsaicin? SNRI? Cannabiroids????

(12) Palliative Sedation
- For intractable (not merely difficult to treat) pain or suffering in end-of-life period
- Propofol? Midazolam? Ketamine? Barbiturates?

Figure 23.2 *Considerations for treating pain in children with serious illness.* Used with permission from Stefan Friedrichsdorf, Benioff Children's Hospitals in Oakland and San Francisco, University of California at San Francisco (UCSF).

- A person's report of an experience as pain should be respected.
- Although pain usually serves an adaptive role, it may have adverse effects on function and social and psychological well-being.
- Verbal description is only one of several behaviors to express pain; inability to communicate does not negate the possibility that a human or a non-human animal experiences pain.

To successfully treat pain in a pediatric patient with serious illness it is paramount to take a detailed history, including medication history, and perform a comprehensive clinical exam. Based on the outcome of these evaluations, medical tests may be ordered if they might guide further treatment options. Most children with serious illnesses experience different distinct and at times overlapping entities of pain pathophysiologies concurrently and/or subsequently, thus explaining the need of protocols providing multimodal analgesia (Figure 23.3).[8] These pain pathophysiologies include

- *Acute somatic pain* arises from the activation of nociceptors (peripheral nerve endings) caused by tissue injury that transmits noxious stimulation. Examples include chemotherapy-induced mucositis, open wounds, occult fractures, hip dysplasia, corneal abrasions, dental abscesses.
- *Total pain:* Cicely Saunders in the 1960s saw a broader view than the IASP definition, acknowledging the impact of spiritual and psychosocial aspects on the pain experience, coining the term "total pain," which includes suffering that encompasses all of a child's physical, psychological, social, spiritual, and practical struggles.[44] This is particularly true for children with palliative care needs, for whom the onset of pain may represent the relentless progression of a life-limiting or life-threatening disease.[45] For a more detailed review of the subject, please refer to the excellent article by Warlow and Hain.[45]

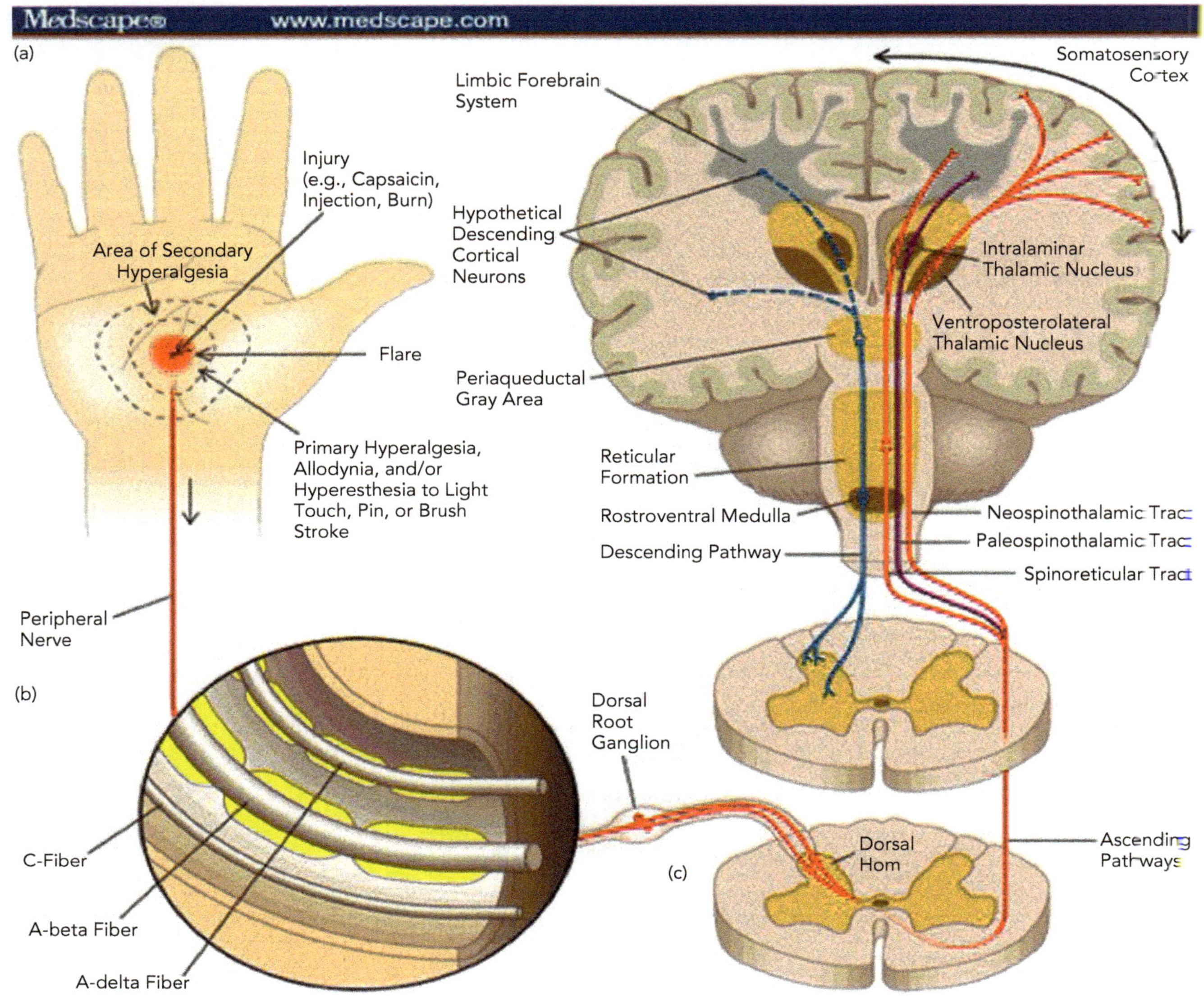

Figure 23.3 Pain pathways. From www.medscape.org/viewarticle/460306_2

- *Neuropathic pain* results from injury to or dysfunction of the somatosensory system. Examples include chemotherapy-induced neuropathy, phantom limb pain, or neurodegenerative disorders. *Central pain* is caused by a lesion or disease within the central somatosensory nervous system.
- *Visceral pain* results from the activation of nociceptors of the thoracic, pelvic, or abdominal viscera. Examples include bladder spasms, pancreatitis, or intrahepatic tumors.
- *Chronic pain* is usually described as pain beyond expected time of healing. Examples include functional abdominal pain, primary headaches, medication overuse headaches, and widespread musculoskeletal pain. A significant subset of children with serious illness also experience chronic pain in addition to their acute, neuropathic, visceral, and total pain. Of note, 20% of children develop chronic postsurgical pain (CPSP) after major surgery.[46]

STEP 2: TREAT UNDERLYING CAUSES

When a child with serious illness presents with a distressing symptom such as unrelieved pain, and this is concurrent with all other areas in pediatrics, it is key to identify and treat the underlying disease process as long as this is feasible and within the goals of care for the individual child and family. The aim is to identify and appropriately address comorbidities which may contribute to the pain experience, such as feeding intolerance, visceral hyperalgesia, fluid overload, constipation, spasticity/contractures, nausea, vomiting, reflux, untreated anxiety, depression or other mental health disorders, sleep disturbance, hypoactive/hyperactive delirium, medication withdrawal, and/or a seizure disorder. A sudden paralysis of the legs, possibly coinciding with loss of bladder and stool control may be indicative of tumor growth within the spinal canal and then might constitute a palliative emergency. This might be addressed with glucocorticosteroids such as dexamethasone, radiation, and/or neurosurgery, increasing the chance for the pediatric patient to return to improved or even normal functioning for a period.

STEP 3: INTEGRATIVE ("NONPHARMACOLOGICAL") THERAPIES

Many integrative medicine modalities have proven helpful in preventing and treating pain in children with serious illness. These modalities are sometimes also referred to as "nonpharmacologic" or "complementary alternative medicine" (CAM). These integrative modalities can be offered to both the sick child and caregivers and siblings to manage the child's as well as their family's distressing symptoms. The modalities need to be adapted to the age, disease progression, and special needs of the child.

In infants and neonates, these modalities include breastfeeding, non-nutritive sucking with sucrose 24%, and skin-to-skin contact.[25,26,47,48] In toddlers, school children, and young adults, age-appropriate effective integrative modalities for include aromatherapy, distraction, abdominal breathing, progressive muscle relaxation, biofeedback, hypnosis, yoga, acupressure, acupuncture, transcutaneous electrical nerve stimulation (TENS), Reiki, music, and massage.[37,49–60] Many of these active mind-body techniques may be effective by decreasing pain, distressing symptoms and anxiety through involvement of several mechanisms simultaneously within the analgesic neuraxis.[58,61–64]

Mind-body techniques such as distraction and guided imagery, which can be taught to the child and/or caregivers appear to modulate the release of endogenous opioids from the periaqueductal and periventricular gray regions to disinhibit descending inhibitory pathways of the brainstem to modulate pain at the supraspinal level.[65–71]

STEP 4: SOCIAL WORK, PSYCHOLOGY, CHAPLAINCY, AND CHILD LIFE

As described elsewhere in this book, advanced specialist PPC can only be provided by an interdisciplinary clinical care team; a lone physician or a sole nurse practitioner is not empowered nor able to provide comprehensive excellent pain assessment and treatment for children with serious advanced illness.

SOCIAL WORK

Most established PPC teams include clinical social workers who provide or coordinate supportive counseling, parent guidance, and psychoeducation including for emotional or existential pain assessment and treatment. In addition, they empower those involved to set appropriate limits and expectations. Families facing uncertainty in light of their child's serious illness have access to these social workers, who then can help in processing the experience of the complex journey. They can provide assessments as to, for example, whether the 24-hour care of a child at home is no longer sustainable for the parents or caregivers. They then can identify possible sources of respite care, including volunteer support, home care nursing, inpatient hospitalization, and/or referral to a free-standing hospice house or unit.

REHABILITATION

Physical therapy is advocated in the literature as an adjunctive modality with favorable outcomes in the prevention and treatment of pain in children with medical complexity.[72] The physical therapist is the movement specialist on the interprofessional PPC team. Given the inextricable link between pain and movement, the physical therapist is optimally positioned to offer movement as analgesia in a preventative, restorative, supportive, or palliative context in accordance with the individual needs of a child and their family.[73]

Conventional physical therapy may consist of activity modification, exercises to improve range of motion and strength, and the application of passive electrotherapeutic modalities such as transcutaneous electrical nerve stimulation (TENS), interferential current (IFC), or thermal agents.[73] However, contemporary thinking in physical therapy suggests an active movement-based approach that considers both cortical and peripheral intervention targets along a movement therapy continuum is preferred.[74,75]

Malfliet et al. (2017) suggest that altered cortical processing may underpin the complex pain presentations in children with serious illness. Indeed, the recognition of the relationship of maladaptive cortical processing and pain suggests that a *movement without moving* approach, with the brain as the primary therapeutic target, be considered in physical therapy intervention. Perceptual manipulation using graded motor imagery, including implicit motor imagery, explicit motor imagery, and mirror visual feedback, permits novel stimulation of cortical regions associated with pain and movement thereby providing the child with pain-free brain-based movement which has been shown to reduce pain.[74] Furthermore, virtual and augmented reality may offer additional cortically based movement intervention that can be effective in modulating pain perception in both acute and complex pain presentations.[75]

Brain-based movement interventions can be progressed to active foundational movement approaches, such as physical activity promotion, which are shown to decrease pain sensitivity via central inhibitory mechanisms.[76,77] Physical activity interventions yield optimal outcomes when tailored to the individual goals of the child and designed on a foundation of pain neuroscience education that targets maladaptive pain cognitions and fear of movement.[75,76]

Graded exposure to goal-directed physical activity can offer the child access to new and novel sensations, decrease the risk of negative mental health sequelae associated with medical complexity, and empower the child and their parents in the management of their condition.[78]

Movement-based physical therapy offers a simple and cost-effective suite of therapeutic options that can improve interprofessional palliative care for children. Well-designed systematic evaluation of movement-based physical therapy approaches are needed to enable strong clinical recommendations in the prevention and treatment of pain in children with medical complexity.

PSYCHOLOGICAL AND PSYCHIATRIC INTERVENTIONS

Pain is not only a common symptom in children with serious illness, it is also among the most feared.[2,79–81] Fear is a central affective component of pain,[82] and rarely is this fear greater than when pain is experienced in the context of a life-threatening illness. Fears of disease progression and death also contribute to the experience of pain and can increase suffering in children with serious illness. Psychological interventions can be used, among many things, to address the fear and distress that pain and illness cause the child and their family, in turn impacting both pain management as well as the child's emotional and sensory experience of pain. Psychotherapeutic interventions are particularly useful to address comorbid mental health issues[83–85] and suicidality[86] that can arise as a result of living with persistent pain and illness. Interestingly, while research in pediatric populations often falls behind that of adults, the recommendation to integrate psychological and psychiatric interventions into pain management has been especially embraced in pediatric populations.[87]

Numerous approaches fit within the boundaries of psychological and psychiatric interventions for PPC, which are often used in combination. This includes guided imagery and breathing, psychoeducation, hypnosis, distraction, progressive muscle relaxation, biofeedback, and cognitive restructuring. Distraction is the most supported approach in children with serious illness, although it has been mostly studied within the context of cancer-related procedural pain and less well in other illnesses. Nonetheless, it is easily employed in broad procedural settings and can work well across a variety of ages and temperaments.[88] Several systematic reviews[89–92] show large effect sizes for distraction as an intervention for procedural pain in children, including several recent studies that support virtual reality–based distraction approaches.[93]

Cognitive strategies, such as restructuring, are better studied in adult populations but are also commonly used with youth. These techniques are particularly important to address how the young patient interprets and makes sense of their pain. For example, a child with cancer may interpret pain as indicating a progression of their disease, fueling further distress.[94,95] Through cognitive restructuring, the child is encouraged to consider alternative, less-threatening interpretations, for example that the pain is a result of treatment targeting the disease. This, in turn, may reduce the distress caused by the pain as well as the perceived need for pharmacologic pain control. Importantly, the goals of cognitive restructuring can change over the course of the child's disease—at later stages the focus may be on challenging different cognitions, such as "there is nothing I can do to control my pain." The most appropriate strategy will also shift according to the course of disease and the child's age—breathing techniques and distraction will be more appropriate for younger children and those with cognitive limitations due to more advanced disease.

As multiple psychological factors contribute to the child's pain experience, multiple actors are also involved in its treatment. Parents play a critical role in shaping the child's response to and management of pain[91,96–98] and are thus commonly integrated into intervention. The child's attitudes and behavioral responses toward pain are often learned by observing and modeling the parent.[99] Thus, the parent's own interpretations of the child's pain could also be usefully addressed through cognitive restructuring. The parent also directly influences the management of the child's pain in their interaction with the healthcare system, for example by communicating increases in the child's pain to the medical team. One salient challenge faced by parents is managing empathic distress as a result of seeing their child in pain.[100,101] Psychological practitioners can work with parents on coping strategies to help them manage their distress, thus reducing the distress observed by the child and enabling more adaptive empathic care.[102]

In addition to mental health professionals, other members of the child's clinical team also influence the child's pain experience via psychological mechanisms. Innovative research, again largely in adults, has revealed that a good therapeutic relationship can enhance placebo analgesia and thus reduce pain through psychological mechanisms (e.g., by reducing expectations of pain) and physiological pathways (e.g., by engaging the endogenous opioid system).[103] Psychological factors are also important in the effective delivery of pharmacological treatments, particularly when considered in a developmental context. For example, a teenager receiving morphine to control disease-related pain may feel uncomfortable reporting the side effect of constipation-related pain to a treating physician. Without being sensitive to these developmental considerations, the child's overall pain experience will be poorly managed regardless of the availability of effective analgesics.

Psychological and psychiatric interventions are a vital part of our toolkit for effective pain management in PPC and are a cornerstone of shifting from a disease-centered to a child- and family-centered model of care. As precision in pharmacological treatment of pain grows, we need equal precision in the assessment and treatment of psychological factors that are integral to the child's pain experience.

CHAPLAINCY

Chaplaincy provides spiritual care and supports to enhance coping in times of crisis, stress, or illness. Spirituality, religion, or life philosophy play an important role in the lives of most verbal patients receiving PPC, as well as their families. A link between spiritual coping and quality of life in adolescents with serious illness has been described.[104] Spirituality screening tools, such as the Faiths or Beliefs, Importance or Influence, Community, Address these issues (FICA) have been successfully implemented into clinical PPC[105] and should be considered part of a comprehensive pain assessment.

CHILD LIFE

Child life specialists work with children as well their parents and siblings in medical settings whether inpatient, outpatient, or at home to help them cope with the challenges of hospitalization, serious illness, and disability. Child life specialists provide children with age-appropriate preparation for painful and/or anxiety-provoking medical procedures and pain treatment/prevention, and they teach coping strategies by engaging in age-appropriate play and self-expression activities. When dealing with children with advanced serious illness, they can offer information, support, and guidance to parents, family members, and classmates (when visiting schools) and can engage siblings in memory-making activities.

STEP 5: BASIC ANALGESIA AND OPIOIDS

BASIC ANALGESIA

Basic (or simple) analgesics include acetaminophen (paracetamol), nonsteroidal anti-inflammatory drugs (NSAIDs), and cyclooxygenase-2 (COX-2) inhibitors. In some countries dipyrone (metamizole) is included as a basic analgesia.[106] See Tables 23.1 and Table 23.6 for recommended dosing.

Due to the antipyretic property of all basic analgesics, in neutropenic and/or immunocompromised patients, these medications may suppress fever as an early sign of sepsis and as such should only be administered in close collaboration with the primary team (e.g., oncologist, transplant clinician)

"By the clock" dosing. When pain is constantly present, administration of both basic analgesia and an opioid should usually be scheduled "around-the clock" (e.g., acetaminophen every 6 hours scheduled and morphine every 4 hours scheduled). As-needed prescriptions only (without scheduled analgesia) often do not reach the patient, and "PRN" ("pro re nate" or "as-needed") is often translated into "patient receives nothing," with 69% of hospitalized pediatric patients for whom analgesics had been ordered not receiving a single dose in one study.[107]

TABLE 23.1 Basic analgesia for children older than 6 months

MEDICATION (ROUTE OF ADMINISTRATION)	PEDIATRIC DOSE	MAXIMAL DOSE	DOSING INTERVAL	COMMENT
Acetaminophen/Paracetamol				
Acetaminophen/ Paracetamol (PO/PR)	10–15 mg/kg	6–24 months = 60 mg/kg/day >2 years: 90 mg/kg/day [max. 650 mg q6h]	q6h	
Acetaminophen/ Paracetamol (IV)	<10 kg = 7.5 mg/kg	30 mg/kg/day	q6h	Due to high price use only if enteral, rectal, or oral administration is contraindicated; reevaluate daily
	1–2 yrs = 15 mg/kg;	60 mg/kg/day	q6h	
	>2 yrs (<50 kg) = 15 mg/kg	75 mg/kg/day	q6h	
	>13 yrs (>50 kg) = 1,000 mg	4000 mg/day	q6h	
Nonsteroidal anti-inflammatory drugs (NSAIDs)				
Ibuprofen (PO)	5–10 mg/kg	400–600 mg/dose (2,400 mg/day)	q6h	
Ibuprofen-Sodium (PO) 256 mg tablet = 200 mg ibuprofen	5 (–10) mg/kg	200–(400) mg/dose	q6h	Fast-acting, compared to regular ibuprofen: onset after 10 minutes, lasts longer, and only half the dose is required
Ketorolac (IV)	6–24 months = 0.25 mg/kg	30 mg/dose	q6h	Recommend dosing no longer than 5 days
	>2 yrs = 0.5 mg/kg	30 mg/dose	q6h	Recommend dosing no longer than 5 days
Naproxen (PO)	5–6 mg/kg	250–375 mg/dose	q12h	
COX-2 inhibitor				
Celecoxib (PO)	1–2 mg/kg	100 mg	q12–24h	If classic NSAIDs are contraindicated; safety and efficacy has been established only in children ≥2 years and for a maximum of 6 months of treatment in JRA

IV, intravenous; PO, by mouth (or enterally via gastric/jejunal tube); PR, rectally; q6h, every 6 hours

q8h, every 8 hours; q12h, every 12 hours; q12–24h, every 12–24 hours.

Used with permission from Stefan Friedrichsdorf, Benioff Children's Hospitals in Oakland and San Francisco, University of California at San Francisco (UCSF).

ACETAMINOPHEN (PARACETAMOL)

Acetaminophen is generally well-tolerated in pediatrics and lacks gastrointestinal and hematological side effects. The mechanisms of antinociception of this commonly administered analgesic remain unclear and seem to include the stimulation of descending (inhibiting) serotonergic pathways, which are possibly endocannabinoid-dependent, through COX-2 inhibition, nitric oxide (NO) synthesis blockade, and interaction with supraspinal calcium (Ca(v)3.2) channels.[108,109] Significant hepatotoxicity[110] is rare with standard dosing, but careful attention to dosing is paramount to avoid toxicity. The liver enzymes aminotransferase (AST) and alanine aminotransferase (ALT) and gamma-glutamyl transferase can increase with normal doses of acetaminophen; although those changes are probably unimportant in the absence of functional or synthetic liver impairment.[111,112] Acetaminophen appears to be opioid-sparing and works synergistically with opioids at normal opioid starting doses, but with high-dose opioids does not seem to add benefit.[113] Intravenous (IV) acetaminophen does not offer a benefit over enteral administration and should only be considered when enteral or rectal administration is not feasible. In the United States, after a recent price rise of 240% ($40 for 1,000 mg), the cost of IV acetaminophen is artificially inflated when compared to the enteral forms.[114]

NONSTEROIDAL ANTI-INFLAMMATORY DRUGS

NSAIDs, such as ibuprofen, naproxen, ketorolac, and meloxicam display an equianalgesic effect; in other words, in principle, one NSAID doesn't provide better analgesia than another. Due to differences in pharmacokinetics, pharmacodynamics, and pharmacogenetics, there are of course interindividual variabilities. Ibuprofen is usually preferred because it carries the least gastrointestinal side effects among NSAIDs that are nonselective for COX-2.

NSAIDs should be used with caution in individuals with renal impairment and in patients with a history or risk of bleeding, including risk of gastrointestinal bleeding or ulcers, as this group of medication inhibits platelet aggregation. Ketorolac has the advantage of IV administration, but, due to higher risks of side effects in children, should be rotated to oral ibuprofen as soon as tolerated.

Compared to standard ibuprofen, the salt formulation (ibuprofen sodium), which is available over the counter in the United States and other countries, has a faster analgesic onset (within 10 minutes), only requires 50% of the dose, and has a longer duration of action.[115]

COX-2 INHIBITOR

Celecoxib (a COX-2 much more than a COX-1 inhibitor) is commonly used in children with serious illness when classical NSAIDs are contraindicated (e.g., due to increased bleeding risks or gastrointestinal side effects). Celecoxib can be compounded into a liquid, thus easing administration in children, and a short course of COX-2 inhibitors can be safely used even in individuals who are undergoing surgery.[116] It is yet unclear whether COX-2 inhibitors display a better cardiovascular risk profile or less renal toxicity compared to classic NSAIDs, as suggested by single studies.[117,118]

DIPYRONE

Dipyrone (metamizole) has an analgesic, spasmolytic, and antipyretic effects and is used to treat pediatric pain in many parts of the world.[106] Due to a possible risk of agranulocytosis with the use of this medication, it has been banned in the United States and several other countries. The analgesic efficacy of IV dipyrone appears similar to that of IV acetaminophen (paracetamol).[106] There is no evidence to support that dipyrone is equivalent or even superior to NSAIDs in pediatric pain.[106]

OPIOIDS

Opioids are indicated in children with serious illness for both medium to severe acute pain due to tissue injury as well as in the treatment of dyspnea. Morphine remains the "gold standard," but other "strong" opioids, such as fentanyl, oxycodone, hydromorphone, diamorphine (in the UK only), and methadone are equally effective in their respective analgesic effects.

Opioid-associated side effects (e.g., constipation, pruritus, and nausea) should be anticipated and treated accordingly. For pediatric opioid starting doses, see Table 23.3; for usual patient-controlled-analgesia (PCA) pump starting doses see Table 23.4.

Opioid rotation may be necessary if tolerance develops or dose-limiting opioid toxicity occurs. A switch from one opioid to another is often accompanied by a change in the balance between analgesia and side effects.[134] A favorable change in opioid side-effect profile may be experienced if there is less cross-tolerance at the opioid receptors mediating analgesia than at those mediating adverse effects. If rotating opioids because of decreasing effectiveness or limiting side effects (i.e., because of incomplete cross-tolerance), the clinician can consider starting at around 50% of the equianalgesic dose and titrating to effect. However, the required decrease for incomplete cross-tolerance may be higher or lower, depending on the clinical context of the individual patient.[135]

"By the clock" dosing. When pain is constantly present, administration of basic both analgesia and opioid should usually be scheduled "around-the-clock" (e.g., acetaminophen every 6 hours scheduled and morphine every 4 hours scheduled).[107]

"Weak" Opioids

"Weak" opioids display an analgesic ceiling effect; in other words, an increase in dose does not result in increased analgesia beyond a certain dose. This group includes mixed agonist/antagonist, partial opioid agonists, and multimechanism analgesics. With the explicit exception of tramadol, and possibly buprenorphine, this group of opioids can not usually be recommended in PPC.

Mixed agonist/antagonist (such as nalbuphine and butorphanol) agents can precipitate withdrawal symptoms when used in opioid-tolerant patients. Tapentadol, a mu

TABLE 23.2 Common opioid myths

MYTH	FACT
Addiction Opioids administered for acute pain or dyspnea cause opioid-use disorder (formerly known as "addiction").	**There is scant evidence to support the existence of an epidemic of addiction and deaths due to appropriate use of prescribed opioids.**[119] Appropriate medical use of prescription opioids in adolescence is NOT associated with substance use disorder in adulthood.[120] The current "opioid crisis" in the United States, according to Krane et al., is more one of deaths from illicit drugs than from prescription opioids and more about deaths from illicit use of prescriptions than from medical use of prescription opioids. [119] We have an epidemic of substance use disorder (SUD) embedded in a complicated matrix of despair and hopelessness across the United States, which correlates closely with socioeconomic factors such as unemployment, poor education, availability of illicit street and diverted prescription opioids, genetic predisposition to SUD, and psychiatric morbidity.
"Getting high" Kids misuse opioids because they want to get high	**Most teenagers are misusing opioids due to unrelieved pain and untreated mental health.** Nineteen percent of adolescents take their prescribed opioids other than prescribed[121] (higher dose, frequency etc.) and thus "misuse opioids." The vast majority of adolescents do so because of unrelieved pain (4 in 5), followed by insomnia and anxiety. Yet only about 11–35% of those (i.e., 1–3 out 50) do so to "get high".[122–124] As a result, safe opioid prescribing for the correct indications only (i.e., not for treating insomnia, mental health concerns, and chronic pain) is warranted.
Medication "too strong"	The opioid "strength" is dose-related. A low dose of an opioid would be weaker than ibuprofen and a higher dose stronger.
Opioids are "masking symptoms"	Opioids do not affect the clinical evaluation of patients with acute abdominal pain[125] and opioids after major cranial surgery in children do *not* result in altered mental status nor respiratory depression.
Opioids cause oversedation/ respiratory depression	While an opioid dose carries a significant dose-related risk of respiratory depression in a patient without acute pain, this is far less so when given for acute pain or dyspnea (using starting doses and titrating to effect).
Opioids are effective for chronic pain, and the higher the pain number in a seriously ill child with chronic pain, the higher the opioid dose that should be given	Opioids should *not* be administered to pediatric patients with chronic pain without tissue injury[126] (i.e., for pain that extends beyond the expected time of healing which hence lacks the acute warning function of physiological nociception), even when they have an underlying serious illness. Opioids administered for chronic pain have low long-term efficacy, a poor safety profile, and commonly a worse clinical outcome.[127–133] On the other hand, in persistent pain conditions (i.e., long-lasting and/or repetitive nociceptive pain caused by tissue injury, such as in children with junctional epidermolysis bullosa, osteogenesis imperfecta, or advanced metastasized bone tumors), opioids usually do play an important role in long-term analgesic management.
Opioids do not cause constipation	Constipation is the only side effect which will not resolve over time. Hence the clinical saying: "The hand which prescribes an opioid without a bowel regimen is the hand which will disimpact the patient."
My favorite opioid will work for most of my patients for most of their pains	Up to 40% of pediatric patients will not achieve good analgesia without dose-limiting adverse effects on any given opioid. Opioid rotation may be necessary if tolerance develops or dose-limiting opioid toxicity occurs.

(delta, kappa)-receptor agonist and a norepinephrine reuptake inhibitor is a close chemical and structural relative of tramadol and so far, it is unclear whether it has any advantage over tramadol.[136] The high price and no current pediatric data make it an unlikely choice due to inexpensive, safe, and efficacious alternatives.

CODEINE

Codeine can no longer be recommended due to pediatric deaths, especially in cytochrome P450 2D6 ultra-rapid metabolizers, and it has become obsolete.[137–143] Of note, in low-income countries where morphine might not be available, the use of codeine may be supported if no other strong opioids are available.

Codeine's ability to provide effective analgesia through its active metabolite, morphine, via the cytochrome P450 2D6 (CYP2D6) system is limited in both "poor" as well as "intermediate" metabolizers (more than one-third of patients). Commonly observed side effects of codeine include nausea, vomiting, constipation, pruritus, and urinary retention. Clinical experience suggests that codeine causes more nausea and vomiting than any other standard analgesic in children.[144]

HYDROCODONE

Hydrocodone (dihydrocodeinone) is usually not available outside the United States, but in the United States is by far the single most commonly prescribed opioid. Like codeine, it appears that hydrocodone is an inactive pro-drug, and the main analgesic effect results from the metabolite hydromorphone.[145] CYP2D6 ultra-rapid metabolizer (similar to codeine's metabolism into morphine) have a much higher risk of respiratory depression, and pediatric death have occurred.[146,147] As such, hydrocodone (analogue to codeine) cannot be recommended for use in pediatrics.

TRAMADOL

Tramadol, a multimechanistic analgesic, on the other hand, continues to play a key role not only in outpatient surgery (e.g., more than 6,000 pediatric tramadol scripts were filled at Children's Minnesota in 2018 in part due to its relative safe respiratory profile), but also in treating episodes of inconsolability in children with progressive neurologic, metabolic, or chromosomally based conditions with impairment of the CNS. Surprisingly, and not well based on scientific evidence, the US Food and Drug Administration (FDA) issued a warning against pediatric use of tramadol and cited the data of three children who have died worldwide in the previous 49 years, therefore actually making it far safer than any other opioid. Unfortunately, this warning may place children at greater risk for unrelieved pain and other distressing symptoms by encouraging clinicians to either use strong opioids in the outpatient setting with a higher risk of respiratory depression or not using opioids at all.[148]

Tramadol is a multimechanistic analgesic commonly used worldwide for pediatric pain management and palliative care.[149–152] Studies examining efficacy and safety of this medication have been conducted worldwide, and results support its use in children.[141,153–163] The analgesic potency of tramadol falls somewhere between ibuprofen and morphine.[164] Although only commercially available in tablet form in the United States, an oral suspension may be compounded into a stable and inexpensive liquid.[165] Outside the United States, both IV and liquid tramadol are readily available. Although tramadol is metabolized into the more potent O-desmethyltramadol, tramadol (unlike codeine) itself appears to be a potent analgesic.

For poor CYP2D6 metabolizers, the parent compound tramadol remains active; hence, those individuals experience no decrease or only a slightly diminished analgesic effect, possibly supported by parallel CYP3A4 metabolism.[164] Data suggest that tramadol administration may result in fewer side effects than with full mu-opioid agonists,[166] and tramadol appears far safer than codeine when it comes to risk of respiratory depression. One study examining statewide poison control center data in the United States[167] reported no respiratory depression in children younger than 6 years who ingested 10/mg/kg or less (up to 5–10 times the recommended dose); however, 2 out of 87 (2%) adults in the sample did experience respiratory depression.

Notably, tramadol has been shown to be particularly helpful in treating neuropathic pain and visceral hyperalgesia[7] presenting as episodes of inconsolability in children with neurologic, metabolic, or chromosomally based condition with impairment of the CNS, such as mitochondropathies.

TEAM REFLECTION

Fourteen-month-old Ella (weight 9.2 kg) was repeatedly hospitalized at a children's hospital with an underlying mitochondropathy and progressive neuromuscular disorder, which a decade later was diagnosed with the rare genetic disorder (RTD-2/BVVLS) Brown-Vialetto-Van Laere syndrome. She was now admitted due to increased frequency and duration of significant episodes of pain and inconsolability associated with vomiting and central apnea, requiring frequent bagging at home. A thorough clinical examination and workup, including laboratory investigations, extensive imagery, and esophago-gastro-duodenoscopy could not reveal an underlying pathology explaining her distressing symptoms.

The basic analgesics ibuprofen and acetaminophen were only moderately helpful for her episodes of pain and discomfort, and the primary and specialist teams had been understandably reluctant about the use of opioids in a child without a clear tissue injury in light of her enigmatic frequent apnea episodes.

After consulting the pediatric pain and palliative care team, Ella was started on 1 mg/kg tramadol every 6 hours by mouth. Within half a day she showed a dramatic improvement of her distressing symptoms. Her frequent vomiting episodes, which had already lasted over several months, resolved completely. Her episodes of pain and inconsolability went down from several hour-long daily episodes to less than one per week. Ella's apnea attacks stopped.

Over the next years Ella continued to present to the palliative care clinic as a complex patient with global motor-neurodevelopmental delay, visual loss, neurogenic bowel and bladder, feeding intolerance with visceral hyperalgesia, and dysautonomia, and she required additional basic and adjuvant analgesia (such as celecoxib, gabapentin, nortriptyline, clonidine) for good symptom control. She is gaining milestones (improving her sign-language, writes, walks). Repeated trials of slowly decreasing tramadol (or switching to morphine or oxycodone) resulted in increased pain episodes, vomiting, and increased apnea. At age of 15, at a weight of 41 kg, she is currently on 60 mg tramadol three times per day plus an as-needed dose of 60 mg, which she requires about once per week.

Buprenorphine

This opioid displays a somewhat unique pharmacology compared to other agents in its class. As a partial mu-opioid receptor agonist with long duration of action, it can cause an "opioid blockade." It is also a delta-opioid receptor antagonist and a kappa-opioid (partial agonist) receptor antagonist (i.e., possibly less likely to cause psychomimetic effects such as dysphoria/hallucinations). The main liver metabolite norbuprenorphine, however, is a partial kappa-agonist and a full mu- and delta-opioid receptor agonist, and as such might be antagonized by buprenorphine.[168,169] In the United States, transdermal patches are available at comparatively low doses only—5, 10, and 20 mcg/hr—whereas in most other countries (e.g., the United Kingdom), patches are available that release 35, 52.5 and 70 mcg/hr buprenorphine. In practice, buprenorphine might be useful in children with mild to moderate pain with nonmalignant life-limiting conditions, especially when there is concern of opioid-induced constipation.

"Strong" Opioids

This group are full mu-opioid receptor agonists, with methadone representing additionally a multimechanistic analgesic. Morphine, fentanyl, oxycodone, hydromorphone (in the UK only: diamorphine), and methadone are very effective in providing analgesia (and treatment of dyspnea at end of life) at equianalgesic doses (see Tables 23.3, 23.4, and 23.6 for starting doses). One opioid per se is not necessarily "more effective" or "stronger" than another. In fact, at equianalgesic doses, all strong opioids are expected to be equally effective in reducing pain. Having said this, in pediatric patients with serious illness, an opioid rotation is indicated in up to 40% of the cases when tolerance develops or dose-limiting opioid side effects occur (e.g., unrelieved pain with respiratory depression and/or nausea).[135] A switch from one opioid to another is often accompanied by a change in the balance between analgesia and side effects,[134] taking advantage of incomplete cross-tolerance.

Opioid-associated side effects, especially constipation, but also pruritus, nausea, and urinary retention should be anticipated and treated accordingly. In the scenario of severe adverse effects, such as opioid-induced respiratory depression, treatment options include reducing (or briefly pausing) the opioid dose (in case of adequate analgesia) or rotating the opioid (if inadequate analgesia) at equianalgesic doses, minus a decrease for incomplete cross-tolerance. That reduction often is around 50%; however, in individual case it may be much higher or lower.[135]

The choice of an opioid is often simply dictated by availability (many low- to medium-income countries have limited or no access to opioids in general), but also sometimes by cognitive bias by clinicians, institutional leadership, and regulators.

MORPHINE

Morphine is considered the gold standard for analgesia against which all other opioids are compared. Routes of administration include oral, sublingual, IV, intramuscular, subcutaneous, intrathecal, and epidural. Morphine is also effective topically in open wounds.[170] See Tables 23.3, 2.4, and 23.6 for typical starting doses, which must be titrated to effect.

Morphine is metabolized by liver glucuronyl-transferase into "the good guy" morphine-6 glucuronide (M6G) and "the bad guy" morphine-3 glucuronide (M3G). M6G is a much stronger analgesic (40–100 times stronger) and displays adverse effects including nausea, vomiting, sedation,

TABLE 23.3 Opioid starting doses for children with acute pain older than 6 months

MEDICATION (ROUTE OF ADMINISTRATION)	PEDIATRIC DOSE	MAXIMAL DOSE	DOSING INTERVAL	COMMENT
Partial mu-receptor agonists ("weak opioid")				
Tramadol (PO, SL, PR)	0.5–1 mg/kg (max 2 mg/dose)	25–50 mg (max. 100 mg)/dose	q4–6h	Analgesic ceiling effect: max. 8 mg/kg/day (>50 kg: max. of 400 mg/day)
Full mu-receptor agonists ("strong opioids")				
Morphine (PO, SL, PR)	0.15–0.3 mg/kg	7.5–15 mg/dose	q4h	
Morphine (IV, SC)	0.05–0.1 mg/kg	2.5–5 mg/dose	q4h	
Oxycodone (PO, SL, PR)	0.15–0.3 mg/kg	7.5–15 mg/dose	q6h	Oxycodone can be administered every 6 hours due to longer half-life; alternatively may be given every 4 hours: 0.1–0.2 mg/kg q4h (max. 5–10 mg q4h)
Fentanyl (IV, SC, SL, transdermal, buccal)	0.5–1 mcg/kg	25–50 mcg	n/a	Due to short half-life, consider starting continuous infusion 0.5–1 mcg/kg/hr (max. 50 mcg/hr), if scheduled analgesia required
Hydromorphone (PO, SL, PR)	40–60 mcg/kg	2,000–3,000 mcg (= 2–3 mg)	q4h	
Hydromorphone (IV, SC)	10–20 mcg/kg	0.5–1 mg	q4h	
Multimechanistic full mu-receptor agonists ("strong opioid")				
Methadone (PO, PR, SL)	0.05–0.1 mg/kg	2.5–5 mg	q8–12h	Methadone should not be prescribed by those unfamiliar with its use! Its effects should be closely monitored for several days, particularly when it is first started and after any dose changes.
Methadone (IV, SC)	0.04–0.08 mg/kg	2–4 mg	q8–12h	Whereas in pediatrics, due to high bioavailability, about 80% of the enteral dose appears to be the equianalgesic IV dose (e.g., 1 mg PO = 0.8 mg IV), adult recommendations suggest 50% conversion (e.g., 1 mg PO = 0.5 mg IV)

Dosing range: Younger children with smaller pain *start* on the lower end of the range, older children with severe pain *start* on the higher end of the dosing range; doses are then titrated to effect.

Maximum per kg dose capped at 50 kg body weight.

For strong opioids: Rescue ("breakthrough" or "PRN") dose equals 10% of total daily dose.

IV, intravenous; PO, by mouth (or enterally via gastric/jejunal tube); SL, sublingually; PR, rectally; q4h, every 4 hours; q6h, every 6 hours.

Used with permission from Stefan Friedrichsdorf, Benioff Children's Hospitals in Oakland and San Francisco, University of California at San Francisco (UCSF).

TABLE 23.4

PCA DOSE	MAX. PCA DOSE (FOR PATIENTS >50 KG)	CONTINUOUS INFUSION (BASAL RATE)	MAX. CONTINUOUS INFUSION (FOR PATIENTS >50 KG)	LOCK-OUT TIME	NUMBER OF MAX. BOLUSES
Morphine					
10–20 mcg/kg	500–1,000 mcg (= 0.5–1 mg)	10–20 mcg/kg/hour	500–1,000 mcg (= 0.5–1 mg)/hour	5–10 minutes	4–6 boluses/hour
Fentanyl					
0.5–1 mcg/kg	25–50 mcg	0.5–1 mcg/kg/hour	25–50 mcg/hour	5–10 minutes	4–6 boluses/hour
Hydromorphone					
2–4 mcg/kg	100–200 mcg	2–4 mcg/kg/hour	100–200 mcg/hour	5–10 minutes	4–6 boluses/hour

Starting doses for patient (or nurse)-controlled analgesia (PCA) pumps for children in acute pain older than 6 months.

Dosing range: Younger children with smaller pain start on the lower end of the range, older children with severe pain start on the higher end of the dosing range, doses will then be titrated to effect with escalation usually in (33–)50% increments both for continuous and PCA bolus dose.

PCA dose usually equals continuous infusion (might differ in individual patients).

Maximum per kg dose capped at 50 kg body weight.

Consider adding low-dose naloxone infusion 0.5–2 mcg/kg/hr (max. 25–100 mcg/hr) to treat potential opioid-induced side effects, such as pruritus, nausea, constipation, urinary retention, hallucinations.

Used with permission from Stefan Friedrichsdorf, Benioff Children's Hospitals in Oakland and San Francisco, University of California at San Francisco (UCSF)

and respiratory depression. M3G is not an analgesic but is a mu-opioid antidote with unique adverse effects, especially hyperexcitability and neurotoxicity. The ratio of M6G/M3G thereby defines the analgesia-to-adverse effect profile in individual children. Both metabolites need to be excreted by the kidney, and children in renal failure have a higher risk of unwanted side effects. Fentanyl or methadone, neither of which is excreted renally, is likely to be a better choice in this scenario.

In standard practice, morphine is most commonly administered via the oral or IV routes. Following oral dosing, morphine has a significant first-pass metabolism in the liver. The currently accepted oral-to- IV potency ratio for morphine is 1:3.[171] Therefore, the usual practice when converting oral morphine to IV is to divide the oral dose by 3 (i.e., 3 mg oral morphine equals 1 mg IV morphine). Morphine is available orally as a concentrated solution, immediate-release tablets, and sustained-release tablets and sachets (the latter not available in the United States).

Renal impairment. M3G does not possess analgesic properties, but is instead nociceptive, does not bind to opioid receptors, and may be responsible for some of the adverse CNS effects such as myoclonus. M3G and M6G are excreted by the kidneys, and their elimination is directly related to creatinine clearance. In patients with renal compromise, M3G and M6G may accumulate in the blood and cerebrospinal fluid, leading to unwanted toxicity (M6G may cause oversedation, pruritus, nausea, etc.; M3G may cause increased nociception, hyperexcitability). Morphine should therefore be administered with caution to patients with renal impairment.

Liver impairment. Only with severe liver failure (e.g., as shown by increased prothrombin time) does morphine's half-life substantially increase, making opioid induced-side effects are more likely.

Morphine in neonates. Morphine appears safe and efficacious in full-term neonates; however, starting doses are usually lower compared to those used in older children. Long-term neurodevelopmental outcome years after former preterm or term babies are exposed to continuous morphine or fentanyl infusion displayed no adverse effects of the opioids on intelligence, motor function, or behavior.[172–175]

Opioid pharmacokinetics and pharmacodynamics in neonates and young infants (up to 6 months of life) require one to administer lower starting doses than in older children. This principle is based on the following:

1. Infants display delayed maturation of hepatic enzyme systems involved in metabolic drug metabolic inactivation. For most opioid analgesics, metabolism matures at approximately 6 months of age.
2. Decreased glomerular filtration and renal tubular secretion result in decreased elimination of opioids and their active metabolites.
3. Decrease levels of alpha-1-acid glycoprotein and albumin translate into decreased plasma protein binding for many drugs and can thus lead to increased concentrations of pharmacologically active unbound drug. The binding of morphine to plasma protein is age-dependent. In premature infants, less than 20% is bound to plasma proteins.[176,177]
4. Within the neonatal period for term infants, the volume of distribution is linearly related to age and body surface area,[176–178] but after the neonatal period the values are approximately the same as in adults.[179,180]
5. As a result of the preceding facts, the morphine elimination half-life in children older than 6 months is 3–4 hours. In full-term infants, the half-life is 7 hours, and in preterm infants 9–10 hours or even up to 20 hours.[179,180] This helps explain why we might schedule morphine every 4 hours in a 1-year-old, but every 6–8 hours in a 1-day-old full-term infant.
6. Infants have immature ventilatory reflexes in response to hypoxia and hypercarbia and are at increased risk of hypoventilation in response to opioids; they therefore require closer observation than older children.

7. However, morphine may not provide adequate analgesia for acute procedural pain among preterm neonates, which is one reason why fentanyl might be a better opioid to manage acute pain in this age group (although it may result in faster development of opioid tolerance).[181] The liver of neonates and young infants (biliary excretion results in small intestine absorption) preferentially produces M3G, with little if any M6G detected.

Therefore, starting doses in very young infants should be reduced to approximately 25% to 30% on a per kilogram basis relative to dosing recommended for older children.

Oxycodone

Oxycodone is a selective mu-opioid receptor agonist, although some animal studies suggest kappa-receptor agonist activity as well.[182] The oral potency ratio of oral oxycodone to morphine is between 1:1 and 2:1.[183] An advantage of oxycodone over morphine is the longer half-life, frequently allowing 6-hour dosing (as oppose to 4-hour with morphine). Renal and hepatic impairment increases oxycodone serum levels.[184]

Hydromorphone

Hydromorphone is another selective mu-opioid receptor agonist. Unlike morphine metabolism, there is no hydromorphone-6-glucuronide (H6G) produced; however, as in morphine, metabolism of the parent compound does result in "the bad guy" hydromorphone-3-glucoronide (H3G). Opioid hyperexcitability has been reported in patients with renal failure taking hydromorphone.[185,186] The normal H3G to hydromorphone plasma ratio is 27:1, but in renal failure it is 100:1.[187]

Fentanyl

Fentanyl is a commonly used opioid for pediatric analgesia prior to painful procedures owing to its rapid onset (about 1 minute) and its brief duration of action (30–45 minutes). It is also used to manage pain in children with cancer, for intra- and postoperative analgesia, in PPC, and for sedation-analgesia in ventilated children in the intensive care unit. Fentanyl provides a good alternative to morphine when tolerance or dose-limiting side effects mandate opioid rotation.[188,189]

Diamorphine

Diamorphine is only available in the United Kingdom, where, after morphine, it is the second most commonly used opioid in pediatrics,[190] administered both intravenously and intranasally.[191–193] Similar to hydromorphone and fentanyl, diamorphine exhibits high lipophilicity.

Methadone

Methadone is an excellent opioid choice in advanced pediatric analgesia and PPC, but it remains underutilized.[194–200] It is a mu-(delta-, kappa)-opioid receptor agonist, an N-methyl-D-aspartate (NMDA)-channel blocker, and a presynaptic blocker of serotonin and norepinephrine reuptake. As such, it is a multimechanistic agent and its effect mimics "three-drugs-in-one": e.g., morphine, ketamine, and amitriptyline. Advantages include methadone's long half-life (allowing every 8- to 12-hour dosing), high effectiveness in complex pain conditions, decreased incidence of constipation, lack of active metabolites, and safe usage in renal failure and in stable liver disease. Cross-tolerance is believed to be avoided secondary to its activity at NMDA receptors.[201,202]

There are several disadvantages, however, including wide dosing variation, a long half-life (which may lead to accumulation, making quick titration difficult), and a more complex equianalgesic conversion, which requires longer and closer patient observation than with other opioids. Methadone displays typical opioid-induced side effects such as sedation, nausea, constipation, and, at higher doses, opioid-induced neurotoxicity (including myoclonus, hallucinations, nightmares); respiratory depression has been described, with some case reports of hypoglycemia.[203,204] Usual starting doses for opioid naïve children at the UCSF Benioff Children's Hospitals Center for Pediatric Pain, Palliative and Integrative Medicine are 0.05–0.1 mg/kg/dose (max 2.5–5 mg orally every 8–12 hours).

Despite its advantages, conversion to methadone remains complicated in pediatric patients. There are significant problems with adult-based conversion tables used in pediatrics,[135,194,199] including tremendous interindividual variability in relative potency estimates, tolerance development with repetitive dosing (dose reduction of 25–75% or more for incomplete cross-tolerance is often inadequately portrayed), the erroneous assumption that relative potency ratios remain irrespective of level of opioid, and no accounting for unidirectional cross-tolerance nor for the possibility of active metabolite accumulation.

The oral-to-parenteral potency ratio of methadone is approximately 1:5 to 2:1. In clinical practice, in adult medicine 10 mg of oral methadone would usually be rotated to 5 mg IV methadone (and 5 mg IV methadone to 5 mg PO methadone). In pediatrics, due to the high bioavailability, withdrawal is not uncommon using this approach, and, as such at our institution we are using "The pediatric 80% approach" (i.e., 10 mg PO methadone = 8 mg IV methadone and 8 mg IV methadone = 10 mg PO methadone).

Methadone has a long and variable half-life. Following single parenteral doses, its potency is similar to that of morphine. In children receiving postoperative analgesia, methadone produced a more prolonged analgesia than morphine.[79,80] Because of its prolonged half-life, methadone has a risk of delayed sedation and overdose occurring several days after initiating treatment. Methadone should not be prescribed by those unfamiliar with its use. Its effects should be closely monitored for several days, particularly when it is first started and after any dose changes.[194,205–207] Given the prolonged half-life, when titrating methadone in an outpatient at home, it is recommended to increase the dose only every 3 days while closely monitoring daily for signs of oversedation.

Breakthrough or rescue dose while on methadone. Depending on the clinical scenario, patients with serious illness and acute pain may use fast-acting strong opioids (e.g., morphine) or methadone for breakthrough pain. Either way, it is always required to state the frequency (e.g., take every 3 hours as needed for medium-severe pain and no signs of oversedation) plus the total number of breakthrough doses allowed per day (e.g., methadone every 4 hours PRN with a maximum of two doses in 24 hours; call prescribing clinician service if unrelieved pain after 2 PRN doses).

OPIOIDS FOR CHRONIC PAIN

Opioids should *not* be administered to pediatric patients with primary pain disorders[126]; that is, chronic pain that extends beyond the expected time of healing and that hence lacks the acute warning function of physiological nociception, even in the presence of an underlying serious illness. Opioids may be more likely to cause more harm than benefit in the treatment of primary pain disorders, which include conditions such as primary headaches (tension headaches/migraines and medication-overuse headaches), chronic musculoskeletal pain/fibromyalgia, chronic sickle cell pain (pain that extends beyond the expected time of acute vaso-occlusive crisis), and functional abdominal pain/centrally mediated abdominal pain syndrome. Opioids administered for primary pain disorders have low long-term efficacy, a poor safety profile, and, commonly, a worse clinical outcome.[127–133] On the other hand, in persistent pain conditions (i.e., long-lasting and/or repetitive nociceptive pain caused by tissue injury, as in children with junctional epidermolysis bullosa, osteogenesis imperfecta, or advanced metastasized bone tumors; e.g., Ewing sarcoma) opioids usually do play an important role in long-term analgesic management.

BREAKTHROUGH PAIN IN CHILDREN

Breakthrough or rescue doses (PRN) are additional doses of opioid incorporated into the analgesic regime to allow for additional analgesia if required by the patient. Breakthrough doses of opioid may be calculated as approximately 10% of the total daily opioid requirement and may be administered by any route of administration every 1–3 hours.[208] As mentioned earlier, especially in an outpatient setting, the maximum number of breakthrough doses per day must be ordered. In other words, "every 1 hour as needed" should not translate into 24 breakthrough doses in 24 hours, but rather "if requiring more than 3 breakthrough doses in 24 hours, call prescribing clinical service." Given the frequency with which additional analgesia may be required for severe pain; it may be convenient for some children to self-administer breakthrough opioid doses using a Patient-controlled analgesia (PCA) device. A prospective study determined the prevalence, characteristics, and impact of breakthrough pain in children with cancer.[209] Twenty-seven pediatric inpatients with cancer aged 7–18 years who had severe pain requiring treatment with opioids participated in this study. The children responded to a structured interview, the Breakthrough Pain Questionnaire for Children, designed to characterize breakthrough pain in children. Measures of pain, anxiety, and depressed mood were completed. Fifty-seven percent of the children experienced one or more episodes of breakthrough pain during the preceding 24 hours, each episode lasting seconds to minutes, occurring three or four times a day, and most commonly characterized as sharp and shooting by the children. Younger children, those 7–12 years, had a significantly higher risk of experiencing breakthrough pain compared to teenagers. No statistical difference could be shown between children with and without breakthrough pain in regard to anxiety and depression. The most effective treatment of an episode of breakthrough pain was a PCA opioid bolus dose. Further studies of breakthrough pain in children and more effective treatment strategies in this age group are necessary.

ADJUVANT ANALGESIA

Adjuvant analgesics may improve pain control either in addition to basic analgesia and/or opioids, or they may also act as primary analgesics, especially in neuropathic and visceral pain treatment.[210,211] This heterogenic group includes gabapentinoids[212,213] (such as gabapentin, pregabalin), alpha-2-adrenergic agonists[214–216] (such as clonidine or dexmedetomidine), low-dose tricyclic antidepressants (TCAs, such as amitriptyline or nortriptyline), NMDA channel blockers (such as low-dose ketamine[217,218]), and sodium-channel blockers (such as lidocaine[219–223]). See Table 23.6 for dosing recommendations.

STEP 6: GABAPENTINOIDS AND/OR TRICYCLIC ANTIDEPRESSANTS

A meta-analysis showed gabapentinoids to be efficacious in the control of neuropathic pain in adults of various etiologies with a number needed to treat (NNT) of 2.9–3.9.[210] Gabapentinoids are alpha-2-delta ligands, locking on a voltage-gated calcium-channel at the presynaptic nerve terminal (first neuron) at the level of the dorsal horn, resulting in decreased release of pain transmitters, such as glutamate, norepinephrine, and substance P. Gabapentin (NNT: 6.3; number needed to harm [NNH]: 25.6) appears to be slightly more effective than pregabaline (NNT: 7.7; NNH: 13.9), which seems more effective than extended-release gabapentin (NNT 8.3; NNH 31.9).[210] Adult data and pediatric experience suggest that a significant number of patients who experience inadequate analgesia from pregabaline benefit from gabapentin, and vice versa. Conversion from gabapentin to pregabalin is around 6:1, meaning 300 mg gabapentin three times a day (i.e., 900 mg/day) equals pregabalin 75 mg twice a day (i.e., 150 mg/day).[19] To avoid pain or precipitating seizures, these anticonvulsants should be weaned over a period of 1–2 weeks.

GABAPENTIN

An initial low starting dose is 2 mg/kg/dose (max. 100 mg/dose) once at night, titrated to 6 mg/kg/dose (i.e., 300 mg/dose for patients >50 kg) three times a day. For mild to medium neuropathic pain, the titration may take up to 2 weeks to avoid side effects. For severe pain, the titration may be significantly faster (1–3 days). If analgesia is inadequate, the dose may be titrated in steps up to 12 mg/kg/dose (max. 600 mg/dose) three times a day, then up to 18 mg/kg/dose (max. 900 mg/dose) three times a day, and finally up to 24 mg/kg/dose (max. 1,200 mg/dose) three times a day. Gabapentin (as

TABLE 23.5 Adjuvant analgesia for infants, children, and adolescents

MEDICATION (ROUTE OF ADMINISTRATION)	PEDIATRIC DOSE	MAX. DOSE (FOR PATIENTS >50 KG)	DOSING INTERVAL	COMMENTS/SIDE EFFECTS
Gabapentinoids				
Gabapentin (PO)	6 mg/kg (titrated up to 24 mg/kg)	300 mg (titrated up to 1,200 mg) TID	TID	In school-aged children may start at lower doses to reduce risk of initial sedation Can NOT be administered rectally (missing active transporter = no absorption) Infants <1 year: 4.5 mg/kg/dose q6h (titrated to effect to max. of 18 mg/kg/dose)
Pregabalin (PO)	1 mg/kg (titrated up to 6 mg/kg)	50 mg (titrated up to 300 mg) BID	BID	Rotation from gabapentin, if distressing side effects or inadequate analgesia Can NOT be administered rectally (missing active transporter = no absorption) In school–age children may start at lower doses to reduce risk of initial sedation No data for infants
Alpha–agonists				
Dexmedetomidine (IV)	0.2 (titrate to max. 2) mcg/kg/hour	10 (titrate to max. 100) mcg/hour	Continuous infusion	
Clonidine (PO, transdermal)	1–3 mcg/kg	50–150 mcg	q4–6h	Transdermal application usually 1:1 conversion to total daily enteral dose
NMDA–channel blocker				
Low–dose ketamine (IV)	1 mcg/kg/minute [= 60 mcg/kg/hour] (titrated to 5 mcg/kg/minute [= 300 mcg/kg/hour])	3 mg/hour (titrated to 15 mg/hour)	Continuous infusion	Conversion to PO ketamine 1:1 (i.e., divide total daily dose by 6 and administer q4h PRN or scheduled)
Tricyclic antidepressants (TCA)				
Amitriptyline (PO)	0.1 mg/kg (titrated to max. 0.5 mg/kg)	5 mg (titrated to max. 25 mg)	qhs	Despite the name, medication NOT potent as an antidepressant Consider EKG to rule out qTc–prolongation Tertiary amine TCA; stronger anticholinergic side effects (including inducing sleep) than nortriptyline For infants >3 months
Nortriptyline (PO)	0.1 mg/kg (titrated to max. 0.5 mg/kg)	5 mg (titrated to max. 25 mg)	qhs	Despite the name, medication NOT potent as an antidepressant Consider EKG to rule out qTc–prolongation For infants >3 months

IV, intravenous; PO, by mouth (or enterally via gastric/jejunal tube); PR, rectally; TID, three times per day; BID, twice per day; q6h, every 6 hours; q8h, every 8 hours; q12h, every 12 hours; q12–24h, every 12–24 hours; NMDA, N-methyl-D-aspertate; qhs, once at night.

Used with permission from Stefan Friedrichsdorf, Benioff Children's Hospitals in Oakland and San Francisco, University of California at San Francisco (UCSF).

oppose to pregabalin) has nonlinear bioavailability, meaning that dose increases close to the maximum dose may have less effect. Side effects include lethargy, ataxia, nystagmus, dizziness, thought disorder, hallucinations, headache, peripheral edema, and myalgia; these side effects appear to be mitigated by slow dose escalation. Especially gabapentin and, to a lesser degree, pregabalin are commonly used in pediatric chronic pain management. There have been no pediatric randomized controlled trials (RCTs) and only a few case reports published[212,213] (see Table 23.5 for starting doses of adjuvant analgesia).

PREGABALIN

Pregabalin should be considered a second choice if gabapentin is ineffective or displays side effects. Safety and efficacy are not established in pediatric patients, and there is no accepted pediatric dosing. Experience and anecdotal evidence suggest the following for older children and teenagers: an initial starting dose 0.5 mg/kg/dose (max. 50 mg/dose) once at night slowly titrated to 1.5 mg/kg/dose (max. 75 mg/dose) every 12 hours twice a day. For mild to medium neuropathic pain, the titration may take up to 2 weeks to avoid side effects. For severe pain, the titration may be significantly faster (2–3 days). If analgesia is inadequate, the dose may be titrated in steps up to 3 mg/kg/dose (max. 150 mg/dose) twice a day, then up to 4.5 mg/kg/dose (max. 225 mg/dose) twice a day, and finally up to 6 mg/kg/dose (max. 300 mg/dose) twice a day.

Possible side effects of pregabalin include blurred vision, life-threatening angioedema (take precautions if prescribing angiotensin converting enzyme [ACE] inhibitors concurrently), dizziness, somnolence, and weight gain.

TABLE 23.6 Analgesia for neonates and infants 0–6 months of age

BASIC ANALGESIA				
DRUG	**ROUTE**	**PEDIATRIC DOSE (AGE)**	**MAXIMAL DOSE**	**DOSING INTERVAL**
Ibuprofen[a]	PO	5–10 mg/kg (Infants 3–6 months)	40 mg/kg/day	6–8 hrs
Acetaminophen	PO, PR	5–10 mg/kg (Neonates 0–30 days) 10 mg/kg (Infants 1–3 months) 10–15 mg/kg (Infants 3–6 months)	20–40 mg/kg/day 40 mg/kg/day 40–60 mg/kg/day	4–6 hrs (maximum 4 doses/day)
Acetaminophen[b]	IV	<10 kg = 7.5 mg/kg	30 mg/kg/day	6 hrs
Opioids				
Morphine	PO/PR/SL	0.075–0.15 mg/kg (neonates 0–30 days) 0.08 0.2 mg (infants 1–12 months)		6 hrs
0.08–0.2 mg/kg (infants 1–6 months)				4–6 hrs
Morphine[d]	IV/SC[c]	0.025–0.05 mg/kg (neonates 0–30 days) 0.08 – 0.2 mg (infants 1–12 months)		6 hrs
0.1 mg/kg (infants 1–6 months) 0.1 mg (infants 1–6 months) 0.1 mg (infants 1–6 months)				6 hrs
Infusion (with PCA bolus of same dose): 0.005–0.01 mg/kg/hr (neonates 0–30 days) 0.01–0.03 mg/kg/hr (Infants 1–6 months)				
Fentanyl[d]	IV/SC[c]	1–2 mcg/kg (neonates and infants 0–12 months) 0.08 – 0.2 mg (Infants 1–12 months)		2–4 hrs
Infusion (with PCA bolus of same dose): 0.5–1 mcg/kg/hr (Neonates and Infants 0–6 months)				
Oxycodone	PO/PR/SL	0.05–0.125 mg/kg (infants 1–6 months)		4–6 hrs

[a]For infants <3 months consult Pain Service.

[b]ONLY if rectal or oral administration is contraindicated; reevaluate daily.

[c] Administer IV slowly over at least 5 minutes.

[d] The intravenous doses for neonates are based on acute pain management and sedation dosing information. Lower doses are required for non-ventilated neonates.

Adapted with permission from World Health Organization. *WHO guidelines on the pharmacological treatment of persisting pain in children with medical illnesses.* Geneva: WHO Press; 2012.

TRICYCLIC ANTIDEPRESSANTS

TCAs are among the best-studied adjuvant analgesics that show efficacy in treating neuropathic pain. TCAs are not effective in treating anxiety in children and teens[224] and therefore should not play a role in treating anxiety or depression in a child in palliative care. Amitriptyline and nortriptyline, which have been extensively studied, block reuptake of serotonin and norepinephrine, which possibly stimulates descending inhibiting pathways stemming from the periaqueductal gray, and they may also block the NMDA receptor. In addition, opioid analgesia might be improved with concurrent TCA administration via a serotoninergic mechanism at the brainstem. Adverse effects of all TCAs include arrhythmia and anticholinergic/antihistamine effects, such as dry mouth, constipation, urinary retention, blurred vision, and sedation. Nortriptyline (a secondary amine) may be better tolerated than amitriptyline (a tertiary amine) because it has fewer anticholinergic side effects.

Amitriptyline and nortriptyline show some efficacy in treating adult neuropathic pain[210]; however, despite the fact that they are commonly used in children, there are no pediatric RCTs.[225,226] Amitriptyline has a NNT of 3.6 and a NNH of 13.4 and has not shown a dose-response effect.[210]

Dose recommendations are the same for both amitriptyline and nortriptyline. Both are available in liquid form and are usually started at 0.1 mg/kg by mouth at bedtime (adult dose 5 mg) and increased to a maximum of 0.4–0.5 mg (max. 20–25 mg once at night). Experience has shown that increasing beyond that dose does not appear to result in increased analgesic effect. It may take 1–2 weeks to titrate up to an effective dose and to determine if the analgesic therapy is working; however, the induction of sleep will start much sooner. An electrocardiogram (ECG) to rule out QTc-prolongation/Wolff-Parkinson-White (WPW) syndrome prior to initiation is recommended.

Overall, the efficacy of TCAs and gabapentinoids appears equal.[210] If a single adjuvant appears ineffective and there are no contraindications in the individual pediatric or adult patient, a combination of a medication from each group is recommended since their mechanism of action is synergistic.

STEP 7: ALPHA-AGONISTS

Alpha-2-adrenergic agonists such as clonidine or dexmedetomidine can be effective adjuvant analgesics for both nociceptive and neuropathic pain.[214,216,227–231] They act at the spinal cord in two ways. First, they act on the same neurons in the cord and lead to the same intracellular events as opioids, but they act through a different receptor: the 2-adrenergic and -opioid receptors activate the same potassium channel via inhibitory G proteins. Thus, it is likely that they enhance the anti-nociceptive effects of opioids. In addition, alpha-2-adrenergic agonists decrease sympathetic outflow involved with neuropathic pain and hyperarousal.[232] Clonidine can be given orally, transdermally, or intraspinally. Side effects include lethargy, dry mouth, and hypotension. Dexmedetomidine can also be an effective adjuvant, leading to opioid-sparing. It carries the advantage of not affecting respiration. However, potential side effects include hypotension and bradycardia, leading most institutions to restrict its use to intensive care units. Dose recommendations are, for dexmedetomidine (0.2–2 mcg/kg/hr IV), to a maximum of 100 mcg/hr; clonidine (starting dose 1–3 mcg/kg; max. 50–150 mcg per dose every hour to every 6 hours, titrated to effect, PO or transdermal).

STEP 8: NMDA CHANNEL BLOCKER

NMDA channels may be involved in the spinal neural circuitry that leads to a neuropathic pain state of resistance to higher dose opioids. At a normal resting level, the NMDA channel is blocked by magnesium. Increased excitation, including strong pain stimuli, may open the NMDA channel, producing hyperexcitability of dorsal root neurons, leading to central sensitization (i.e., amplification of neural signaling within the CNS that elicits pain hypersensitivity), wind-up phenomenon, and memory of pain. NMDA receptor antagonists, such as ketamine, methadone, and levorphanol (possibly dextromethorphan and amantadine), which block the channel, can help prevent this phenomenon, leading to decreased opioid resistance, improved hyperalgesia, and improved allodynia.

Ketamine is an NMDA-receptor antagonist, but it possesses other actions which may contribute to its analgesic effect, including a mu-, delta-, and kappa-opioid–like effect; interactions with calcium and sodium channels; cholinergic transmission; and noradrenergic and serotonergic reuptake inhibition. Ketamine is effective for pediatric neuropathic pain in low (i.e., subanesthetic) doses, both alone or in combination with opioids. Ketamine is unique among anesthetic agents in that it does not depress respiratory and cardiovascular systems. In low analgesic doses, the typical anesthetic-dose side effects of ketamine (nystagmus, lacrimation, tachycardia, and altered sensorium) are not usually seen, though pediatric data are limited. There is evidence of significant opioid reduction and improved analgesia following initiation of low-dose ketamine.[218,233] Low-dose ketamine has been described as effective in burn patients.[234]

Analgesic (subanesthetic) ketamine dosing includes the following: IV: 1–5 mcg/kg/min (equivalent to 0.06–0.3 mg/kg/hr), with maximum of 3–15 mg/hr IV; PO: 0.2–0.5 mg/kg three or four times a day or as needed. Ketamine may also be administered subcutaneously, sublingually, intranasally, rectally, or spinally). In the United States, ketamine is only available as a racemic mixture [S(+)-enantiomer (providing analgesia, general anesthesia); R(-)-enantiomer (causing bronchodilatation, nightmares)]. In most other countries, ketamine-S [S(+)-enantiomer] is also available, reducing the required dose by 40–50%.

NMDA-receptor antagonists depress central sensitization to painful stimuli. Dextromethorphan, dextrorphan, ketamine, memantine, and amantadine, among others, have been shown to have NMDA-receptor antagonist activities. The clinical usefulness of some of these medications is however compromised by a high adverse side effect to analgesic ratio.

Dosing recommendations for oral ketamine are more provisional. Most of the available information about oral and/or parenteral ratios in pediatrics is based on single doses for preoperative or preprocedural sedation, and these ratios probably do not account adequately for accumulation of the active metabolite, norketamine, with chronic dosing. Our clinical impression is that with chronic dosing, some patients report benefit from dosing of oral ketamine (i.e., swallowing the IV formulation) in a dose range of 1:1 (e.g., 3 mg/hour IV = 12 mg every 4 hours scheduled orally or as needed).

STEP 9: SODIUM CHANNEL BLOCKER

Another adjuvant analgesia that appears to be effective for neuropathic pain in selective patients is IV lidocaine,[219,235] including for the treatment of background or procedural burn pain.[236] Side effects of IV lidocaine include allergic reaction (serious, but rare) and dose-related numbness around the mouth, dizziness, slurring of speech, hallucinations, muscle twitches, and seizures.[223]

STEP 10: REGIONAL ANESTHESIA AND INTERVENTIONAL PAIN THERAPIES

Regional anesthesia is one of the most effective analgesic modalities because it minimizes systemic side effects, improves quality of life, and can assist with opioid reduction.[237–246] Regional anesthesia is the practice of injecting a local anesthetic near a nerve or group of nerves in order to block pain conduction. It is most commonly used perioperatively when a focal part of the body is operated upon (e.g., numbing the brachial plexus for arm surgery). It can provide analgesia to a specific nerve (e.g., femoral nerve) or to a plexus of nerves (brachial plexus). An expansion of regional anesthesia places a catheter near the desired nerve (or plexus) in order to run local anesthetic medication continuously for a period of time. If the patient experiences breakthrough pain while receiving the continuous infusion of the local anesthetic, a patient-controlled function can allow the patient to give themselves an additional dose of medication as needed (patient controlled regional anesthesia [PCRA]). Patients can also be sent home with a nerve catheter connected to a pump containing local anesthetic so the infusion can be continued in the home setting for short durations. This has been found to be safe

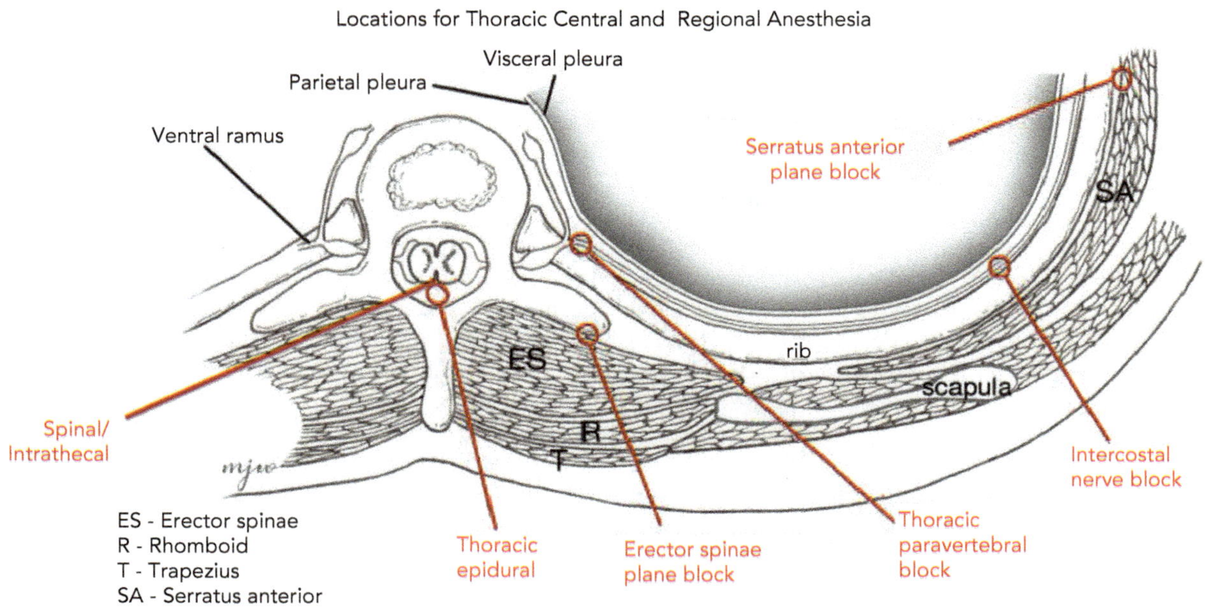

Figure 23.4 *Locations for thoracic central and regional anesthesia.*

and effective for postoperative pain management in pediatric patients[247,248] with case studies showing it effective for pediatric oncologic pain.[249,250]

A further expansion of regional anesthesia is the practice of delivering additional medications and/or therapies near the nerve, such as steroids (to aid in reducing inflammation) or denaturing/neurolytic compounds or thermal heat (to destroy the nerve) (Figures 23.4 and 23.5). These techniques are called *interventional pain therapies* and can be successful at treating pain from nerves and tissues that are compromised due to tumor invasion or other structural disruption. Anesthesiologists are commonly trained in regional anesthesia procedures for use perioperatively; additional education and training is usually obtained to perform interventional pain techniques.

Another form of analgesia, called *central neuraxial analgesia*, can be helpful when attempting to treat larger areas

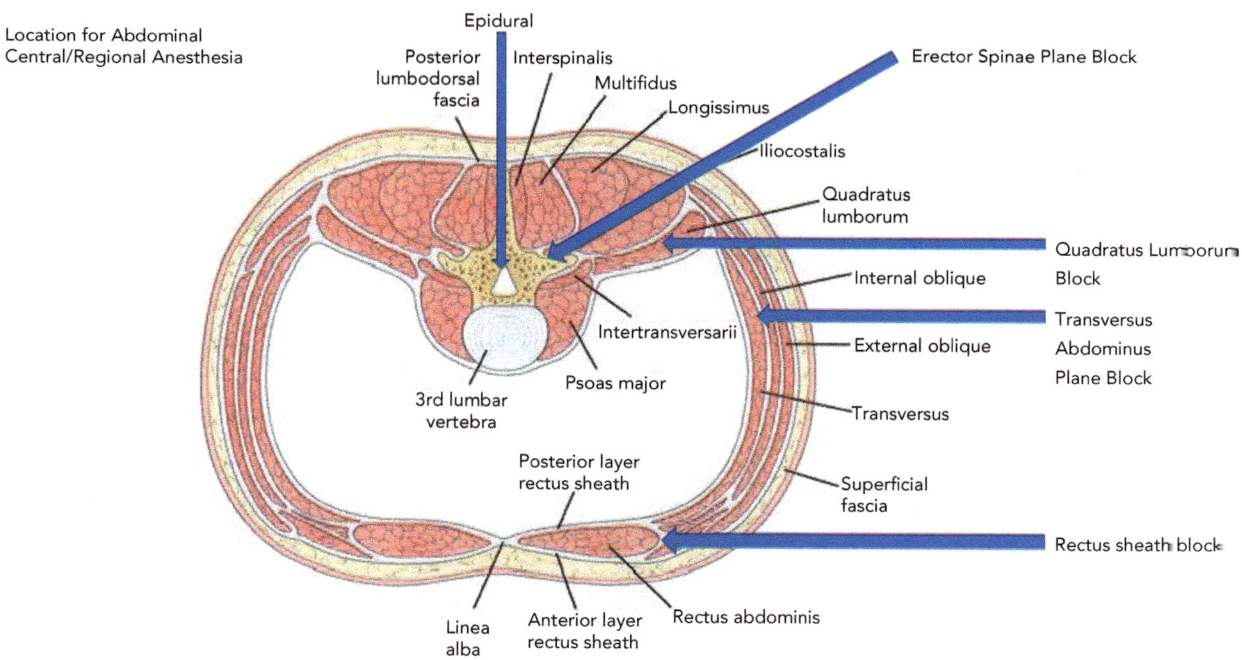

Figure 23.5 *Location for abdominal central/regional anesthesia.*

of the body (i.e., thorax, abdomen/pelvis). This technique involves inserting a catheter into the epidural or intrathecal space to provide a combination of medications that interact with the spinal interneurons involved in pain transmission. Medications commonly placed in these infusions include local anesthetics, opioid medications, alpha-agonists (clonidine), baclofen, and other medications. Catheters can be placed percutaneously for a temporary period (weeks), or they can be tunneled and used for a longer period of time. An advanced method of medication delivery to the intrathecal space is the *intrathecal pump.* It can be surgically implanted in patients and can continuously deliver medications into the spinal fluid for an infinite duration. This therapy has been found to be helpful in treating pain in pediatric patients with solid tumors.[10]

Unfortunately, there are several barriers to the use of regional anesthesia and interventional techniques in PPC patients. Barriers fall into one of four broad categories: patient factors, provider factors, logistical issues, and education.[10] Patient-related barriers to the use of these therapies include patient knowledge and willingness to undergo the procedure and patient candidacy issues (critically ill, coagulopathic, structural issues). Provider-related barriers include the relative paucity of pediatric pain physicians trained to provide these pain therapies and often the inability to access adult pain physicians for this expertise. Logistical factors include difficulty with access to medications, equipment, and providers 24/7 for in-home/in-hospice patients. Educational factors include a lack of literature on the use of regional anesthesia for PPC and reduced general knowledge of this therapy in the pediatric medical community.

Pain nerve fibers course through the body alongside other nerve fibers that control sensation, proprioception, sympathetic function, and motor function. Because of this proximity, there are significant side effects that may occur when a numbing or denaturing agent is applied to a nerve. These side effects include motor weakness, orthostatic hypotension, altered light touch and temperature sensation, urinary retention, and fecal incontinence.[244] These side effects are important to disclose to the patient prior to the procedure, and it is important that other members of the healthcare team are aware of these issues.

The benefits of regional/central anesthesia and interventional pain treatments include[244–249] significantly improved pain control, improved mobility and participation in physical therapy, and improved respiratory mechanics. Another important benefit is reduction of opioid burden and therefore opioid side-effects like sedation, nausea, constipation, urinary retention, delirium, and pruritis. Perhaps the greatest benefit is the improved quality of life and patient satisfaction found with this method of pain treatment. Indeed, this pain treatment method allows for the end-of-life patient to be awake and able to participate in conversations and experiences with clinicians and family (Figure 23.6).

STEP 11: OTHER ADJUVANTS

POTENTIAL CO-ANALGESICS

Other adjuvants or co-analgesics in the treatment of pain in children with serious illness, depending on the clinical scenario, may include muscle relaxants (such as baclofen or cyclobenzaprine), bisphosphonates (such as pamidronate), antispasmodics (such as hyoscine butyl bromide [not available in the United States], hyoscyamine, oxybutynin), botulinum-toxin A (for spasticity or localized neuropathic pain), topical capsaicin, a serotonin-norepinephrine reuptake inhibitor (SNRI,) or anti-tumor necrosis-factor (TNF) α agents (e.g., adalimumab, etanercept, infliximab).

LOW-DOSE PROPOFOL

Propofol is an anesthetic with unknown clinical mechanism, which can cause general anesthesia and respiratory depression. In end-of-life scenarios with otherwise intractable pain and/or nausea we have successfully utilized low-dose propofol, titrated to a dose below mild sedation (e.g., starting dose 0.5–1 mg/kg/hour = 8–16 mcg/kg/minute).[251] At higher doses it may be considered for palliative sedation.

CANNABIS AND CANNABINOIDS

Evidence of clinical efficacy? Despite promising results in rodents, preclinical trials, and anecdotal case series, cannabis and medical marijuana (including cannabidiol [CBD] and tetrahydrocannabinol [THC]) lack any evidence to support its use for treatment of pain in humans.[252,253] There is no evidence for clinical efficacy in treating neuropathic pain,[210] cancer pain,[254] chronic non-cancer pain,[255] or pediatric pain.[256] While pediatric evidence for benefit was strongest for chemotherapy-induced nausea and vomiting, with increasing evidence of benefit for epilepsy, there is *no pediatric evidence* to support use for neuropathic pain, headaches, migraines, spasticity, posttraumatic stress disorder (PTSD), Tourette syndrome, anxiety, autism, depression, or cancer, nor do these agents show anti-inflammatory effects.[256]

Evidence of clinical harm? The updated American Academy of Pediatrics policy opposes marijuana use,[257] citing lack of research and potential harms including correlation with mental illness,[258] testicular cancer,[259–261] decline in IQ,[262,263] and increased risk of addiction.[264]

With no evidence for efficacy, and strong evidence for harm, like any other medication or intervention cannabinoids are not indicated as an analgesic. In our clinical practice, we do not support the use of marijuana (or medical cannabis) for a child with a primary pain disorder and a normal life expectancy. However, in children with life-limiting conditions, the administration of medical cannabis might be requested by patients and their parents, and certainly may be considered on a case-by-case basis weighing risks and benefits. It is important to watch carefully for side effects, which are not uncommon (including pancreatitis, psychosis, etc.).

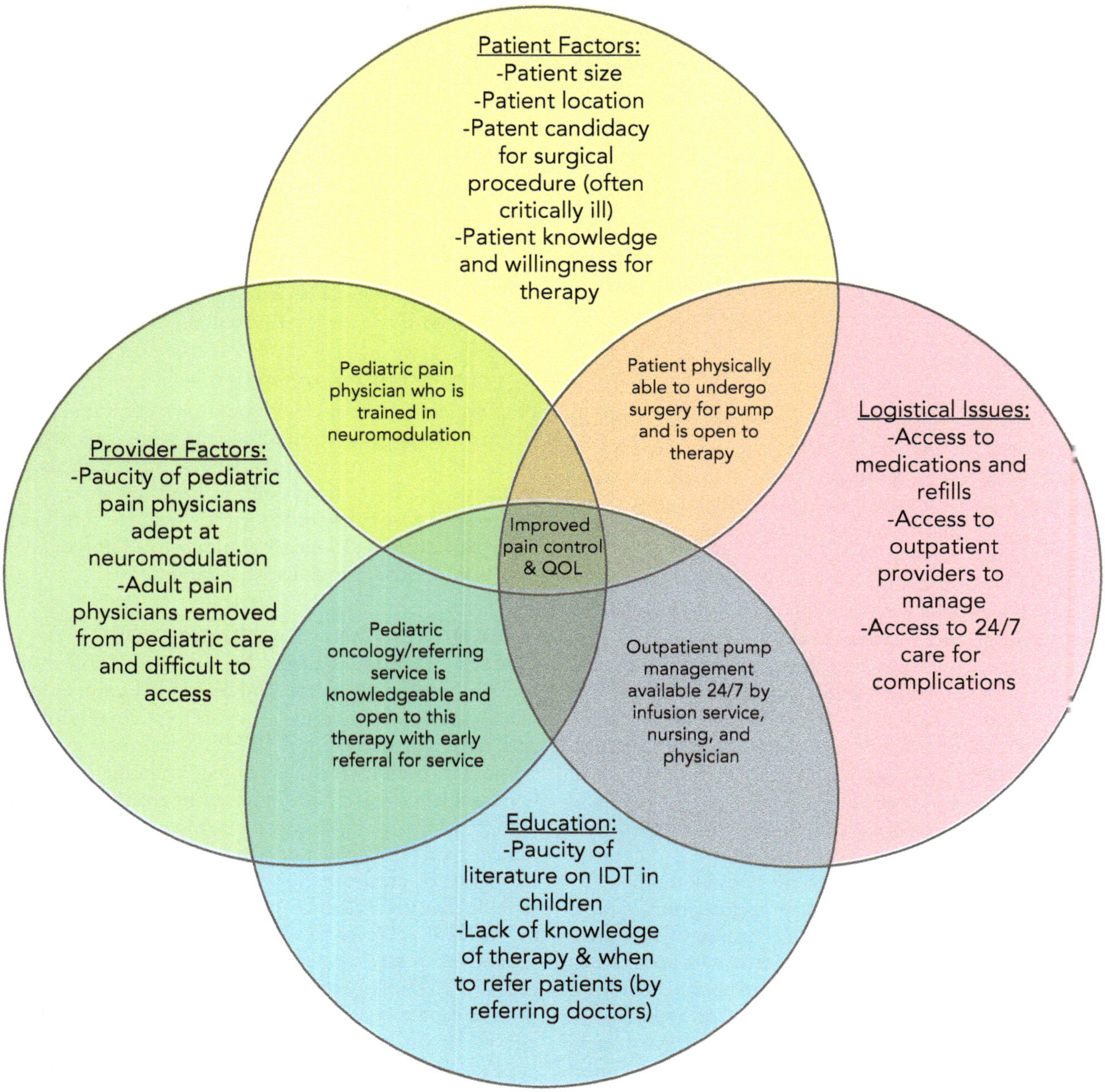

Figure 23.6 *Considerations and obstacles for implementing intrathecal drug therapies (IDT) in children with serious illness.*

STEP 12: PALLIATIVE SEDATION

Ultimately, the goal of PPC clinicians who provide advanced symptom treatment is to maximize quality of life by successfully managing distressing symptoms. Occasionally, even after exhausting all advanced treatment strategies, including those listed in Figure 23.2, adequate symptom control may not possible or attainable and palliative sedation might be considered. See Chapter 27 for additional details.

"Intractable" should not be confused with merely "difficult to treat." The goal is to alleviate the child's suffering. It is vital to recognize when palliative sedation is truly indicated and when further attempts at advanced symptom treatment need to be made. The use of sedation for refractory pain generally assumes that therapies beyond the conventional have been used or are impractical and that there is no acceptable means of providing analgesia without compromising consciousness. Given the principles of pain management outlined earlier, this is an extremely rare practice in pediatrics.

In addition, this is not a decision made solely by the medical team. Including the patient, when possible, and the family in the decision-making process is vital. Following the involvement of an interdisciplinary team including PPC specialists and experts in the underlying condition, as well as an ethics team, palliative sedation might be considered a valuable and efficacious intervention for refractory suffering at the end of life.

Palliative sedation has been mistakenly criticized as a form of euthanasia. Euthanasia has the deliberate aim of ending a patient's life at the request of the patient to avoid or end intolerable suffering. Palliative sedation aims to relieve suffering using the lowest doses of medications necessary. The difference primarily lies in the intent of the clinicians. When instituting palliative sedation, doses are slowly titrated upward until symptoms are controlled. Transient respite sedation may be considered earlier in the illness trajectory to provide temporary relief while waiting for more effective analgesic therapies to take effect.

The doctrine of *double effect* is often used to explain that an action is permissible even if it causes serious harm, such as death, if the intent of the action is to promote a good end, such as control of pain.

It appears that established PPC programs in large US tertiary centers usually utilize palliative sedation less than once per year, according to personal conversations. Depending on goals of care (e.g., sedation at night only, short-term sedation to allow for family to gather and say good-bye), usually short-acting agents, such as propofol, midazolam, dexmedetomidine, ketamine, and/or short-acting opioids are employed. Longer acting agents, such as barbiturates, diazepam, or methadone may be considered during end of life, when titration of the level of sedation is not anticipated.

CONCLUSION

The effective prevention and treatment of pain in children and adolescents with life-limiting diseases often requires intensive "multimodal" pain control. Safe multimodal analgesia[10] may include one, several, or all of the following approaches: pharmacology (e.g., simple analgesia and/or opioids and/or adjuvant analgesia), anesthetic interventions (e.g., neuraxial analgesia, nerve blocks), chaplaincy (addressing spirituality), social work, rehabilitation (e.g., physical therapy, occupational therapy, sleep hygiene), psychotherapy (e.g., cognitive behavioral therapy), and age-appropriate positioning and integrative (nonpharmacological) therapies, such as breathing techniques, self-hypnosis, and distraction. As a consequence, the need for sedation to reduce conscious awareness, even in the setting of difficult to pain, should be an extremely rare entity in pediatric clinical pain management practice.

Also, it is inappropriate to perform elective painful procedures (such as wound dressing changes, blood draws, IV cannulations, injections, lumbar punctures, etc.) in children without evidence-based treatments to avoid or minimize pain.

Underlying pain pathologies in the largest PPC group, nonverbal children with progressive neurologic, metabolic, or chromosomally based conditions, where the CNS is impaired, often remain enigmatic. One might speculate that many of these children may have not one, but several underlying conditions simultaneously: acute somatic nociceptive pain (such as otitis media), visceral pain (such as bladder spasms, constipation), chronic postoperative pain,[265–268] autonomic disorders,[269] chronic pain beyond the expected time of healing or primary pain disorder (such as primary headaches, centrally mediated abdominal pain syndrome, chronic musculoskeletal pain),[126,270–273] medication overuse headaches,[274] visceral hyperalgesia,[275] psycho-social-spiritual pain, and/or neuropathic pain.[269,276–278]

Nearly all research regarding assessment and treatment of pain and distressing symptoms in children with serious illness is undertaken in pediatric oncology. It is paramount that research and knowledge translation to achieve symptom control spreads out to reach children with non-cancer conditions as well.

ACKNOWLEDGMENTS

We would like to thank the authors of this chapter in the first edition John J. Collins, Charles B. Berde, and Judith A. Frost.

REFERENCES

1. Feudtner C, Kang TI, Hexem KR, et al. Pediatric palliative care patients: A prospective multicenter cohort study. *Pediatrics* 2011;127(6):1094–1101.
2. Wolfe J, Grier HE, Klar N, et al. Symptoms and suffering at the end of life in children with cancer. *N Engl J Med.* 2000;342(5):326–333.
3. Wolfe J, Hammel JF, Edwards KE, et al. Easing of suffering in children with cancer at the end of life: Is care changing? *J Clin Oncol.* 2008;26(10):1717–1723.
4. Friedrichsdorf SJ, Postier A, Dreyfus J, Osenga K, Sencer S, Wolfe J. Improved quality of life at end of life related to home-based palliative care in children with cancer. *J Palliat Med.* 2015;18(2):143–150.
5. Wolfe J, Orellana L, Ullrich C, et al. Symptoms and distress in children with advanced cancer: Prospective patient-reported outcomes from the PediQUEST study. *J Clin Oncol.* 2015;33(17):1928–1935.
6. Hechler T, Blankenburg M, Friedrichsdorf SJ, et al. Parents' perspective on symptoms, quality of life, characteristics of death and end-of-life decisions for children dying from cancer. *Klinische Padiatrie.* 2008;220(3):166–174.
7. Friedrichsdorf SJ, Postier AC, Andrews GS, Hamre KE, Steele R, Siden H. Pain reporting and analgesia management in 270 children with a progressive neurologic, metabolic or chromosomally based condition with impairment of the central nervous system: Cross-sectional, baseline results from an observational, longitudinal study. *J Pain Res.* 2017;10:1841–1852.
8. Friedrichsdorf SJ, Goubert L. Pediatric pain treatment and prevention for hospitalized children. *Pain Rep.* 2020;5(1):e804.
9. Michelson JD, Addante RA, Charlson MD. Multimodal analgesia therapy reduces length of hospitalization in patients undergoing fusions of the ankle and hindfoot. *Foot Ankle Int.* 2013;34(11):1526–1534.
10. Friedrichsdorf SJ. Prevention and treatment of pain in hospitalized infants, children, and teenagers: From myths and morphine to multimodal analgesia. In *Pain 2016: Refresher Courses. 16th World Congress on Pain.* IASP Press; 2016:309–319.
11. Friedrichsdorf SJ, Remke S, Hauser J, et al. Development of a pediatric palliative care curriculum and dissemination model: Education in Palliative and End-of-Life Care (EPEC) pediatrics. *J Pain Symptom Manage.* 2019.
12. Defrin R, Amanzio M, de Tommaso M, et al. Experimental pain processing in individuals with cognitive impairment: Current state of the science. *Pain.* 2015;156(8):1396–1408.

13. Voepel-Lewis T, Malviya S, Tait AR, et al. A comparison of the clinical utility of pain assessment tools for children with cognitive impairment. *Anesth Analg.* 2008;106(1):72–78.
14. Malviya S, Voepel-Lewis T, Burke C, Merkel S, Tait AR. The revised FLACC observational pain tool: Improved reliability and validity for pain assessment in children with cognitive impairment. *Paediatr Anaesth.* 2006;16(3):258–265.
15. Hunt A, Goldman A, Seers K, et al. Clinical validation of the paediatric pain profile. *Dev Med Child Neurol.* 2004;46(1):9–18.
16. Hunt A, Wisbeach A, Seers K, et al. Development of the paediatric pain profile: Role of video analysis and saliva cortisol in validating a tool to assess pain in children with severe neurological disability. *J Pain Symptom Manage.* 2007;33(3):276–289.
17. Breau LM, McGrath PJ, Camfield CS, Finley GA. Psychometric properties of the non-communicating children's pain checklist-revised. *Pain.* 2002;99(1-2):349–357.
18. Ledowski T, Reimer M, Chavez V, Kapoor V, Wenk M. Effects of acute postoperative pain on catecholamine plasma levels, hemodynamic parameters, and cardiac autonomic control. *Pain.* 2012;153(4):759–764.
19. Friedrichsdorf SJ, Postier A, Eull D, et al. Pain outcomes in a US children's hospital: A prospective cross-sectional survey. *Hosp Pediatr.* 2015;5(1):18–26.
20. Postier AC, Eull D, Schulz C, et al. Pain experience in a US children's hospital: A point prevalence survey undertaken after the implementation of a system-wide protocol to eliminate or decrease pain caused by needles. *Hosp Pediatr.* 2018;8(9):515–523.
21. Friedrichsdorf SJ, Eull D, Weidner C, Postier A. A hospital-wide initiative to eliminate or reduce needle pain in children using lean methodology. *Pain Rep.* 2018;3(Suppl 1):e671.
22. Taddio A, Pillai Riddell R, Ipp M, et al. Relative effectiveness of additive pain interventions during vaccination in infants. *CMAJ.* 2016.
23. Lunoe MM, Drendel AL, Levas MN, et al. A randomized clinical trial of jet-injected lidocaine to reduce venipuncture pain for young children. *Ann Emerg Med.* 2015;66(5):466–474.
24. Lunoe MM, Drendel AL, Brousseau DC. The use of the needle-free jet injection system with buffered lidocaine device does not change intravenous placement success in children in the emergency department. *Acad Emerg Med.* 2015;22(4):447–451.
25. CHEO Be Sweet to Babies research team, University of Ottawa School of Nursing. Be sweet to babies. 2014. http://www.cheo.on.ca/en/BeSweet2Babies
26. Shah PS, Herbozo C, Aliwalas LL, Shah VS. Breastfeeding or breast milk for procedural pain in neonates. *Cochrane Database Syst Rev.* 2012;12:CD004950.
27. Stevens B, Yamada J, Campbell-Yeo M, et al. The minimally effective dose of sucrose for procedural pain relief in neonates: A randomized controlled trial. *BMC Pediatr.* 2018;18(1):85.
28. Gray L, Garza E, Zageris D, Heilman KJ, Porges SW. Sucrose and warmth for analgesia in healthy newborns: An RCT. *Pediatrics.* 2015;135(3):e607–614.
29. Gray L, Lang CW, Porges SW. Warmth is analgesic in healthy newborns. *Pain.* 2012;153(5):960–966.
30. Campbell-Yeo M, Johnston C, Benoit B, et al. Trial of repeated analgesia with Kangaroo Mother Care (TRAKC Trial). *BMC Pediatr.* 2013;13:182.
31. Campbell-Yeo ML, Johnston CC, Joseph KS, et al. Co-bedding between preterm twins attenuates stress response after heel lance: Results of a randomized trial. *Clin J Pain.* 2014;30(7):598–604.
32. Johnston C, Campbell-Yeo M, Fernandes A, Inglis D, Streiner D, Zee R. Skin-to-skin care for procedural pain in neonates. *Cochrane Database Syst Rev.* 2014;1:CD008435.
33. Campbell-Yeo ML, Disher TC, Benoit BL, Johnston CC. Understanding kangaroo care and its benefits to preterm infants. *Pediatric Health Med Ther.* 2015;6:15–32.
34. Benoit B, Campbell-Yeo M, Johnston C, Latimer M, Caddell K, Orr T. Staff nurse utilization of kangaroo care as an intervention for procedural pain in preterm infants. *Adv Neonatal Care.* 2016;16(3):229–238.
35. Campbell-Yeo M, Johnston CC, Benoit B, et al. Sustained efficacy of kangaroo care for repeated painful procedures over neonatal intensive care unit hospitalization: A single-blind randomized controlled trial. *Pain.* 2019.
36. Karlson K, Darcy L, Enskär K. The use of restraint is never supportive. Poster presented at the Nordic Society of Pediatric Hematology/Oncology (NOPHO) 34th Annual meeting 2016 and 11th Biannual Meeting of Nordic Society of Pediatric Oncology Nurses (NOBOS); May 27–31, 2016; Reykjavik, Iceland.
37. Uman LS, Birnie KA, Noel M, et al. Psychological interventions for needle-related procedural pain and distress in children and adolescents. *Cochrane Database Syst Rev.* 2013(10):CD005179.
38. Schechter NL, Allen DA, Hanson K. Status of pediatric pain control: A comparison of hospital analgesic usage in children and adults. *Pediatrics.* 1986;77(1):11–15.
39. Broome ME, Richtsmeier A, Maikler V, Alexander M. Pediatric pain practices: A national survey of health professionals. *J Pain Symptom Manage.* 1996;11(5):312–320.
40. Zier JL, Liu M. Safety of high-concentration nitrous oxide by nasal mask for pediatric procedural sedation: Experience with 7802 cases. *Pediatr Emerg Care.* 2011;27(12):1107–1112.
41. Friedrichsdorf SJ. Nitrous gas analgesia and sedation for lumbar punctures in children: Has the time for practice change come? *Pediatr Blood Cancer.* 2017;64(11).
42. Livingston M, Lawell M, McAllister N. Successful use of nitrous oxide during lumbar punctures: A call for nitrous oxide in pediatric oncology clinics. *Pediatr Blood Cancer.* 2017;64(11).
43. IASP. IASP Announces Revised Definition of Pain. 2020. https://www.iasp-pain.org/PublicationsNews/NewsDetail.aspx?ItemNumber=10475.
44. Richmond C. Dame Cicely Saunders. *BMJ* 2005;331(7510):238.
45. Warlow TA, Hain RDW. 'Total pain' in children with severe neurological impairment. *Children (Basel).* 2018;5(1).
46. Rabbitts JA, Fisher E, Rosenbloom BN, Palermo TM. Prevalence and predictors of chronic postsurgical pain in children: A systematic review and meta-analysis. *J Pain.* 2017;18(6):605–614.
47. Stevens B, Yamada J, Ohlsson A, Haliburton S, Shorkey A. Sucrose for analgesia in newborn infants undergoing painful procedures. *Cochrane Database Syst Rev.* 2016;7:CD001069.
48. Gao H, Gao H, Xu G, et al. Efficacy and safety of repeated oral sucrose for repeated procedural pain in neonates: A systematic review. *Int J Nurs Stud.* 2016;62:118–125.
49. Bussing A, Ostermann T, Ludtke R, Michalsen A. Effects of yoga interventions on pain and pain-associated disability: A meta-analysis. *J Pain.* 2012;13(1):1–9.
50. Evans S, Moieni M, Taub R, et al. Iyengar yoga for young adults with rheumatoid arthritis: Results from a mixed-methods pilot study. *J Pain Symptom Manage.* 2010;39(5):904–913.
51. Vas J, Santos-Rey K, Navarro-Pablo R, et al. Acupuncture for fibromyalgia in primary care: A randomised controlled trial. *Acupunct Med.* 2016.
52. Verkamp EK, Flowers SR, Lynch-Jordan AM, Taylor J, Ting TV, Kashikar-Zuck S. A survey of conventional and complementary therapies used by youth with juvenile-onset fibromyalgia. *Pain Manag Nurs.* 2013;14(4):e244–250.
53. Kuttner L, Friedrichsdorf SJ. Hypnosis and palliative care. In *Therapeutic Hypnosis with Children and Adolescents.* 2nd ed. Crown House Publishing; 2013:491–509.
54. Hunt K, Ernst E. The evidence-base for complementary medicine in children: A critical overview of systematic reviews. *Arch Dis Child.* 2011;96(8):769–776.
55. Evans S, Tsao JC, Zeltzer LK. Complementary and alternative medicine for acute procedural pain in children. *Altern Ther Health Med.* 2008;14(5):52–56.
56. Richardson J, Smith JE, McCall G, Pilkington K. Hypnosis for procedure-related pain and distress in pediatric cancer patients: A systematic review of effectiveness and methodology related to hypnosis interventions. *J Pain Symptom Manage.* 2006;31(1):70–84.

57. Friedrichsdorf SJ, Kohen DP. Integration of hypnosis into pediatric palliative care. *Ann Palliat Med.* 2018;7(1):136–150.
58. Evans S, Tsao JC, Zeltzer LK. Paediatric pain management: Using complementary and alternative medicine. *Rev Pain.* 2008;2(1):14–20.
59. Xiang A, Cheng K, Shen X, Xu P, Liu S. The immediate analgesic effect of acupuncture for pain: A systematic review and meta-analysis. *Evid Based Complement Alternat Med.* 2017;2017:3837194.
60. Friedrichsdorf S, Kuttner L, Westendorp K, McCarty R. Integrative pediatric palliative care. In Culbert TP, Olness K, eds. *Integrative Pediatrics.* Oxford University Press; 2010:569–593.
61. Kohen DP, Olness KN. *Hypnosis and Hypnotherapy with Children.* 4th ed. Routledge, Taylor & Francis; 2011.
62. Stubberud A, Varkey E, McCrory DC, Pedersen SA, Linde M. Biofeedback as prophylaxis for pediatric migraine: A meta-analysis. *Pediatrics.* 2016;138(2).
63. Kovacic K, Hainsworth K, Sood M, et al. Neurostimulation for abdominal pain-related functional gastrointestinal disorders in adolescents: A randomised, double-blind, sham-controlled trial. *Lancet Gastroenterol Hepatol.* 2017;2(10):727–737.
64. Baeumler PI, Fleckenstein J, Benedikt F, Bader J, Irnich D. Acupuncture-induced changes of pressure pain threshold are mediated by segmental inhibition: A randomized controlled trial. *Pain.* 2015;156(11):2245–2255.
65. Hemington KS, Coulombe MA. The periaqueductal gray and descending pain modulation: Why should we study them and what role do they play in chronic pain? *J Neurophysiol.* 2015:jn 00998 02014.
66. Valet M, Sprenger T, Boecker H, et al. Distraction modulates connectivity of the cingulo-frontal cortex and the midbrain during pain: An fMRI analysis. *Pain.* 2004;109(3):399–408.
67. Tracey I, Ploghaus A, Gati JS, et al. Imaging attentional modulation of pain in the periaqueductal gray in humans. *J Neurosci.* 2002;22(7):2748–2752.
68. Derbyshire SW, Osborn J. Modeling pain circuits: How imaging may modify perception. *Neuroimaging Clin N Am.* 2007;17(4):485–493, ix.
69. Bingel U, Wanigasekera V, Wiech K, et al. The effect of treatment expectation on drug efficacy: Imaging the analgesic benefit of the opioid remifentanil. *Sci Transl Med.* 2011;3(70):70ra14.
70. Yu R, Gollub RL, Spaeth R, Napadow V, Wasan A, Kong J. Disrupted functional connectivity of the periaqueductal gray in chronic low back pain. *Neuroimage Clin.* 2014;6:100–108.
71. Giordano J. The neurobiology of nociceptive and anti-nociceptive systems. *Pain Physician.* 2005;8(3):277–290.
72. Malfliet A, Leysen L, Pas R, et al. Modern pain neuroscience in clinical practice: Applied to post-cancer, paediatric and sports-related pain. *Braz J Phys Ther.* 2017;21(4):225–232.
73. Baravid E, Covarrubias N, Tribuzio B, Liao S. The benefits of rehabilitation for palliative care patients. *Am J Hosp Palliat Care.* 2015;32(1):34–43.
74. Ramsey LH, Karlson CW, Collier AB. Mirror therapy for phantom limb pain in a 7-year-old male with osteosarcoma. *J Pain Symptom Manage.* 2017;53(6):e5–e7.
75. Harrison LE, Pate JW, Richardson PA, Ickmans K, Wicksell RK, Simons LE. Best-evidence for the rehabilitation of chronic pain Part 1: Pediatric pain. *J Clin Med.* 2019;8(9).
76. Caes L, Fisher E, Clinch J, Eccleston C. Current evidence-based interdisciplinary treatment options for pediatric musculoskeletal pain. *Curr Treatm Opt Rheumatol.* 2018;4(3):223–234.
77. Sluka KA, Frey-Law L, Hoeger Bement M. Exercise-induced pain and analgesia? Underlying mechanisms and clinical translation. *Pain.* 2018;159 (Suppl 1):S91–S97.
78. Snaman JM, Baker JN, Ehrentraut JH, Anghelescu DL. Pediatric oncology: Managing pain at the end of life. *Paediatr Drugs.* 2016;18(3):161–180.
79. Jalmsell L, Kreicbergs U, Onelov E, Steineck G, Henter JI. Symptoms affecting children with malignancies during the last month of life: A nationwide follow-up. *Pediatrics.* 2006;117(4):1314–1320.
80. Hechler T, Blankenburg M, Friedrichsdorf SJ, et al. Parents' perspective on symptoms, quality of life, characteristics of death and end-of-life decisions for children dying from cancer. *Klin Padiatr.* 2008;220(3):166–174.
81. Feudtner C, Kang TI, Hexem KR, et al. Pediatric palliative care patients: A prospective multicenter cohort study. *Pediatrics.* 2011;127(6):1094–1101.
82. Merskey H Albe Fessard D, Bonica JJ, Carmon A, et al. Pain terms: A list with definitions and notes on usage. Recommended by the IASP subcommittee on taxonomy. *Pain.* 1979;6(3):249.
83. Kurtz BP, Abrams AN. Psychiatric aspects of pediatric cancer. *Child Adolesc Psychiatr Clin N Am.* 2010;19(2):401–421, x-xi.
84. Nathan PC, Nachman A, Sutradhar R, et al. Adverse mental health outcomes in a population-based cohort of survivors of childhood cancer. *Cancer.* 2018;124(9):2045–2057.
85. Steif BL, Heiligenstein EL. Psychiatric symptoms of pediatric cancer pain. *J Pain Symptom Manage.* 1989;4(4):191–196.
86. Recklitis CJ, Diller LR, Li X, Najita J, Robison LL, Zeltzer L. Suicide ideation in adult survivors of childhood cancer: A report from the Childhood Cancer Survivor Study. *J Clin Oncol.* 2010;28(4):655–661.
87. Kazak AE, Penati B, Brophy P, Himelstein B. Pharmacologic and psychologic interventions for procedural pain. *Pediatrics.* 1998;102(1 Pt 1):59–66.
88. McGrath PJ, Stevens BJ, Walker SM, Zempsky WT, eds. *Oxford Textbook of Paediatric Pain.* Oxford University Press; 2013.
89. Powers SW. Empirically supported treatments in pediatric psychology: Procedure-related pain. *J Pediatr Psychol.* 1999;24(2): 131–145.
90. Demore MaC, Lindsey L. Distraction for pediatric immunization pain: A critical review. *J Clin Psychol Med Settings.* 2005;12:281–291.
91. Chambers CT, Craig KD, Bennett SM. The impact of maternal behavior on children's pain experiences: An experimental analysis. *J Pediatr Psychol.* 2002;27(3):293–301.
92. Uman LS, Chambers CT, McGrath PJ, Kisely S. A systematic review of randomized controlled trials examining psychological interventions for needle-related procedural pain and distress in children and adolescents: An abbreviated Cochrane review. *J Pediatr Psychol.* 2008;33(8):842–854.
93. Mahrer NE, Gold JI. The use of virtual reality for pain control: A review. *Curr Pain Headache Rep.* 2009;13(2):100–109.
94. Heathcote LC, Eccleston C. Pain and cancer survival: A cognitive-affective model of symptom appraisal and the uncertain threat of disease recurrence. *Pain.* 2017;158(7):1187–1191.
95. Tutelman PR, Chambers CT, Urquhart R, et al. When "a headache is not just a headache": A qualitative examination of parent and child experiences of pain after childhood cancer. *Psychooncology.* 2019;28(9):1901–1909.
96. Caes L, Goubert L, Devos P, Verlooy J, Benoit Y, Vervoort T. The relationship between parental catastrophizing about child pain and distress in response to medical procedures in the context of childhood cancer treatment: A longitudinal analysis. *J Pediatr Psychol.* 2014;39(7):677–686.
97. Caes L, Vervoort T, Devos P, Verlooy J, Benoit Y, Goubert L. Parental distress and catastrophic thoughts about child pain: Implications for parental protective behavior in the context of child leukemia-related medical procedures. *Clin J Pain.* 2014;30(9):787–799.
98. Rabbitts JA, Groenewald CB, Tai GG, Palermo TM. Presurgical psychosocial predictors of acute postsurgical pain and quality of life in children undergoing major surgery. *J Pain.* 2015;16(3):226–234.
99. Stone AL, Wilson AC. Transmission of risk from parents with chronic pain to offspring: An integrative conceptual model. *Pain.* 2016;157(12):2628–2639.
100. Simons LE, Goubert L, Vervoort T, Borsook D. Circles of engagement: Childhood pain and parent brain. *Neurosci Biobehav Rev.* 2016;68:537–546.

101. Penner LA, Cline RJ, Albrecht TL, et al. Parents' empathic responses and pain and distress in pediatric patients. *Basic Appl Soc Psych.* 2008;30(2):102–113.
102. Rancourt KM, Chorney JM, Kain Z. Children's immediate postoperative distress and mothers' and fathers' touch behaviors. *J Pediatr Psychol.* 2015;40(10):1115–1123.
103. Jensen K, Kelley JM. The therapeutic relationship in psychological and physical treatments, and their placebo controls. *Psychol Conscious.* 2016;3(2):132–145.
104. Grossoehme DH, Szczesniak R, McPhail GL, Seid M. Is adolescents' religious coping with cystic fibrosis associated with the rate of decline in pulmonary function? A preliminary study. *J Health Care Chaplain.* 2013;19(1):33–42.
105. Borneman T, Ferrell B, Puchalski CM. Evaluation of the FICA tool for spiritual assessment. *J Pain Symptom Manage.* 2010;40(2):163–173.
106. de Leeuw TG, Dirckx M, Gonzalez Candel A, Scoones GP, Huygen F, de Wildt SN. The use of dipyrone (metamizol) as an analgesic in children: What is the evidence? A review. *Paediatr Anaesth.* 2017;27(12):1193–1201.
107. Howard RF. Current status of pain management in children. *JAMA.* 2003;290(18):2464–2469.
108. Mallet C, Daulhac L, Bonnefont J, et al. Endocannabinoid and serotonergic systems are needed for acetaminophen-induced analgesia. *Pain.* 2008;139(1):190–200.
109. Kerckhove N, Mallet C, Francois A, et al. Ca(v)3.2 calcium channels: The key protagonist in the supraspinal effect of paracetamol. *Pain.* 2014;155(4):764–772.
110. Heubi JE, Barbacci MB, Zimmerman HJ. Therapeutic misadventures with acetaminophen: Hepatoxicity after multiple doses in children. *J Pediatr.* 1998;132(1):22–27.
111. Watkins PB, Kaplowitz N, Slattery JT, et al. Aminotransferase elevations in healthy adults receiving 4 grams of acetaminophen daily: A randomized controlled trial. *JAMA.* 2006;296(1):87–93.
112. van der Marel CD, Peters JW, Bouwmeester NJ, Jacqz-Aigrain E, van den Anker JN, Tibboel D. Rectal acetaminophen does not reduce morphine consumption after major surgery in young infants. *Br J Anaesth.* 2007;98(3):372–379.
113. Israel FJ, Parker G, Charles M, Reymond L. Lack of benefit from paracetamol (acetaminophen) for palliative cancer patients requiring high-dose strong opioids: A randomized, double-blind, placebo-controlled, crossover trial. *J Pain Symptom Manage.* 2010;39(3):548–554.
114. Johnson CY. The growing case against IV Tylenol, once seen as a solution to the opioid crisis. *The Washington Post* 2018.
115. Moore RA, Derry S, Straube S, Ireson-Paine J, Wiffen PJ. Faster, higher, stronger? Evidence for formulation and efficacy for ibuprofen in acute pain. *Pain.* 2014;155(1):14–21.
116. Teerawattananon C, Tantayakom P, Suwanawiboon B, Katchamart W. Risk of perioperative bleeding related to highly selective cyclooxygenase-2 inhibitors: A systematic review and meta-analysis. *Semin Arthritis Rheum.* 2017;46(4):520–528.
117. Nissen SE, Yeomans ND, Solomon DH, et al. Cardiovascular safety of Celecoxib, Naproxen, or Ibuprofen for arthritis. *N Engl J Med.* 2016;375(26):2519–2529.
118 . Sondergaard KB, Weeke P, Wissenberg M, et al. Non-steroidal anti-inflammatory drug use is associated with increased risk of out-of-hospital cardiac arrest: A nationwide case-time-control study. *Eur Heart J Cardiovasc Pharmacother.* 2016.
119. Krane EJ, Weisman SJ, Walco GA. The national opioid epidemic and the risk of outpatient opioids in children. *Pediatrics.* 2018;142(2).
120. McCabe SE, Veliz P, Schulenberg JE. Adolescent context of exposure to prescription opioids and substance use disorder symptoms at age 35: A national longitudinal study. *Pain.* 2016;157(10):2173–2178.
121. McCabe SE, West BT, Boyd CJ. Medical use, medical misuse, and nonmedical use of prescription opioids: Results from a longitudinal study. *Pain.* 2013;154(5):708–713.
122. Voepel-Lewis T, Boyd CJ, McCabe SE, et al. Deliberative prescription opioid misuse among adolescents andemerging adults: Opportunities for targeted interventions. *J Adolesc Health.* 2018;63(5):594–600.
123. McCabe SE, West BT, Cranford JA, et al. Medical misuse of controlled medications among adolescents. *Arch Pediatr Adolesc Med.* 2011;165(8):729–735.
124. McCabe SE, West BT, Boyd CJ. Motives for medical misuse of prescription opioids among adolescents. *J Pain.* 2013;14(10):1208–1216.
125. Ranji SR, Goldman LE, Simel DL, Shojania KG. Do opiates affect the clinical evaluation of patients with acute abdominal pain? *JAMA.* 2006;296(14):1764–1774.
126. Schechter NL. Functional pain: Time for a new name. *JAMA Pediatrics.* 2014;168(8):693–694.
127. Chapman CR, Lipschitz DL, Angst MS, et al. Opioid pharmacotherapy for chronic non-cancer pain in the United States: A research guideline for developing an evidence-base. *J Pain.* 2010;11(9):807–829.
128. Chapman CR, Davis J, Donaldson GW, Naylor J, Winchester D. Postoperative pain trajectories in chronic pain patients undergoing surgery: The effects of chronic opioid pharmacotherapy on acute pain. *J Pain.* 2011;12(12):1240–1246.
129. Elliott JA, Horton E, Fibuch EE. The endocrine effects of long-term oral opioid therapy: A case report and review of the literature. *J Opioid Manag.* 2011;7(2):145–154.
130. Chaparro LE, Furlan AD, Deshpande A, Mailis-Gagnon A, Atlas S, Turk DC. Opioids compared with placebo or other treatments for chronic low back pain: An update of the Cochrane Review. *Spine (Phila Pa 1976).* 2014;39(7):556–563.
131. Ashworth J, Green DJ, Dunn KM, Jordan KP. Opioid use among low back pain patients in primary care: Is opioid prescription associated with disability at 6-month follow-up? *Pain.* 2013;154(7):1038–1044.
132. Scherrer JF, Salas J, Lustman PJ, Burge S, Schneider FD, Residency Research Network of Texas I. Change in opioid dose and change in depression in a longitudinal primary care patient cohort. *Pain.* 2015;156(2):348–355.
133. Chen L, Vo T, Seefeld L, et al. Lack of correlation between opioid dose adjustment and pain score change in a group of chronic pain patients. *J Pain.* 2013;14(4):384–392.
134. Drake R, Longworth J, Collins JJ. Opioid rotation in children with cancer. *J Palliat Med.* 2004;7(3):419–422.
135. Friedrichsdorf SJ. From Coke to Pepsi to Mountain Dew? Rotating opioids in advanced pediatric palliative care. *AAHPM Winter Quarterly Clinical Pearls* 2014;15(4):8–9.
136. Prommer EE. Tapentadol: An initial analysis. *J Opioid Manag.* 2010;6(3):223–226.
137. Koren G, Cairns J, Chitayat D, Gaedigk A, Leeder SJ. Pharmacogenetics of morphine poisoning in a breastfed neonate of a codeine-prescribed mother. *Lancet.* 2006;368(9536):704.
138. Ciszkowski C, Madadi P, Phillips MS, Lauwers AE, Koren G. Codeine, ultrarapid-metabolism genotype, and postoperative death. *N Engl J Med.* 2009;361(8):827–828.
139. Kelly LE, Rieder M, van den Anker J, et al. More codeine fatalities after tonsillectomy in North American children. *Pediatrics.* 2012;129(5):e1343–1347.
140. Friedrichsdorf SJ, Nugent AP, Strobl AQ. Codeine-associated pediatric deaths despite using recommended dosing guidelines: Three case reports. *J Opioid Manag.* 2013;9(2):151–155.
141. Friedrichsdorf SJ, Postier AC, Foster LP, et al. Tramadol versus codeine/acetaminophen after pediatric tonsillectomy: A prospective, double-blinded, randomized controlled trial. *J Opioid Manag.* 2015;11(4):283–294.
142. Chidambaran V, Sadhasivam S, Mahmoud M. Codeine and opioid metabolism: Implications and alternatives for pediatric pain management. *Curr Opin Anaesthesiol.* 2017;30(3):349–356.

143. FDA. Codeine and tramadol medicines: Drug safety communication—restricting use in children, recommending against use in breastfeeding women. 2017. https://www.fda.gov/Safety/MedWatch/SafetyInformation/SafetyAlertsforHumanMedicalProducts/ucm554029.htm?source=govdelivery&utm_medium=email&utm_source=govdelivery
144. Moir MS, Bair E, Shinnick P, Messner A. Acetaminophen versus acetaminophen with codeine after pediatric tonsillectomy. *Laryngoscope.* 2000;110(11):1824–1827.
145. Singla A, Sloan P. Pharmacokinetic evaluation of hydrocodone/acetaminophen for pain management. *J Opioid Manag.* 2013;9(1):71–80.
146. Morrow PL, Faris EC. Death associated with inadvertent hydrocodone overdose in a child with a respiratory tract infection. *Am J Forensic Med Pathol.* 1987;8(1):60–63.
147. Madadi P, Hildebrandt D, Gong IY, et al. Fatal hydrocodone overdose in a child: Pharmacogenetics and drug interactions. *Pediatrics.* 2010;126(4):e986–989.
148. Friedrichsdorf SJ. From tramadol to methadone: Opioids in the treatment of pain and dyspnea in pediatric palliative care. *Clin J Pain.* 2019;35(6):501–508.
149. Pruskowski J, Arnold RM. Tramadol in palliative care #290. *J Palliat Med.* 2015;18(5):461–462.
150. Moore RA, McQuay HJ. Single-patient data meta-analysis of 3453 postoperative patients: Oral tramadol versus placebo, codeine and combination analgesics. *Pain.* 1997;69(3):287–294.
151 Bamigbade TA, Langford RM. Tramadol hydrochloride: An overview of current use. *Hosp Med.* 1998;59(5):373–376.
152 Bamigbade TA, Langford RM. The clinical use of tramadol hydrochloride. *Pain Rev.* 1998(5):155–182.
153. Finkel JC, Rose JB, Schmitz ML, et al. An evaluation of the efficacy and tolerability of oral tramadol hydrochloride tablets for the treatment of postsurgical pain in children. *Anesth Analg.* 2002;94(6):1469–1473.
154. Rose JB, Finkel JC, Arquedas-Mohs A, Himelstein BP, Schreiner M, Medve RA. Oral tramadol for the treatment of pain of 7–30 days' duration in children. *Anesth Analg.* 2003;96(1):78–81.
155. Ozalevli M, Unlugenc H, Tuncer U, Gunes Y, Ozcengiz D. Comparison of morphine and tramadol by patient-controlled analgesia for postoperative analgesia after tonsillectomy in children. *Pediatr Anaesth.* 2005;15(11):979–984.
156. Hullett BJ, Chambers NA, Pascoe EM, Johnson C. Tramadol vs morphine during adenotonsillectomy for obstructive sleep apnea in children. *Pediatr Anaesth.* 2006;16(6):648–653.
157. Rodriguez RF, Castillo JM, Castillo MP, et al. Hydrocodone/acetaminophen and tramadol chlorhydrate combination tablets for the management of chronic cancer pain: A double-blind comparative trial. *Clin J Pain.* 2008;24(1):1–4.
158. Moyao-Garcia D, Hernandez-Palacios JC, Ramirez-Mora JC, Nava-Ocampo AA. A pilot study of nalbuphine versus tramadol administered through continuous intravenous infusion for postoperative pain control in children. *Acta Biomed.* 2009;80(2):124–130.
159. Murphy JD, Yan D, Hanna MN, et al. Comparison of the postoperative analgesic efficacy of intravenous patient-controlled analgesia with tramadol to intravenous patient-controlled analgesia with opioids. *J Opioid Manag.* 2010;6(2):141–147.
160. Rauers NI, Stuber F, Lee EH, et al. Antagonistic effects of ondansetron and tramadol? A randomized placebo and active drug-controlled study. *J Pain.* 2010;11(12):1274–1281.
161. Uysal HY, Takmaz SA, Yaman F, Baltaci B, Basar H. The efficacy of intravenous paracetamol versus tramadol for postoperative analgesia after adenotonsillectomy in children. *J Clin Anesth.* 2011 23(1):53–57.
162. Alencar AJ, Sanudo A, Sampaio VM, Gois RP, Benevides FA, Guinsburg R. Efficacy of tramadol versus fentanyl for postoperative analgesia in neonates. *Arch Dis Child Fetal Neonatal Ed.* 2012;97(1):F24–29.
163. Ayatollahi V, Behdad S, Hatami M, Moshtaghiun H, Baghianimoghadam B. Comparison of peritonsillar infiltration effects of ketamine and tramadol on post tonsillectomy pain: A double-blinded randomized placebo-controlled clinical trial. *Croat Med J.* 2012;53(2):155–161.
164. Hain RD, Miser A, Devins M, Wallace WH. Strong opioids in pediatric palliative medicine. *Paediatr Drugs.* 2005;7(1):1–9.
165. Allen LV J. Tramadol hydrochloride 5mg/mL oral liquid. *Int J Pharm Compd* 2006;10(4):307.
166. Desmeules JA. The tramadol option. *Eur J Pain.* 2000;4(Suppl A):15–21.
167. Marquardt KA, Alsop JA, Albertson TE. Tramadol exposures reported to statewide poison control system. *Ann Pharmacother.* 2005;39(6):1039–1044.
168. Huang P, Kehner GB, Cowan A, Liu-Chen LY. Comparison of pharmacological activities of buprenorphine and norbuprenorphine: Norbuprenorphine is a potent opioid agonist. *J Pharmacol Exp Ther.* 2001;297(2):688–695.
169. Yassen A, Kan J, Olofsen E, Suidgeest E, Dahan A, Danhof M. Mechanism-based pharmacokinetic-pharmacodynamic modeling of the respiratory-depressant effect of buprenorphine and fentanyl in rats. *J Pharmacol Exp Ther.* 2006;319(2):682–692.
170. Jacobsen J. Topical opioids for pain #185. *J Palliat Med.* 2009;12(4):380–381.
171. Cherny NI, Foley KM. Nonopioid and opioid analgesic pharmacotherapy of cancer pain. *Otolaryngol Clin North Am.* 1997;30(2):279–306.
172. McPherson C, Haslam M, Pineda R, Rogers C, Neil JJ, Inder TE. Brain injury and development in preterm infants exposed to fentanyl. *Ann Pharmacother.* 2015;49(12):1291–1297.
173. Steinhorn R, McPherson C, Anderson PJ, Neil J, Doyle LW, Inder T. Neonatal morphine exposure in very preterm infants-cerebral development and outcomes. *J Pediatr.* 2015;166(5):1200–1207 e1204.
174. MacGregor R, Evans D, Sugden D, Gaussen T, Levene M. Outcome at 5–6 years of prematurely born children who received morphine as neonates. *Arch Dis Child Fetal Neonatal Ed.* 1998;79(1):F40–43.
175. de Graaf J, van Lingen RA, Valkenburg AJ, et al. Does neonatal morphine use affect neuropsychological outcomes at 8 to 9 years of age? *Pain.* 2013;154(3):449–458.
176. McRorie TI, Lynn AM, Nespeca MK, Opheim KE, Slattery JT. The maturation of morphine clearance and metabolism. *Am J Dis Child.* 1992;146(8):972–976.
177. Bhat R, Chari G, Gulati A, Aldana O, Velamati R, Bhargava H. Pharmacokinetics of a single dose of morphine in preterm infants during the first week of life. *J Pediatr.* 1990;117(3):477–481.
178. Pokela ML, Olkkola KT, Seppala T, Koivisto M. Age-related morphine kinetics in infants. *Dev Pharmacol Ther.* 1993;20(1-2):26–34.
179. Stanski DR, Greenblatt DJ, Lowenstein E. Kinetics of intravenous and intramuscular morphine. *Clin Pharmacol Ther.* 1978;24(1):52–59.
180. Olkkola KT, Maunuksela EL, Korpela R, Rosenberg PH. Kinetics and dynamics of postoperative intravenous morphine in children. *Clin Pharmacol Ther.* 1988;44(2):128–136.
181. Carbajal R, Lenclen R, Jugie M, Paupe A, Barton BA, Anand KJ. Morphine does not provide adequate analgesia for acute procedural pain among preterm neonates. *Pediatrics.* 2005;115(6):1494–1500.
182. Nielsen CK, Ross FB, Lotfipour S, Saini KS, Edwards SR, Smith MT. Oxycodone and morphine have distinctly different pharmacological profiles: Radioligand binding and behavioural studies in two rat models of neuropathic pain. *Pain.* 2007;132(3):289–300.
183. Kalso E. How different is oxycodone from morphine? *Pain.* 2007;132(3):227–228.
184. Kaiko R, Benziger D, Cheng C, Hou Y, Grandy R. Clinical pharmacokinetics of controlled-release oxycodone in renal impairment. *Clinical Pharm Ther.* 1996;59(1):130.

185. Babul N, Darke AC. Putative role of hydromorphone metabolites in myoclonus. *Pain.* 1992;51(2):260–261.
186. Davis M, Wilcock A. Modified release opioids. *Eur J Palliat Care.* 2001(8):142–146.
187. Babul N, Darke AC, Hagen N. Hydromorphone metabolite accumulation in renal failure. *J Pain Symptom Manage.* 1995;10(3):184–186.
188. Cherny NJ, Chang V, Frager G, et al. Opioid pharmacotherapy in the management of cancer pain: A survey of strategies used by pain physicians for the selection of analgesic drugs and routes of administration. *Cancer.* 1995;76(7):1283–1293.
189. Goodarzi M. Comparison of epidural morphine, hydromorphone and fentanyl for postoperative pain control in children undergoing orthopaedic surgery. *Paediatr Anaesth.* 1999;9(5):419–422.
190. Hewitt M, Goldman A, Collins GS, Childs M, Hain R. Opioid use in palliative care of children and young people with cancer. *J Pediatr.* 2008;152(1):39–44.
191. Kidd S, Brennan S, Stephen R, Minns R, Beattie T. Comparison of morphine concentration-time profiles following intravenous and intranasal diamorphine in children. *Arch Dis Child.* 2009;94(12):974–978.
192. Telfer P, Criddle J, Sandell J, Davies F, Morrison I, Challands J. Intranasal diamorphine for acute sickle cell pain. *Arch Dis Child.* 2009;94(12):979–980.
193. Kendall JM, Reeves BC, Latter VS; Nasal Diamorphine Trial Group. Multicentre randomised controlled trial of nasal diamorphine for analgesia in children and teenagers with clinical fractures. *BMJ.* 2001;322(7281):261–265.
194. Fife A, Postier A, Flood A, Friedrichsdorf SJ. Methadone conversion in infants and children: Retrospective cohort study of 199 pediatric inpatients. *J Opioid Manag.* 2016;12(2):123–130.
195. Friedrichsdorf S, Kang T. The management of pain in children with life-limiting illnesses. *Pediatr Clin North Am.* 2007;54(5):645–672.
196. Berde C, Sethna N, Holzman R. Pharmacokinetics of methadone in children and adolescents in the peri-operative period. *Anesthesiology.* 1987;67:A519.
197. Williams PI, Sarginson RE, Ratcliffe JM. Use of methadone in the morphine-tolerant burned paediatric patient. *Br J Anaesth.* 1998;80(1):92–95.
198. Chana SK, Anand KJS, Rutter N. Can we use methadone for analgesia in neonates? *Arch Dis Child Fetal Neonatal Ed.* 2001;85(2):79F–81.
199. Davies D, DeVlaming D, Haines C. Methadone analgesia for children with advanced cancer. *Pediatr Blood Cancer.* 2008;51(3):393–397.
200. Anghelescu DL, Faughnan LG, Hankins GM, Ward DA, Oakes LL. Methadone use in children and young adults at a cancer center: A retrospective study. *J Opioid Manag.* 2011;7(5):353–361.
201. Mercadante S, Caraceni A. Conversion ratios for opioid switching in the treatment of cancer pain: A systematic review. *Palliat Med.* 2011;25(5):504–515.
202. Toombs JD, Kral LA. Methadone treatment for pain states. *Am Fam Physician.* 2005;71(7):1353–1358.
203. Moryl N, Pope J, Obbens E. Hypoglycemia during rapid methadone dose escalation. *J Opioid Manag.* 2013;9(1):29–34.
204. Flory JH, Wiesenthal AC, Thaler HT, Koranteng L, Moryl N. Methadone use and the risk of hypoglycemia for inpatients with cancer pain. *J Pain Symptom Manage.* 2016;51(1):79–87 e71.
205. Madden K, Bruera E. Very-low-dose methadone to treat refractory neuropathic pain in children with cancer. *J Palliat Med.* 2017;20(11):1280–1283.
206. Mercadante S, Bruera E. Methadone as a first-line opioid in cancer pain management: A systematic review. *J Pain Symptom Manage.* 2018;55(3):998–1003.
207. Friedrichsdorf SJ. From tramadol to methadone: Opioids in the treatment of pain and dyspnea in pediatric palliative care. *Clin J Pain.* 2019.
208. Cherny NI, Foley KM. Nonopioid and opioid analgesic pharmacotherapy of cancer pain. *Hematol Oncol Clin North Am.* 1996;10(1):79–102.
209. Friedrichsdorf S, Finney D, Bergin M, Stevens M, Collins J. Breakthrough pain in children with cancer. *J Pain Symptom Manage.* 2007;34(2):209–216.
210. Finnerup NB, Attal N, Haroutounian S, et al. Pharmacotherapy for neuropathic pain in adults: A systematic review and meta-analysis. *Lancet Neurol.* 2015;14(2):162–173.
211. Friedrichsdorf SJ, Nugent AP. Management of neuropathic pain in children with cancer. *Curr Opin Support Palliat Care.* 2013;7(2):131–138.
212. Hauer JM, Solodiuk JC. Gabapentin for management of recurrent pain in 22 nonverbal children with severe neurological impairment: A retrospective analysis. *J Palliat Med.* 2015;18(5):453–456.
213. Edwards L, DeMeo S, Hornik CD, et al. Gabapentin use in the neonatal intensive care unit. *J Pediatr.* 2016;169:310–312.
214. Horvath R, Halbrooks EF, Overman DM, Friedrichsdorf SJ. Efficacy and safety of postoperative dexmedetomidine administration in infants and children undergoing cardiac surgery: A retrospective cohort study. *J Pediatr Intensive Care.* 2015(3):138–145.
215. Burns J, Jackson K, Sheehy KA, Finkel JC, Quezado ZM. The use of dexmedetomidine in pediatric palliative care: A preliminary study. *J Palliat Med.* 2017;20(7):779–783.
216. Chrysostomou C, Schulman SR, Herrera Castellanos M, et al. A phase II/III, multicenter, safety, efficacy, and pharmacokinetic study of dexmedetomidine in preterm and term neonates. *J Pediatr.* 2014;164(2):276–282 e271–273.
217. Kajiume T, Sera Y, Nakanuno R, et al. Continuous intravenous infusion of ketamine and lidocaine as adjuvant analgesics in a 5-year-old patient with neuropathic cancer pain. *J Palliat Med.* 2012;15(6):719–722.
218. Finkel J, Pestieau S, Quezado Z. Ketamine as an adjuvant for treatment of cancer pain in children and adolescents. *J Pain.* 2007;8(6):515–521.
219. Peixoto RD, Hawley P. Intravenous lidocaine for cancer pain without electrocardiographic monitoring: A retrospective review. *J Palliat Med.* 2015;18(4):373–377.
220. Seah DSE, Herschtal A, Tran H, Thakerar A, Fullerton S. Subcutaneous lidocaine infusion for pain in patients with cancer. *J Palliat Med.* 2017;20(6):667–671.
221. Wallace MS, Lee J, Sorkin L, Dunn JS, Yaksh T, Yu A. Intravenous lidocaine: Effects on controlling pain after anti-GD2 antibody therapy in children with neuroblastoma: A report of a series. *Anesth Analg.* 1997;85(4):794–796.
222. Massey GV, Pedigo S, Dunn NL, Grossman NJ, Russell EC. Continuous lidocaine infusion for the relief of refractory malignant pain in a terminally ill pediatric cancer patient. *J Pediatr Hematol Oncol.* 2002;24(7):566–568.
223. Ferrini R, Paice JA. How to initiate and monitor infusional lidocaine for severe and/or neuropathic pain. *J Support Oncol.* 2004;2(1):90–94.
224. Wang Z, Whiteside SPH, Sim L, et al. Comparative effectiveness and safety of cognitive behavioral therapy and pharmacotherapy for childhood anxiety disorders: A systematic review and meta-analysis. *JAMA Pediatrics.* 2017;171(11):1049–1056.
225. Bahar RJ, Collins BS, Steinmetz B, Ament ME. Double-blind placebo-controlled trial of amitriptyline for the treatment of irritable bowel syndrome in adolescents. *J Pediatr.* 2008;152(5):685–689.
226. Saps M, Youssef N, Miranda A, et al. Multicenter, randomized, placebo-controlled trial of amitriptyline in children with functional gastrointestinal disorders. *Gastroenterology.* 2009;137(4):1261–1269.
227. Brummett CM, Trivedi KA, Dubovoy AV, Berland DW. Dexmedetomidine as a novel therapeutic for postoperative pain in a patient treated with buprenorphine. *J Opioid Manag.* 2009;5(3):175–179.
228. Roberts SB, Wozencraft CP, Coyne PJ, Smith TJ. Dexmedetomidine as an adjuvant analgesic for intractable cancer pain. *J Palliat Med.* 2011;14(3):371–373.

229. O'Mara K, Gal P, Wimmer J, et al. Dexmedetomidine versus standard therapy with fentanyl for sedation in mechanically ventilated premature neonates. *J Pediatr Pharmacol Ther.* 2012;17(3):252–262.
230. O'Neil T, Rodgers PE, Shultz C. Dexmedetomidine as adjuvant therapy for acute postoperative neuropathic pain crisis. *J Palliat Med.* 2014;17(10):1164–1166.
231. Aydogan MS, Korkmaz MF, Ozgul U, et al. Pain, fentanyl consumption, and delirium in adolescents after scoliosis surgery: Dexmedetomidine vs midazolam. *Paediatr Anaesth.* 2013;23(5):446–452.
232. Funai Y, Pickering AE, Uta D, et al. Systemic dexmedetomidine augments inhibitory synaptic transmission in the superficial dorsal horn through activation of descending noradrenergic control: An in vivo patch-clamp analysis of analgesic mechanisms. *Pain.* 2014;155(3):617–628.
233. Assouline B, Tramer MR, Kreienbuhl L, Elia N. Benefit and harm of adding ketamine to an opioid in a patient-controlled analgesia device for the control of postoperative pain: Systematic review and meta-analyses of randomized controlled trials with trial sequential analyses. *Pain.* 2016;157(12): 2854–2864.
234. Norambuena C, Yanez J, Flores V, Puentes P, Carrasco P, Villena R. Oral ketamine and midazolam for pediatric burn patients: A prospective, randomized, double-blind study. *J Pediatr Surg.* 2013;48(3):629–634.
235. Krane E, Leong M, Golianu B, Leong Y. Treatment of pediatric pain with nonconventional analgesics. In Schechter N, Berde C, Yaster M, eds. *Pain in Infants, Children, and Adolescents.* Lippincott Williams & Wilkins; 2003:225–240.
236. Wasiak J, Mahar PD, McGuinness SK, et al. Intravenous lidocaine for the treatment of background or procedural burn pain. *Cochrane Database Syst Rev.* 2014(10):CD005622.
237. Sen IM, Sen RK. Regional anesthesia for lower limb burn wound debridements. *Arch Trauma Res.* 2012;1(3):135–136.
238. Cuignet O, Mbuyamba J, Pirson J. The long-term analgesic efficacy of a single-shot fascia iliaca compartment block in burn patients undergoing skin-grafting procedures. *J Burn Care Rehabil.* 2005;26(5):409–415.
239. Bussolin L, Busoni P, Giorgi L, Crescioli M, Messeri A. Tumescent local anesthesia for the surgical treatment of burns and postburn sequelae in pediatric patients. *Anesthesiology.* 2003;99(6):1371–1375.
240. Hernandez JL, Savetamal A, Crombie RE, et al. Use of continuous local anesthetic infusion in the management of postoperative split-thickness skin graft donor site pain. *J Burn Care Res.* 2013;34(4):e257–262.
241. Shank ES, Martyn JA, Donelan MB, Perrone A, Firth PG, Driscoll DN. Ultrasound-guided regional anesthesia for pediatric burn reconstructive surgery: A prospective study. *J Burn Care Res.* 2016;37(3):e213–217.
242. Cuignet O, Pirson J, Boughrouph J, Duville D. The efficacy of continuous fascia iliaca compartment block for pain management in burn patients undergoing skin grafting procedures. *Anesth Analg.* 2004;98(4):1077–1081.
243. Rork JF, Berde CB, Goldstein RD. Regional anesthesia approaches to pain management in pediatric palliative care: A review of current knowledge. *J Pain Symptom Manage.* 2013;46(6): 859–873.
244. Burns DA. Using Regional Anesthesia to Manage Pediatric Acute Pain. 10th Pediatric Pain Master's Class; 2017. Minneapolis, MN.
245. Anghelescu DL, Faughnan LG, Baker JN, Yang J, Kane JR. Use of epidural and peripheral nerve blocks at the end of life in children and young adults with cancer: The collaboration between a pain service and a palliative care service. *Paediatr Anaesth.* 2010;20(12):1070–1077.
246. Conn M, Borucki A, Spencer R, Goldsby R, Poree L. Intrathecal drug delivery therapy for pediatric cancer pain: Two case reports and limits to access. Poster presented at the North American Neuromodulation Society 23rd Annual Meeting; 2020. Las Vegas, NV.
247. Gurnaney H, Kraemer FW, Maxwell L, Muhly WT, Schleelein L, Ganesh A. Ambulatory continuous peripheral nerve blocks in children and adolescents: A longitudinal 8-year single center study. *Anesth Analg.* 2014;118(3):621–627.
248. Anghelescu DL, Harris BL, Faughnan LG, et al. Risk of catheter-associated infection in young hematology/oncology patients receiving long-term peripheral nerve blocks. *Paediatr Anaesth.* 2012;22(11):1110–1116.
249. Pacenta HL, Kaddoum RN, Pereiras LA, Chidiac EJ, Burgoyne LL. Continuous tunnelled femoral nerve block for palliative care of a patient with metastatic osteosarcoma. *Anaesth Intensive Care.* 2010;38(3):563–565.
250. Burgoyne LL, Pereiras LA, Bertani LA, et al. Long-term use of nerve block catheters in paediatric patients with cancer related pathologic fractures. *Anaesth Intensive Care.* 2012;40(4):710–713.
251. Hooke MC, Grund E, Quammen H, Miller B, McCormick P, Bostrom B. Propofol use in pediatric patients with severe cancer pain at the end of life. *J Pediatr Oncol Nurs.* 2007;24(1): 29–34.
252. Hill KP. Medical marijuana for treatment of chronic pain and other medical and psychiatric problems: A clinical review. *JAMA.* 2015;313(24):2474–2483.
253. Deshpande A, Mailis-Gagnon A, Zoheiry N, Lakha SF. Efficacy and adverse effects of medical marijuana for chronic noncancer pain: Systematic review of randomized controlled trials. *Can Fam Physician.* 2015;61(8):e372–381.
254. Boland EG, Bennett MI, Allgar V, Boland JW. Cannabinoids for adult cancer-related pain: Systematic review and meta-analysis. *BMJ Support Palliat Care.* 2020;10(1):14–24.
255 . Stockings E, Campbell G, Hall WD, et al. Cannabis and cannabinoids for the treatment of people with chronic noncancer pain conditions: A systematic review and meta-analysis of controlled and observational studies. *Pain.* 2018;159(10): 1932–1954.
256. Wong SS, Wilens TE. Medical cannabinoids in children and adolescents: A systematic review. *Pediatrics.* 2017;140(5).
257. Ammerman S. Updated AAP policy opposes marijuana use, citing potential harms, lack of research. AAP News. 2015. http://aapnews.aappublications.org/content/early/2015/01/26/aapnews.20150126-1
258. Casadio P, Fernandes C, Murray RM, Di Forti M. Cannabis use in young people: The risk for schizophrenia. *Neurosci Biobehav Rev.* 2011;35(8):1779–1787.
259. Daling JR, Doody DR, Sun X, et al. Association of marijuana use and the incidence of testicular germ cell tumors. *Cancer.* 2009;115(6):1215–1223.
260. Trabert B, Sigurdson AJ, Sweeney AM, Strom SS, McGlynn KA. Marijuana use and testicular germ cell tumors. *Cancer.* 2011;117(4):848–853.
261. Lacson JC, Carroll JD, Tuazon E, Castelao EJ, Bernstein L, Cortessis VK. Population-based case-control study of recreational drug use and testis cancer risk confirms an association between marijuana use and nonseminoma risk. *Cancer.* 2012;118(21):5374–5383.
262. Meier MH, Caspi A, Ambler A, et al. Persistent cannabis users show neuropsychological decline from childhood to midlife. *Proc Natl Acad Sci U S A.* 2012;109(40):E2657–2664.
263. Moffitt TE, Meier MH, Caspi A, Poulton R. Reply to Rogeberg and Daly: No evidence that socioeconomic status or personality differences confound the association between cannabis use and IQ decline. *Proc Natl Acad Sci U S A.* 2013;110(11): E980–982.
264. Meier MH, Hall W, Caspi A, et al. Which adolescents develop persistent substance dependence in adulthood? Using

population-representative longitudinal data to inform universal risk assessment. *Psychol Med.* 2016;46(4):877–889.
265. Fortier MA, Chou J, Maurer EL, Kain ZN. Acute to chronic postoperative pain in children: Preliminary findings. *J Pediatr Surg.* 2011;46(9):1700–1705.
266. Sieberg CB, Simons LE, Edelstein MR, et al. Pain prevalence and trajectories following pediatric spinal fusion surgery. *J Pain.* 2013;14(12):1694–1702.
267. Page MG, Stinson J, Campbell F, Isaac L, Katz J. Identification of pain-related psychological risk factors for the development and maintenance of pediatric chronic postsurgical pain. *J Pain Res.* 2013;6:167–180.
268. Noel M, Rabbitts JA, Tai GG, Palermo TM. Remembering pain after surgery: A longitudinal examination of the role of pain catastrophizing in children's and parents' recall. *Pain.* 2015;156(5):800–808.
269. Nickel FT, Seifert F, Lanz S, Maihofner C. Mechanisms of neuropathic pain. *Eur Neuropsychopharmacol.* 2012;22(2):81–91.
270. Goodman JE, McGrath PJ. The epidemiology of pain in children and adolescents: A review. *Pain.* 1991;46(3):247–264.
271. Hechler T, Dobe M, Zernikow B. Commentary: A worldwide call for multimodal inpatient treatment for children and adolescents suffering from chronic pain and pain-related disability. *J Pediatr Psychol.* 2010;35(2):138–140.
272. King S, Chambers CT, Huguet A, et al. The epidemiology of chronic pain in children and adolescents revisited: A systematic review. *Pain.* 2011;152(12):2729–2738.
273. Friedrichsdorf SJ, Giordano J, Desai-Dakoji K, Warmuth A, Schulz CA. Chronic pain in children and adolescents: Diagnosis and treatment of primary pain disorders in head, abdomen, muscles and joints. *Children (Basel).* 2016;3(4):E42.
274. Lauwerier E, Paemeleire K, Van Damme S, Goubert L, Crombez G. Medication use in patients with migraine and medication-overuse headache: The role of problem-solving and attitudes about pain medication. *Pain.* 2011;152(6):1334–1339.
275. Di Lorenzo C, Youssef NN, Sigurdsson L, Scharff L, Griffiths J, Wald A. Visceral hyperalgesia in children with functional abdominal pain. *J Pediatr.* 2001;139(6):838–843.
276. Walco GA, Dworkin RH, Krane EJ, LeBel AA, Treede RD. Neuropathic pain in children: Special considerations. *Mayo Clin Proc.* 2010;85(3 Suppl):S33–41.
277. Cohen SP, Mao J. Neuropathic pain: Mechanisms and their clinical implications. *BMJ.* 2014;348:f7656.
278. Chu C, Levine E, Gear RW, Bogen O, Levine JD. Mitochondrial dependence of nerve growth factor-induced mechanical hyperalgesia. *Pain.* 2011;152(8):1832–1837.

24 | RESPIRATORY SYMPTOMS

ROSE SHARPE, MEGAN JORDAN, RAYMOND BARFIELD, SARAH GALL, MARGARITA BIDEGAIN, KRISTEN LAKIS, RENEE BARTLE, AND EMILY LAYOK

Breath is the finest gift of nature. Be grateful for this wonderful gift.

AMIT RAY[3]

INTRODUCTION

Respiratory symptoms in children are common and are one of the most distressing symptoms to patients, parents, and caregivers. They occur in 25.6% of children with progressive genetic, metabolic, or neurological conditions.[1,2,4] Systemic problems, such as weakness of the respiratory musculature, are seen with Duchenne muscular dystrophy, spinal muscular atrophy, or cystic fibrosis (discussed in Chapter 31). Localized problems such as airway abnormalities, swallowing difficulties, aspiration of secretions, or pneumonia may cause breathing difficulties. Metastases of tumors can cause widespread disease in the entire thorax, pleural effusions, pneumothorax, or airway compression. As children near the end of life, it is common to see the development of abnormal breathing patterns such as apnea, dyspnea, or Cheyne-Stokes respirations and difficulties with cough and secretion management.[5] Respiratory symptoms at the end of life tend to be one of the most distressing and leave a lasting impact on those who witness them.

Respiratory management in children is complex. There are many interventions both invasive and noninvasive that can be offered to provide support and comfort. Not being able to breathe normally is frightening to both the child and the caregiver. Care for the child will need to involve the coordinated efforts of the interdisciplinary team. The members may vary depending on the institution, but typically include a physician, nurse, social worker, child life specialist, chaplain, psychiatrist and/or psychologist, and respiratory therapist (see Table 24.1). The team collaborates to help support and empower the child and family through times that can be difficult and anxiety producing. It is important to consider not only the child and family's physical needs, but also their spiritual and psychosocial needs.

This chapter examines common respiratory symptoms with emphasis on those seen in advanced illness including end of life, management of these symptoms by the interdisciplinary team, and how advance care planning can help ease the distress of making decisions "in the moment" when respirations can no longer be sustained outside of the intensive care unit (ICU). Discharges to palliative care or hospice do not typically occur from ICUs. However, this is becoming more common with medical interventions that extend life. Challenges related to respiratory support during the transition from the ICU to home will also be explored.

CLINICAL VIGNETTE

Samuel was a 17-year-old patient with a rare, metastatic cancer called clear cell sarcoma. He was passionate about literature and theater. He loved to read and re-read the novel *The Life of Pi*[6] because Pi was lost at sea in a lifeboat with a tiger and Pi masters and trains the tiger. Samuel knew what it was to be lost, but he was unable to master the tiger of his cancer. His parents were able to pay for every available treatment, including radical surgical resection of tumors in Europe. But the cancer progressed relentlessly. As he approached the end of his life, Samuel's respiratory agony increased because of uncountable pulmonary metastases. He was in the hospital, but he frequently asked to be alone. His parents would sit outside his room, searching the internet for new treatments. His father asked the palliative care physician to visit with him, just in case there were options available to make him more comfortable. Samuel agreed to meet. The palliative care physician sat with him quietly for almost half an hour before saying anything. He finally asked, "Samuel, what do you need right now?" Speaking in broken sentences, a few words at a time, Samuel answered, "I would be so much better if I could just cry. But I cannot breathe in enough air to cry. All I want is to cry one time, and I will be OK." The palliative care physician assembled a team that included Samuel's nurse and respiratory therapist, and, with a combination of opioids, anxiolytics, oxygen, diuretics, and beta-agonists, Samuel was able to breathe in enough to cry. When he finished, his parents agreed to focus on comfort care. Samuel was given

TABLE 24.1 Respiratory interdisciplinary care team

INTERDISCIPLINARY TEAM MEMBER	INTERVENTIONS
Respiratory therapist	Assessment of the patients' current respiratory status and home therapies the patient and family are utilizing. Airway management (invasive and noninvasive interventions), nebulizer treatments, assistance with cough assist, and other respiratory therapies prescribed. Makes recommendations regarding any changes to therapies to the interdisciplinary team in order to optimize respiratory health. Educate the patient and family on respiratory therapies and equipment as needed.
Nurse	Assessment and management of respiratory symptoms; use of nonpharmacological interventions such as positioning and play as well as pharmacological interventions to provide comfort for respiratory symptoms; maintains hygiene of patient and environment; provides anticipatory guidance to child and family as needed.
Physician	Assessment and identification of respiratory symptoms; recommendation of nonpharmacologic and pharmacological interventions for management of distressing symptoms as needed.
Child life specialist	Assessment of coping of patient and family secondary to changes in respiratory status; provide coping interventions through play; offer nonpharmacological interventions for distraction, normalization, and familiarization of medical setting.
Psychiatrist/psychologist	Assessment and management of psychiatric symptoms related to respiratory distress such as anxiety and depression with pharmacological interventions (provided by a psychiatrist) or psychotherapy interventions that may include techniques such as cognitive-behavioral strategies, mindfulness, or relaxation training (provided by psychiatrist or psychologist)
Chaplain	Assessment of patient and family's religion and spirituality, paying particular attention to its impact on coping with change in respiratory status, health outcomes, and decision-making; chaplains also provide spiritual-emotional support during periods of crisis.
Clinical social worker	Assessment of coping of both patient and family during change in respiratory status; offer nonpharmacological interventions for distress, anxiety, and depression; assessment of values and spiritual beliefs on complex medical decisions; assistance to identify resources.

relief from his respiratory distress, and 2 days later he died peacefully, surrounded by people who loved him.

DYSPNEA

Dyspnea is "a subjective experience of breathing discomfort that consists of qualitatively distinct sensations that vary in intensity."[7] This experience is affected by physiological, psychological, social, and environmental factors and can be found in patients of all ages with a variety of illnesses. The prevalence of dyspnea in pediatric patients with life-threatening conditions varies from 21% to 80%.[8] Dyspnea has been identified to cause a substantial or great deal of suffering by parental report in pediatric patients with cancer and heart disease at the end of life.[9,10] The causes of dyspnea (Table 24.2) vary widely and can occur due to the malformation or malfunction of different organ systems or the presence of psychological distress such as anxiety and depression.

The assessment of dyspnea in the pediatric population often includes the evaluation of both subjective and objective elements. Physical signs that may indicate the presence of dyspnea include increased respiratory rate, pursed lip breathing, gasping, and use of accessory muscles, recognized through obvious retractions.[11,12] The presence of labored breathing may not fully characterize the patient's experience or may only occur during times of stress, such as feeding for neonates or exertion in older children and adolescents.[8,12] Self-report of this subjective sensation is often difficult in pediatrics given lack of communication skills in neonates, young children, and those with severe neurologic impairment.[8] Therefore, assessment of dyspnea often requires collaboration with parents to assess triggers and response to exertion. Tools to measure dyspnea in children are limited and most are validated for patients older than 6 years who have cystic fibrosis. These include "modified Borg Scale," "Visual Analog Scale," and "Dalhousie Dyspnea Scale," which can also be used in children with asthma. They have been found to be more effective when combining verbal and pictorial descriptions.[8,13] Dyspnea assessment, as with all symptoms in palliative care, requires careful history-taking and physical examination to determine the possible underlying etiologies

TABLE 24.2 Causes of dyspnea

PATHOPHYSIOLOGY	DISEASE EXAMPLES
Respiratory muscle weakness	Muscular dystrophies
Fixed or intermittent airway obstruction	Asthma, congenital anomalies of airway, tumor compression
Intrathoracic lung parenchyma abnormalities	Aspiration, cystic fibrosis, pneumonia, pulmonary edema, pulmonary hemorrhage, tumor
Intrathoracic extra-parenchymal abnormalities	Hemothorax, pleural effusion, pneumothorax
Blood gas abnormalities	Genetic and metabolic disease, infection, renal failure
Decreased blood supply	Anemia, cardiac disease, congenital vascular anomalies, pulmonary embolism, superior vena cava obstruction

TABLE 24.3 Respiratory symptoms management

SYMPTOMS	MEDICATION	DOSING	COMMENTS
Dyspnea	*Opioids:*		
	Morphine	0.02–0.05 mg/kg/dose IV 0.06–0.15 mg/kg/dose PO	¼ to ½ dose used for analgesia
	Oxycodone	0.04–0.1 mg/kg/dose PO	
	Hydromorphone	0.005–0.01 mg/kg/dose IV 0.01–0.02 mg/kg/dose PO	
	Fentanyl	0.5–1 mcg/kg/dose IV 1.5 mcg/kg/dose IN	
	Benzodiazepines:		
	Lorazepam	0.02–0.05 mg/kg/dose IV/PO	
	Midazolam	0.05–0.1 mg/kg/dose IV	
		0.06–0.12 mg/kg/hour continuous infusion	1–2 mcg/kg/min; titrate to desired effect
		0.2 mg/kg/dose IN	Administer with intranasal lidocaine to reduce burning sensation
Secretions	*Anticholinergics:*		
	Glycopyrrolate	4–10 mcg/kg/dose IV q4h (max. 0.2 mg/dose) 40–100 mcg/kg/dose PO q6–8h	Does not cross blood–brain barrier
	Scopolamine patch	6 mcg/kg/dose Patients 8–15 kg – ½ patch q72h Patients> 15 kg –1 patch q72h	Do NOT cut the patch, leave portion of the original adhesive on patch is dose is < 1 patch
	Atropine ophthalmic drops	1–2 gtts SLq2–4h	Mixed evidence of effectiveness
	Hyoscamine	Weight-based dosing	Max 6 doses per day
	Mucolytics:		
	Nebulized saline solution	0.9% normal saline solution	Administered via nebulizer
	Guaifenesin	Patients age 2–6 years 50–100 mg q4h Patients age 6–12 years 100–200 mg q4h Patients age >12 years 200–400 mg q4h	Only recommended in children >2 years old
	Acetylcysteine 10% solution	Infants 2–4 mL q6–8h Children/adolescents 6–10 mL q6–8h	Patient should receive bronchodilator 10–15 mins prior to acetylcysteine neb

of this symptom and the impact of dyspnea on the patient's quality of life.

Modalities that target reversing or improving the underlying etiology for dyspnea are the first step in management of this symptom if these interventions are concordant with patient and family goals of care. Management for dyspnea is best provided in a calm environment, which will help minimize any associated anxiety. The treatment strategies for dyspnea are a combination of pharmacologic (Table 24.3), psychosocial, psychological, and mechanical interventions (Box 24.1) that should be escalated to match the intensity of the symptom.[11,12] Education should be provided to the patient and family about options for dyspnea management strategies, as well as consistent reevaluation of the patient's dyspnea with each intervention.[14]

A Cochrane review of adults with dyspnea showed that interventions such as mechanical vibration of the chest wall, electrical stimulation of leg muscles, walking aids, and breathing training helped relieve shortness of breath; there have been mixed results for acupuncture and acupressure.[15] There is insufficient evidence to assess relaxation, cognitive-behavioral strategies, and distraction for the management of dyspnea.[7,15,16] Many children respond well to deep breathing, bubbles, and use of a pinwheel to help control breathing when they are feeling anxious and short of breath. Use of a fan to direct air movement over the face has been observed to reduce dyspnea.[7,14] Appropriate positioning, especially for patients with neuromuscular disorders can help reduce dyspnea and orthopnea.

BOX 24.1 NONPHARMACOLOGIC DYSPNEA MANAGEMENT

- Calm environment
- Breathing training
- Guided imagery
- Walking aids
- Positioning
- Fan
- Oxygen
- Medical air
- Airway clearance therapy
- Noninvasive positive pressure ventilation
- Tracheostomy

In patients with hypoxemia, use of oxygen is appropriate, but very few studies regarding this intervention have been done systematically in patients with life-threatening illnesses.[8] A 2011 randomized control trial in adults evaluated oxygen versus medical air for non-hypoxemic palliative care patients and found that neither gas was superior in improving quality of life or relieving shortness of breath.[14] Patients and families often find comfort in having access to oxygen, especially in the home setting, as this provides them a sense of self-control in managing shortness of breath. Some pediatric patients with neuromuscular weakness or airway anomalies may benefit from the use of airway clearance therapy to aid with secretion management, noninvasive ventilation (NIV), or even mechanical ventilation via tracheostomy. A conversation about goals of care should be held with the patient and family prior to initiation of these life-altering interventions. Time-limited trials of NIV are possible to assess for improvement in dyspnea. In the setting of reversible illness, some families may also consider intubation; however, the decision to discontinue ventilatory support may be more difficult for families.[12]

Opioids are the primary medication used to manage dyspnea in patients with advanced illness.[17] Sometimes medical personnel and parents are fearful of respiratory depression and the possibility of accelerated death with opioid therapy. However, studies have shown improvement in respiratory rate and dyspnea control without iatrogenic hypoventilation or hypoxia. Education, careful observation, and appropriate dosing can alleviate this inappropriate fear of opioid use.[8,12,14] The typical starting dose of opioids for the management of dyspnea is one-quarter to one-half of the dose used for pain (Table 24.3), and this dose can be increased as needed for symptom relief. In adults there is evidence for use of low-dose sustained-released morphine for treatment of chronic refractory shortness of breath in the setting of advanced progressive disease.[18] Oral opioid preparations are preferred to intravenous for management of chronic dyspnea.[8,12] Intranasal fentanyl is a safe and effective medication for management of acute respiratory distress in children with life-limiting conditions.[19] There is no evidence to support the use of inhaled opioids.[17]

Benzodiazepines are not meant to serve as a stand-alone therapy to manage dyspnea in children.[12] A meta-analysis of studies assessing the use of benzodiazepines in adults with advanced illness showed no improvement in shortness of breath.[20] They can be used to treat comorbid anxiety, which may help improve dyspnea.[7,14] Benzodiazepines should be considered in refractory dyspnea that is not improving despite various treatments. Other medications that may also provide relief of associated symptoms include mucolytics, bronchodilators, diuretics, anticholinergics, and steroids. Steroids can be a double-edged sword, reducing airway inflammation but also carrying the risk of weakening respiratory muscles, and they should be used with caution.[7]

Child life specialists work closely with patients who have respiratory compromise secondary to chronic illnesses or nearing the end of life. They collaborate with other members of the psychosocial team, including psychiatry, psychology, chaplains, and social work to develop nonpharmacological coping and symptom management plans for these patients.[21] Child life specialists begin relationships with patients through play to establish friendly rapport with the patient and to earn the patient's trust, to allow assessment of the patient's developmental stage and establish an appropriate teaching plan or intervention.

For patients with respiratory compromise an effective activity for improving lung capacity and to help with coping is blowing bubbles. Blowing bubbles has many benefits including simple stress relief, promoting normalization, supporting development, and, most importantly, helping one to breathe deeply and steadily. Bubbles are a familiar and fun visual to show a child how they can control their breathing. A child life specialist can then help the child to replicate this sensation when they are not blowing bubbles to help control their breathing.[22]

Guided imagery can be extremely beneficial for patients with chronic respiratory symptoms. Not only does it encourage a patient to be distracted for a moment, but it helps to regulate their body and breathing, provides a sense of control over their body in an environment where they have little control, and allows them to better manage their distress.[22] These exercises can be done with family or the patient's nurse as well as through technology. There are a variety of applications for cellphones, computers, and tablets that promote and assist with guided imagery, guided visualizations for deep breathing, and meditation that can provide benefits to many patients.[23] Through an established trusting relationship, play, and developmentally appropriate education, child life specialists can help patients understand their breathing during challenging times.

Psychologists or psychiatrists in conjunction with the interdisciplinary team can assist patients who experience anxiety which can lead to respiratory difficulties by incorporating cognitive-behavioral therapy (CBT). CBT has been associated with improvements in quality of life in patients with anxiety.[24] Social workers can also assist with helping patients gain distress tolerance skills, develop relaxation techniques, and utilize guided imagery skills. The social worker is also attentive to the family system and can help them think through complex decision-making.

Some families find benefit from spiritual support. Chaplains can provide spiritual resources, assist with stress management, and can help with traditional rituals. If anxiety can't be managed with these interventions, the addition of an anxiolytic may be helpful to manage anxious behavior leading to dyspnea. These medications can be prescribed by the psychiatrist or the patient's primary provider.

COUGH

Cough interferes with activities as basic as eating and sleeping and can also contribute to social isolation by discouraging affected individuals from engaging in public events. Moreover, cough leads to fatigue, abdominal or chest pain, and even vomiting and rib fractures. Persistent cough is a serious problem affecting quality of life that healthcare professionals sometimes underestimate. Our understanding of triggers such as afferent sensory nerves originating in the upper airway,[25] TRPV1 receptors and TRPA1 receptors,[26] has improved. Unfortunately, preliminary studies in adults have not shown clinical effectiveness of therapies targeted to these pathways.

Identification of underlying pathology is important in treating cough in those diagnosed with serious and life-threatening illnesses. Overt and silent aspirations are clear triggers of chronic cough and can be treated with pro-motility agents and thickened-consistency diets. Cough due to anatomic excitation of contributory reflexes and nerves, often found in malignancy, can sometimes be treated with surgery, chemotherapy, and radiotherapy, both external beam and brachytherapy. Many patients with life-threatening illness are also vulnerable to infection and fluid overload, which can be treated with antibiotics and diuretics, if so aligned with the patient's and/or caregiver's goals.

Cough may respond to N-methyl-d-aspartate (NMDA) receptor antagonists, such as dextromethorphan.[27] This is often available in low-dose formulations in over-the-counter cough preparations. Suppression of cough can also be achieved with systemic agents such as opioids. Recently, and especially in adults with lung cancer, there has been an increasingly recognized role of speech therapy, which teaches patients strategies to control cough, identify triggers of cough, and receive training in oral hygiene.[28] Even more recently, a randomized controlled trial in adults showed even greater efficacy of pregabalin and speech therapy together for chronic cough.[29] Very few studies in pediatric patients exist, but several studies have concluded that demulcents, particularly honey, can be useful in this population.[30]

SECRETIONS

Suctioning is the first line treatment for airway maintenance in children with excessive or difficult to manage secretions. In-home portable suction equipment is easily provided. Deep suctioning is thought to cause discomfort in patients; thus, this is generally avoided at end of life.

Excessive, thin secretions can be controlled by a variety of anticholinergic medications, although the evidence for these strategies is quite weak (Table 24.3).[31] Within this class of medications, the one least likely to cross the blood–brain barrier is glycopyrrolate. Other agents commonly used to thicken or dry secretions include atropine ophthalmic drops administered orally, hyoscyamine, and scopolamine. These medications need to be carefully titrated to avoid causing excessive dry mouth and so that the secretions do not become too thick. If this complication arises, secretions may become much harder to move within the airways, leading to the formations of large, solid mucous plugs, which can then worsen the child's respiratory symptoms. Additionally, families and caregivers also need to be alert to other anticholinergic symptoms, such as urinary retention, which sometimes requires indwelling urinary catheterization and may cause worsening constipation.

Children with sialorrhea, in particular those with neurologic disorders, may require more intensive therapies given the impact of this symptom on their quality of life. Therapies such as botulinum toxin A injections (BtA) and salivary gland surgery may be good options for intervention. Botulinum toxin A has many clinical applications but has gained popularity as a treatment for saliva management. Injections are typically administered with the use of local anesthesia or done under general anesthesia in conjunction with other procedures. A saliva control clinic in the United Kingdom found effective responses to BtA in 61% of their patients with a mean duration of efficacy of 4 months, with a range of 2 weeks to 18 months. Sixteen percent of children developed complications which included dysphagia (16%) and xerostomia (3%), and a further 4% developed thick, sticky secretions.[32] Another smaller study showed that 80% of caregivers noted an improvement in the child's quality of life after botulinum toxin (Botox) treatment of sialorrhea.[33] If all forms of pharmacotherapy including BtA are not effective, surgery can be considered especially if the child is having issues with aspiration. Salivary gland surgery, which comprises of either submandibular duct transfer with excision of sublingual glands for children not at risk for aspiration or bilateral submandibular excision with bilateral parotid duct ligation for children with known aspiration risk, was an effective intervention for sialorrhea in 88% of the children at a saliva control clinic.[32]

In advanced illness, the focus is most frequently on drying secretions. There are times, however, when thinning secretions is most helpful to patients. This is often the case when patients have infection or tumor leading to cough and difficulty expectorating their mucus and secretions. In these situations, thinning or emulsifying secretions with mucolytics makes it easier for patients to expectorate (Table 24.3). Normal saline nebulizer treatments and guaifenesin therapies are most commonly used. A less common and costlier alternative is aerosolized acetylcysteine.

PULMONARY HEMORRHAGE

Pulmonary hemorrhage presents with a clinical spectrum ranging from blood-tinged sputum to sudden, life-threatening hemoptysis. In the pediatric population, significant pulmonary hemorrhage commonly arises from complications of advanced lung disease, sepsis, or end-stage liver disease. Bleeding is exacerbated by coagulopathies and thrombocytopenia. Pediatric oncology patients experience pulmonary hemorrhage as a result of both invasive disease and the treatment for disease, including radiation and chemotherapeutic agents such as cyclophosphamide, busulfan, and bleomycin.[34] Patients who have had hematopoietic stem cell transplantation are particularly vulnerable to both infectious and noninfectious causes of lung injury that can lead to intraparenchymal bleeding.[35] Diffuse alveolar hemorrhage in these patients has a particularly high mortality rate.[36] Beyond these specific causes, pulmonary hemorrhage can be seen in any critically ill patient who is mechanically ventilated. Therapies are generally directed at treatment of underlying infections, correction of coagulopathies and thrombocytopenia, and, in some cases, administration of corticosteroids, activated Factor VII, and aminocaproic acid to stabilize clots and judicious use of positive pressure in intubated patients.[37] But with overwhelming hemorrhage, such interventions are often inadequate to control the bleeding, and they may be inappropriate in the context of end-of-life care where the priority is comfort. Knowing the diseases and treatments associated with increased risk of bleeding can help a team create a plan in light of an individual patient's trajectory and goals of care.

When a patient has a disease or undergoes a treatment known to increase the chance of pulmonary bleeding, anticipatory care can mitigate trauma and avoid unwanted or ineffective interventions.[38] Whether mild or severe, pulmonary hemorrhage can be frightening to patients, families, and healthcare professionals. The possibility of hemorrhage and the plan for intervening should be explained to the patient, if appropriate, based on age and maturity, and to the patient's family and other care providers. The visual impact of bleeding can be profound. To diminish this, patients can wear darker clothing, and darker bed linens and towels can be provided. When patients are alert, pulmonary hemorrhage can cause distress. As with other causes of dyspnea, respiratory distress associated with bleeding can be eased with opioids. During an acute event, a bolus of midazolam given subcutaneously or intravenously can relieve anxiety and reduce a patient's memory of the event.[39] If the bleeding persists, the patient may benefit from a continuous midazolam infusion. It will be important for patient and family to be counseled that this infusion will cause moderate sedation and relief of anxiety for the patient while the medical team continues to manage dyspnea and bleeding.

PLEURAL EFFUSIONS, PNEUMOTHORAX, AND HEMOTHORAX

Many infectious and noninfectious diseases can lead to the accumulation of fluid, air, or blood between the lung and chest wall—pleural effusion, pneumothorax, and hemothorax, respectively. These accumulations may be asymptomatic when they are small, but they can cause significant dyspnea as they enlarge. Decisions about how, and whether, to intervene depend on the child's overall disease trajectory and the goals of care. If a child's underlying disease is very advanced, excellent end-of-life care might lead a team toward conservative medical management of symptoms. On the other hand, if a child is doing relatively well, other options such as surgical intervention or radiation therapy might be appropriate.

Treatment choice should be aligned with the patient's goals of care, and it should be fitting to the clinical realities of the patient's condition. But deciding whether or not an intervention will offer meaningful benefit in these situations is sometimes difficult. For example, when a patient has a malignant pleural effusion in the context of progressive cancer, draining the effusion will not stop it from quickly reaccumulating. Placing a pigtail catheter might provide transient relief, but these catheters are small and they often become clogged with tumor cells. A larger chest tube might drain the effusion more reliably and for a longer period of time, but many patients experience pain at the chest tube site, and the presence of a chest tube can limit a patient's mobility and options for location of treatment. These important aspects of medical and surgical interventions must be anticipated and weighed against the benefits that might be conferred.

Once an effusion is drained, pleurodesis might prevent or slow the reaccumulation. Pleurodesis is a procedure in which foreign materials are placed between the pleural surfaces of the chest wall and the lung to induce inflammation, allowing the two pleural surfaces to permanently adhere to each other. In theory this avoids recurrence of a pneumothorax or pleural effusion. In adult patients, pleurodesis is generally performed thoracoscopically, and talc is used as the material of choice to seal the pleural surfaces together.[40]

A more recent innovation is the insertion of a tunneled catheter for control of malignant pleural effusion. These are increasingly being used for ambulatory adult patients and can often be inserted by a thoracic surgeon as an outpatient procedure.[41] This procedure involves placing a tunneled catheter under the skin and subcutaneous tissue, through the thorax, and into the pleural collection of fluid. The exterior portion of the catheter can then be attached to a sterile collection bottle to perform serial drainages of the effusion as it reaccumulates, to maintain comfort. One study of 250 insertions in adults suggested that this approach is superior compared with talc pleurodesis, due primarily to the avoidance of a days-long hospital admission and long duration of result, usually until patients' deaths.[42] In pediatric palliative care, we often borrow from the experience accumulated in the world of adult medicine. This is certainly true in the case of pulmonary sources of distress. In all cases, the potential impact and benefit of the intervention must be weighed in light of the patient's reality, including the trajectory of the patient's disease and the overall goals of care.

WEAKNESS IN THE RESPIRATORY MUSCULATURE

Breathing difficulties can occur as a result of weakness in the respiratory musculature. Two inherited disease processes that cause severe muscle weakness are spinal muscular atrophy (SMA) and Duchenne muscular dystrophy (DMD).

SMA is a group of severe, genetic neuromuscular diseases that affect the spinal motor neurons. It has an estimated incidence of 1 in every 6,000 to 1 in 10,000 live births.[43] It is caused by a loss or defect of the SMN1 gene. The SMN1 gene is responsible for providing instruction to make the SMN protein, which in turn maintains healthy motor neuron function. With the degeneration of the spinal motor neurons, there is progressive muscle atrophy, weakness, and paralysis.[44]

Included in the atrophy and weakness are the intercostal muscles, resulting in an irregularly bell-shaped chest and an abnormal breathing pattern. Type-1 and Type-2 SMA have the greatest impact on the respiratory system.

Type-1 SMA is the most common (45% of all cases) and most severe; the onset in children has been noted to be between birth and 6 months.[45] Respiratory insufficiency is typically seen at birth and issues may even have been noted prior to birth with reported decreased intrauterine movement (Type-1). Due to the weakness of the respiratory system, a caregiver or clinician may note a weak cry, an irregularly bell-shaped chest, and irregular breathing. The chest wall takes on a bell-shaped appearance resulting from poor expansion of the ribcage. Because of respiratory muscle weakness, the infant is typically seen "belly-breathing" (paradoxical breathing).[45,46] With this type of breathing, the abdomen protrudes and the chest wall flattens on inspiration instead of the chest wall expanding.[43,46] In this case, the infant is utilizing accessory muscles to generate each breath. This pattern of breathing is not effective for long periods of time and can result in respiratory fatigue or failure. Once the respiratory system has reached this point, adjunct therapies may be needed to support the child's breathing. These therapies may include supplemental oxygen or NIV such as bilevel positive airway pressure (BIPAP) or continuous positive airway pressure (CPAP). Children with SMA may also have difficulty swallowing food as well as managing oral secretions due to bulbar (cranial nerves 9–12) dysfunction.[43] Dysphagia may also impact the respiratory system due to aspiration, leading to risk of pneumonia, and can affect nutrition. Providers and families will need to think about feeding tube options for their child to provide long-term nutritional support.

Scoliosis or curvature of the spine is believed to occur with an incidence of 60–90% within the Type-1 and -2 SMA. This can contribute to respiratory compromise since the chest wall is restricted and cannot move in an effective manner and proper lung expansion is inhibited.[44] This, in turn, can lead to areas within the lungs becoming atelectatic. Adjunct therapies may need to be utilized to support the child's breathing. The child, secondary to poor chest movement and a weak cough, may not mobilize pulmonary secretions independently. Assisted cough and postural drainage therapies should be considered part of a proactive care approach. Postural drainage entails placing the child in positions that will encourage secretions to mobilize into the larger airways for removal. Cough assist is a cycle of applied positive and then negative pressure. The positive pressure will assist the child in taking deeper breaths where the negative pressure acts as an artificial cough in order to help remove pulmonary secretions. The strength and function of the child's respiratory system/musculature should also be routinely assessed by pulmonary function testing (PFT), which measures lung volumes, airflow, and gas exchange. A decline or drop in PFT results may reflect a weakening of the respiratory system. When the respiratory system/musculature weakens to a point where the child is having nocturnal hypoxemia or hypoventilation, NIV may be initiated. This may avoid or prolong the need for advanced ventilation strategies, including the need for a tracheostomy.[43]

New therapeutic approaches may have a positive effect not only on survival, but also on respiratory status. Nusinersen has become commercially available after two successful double-blind clinical trials in early- and late-onset SMA.[47] There is evidence that infants with SMA1 may have improved ventilation-free survival at 24 months compared to a historic cohort of patients.[43,49]

DMD is an inherited X-linked genetic disorder with an estimated incidence of 1 in every 3,600–6,000 live male births.[50] With this disease process, the gene codes for the protein dystrophin are deleted or mutated. Dystrophin is made within all muscle cells of the heart and skeletal muscle fibers. It functions to both support and protect muscle fibers. If dystrophin is missing or defective, as in DMD, muscle cells can become damaged and do not work efficiently. Damaged cells will lead to an inflammatory process, which causes even further muscle damage. DMD is more commonly seen in boys, although in rare cases it can affect girls although it is usually milder.[51]

Muscle weakness/atrophy significantly impacts the cardiopulmonary system. Typically, by the child's early teens, respiratory and heart muscles have begun to be altered by the diseases' progression. Cardiac impairments present as cardiomyopathy or cardiac arrhythmias,[52,53] which can impact circulation and thus affect all of the body's tissues and organs that depend on optimal cardiopulmonary function. The respiratory musculature, inclusive of the diaphragm, will also become progressively weaker. This in turn will influence how well the child's chest expands and their ability to cough and clear pulmonary secretions. PFT should be routinely performed to monitor for early signs of respiratory compromise.[51]

Many of these young patients will also have skeletal problems secondary to progressive muscle degeneration and weakness, and postural compensation and contractures/deformities are likely to occur, including scoliosis.[53] This in turn will create respiratory issues since the chest is not able to move optimally. As the individuals' disease progresses, the inability to create a strong cough and take deep enough breaths can lead to other pulmonary complications including atelectasis, retained pulmonary secretions, hypoventilation, and respiratory failure. Postural drainage and cough assist may help to remove pulmonary secretions. If hypoxemia or hypoventilation occur, NIV may be necessary. If a child's respiratory status worsens to the point of respiratory failure in the context of either disease progression or pulmonary infection, mechanical ventilation may be necessary as a temporarily or long-term solution.

There is no known cure for either disease. However, as medical treatments have advanced, life expectancy has increased into young adulthood. Caregivers may have an emotional journey watching their child with a debilitating disease, and the complications that can occur can be overwhelming. As the function of the respiratory systems declines, there should be ongoing discussions between the interdisciplinary team, the caregiver(s), and the child/young adult regarding immediate and long-term goals with respect to quality of life and acceptable forms of intervention.

NONINVASIVE VENTILATION

NIV includes face mask, nasal mask, Oxy-Hood, high flow nasal cannula (HFNC), CPAP, and BIPAP. HFNC, CPAP, and BIPAP are more commonly seen in children, thus discussion will focus on these. There are indications for use of NIV in infants and children with both acute and chronic conditions. The use of NIV is growing. In infants, NIV can be used for alveolar recruitment, post-extubation, hypotonia with respiratory insufficiency, conditions associated with a loss of lung volume, and obstructive airway disease (e.g., tracheomalacia, bronchomalacia, and laryngomalacia). NIV is indicated in children for respiratory insufficiency associated with acute lung injury, pneumonia, asthma, bronchitis, pulmonary edema associated with renal or cardiac failure, cystic fibrosis, neuromuscular disease, neurologic disorders associated with respiratory depression, chest wall deformities, post-extubation, and obstructive sleep apnea.[54–56] These examples represent only a few indications. Noninvasive positive pressure ventilation (NIPPV) is used in children with chronic hypoventilation secondary to muscular weakness as seen in muscular dystrophy and spinal muscular atrophy.[57] There are contraindications to noninvasive respiratory support, including if the child had previous unsuccessful NIV or CPAP, frequent and severe apneas, tracheoesophageal fistula, craniofacial abnormalities that may prevent application, untreated pneumothorax, or neuromuscular disorders associated with severe respiratory depression. NIV support is not effective in children with moderate to severe acute respiratory distress (ARDS) with respiratory failure, untreated pneumothorax, facial injuries, traumatic injuries, burns, risk of aspiration, severe hemodynamic compromise, patients undergoing upper gastrointestinal tract surgeries, or those with increased intracranial pressure.[58] While there are interventions that can provide life-sustaining care, this care may not be appropriate for every family.

HFNC is a form of NIV. It delivers a mixture of air and oxygen via a plastic tubing and sits inside the nostrils.[59] The definition of high flow varies with the age of the patient and is not universal. Flows greater than or equal to 1 liter per minute (LPM) is considered high flow in neonatal patients, but flow ranges for older children are not well established in literature. Flows greater than or equal to 3 LPM meet criteria for high flow in toddlers, and flows greater than or equal to 5 LPM is considered high flow in older children. The assumed benefits of HFNC are realized from maximum mucociliary clearance, reduced inflammatory reactions, inhibition of the bronchoconstrictor reflex, reduced airway resistance, and a variable degree of washout of the nasopharyngeal dead space, but the evidence for positive pressure delivery with HFNC is mixed and highly variable.[58] All forms of noninvasive respiratory support require adequate humidification to prevent drying of the mucus membranes.

Among the greatest challenges with use of NIV in infants and children are the interfaces and delivery devices. Patient interfaces and headgear have expanded and include a wider variety of total face masks, nasal masks, nasal pillows, and, most recently, cloth masks.[58] Clinicians should be mindful that despite improved masks patients may not tolerate the excessive flow associated with NIV. It may be necessary to consider both nonpharmacological and pharmacological interventions for anxiety management which could help to improve adherence.[57] The facial areas will need close monitoring for skin breakdown and pressure ulcers. A pulse oximeter and a cardiac monitor are recommended for all forms of oxygen. Close monitoring of oxygen saturations will be needed, but this may change as the child nears death. Transition toward end of life may indicate another discussion point where clinician and family will need to decide if NIV is helpful or if it is causing discomfort. Loving families may decide to continue this intervention while others may decide to stop it.

Recent evidence advocating for less invasive ventilation has been a catalyst to increase the study and use of CPAP in infants and pediatric patients. CPAP refers to the administration of continuous positive airway pressure during all phases of the respiratory cycle of a spontaneously breathing patient. CPAP is used in patients with hypoxemia related to alveolar collapse or symptoms of obstructive sleep apnea or upper airway collapse.[57] In the case of a patient with a viral illness in which the patient needs a limited period for recovery, CPAP or another source of NIV may be appropriate, although not without discomfort from a tight-fitting mask that may be difficult to wear if patient has claustrophobia. The goal of CPAP is to restore adequate functional residual capacity to correct, reverse, or minimize alveolar collapse and reduce the work of breathing because it unloads the work of the inspiratory muscles and allows effective inflation in excess of the opening pressures of the lungs.[58] The level of CPAP required to accomplish this goal will vary depending on the child and the disease process. Infants typically require 5–8 cm of water (cm H_2O), but disorders associated with low lung compliance may require CPAP levels in excess of 10 cm H_2O.[57] Pressure-constant delivery devices are preferred to provide constant pressure and prevent alveolar collapse. When adequate CPAP levels are achieved, the work of breathing improves, and oxygen saturations increase. Weaning from CPAP should start once the disease process is identified and improving. CPAP can also be used nocturnally for the treatment of obstructive sleep apnea.[56,58] Weaning from CPAP typically involves transition to HFNC or nasal cannula.

BIPAP is a form of noninvasive positive pressure ventilation that allows unrestricted spontaneous breathing at any moment of the ventilatory cycle. Depending on spontaneous breathing activity, it can be subdivided into no spontaneous breathing continuous (CMV)-BIPAP or spontaneous breathing at a lower pressure level intermittent (IMV)-BIPAP.[60] It is often used in the treatment of lung disease and respiratory weakness. It provides both inspiratory and expiratory pressure. It is commonly used in pediatrics for the treatment of impending respiratory failure, acute or chronic respiratory insufficiency secondary to pulmonary disease, neuromuscular disease, airway obstruction, infectious process, or post-extubation management to avoid intubation or reintubation.[54]

Over the past 20 years the use of NIV has led to a 5- to 15-fold increase in the use of mechanical ventilation worldwide. The worldwide prevalence ranges from 2.1 to 13.7/100,000 in children.[61–69] NIV is considered the standard of care for a range of medical conditions which lead to sleep-disordered breathing and chronic respiratory insufficiency or failure, with a greater proportion of those starting on home mechanical ventilation surviving to adulthood.[62,70]

Many children who require NIV are medically complex. This includes children with chronic conditions that affect multiple body systems or progressive conditions associated with deteriorating health with limitations on life expectancy and dependence on technology.[71] Caregiving for this cohort of children is indeed challenging. Caregivers often reported sleep deprivation and financial and social hardships.[72]

INVASIVE VENTILATION

INTUBATION

If NIV becomes ineffective or intolerable, then the next step is endotracheal intubation. Intubation can provide stability for the patient who is experiencing respiratory distress and offer recovery while other interventions are used to maximize respiratory status.[73] This intervention requires thoughtful consideration and discussion as endotracheal intubation and mechanical ventilation can be damaging to the lungs. Will this intubation allow time to rest and heal, for the child to return to baseline? Intubation can also make interaction and meaningful time with family difficult because of the need for sedation to allow tolerance of the endotracheal tube. Frequent conversations should occur between the medical team and family. The patient's and family's goals should be at the forefront of conversations. In the case of progressive disease, it is likely that even if the child recovers from this acute event they may need intubation again in the future. Therefore, it is an important conversation to have with the child's family. If intubation were to occur again and no recoverable condition is found, it may be reasonable to discuss a time-limited trial on the ventilator. Endotracheal intubation is not meant to be a long-term solution but it can be a bridge to another intervention like a tracheostomy. It will be important to discuss all options with the caregiver/family.[73]

TRACHEOSTOMY

The past decade has seen an increase in the number of tracheostomies performed in children. Children with tracheotomies represent a very complex cohort of patients with sustained reliance on the tracheostomy and related medical technology for long-term survival. While it is commonly performed in the adult population, it is less common in pediatrics because no consensus exists determining how long a child should remain endotracheally intubated.[74]

Tracheostomies have been increasingly performed in children with complex and chronic conditions, for management of upper airway obstruction, prolonged ventilation, abnormal ventilatory drive, and irreversible neuromuscular conditions.[75–79] More than 50% of children who receive a tracheostomy are under the age of 1 at the time of placement.[80] Decannulation rates in this population of children range from 28% to 51%, with the average time for tracheostomy remaining in place for 2 years.[81–87] Tracheostomy is performed more frequently in children with chronic conditions including those with neurological impairment, congenital heart and lung disease, upper airway anomalies (either congenital or acquired secondary to prolonged intubation), or with a need for prolonged ventilation secondary to respiratory failure.[76] While tracheostomies provide life-saving options for some children, it is not without difficulties. Once the child progresses past the possible complications of pneumothorax, pneumomediastinum, hemorrhage, tissue injury, and pulmonary edema, accidental decannulation and mucus plugging can remain ongoing challenges for the child and family.[74] For children who have chronic ventilator dependence who are preparing for discharge from acute care to the community, challenges exist as there are no clinical practice guidelines available to healthcare professionals to ensure a safe hospital discharge and community management.[88] Despite the mandate for national action by the Institute of Medicine in 2003 for children with special healthcare needs, there are no evidence-based guidelines for this complex subgroup of technology-dependent children.[89] Current recommendations for hospital discharge include an awake, trained caregiver present at all times and at least two trained family caregivers specifically for the child's care because a single caregiver will rarely be able to shoulder the burden of care. Standardized equipment for monitoring, emergency preparedness, and airway clearance also must be a part of the discharge plan. These children often have several specialists involved in their care and benefit from having a medical home. The American Thoracic Society recommends a comprehensive medical home co-managed by the generalist and respiratory subspecialist. While care for this group of children may seem challenging for practitioners, families and patients see the benefits of care in the home setting.[88] Although care at home can be beneficial, it also has many challenges. Children often qualify for home health nursing, which allows families to work, care for other children, and allow time to coordinate care for the child. However, availability of nursing care can be limited, especially in rural communities. This shortage often leaves families providing around the clock care themselves, which leads to fatigue and financial hardship (Figure 24.1).

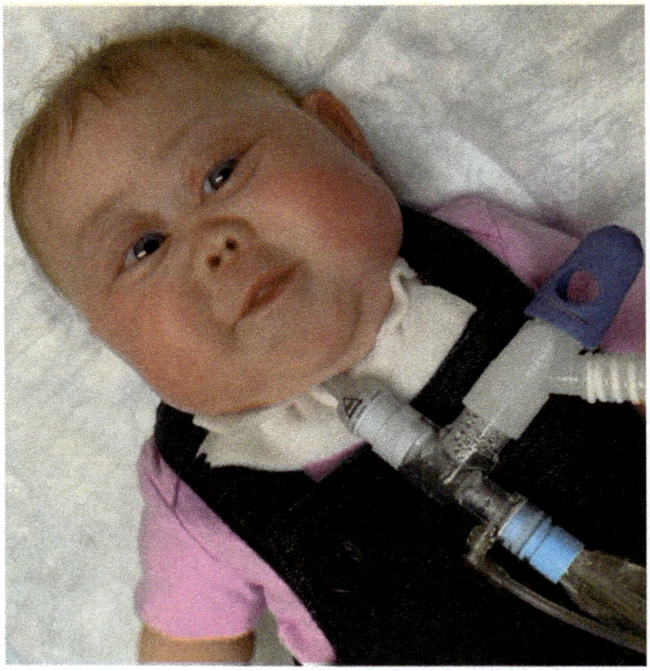

Figure 24.1 Parenting a child with holoprosencephaly and a tracheostomy.

Family Reflection

Parenting a Child with Holoprosencephaly and a Tracheostomy: A Parental Perspective

My daughter was diagnosed with semi-lobar holoprosencephaly, a condition in which the forebrain fails to divide. When she was born, my daughter struggled with breathing on her own, thus resulting in assistance from the vent hood and trumpet. When these options failed her, tracheostomy seemed to be our last resort a month and a half later. We were devastated by the idea of needing a tracheostomy. My husband and I were pained by the thought that we may never hear our daughter's voice or cry. It was a very depressing thing for us to consider. However, we couldn't bear the thought of anything bad happening to our child in the time that it would take for us to decide what would be best. After a fair amount of research and weighing the pros and cons, we reached the conclusion that the tracheostomy would be the best option for our baby girl. After the surgery, we immediately noticed drastic changes in her personality. She looked happier and healthier. While everything seemed better after the surgery, I believe the decision would have been much easier to make had the subject been presented to us as a more positive thing, as something that we shouldn't dread. Learning to care for a baby with a tracheostomy was scary in the beginning. Nevertheless, after education from the respiratory therapists and nurses along with some hands-on experience, it no longer seemed intimidating. By the time I reached my third trach change, I had grown confident. It was a task that needed to be done quick, clean, and correct. My partner and I felt more comfortable knowing that we could be completely hands-on. We knew that if anything should go wrong, we had a team of people who would step in and work alongside us to fix the situation. We appreciated the involvement of the palliative care team as they helped us to determine our goals, validated our concerns, and helped us frame our questions. I wish we could have walked into the situation more open-minded and aware a tracheostomy could be beneficial to her, rather than taking something away from her. I wish I had understood that I wasn't being selfish; I was paving the way for a healthy and happy little girl.

SPECIAL CONSIDERATIONS IN INFANTS WITH RESPIRATORY SYMPTOMS

There were 22,341 infant deaths in the United States in 2017, or 579.3 deaths per 100,000, with the majority of deaths due to congenital malformations (21% or 119.2 deaths per 100,000).[90–92] Greater technological advances in prenatal screening and diagnostic testing has led to an increased detection of congenital anomalies early in pregnancy and contributed to changes in parental and providers' attitudes. For instance, infants with trisomy 13 (Patau syndrome) or 18 (Edwards syndrome) have conditions associated with high early mortality and severe cognitive impairment, but some families and providers are opting for life-sustaining interventions.[93] Increased survival beyond the first year of life and even decades has been reported in infants with Trisomy 13 or 18 who undergo surgical interventions. However, overall mortality remains high, and surgeries are often considered only in carefully selected infants, when it is in line with goals of care to allow for a better quality of life and possible discharge home.[94–96] This shift in parental and providers' attitudes has been associated with longer neonatal ICU (NICU) stays and increased use of medical technology allowing children with previously considered "fatal" illnesses to live longer and highlighting the need for increased involvement of palliative and hospice care teams for symptom management, goals of care, and family and provider support.[4,97,98]

Infants requiring respiratory support at home are particularly complicated to discharge as the equipment is not always available in the same format in the community as it is in the hospital. For example, it may be challenging to provide HFNC with appropriate prong sizes and blenders to titrate oxygen levels; thus, the infant should transition to the respiratory format that will be available in the community before discharge. Finding equipment that will fit the infant's face may also present challenge if the child weighs less than 2.5 kilograms. Consultation with the outpatient respiratory therapist is ideal prior to discharge home. Other barriers that infants may encounter are local hospice providers and pediatricians who may not be comfortable with end-of-life symptom management for small infants. Pediatric palliative care teams can provide guidance for symptom management to assist the local medical team with keeping the infant and family at home if this is in line with the family's goals.

ADVANCE CARE PLANNING

A significant burden of respiratory symptoms often heralds the realization that a child is seriously ill. However, the technical and medical supports available to ease breathing can mask the gravity of the situation. It is not uncommon for caregivers of chronically ill children to focus on how the patient is being ventilated when the child becomes more ill. At these times, the underlying disease and its potential for worsening may seem less obvious to parents than the limitations of the mechanical ventilation. Often, there is an element of shock when children with chronic illness and profound respiratory compromise succumb to their disease. DeCourcey and colleagues identify early conversations "whereby patients, their families, and their healthcare providers reflect on patient and family goals and discuss how these should inform medical care, ideally after an exploration of their needs, values, strengths, hopes, and worries" as critical.[99] These conversations, also known as pediatric advance care planning (pACP), are the gold standard for serious illness care.

Clinicians may feel apprehensive about conversations with families whose child is experiencing respiratory decompensation and who are considering increased respiratory support. These conversations should begin with an understanding of the family's goals for their child. Escalating respiratory support will likely sustain life but may increase suffering, both in terms of the intervention itself as well as the quality of life it prolongs for the child.[73] It is important for providers to have open, honest communication with patients and families regarding known disease progression. However, it is not always possible to accurately predict how long children with life-limiting conditions will live or what dying may be like for them. It will be important to understand how the patient/family defines suffering. These conversations may take place over a short period of time or even years depending on the child's condition. Families may choose to maximize nutrition, physical therapy, and take active steps to prevent respiratory infections and manage secretions with suctioning and cough assist.[100] Respiratory decline may be temporarily postponed, but it is difficult to prevent. If decline occurs, NIV can be used in infants and children with acute and chronic conditions associated with impaired respiratory drive, inadequate lung inflation, and altered gas exchange resulting in respiratory insufficiency or failure.[57] However, there should be open dialogue with patient and family regarding how much respiratory support will be acceptable for them.

During these pACP conversations, parents are often given choices for their children that they feel unprepared to make. Decisions regarding placement of a tracheostomy can be life-changing for both the child and family. It may alter who serves as primary caregiver for the patient, the parents' ability to work, and the family's ability to continue their current lifestyle. The discussion with families should include important physiological explanations including why the child is not able to breathe on their own as well as the fact that the child will lack the ability to vocalize initially and, at times, long-term; thus caregivers will not be able to hear their child cry or speak. This can be quite distressing for families. However, depending on the child's physiology it is possible that work with speech therapy and a speaking valve may make speech possible. A tracheostomy allows families to see their child's entire face, sometimes for the first time in months as it may have been previously covered with tape to keep the endotracheal tube in place or a face mask or nasal cannula from NIV. Having the face free allows for improved comfort, social interaction, and more freedom to pursue therapies.

While the medical team does its best to prepare parents to make decisions that are in alignment with the child and family's goals of care, it is often difficult to realize the caregiver commitments until the family is at home. There are several online sites that can provide parents with information about tracheostomies, often from parents who have had to make the same difficult decision. The Courageous Parents Network is an excellent resource that provides guidance for providers and parents, videos of parents who decided that a tracheostomy was the right choice for them, and videos from families that decided to forgo tracheostomy. The child tracheostomy decision guide provides helpful information that can help guide discussions with providers. The web address is https://courageousparentsnetwork.org/guides/child-tracheostomy-decision-guide.[101] There are various guides that can be found on tracheostomy care, but guidance and care of the child's tracheostomy should originate from the institution that will be providing ongoing care for the child and family.

Although decisions about interventions to manage respiratory compromise are often made by parents, pediatric patients' preferences regarding advance care planning are receiving increasing attention in research and practice. Both providers and parents may be concerned about including a pediatric patient in advance care planning for fear of stripping the patient of hope or overwhelming them with information.[102] Nonetheless, the benefits of including pediatric patients in conversations about diagnosis, treatment, and prognosis have been well-documented.[103,104] It is critical to utilize developmentally appropriate tools and be sensitive to emotions that may surface including fear, guilty, anger, denial, and surprise. A variety of developmentally appropriate discussion guides are available to facilitate patient involvement in decisions (see Table 24.4). These guides address topics including mechanical ventilation, strategies for providing comfort in face of changing or limited treatment options, and preparation for end of life.

ABNORMAL BREATHING PATTERNS AT THE END OF LIFE

As death draws nearer, there will be noticeable changes in the child's breathing. The respiratory rate may transition from normal to a series of rapid breaths followed by no breathing at all (apnea). This event is referred to as *Cheyne-Stokes breathing*.[5] This can happen for an extended period of time (sometimes weeks) before death occurs. The patient's mouth may become dry during this period; moistening the mouth with wet

TABLE 24.4 Advance care planning resources

RESOURCE	DESCRIPTION
My Wishes	A discussion guide for children regarding serious illness care. Available in Spanish.
Voicing My Choices	A discussion guide for adolescents and young adults regarding serious illness care. Available in Spanish.
Courageous Parents Network	An online portal of resources for parents making decisions regarding serious illness care. Includes videos, decision guides, and information sheets.
Child Tracheostomy Decision Guide	A decision guide for caregivers considering tracheostomy for their child.
Seattle Children's Decision-Making Tool	A discussion guide for healthcare providers and families faced with complex medical decisions.

sponges or ice chips as tolerated may provide comfort. There may be times when breathing becomes shallower and more labored. This may be worsened if the patient is feeling anxious. A loved one's presence, a calm environment, music, or integrative therapies may be helpful. If anxiety persists, an anxiolytic may be helpful. It will be important to counsel families about changing respiratory patterns near the end of life as apnea can continue for an extended period of time, giving the impression that death has occurred; then the patient resumes breathing, and this can be anxiety-producing for family.

Patients may develop noisy breathing as a result of the movement of secretions in an uncontrolled airway secondary to neurologic deterioration as they lose consciousness prior to death. Use of the term "death rattle" should be discouraged as this is distressing to caregivers and families. Positioning the patient on their side or elevating the head of the bed can be helpful.[5] An adult study suggested that a higher amount of fluid intake before death may be associated with terminal restlessness during the last 24 hours of life and concluded that providing dying patients with artificial fluid may not be beneficial.[105] It is also appropriate to assess the benefit of artificial nutrition and hydration, as this may be contributing to the development of terminal secretions. Pharmacologic intervention with anticholinergic agents can reduce saliva and bronchial mucous, which can reduce the intensity of secretions.[106] While there is no evidence that secretions cause discomfort for the patient, the sounds associated with this condition can be extremely distressing for caregivers. Anticipatory guidance and reassurance that this condition is not causing pain is very helpful for both providers and loved ones.

CONCLUSION

Clinicians are often anxious about having difficult discussions with families about their child's declining respiratory status and whether escalating respiratory support is the right next step for their child. These conversations should begin with an understanding of the patient's and family's goals. It should also include discussion of managing respiratory symptoms through nonpharmacologic techniques, use of technology, and medication management, which are guided by the goals of the patient and family. These are not one-time conversations. In some cases, these conversations may occur over many years. It may be necessary to adjust the goals depending on the disease progression. The interdisciplinary team approach is invaluable to patients and families as they determine goals at each decision-making point. Advance care planning using available tools may be helpful to the child and family to empower them to prioritize what is important to them. These important discussions may prevent them from having to make critical decisions "in the moment" when escalating respiratory support may sustain life but also may increase suffering and prolong the inevitable.[73]

ACKNOWLEDGMENTS

We would like to thank David J. Casarett, MD, MA, Chief of Palliative Care, Professor of Medicine, Duke University and Health System, for his review of this manuscript.

REFERENCES

1. Brinkman JE, Sharma S. Physiology, respiratory drive. StatPearls. 2019. https://www.ncbi.nlm.nih.gov/books/NBK482414/. Updated May 9, 2021.
2. McConnell A. *Respiratory Muscle Training*. Churchill Livingstone; 2013.
3. Ray A. *Meditation: Insights and Inspirations*. Inner Light Publishers 2010.
4. Rapoport A, Shaheed J, Newman C, Rugg M, Steele R. Parental perceptions of forgoing artificial nutrition and hydration during end-of-life care. *Pediatrics*. 2013;131(5):861–869.
5. Lamers W. Signs of approaching death. 2017. https://hospicefoundation.org/Hospice-Care/Signs-of-Approaching-Death
6. Martel Y. *Life of Pi*. Harcourt; 2001.
7. Dyspnea. Mechanisms, assessment, and management: A consensus statement. American Thoracic Society. *Am J Respir Crit Care Med*. 1999;159(1):321–340.
8. Pieper L, Zernikow B, Drake R, Frosch M, Printz M, Wager J. Dyspnea in children with life-threatening and life-limiting complex chronic conditions. *J Palliat Med*. 2018;21(4):552–564.
9. Blume ED, Balkin EM, Aiyagari R, et al. Parental perspectives on suffering and quality of life at end-of-life in children with advanced heart disease: An exploratory study. *Pediatr Crit Care Med*. 2014;15(4):336–342.
10. Wolfe J, Grier HE, Klar N, et al. Symptoms and suffering at the end of life in children with cancer. *N Engl J Med*. 2000;342(5):326–333.
11. Houlahan KE, Branowicki PA, Mack JW, Dinning C, McCabe M. Can end of life care for the pediatric patient suffering with escalating and intractable symptoms be improved? *J Pediatr Oncol Nurs*. 2006;23(1):45–51.
12. Robinson WM. Palliation of dyspnea in pediatrics *Chron Respir Dis*. 2012;9(4):251–256.
13. Schweitzer C, Marchal F. Dyspnoea in children. Does development alter the perception of breathlessness? *Respir Physiol Neurobiol*. 2009;167(1):144–153.

14. Kamal AH, Maguire JM, Wheeler JL, Currow DC, Abernethy AP. Dyspnea review for the palliative care professional: Treatment goals and therapeutic options. *J Palliat Med.* 2012;15(1):106–114.
15. Bausewein C, Booth S, Gysels M, Higginson I. Non-pharmacological interventions for breathlessness in advanced stages of malignant and non-malignant diseases. *Cochrane Database Syst Rev.* 2008(2):CD005623.
16. Anbar RD. Self-hypnosis for management of chronic dyspnea in pediatric patients. *Pediatrics.* 2001;107(2):E21.
17. Barnes H, McDonald J, Smallwood N, Manser R. Opioids for the palliation of refractory breathlessness in adults with advanced disease and terminal illness. *Cochrane Database Syst Rev.* 2016;3:CD011008.
18. Currow DC, Ekstrom M, Abernethy AP. Opioids for chronic refractory breathlessness: Right patient, right route? *Drugs.* 2014;74(1):1–6.
19. Pieper L, Wager J, Zernikow B. Intranasal fentanyl for respiratory distress in children and adolescents with life-limiting conditions. *BMC Palliat Care.* 2018;17(1):106.
20. Simon ST, Higginson IJ, Booth S, Harding R, Weingartner V, Bausewein C. Benzodiazepines for the relief of breathlessness in advanced malignant and non-malignant diseases in adults. *Cochrane Database Syst Rev.* 2016;10:CD007354.
21. Association of Child Life Professionals. The case for child life. Association of Child Life Professionals. 2018. https://www.childlife.org/the-child-life-profession/the-case-for-child-life.
22. Lowry G. *Following Imagination: Activities That Move Create and Play with Guided Imagery.* Practical Parenting Solutions; 2010.
23. Abou-Assi E. 9 free and helpful apps for children with anxiety. https://www.myautism.org/9-free-helpful-apps-children-anxiety/#. 2017.
24. Hofmann SG, Wu JQ, Boettcher H. Effect of cognitive-behavioral therapy for anxiety disorders on quality of life: A meta-analysis. *J Consult Clin Psychol.* 2014;82(3):375–391.
25. Chamberlain SA, Garrod R, Douiri A, et al. The impact of chronic cough: A cross-sectional European survey. *Lung.* 2015;193(3):401–408.
26. Bonvini SJ, Birrell MA, Smith JA, Belvisi MG. Targeting TRP channels for chronic cough: From bench to bedside. *Naunyn Schmiedebergs Arch Pharmacol.* 2015;388(4):401–420.
27. Canning BJ. Central regulation of the cough reflex: Therapeutic implications. *Pulm Pharmacol Ther.* 2009;22(2):75–81.
28. Vertigan AE, Gibson PG. The role of speech pathology in the management of patients with chronic refractory cough. *Lung.* 2012;190(1):35–40.
29. Vertigan AE, Kapela SL, Ryan NM, Birring SS, McElduff P, Gibson PG. Pregabalin and speech pathology combination therapy for refractory chronic cough: A randomized controlled trial. *Chest.* 2016;149(3):639–648.
30. Paul IM, Beiler J, McMonagle A, Shaffer ML, Duda L, Berlin CM, Jr. Effect of honey, dextromethorphan, and no treatment on nocturnal cough and sleep quality for coughing children and their parents. *Arch Pediatr Adolesc Med.* 2007;161(12):1140–1146.
31. Wee B, Hillier R. Interventions for noisy breathing in patients near to death. *Cochrane Database Syst Rev.* 2008(1):CD005177.
32. Montgomery J, McCusker S, Lang K, et al. Managing children with sialorrhoea (drooling): Experience from the first 301 children in our saliva control clinic. *Int J Pediatr Otorhinolaryngol.* 2016;85:33–39.
33. Khan WU, Campisi P, Nadarajah S, et al. Botulinum toxin A for treatment of sialorrhea in children: An effective, minimally invasive approach. *Arch Otolaryngol Head Neck Surg.* 2011;137(4):339–344.
34. Elbahlawan L, Rains KJ, Stokes DC. Respiratory care considerations in the childhood cancer patient. *Respir Care.* 2017;62(6):765–775.
35. Klein OR, Cooke KR. Idiopathic pneumonia syndrome following hematopoietic stem cell transplantation. *J Pediatr Intensive Care.* 2014;3(3):147–157.
36. Heggen J, West C, Olson E, et al. Diffuse alveolar hemorrhage in pediatric hematopoietic cell transplant patients. *Pediatrics.* 2002 109(5) 965–971.
37. Elbahlawan L, Srinivasan A, Morrison RR. A critical care and transplantation-based approach to acute respiratory failure after hematopoietic stem cell transplantation in children. *Biol Blood Marrow Transplant.* 2016;22(4):617–626.
38. Bidet G, Daoust L, Duval M, et al. An order protocol for respiratory distress/acute pain crisis in pediatric palliative care patients: Medical and nursing staff perceptions. *J Palliat Med.* 2016;19(3):306–313.
39. Navigante AH, Cerchietti LC, Castro MA, Lutteral MA, Cabalar ME. Midazolam as adjunct therapy to morphine in the alleviation of severe dyspnea perception in patients with advanced cancer. *J Pain Symptom Manage.* 2006;31(1):38–47.
40. Epelbaum O, Rahman NM. Contemporary approach to the patient with malignant pleural effusion complicating lung cancer. *Ann Transl Med.* 2019;7(15):352.
41. Desai NR, Lee HJ. Diagnosis and management of malignant pleural effusions: State of the art in 2017. *J Thorac Dis.* 2017;9(Suppl 10): S1111–S1122.
42. Tremblay A, Michaud G. Single-center experience with 250 tunnelled pleural catheter insertions for malignant pleural effusion. *Chest.* 2006;129(2):362–368.
43. D'Amico A, Mercuri E, Tiziano FD, Bertini E. Spinal muscular atrophy. *Orphanet J Rare Dis.* 2011;6:71.
44. Mercuri E, Finkel RS, Muntoni F, et al. Diagnosis and management of spinal muscular atrophy: Part 1: Recommendations for diagnosis, rehabilitation, orthopedic and nutritional care. *Neuromuscul Disord.* 2018;28(2):103–115.
45. Arnold WD, Kassar D, Kissel JT. Spinal muscular atrophy: Diagnosis and management in a new therapeutic era. *Muscle Nerve.* 2015;51(2):157–167.
46. Tisdale S, Pellizzoni L. Disease mechanisms and therapeutic approaches in spinal muscular atrophy. *J Neurosci.* 2015;35(23):8691–8700.
47. Neil EE, Bisaccia EK. Nusinersen: A novel antisense oligonucleotide for the treatment of spinal muscular atrophy. *J Pediatr Pharmacol Ther.* 2019;24(3):194–203.
48. Michelson D, Ciafaloni E, Ashwal S, et al. Evidence in focus: Nusinersen use in spinal muscular atrophy: Report of the Guideline Development, Dissemination, and Implementation Subcommittee of the American Academy of Neurology. *Neurology.* 2018;91(20):923–933.
49. Sansone VA, Pirola A, Albamonte E, et al. Respiratory needs in patients with Type 1 spinal muscular atrophy treated with Nusinersen. *J Pediatr.* 2020 Apr; 219:223–228e4. doi:10.1016/j.jpeds.2019.12.047
50. Bushby K, Finkel R, Birnkrant DJ, et al. Diagnosis and management of Duchenne muscular dystrophy, part 1: Diagnosis, and pharmacological and psychosocial management. *Lancet Neurol.* 2010;9(1):77–93.
51. National Institute of Health. Duchenne muscular dystrophy. Genetic and Rare Disease Information Center. 2017. https://rarediseases.info.nih.gov/diseases/6291/duchenne-muscular-dystrophy
52. Bushby K, Finkel R, Birnkrant DJ, et al. Diagnosis and management of Duchenne muscular dystrophy, part 2: Implementation of multidisciplinary care. *Lancet Neurol.* 2010;9(2):177–189.
53. Mah JK. Current and emerging treatment strategies for Duchenne muscular dystrophy. *Neuropsychiatr Dis Treat.* 2016;12:1795–1807.
54. Basnet S, Mander G, Andoh J, Klaska H, Verhulst S, Koirala J. Safety, efficacy, and tolerability of early initiation of noninvasive positive pressure ventilation in pediatric patients admitted with status asthmaticus: A pilot study. *Pediatr Crit Care Med.* 2012;13(4):393–398.
55. de Miguel-Diez J, Jimenez-Garcia R, Hernandez-Barrera V, et al. National trends in hospital admissions for asthma exacerbations among pediatric and young adult population in Spain (2002–2010). *Respir Med.* 2014;108(7):983–991.
56. Teague GW, Thompson-Batt D. Non-invasive mechanical ventilation of the infant and children. In Walsh BK, ed. *Neonatal and Pediatric Respiratory Care.* 4th ed. Elsevier; 2015:287–299.
57. Fedor KL. Noninvasive respiratory support in infants and children. *Respir Care.* 2017;62(6):699–717.
58. Loh LE, Chan YH, Chan I. Noninvasive ventilation in children: A review. *J Pediatr (Rio J).* 2007;83(2 Suppl):S91–99.
59. Mayfield S, Jauncey-Cooke J, Hough JL, Schibler A, Gibbons K, Bogossian F. High-flow nasal cannula therapy for respiratory support in children. *Cochrane Database Syst Rev.* 2014(3):CD009850.

60. Hormann C, Baum M, Putensen C, Mutz NJ, Benzer H. Biphasic positive airway pressure (BIPAP)--a new mode of ventilatory support. *Eur J Anaesthesiol.* 1994;11(1):37–42.
61. Amin R, Sayal P, Syed F, Chaves A, Moraes TJ, MacLusky I. Pediatric long-term home mechanical ventilation: Twenty years of follow-up from one Canadian center. *Pediatr Pulmonol.* 2014;49(8):816–824.
62. Chatwin M, Tan HL, Bush A, Rosenthal M, Simonds AK. Long term non-invasive ventilation in children: Impact on survival and transition to adult care. *PLoS One.* 2015;10(5):e0125839.
63. Edwards EA, Hsiao K, Nixon GM. Paediatric home ventilatory support: The Auckland experience. *J Paediatr Child Health.* 2005;41(12):652–658.
64. Gonzalez Cortes R, Bustinza Arriortua A, Pons Odena M, et al. [Domiciliary mechanical ventilation in children: A Spanish multicentre study]. *An Pediatr (Barc).* 2013;78(4):227–233.
65. Goodwin S, Smith H, Langton Hewer S, et al. Increasing prevalence of domiciliary ventilation: Changes in service demand and provision in the South West of the UK. *Eur J Pediatr.* 2011;170(9):1187–1192.
66. McDougall CM, Adderley RJ, Wensley DF, Seear MD. Long-term ventilation in children: Longitudinal trends and outcomes. *Arch Dis Child.* 2013;98(9):660–665.
67. Nathan AM, Loo HY, de Bruyne JA, et al. Thirteen years of invasive and noninvasive home ventilation for children in a developing country: A retrospective study. *Pediatr Pulmonol.* 2017;52(4):500–507.
68. Sovtic A, Minic P, Vukcevic M, Markovic-Sovtic G, Rodic M, Gajic M. Home mechanical ventilation in children is feasible in developing countries. *Pediatr Int.* 2012;54(5):676–681.
69. Wallis C, Paton JY, Beaton S, Jardine E. Children on long-term ventilatory support: 10 years of progress. *Arch Dis Child.* 2011;96(11):998–1002.
70. Castro-Codesal ML, Dehaan K, Featherstone R, et al. Long-term non-invasive ventilation therapies in children: A scoping review. *Sleep Med Rev.* 2018;37:148–158.
71. Cohen E, Kuo DZ, Agrawal R, et al. Children with medical complexity: An emerging population for clinical and research initiatives. *Pediatrics.* 2011;127(3):529–538.
72. Thomson J, Shah SS, Simmons JM, et al. Financial and social hardships in families of children with medical complexity. *J Pediatr.* 2016;172:187–193 e181.
73. Macauley R. To trach or not to trach, that is the question. *Paediatr Respir Rev.* 2019;29:9–13.
74. Watters KF. Tracheostomy in infants and children. *Respir Care.* 2017;62(6):799–825.
75. Arcand P, Granger J. Pediatric tracheostomies: Changing trends. *J Otolaryngol.* 1988;17(2):121–124.
76. Berry JG, Graham RJ, Roberson DW, et al. Patient characteristics associated with in-hospital mortality in children following tracheotomy. *Arch Dis Child.* 2010;95(9):703–710.
77. Goldenberg D, Ari EG, Golz A, Danino J, Netzer A, Joachims HZ. Tracheotomy complications: A retrospective study of 1130 cases. *Otolaryngol Head Neck Surg.* 2000;123(4):495–500.
78. Graf JM, Montagnino BA, Hueckel R, McPherson ML. Pediatric tracheostomies: A recent experience from one academic center. *Pediatr Crit Care Med.* 2008;9(1):96–100.
79. Liu C, Heffernan C, Saluja S, et al. Indications, hospital course, and complexity of patients undergoing tracheostomy at a tertiary care pediatric hospital. *Otolaryngol Head Neck Surg.* 2014;151(2):232–239.
80. Berry JG, Graham DA, Graham RJ, et al. Predictors of clinical outcomes and hospital resource use of children after tracheotomy. *Pediatrics.* 2009;124(2):563–572.
81. Carron JD, Derkay CS, Strope GL, Nosonchuk JE, Darrow DH. Pediatric tracheotomies: Changing indications and outcomes. *Laryngoscope.* 2000;110(7):1099–1104.
82. de Trey L, Niedermann E, Ghelfi D, Gerber A, Gysin C. Pediatric tracheotomy: A 30-year experience. *J Pediatr Surg.* 2013;48(7):1470–1475.
83. French LC, Wootten CT, Thomas RG, Neblett WW, 3rd, Werkhaven JA, Cofer SA. Tracheotomy in the preschool population: Indications and outcomes. *Otolaryngol Head Neck Surg.* 2007;137(2): 280–283.
84. Leung R, Berkowitz RG. Decannulation and outcome following pediatric tracheostomy. *Ann Otol Rhinol Laryngol.* 2005;114(10): 743–748.
85. Mahadevan M, Barber C, Salkeld L, Douglas G, Mills N. Pediatric tracheotomy: 17-year review. *Int J Pediatr Otorhinolaryngol.* 2007;71(12):1829–1835.
86. Ozmen S, Ozmen OA, Unal OF. Pediatric tracheotomies: A 37-year experience in 282 children. *Int J Pediatr Otorhinolaryngol.* 2009;73(7):959–961.
87. Tantinikorn W, Alper CM, Bluestone CD, Casselbrant ML. Outcome in pediatric tracheotomy. *Am J Otolaryngol.* 2003;24(3): 131–137.
88. Sterni LM, Collaco JM, Baker CD, et al. An official American Thoracic Society Clinical practice guideline: Pediatric chronic home invasive ventilation. *Am J Respir Crit Care Med.* 2016;193(8):e16–35.
89. Institute of Medicine. *Priority Areas for National Action: Transforming Health Care Quality*. National Academies Press; 2003.
90. Ely DM DA. Infant mortality in the United States, 2017: Data from the period linked birth/infant death file. National Center for Health Statistics. National Vital Statistics Report web site. 2019. https://www.cdc.gov/nchs/data/nvsr/nvsr68/nvsr68_10-508.pdf
91. Garten L, Ohlig S, Metze B, Buhrer C. Prevalence and characteristics of neonatal comfort care patients: A single-center, 5-year, retrospective, observational study. *Front Pediatr.* 2018;6:221.
92. Hoell JI, Warfsmann J, Distelmaier F, Borkhardt A, Janssen G, Kuhlen M. Challenges of palliative care in children with inborn metabolic diseases. *Orphanet J Rare Dis.* 2018;13(1):112.
93. Carey JC. Attitudes of neonatologists toward delivery room management of confirmed trisomy 18: Potential factors influencing a changing dynamic. *Pediatrics.* 2009;123(3):e547–548 author reply e549.
94. Nelson KE, Rosella LC, Mahant S, Guttmann A. Survival and surgical interventions for children with trisomy 13 and 18 *JAMA.* 2016;316(4):420–428.
95. Peterson JK, Kochilas LK, Catton KG, Moller JH, Setty SP. Long-term outcomes of children with trisomy 13 and 18 after congenital heart disease interventions. *Ann Thorac Surg.* 2017;103(6):1941–1949.
96. Spierson H, Masood Y, Craigie RJ, Edi-Osagie N. Trisomy 18: Palliative surgical intervention. *Arch Dis Child.* 2018;103(10):1001.
97. Craig F, Mancini A. Can we truly offer a choice of place of death in neonatal palliative care? *Semin Fetal Neonatal Med.* 2013;18(2):93–98.
98. Pallotto I, Lantos JD. Treatment decisions for babies with trisomy 13 and 18. *HEC Forum.* 2017;29(3):213–222.
99. DeCourcey DD, Silverman M, Oladunjoye A, Wolfe J. Advance care planning and parent-reported end-of-life outcomes in children, adolescents, and young adults with complex chronic conditions. *Crit Care Med.* 2019;47(1):101–108.
100. Hawkins SM, Jensen EL, Simon SL, Friedman NR. Correlates of pediatric CPAP adherence. *J Clin Sleep Med.* 2016;12(6): 879–884.
101. Courageous Parents Network. Child tracheostomy decision guide. 2018. https://courageousparentsnetwork.org/guides/child-tracheostomy-decision-guide
102. Cousino MK, Schumacher KR, Magee JC, et al. Communication about prognosis and end-of-life in pediatric organ failure and transplantation. *Pediatr Transplant.* 2019;23(3):e13373.
103. Curtin KB, Watson AE, Wang J, Okonkwo OC, Lyon ME. Pediatric advance care planning (pACP) for teens with cancer and their families: Design of a dyadic, longitudinal RCCT. *Contemp Clin Trials.* 2017;62:121–129.
104. Wiener L, Zadeh S, Wexler LH, Pao M. When silence is not golden: Engaging adolescents and young adults in discussions around end-of-life care choices. *Pediatr Blood Cancer.* 2013;60(5):715–718.
105. Lokker ME, van der Heide A, Oldenmenger WH, van der Rijt CCD, van Zuylen L. Hydration and symptoms in the last days of life. *BMJ Support Palliat Care.* 2019.
106. Clark K, Butler M. Noisy respiratory secretions at the end of life. *Curr Opin Support Palliat Care.* 2009;3(2):120–124.

25 | GASTROINTESTINAL SYMPTOMS

KEVIN MADDEN AND MARGARET M. MAHON

Digestion, of all the bodily functions, is the one which exercises the greatest influence on the mental state of an individual.

JEAN-ANTHELME BRILLAT-SAVARIN

INTRODUCTION

Symptoms involving the gastrointestinal (GI) tract, including nausea, vomiting, diarrhea, and constipation are common throughout childhood and occur for a wide range of reasons in healthy children as well as in those with underlying diseases. When caring for a child in the context of serious illness, these symptoms may be of important clinical significance; thus, diagnosing their source and identifying a treatment strategy are critical. Approximately 1 in 10 children receiving specialty palliative care have a primary GI condition[1] while children with other primary life-limiting or life-threatening illnesses suffer from bothersome GI symptoms that are severe enough to warrant visits to the emergency department.[2] Anticipating such eventualities with the family can make even emergencies less stressful.

Parents or other caregivers are often the first to become aware of a child's symptoms, either through observation or through the child's disclosure. Parents and often the children themselves are the experts in how *this* disease, treatment, and side effect affect *this* child. Symptom burden is not just determined by the severity of a symptom, but also by the extent to which it interferes with a child's quality of life.[3,4] One of the hallmarks of pediatric palliative care is collaboration with families to anticipate and recognize the needs of the child and then help the family provide effective symptom relief. In this chapter, we describe the assessment and management of pediatric GI conditions that are likely to be seen by palliative care providers. The crux of this care is interdisciplinary, and different interventions may be initiated, either individually or in combination, along the trajectory of a child's illness.

Clinical Vignette

A 16-year-old girl with cystic fibrosis (CF) and advanced but stable lung disease was hospitalized with severe abdominal pain, nausea, and anorexia following viral gastroenteritis. There was an initial belief that she might have a partial bowel obstruction, but this was ruled out after multiple investigations failed to show any significant organic factors. She adamantly denied anxiety or depressive symptoms.

Her gastrointestinal symptoms did not improve with standard psychological and pharmacologic strategies, and her lung function began to deteriorate further secondary to weight loss and immobility. A meeting involving the teen, her parents, and the psychosocial team provided a forum for the child and her parents to discuss the young woman's condition and the family's understanding in the context of social supports and spiritual beliefs. The teen knew that she would likely die from her condition, though hoped not soon. The family had always known CF was a terminal diagnosis but hoped for decades more. It was distressing for all to realize that they likely did not have as much time as they hoped for. The family was able to speak openly about their fears and anxieties about death. The young woman realized that her symptoms represented a terminal illness and that her death might be sudden and unexpected. She made clear that she wanted to make sure that her family would be present, as she previously had been reluctant to discuss these matters with her parents, believing they would be disappointed in her.

These revelations opened the way for her primary pediatrician to later that week discuss the likely modes of death from CF and the expectation that her death was not imminent, given proper nutrition and mobilization. The pediatrician also promised to talk openly and honestly with her when her lung function declined to the point that her death was near. Within several days the young woman was eating well, mobilizing, communicating more openly with her family, and her pain levels were manageable. She lived with a good quality of life for an additional 14 months before dying at home with her family present.

SYMPTOMS OF THE MOUTH AND THROAT

MOUTH CARE

The care of a child's mouth is an essential element of a child's overall care and one in which an informed child and family can take a lead role. This can be associated with an improved quality of life, create a sense of control, and prevent mouth care from being overlooked. This aspect of palliative care for children has been well-documented[5] for children with cancer, with many of these recommendations also applicable to children with a life-limiting illness or life-threatening illness of nonmalignant origins.

Most problems are diagnosed with a good history and an examination of the mouth. Many oral assessment tools have been reviewed,[5] but only Eiler's Oral Assessment Guide[6] is user-friendly and appropriate for everyday clinical use in children and adults. This guide covers the assessment of voice, ability to swallow, lips, tongue, saliva, mucous membrane, gingival, and teeth or dentures.

Several possible conditions or symptoms may require management, including

- Poor oral hygiene
- Oral candidiasis
- Mouth ulceration, including mucositis
- Xerostomia, or dry mouth

TREATMENT: INTEGRATIVE AND SUPPORTIVE THERAPIES

The mainstay of preventing the development of mouth problems is the twice-daily routine of careful and gentle cleaning of the teeth and gums with a fluoride toothpaste.[5] This should apply to all cooperative children, including those with severe disabilities. In the unconscious or less cooperative child, mouth-care sponges dipped in mouthwash can be applied to the gums and teeth to keep the mouth moist. Cocoa butter, cream, or soft white paraffin can be applied to the lips to prevent dryness and cracking.

For children with a life-limiting illness or a life-threatening illness, a regular dental review and oral assessment by a dentist with specific experience and training in pediatrics, and often specializing in conditions such as cerebral palsy, autism, or cancer, should be a standard of care. Ongoing evaluation and management by a dental specialist is likely to vary across the trajectory of the child's condition. For children in the advanced stages of illness, routine dental appointments may not be as crucial.

XEROSTOMIA

Xerostomia, or dry mouth, is very common across the course of many serious illnesses. This symptom can cause significant distress at a level similar to pain. Dry mouth results from a reduction in saliva secretion, especially the serous component. This can lead to difficulties with eating and speaking, contribute to anorexia, cause an altered sense of taste (dysgeusia), and can increase the risk of oral infections.

AN APPROACH TO THE CHILD WITH XEROSTOMIA

Evaluation requires a review of the possible causes, including a thorough review of medications. The list of medications implicated with xerostomia is large, but anticholinergics, tricyclic antidepressants, antipsychotics, anticonvulsants, antihistamines, and diuretics are the most common causes. It is imperative to inquire whether the parents are administering any alternative, homeopathic, or complementary therapies.

TREATMENT

Specific etiologies should be managed in the context of the child's current health status and goals of care. For example, if xerostomia is due to a medication, everything from dose reduction to rotating to a similar medication in the same class without the particular side effect to discontinuing the offending class of medications altogether should be considered. In the case of dehydration, the underlying reason could be corrected and the oral fluid intake of the child increased, if consistent with the goals of care. Similarly, the use of subcutaneous and intravenous fluid administration could be considered if aligned with the overall goals of care of the child and the family. The prevalence of xerostomia in the last week of life is about 40%[7]; it can be managed with artificial saliva, although anecdotally many children find the taste and consistency of artificial saliva to be more bothersome than the sensation that accompanies xerostomia.

DYSPHAGIA

Dysphagia is difficulty swallowing, in contrast to odynophagia, which is painful swallowing. These conditions might occur independently or together and can occur in children who are relatively well. While seemingly simple, swallowing is a complex, highly coordinated process that begins in the cerebrum and ends with the coordination of the oral, pharyngeal, and esophageal musculature. Dysphagia can occur when the nerves along the pathway do not function properly. This may be caused by a variety of conditions: hypoxic-ischemic encephalopathy, metabolic disorders, medications, pain, and deconditioning of the musculature from lack of use over a sustained period are all common etiologies. Many parents of children who suffer from dysphagia benefit from education about how deceptively complicated this process is, as, for most of us, swallowing is a subconscious process.

AN APPROACH TO THE CHILD WITH DYSPHAGIA

Dysphagia can occur due to progression of underlying disease process, treatment of the underlying disease, surgical interventions, radiotherapy, chemotherapy, and medications. For example, damage to the brain and central nervous system (CNS) from cerebral palsy, neurodegenerative disorders, metabolic disorders, brain tumors, or congenital and genetic disorders can impair the ability to swallow normally and safely. Structural problems secondary to obstruction or infiltration or compression from solid tumors of the head and neck can disrupt the normal swallowing process. The progressive weakening and deconditioning of skeletal muscle from muscular dystrophy (MD) can make it challenging for these children to swallow. And perhaps the overall most common cause of dysphagia in children is actually a secondary dysphagia that stems from significant pain due to the treatment of cancer from radiation or chemotherapy.

The overall prevalence of dysphagia in children receiving specialty palliative care is unknown, likely reflective of the diverse patient population served. For children with MD, the prevalence approaches 100%; for others it varies widely depending on the underlying etiology. The prevalence of dysphagia during the last month of life, however, affects about one-quarter to one-third of dying children,[7,8] and in the advanced cancer population the prevalence increases over time.[8]

PHYSICAL EXAM AND DIAGNOSTIC TESTS

Evaluation of dysphagia and other throat symptoms requires a holistic approach that goes beyond the observation of feeding.[9] The symptoms most likely to be associated with dysphagia are a wet voice, wet breathing, and cough.[10] Age and neurological status influence the significance of these clinical markers. Despite the association between clinical symptoms such as coughing during feeds, changes in voice, and color changes while feeding, the ability to clinically detect dysphagia is low and studies comparing a therapist's judgment to a videofluoroscopic swallowing study (VFSS) had both low sensitivity and specificity.[11]

As with any intervention in children with serious illness receiving specialty palliative care, however, one must carefully balance the benefits of eating and drinking with the risk of aspiration. In the case in which a child and family do not want to assume the risk of aspiration, the pleasure of taste is often overlooked. Oral foam care brushes can be dipped in any beverage and many foods. When gently placed in the mouth, it can bring great pleasure and improve the quality of life of a child who may not have tasted anything for days to weeks to months. There is also an appreciable benefit for the parent, who can feel reassured that they are continuing to provide loving attention and enhancing their child's quality of life.

Symptoms that may indicate the presence of dysphagia include

Infants with poor coordination of suck and swallow	Back arching
The presence of drooling, vomiting, and/or coughing	Inability to coordinate breathing
A feeling that food or liquids are sticking in the throat or esophagus	Difficulty in chewing food
Trying to swallow a single mouthful of food several times	Discomfort in the throat or chest
Wet or raspy sounding voice during or after feeding	Gagging
Food or liquids coming out of the nose during or after feeding	Recurrent pneumonia
Color change during feeding, such as becoming blue or pale	Change in voice before or after eating; tiredness or shortness of breath during feeding

Several investigations can be undertaken to provide more information to guide diagnosis and management of the child's condition. These include

- Videofluoroscopic swallowing studies
- Barium swallow/upper GI series
- Endoscopy
- Esophageal manometry
- Laryngoscopy

If the child is approaching end of life, further evaluation should be considered if the investigation is likely to change the child's comfort or are consistent with the goals of care. The appropriateness of these assessments depends on what course of action is being contemplated and must be individualized to the child and his or her situation. If a single study were used to determine the presence of dysphagia and aspiration, then VFSS, in which a series of x-rays examine the child's swallow after the child takes a small amount of liquid or solid containing barium, would likely be the most informative while also causing the least discomfort for the child.

TREATMENT: INTEGRATIVE AND SUPPORTIVE THERAPIES

The extent to which dysphagia is managed depends on the stage of the child's illness and the goals of the child and the family. Speech therapists bring a level of knowledge and experience that is invaluable in the assessment and treatment of dysphagia. (In some institutions, this role may be assumed by occupational therapists, or sometimes a collaborating dietician.) They can provide specific exercises to improve coordination and muscle strength or suggest individualized strategies to compensate for impaired swallowing function and enhance the ease and safety of oral intake.[12]

Some therapists who are not typically a part of the palliative care team and are not used to working in the context of changing goals of care may be uncomfortable with modifying recommendations. Explaining the necessity for changing goals of care when a child is at end of life may allow the therapist to become more engaged in the child's care.

TREATMENT: PHARMACOLOGIC THERAPIES

Underlying causes of dysphagia that may be amenable to treatment include xerostomia, concomitant infection of the oropharyngeal cavity, pain, gastroesophageal reflux disease (GERD), and, in rare circumstances, anxiety, fear, and depression. Dysphagia from oropharyngeal neutropenic mucositis and thrush due to *Candida albicans* usually require additional medications to effectively treat. Treatment of the underlying odynophagia—opioids for mucositis and antifungal medications for thrush—usually result in less pain and improved swallowing.

Children at end of life with dysphagia that is unaccompanied by odynophagia (such as seen with or thrush) may not benefit from treatment. The exception would be a procedure that could reverse a process or improve quality of life, such as radiotherapy to shrink a tumor mass or widen a stricture. Treatment-related dysphagia may be caused by a medication or other treatment. If medication-related, the medication should be rotated or discontinued. In other conditions, dysphagia may be irreversible, in which case the focus should be on alleviation of the symptom. If death is close, interventions that promote comfort, including opioids, orally or intravenously, perhaps with patient-controlled analgesia (PCA) should be considered.

ANOREXIA AND CACHEXIA

At its simplest, anorexia is a loss of appetite. It is a common clinical symptom in children with life-limiting and life-threatening illnesss.[1,7,13,14] The rituals around the provision of food are deeply embedded in religious, familial, and sociocultural belief systems, allowing anorexia to permeate almost all aspects of a child's life. Children may feel excluded and isolated from social activities that involve food, such as family gatherings, birthday parties, and events at school. Despite their intentions and often astonishing efforts, caregivers can feel powerless in their ability to enhance their child's appetite.

Most research on anorexia is in children with cancer, where it is consistently one of the top five most prevalent symptoms.[15–17] Anorexia is present in one-quarter of these patients, usually as a consequence of chemotherapy or radiation therapy but can also arise from pain, dysphagia, depression, or severe constipation. Almost all children with anorexia[15,18] and their caregivers[19] experience high levels of distress caused by their change in appetite. Yet for children with cancer referred to a specialized palliative care team, anorexia was the most common symptom identified by patient-reported outcome tools that was not previously diagnosed or treated by the referring oncology service.[17] This finding serves to underscore the importance of systematic symptom assessment of children receiving specialized palliative care. If a child's cancer is advanced, the frequency of anorexia increases to almost one-third of children in the last 12 weeks of life.[15]

Cachexia comes from the Greek words *kakós* and *hexis*, which translates to "bad condition." It is a condition of involuntary weight loss and is defined medically as "a complex metabolic syndrome associated with underlying illness and characterized by loss of muscle with or without loss of fat mass."[20] Cachexia is usually associated with anorexia in a complex state of advanced protein-calorie malnutrition recognized as anorexia-cachexia syndrome. Growth failure may be the initial manifestation of anorexia-cachexia syndrome in children rather than weight loss. For many parents, the sight of their child visibly losing weight may intensify feelings of helplessness and failure as parents and lead to misunderstanding and blame within the extended family.

The process of anorexia-cachexia syndrome is complicated, but it is clear that anorexia alone is inadequate for the syndrome to develop. In normal circumstances, the reduced caloric intake from anorexia results in a loss of fat stores, which stimulates an adaptive response to maintain the fat stores. This response is driven by declining levels of leptin, a hormone secreted by adipose tissue. The consequence of low levels of leptin in the brain is for the hypothalamus to increase orexigenic signals such as neuropeptide-Y (NPY) to stimulate appetite, repress energy expenditure, and decrease anorexigenic signals, corticotrophin-releasing factor, and melanocortin to achieve the same effect.[21]

There is increasing evidence that the cachectic process is established by an acute phase response mediated by several cytokines of which tumor necrosis factor-alpha, interleukin-1, interleukin-6, and interferon-gamma have been implicated. The evidence suggests that these cytokines stimulate the expression and release of leptin and mimic the hypothalamic negative feedback signaling from leptin, which in turn prevents the standard compensatory mechanisms that are typically initiated in the face of reduced food intake and decreasing weight.

This abnormal response was observed in a study[22] that reported on the possible role of leptin and NPY levels as prognostic indicators in children with cancer. The study revealed a mean NPY level of 82.32 pmol/L and mean leptin level of 6.60 ng/mL at diagnosis in children who achieved complete remission versus a mean NPY and leptin level of 430.16 pmol/L and 0.192 ng/mL, respectively in those children who died of their disease during the follow-up period. Furthermore, the mean NPY level declined and the mean leptin level increased during chemotherapy in the children studied. Other hallmark features of anorexia-cachexia syndrome include hypermetabolism and changes in the metabolism of carbohydrates, proteins, and fats.

PHYSICAL EXAM AND DIAGNOSTIC TESTS

While there are no specific diagnostic criteria for anorexia-cachexia syndrome, knowledge of the underlying disease process, clinical history, and focused physical examination allows for an accurate clinical diagnosis. Body weight, skinfold thickness, and body composition can aid in the confirmation of the diagnosis if needed, although they are often not necessary. Anorexia or cachexia may be a part of a lifelong illness. For example, children with chronic kidney disease have a risk of protein energy wasting or of cachexia.[23] If a child is at the end of life, if goals of care are focused on comfort, the child and family may decide against additional procedures, which may allow the child to remain at home.

Body weight can be useful in monitoring the rate of deterioration either by detecting a frank weight loss or failure to grow over time. A rapid decline in weight may be suggestive of a change in fluid balance. If consistent with the child's and family's goals, it may be reasonable to intervene and correct the problem.

Extensive laboratory tests evaluating nutritional depletion are of limited value[24] and can often stir a great deal of anxiety and apprehension in children and young people. They, therefore, cannot be recommended as routine. Albumin is the most common laboratory value checked because of its low cost and accuracy when liver and renal disease are absent.[25] However, testing for potentially reversible causes such as hypercalcemia are warranted if the child's underlying diagnosis, history, and physical exam are suggestive of electrolyte abnormalities.

While the presence of anorexia-cachexia syndrome in children with advanced cancer may suggest an unavoidable deterioration to death, anorexia and cachexia together or alone can represent several readily correctable causes that should be kept in mind during an assessment. Consideration needs to be given to

- Adverse effects of medication
- Dehydration
- Mouth problems, such as oral thrush, xerostomia
- Dysphagia, GERD, constipation, intestinal obstruction
- Infection
- Nausea and vomiting
- Pain
- Psychological factors, such as anxiety, fear, depression

TREATMENT: INTEGRATIVE AND SUPPORTIVE THERAPIES

Management of anorexia-cachexia syndrome should begin with a preemptive acknowledgment that this process is not unexpected. Providing information and education to the child and family is essential, and its importance should not be underestimated. Creating an environment of trust and transparency allows for anticipatory exploration of the emotional and spiritual meanings of anorexia-cachexia syndrome to the child and family. Such discussion then facilitates the disclosure of commonly held misconceptions that might otherwise be left unaddressed. For example, the belief that it is necessary to feed a child in the face of reduced food intake stems from instinctive, primal, and deeply powerful feelings about the parental role to protect and nurture. Another common belief, borne of a sense of frustration and helplessness, is that relentless, progressive weight loss and failure to grow mean that their child is receiving inadequate care. Addressing these emotionally loaded misconceptions mitigates at least one measure of parental distress. Across each of these situations is the common misunderstanding (including by healthcare providers) that calories can prolong life. Cancer cachexia is much more than a lack of calories. Rather, it is an immunological syndrome in which the uptake of nutrients is blocked by the immunological situation in which the tumor places the body.

Anticipatory guidance, as in the previous examples, facilitates the development of empowering strategies for both the child and family. While these approaches are unlikely to improve survival, they do enhance the quality of life and feelings of comfort for the child and family. Strategies that may increase food intake include

- Offering the child favorite foods based on pleasure, not on "should" and "ought"
- Eliminating dietary restrictions
- Reducing portion sizes and increasing the number of meals
- Making food look more enticing
- Avoiding disliked foods

It is crucial to counsel parents that there is evidence[26] that hypercaloric feeding does not increase lean tissue or skeletal muscle[20] mass, and there is no significant improvement in survival.

Psychological, emotional, and spiritual issues include[24]

- Encouraging child and family interaction to reduce psychological distress
- Helping the family to distinguish between things they can and cannot control (e.g., helping their child find comfort vs. halting disease progression)
- Exploring what the child's not eating and losing weight means to the family. This discussion may provide better understanding of their distress, as well as added opportunity to clarify misconceptions.
- Assessing the impact of symptoms on the child and family
- Assessing the quality of life of the child and family

TREATMENT: PHARMACOLOGICAL THERAPIES

Pharmacologic management of anorexia-cachexia syndrome is adjunctive to the integrative and supportive measures highlighted previously. Data suggest that both anorexia and weight loss occur in high frequency and respond poorly to treatment in children and young people with progressive malignant disease.[8] Many extant pharmacologic agents are not successful in alleviating the symptoms, though a large number of existing and experimental agents have been reported to be helpful. Data supporting the use of medications to manage anorexia and cachexia are limited in adults and nonexistent in children. Arguably, the most studied drugs are those of the progestational group, most prominently megestrol acetate. A Cochrane review[27] found that megestrol acetate improved appetite and weight gain in adult patients with cancer. It did not, however, improve muscle mass or the tissue lost in cachexia, and the weight gain was mainly due to increases in body fat. No overall conclusion could be drawn on quality of life because of statistical and clinical heterogeneity. Similarly, patient numbers and methodological shortcomings allowed no recommendations to be made about megestrol acetate use in patients with AIDS or other underlying pathologies.

Cyproheptadine hydrochloride has been used in children with cancer and cancer treatment–related cachexia and was shown[28] to improve average weight gain. The main side effect was drowsiness. In a systematic review, cyproheptadine has been helpful in achieving weight gain for some children of all ages and across a range of conditions.[29] These findings did *not,* however, apply to children with HIV, cancer, or other progressive diseases and so while it is recommended and used in children receiving specialty palliative care, the child's and parental expectations must be tempered with accurate anticipatory guidance that it may not be as helpful as they hope for.

Megestrol acetate has been trialed in a small number of children with cachexia due to cancer,[30–32] CF,[33,34] and HIV disease[35] and has been reported to improve nutritional status by increasing appetite and weight. Additionally, adverse effects were significant, including most children developing adrenal suppression and one child manifesting clinical hypoadrenalism with hemodynamic collapse requiring ionotropic support.[31] This effect was shown to be transient[32] as a normal adrenocorticotropic hormone (ACTH) stimulation test was returned once megestrol acetate was discontinued.

OTHER INTERVENTIONS: FEEDING DEVICES AND TOTAL PARENTERAL NUTRITION

If integrative and pharmacotherapy are not effective and the goal of care is to optimize the child's function and nutritional status, the child may benefit from nutrition supplied through an alternative route. Nutrition may be administered through an enteral feeding device such as a nasogastric (NG), nasoduodenal (ND), nasojejunal (NJ) gastric (GT), gastrojejunal (GJ), or jejunal (J) tubes. Gastric feeding devices can further be characterized by whether they were placed endoscopically or surgically, and this will be discussed later. Multiple professional organizations[33,36] support nutritional support for neurologically impaired children via enteral tube feedings and recommend that they be initiated early in children who are unable to feed orally or who cannot achieve sufficient oral intake to maintain adequate nutritional or hydration status. These devices are very common, as a survey study of six large pediatric palliative care programs in the United States and Canada revealed that almost half of all children receiving specialty palliative care had a GT.[1]

There are distinctions to each route of feeding. Both NG and GT are commonly used to feed or administer medication in children with complex chronic conditions when there are risks with oral intake. While NG or NJ tube feedings have historically been reserved for short-term nutritional intervention and GT or GJ tube feedings for circumstances where long-term nutritional rehabilitation is required,[33] each child's situation is unique. Providers should be flexible, mindful, and fluid in making recommendations that would help children and their families achieve their goals in the context of their illness.

NG tubes require the insertion of a silicone-based tube into the nasopharyngeal airway with an end in the stomach. In the case of NJ tubes, they end in the jejunum. The success of placement can be evaluated by the drawing back of acidic stomach contents in the case of an NG or by radiological visualization with NJ tubes. The long-term use of the nasopharyngeal route is associated with the development of ulceration and possible perforation of the nasal septum. It is prudent to closely monitor the duration of use, and, with consideration given to the context of the child and their illness, review whether a more permanent device should be placed in the stomach.

Tubes that enter the stomach can be placed either via a percutaneous endoscopic route by a pediatric gastroenterologist or surgically by a pediatric general surgeon. After its introduction in the 1980s, the percutaneous endoscopic gastrostomy (PEG) tube quickly became one of the most preferred methods due to its minimally invasive nature, speed, and low cost when compared to a surgical gastrostomy tube. Furthermore, there were fewer complications and a shorter duration of post-placement antibiotics in the PEG group compared to the surgically placed group.[37] In patients with complex anatomy (scoliosis, malrotation, situs inversus) it may be advisable to proceed with a surgically placed GT to ensure proper placement.

Where a GT terminates—in the stomach, duodenum, or jejunum—largely depends on the precise reason a tube is being placed in the first place. For children who need the administration of medications and delivery of sufficient nutrition and hydration but lack significant GERD or delayed gastric emptying, a true gastrostomy that ends in the stomach should suffice. For children with significant GERD, more complex gastrointestinal pathology, or other gastrointestinal comorbidities, a duodenal or jejunal tube is likely to be more beneficial.

The location of the distal end of a duodenal or jejunal tube allows for the post-pyloric delivery of enteral nutrition, thereby minimizing the risk that contents could propel backward into the esophagus. Medications cannot be given through the jejunal part of the feeding tube, but rather go through the gastric port. Duodenal and jejunal tubes, however, are rife with potential limitations and complications, and so the decision of where a GT should terminate is a nuanced one. Enteral nutrition cannot be given via bolus feeds into the duodenum or jejunum as the intestines do not have the same capacity as the stomach to handle larger volumes of food. Food must be delivered as a continuous infusion, which increases the amount of medical technology and equipment to maintain, travel with, and troubleshoot. Additionally, given the tube's location in the intestine, it must be placed—and replaced when dislodged or accidentally removed—at a medical facility with proper placement confirmed by direct visualization.

The delivery of nutrition and hydration by a feeding tube has been consistently associated with an improvement in mean percent ideal body weight for height-age,[38,39] a parental perception of improved mood of the child,[39] and a significant improvement in caregiver quality of life at 6 months and 12 months after GT insertion[40] with no significant increased financial burden.[41] The lack of well-designed randomized controlled trials[42] in children with cerebral palsy who have feeding devices—and who represent a large proportion of patients receiving specialty palliative care—highlights the uncertainty involved in the decision-making process. Unfortunately, improvements in the child's health-related quality of life decline after 12 months.[43] Some studies have demonstrated an association between feeding tubes and an increased risk of death, with many complications reported, including potential for increased gastroesophageal reflux and aspiration into the lungs.[39] Children with jejunostomy tubes are at an increased risk for GERD and intestinal perforation, as well as frequent dislodging that requires anywhere from one to three tube replacements per year, depending on age.[44] Older children are more likely to need more frequent replacements than younger children, while younger children are more likely to suffer an intestinal perforation.[45]

The phrase that many parents of children with a life-limiting or life-threatening illness use to succinctly capture their goals is for their child to "live as long as possible, as well as possible." This accounts for both extending life and maintaining or enhancing the quality of life—the two are not mutually exclusive and can be interdependent. When the use of feeding devices does not meet the goal of providing sufficient nutrition to sustain growth, families will often inquire about total parenteral nutrition (TPN). The request stems from a desire to extend their child's life without sacrificing their child's quality of life. Yet the traditional view is that, in most cases, long-term provision of TPN does not extend nor improve the quality of life, with the exception of children who have intestinal failure. Compounding this sentiment is that there are no clear consensus guidelines from the North American Society for Pediatric Gastroenterology, Hepatology and Nutrition or the European Society for Paediatric Gastroenterology Hepatology and Nutrition that address the unique needs of these patients. While some data in adult cancer patients demonstrate no improvement in quality of life[46] with the use of TPN, other studies suggest that the use of TPN is associated with both an improved quality of life[47–50] and an extension of life.[51,52] Evidence is emerging that the use of home TPN in children does not adversely affect the quality of life when compared to children with enteral feeding devices,[53] and the long-term health-related quality of life of pediatric intestinal failure patients receiving home TPN is similar to that of healthy peers.[54] As children with complex chronic conditions live increasingly longer lives and medical technology becomes progressively available, transportable, and efficient, the question of home TPN will likely become increasingly relevant to palliative care providers, the subspecialists who manage TPN, and the children and families who may benefit from this therapeutic intervention.

The decision to initiate artificial nutrition and hydration is not an easy one and should be viewed as we view other technological interventions that sustain life, such as mechanical ventilators or dialysis. For those deciding to pursue a feeding device for their child, proper care of all feeding devices is essential and is well-described in the literature,[55] along with best practice guidelines.[56] The issue of forgoing artificial nutrition and hydration is more comprehensively addressed in Chapter 14 "Advanced Care Planning Along the Continuum" and Chapter 27 "Easing Distress When Death Is Near."

There is minimal pediatric data in the management of visceral hyperalgesia.[57] A trial of changing the formula type or route of administration should be considered. If these are not effective, decreasing the volume of feeds may be helpful. Such a suggestion may elicit parental anxiety, and potentially resistance, governed by a fear of "starving" the child. Reassurance that the goal is to improve distressing symptoms by decreasing the feeding volume may mitigate some of the distress, as well as the proposal of a "time-limited trial," such as reducing daily feeding volume by 25–50% for 3 days to establish treatment effectiveness and foster parental rapport.

When these strategies are not as effective as hoped for, the addition of a gabapentinoid (gabapentin, pregabalin) or a tricyclic antidepressant can be helpful. Due to their efficacy in refractory neuropathic pain, one may consider duloxetine or methadone[58] in particularly challenging cases. The use of other opioids is reserved for children approaching the end of life. For further discussion of management of visceral hyperalgesia, see Chapter 19, "Neurological Symptoms."

NAUSEA AND VOMITING

Nausea is best thought of as the feeling or sensation of impending emesis, often accompanied by sialorrhea, eructation, and dizziness.[59] The word itself derives from the Greek *nausia,* meaning "seasickness" (*naus,* ship). Nausea is to be distinguished from emesis (vomiting) itself, which is a coordinated series of sensory-motor reflexes that can occur because of or in the absence of nausea.

Nausea is incredibly burdensome and disruptive to children. In a study of adolescents and young adults (AYAs) with cancer, nausea was extremely intrusive, with a severity of moderate or greater more than 80% of the time it was experienced.[3] These AYAs described nausea as a priority symptom based on the degree to which it affected physical and emotional functioning and how much it impeded independence.[3] The authors also found the AYA might not report the symptom, emphasizing the need for a structured approach to history and physical.[3] Furthermore, nausea is a unique predictor of a child's social disability and correlates with lower academic and social functioning.[60] Children with nausea have significantly more school absences than other children, and nausea leads to decreased overall quality of life and functional disability.[60]

Vomiting, as distinguished from nausea, involves the "forceful retrograde expulsion of stomach contents through the oral cavity."[61] Vomiting is also differentiated from regurgitation, a related phenomenon that consists of the expulsion of esophageal contents but without the coordinated airway closure of the vomiting reflex.

Vomiting is not always preceded by nausea. Furthermore, the central pathways of nausea and vomiting differ.[62] Causes of vomiting may be from within or outside of the GI tract. Factors of the GI tract leading to vomiting include GI infections (e.g., gastroenteritis, hepatitis), anatomic insults (e.g., intussusception, surgical adhesions), mucosal injuries (e.g., chronic granulomatous disease, inflammatory bowel disease), GI motility disorders (e.g., paralytic ileus, gastroparesis), visceral GI disorders (e.g., pancreatitis, cholecystitis), and other factors.[63] External factors include infection or inflammation, disease (e.g., chronic granulomatous disease, otitis media, pyelonephritis), endocrine derangements (e.g., carcinoid syndrome, diabetic ketoacidosis), metabolic derangements (e.g., urea cycle defects, storage disease), genitourinary disorders (e.g., uremia, hydronephrosis secondary to ureteropelvic obstruction), or neurologic disorders (e.g., hydrocephalus, concussion).[63]

It is essential to distinguish between chronic and acute nausea. Chronic nausea may not be constant, but it is recurrent and frequent, lasting for more than 1 month. Common causes include pancreatitis, GERD, or gastroparesis. Chronic nausea might also be due to pregnancy, sometimes lower on the differential list of a young woman with a serious illness than it would be for a healthier female. The neurologic pathways of acute and chronic nausea are different; the central pathway of chronic nausea is similar to the pathway for chronic pain, which expands the repertoire of treatments for nausea to include those used for neuropathic pain, such as gabapentinoids.[62]

Multiple afferent and efferent pathways lead to the symptom of nausea and the effect of emesis (see Figure 25.1). There are four primary pathways: the cerebral cortex, the area postrema (that contains the chemoreceptor trigger zone [CTZ]), neuronal pathways within the vestibular nuclei, and vagal afferents from the upper gut.[64,65] Stimulation of chemoreceptors and stretch receptors in the GI tract stimulate vagal afferents of the sympathetic nervous system.

All of these pathways are coordinated through the vomiting center (VC), which is located in the medulla oblongata. The VC is a convergence area formed by several anatomically distinct structures. The medulla contains muscarinic and histamine receptors.[66] The VC is mostly inside the blood–brain barrier. It receives stimulation from the CNS, including the cerebral cortex (psychological factors, including anticipation) and sensory organs, vestibular components, and the GI tract, including chemicals that affect the CTZ.[67] The CTZ contains dopamine and serotonin receptors.[66] Impulses from the VC stimulate the smooth muscles of the GI system, thereby initiating and controlling the act of emesis.

The CTZ is a part of the VC, however, the CTZ is outside the blood–brain barrier in the *area postrema*. Therefore, the CTZ can detect the chemical substances that can induce nausea and vomiting.[68]

AN APPROACH TO THE CHILD WITH NAUSEA

Identifying the underlying cause(s) of nausea and vomiting typically is useful for selecting the therapeutic option. Although the causes of nausea and vomiting are often multifactorial, an etiology-based approach allows identification of a primary neurotransmitter pathway, which, in turn, facilitates informed decision-making about the most useful neurotransmitter antagonist with which to initiate treatment. The most robust supportive data for the etiology-based approach are found in the treatment of chemotherapy- or radiation-related nausea and vomiting and the treatment for malignant bowel obstruction.

HISTORY

While history typically focuses on proximal causes (i.e., identifying contemporaneous factors that occurred around the time of nausea), the context of the child's underlying disease allows examination of interactive factors. Therefore, the history of nausea and vomiting focuses on potential causes.

Nausea and vomiting are common in many chronic and severe illnesses resulting from disease and treatment; however, more is known about how to treat these symptoms arising from treatment than from disease.[69] Nausea and vomiting occur not just from the GI tract, but also the CNS, and

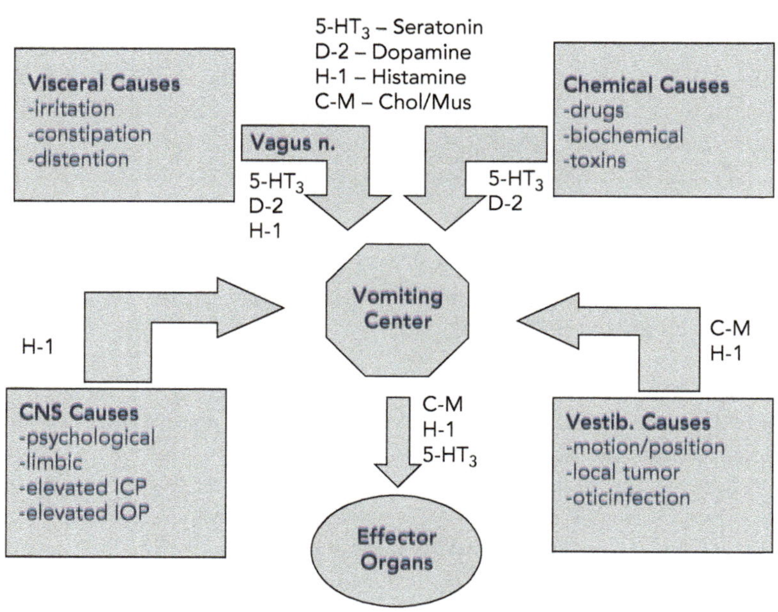

Figure 25.1 Causes, pathways, and neurotransmitters for nausea and vomiting. Used with permission from Harrison CM. A practical approach to nausea and vomiting. In Mahon M, ed. lecture ed2015.

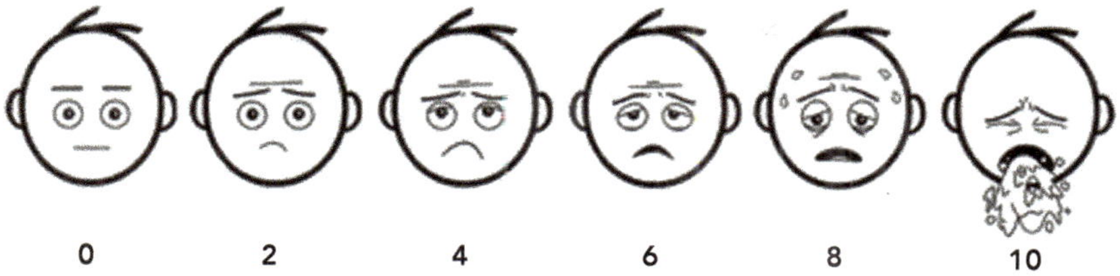

Figure 25.2 Nausea scale.

include vestibular, otic, and metabolic factors.[65] Furthermore, the anticipation of nausea and vomiting can itself cause nausea and vomiting. Understanding these factors can guide history and assessment.

Symptoms are subjective experiences. Therefore, a child's characterization is essential. One tool commonly used is aptly called the Baxter Retching Faces Scale (BARF) scale (Figure 25.2).[70] The scale is sometimes called the Baxter Animated Retching Faces scale. The BARF scale is a 0–10 scale with six faces; the child is asked to identify which face best represents the current experience of nausea. The scale has been validated with emergency department and postoperative samples of children. In assessing the utility of the scale in children with postoperative nausea and vomiting and postdischarge nausea and vomiting, Watcha and colleagues found the tool useful for children in these groups, with a clinically relevant score difference of 1.47/10.[71] The authors also found that clinically relevant nausea was common; however, the presence of nausea did not predict whether the child would be treated with an antiemetic. Only the presence of emesis predicted the administration of antiemetics.[71]

PHYSICAL EXAM AND DIAGNOSTIC TESTS

The physical and laboratory examination, like the history, should consider the multifactorial causes of nausea and vomiting. This should include a physical exam and lab findings that are affected by the underlying disease or injury and those that are separate.

TREATMENT: INTEGRATIVE AND SUPPORTIVE THERAPIES

Nonpharmacologic interventions are crucial in the management of nausea and vomiting. Children are often aware of which foods or beverages they will be more likely to tolerate. This is a critical opportunity for children to learn to "listen to their bodies." Though not uniformly effective, a small amount (one bite, one sip) of what the child "feels like" having is a good test. If the child can tolerate oral intake, small meals taken more frequently are more likely to stay where they are intended. Avoid strong odors and flavors, which also includes food and drink that visitors might bring in. For example, the smell of a parent's coffee or grilled vegetables might trigger nausea and vomiting. Some children do better if someone is there with them, either for company or distraction. Triggers for nausea and vomiting vary widely between children.

Therapies including behavioral techniques, hypnosis, acupuncture, acupressure, and aromatherapy (anecdotally) have been shown to be efficacious in managing nausea and vomiting in children.[4,72–74] Professionals from dietetics, social work, psychology, child life, rehabilitation, and education provide different perspectives to shaping the child's care.[73,75] Behavioral therapies may also help.[4,72,73] Hypnosis and guided imagery may be particularly helpful with anticipatory nausea and vomiting.[73,76] Acupuncture may also be beneficial for this symptom; however, may not be permitted if a child is neutropenic or thrombocytopenic. Choksi and colleagues studied the integration of acupuncture into the care of children with cancer: 52% of the children chose to accept acupuncture, and 51% of participants sought treatment for nausea.[77] The authors found "no increased incidence of adverse events in children with thrombocytopenia . . . or neutropenia." Still, institutions and treatment teams may have preferences for levels below which they do not want a child to receive acupuncture, for example, no acupuncture for a child with fewer than 50,000 platelets.[77]

Sea-bands (acupressure wrist bands) use traditional Chinese medicine techniques to provide pressure to the P6 acupoint on the ventral surface of the wrist to alleviate nausea and vomiting.[78] Children can be taught to apply their own bands. While Sea-bands are helpful in some instances of nausea and vomiting, they are not beneficial for children with chemotherapy-induced nausea and vomiting (CINV) receiving highly emetogenic chemotherapy.[78]

Although aromatherapy is sometimes recommended for nausea and vomiting, the evidence to support its efficacy is limited. In a Cochrane review specific to postoperative nausea and vomiting, aromatherapy was found to be no more effective than placebo.[79]

TREATMENT: PHARMACOLOGIC THERAPIES

Five neurotransmitter receptors account for the majority of activity that mediates nausea and vomiting. The most important receptors include serotonin ($5HT_3$), dopamine (D_2), acetylcholine muscarinic (M_1 or M_3, M_4, or M_5), histamine (H_1), or neurokinin (NK_1).[64,72,80] The goal of treatment of nausea and vomiting is to antagonize the predominant neurotransmitter of the most likely pathway leading to nausea and vomiting. Most of what is known about the efficacy of neurotransmitter antagonism in children is based on research with chemotherapy-induced nausea and vomiting and postoperative nausea and vomiting.

Understanding vomiting pathways is clinically useful for choosing antagonists in symptom management, or at least the initial antiemetic that which is most likely to be effective.

Not uncommonly, more than one antiemetic is necessary to quell the child's symptoms. If another antiemetic is required, choose one from a different receptor antagonist class. This is often empiric. Even in the management of CINV, there is a lack of consensus about optimal management.[81] Please see Table 25.1 for medications for the treatment of nausea and vomiting.

Serotonin ($5HT_3$) receptors are located in the area postrema. Serotonin antagonists (e.g., ondansetron or granisetron) block serotonin viscerally (causes such as distention or GI irritation) with vagal transmission and centrally at the CTZ.[82] The CTZ is stimulated by chemical causes, such as anesthesia or chemotherapy. These receptors respond to many cancer-directed chemotherapy drugs and uremia, producing nausea and vomiting. Therefore, serotonin antagonists are typically the first line for CINV, postop nausea and vomiting, or nausea and vomiting as a side effect of other potential toxins or GI stimulants. In some patients who do not have benefit from ondansetron, rotating to granisetron may be beneficial. Antiserotonergic agents are also used following bone marrow transplant, which is typically accompanied by a chemotherapeutic conditioning regimen. Serotonin antagonism has been recommended as the second line in the management of pediatric gastroenteritis after hydration.[67] Serotonin antagonism is also indicated before and after radiation therapy.[83]

Dopamine type 2 (D_2)-receptors in the area postrema are stimulated by emetogenic substances such as calcium, uremia products, opioids, and digoxin. Dopamine receptors are also found throughout the gastrointestinal system. Dopamine antagonists (e.g., metoclopramide, haloperidol) are commonly used to treat nausea and vomiting in children, including CINV. The dopamine receptor antagonist metoclopramide is active in the area postrema. It also acts as a gastrointestinal prokinetic, prompting gastric emptying and increasing the tone of the lower esophageal sphincter by blocking GI dopamine receptors. Metoclopramide stimulates gastric cholinergic receptors.[84]

Side effects, including sedation, sometime limit the use of dopamine antagonists, but extrapyramidal effects are the symptom to be most wary of.[81] Extrapyramidal side effects are more likely with metoclopramide than with other antidopaminergic drugs.[75] Prokinetics (e.g., metoclopramide) should not be administered concurrently with antimuscarinic agents, such as diphenhydramine or scopolamine, as anticholinergic agents block the final common pathway of prokinetic agents. The concurrent administration of diphenhydramine and metoclopramide to prevent extrapyramidal effects, as practiced in some centers, will, therefore, result in the loss of metoclopramide's prokinetic effect but not its antiemetic effect. The concurrent intravenous administration of dopamine antagonists with 5-HT_3-receptor antagonists increases the risk of cardiac arrhythmia.[82] For patients with refractory nausea, especially CINV, a dopamine antagonist may be added as a second-line agent, in addition to an antiserotonergic.[76,83]

As is true with all symptom medications, a lack of benefit from one class often leads to rotation to medicine from another group of antiemetics. Rather than rotation, if a child has incomplete relief of nausea and vomiting, it is better to add medication from another antiemetic class.[85]

Mu-1 and mu-2-opioid receptors are found in the CTZ.[86] The emetogenic action of opioids is believed to be mediated through mu-2 receptor stimulation, which, in turn, potentiates the release of dopamine. For some children, this release of dopamine stimulates nausea and vomiting. Unexpectedly, however, a child who experiences emesis with a low or standard opioid dose may not experience nausea and vomiting with a higher opioid dose. This is due to the action of the higher opioid doses "at receptor sites deeper in the medulla."[86]

Histamine receptors are present at multiple sites. There are histamine receptors in the inner ear, in the CTZ in the area postrema, and in the VC in the vestibular nucleus. Nausea can result from disturbances to the vestibular system that comprises semicircular canals and otolith organs. The vestibular system is responsible for balance sensation and movements. Histamine mediates the transmission of nausea via the vagus nerve.

Histamine antagonists (e.g., diphenhydramine, promethazine) are often over-the-counter medications for the prevention or treatment of motion sickness, including nausea and vomiting, as well as for vertigo. Antihistamines are often sedating. Unfortunately, antihistamines are sometimes administered for sedation effect, rather than for the antihistamine effect. There are a few nonsedating antihistamines, such as loratadine or cetirizine; however, these medications are less beneficial in alleviating nausea and vomiting.

Acetylcholine works to increase gut motility and secretions, as well as stimulate nausea. Anticholinergics block muscarinic receptors and inhibit cholinergic transmission from the vestibular system to the VC.

Muscarinic acetylcholine receptors are G protein-coupled receptors that are found throughout the body, within and outside of the CNS. They are a part of most physiologic processes.[87] Motion sickness, nausea, and vomiting caused by motion is mediated in different areas of the brainstem, including the area postrema, the vagal nuclear complex, the VC, and the vestibular complex.[88] Anticholinergics/antimuscarinics are most often used to treat nausea and vomiting due to vestibular stimulation (e.g., meclizine, dimenhydrinate).

There are few pediatric studies of either antihistamines or anticholinergic/antimuscarinics in pediatric populations. As with other pediatric medications, their use is sometimes empirical.

NK1 antagonists. Substance P activates the neurokinin 1 (NK1) receptor. A newer antiemetic class is that of NK1 antagonists. Substance P is found through the central and peripheral nervous systems, though it is more concentrated in some parts than in others. It is also found in the GI tract. Substance P has a role in emesis, as well as in inflammatory and immune responses, cancer, pain, and other factors.[89] Substance P is ubiquitous in the CNS, although it is found in higher concentrations in some parts more than others. One part that that deals with pain is the Rexed lamina II of the spinal cord's dorsal horn. The other part is the CTZ. Various

TABLE 25.1 Medications in the treatment of nausea and vomiting

RECEPTOR ACTIVITY	MEDICATION	DOSE	ROUTE OF ADMINISTRATION	COMMENTS AND SIDE EFFECTS
5-HT_3-receptor antagonists	Ondansetron (Zofran)	0.1–0.2 mg/kg q6–8h; max. 4–8 mg/dose	IV, PO, SL	Headache, constipation
	Granisetron (Kytril)	0.01–0.05 mg/kg q8h; max. 3 mg/dose	IV, PO, transdermal patch	Headache, constipation
5-HT_2-receptor antagonist/ Dopamine(D_2)- receptor antagonists	Olanzapine (Zyprexa)	1.25–2.5 mg PO q6h prn; titrate up to max 20 mg/daily	PO	May also help with anxiolysis and insomnia
Dopamine(D_2)- receptor antagonists	Metoclopramide (Reglan)	0.15–0.3 mg/kg (max. 10–15 mg) q6h	IV, PO, PR	Extrapyramidal side effects. Contraindicated suspected/ known bowel obstruction
	Haloperidol (Haldol)	0.01–0.1 mg/kg q12h (slowly titrated to max. of 1–2 mg/ kg, max. 100 mg/dose)	IV, PO	Extrapyramidal side effects.
	Domperidone	0.2–0.4 mg/kg q4–8h; max. 10 mg	PO, PR	Does not cross blood–brain barrier, no extrapyramidal side effects
Histamine (H_1)/muscarinic acetylcholine (ACh_m) receptor antagonists	Dimenhydrinate (Dramamine)	1–2 mg/kg q8h IV; 2–5 mg/ kg q6–12h	IV, PO, PR	Anticholinergic side effects including constipation, sedation
	Hydroxyzine	2 mg/kg/day divided q6–8h, max. 100 mg/dose	PO	Anticholinergic side effects
	Diphenhydramine (Benadryl)	0.5–1 mg/kg q6h (max. 50 mg)	PO, IV	Anticholinergic side effects, including significant sedation
	Promethazine (Phenergan)	0.2–0.5 mg/kg q6h	IV, PO	Anticholinergic side effects, including significant sedation; avoid when also using dopamine(D_2)- receptor antagonists
	Scopolamine (Transdermal Scop)	0.01 mg mg/kg q6h IV; Patch: 0.33 mg/24h or 0.5 mg/24h: > 10 years q72h	IV, transdermal	Antimuscarinic, not an antihistamine. Anticholinergic side effects
Dopamine(D_2)- and histamine (H_1)/muscarinic acetylcholine (ACh_m) receptor antagonists	Chlorpromazine (Thorazine)	PO, PR: 0.5–2 mg/kg; IV: 0.25–1 mg/kg slow infusion	PO, PR, IV	Phenothiazine: psychotropic effect. Extrapyramidal and anticholinergic side effects, agranulocytosis
	Prochlorperazine (Compazine)	0.1–0.2 mg/kg q8h	PO	Phenothiazine: psychotropic effect. Extrapyramidal and anticholinergic side effects, agranulocytosis
Neurokinin-1 receptor antagonists	Aprepitant (Emend)	>12 years preoperative dose 40 mg (not per kg) once 125 mg (not per kg once, then 80 mg once per day during chemotherapy)	PO	Chemotherapy-associated nausea. Side effects: Constipation, headaches, fatigue, sinus tachycardia
Cannabinoid (CB_1) receptor agonist	Nabilone (Cesamet)	Adult dose: 1–2 mg BID	PO	May stimulate appetite Side effects: dizziness, dysphoria, hallucinations, arterial hypotension
	Dronabinol (Marinol)	5 mg/m^2 q2–4h, max. 4–6 doses/day	PO	Dizziness, dysphoria, hallucinations, arterial hypotension

toxins that float through the cerebrospinal fluid (CSF), such as chemotherapy agents, especially platinum-based chemotherapy agents, stimulate the production of substance P in the CTZ. This, in turn, stimulates the production of neurokinins. Therefore, this neuropeptide soup then potentiates the action of excitatory neurotransmitters, such as glutamate, increasing the rate of activity in the CTZ. This results in a continuous sensation of nausea and a desire to vomit.

A newer class of antiemetics has been designed to block the action of substance P and neurokinins: NK1 antagonists.[90] NK1 antagonists work primarily at the nucleus tractus solitaries and areas of reticular blocking receptors.[65] In addition to antiemetic properties, NK1 antagonists have anxiolytic and antidepressant properties.[91] The biochemistry and structure of NK1 remains incompletely understood.[89] NK1 antagonists are less effective at preventing nausea and more effective at preventing vomiting.[65]

Aprepitant, an NK1 antagonist, works by crossing the blood–brain barrier. Its use with children is increasing, typically in combination with an antiserotonergic.[75] As mentioned previously, the CTZ is located in the area postrema, one of the few places in the CNS where there is *no* blood–brain barrier. This area of neurotransmitters and antagonism is relatively new. Dysgeusia has been recognized as a side effect of NK1 antagonists and may limit their use in children undergoing treatment for cancer.[90] Those who take oral feeds while on aprepitant had increased nausea and pain scores.[91,92]

Cannabinoids. The cannabinoid receptor CB_1 is found in the CNS, mainly in the periaqueductal gray and the rostral ventromedial medulla, as well as in the peripheral nervous system. Stimulation of this receptor leads to suppression of the release of intestinal neurotransmitters. Cannabinoids are therefore sometimes used as a treatment for nausea and vomiting, though they are distinct from "medical marijuana." The US Food and Drug Administration (FDA) has approved two cannabis-derived medications for the treatment of nausea and vomiting: dronabinol and nabilone. Both of these medications are synthetic delta-9-tetrahydrocannabinol (THC). The National Academies for Science, Engineering, and Medicine[93] (NASEM) found substantial or conclusive evidence of benefit for CINV.[93] The antiemetic effect likely occurs because of the impact of the medication on the cannabinoid receptor system, the CB1 receptor.[94,95] Both dronabinol and nabilone are approved for CINV,[95–97] though neither is recommended as a first-line antiemetic.[98] Both have been used in the care of children; however, the benefit was low and side effects frequent.[94,99] It is not uncommon for patients who are started on a THC derivative to discontinue use due to side effects, including dizziness, drowsiness, and other symptoms.[100] The range in effects and side effects may also result from variability in pharmacokinetics and absorption.[100] More research in this area is needed.[93,101]

The benefits of "medical marijuana" are poorly documented for children.[102] Regardless, many families pursue its use, sometimes because they believe it is a "natural" substance, so is less likely to cause harm, and sometimes because they are frustrated with the persistence of the child's symptoms despite traditional medical interventions. Children are given cannabis with food into which cannabis has been baked ("edibles"), oil, vaporized cannabis, or by smoking it.[102] A challenge of medical cannabis is that, because it does not come in standardized doses, it is unclear how much cannabis the child is getting. Many parents might also inquire about the use of the nonpsychotropic cannabinoid, cannabidiol (CBD). While seemingly benign, CBD dramatically alters the metabolism of medications, including methadone,[103] and so children are at high risk for developing clinically significant drug-drug interactions.

Steroids are beneficial for a plethora of symptoms, including nausea and vomiting. For children on a treatment protocol, steroids may be contraindicated. Children with increased intracranial pressure (ICP) due to trauma or space-occupying lesion may benefit from steroids. The specific dynamics of how increased ICP leads to vomiting, with or without nausea remain incompletely understood.[104] The mechanics of how ICP leads to nausea and vomiting might vary by grade and disease severity.[104] This means the need for a steroid is likely to vary, even as the child's disease changes. Corticosteroids also inhibit prostaglandin synthesis, further contributing to antiemesis. Dexamethasone is commonly used for symptom management. Side effects of steroids include mood swings and weight gain, so the cost versus benefit must be continuously evaluated.

Atypical antipsychotics (e.g., olanzapine) have been recommended in adults for the prevention of CINV.[105] Olanzapine works on multiple neurotransmitters, including dopamine (D_{1-4}), serotonin ($5HT_{2a, 2c}$, $5HT_3$, $5HT_6$), histamine (H_1), "catecholamines at alpha 1 adrenergic receptors, [and] acetylcholine at muscarinic receptors."[106] Olanzapine is recommended (typically with other antiemetics) for children who are receiving highly emetogenic chemotherapy; for those for whom olanzapine is contraindicated, metoclopramide should be added.[107]

Subcutaneous infusions. If emesis limits absorption, medication should be administered parenterally.[69] If intravenous access is difficult, consider a subcutaneous infusion. This might be helpful if the child's nausea and vomiting are persistent, or if they have difficulty swallowing, are delirious or have a large pill burden. Subcutaneous infusions are inexpensive, typically well-tolerated, and are practical for home use. The blood levels of medications administered subcutaneously are comparable to those given intravenously. Furthermore, multiple agents of compatible fluids can be delivered in a single infusion. For example, an antiemetic, an opioid, and a steroid can be given in one infusion. Medications that should *not* be given in combination include chlorpromazine, diazepam, and phenytoin.

SUMMARY

Nausea and vomiting are common, dreaded, and complex symptoms. Understanding the pathways and neurotransmitters that lead to nausea and vomiting guides the interventions. Pharmacologic and nonpharmacologic measures should be considered. Evidence for the management of nausea and vomiting not related to chemo is weak.[72] When addressing pharmacy, start with a single agent, adding as necessary, preferably a medication that antagonizes a different neurotransmitter. Consider that several antiemetics antagonize more than one neurotransmitter. When determining whether the medication should be scheduled (e.g., before a specific medication), around the clock, or as needed, consider the cause. Also, one should consider what has worked for the child in similar circumstances in the past. The child and family are often the best guides.

Please refer to Box 25.1 for the nausea and vomiting treatment algorithm.

BOX 25.1 NAUSEA AND VOMITING TREATMENT ALGORITHM

There is no one treatment algorithm for nausea and vomiting. The cause or likely cause will determine first-line therapies. These are general guidelines to consider when initiating antiemetic treatment for children

- Establish the probable cause
  - Eliminate or reduce if possible
- Simple nausea can be treated with over-the-counter medications
- Consider the neural pathways, neurotransmitters/receptors involved (see Table 25.1)
- Select a class of antiemetic that antagonizes those neurotransmitters
- Take most medications after meals
  - If the cause is chemical (e.g., chemotherapy), one is likely to start with a $5HT_3$ antagonist, such as ondansetron or granisetron.
  - If the cause is not evident, consider a serotonin and dopamine antagonist simultaneously[4,72]
  - Vertigo: antihistamine/anticholinergic[72]
- Medications are typically antagonistic for one class of receptors but often show antagonism toward other classes of receptors.
- In an emergency: Prefer "portmanteau" drugs
  - Haloperidol: antidopaminergic
  - Metoclopramide: prokinetic, CTZ blocking
  - Methotrimeprazine: anticholinergic, sedation, analgesia
  - Dimenhydrinate: H_1 and Ach-receptor antagonist
- Using multiple antiemetics for children receiving chemotherapy puts them at greater risk for changes in the way food tastes[90]

In situations where the etiology of nausea and vomiting remains elusive, an empiric approach may be taken:

- Start: metoclopramide, q8h
  - Dual effect: gastric stasis and CTZ
- If not sufficient, add
  - Haloperidol q8h around the clock (atc), or
  - Chlorpromazine q8h atc
  - Ondansetron q12h
- If a third drug is needed: add an antihistamine
  - Hydroxyzine mg q8h atc or diphenhydramine
  - May prevent dystonia from dopamine antagonists
- If not satisfactory: add corticosteroid
  - Dexamethasone qAM

CONSTIPATION

Constipation is a decrease in the passage of stool, both in frequency and volume; the stool is typically small, hard, and lumpy. Constipated stools are often difficult to pass and painful. Sometimes the child has a feeling that evacuation was incomplete, called *rectal tenesmus*.[108]

Constipation is common in children. Approximately 12% of children experience constipation, and about 25% of pediatric GI visits are due to constipation, typically functional constipation.[109] Functional constipation, now called "disorders of gut–brain interaction,"[110] cannot be explained by physiologic abnormalities, including biochemical or structural changes.[111] These children are likely to have multiple comorbidities, such as anxiety, or asthma.[112] Constipation is also common in children undergoing treatment for serious illness, resulting from the effects of disease or treatment, but it is often underrecognized and undertreated.[113]

AN APPROACH TO THE CHILD WITH CONSTIPATION

Constipation in children with a serious illness may be affected by comorbidities or preexisting conditions.[114] Constipation is often a symptom of an underlying disorder; it may be caused by decreased mobility, insufficient dietary fiber, diminished fluid intake, or slow motility of waste material through the large intestine. Medications, foods, or disease may cause constipation. Disease-related causes might include obstruction (e.g., tumor inside, or external to but compressing the intestine), neurologic (e.g., spinal cord involvement), or electrolyte imbalance (e.g., hypercalcemia).

Constipation often leads to other symptoms, including abdominal pain, bloating, or feelings of fullness, nausea, and vomiting. Too often, constipation is missed or misdiagnosed because of diarrhea. A diagnosis of constipation requires a thorough, albeit relatively simple history. The verification of constipation typically can be accomplished with a plain x-ray and does not require advanced imaging.[115] Often, radiologists do not comment on radiographic fecal burden,[115] so it is vital to identify the concern for constipation in the radiology order.

Opioids are a common cause of constipation. Opioid-induced constipation (OIC) occurs because opioid receptors exist in the gut, second in number only to the CNS. There are "mu receptors in the stomach and small intestine, and mu receptors located in the small intestine and proximal colon,"[116] so opioids that bind to mu receptors in the CNS also bind to mu receptors in the gut, causing OIC. When opioids are prescribed for a child, a bowel regimen should always be prescribed simultaneously unless there is a compelling reason not to do so.

HISTORY

All children seeing a palliative care provider should be screened for constipation. Children are often reluctant to discuss their bowel movements and patterns. It is the responsibility of nurses, physicians, and others taking care of children to ask the questions routinely, emphasizing that we ask all children and families about bowel function. Once the questioning is part of the visit routine, the topic can become routine for the child. Whenever possible, it is essential to ask the child directly, as the parent may not be aware of this "intimate" detail.

The history should start with what is "normal" for this child. How often does the child have a bowel movement? What is the color and consistency of a regular bowel movement? With some disorders, such as CF, an unusual fecal odor may be typical. That odor may be embarrassing for the child, limiting their ability to have bowel movements at school or other more public locations. If the child has spina bifida or CF, then the baseline is likely to be different from that of most children. If the child has cancer, "normal" will vary depending on whether it was a time of treatment and whether the treatment is chemotherapy, immunotherapy, transplant, or something else. If the child is receiving chronic opioids, they may have OIC at baseline with exacerbations during times of crisis with increased opioid use. Ask the child. Normalize it.

In addition to frequency, ask about consistency. The Bristol Stool Scale can be used for visual images, if necessary.[117] It has been used in practice and in research to characterize types of stool. It is a 1–7 scale, in which types 1 and 2 indicate constipation, and type 7 indicates watery stool. It has been used as a part of the diagnostic workup for irritable bowel syndrome and Crohn's disease.[117] Most children can talk about consistency with reasonable specificity. "Is it formed, is it soft, is it hard?" This leads to asking about ease of passage. "Do you have to push hard?" Or urgency or fecal incontinence. "Does it ever come out even before you get to the toilet?"

Similarly, children can be specific about color, for example, light brown, dark brown, yellow, green, white. Ask about odor, and if they have noticed any change in smell. This may be a sign of an infection or result from the management of an infection. Alternatively, a strong odor with diarrhea and soiling might indicate constipation with overflow incontinence. Finally, ask about tenesmus. "Do you ever feel like there's more, but you can't get it out?" Of course, with older children, you can use the term "incomplete emptying." If you keep the discussion objective, most children will, too. Some, however, might see if they can "gross you out."

Many medications can contribute to constipation. Besides opioids, other medication offenders include tricyclic antidepressants, anticholinergics, antacids, calcium supplements, calcium channel blockers, diuretics, and iron supplements,[118] as well as phenothiazines, antihistamines, and diuretics.

PHYSICAL EXAM

Assessment for constipation includes a thorough physical exam, with a focus on the abdominal exam and, in some cases, a rectal exam. The abdominal exam should include assessment for distention and tenderness. Palpation can reveal hard, palpable stool in the ascending, descending, or sigmoid colon. Palpation of constipated stool may be easier to detect in a thinner child; however, firmness in any quadrant or region should be noted. The exam should also assess for bladder distention, which may indicate a concomitant or contributing problem.

When including a rectal exam use the fifth finger in small children. The exam should reveal whether there is stool in the vault and its consistency. The rectal exam can also reveal fissures or hemorrhoids. If, however, the child has neutropenia or thrombocytopenia, the rectal exam should be deferred. The neurologic exam is also essential. The examiner should attend to sphincter tone and lower extremity motor weakness or paresthesias.

Alterations in lab values may point to a cause of constipation. Pay attention to thyroid function and electrolyte levels (e.g., hypokalemia, hypercalcemia). In addition to opioids, other medications, including those used to treat nausea and vomiting, may cause constipation.

Constipation should be managed with a stepwise approach.[119] Prevention is ideal, but the management of the existing syndrome is frequently necessary. Treatments for prevention and alleviation are often similar, though medication frequency and the dose may vary.

As with most of palliative care, the cause should be identified and, whenever possible, treated. This might include addressing physical causes, such as weakness or decreased abdominal tone. Posture and positioning while defecating can affect results. Bathroom access may be a problem, including privacy. Even psychological factors such as depression are sometimes related to bowel function, including constipation, in part due to activity and dietary choices. Please see Table 25.2 for medications for the treatment of constipation.

TREATMENT: INTEGRATIVE AND SUPPORTIVE THERAPIES

Nonpharmacological therapies are the first step to the management of constipation, though this might not be sufficient with opioid use. Adequate fiber and fluids are essential, as is establishing a routine.[120] This is sometimes more difficult for children who are in school. Hospitalized children may also have difficulty with structure and privacy. Taking time for attempting a bowel movement after meals, especially after breakfast, is most likely to promote success.

Increased activity promotes intestinal movement. If possible, physical therapy, recreation therapy, or child life may help the child engage in movement that is enjoyable for him. Increasing oral fluid intake is often helpful. Work with the child to identify a repertoire of beverages (not diuretics) because increased fluid intake can increase the chance of laxation. Increasing dietary fiber can usually be done without substantially changing the child's diet. The involvement of a dietician working with the child and family may yield a broader range of dietary options. Some children enjoy prune juice or prunes.

Teaching the child to assume a squatting position to help manage and prevent constipation may facilitate laxation; this is widely practiced in Asia and Africa.[121] Given their smaller

TABLE 25.2 Medications in the treatment of constipation

CLASS	MEDICATION	DOSE	ROUTE OF ADMINISTRATION	COMMENTS AND SIDE EFFECTS
Liquid osmotic laxatives	Lactulose (Enulose) 15g/10 mL	Infants: 0.8–3.5 mL (not per kg) TID Children: 10–30 mL (not per kg) TID	PO	Dose titration to effect beyond these doses possible. Side effects: bloating, cramping, diarrhea, nausea, abdominal pain
	Polyethylene glycol 3350 (Miralax)	8.5–17 g dissolved in 120–240 mL fluid (water, soda, juice) once per day	PO	Side effects: diarrhea, nausea, abdominal pain
	Milk of Magnesia	2–6 yrs: 400–1,200 mg/day 6–12 yrs: 1,200–2,400 mg/day >12 yrs: 2,400–4,800 mg/day	PO	Contraindicated in renal insufficiency
Surfactant laxatives	Docusate sodium (Colace)	>3 yrs: 10–40 mg/day divided in 1–4 doses 3–6 yrs: 20–60 mg/day divided in 1–4 doses 6–12 yrs: 40–120 mg/day divided in 1–4 doses >12 yrs: 50–200 mg/day divided in 1–4 doses	PO	Side effects: diarrhea, nausea, abdominal pain
Stimulants	Senna	Standardized Senna Concentrate 1–5 yrs: 109–218 mg (not per kg) qHS 5–15 yrs: 218–436 mg (not per kg) qHS Sennoside 6 mo–2 yrs: 3.75 mg (not per kg) qHS 3–10 yrs: 7.5–15 mg (not per kg) qHS >10 yrs: 15–30 mg (not per kg) qHS	PO (also as tea), PR	Side effects: nausea, abdominal pain, cramping
	Bisacodyl	6–11 yrs: 5 mg (not per kg) once daily >12 yrs: 5–15 mg (not per kg) once daily	PO, PR	Side effects: nausea, abdominal pain, cramping
Mu receptor antagonists	Methylnaltrexone	0.15 mg/kg q48h; max 8–12 mg	IV, SC	

size or weakness with serious or advanced illness, the use of a footstool can approximate a squatting position.[121]

Other measures that may be helpful with children include acupuncture or acupressure. Abdominal massage, rubbing in slow, clockwise circles can also promote laxation. The child can be taught to do this for herself. Biofeedback may be helpful for constipation and other defecation disorder.[122]

Manual disimpaction may be necessary if the child has abdominal pain and the rectal exam reveals hard stool in the ampulla. Suppositories and enemas (perhaps done serially) might make disimpaction easier. Disimpaction can be very uncomfortable. Premedication is often ideal. For some children, a small dose of a benzodiazepine might make the process easier. The provider must use extra lubrication (a water-soluble gel) to minimize discomfort.

TREATMENT: PHARMACOLOGICAL THERAPIES

When medications are necessary, over-the-counter management is possible for many children, both those who are healthy and those with underlying illness or injury. *Laxatives* are typically the first line of therapy. Types of laxatives include stool softeners, osmotic laxatives, lubricants laxatives, and stimulant laxatives. Understanding the cause of constipation can help identify a starting point, although the inability to specify the cause may necessitate an empirical approach.

Stool softeners, also called *emollient laxatives* or *surfactants* are anionic surfactants that work by pulling water and fat into the stool, lowering the surface tension, thus "softening" the stool. This makes it easier to pass. Docusate is an emollient laxative with a surfactant that comes in pills or liquids formulations. Some children do not like the taste, but children who do well with pills generally tolerate docusate. Stool softeners may be combined with other laxatives, for example, a stimulant, for better effect. An example of this is docusate/senna.

Osmotic laxatives pull water in to soften the stool and thereby ease its passage. The colon does not absorb osmotic laxatives. Increased water also increases stool size, which stimulates the intestinal wall, thereby inducing bowel movements.[123] Osmotic laxatives typically work quickly. They are also used for bowel preparation for colonoscopy. Oral osmotic laxatives include polyethylene glycol (Miralax), magnesium hydroxide (Milk of Magnesia), and lactulose. Glycerin suppositories are also osmotic. Lactulose requires a prescription.

Polyethylene glycol, a commonly used osmotic laxative, is biologically inert, minimally absorbed, and does not influence the transit of other solutes.[111] To work effectively, polyethylene glycol requires that the child drink a particular volume of oral fluids, depending on the child's size.

Magnesium hydroxide should not be used in children with kidney disease.[124] A Cochrane review found that the level of evidence is low or very low to support the recommendation of an osmotic laxative, but that polyethylene glycol might be superior.[125] Many clinicians perceive lactulose as a better laxative, often prescribing it for severe constipation. The Cochrane review, however, found "no evidence to suggest that lactulose is superior to the other agents studied."[125] Side effects of lactulose include flatulence, nausea, diarrhea, abdominal pain, fecal incontinence, and headache.[111,125]

Psyllium is another stool softener that swells and increases the size of the fecal mass. The larger size of the fecal mass can stimulate the defecation reflex. It, too, is safe for children. Laxatives that start as a powder should never be taken in that form, as that can cause esophageal obstruction. Follow package directions and, ideally, follow with another glass of liquid. Psyllium should not be taken with other medications as it can impair their absorption.

Stimulant laxatives are motility agents that work by stimulating the muscles in the intestinal wall to contract to move stool forward.[111] In other words, stimulant laxatives irritate the bowl to increase peristalsis. They also reduce absorption from the stool into the colon.[116] Stimulant laxatives include sennosides (oral) or bisacodyl (oral or suppository). Castor oil, another stimulant laxative, breaks down into the fatty acid ricinoleic acid which activates smooth muscle, creating a calcium surge that stimulates propulsion.[126]

Side effects of stimulant laxatives include dehydration and electrolyte imbalance. Stimulant laxatives are typically the second line of therapy, used for children who do not respond to nonpharmacologic interventions or osmotic laxatives.[124] They should not be used regularly or routinely; regular use can promote dependence due to the development of hypoperistalsis. Always check bowel sounds before administration of a stimulant laxative; bowel rupture can occur if the child has an obstruction.

Lubricant laxatives line the intestine, preventing water from being absorbed from the stool into the bowel. This maintains the stool's softness. Mineral oil is an example of a lubricant laxative that was suggested as an effective laxative in a Cochrane review.[125] The regular use of mineral oil is discouraged, however, as it can impede the absorption of nutrients and fat-soluble vitamins. It should not be given if the child is nauseated, nor before bedtime as aspiration of the oil can occur.

If the administration of laxatives is inadequate to promote regular laxation, or if the side effects limit treatment, additional therapies may be necessary. If slow transit time is suspected, a prokinetic may be helpful. This might include a prokinetic or a prosecretory agent.[119,127]

Prokinetics work by increasing lower esophageal sphincter tone and increasing gastric motility to promote gastric emptying.[128] Cisapride was a commonly used prokinetic agent, but it was taken off the market due to cardiac side effects.[128] Metoclopramide is an effective prokinetic; however, extrapyramidal symptoms (EPS) can limit its use. It is contraindicated in children younger than 1 year, and its use should be limited in children younger than 5 years.[129] In addition to EPS, other side effects include diarrhea and sedation, though all of these effects are reversible and without long-term significance.[129] The addition of metoclopramide to polyethylene glycol may not be more efficacious than polyethylene glycol alone.[130]

Prosecretory agents work by stimulating intestinal chloride secretion as a means to increase intestinal secretions.[131] Two prosecretory agents are lubiprostone and linaclotide. Linaclotide (Linzess) has recently been the subject of a forceful marketing campaign so that parents may be asking for it by name. These medications have not been evaluated for use in children.

Probiotics for children and adults also have received a lot of attention in the lay media and are heavily advertised. Probiotics are available in foods (e.g., added into cottage cheese, or occurring naturally in yogurt or fermented foods) and as over-the-counter supplements. In a careful review of meta-analyses and systematic reviews, Harris and colleagues found no benefit of probiotic in the frequency of children's defecation.[132] One exception is that probiotics might be helpful for children with CF and inherently altered GI function and flora, though the evidence is limited.[133]

Suppositories and *enemas* may be helpful for some children. Glycerin suppositories (see earlier discussion of osmotic laxatives) promote defecation by softening and lubricating. Suppositories can also provide rectal stimulation to encourage defecation. As with adults, children may be reluctant to accept a suppository or enema. It is often more the idea of *rectal* medications that is discomfiting than a history of unpleasant experiences. Maintaining privacy and negotiating for the time of the intervention can help. Rectal administration is contraindicated in a child with thrombocytopenia; often, 50,000 platelets/microliter is used as a cutoff and is not recommended for children with neutropenia. It is important to consider volume when choosing an enema for a child; if possible, use a pediatric formulation to ensure a safe volume.

In a study comparing the efficacy of KLYX enemas (docusate sodium and sorbitol 70%) and suppositories containing free fatty acids (FFAs) in children in the emergency department, the FFA suppositories were as effective as the enema in laxation and symptom relief.[134] The authors posited that the suppository is perceived as less invasive than an enema for the child.

The need for a bowel regimen is lifelong in people with spinal cord injuries and spina bifida. In a study of children with spina bifida, Choi and colleagues found that bowel issues, including constipation and fecal incontinence affect the quality of life not only of children but also of their caregivers.[135] In some pediatric institutions, children's caregivers are asked to continue the bowel and bladder care they had provided to children at home, "because they know it better." When children with chronic bowel needs are hospitalized, it is an opportunity to provide respite for caregivers. The child and parent are often eager to give suggestions about how the routine should best be done for *this* child.

OPIOID-INDUCED CONSTIPATION

Opioid-induced bowel dysfunction is a ubiquitous set of side effects associated with opioid use; common symptoms include not only constipation, but also abdominal pain, bloating, gastroesophageal reflux, nausea, and vomiting.[116] Up to 70–97% of chronic opioid users have OIC, even though daily oral morphine equivalents for most respondents was 50 mg/day or less.[113,136] Many of the GI side effects resolve after a few days on the opioid or are managed with opioid rotation; not true for OIC. OIC is the most common side effect of opioids and has significant deleterious effects on quality of life.[127] Every child on an opioid should have a prescription for a bowel regimen. The American Gastroenterological Association (AGA) has developed guidelines for the management of OIC.[116] Though the guidelines were written for adults, the principles do apply to many aspects of pediatric care.

Management of OIC requires the same tools as constipation from other causes. Many seriously ill children will have reasons for constipation in addition to opioids. Do a complete history, as described earlier, considering physical causes, concurrent medication use, activity level, and the child's experience of constipation in the past. "In patients with OIC, the AGA recommends laxatives as first-line agents."[116] Initial laxatives might include stool softener and osmotic stimulant, with lubricant agent.[137] If nonpharmacologic management coupled with laxatives is not beneficial, a prokinetic should be added.[127]

For patients with OIC, peripherally acting mu-opioid receptor agonists have been approved for OIC, and the AGA recommends these if the preceding interventions have not led to a regular bowel routine. More recently, peripherally acting mu-opioid receptor agonists (PAMORA) have been approved for OIC, especially OIC that is refractory to laxatives.[122,137] PAMORAs act peripherally in the GI tract.[121] Common PAMORAs have been IV (methylnaltrexone) or, more recently, oral (methylnaltrexone, alvimopan, naldemedine, naloxone). Recent guidelines have described the strength of supportive evidence for two oral medications, alvimopan and methylnaltrexone, as weak or nonexistent.[121] In one meta-analysis, people who use a PAMORA have more frequent bowel movements than those who received a placebo, as well as better quality of life; however, they also had more adverse events.[138] Methylnaltrexone IV should be given every other day or every third day, and only rarely should its use be increased.[139] The level of evidence for the use of methylnaltrexone is low.[139]

PAMORAs are not first-line medications and should only be introduced after routine bowel regimens have been tried for a period of time likely to provide benefit. The data about PAMORAs in children remain limited, although in one study with 27 children, 63% had a bowel movement within 24 hours of administration.[140] It is essential that providers follow the administration recommendations and do not, as some have done, recommend a daily administration of a PAMORA with no end specified.

PAMORAs are not recommended in people with advanced illness.[141] Pediatric use is not recommended for methylnaltrexone, naloxegol, alvimopan, or naldemedine.

Lubiprostone is a chloride channel activator;[142] it works by allowing the intestine to pull in water and sodium to increase colonic peristalsis.[143] Lubiprostone has been successfully used to treat functional constipation in children. This is important to consider in the context of children with serious illness as idiopathic constipation can be an unrelated comorbidity. In a study exploring side effects, nausea was significantly more common in Western children than in East Asian children.[144] Lubiprostone has been used for OIC in children, but limited research exists about its use in children.

Please refer to Box 25.2 for the constipation treatment algorithm.

BOX 25.2 CONSTIPATION TREATMENT ALGORITHM

- General history, focus on bowels
- Abdominal exam
- Rectal assessment
- Medication review
- When constipated
  - Dietary/fluids
    - Popsicles
    - Clear drinks
    - Gelatin desserts
  - Other approaches
    - Small frequent meals
    - Consider what the child has a taste for
- Constipation is a symptom of an underlying disorder. Consider and treat the cause
- Reduce or eliminate medications that can cause or contribute to constipation, including opioids, antihistamines, NSAIDs, antacids, iron, benzodiazepines, and diuretics
- If necessary, choose a medication based on the presumed cause
  - The oral route is preferable
  - The rectal route might be necessary; normalize it
    - Avoid the rectal route in thrombocytopenic children

SPECIAL CONSIDERATIONS

Some diseases have specific bowel considerations that should be taken into account. In addition to spina bifida and spinal cord injury (discussed earlier), CF (see Chapter 31 for more details) and MD (see Chapter 19 for more details) require different approaches.

CF is an autosomal recessive disorder that affects multiple organ systems, including the lungs and GI tract. Children with CF are likely to have frequent respiratory infections and GI inflammation associated with intestinal dysbiosis.[133] With significant infections, normal "good" gut bacteria decreases. Because of this change in normal flora, probiotics might be beneficial for children with CF. The introduction of probiotics should only be undertaken with the advice of a provider.

Pancreatic enzymes are used to replace deficiencies in children with CF. Pancreatic enzyme replacement therapy (PERT), such as pancrelipase, allows children with CF to digest food and absorb nutrients. These enzymes are typically taken about an hour before eating. Adherence to clinical guidelines can lead to significant improvements in weight, height, and body mass index (BMI) z-scores.[145]

Constipation and distal intestinal obstruction syndrome (DIOS) are common in children with CF. DIOS differs from constipation in that it is a combination of feces and mucous that adheres to the intestinal wall, causing a blockage.[146]

Muscular dystrophy is a group of at least 30 inherited disorders, each of which leads to progressive weakness and skeletal muscle degeneration.[147] The genetic variations differ between types of MD, but each leads to an impairment in the child's ability to produce dystrophin, a cytoskeletal protein.[148] Duchenne's MD is the most common form, primarily affecting boys, with an age of onset typically by 5 years and an expected survival of about 35 years. Muscular dystrophy is a multisystem disease.[149] GI disorders in some of the MDs include dysmotility, feeding intolerance, and constipation,[150,151] although GI transit time is not impaired in children with MD.[151] GI issues, especially constipation, are frequently underrecognized, and hence, inadequately treated.[151–153] The regimens described earlier typically can be used to manage intestinal dysfunction in children with MD, but, because of their higher risk, the need for ongoing assessment is crucial.

DIARRHEA

The cause and effects of diarrhea vary tremendously around the world. Infectious diarrhea is prevalent in developing countries, where diarrhea contributes to 12–18% of the deaths of children under 5 years of age[154,155] and is the fourth leading cause of under-5 deaths.[156] The causes of diarrhea include viruses, bacteria, and parasites; these organisms impede GI functioning, especially secretion and absorption.[156] In developed countries, the causes of diarrhea differ, and the mortality is strikingly less. The most common cause is viral. Regardless, when it does occur, especially in children with serious underlying illnesses, it can be an emergency.

Most children get diarrhea at some point. Diarrhea can occur from disease (e.g., CF, irritable bowel), treatment (e.g., antibiotics, chemotherapy), or normal childhood activities (e.g., eating too much frosting and inducing a dumping syndrome). In children living with illness, diarrhea can have different causes. For example, in children with cancer, diarrhea may be related to the specific cancer or treatment of the cancer. Other common causes of diarrhea in children living with serious illness or injury include gastroenteritis, malabsorption, laxative overuse, overflow around constipated stool or fecal impaction, radiation therapy, or concurrent illness, such as colitis. Cancer has been identified as an independent risk factor for *Clostridium difficile*-associated colitis in hospitalized children although infectious diarrhea in children with cancer could also be from adenovirus, astrovirus, or norovirus.[157]

Diarrhea includes at least an increased frequency of stools and, more often, the occurrence loose or watery stools; the child may or may not have concurrent symptoms of abdominal cramps, nausea, vomiting, or fever.[158] Bowel movements are more frequent and more liquid because the colon does not reabsorb enough water. Diarrhea is a defense mechanism as the body tries to eliminate toxins and pathogens, which might include medications or infections. Diarrhea is common but can become serious if it leads to dehydration, electrolyte imbalance,[158] or an acid–base imbalance.

What constitutes a "normal" pattern of bowel movements varies with the age of the child, so an assessment of diarrhea must consider the child's baseline. Consider the frequency, consistency, and color. In infants, the variability is also based on whether the child is being breastfed.

Viral gastroenteritis, an intestinal infection, is the most common cause of diarrhea. (NB: "stomach flu" is a distinct misnomer.) This diarrhea may be enterotoxic—caused by an organism that secretes toxins—and lead to a secretory diarrhea. Gastroenteritis may also be cytotoxic, caused by medications such as chemotherapy, or by radiation that causes epithelial damage.[159]

Viral gastroenteritis includes watery diarrhea but is often accompanied by abdominal cramping, nausea, vomiting, and occasionally fever. Viral gastroenteritis typically occurs as a result of contact or by ingesting food or drink that have been contaminated. Symptoms begin 0.5 to 5 days after exposure and persist for 3–7 days. Because of their different fluid volume, children, especially infants and those with compromised immune systems, can rapidly become dehydrated and experience fluid and electrolyte imbalance. They might become seriously ill in a short period. There is no treatment for viral gastroenteritis. Prevention, primarily with handwashing, is crucial.

There are multiple other causes of infectious diarrhea, more likely to occur in developing countries. Indirect mechanisms of infectious diarrhea involve hormones and neurotransmitters that affect GI regulation, as well as inflammatory changes.[160]

Diarrhea can have its complications. Because of its frequency, *C. difficile* (*C diff*) s a good exemplar. *C diff* is the most common cause of hospital-acquired diarrhea.[161] Usually, children older than 2 years are screened after they have had three or more loose stools in 24 hours, though the level of evidence for this recommendation is weak and of very low quality.[162] Guidelines from the Infectious Diseases Society of America (IDSA) now include pediatric considerations. Specifically, they recommended that children not be screened unless their diarrhea is prolonged or worsening, *and* the child has risk factors such as a compromised immune status or exposure that would increase risk, such as antibiotics or hospitalization.[162] This reminds us of the importance of antibiotic stewardship. If antibiotics are necessary, they should be chosen based on local epidemiology and discontinued as soon as possible.[162] Though the evidence is weak, metronidazole or vancomycin is recommended for the treatment of first or first recurrence of *C diff* infection.[162] Children with *C diff* are at risk for pseudomembranous colitis, which occurs when *C diff* overgrowth leads to inflammation or swelling of the colon.

There are four major types of diarrhea. *Osmotic diarrhea* occurs when solutes remain in the intestine, producing an osmotic effect.[159,163] Because water is not absorbed, this water is passed as diarrhea. Causes include lactose intolerance, fat malabsorption, dumping syndrome following GI surgery, or certain medications, such as sorbitol or antacids.[159]

The small intestine typically contains a lot of water before it is absorbed. If the water is not absorbed, secretory diarrhea may develop. Specifically, *secretory diarrhea* occurs when electrolytes or salts are secreted into the intestine, typically due to toxins, such as bacteria, viruses, caffeine, laxatives, medications, or increased bile acids.[163,164] In developing countries, cholera is a common cause of diarrhea, too often fatal.[164]

The gastrointestinal barrier is a permeable border that separates the environment outside of the body from the internal environment.[165] Chronic inflammatory conditions can occur when this barrier is interrupted.[165] One effect of the gastrointestinal barrier being interrupted is that the mechanism of water absorption becomes impaired.[164] Graft versus host disease (GVHD) can also cause diarrhea.[166] The GI lining cannot regenerate quickly, thus leaving the endothelium more susceptible to infection. Patients with GVHD are therefore vulnerable for both secretory and infections diarrhea. *Inflammatory* and *infectious diarrhea* occur when bacteria, viruses, or protozoa cause an interruption to the GI barrier. White blood cells are activated, leading to inflammation. Epithelial cells are damaged or killed, then replaced by immature cells that are incapable of aiding the absorption of nutrients and water.[164] This leads to diarrhea.

Diarrhea due to impaired motility occurs when changes in transit time mean that nutrients and water do not have enough time to be absorbed.[164] Though this altered transit time can lead to diarrhea, it is not clear if it is a unique cause or more an effect of other types of diarrhea.

TREATMENT: INTEGRATIVE AND SUPPORTIVE THERAPIES

Diarrhea has many causes and many mechanisms. Despite this variation, treatments for diarrhea are similar. As with most of palliative care, whenever possible, identify the cause. If possible, eliminate or modify the reason. If the cause cannot be removed (e.g., a course of antibiotics, chemotherapy, or radiation), medications might be necessary (see later discussion). Please see Table 25.3 for medications for the treatment of diarrhea.

It is crucial to identify whether the child is currently dehydrated. If possible, oral rehydration at home should be attempted. Breastfeeding infants should continue to breastfeed.[158,167] Even in hospitalized children, oral rehydration therapy (ORT) is preferable as first-line treatment. There is no greater need for IV rehydration in children who have first used ORT in the outpatient setting; in the emergency department, children started with ORT have about a 4% risk of needing IV rehydration.[168]

If the child has diarrhea due to infection, the child should be supported. The goal is not to stop the diarrhea, but to replace what the child has lost or will lose.[168] They should be encouraged to increase fluid intake to 8–10 glasses a day and to take small, frequent meals.[163] Asking the child what she wants to eat is often a good indicator of what she will tolerate. Complex carbohydrates are often well-tolerated.[158] Encourage foods that might decrease diarrhea (lower fat, lower sugar), and avoid foods that might promote diarrhea (higher sugar drinks, high-fiber foods, fatty foods).[163] Most children can continue an age-appropriate diet, including the intake of regular milk.[158]

For decades, the bananas, rice, applesauce, and tea (or toast) (BRAT) diet has been recommended. One of the challenges of the BRAT diet is that it is restrictive, excluding foods that the child might prefer to eat. No research has been done to support any advantage of the BRAT diet, including the absence of a need for absolute exclusion of milk.[167] Children should eat what they can tolerate.

As a rule, antimotility agents should be avoided. As my mother would say, "better an empty house than an unwelcome guest." Diarrhea often happens because of the harmful bacteria, viruses, or toxins. Slowing motility may mean the retention of deleterious substances, thus prolonging the disease and its adverse effects.[167]

Dehydration looks different at different ages. Look for dry lips and a dry mouth. Monitor the frequency of wet diapers and note any decrease. If a child of any age goes 6 hours without voiding, the child is likely dehydrated.[168] In

TABLE 25.3 Medications in the treatment of diarrhea

MEDICATION	DOSE	ROUTE OF ADMINISTRATION	COMMENTS AND SIDE EFFECTS
Loperamide (Imodium)	0.03–0.27 mg/kg TID	PO	Bloating, constipation; occasionally, central nervous side effects (especially in infants); inhibitors of P-glycoprotein (such as ketoconazole, omeprazole, quinidine, verapamil) allow loperamide to cross the blood–brain barrier and as a result manifest central opioid effects
Bismuth subsalicylate - (Pepto-Bismol)	15–25 mg/kg 5–6 times/day	PO	Limited pediatric data, caution: Reye's syndrome; stool colored black
Cholestyramine (Questran)	0–6 years: 1–2 g BID (–QID) >6 years: 2–4 g BID (–QID)	PO	Few documented adverse effects; dose NOT per kg
Octreotide (Sandostatin)	Starting dose: 1–2 mg/kg BID–TID, titration to effect to >10 mg/kg/dose	IV, SC	Limited pediatric evidence; side effects: nausea, worsening of preexisting arterial hypertonus; cholelithiasis, gallbladder hypercontractility

infants, note the absence of tears with crying. Most children who have diarrhea do not need lab tests unless diarrhea persists for more than a few days or if the child becomes notably dehydrated.

TREATMENT: PHARMACOLOGICAL THERAPIES

Most children with diarrhea will *not* need medications. In some cases, antibiotics might be necessary to treat the infection. Some children with diarrhea have nausea and vomiting, so treatment of that symptom may be required. As with nausea and vomiting, probiotics are unlikely to provide benefit.[132,158] One group of researchers to recommend specific probiotic strains, specifically *Lactobacillus rhamnosis* GG (LGG) and *Saccharomyces boulardii* may be beneficial for children with gastroenteritis as a supplement to ORT.[160]

The specific action of antidiarrheals depends on the cause and type of diarrhea (see earlier discussion). Identify the type of diarrhea to interfere with that cause, influencing ion absorption, secretion, permeability, and other factors of the intestinal environment.[169]

Opioids and opioid-similar medication are mu-receptor opioid agonists, used for moderate to severe diarrhea. They act locally on the GI tract opioid receptors, slowing peristalsis, allowing time for additional water reabsorption from the colon and the development of more solid stools. It also increases the anal sphincter tone. They also have an antisecretory effect. These medications are well-absorbed from the gastrointestinal tract, are almost entirely metabolized by the liver, and are excreted via the bile. These medications include loperamide (Imodium), which is chemically similar to opioids and haloperidol; it does not cross the blood–brain barrier.[170] Loperamide should not be used in children younger than 2 years.

Other opioid antidiarrheals include camphorated opium tincture (Paregoric), difenoxin with atropine (Motofen), and diphenoxylate with atropine (Lomotil). In this case, opioids are combined with atropine to discourage overuse of these drugs. Side effects are the same as opioids used for other indications and can include drowsiness, nausea, dizziness, and constipation. Opioid antidiarrheals should not be used if diarrhea is due to bacteria or toxins; decreased motility will allow the infection to worsen.

Bismuth-containing antidiarrheals work topically on the GI mucosa, providing localized coating effects, absorption of toxins, with some antisecretory and antimicrobial effects. The presence of salicylate means that bismuth subsalicylate should be avoided in children with viral infections. Side effects include constipation, nausea, and tinnitus.

Cholestyramine works by binding intestinal bile acids, increasing fecal elimination, and preventing reabsorption.[171] The primary indication is hypercholesterolemia, as well as for pruritis in people with liver failure. It has been used for children with chronic diarrhea. Cholestyramine has no systemic absorption.[171] It is typically not used in children younger than 6 years of age.

Octreotide has been used off label, outside of FDA approval, in refractory diarrhea associated with chemotherapy, GVHD, and AIDS-associated diarrhea due to cryptosporidium.[172] There is a paucity of data allowing the recommendation of octreotide for use with children, especially those under 6 years of age. Serious adverse effects, including hypoxia, necrotizing enterocolitis, and death are recorded, though children in these studies have severe comorbidities.[172]

Simethicone is used to alleviate symptoms of gas in the stomach and intestines. It is sometimes combined with antacids or antidiarrheals to treat gas pain that may be associated with diarrhea. It works by breaking larger bubbles into smaller ones by reducing surface tension.

SKIN CARE FOR CHILDREN WITH DIARRHEA

Peri-rectal skin irritation is common in children with diarrhea. This occurs for several reasons. The stool is irritating because of the bacteria, and diarrhea is abrasive because the enzymes that help in food digestion can be present and will act on the skin. Soap can also be drying and irritating. Toilet paper and the friction from wiping can also be irritating.

Skin breakdown often can be prevented with frequent hygiene, but with severe diarrhea, skin irritation is common. In this case, barrier creams such as zinc oxide can protect the child's skin from further damage and allow healing.

Please refer to Box 25.3 for the diarrhea treatment algorithm.

BOWEL OBSTRUCTION

Across ages, of those hospitalized for acute abdominal pain, 15% have a bowel obstruction, and 20% of those require surgery.[173] In children, an obstruction may be caused by disease,

BOX 25.3 DIARRHEA TREATMENT ALGORITHM

- The cause of diarrhea should be identified and treated if possible
- Be aware of fluid and electrolyte loss if diarrhea is severe, prolonged, or if the child is an infant or medically fragile
- Supplemental hydration and electrolytes may be required; assess fluid status and electrolyte levels
- Type of antidiarrheal drug chosen will depend on the identified cause
- Categories used include opioids and related, bismuth, bulk-forming
- Treatment depends on severity and etiology
- Medications for simple diarrhea: OTC
  - Loperamide
  - Bismuth compounds
  - Psyllium preparations
  - Probiotic supplements for certain populations
- Opioids for severe diarrhea
  - Most effective
  - Slow peristalsis

hernia, congenital anomalies, surgical complications, ileus, infection, medication side effects (especially opioids), and other causes.

Bowel obstruction is a "mechanical or functional obstruction to the normal passage of products of digestion. It may be partial or complete, involve the small bowel or the large bowel, high grade (with bowel ischemia) or low grade (with intact blood supply), high level (up to the distal ileum) or low level (colonic obstruction)."[174] An obstruction can occur anywhere along the length of the intestine. It may be within the lumen or extraluminal. The blockage may be partial or complete. More severe cases involve intestinal ischemia. Bowel obstruction can be associated with significant morbidity.[175,176] An excellent history to consider risk factors is essential. In children who have had small bowel surgery, the risk for obstruction is greatest in the first year following surgery.[176]

Intussusception occurs when the intestine telescopes on itself. Intussusception is the leading cause of obstruction in children aged 3 months to 3 years.[177]

Pseudo-obstruction is a disorder of motility, not of obstruction. It is difficult to diagnose and can be fatal.[178] Pseudo-obstruction is "characterized by an impairment of coordinated propulsive activity in the gastrointestinal tract mimicking mechanical intestinal obstruction."[179] Pseudo-obstruction occurs because of the altered functioning of nerves and muscles, impeding the normal movement of food and fluid through the GI tract.

HISTORY

The presentation of bowel obstruction varies based on the location of the obstruction. Pain is almost always present; note whether it is continuous or episodic. The child's pain is often cramping, though with a more distal obstruction the pain may be described as deep. The child might have nausea with or without vomiting; vomiting is more common with small intestine obstruction. This makes sense: if the blockage is higher, the path of escape is emesis. If the blockage is lower, the child is more likely to have bowel symptoms. The child with obstruction may have constipation, but if severe, may have diarrhea around the constipated stool.

The symptoms of intussusception typically include pain (severe, intermittent), distention, emesis, and often, rectal bleeding.[177] Diagnosis is confirmed with ultrasound.[177] The symptoms of pseudo-obstruction are similar and include pain, distention, nausea, vomiting, constipation, or diarrhea.[180]

PHYSICAL EXAM AND DIAGNOSTIC STUDIES

The abdomen is often distended, with or without a palpable mass. The abdomen may be tympanic, and bowel sounds may be high-pitched. None of these findings is essential for a diagnosis of bowel obstruction.

Imaging is an essential tool for diagnosing bowel obstruction and may involve x-rays, dye studies, ultrasound, or computed tomography (CT).[174] An abdominal x-ray can demonstrate bowel distention and gas-fluid levels for small bowel obstruction. Flat plates are less sensitive for a low grade or partial obstruction. A CT scan might provide more information about concurrent/causative disease and will guide decision-making about intervention: observation, surgery, endoscopy, or pharmacological. The use of contrast offers information about the location and extent of the obstruction and also will provide information about motility. Gadolinium side effects are rare (<3%) and are less common in children who are sedated.[181] When they do occur, typical side effects are nausea and vomiting.[181] In children who need frequent studies (e.g., children with cancer), the child's apprehension about side effects might make future studies more difficult.[181] Barium is sometimes used and provides a good definition, but it can lead to impaction. Gastrografin is not only used as a contrast medium, but it is also used for therapeutic enema. Consult with radiology who can advise which physical exam factors and clinical considerations should affect the choice of a contrast medium. Esophagogastroduodenoscopy (EGD) may be indicated for some cases of upper GI obstruction.[182]

TREATMENT: INTEGRATIVE AND SUPPORTIVE THERAPIES

Intestinal obstruction is sometimes challenging to identify, but time is essential.[183] Children with a bowel obstruction can become ill quickly, necessitating rapid surgical intervention, though this is the exception. In most children with bowel obstruction, the preferred intervention is nonoperative management,[184] including the correction of electrolyte imbalance, gastric decompression, and fluid resuscitation, with close monitoring of the abdominal exam for 1–2 days.[176] If nasogastric decompression is not possible, a PEG tube may be placed. In one sample, 12% of children required emergency surgery, and the rest received nonoperative management, which was successful in 54% of cases.[184] If possible, a laparoscopic approach is preferred, but an open approach is sometimes necessary.[176] Infants were at significantly greater risk of needing surgical intervention.[150]

In some children, operative management is not possible. In those cases, the approach is focused on improving comfort. This focus on symptom management can improve both comfort and quality of life.[185] This may require patient-controlled analgesia; children have been successfully sent home with follow-up.[185]

Treatment of intussusception is typically done with a pneumatic or hydrostatic enema.[186] Intussusception may recur. If the intussusception does recur, but the child does not have peritoneal signs, the enema is repeated.[177] Peritoneal signs are pronounced, and include pain, rebound tenderness, guarding, and decreased abdominal sounds.

Treatment of pseudo-obstruction is complicated, with too few treatment options.[178] The goal is the restoration of normal intestinal motility, but this is difficult to obtain. No specific medication is recommended to treat pseudo-obstruction.[179] Treatment almost always involves surgery, with extensive nutrition support.[178]

Initially, oral feeding can continue in cases of partial or intermittent obstruction. The child should be permitted small, frequent meals, using a low-residue, low-fiber diet. Complete and continuous obstructions do not preclude oral intake with a trial of occasional, small snacks and sips allowable. When nonoperative management is the path, oral hydration is often not possible. Initially, IV hydration is used. If the condition persists, TPN may be necessary.

TREATMENT: MANAGEMENT OF ASSOCIATED SYMPTOMS

Nausea and vomiting are very common in children with bowel obstruction. Frequently used medications include antisecretory and antiemetic agents. In the case of complete obstruction, prokinetic agents should be avoided. If the child has a partial obstruction without colic, a prokinetic such as metoclopramide might be tried, though the dose should be low and the child should be closely monitored for worsening symptoms. If this occurs, the prokinetic should be stopped.[69] Either an NG or a PEG tube can be very helpful for symptom management, especially nausea and vomiting.

Pain may be the initial symptom in children with bowel obstruction. The pain is often a colic or spasm pain. In this case, a muscarinic agent such as hyoscyamine may be helpful. More severe pain necessitates the use of an opioid. If the child has concurrent kidney injury, morphine and hydromorphone should be avoided due to the risk of accumulation of neuroexcitatory metabolites. Corticosteroids may be used for symptom management, and their anti-inflammatory and anti-secretory effect might, in a few cases, help with the resolution of the obstruction.[187]

Constipation can cause bowel obstruction and should be considered in children with a history of constipation or at risk for constipation (e.g., the child on opioids). Because the stool burden is sometimes not commented on the review of radiographs, the x-ray request should ask specifically about the stool burden. With a partial obstruction, a stool softener at a low dose (to avoid colic) may relieve constipation and symptoms.

Octreotide is a somatostatin analogue that, among other effects, slows intestinal motility, decreasing gastric acid secretion and increasing mucous production.[188] Decreasing the fluid volume may reduce the symptom burden of children with bowel obstruction. In children with pseudo-obstruction, octreotide is advantageous in improving the ability of children who are TPN-dependent to tolerate oral feeds.[189]

Please refer to Box 25.4 for the bowel obstruction treatment algorithm.

BOX 25.4 BOWEL OBSTRUCTION TREATMENT ALGORITHM

- Diagnosis:
  - History:
    - Previous surgery
    - Advanced cancer
    - Inflammatory bowel disease
    - Abdominal XRT
  - Symptoms:
    - Crampy, colicky abdominal pain
    - Bloating
    - Nausea and vomiting
    - Inability to pass stool or flatus
  - Signs:
    - Abdominal tenderness, usually generalized
    - Bowel sounds: high-pitched or absent (in paralytic ileus)
  - Radiographic:
    - Plain abdominal film (initial study of choice)
    - CT scan (may be needed for surgical management)
    - Contrast studies (may be needed for surgical management)
  - Laboratory:
    - Complete metabolic panel
    - Complete blood count
  - Differential diagnosis:
    - Paralytic ileus
      - Postoperative
      - Opioid-induced
    - Severe constipation
  - Initial management:
    - Surgical consultation
    - Volume repletion and electrolyte correction
    - Bowel decompression
      - NG tube (if consistent with goals of care, especially the child's comfort)
      - Venting gastrostomy
      - Bowel stent (if stentable location identified)
    - Medical management:
      - Antisecretory agents
      - Anticholinergics
      - Antiemetics (haloperidol is the first-choice antiemetic in this setting)
      - Pro-kinetics (for partial obstruction; avoid if an obstruction is complete or if colicky pain is prominent)
      - Corticosteroids (reduces bowel edema and inflammation)

CONCLUSION

GI symptoms are common and intrusive. While knowledge about managing these symptoms has increased dramatically in recent decades, much still remains to be learned to allow children to live better. Nausea, vomiting, anorexia, and constipation remain incompletely managed. The burden of these symptoms sometimes impedes the pursuit of additional disease-focused therapies. More research is needed about medications and other interventions. Children will almost certainly benefit from further research into integrative therapies. Perhaps most importantly, clinicians must be aware of the burden of GI symptoms, which should always be included in a review of symptoms so they can be intensively treated.

FAMILY REFLECTION

My son had endured so much suffering during the treatment of cancer. People who have not had cancer, or known someone with cancer, know about the relentless fatigue, the literal gut-wrenching nausea and vomiting, the losing of hair. He had all of that. We were not prepared for the tortuous pain of mucositis. The cracked, bleeding lips; the ulcers that ravaged his mouth, tonsils, and throat; the deep burning in his chest; the ever-present sharp pains in his stomach. Forget about food—water caused so much pain that he didn't even want drops of it. The opioid pain medication dulled the pain, but never relieved it enough so he could eat or drink, and we teetered between uncontrolled pain and being sedated from the treatment of the pain. The supportive [palliative care] team was trying to walk a tight-rope with the medication, but it became an existential nightmare—nobody could tell us when the pain would get better, just that it would. It was then that my son and I saw how the supportive care team *really* functioned. The social worker was able to help my son manage the confusing feelings he was having—anger, sadness, loneliness. She helped me with those feelings, too, but I found the chaplain to be who I really looked to for reassurance that there would be a day when the pain would go away and not just the physical pain my son had. The deep pain a parent feels when they feel helpless to protect their child. My son and I created a motto whenever we felt hopeless: "Who can help? Supportive Care can help!"

REFERENCES

1. Feudtner C, Kang TI, Hexem KR, et al. Pediatric palliative care patients: A prospective multicenter cohort study. *Pediatrics*. 2011;127(6):1094–101. doi:10.1542/peds.2010-3225
2. Gaucher N, Humbert N, Gauvin F. P045: What do we know about pediatric palliative care patients who consult the emergency department? *CJEM*. 2016;18(S1):S93–S94. doi:10.1017/cem.2016.221
3. Linder LA, Stegenga K, Erickson J, et al. Priority symptoms, causes, and self-management strategies reported by AYAs with cancer. *J Pain Symptom Manage*. 2019;58(5):774–783. doi:10.1016/j.jpainsymman.2019.07.008
4. National Comprehensive Cancer Network. NCCN Clinical practice guidelines in oncology. 2020. https://www.nccn.org/guidelines/guidelines-detail?category=3&id=1454
5. Coulson S. Mouth care in children with cancer. *Paediatr Nurs*. 2007;19(4):18.
6. Eilers J, Berger AM, Petersen MC. Development, testing, and application of the oral assessment guide. *Oncol Nurs Forum*. 1988;15(3): 325–330.
7. Drake R, Frost J, Collins JJ. The symptoms of dying children. *J Pain Symptom Manage*. 2003;26(1):594–603.
8. Goldman A, Hewitt M, Collins GS, Childs M, Hain R, United Kingdom Children's Cancer Study Group/Paediatric Oncology Nurses' Forum Palliative Care Working Group. Symptoms in children/young people with progressive malignant disease: United Kingdom Children's Cancer Study Group/Paediatric Oncology Nurses Forum survey. *Pediatrics*. 2006;117(6):e1179–1186. doi:10.1542/peds.2005-0683
9. Arvedson JC. Assessment of pediatric dysphagia and feeding disorders: Clinical and instrumental approaches. *Dev Disabil Res Rev*. 2008;14(2):118–127. doi:10.1002/ddrr.17
10. Weir K, McMahon S, Barry L, Masters IB, Chang AB. Clinical signs and symptoms of oropharyngeal aspiration and dysphagia in children. *Eur Respir J*. 2009;33(3):604–611. doi:10.1183/09031936.00090308
11. DeMatteo C, Matovich D, Hjartarson A. Comparison of clinical and videofluoroscopic evaluation of children with feeding and swallowing difficulties. *Dev Med Child Neurol*. 2005;47(3):149–157. doi:10.1017/s0012162205000289
12. Brooks L. Treatment for dysphagia: A speech language pathologist's perspective. In Ongkasuwan J, Chiou EH, eds. *Pediatric Dysphagia: Challenges and Controversies*. Springer; 2018: 147–161.
13. Santucci G, Mack JW. Common gastrointestinal symptoms in pediatric palliative care: Nausea, vomiting, constipation, anorexia, cachexia. *Pediatr Clin North Am*. 2007;54(5):673–689.
14. Wolfe J, Grier HE, Klar N, et al. Symptoms and suffering at the end of life in children with cancer. *N Engl J Med*. 2000;342(5):326–33. doi:10.1056/NEJM200002033420506
15. Wolfe J, Orellana L, Ullrich C, et al. Symptoms and distress in children with advanced cancer: Prospective patient-reported outcomes from the PediQUEST study. *J Clin Oncol*. 2015;33(17):1928.
16. Collins JJ, Byrnes ME, Dunkel IJ, et al. The measurement of symptoms in children with cancer. *J Pain Symptom Manage*. 2000;19(5):363–77.
17. Madden K, Magno Charone M, Mills S, et al. Systematic symptom reporting by pediatric palliative care patients with cancer: A preliminary report. *J Palliat Med*. 2019;22(8):894–901.
18. Jalmsell L, Kreicbergs U, Onelöv E, Steineck G, Henter J-I. Symptoms affecting children with malignancies during the last month of life: A nationwide follow-up. *Pediatrics*. 2006;117(4):1314–1320.
19. Poole K, Froggatt K. Loss of weight and loss of appetite in advanced cancer: A problem for the patient, the carer, or the health professional? *Palliat Med*. 2002;16(6):499–506.
20. Evans WJ, Morley JE, Argilés J, et al. Cachexia: A new definition. *Clin Nutr*. 2008;27(6):793–799. doi:10.1016/j.clnu.2008.06.013
21. Inui A. Cancer anorexia-cachexia syndrome: Current issues in research and management. *CA Cancer J Clin*. 2002;52(2):72–91.
22. Çağlar K, Kutluk T, Varan A, et al. Leptin and neuropeptide Y plasma levels in children with cancer. *J Pediatr Endocrinol Metabol*. 2005;18(5):485–490.
23. Mak RH, Cheung WW, Zhan J-Y, Shen Q, Foster BJ. Cachexia and protein-energy wasting in children with chronic kidney disease. *Pediatr Nephrol*. 2012;27(2):173–181.
24. Mason P. Anorexia-cachexia: The condition and its causes. *Pharm J*. 2007;
25. Inui A. Feeding-related disorders in medicine, with special reference to cancer anorexia-cachexia syndrome. *Rinsho Byori*. 2006;54(10): 1044–1051.
26. Kotler DP. Cachexia *Ann Intern Med*. 2000;133(8):622–634.
27. Ruiz Garcia V, López-Briz E, Carbonell Sanchis R, Gonzalvez Perales JL, Bort-Martí S. Megestrol acetate for treatment of anorexia-cachexia syndrome. *Cochrane Database Syst Rev*. 2013;(3) doi:10.1002/14651858.CD004310.pub3
28. Couluris M, Mayer JL, Freyer DR, Sandler E, Xu P, Krischer JP. The effect of cyproheptadine hydrochloride (periactin) and megestrol acetate (megace) on weight in children with cancer/treatment-related cachexia. *J Pediatr Hematol Oncol*. 2008;30(11):791–797. doi:10.1097/MPH.0b013e3181864a5e
29. Harrison ME, Norris ML, Robinson A, Spettigue W, Morrissey M, Isserlin L. Use of cyproheptadine to stimulate appetite and body weight gain: A systematic review. *Appetite*. 2019;137:62–72.
30. Azcona C, Castro L, Crespo E, Jimenez M, Sierrasesumaga L. Megestrol acetate therapy for anorexia and weight loss in children with malignant solid tumours. *Aliment Pharmacol Ther*. 1996;10(4): 577–586. doi:10.1046/j.1365-2036.1996.25166000.x
31. Orme LM, Bond JD, Humphrey MS, et al. Megestrol acetate in pediatric oncology patients may lead to severe, symptomatic adrenal suppression. *Cancer*. 2003;98(2):397–405.
32. Meacham LR, Mazewski C, Krawiecki N. Mechanism of transient adrenal insufficiency with megestrol acetate treatment of cachexia in

children with cancer. *J Pediatr Hematol Oncol*. 2003;25(5):414–417. doi:10.1097/00043426-200305000-00013
33. Marchand V, Motil KJ, NASPGHAN Committee on Nutrition. Nutrition support for neurologically impaired children: A clinical report of the North American Society for Pediatric Gastroenterology, Hepatology, and Nutrition. *J Pediatr Gastroenterol Nutr*. 2006;43(1):123–135. doi:10.1097/01.mpg.0000228124.93841.ea
34. Eubanks V, Koppersmith N, Wooldridge N, et al. Effects of megestrol acetate on weight gain, body composition, and pulmonary function in patients with cystic fibrosis. *J Pediatr*. 2002;140(4):439–444. doi:10.1067/mpd.2002.121936
35. Stockheim JA, Daaboul JJ, Yogev R, Scully SP, Binns HJ, Chadwick EG. Adrenal suppression in children with the human immunodeficiency virus treated with megestrol acetate. *J Pediatr*. 1999;134(3):368–370. doi:10.1016/s0022-3476(99)70467-1
36. Romano C, Van Wynckel M, Hulst J, et al. European Society for Paediatric Gastroenterology, Hepatology and Nutrition guidelines for the evaluation and treatment of gastrointestinal and nutritional complications in children with neurological impairment. *J Pediatr Gastroenterol Nutr*. 2017;65(2):242–264.
37. Kim J, Lee M, Kim SC, Joo CU, Kim SJ. Comparison of percutaneous endoscopic gastrostomy and surgical gastrostomy in severely handicapped children. *Pediatr Gastroenterol Hepatol Nutr*. 2017;20(1):27–33.
38. Naureckas SM, Christoffel KK. Nasogastric or gastrostomy feedings in children with neurologic disabilities. *Clin Pediatr (Phila)*. 1994;33(6):353–359. doi:10.1177/000992289403300608
39. Sleigh G, Brocklehurst P. Gastrostomy feeding in cerebral palsy: A systematic review. *Arch Dis Child*. 2004;89(6):534–539.
40. Sullivan PB, Juszczak E, Bachlet AM, et al. Impact of gastrostomy tube feeding on the quality of life of carers of children with cerebral palsy. *Dev Med Child Neurol*. 2004;46(12):796–800. doi:10.1017/s0012162204001392
41. Townsend JL, Craig G, Lawson M, Reilly S, Spitz L. Cost-effectiveness of gastrostomy placement for children with neurodevelopmental disability. *Arch Dis Child*. 2008;93(10):873–877. doi:10.1136/adc.2007.133454
42. Gantasala S, Sullivan PB, Thomas AG. Gastrostomy feeding versus oral feeding alone for children with cerebral palsy. *Cochrane Database Syst Rev*. 31 2013;(7):CD003943. doi:10.1002/14651858.CD003943.pub3
43. Mahant S, Friedman JN, Connolly B, Goia C, Macarthur C. Tube feeding and quality of life in children with severe neurological impairment. *Arch Dis Child*. 2009;94(9):668–673. doi:10.1136/adc.2008.149542
44. Campwala I, Perrone E, Yanni G, Shah M, Gollin G. Complications of gastrojejunal feeding tubes in children. *J Surg Res*. 2015;199(1):67–71.
45. Morse J, Baird R, Muchantef K, Levesque D, Morinville V, Puligandla PS. Gastrojejunostomy tube complications—a single center experience and systematic review. *J Pediatr Surg*. 2017;52(5):726–733.
46. Bouleuc C, Anota A, Cornet C, et al. Impact on health-related quality of life of parenteral nutrition for patients with advanced cancer cachexia: Results from a randomized controlled trial. *Oncologist*. 2020;25(5):e843.
47. Tobberup R, Thoresen L, Falkmer UG, Yilmaz MK, Solheim TS, Balstad TR. Effects of current parenteral nutrition treatment on health-related quality of life, physical function, nutritional status, survival and adverse events exclusively in patients with advanced cancer: A systematic literature review. *Crit Rev Oncol Hematol*. 2019;139:96–107.
48. Obling SR, Wilson BV, Pfeiffer P, Kjeldsen J. Home parenteral nutrition increases fat free mass in patients with incurable gastrointestinal cancer. Results of a randomized controlled trial. *Clin Nutr*. 2019;38(1):182–190.
49. Lundholm K, Daneryd P, Bosaeus I, Körner U, Lindholm E. Palliative nutritional intervention in addition to cyclooxygenase and erythropoietin treatment for patients with malignant disease: Effects on survival, metabolism, and function: A randomized prospective study. *Cancer*. 2004;100(9):1967–1977.
50. Cotogni P, De Carli L, Passera R, et al. Longitudinal study of quality of life in advanced cancer patients on home parenteral nutrition. *Cancer Med*. 2017;6(7):1799–1806.
51. Cotogni P, Ossola M, Passera R, et al. Home parenteral nutrition prolongs survival in incurable malnourished cancer patients: A prospective cohort study. SSRN. 2019.
52. Cotogni P, Monge T, Passera R, Brossa L, De Francesco A. Clinical characteristics and predictive factors of survival of 761 cancer patients on home parenteral nutrition: A prospective, cohort study. *Cancer Medicine*. 2020;
53. Tran LC, Lazonby G, Morello R, et al. How good is quality-of-life for children receiving home parenteral nutrition? A pilot study. *Clinical nutrition ESPEN*. 2019;29:119–124.
54. Mutanen A, Kosola S, Merras-Salmio L, Kolho K-L, Pakarinen MP. Long-term health-related quality of life of patients with pediatric onset intestinal failure. *J Pediatr Surg*. 2015;50(11):1854–1858.
55. Northington L, Lyman B, Moore C, Guenter P. Pediatric nasogastric tubes in the home: Recommendations for practice. *Home Healthc Now*. 2018;36(3):148–153.
56. NHS Quality Improvement Scotland. Information and advice provision for parents and carers of nasogastric and gastrostomy fed children. Updated August 2007. http://www.healthcareimprovementscotland.org/previous_resources/best_practice_statement/gastrostomy_nasogastric_advice.aspx
57. Zangen T, Ciarla C, Zangen S, et al. Gastrointestinal motility and sensory abnormalities may contribute to food refusal in medically fragile toddlers. *J Pediatr Gastroenterol Nutr*. 2003;37(3):287–293. doi:10.1097/00005176-200309000-00016
58. Madden K, Bruera E. Very-low-dose methadone to treat refractory neuropathic pain in children with cancer. *J Palliat Med*. 2017;20(11):1280–1283.
59. Balaban CD, Yates BJ. What is nausea? A historical analysis of changing views. *Auton Neurosci*. 2017;202:5–17. doi:https://doi.org/10.1016/j.autneu.2016.07.003
60. Kovacic K, Williams S, Li BUK, Chelimsky G, Miranda A. High prevalence of nausea in children with pain-associated functional gastrointestinal disorders: Are Rome Criteria applicable? *J Pediatr Gastroenterol Nutr*. 2013;57(3):311–315. doi:10.1097/MPG.0b013e3182964203
61. Li BUK, Kovacic, K. Nausea, vomiting, and pyloric stenosis. In Kleinman RE, Goulet O-J, Mieli-Vergani G, Sanderson IR, Sherman PM, Shneider BL, eds. *Walker's Pediatric Gastrointestinal Disease: Physiology, Diagnosis, Management*. 6th ed. People's Medical House; 2018.
62. Singh P, Kuo B. Central aspects of nausea and vomiting in GI disorders. *Curr Treat Options Gastroenterol*. 2016;14(4):444–451. doi:10.1007/s11938-016-0107-x
63. Samprathi M, Jayashree M. Child with vomiting. *Indian J Pediatr*. 2017;84(10):787–791. doi:10.1007/s12098-017-2456-4
64. Hasler WL. Pharmacological causes and treatments of nausea and vomiting. In Koch KL, Hasler WL, eds. *Nausea and Vomiting: Diagnosis and Treatment*. Springer International; 2017: 119–137.
65. Shaikh SI, Nagarekha D, Hegade G, Marutheesh M. Postoperative nausea and vomiting: A simple yet complex problem. *Anesth Essays Res*. 2016;10(3):388–396. doi:10.4103/0259-1162.179310
66. Bhakta AG, Goel R. Causes and treatment of nausea and vomiting. *Prescriber*. 2017;28(7):17–23.
67. Canziani BC, Uestuener P, Fossali EF, et al. Clinical practice: Nausea and vomiting in acute gastroenteritis: Physiopathology and management. *Eur J Pediatr*. 2018;177(1):1–5. doi:10.1007/s00431-017-3006-9
68. MacDougall MR, Sharma S. Physiology, chemoreceptor trigger zone. StatPearls. Updated February 3, 2019. https://www.ncbi.nlm.nih.gov/books/NBK537133/#__NBK537133_dtls__
69. Keeley PW. Nausea and vomiting in palliative care. *Medicine*. 2020;48(1):14–17. doi:https://doi.org/10.1016/j.mpmed.2019.10.009
70. Baxter AL, Watcha MF, Baxter WV, Leong T, Wyatt MM. Development and validation of a pictorial nausea rating scale for children *Pediatrics*. 2011;127(6):e1542. doi:10.1542/peds.2010-1410

71. Watcha MF, Lee AD, Medellin E, Felberg MT, Bidani SA. Clinical use of the pictorial Baxter Retching Faces scale for the measurement of postoperative nausea in children. *Anesth Analg*. 2019;128(6):1249–1255. doi:10.1213/ane.0000000000003850
72. NCCN. Antiemesis. NCCN Guidelines Version 1.2020. Updated 15 2020. NCCN. https://www.nccn.org/professionals/physician_gls/pdf/antiemesis.pdf
73. National Comprehensive Cancer Network. NCCN Guidelines for patients. Nausea and vomiting. 2020. https://www.nccn.org/patients/guidelines/content/PDF/nausea-patient.pdf
74. Weaver MS, Robinson J, Wichman C. Aromatherapy improves nausea, pain, and mood for patients receiving pediatric palliative care symptom-based consults: A pilot design trial. *Palliat Support Care*. 2020;18(2):158–163.
75. Weaver M, Carter B, Keefer P, Korones DN, Miller EG. *Pediatric Palliative Care and Hospice*. 5th ed. Vol 7. *Essential Practices in Hospice & Palliative Medicine*. American Academy of Hospice & Palliative Medicine; 2017.
76. Hesketh PJ, Kris MG, Basch E, et al. Antiemetics: American Society of Clinical Oncology Clinical Practice guideline update. *J Clin Oncol*. 2017;35(28):3240–3261. doi:10.1200/JCO.2017.74.4789
77. Chokshi SK, Ladas EJ, Taromina K, et al. Predictors of acupuncture use among children and adolescents with cancer. *Pediatric Blood & Cancer*. 2017;64(7):e26424. doi:10.1002/pbc.26424
78. Dupuis LL, Sung L, Molassiotis A, Orsey AD, Tissing W, van de Wetering M. 2016 Updated MASCC/ESMO consensus recommendations: Prevention of acute chemotherapy-induced nausea and vomiting in children. *Support Care Cancer*. 2017/01/01 2017;25(1):323–331. doi:10.1007/s00520-016-3384-y
79. Hines S, Steels E, Chang A, Gibbons K. Aromatherapy for treatment of postoperative nausea and vomiting. *Cochrane Database Syst Rev*. 2012 Apr 18;(4):CD007598. doi:10.1002/14651858.CD007598.pub2. Update in: Cochrane Database Syst Rev. 2018 Mar 10;3:CD007598. PMID: 22513952.
80. Denholm L, Gallagher G. Physiology and pharmacology of nausea and vomiting. *Anaesth Intens Care Med*. 2018;19(9):513–516. doi:https://doi.org/10.1016/j.mpaic.2018.06.010
81. Ruggiero A, Rizzo D, Catalano M, Coccia P, Triarico S, Attiná G. Acute chemotherapy-induced nausea and vomiting in children with cancer: Still waiting for a common consensus on treatment. *J Int Med Res*. 2018;46(6):2149–2156. doi:10.1177/0300060518765324
82. Theriot J, Wermuth HR, Ashurst JV. Antiemetic serotonin-5-HT3 receptor blockers. StatPearls. Updated October 29, 2019. https://www.statpearls.com/ArticleLibrary/viewarticle/38853
83. Basch E, Prestrud AA, Hesketh PJ, et al; American Society of Clinical Oncology. Antiemetic use in oncology: Updated guideline recommendations from ASCO. *Am Soc Clin Oncol Educ Book*. 2012;(32):532–540. doi:10.14694/EdBook_AM.2012.32.230
84. ICN Richtlijnwerkgroep. Nausea and vomiting, version 4.0. Integraal Kankercentrum Nederland (KNL). https://www.oncoline.nl/index.php?pagina=/richtlijn/item/pagina.php&id=39044&richtlijn_id=986
85. Smith HS, Cox, Lorraine R, Smith, Benjamin R. Dopamine receptor antagonists. *Ann Palliat Med*. 2012;1(2):6. https://apm.amegroups.com/article/view/1039/1266. doi:10.3978/j.issn.2224-5820.2012.07.09
86. Smith HS, Smith JM, Seidner P. Opioid-induced nausea and vomiting. *Ann Palliat Med*. 2012;1(2):121–129.
87. Saternos HC, Almarghalani DA, Gibson HM, et al. Distribution and function of the muscarinic receptor subtypes in the cardiovascular system. *Physiol Genomics*. 2017;50(1):1–9. doi:10.1152/physiolgenomics.00062.2017
88. Pedigo NW, Brizzee KR. Muscarinic cholinergic receptors in area postrema and brainstem areas regulating emesis. *Brain Res Bull*. 1985; 14(2):169–177.doi:https://doi.org/10.1016/0361-9230(85)90076-0
89. Chen S, Lu M, Liu D, et al. Human substance P receptor binding mode of the antagonist drug aprepitant by NMR and crystallography. *Nat Commun*. 2019;10(1):638. doi:10.1038/s41467-019-08568-5
90. Nolden A, Joseph PV, Kober KM, et al. Co-occurring gastrointestinal symptoms are associated with taste changes in oncology patients receiving chemotherapy. *J Pain Symptom Manage*. 2019;58(5):756–765. doi:https://doi.org/10.1016/j.jpainsymman.2019.07.016
91. Ibrahim MA, Preuss CV. Antiemetic Neurokinin-1 Receptor Blockers. 2021 Feb 17. In: StatPearls [Internet]. Treasure Island (FL): StatPearls Publishing; 2021 Jan–. PMID: 29262116.
92. Jacob D, Busciglio I, Burton D, et al. Effects of NK1 receptors on gastric motor functions and satiation in healthy humans: Results from a controlled trial with the NK1 antagonist aprepitant. *Am J Physiol Gastrointest Liver Physiol*. 2017;313(5):G505–G510. doi:10.1152/ajpgi.00197.2017
93. National Academies of Sciences Engineering, and Medicine. *The Health Effects of Cannabis and Cannabinoids*. National Academies Press; 2017.
94. Elder JJ, Knoderer HM. Characterization of dronabinol usage in a pediatric oncology population. *J Pediatr Pharmacol Ther*. 2015;20(6):462–467. doi:10.5863/1551-6776-20.6.462
95. FDA. FDA approves Valeant's Cesamet. FDA. 24 May 2006. https://www.fdanews.com/articles/87057-fda-approves-valeant-s-cesamet
96. FDA. Marinol: Full prescribing information. FDA. Updated August 2017. Accessed February 4, 2020. https://www.accessdata.fda.gov/drugsatfda_docs/label/2017/018651s029lbl.pdf
97. Turcotte D, Doupe M, Torabi M, et al. Nabilone as an adjunctive to gabapentin for multiple sclerosis-induced neuropathic pain: A randomized controlled trial. *Pain Med*. 2015;16(1):149–159. doi:10.1111/pme.12569
98. Bradford May M, Glode AE. Dronabinol for chemotherapy-induced nause and vomiting unresponsive to antiemetics. *Cancer Manag Res*. 2016;8:49–55.
99. Polito S, MacDonald T, Romanick M, et al. Safety and efficacy of nabilone for acute chemotherapy-induced vomiting prophylaxis in pediatric patients: A multicenter, retrospective review. *Pediatr Blood Cancer*. 2018;65(12):e27374. doi:10.1002/pbc.27374
100. Badowski ME. A review of oral cannabinoids and medical marijuana for the treatment of chemotherapy-induced nausea and vomiting: A focus on pharmacokinetic variability and pharmacodynamics. *Cancer Chemother Pharmacol*. 2017;80(3):441–449. doi:10.1007/s00280-017-3387-5
101. Ho C, MacDougal D. Nabilone for the treatment of nausea and vomiting or anorexia: A review of clinical effectiveness and guidelines. Updated 27 Feb 2019. https://cadth.ca/index.php/nabilone-treatment-nausea-and-vomiting-or-anorexia-review-clinical-effectiveness-and-guidelines
102. Ofir R, Bar-Sela G, Weyl Ben-Arush M, Postovsky S. Medical marijuana use for pediatric oncology patients: Single institution experience. *Pediatr Hematol Oncol*. 2019;36(5):255–266.
103. Madden K, Tanco K, Bruera E. Clinically significant drug-drug interaction between methadone and cannabidiol. *Pediatrics*. 2020;145(6)
104. Sorribes IC, Moore MNJ, Byrne HM, Jain HV. A biomechanical model of tumor-induced intracranial pressure and edema in brain tissue. *Biophys J*. 2019;116(8):1560–1574. doi:https://doi.org/10.1016/j.bpj.2019.02.030
105. Flank J, Schechter T, Gibson P, et al. Olanzapine for prevention of chemotherapy-induced nausea and vomiting in children and adolescents: A multi-center, feasibility study. *Support Care Cancer*. 2018;26(2):549–555.
106. Navari RM. Management of chemotherapy-induced nausea and vomiting in pediatric patients. *Pediatr Drugs*. 2017;19(3):213–222.
107. Flank J, Robinson PD, Holdsworth M, et al. Guideline for the treatment of breakthrough and the prevention of refractory chemotherapy-induced nausea and vomiting in children with cancer. *Pediatr Blood Cancer*. 2016;63(7):1144–1151.
108. National Institute of Diabetes and Digestive and Kidney Diseases. Definition & facts for constipation. NIH. Updated May 2018. https://www.niddk.nih.gov/health-information/digestive-diseases/constipation/definition-facts

109. Tambucci R, Quitadamo P, Thapar N, et al. Diagnostic tests in pediatric constipation. *J Pediatr Gastroenterol Nutr.* 2018;66(4):e89–e98. doi:10.1097/MPG.0000000000001874
110. Schmulson MJ, Drossman DA. What is new in Rome IV. *J Neurogastroenterol Motil.* 2017;23(2):151–163. doi:10.5056/jnm16214
111. Koppen IJN, Broekaert IJ, Wilschanski M, et al. Role of polyethylene glycol in the treatment of functional constipation in children. *J Pediatr Gastroenterol Nutr.* 2017;65(4):361–363. doi:10.1097/mpg.0000000000001704
112. Colman RJ, Rosario NBS, Gutierrez Bonilla A, et al. Prevalence of functional GI disorders among pediatric patients with persistent asthma. *J Digest Dis.* 2018/09/01 2018;19(9):522–528. doi:10.1111/1751-2980.12653
113. Valenta S, Spichiger E, Paul SM, et al. A longitudinal study of predictors of constipation severity in oncology outpatients with unrelieved pain. *J Pain Symptom Manage.* 2020;59(1):9–19.e1. doi:https://doi.org/10.1016/j.jpainsymman.2019.08.027
114. Danly D. *The Compounding Costs of Constipation.* AAHMP; 2019: 6–7.
115. Rangan V. Taking a load off diagnosing constipation: Utility of the plain film. *Dig Dis Sci.* 2019;64(12):3369–3371. doi:10.1007/s10620-019-05878-y
116. Crockett SD, Greer KB, Heidelbaugh JJ, Falck-Ytter Y, Hanson BJ, Sultan S. American Gastroenterological Association Institute guideline on the medical management of opioid-induced constipation. *Gastroenterology.* 2019;156(1):218–226. doi:https://doi.org/10.1053/j.gastro.2018.07.016
117. Chumpitazi BP, Self MM, Czyzewski DI, Cejka S, Swank PR, Shulman RJ. Bristol Stool Form Scale reliability and agreement decreases when determining Rome III stool form designations. *Neurogastroenterol Motil.* 2016;28(3):443–448. doi:10.1111/nmo.12738
118. Kapo J, Hui F, Giddings-Connolly R, et al. *Essentials 4: Nonpain Symptom Management.* 5th ed. vol UNIPAC 4. *Essential Practices in Hospice & Palliative Medicine.* AAHMP; 2017.
119. Vriesman MH, Koppen IJN, Camilleri M, Di Lorenzo C, Benninga MA. Management of functional constipation in children and adults. *Nat Rev Gastroenterol Hepatol.* 2020;17(1):21–39. doi:10.1038/s41575-019-0222-y
120. National Institute of Diabetes and Digestive and Kidney Diseases. Treatment for constipation in children. National Institutes of Health, NIDDK. Updated May 2018. https://www.niddk.nih.gov/health-information/digestive-diseases/constipation-children/treatment
121. Wald A. Update on the management of constipation. *JAMA.* 2019;322(22):2239–2240. doi:10.1001/jama.2019.16029
122. Bharucha AE, Wald A. Chronic constipation. *Mayo Clinic Proceedings.* 2019;94(11):2340–2357. doi:https://doi.org/10.1016/j.mayocp.2019.01.031
123. Mori S, Tomita T, Fujimura K, et al. A randomized double-blind placebo-controlled trial on the effect of magnesium oxide in patients with chronic constipation. *J Neurogastroenterol Motil.* 2019;25(4):563–575. doi:10.5056/jnm18194
124. Texas Children's Hospital. Over-the-counter medications for kids—Part 2: Constipation, gas/indigestion and probiotics. Updated May 8, 2014. https://www.texaschildrens.org/blog/2014/05/over-counter-medications-kids-%E2%80%93-part-2-constipation-gasindigestion-and-probiotics
125. Gordon M, MacDonald JK, Parker CE, Akobeng AK, Thomas AG. Osmotic and stimulant laxatives for the management of childhood constipation. *Cochrane Database Syst Rev.* 2016 Aug 17;2016(8):CD009118. doi:10.1002/14651858.CD009118.pub3. PMID: 27531591; PMCID: PMC6513425.
126. Alookaran J, Tripp J. Castor Oil. 2021 Jul 8. In: StatPearls [Internet]. Treasure Island (FL): StatPearls Publishing; 2021 Jan–. PMID: 31869090.
127. Daniali M, Nikfar S, Abdollahi M. Evaluating naloxegol for the treatment of opioid-induced constipation. *Expert Opin Pharmacother.* 2020;21(8):883–891. doi:10.1080/14656566.2020.1735354
128. Vieira M. Gastroesophageal reflux and prokinetics. In Vandenplas Y, ed. *Gastroesophageal Reflux in Children.* Springer; 2017: 313–320.
129. Lau Moon Lin M, Robinson PD, Flank J, Sung L, Dupuis LL. The safety of metoclopramide in children: A systematic review and meta-analysis. *Drug Safety.* 2016;39(7):675–687. doi:10.1007/s40264-016-0418-9
130. Frazer K, Wells J. What is the role of prokinetic agents in patients with constipation? *Evidence-Based Practice.* 2016;19(4):7. doi:10.1097/01.EBP.0000541191.93721.ca
131. Yang H, Ma T. Luminally acting agents for constipation treatment: A review based on literatures and patents. *Front Pharmacol.* 2017;8:418. doi:10.3389/fphar.2017.00418
132. Harris RG, Neale EP, Ferreira I. When poorly conducted systematic reviews and meta-analyses can mislead: A critical appraisal and update of systematic reviews and meta-analyses examining the effects of probiotics in the treatment of functional constipation in children. *Amer J Clin Nutr.* 2019;110(1):177–195. doi:10.1093/ajcn/nqz071
133. Ananthan A, Balasubramanian H, Rao S, Patole S. Probiotic supplementation in children with cystic fibrosis—a systematic review. *Eur J Pediatr.* 2016;175(10):1255–1266. doi:10.1007/s00431-016-2769-8
134. Ormarsson OT, Asgrimsdottir GM, Loftsson T, Stefansson E, Lund SH, Bjornsson ES. Free fatty acid suppositories are as effective as docusate sodium and sorbitol enemas in treating constipation in children. *Acta Paediatrica.* 2016;105(6):689–694. doi:10.1111/apa.13394
135. Choi EKI, Young Jae; Han, Sang Won. Bowel management and quality of life in children with spina bifida in South Korea. *Gastroenterol Nurs.* 2017;40(3):208–215. doi:https://doi.org/10.1097/SGA.0000000000000135
136. Dekel BGS, Sorella MC, Vasarri A, Gori A, Melotti RM. Opioid-induced constipation in mixed chronic pain patients: Prevalence and predictors analysis. *J Opioid Manag.* 2019;15(5)doi:https://doi.org/10.5055/jom.2019.0527
137. Rao VL, Micic D, Davis AM. Medical management of opioid-induced constipation. *JAMA.* 2019;322(22):2241–2242. doi:10.1001/jama.2019.15852
138. Nishie K, Yamamoto S, Yamaga T, Horigome N, Hanaoka M. Peripherally acting μ-opioid antagonist for the treatment of opioid-induced constipation: Systematic review and meta-analysis. *J Gastroenterol Hepatol.* 2019;34(5):818–829. doi:10.1111/jgh.14586
139. Portenoy RK, Mehta Z, Ahmed E. Prevention and management of side effects in patients receiving opioids for chronic pain. UpToDate. Updated 27 July 2021. https://www.uptodate.com/contents/prevention-and-management-of-side-effects-in-patients-receiving-opioids-for-chronic-pain
140. Novak C, Hogg A, Sue K, Davies D. Peripherally acting μ-opioid receptor antagonists for treatment of opioid-induced constipation in children. *Paediatr Child Health.* 2020; doi:10.1093/pch/pxz165
141. Uritsky TJ. Methylnaltrexone: Peripherally acting μ-opioid receptor antagonist. *J Adv Pract Oncol.* 2019;10(1):62–67.
142. Hyman PE, Di Lorenzo C, Prestridge LL, Youssef NN Ueno R. Lubiprostone for the treatment of functional constipation in children. *J Pediatr Gastroenterol Nutr.* 2014;58(3):283–291.
143. Wilson N, Schey R. Lubiprostone in constipation Clinical evidence and place in therapy. *Ther Adv Chronic Dis.* 2015;5(2):40–50.
144. Sugimoto M, Murata M, Mizuno H. Differences in efficacy and safety of lubiprostone used for idiopathic vs opioid-induced constipation: Meta-analysis of East Asian and Western populations. *J Clin Biochem Nutr.* 2020:19–118.
145. Ruseckaite R, Pekin N, King S, et al. Evaluating the impact of 2006 Australasian Clinical Practice Guidelines for nutrition in children with cystic fibrosis in Australia. *Respiratory Medicine.* 2018/09/01/2018;142:7–14. doi:https://doi.org/10.1016/j.rmed.2018.07.007
146. Green J, Gilchrist, Francis J, Carroll, Will. Interventions for preventing distal intestinal obstruction syndrome (DIOS) in cystic

fibrosis. *Cochrane Database Syst Rev*. 2018;2018(6):CD012619. doi:10.1002/14651858.CD012619.pub2

147 National Institute of Neurological Disorders and Stroke. Muscular dystrophy information page. NINDS. Updated December 17 2019. https://www.ninds.nih.gov/Disorders/All-Disorders/Muscular-Dystrophy-Information-Page

148. Genetics Home Reference. Duchenne and Becker muscular dystrophy. https://medlineplus.gov/genetics/condition/duchenne-and-becker-muscular-dystrophy/. Last updated 18 August 2020.

149. Birnkrant DJ, Bushby K, Bann CM, et al. Diagnosis and management of Duchenne muscular dystrophy, Part 1: Diagnosis and neuromuscular, rehabilitation, endocrine, and gastrointestinal and nutritional management. *The Lancet Neurology*. 2018;17(3):251–267. doi:https://doi.org/10.1016/S1474-4422(18)30024-3

150. Bortolin K, Ceballos Saenz D, Zizzo A, Campbell C. A303 Gastrointestinal manifestations in patients with congenital myotonic dystrophy. *J Canadian Assn Gastroenterol*. 2018;1(suppl_2):434–435. doi:10.1093/jcag/gwy009.303

151. Kraus D, Wong B, Hu S, Kaul A. Gut transit in Duchenne muscular dystrophy is not impaired: A study utilizing wireless motility capsules *J Pediatrics*. 2018;194:238–240. doi:https://doi.org/10.1016/j.jpeds.2017.10.063

152. Brumbaugh D, Watne L, Gottrand F, et al. Nutritional and gastrointestinal management of the patient with Duchenne muscular dystrophy. *Pediatrics*. 2018;142(Supplement 2):S53. doi:10.1542/peds.2018-0333G

153. Kraus D. Wong BL, Horn PS, Kaul A. Constipation in Duchenne muscular dystrophy: Prevalence, diagnosis, and treatment. *J Pediatrics*. 2016;171:183–188. doi:https://doi.org/10.1016/j.jpeds.2015.12.046

154. Chirla SD, Datla S. Efficacy of zinc therapy in acute diarrhea in children. *Int J Contemp Pediatr*. 2018 Nov;5(6):2228–2231. doi:http://dx.doi.org/10.18203/2349-3291.ijcp20184285

155. Kotloff KL. The burden and etiology of diarrheal illness in developing countries. *Pediatr Clin North Am*. 2017;64(4):799–814. doi:https://doi.org/10.1016/j.pcl.2017.03.006

156. Fitzwater S, Shet A, Santosham M, Kosek M. Infectious diarrhea. In Selendy JM, ed. *Water and Sanitation-Related Diseases and the Changing Environment Challenges, Interventions, and Preventive Measures* 2nd ed. John Wiley & Sons; 2017: 65–93.

157. Mhaissen MN, Rodriguez A, Gu Z, et al. Epidemiology of diarrheal illness in pediatric oncology patients. *J Pediatr Infect Dis Soc*. 2016;6(3):275–280. doi:10.1093/jpids/piw050

158. Fleisher GR, O'Ryan MG. Patient education: Acute diarrhea in children (Beyond the basics). Up to date. Updated 29 June 2020. https://www.uptodate.com/contents/acute-diarrhea-in-children-beyond-the-basics?search=Fleisher%20GR,%20O%E2%80%99Ryan%20MG.%20Patient%20education:%20Acute%20diarrhea%20in%20children%20(Beyond%20the%20basics).%20&source=search_result&selectedTitle=2~150&usage_type=default&display_rank=2#H21

159. Krishnamurthy SS, Macaron C. Management of acute chemotherapy-related diarrhea. Updated May 23, 2019. https://www.uptodate.com/contents/management-of-acute-chemotherapy-related-diarrhea#!

160. Guarino A, Ruberto E, Buccigrossi V. Mechanisms of antidiarrheal effect by probiotics. *J Pediatr Gastroenterol Nutr*. 2016;63(1S):S50. doi:10.1097/01.mpg.0000489623.05312.d2

161. Enoch DA, Butler MJ, Pai S, Aliyu SH, Karas JA. Clostridium difficile in children: Colonisation and disease. *J Infection*. 2011;63(2):105–113. doi:https://doi.org/10.1016/j.jinf.2011.05.016

162. McDonald LC, Gerding DN, Johnson S, et al. Clinical practice guidelines for clostridium difficile infection in adults and children: 2017 update by the Infectious Diseases Society of America (IDSA) and Society for Healthcare Epidemiology of America (SHEA). *Clin Infect Dis*. 2018;66(7):e1–e48. doi:10.1093/cid/cix1085

163. Canadian Society of Intestinal Research. Diarrhea and diet. September/October 2003. https://badgut.org/information-centre/health-nutrition/diarrhea-and-diet/

164. vivo.colostate.edu. Pathophysiology of diarrhea. http://www.vivo.colostate.edu/hbooks/pathphys/digestion/smallgut/diarrhea.html

165. Oshima T, Miwa H. Gastrointestinal mucosal barrier function and diseases. *J Gastroenterol*. 2016;51(8):768–778. doi:10.1007/s00535-016-1207-z

166. Morillo-Gutierrez B, Slatter M. Diarrhea post-HSCT. In Rhamani F, Rezaei N, eds. *Pediatric Autoimmunity and Transplantation*. Springer; 2020: 241–245.

167. Akhondi H, Simonsen K. Bacterial diarrhea. StatPearls. Updated February 27, 2020. https://www.ncbi.nlm.nih.gov/books/NBK551643/?report=printable

168. Schenkman N, Spencer E. Is oral rehydration in pediatric patients with gastroenteritis more effective than parenteral rehydration? *Evid Based Pract*. 2019;22(8):1–2. doi:10.1097/ebp.0000000000000618

169. Beat Lutc GM, Maldonado R, Hillard CJ. The endocannabinoid system in guarding against fear, anxiety and stress. *Nat Rev Neurosci*. 2015;16:705–718.

170. National Center for Biotechnology Information. PubChem Compound Summary for CID 3954, Loperamide(1+). Retrieved August 5, 2021 from https://pubchem.ncbi.nlm.nih.gov/compound/Loperamide_1

171. Holland K. Understanding bile acid malabsorption. Healthline. Updated April 19, 2018. https://www.healthline.com/health/bile-acid-malabsorption

172. Debnath D, Cheriyath P. Octreotide. [Updated 2021 May 8]. In: StatPearls [Internet]. Treasure Island (FL): StatPearls Publishing; 2021 Jan-. Available from: https://www.ncbi.nlm.nih.gov/books/NBK544333/?ff=20210608030118&v=2.14.4

173. Catena F, De Simone B, Coccolini F, Di Saverio S, Sartelli M, Ansaloni L. Bowel obstruction: A narrative review for all physicians. *World J Emerg Surg*. 2019;14(1):20. doi:10.1186/s13017-019-0240-7

174. Chandra AA, Mangalhara N, Jaipal U, Agarwal M, Bhandara A. Why no poop? A pictoral essay of radiological diagnosis of pediatric bowel obstruction. Presented at: Electronic Presentation Online System; 2019; Session ECR 2019/C-0270. https://epos.myesr.org/esr/viewing/index.php?module=viewing_poster&task=&pi=146593

175. Fujisaki T, Fujita Y, Mizuta H, et al. Large bowel obstruction caused by urinary retention from benign prostate hyperplasia. *Radiol Case Rep*. 2019;14(2):213–216. doi:https://doi.org/10.1016/j.radcr.2018.10.031

176. Saeman MR, Diesen DL. Laparoscopic lysis of adhesions for pediatric bowel obstruction. In Walsh DS, Ponsky TA, Bruns NE, eds. *The SAGES Manual of Pediatric Minimally Invasive Surgery*. Springer International; 2017: 401–412.

177. Kulaylat AN, Martin KL. Pediatric intussusception. In Docimo S Jr, Pauli EM, eds. *Clinical Algorithms in General Surgery: A Practical Guide*. Springer International; 2019: 525–528.

178. Di Nardo G, Di Lorenzo C, Lauro A, et al. Chronic intestinal pseudo-obstruction in children and adults: Diagnosis and therapeutic options. *Neurogastroenterol Motil*. 2017;29(1):e12945. doi:10.1111/nmo.12945

179. Zenzeri L, Tambucci R, Quitadamo P, Giorgio V, De Giorgio R, Di Nardo G. Update on chronic intestinal pseudo-obstruction. *Curr Opin Gastroenterol*. 2020. Published ahead of print. doi:10.1097/mog.0000000000000630

180. NIDDK. Intestinal pseudo-obstruction. DHHS NIDDK. Updated February 2014. https://www.niddk.nih.gov/health-information/digestive-diseases/intestinal-pseudo-obstruction

181. Neeley C, Moritz M, Brown JJ, Zhou Y. Acute side effects of three commonly used gadolinium contrast agents in the paediatric population. *Br J Radiol*. 2016;89(1063):20160027. doi:10.1259/bjr.20160027

182. Thomson M, Tringali A, Dumonceau J-M, et al. Paediatric gastrointestinal endoscopy: European Society for Paediatric Gastroenterology Hepatology and Nutrition and European Society

of Gastrointestinal Endoscopy guidelines. *J Pediatr Gastroenterol Nutr*. 2017;64(1):133–153. doi:10.1097/mpg.0000000000001408
183. Fukuhara S, Yamaguchi Y. Small bowel obstruction and the role of bedside ultrasonography performed by a pediatric emergency physician: A case report. *J Acute Med*. 2019;9(4):194–197. doi:10.6705/j.jacme.201912_9(4).0006
184. Hyak J, Campagna G, Johnson B, et al. Management of pediatric adhesive small bowel obstruction: Do timing of surgery and age matter? *J Surg Res*. 2019;243:384–390. doi:https://doi.org/10.1016/j.jss.2019.05.061
185. Ghoshal A, Salins N, Damani A, Deodhar J, Muckaden MA. Medical management of pediatric malignant bowel obstruction in a patient with Burkitt's lymphoma and ataxia telangiectasia using continuous ambulatory drug delivery system. *J Pain Palliat Care Pharmacother*. 2016;30(1):44–48. doi:10.3109/15360288.2015.1134748
186. Marsicovetere P, Ivatury SJ, White B, Holubar SD. Intestinal Intussusception: Etiology, diagnosis, and treatment. *Clin Colon Rectal Surg*. 2017;30(1):30–39. doi:10.1055/s-0036-1593429
187. Levine SK, Shega JW. What interventions are effective for relieving acute bowel obstruction in cancer and other conditions? In Goldstein NE, Morrison RS, eds. *Evidence-Based Practice in Palliative Medicine*. WB Saunders; 2013:147–152.
188. Chandran S, Agarwal A, Llanora GV, Chua MC. Necrotising enterocolitis in a newborn infant treated with octreotide for chylous effusion: Is octreotide safe? *BMJ Case Rep*. 2020;13(2):e232062. doi:10.1136/bcr-2019-232062
189. Ambartsumyan L, Flores A, Nurko S, Rodriguez L. Utility of octreotide in advancing enteral feeds in children with chronic intestinal pseudo-obstruction. *Pediatric Drugs*. 2016;18(5):387–392. doi:10.1007/s40272-016-0189-x

26 | DERMATOLOGIC CONDITIONS AND SYMPTOM CONTROL

KIMBERLY A. BOWER, JULIE GOOD, ANKE REINEKE, CRISTINA GORDON, AND MICHELE R. BURDETTE-TAYLOR

Beauty is not in the face; beauty is light in the heart

KAHLIL GIBRAN

INTRODUCTION

Skin disorders are often encountered in seriously ill patients and can have significant physical, emotional, social, and spiritual impact. The skin is the largest organ in the body and accounts for 15% of a person's body weight. It provides protection from the external environment, allowing intimacy through the ability to touch and be touched. The skin is visible to the external world, thus strongly affecting appearance, which in turn impacts social interactions and self-image. Appearance also influences parents' perception of their child's health and well-being. For all of these reasons it is critical to use an interdisciplinary team to take a whole-person approach to the treatment of dermatologic conditions (Table 26.1).

Clinical Vignette

Matt is a 13-year-old boy with hereditary sensory autonomic neuropathy type II. He presents as significantly younger than his stated age and academically is at a first-grade level. His ability to sense pain is very limited, and for this reason he has developed multiple wounds throughout his life. He has also been treated several times for osteomyelitis and has had his left leg amputated below the knee. He was recently admitted to the pediatric intensive care unit (PICU) for sepsis. He is wheelchair bound and incontinent of urine and stool. His appetite is poor and his albumin is 2.5. He has three large Stage III wounds on his coccyx. There is an unpleasant odor coming from the wounds. Matt is very self-conscious and is reluctant to have anyone other than his mother look at his wounds.

Matt lives with his mother, 11-year-old brother, and 9-year-old sister. The family is Catholic and has limited resources. Matt has not attended school for the past year because his mother believes that his wounds get worse when he is at school. He also does not leave the house very frequently because he is self-conscious.

An interdisciplinary care team consisting of a nurse, social worker, spiritual counselor, bereavement counselor, physician, psychiatrist, wound care nurse, and dietitian started working with Matt and his family. A treatment plan for the wounds was devised. The odor from the wounds resolved, and the wounds slowly began to decrease in size. The wound care nurse ensured that Matt had a pressure-relieving mattress on his bed and a pressure-relieving cushion for his wheelchair. The nurse did regular dressing changes while the social worker provided Matt with distraction and emotional support during the procedure. The nurse also educated his mother on wound care and prevention. The dietitian worked with the patient to identify ways to improve his nutritional status. The psychiatrist diagnosed Matt with depression and started him on an antidepressant medication. The social worker helped to identify resources for the family and provided emotional support to the patient and his siblings. The patient's mother worked with a bereavement counselor to address her fear about the possibility of Matt dying prematurely, and the spiritual counselor provided prayer and addressed Matt's mother's questions about why God had made her son sick.

With support from the team Matt's mood improved and he started to leave the house and go on outings more frequently. In fact, he became restless and started to look for any excuse to leave the house. The team started to work with Matt's school on a plan to allow him to return to school.

Given Matt's underlying medical condition, he will always have wounds and a risk of osteomyelitis, sepsis, and death. Matt's medical condition will continue to affect him physically and emotionally. Exacerbation of his physical symptoms will likely cause new emotional and spiritual distress. Matt's siblings will be significantly affected by his illness, and his mother will continue to benefit from help locating resources and from counseling and spiritual

TABLE 26.1 The roles of team members in the treatment of wounds

DISCIPLINE	ROLE
Psychosocial clinician Psychologist Social worker	Identify that there is a wound or that there is emotional distress related to a wound Provide presence and support to the patient and family Assess the emotional impact of the wound on the child Assess the emotional impact of the wound on the child's family members Provide therapy and counseling to the patient Provide therapy and counseling to the family Provide education and support in the patient's school for the child's classmates Provide activity therapies to the patient and family, such as art, music, and play
Child life specialist	Identify that there is a wound or that there is emotional distress related to a wound Provide presence and support to the patient and family Provide activity therapies to the patient and family, such as art, music, and play Prepare the patient for what to expect during a dressing change Provide distraction during a dressing change
Spiritual counselor	Identify that there is a wound or that there is emotional distress related to a wound Provide presence and support to the patient and family Assess whether the wound is causing spiritual distress to the patient Address the spiritual distress that may be caused by the wound Identify and address the spiritual needs of the patient's family Perform spiritual rituals that may support the patient and family
Nurse	Identify that there is a wound or that there is emotional distress related to a wound Provide presence and support to the patient and family Assess the physical signs and symptoms associated with the wound Provide hands-on medical care including dressing changes, medication administration, and repositioning Educate the family about wound care and wound prevention Educate the school nurse about the patient's medical and emotional needs
Certified nurses assistant	Identify that there is a wound or that there is emotional distress related to a wound Provide presence and support to the patient and family Provide repositioning and skin care
Physician	Identify that there is a wound or that there is emotional distress related to a wound Provide presence and support to the patient and family Assess the physical signs and symptoms associated with the wound Provide medical care including dressing changes, medication administration, and repositioning Prescribe a treatment plan
Psychiatrist	Identify that there is a wound or that there is emotional distress related to a wound Provide presence and support to the patient and family Assess the emotional impact of the wound on the child Assess the emotional impact of the wound on the child's family members Make a psychiatric diagnosis such as anxiety disorder or depression Prescribe a treatment plan including medications
Wound care specialist	Identify that there is a wound or that there is emotional distress related to a wound Provide presence and support to the patient and family Make recommendations to the team about the best management plan to treat the wound Provide hands on medical care including dressing changes

support. Matt's story highlights the need for a family-centered interdisciplinary approach to the care of children with chronic medical conditions and wounds.

PSYCHOSOCIAL IMPACT OF DERMATOLOGIC CONDITIONS

Dermatological disorders in seriously ill patients have traditionally been viewed from the perspective of their medical management, with little focus on psychosocial issues. Recent research, even though limited, has shown increased emphasis on their impact on body image, pain, and the comfort of touch and intimacy. The interdisciplinary team's awareness and understanding of these dimensions are crucial if they are to provide optimal and specialized care for these young patients and their families.

BODY IMAGE

Body image is a central part of self-concept and self-esteem and is broadly defined as "the composite of thoughts, values, and feelings that one has for one's physical and personal self at any given time."[1] Patients with obvious differences—or changes—in appearance report that they feel embarrassed, at times experiencing a "loss of self" that prevents them from connecting with their own identity.[2] Children's responses to their own appearance—whether "different" as a defining feature of a disorder or a significant change from their own "normal"—can be highly individual. Influencing factors include whether an affected body part or function is particularly emotionally laden for the child and whether there is visible disfigurement. As a result of physical changes in appearance, others may stare or avoid looking at a child. Thereafter, the child may suffer emotionally and may withdraw socially. Throughout the literature, studies have suggested that altered body image can interfere with daily functioning and has been associated with grief, anxiety, depression, social introversion, social avoidance behaviors, decline in self-esteem, avoidance of intimate relationships, and overall poor quality of life.[3–5]

Cancer is an example of a diagnosis in which both the disease and the treatment frequently lead to changes in physical appearance. Some effects are temporary (e.g., hair loss, presence of central venous catheter) and other can be permanent (e.g., skin changes due to chemotherapy, scars from surgeries). Such body-altering effects of cancer have been reported by adolescents as the worst aspects of living with the disease,[6] especially when others tease or shun them, or engage in other hurtful social interactions. Physical changes due to cancer or its treatment can be devastating to the child's self-image and can place the child at an increased risk for psychological adjustment issues.[7–9] Physical appearance and attractiveness are major issues confronting adolescents, and their body image becomes a central aspect of identity development.[10] The adolescents' sense of self-worth can be affected to such a degree that they may withdraw from their friends and family. Older adolescents facing changes in body image may be less likely to establish intimate relationships.[11]

A skin disorder may similarly affect children's sense of self-competence and self-worth in their relationships with family and friends. Young children rely primarily on their parents and siblings for support, whereas adolescents turn more to their peers, who are in turn influential in their self-definition and self-evaluation. If children or adolescents have diminished social contact in any of their relationships, this may have significant implications on their ability to cope with the skin disease and can have negative effects on their overall quality of life.

Epidermolysis bullosa (EB) is a rare disorder in which "the skin tears apart, blisters, and shears off leading to severe pain, disfigurement, and wounds that may never heal." Negative body image in EB can be related to poor self-esteem, anxiety, and depression.[12] In one study, psychiatric symptoms, particularly depression, anxiety, and behavioral disturbance, were experienced by 80% of patients with EB.[13] It is important to keep in mind that all the psychological responses described may not be simply the result of the skin condition per se, but may be the child's response to the overwhelming impact of living with a life-threatening illness.[14]

FAMILY REFLECTION

"When I reflect on ways in which EB does not affect my daughter, I come up empty. It affects what and how she eats, it affects how she plays, how she walks and runs, how she holds a pen, how we hold her; EB is a thief of both time and money; and a giver of pain, anxiety and sleepless nights. I have often heard EB described as 'the worst disease you've never heard of,' and I honestly don't see that as an exaggeration. For my daughter, EB causes blisters and wounds from head to toe. There has not been a day of her life when we have not had to take a needle to her skin, to drain blisters to keep them from growing; to wrap wounds, to keep them from becoming infected. Not a single day. As an infant it was literal torture what we had to do to her to keep her alive, now as a school age child, she knows the routine, she lets me do what I need to do to keep her healthy. And in a way that's a beautiful thing, we have figured out (for now), how to keep her comfortable during wound care, but it is also really sad as a parent, to know that your 6-year-old has to endure on a daily basis what most adults can't even conceive of. At the end of the day, there is no separating my child from EB, she is who she is in part because of what she has gone through. And thanks to a lot of early intervention, I can say that I am raising an incredibly strong, resilient, and happy child who wants nothing more at the end of the day, then to just be a kid, EB and all."

Becky (mother of Clara, age 6,
who has severe generalized EB simplex)

PAIN

The experience of pain is a crucial consideration in the psychological impact of skin conditions and their treatments. A wound is a constant reminder to children of the traumatic changes that their body has undergone. Clinicians' attentiveness and sensitivity to children's responses during wound care are of paramount importance, as patients often link their depression and anxiety to the experience of pain.[15,16] In children with EB, the pain is associated with frustration, embarrassment, sadness, anxiety, and fear of being hurt.[17] When pain, skin breakdown, and scarring lead to limitation of motion and activity, even therapies with the goal of improving function become implicated in children's overall distress.[18] The critical contribution of expert consultation in pain and symptom management cannot be underestimated for these children.

COMFORT OF TOUCH AND INTIMACY

Regardless of the underlying medical diagnosis, intact skin allows for intimacy and the ability to touch and be touched—a powerful way for a child's family to express their care. Any change in a child's body or body image may compromise that physical closeness, either through the child's own reactions or those of the family. Loss of this intimacy may in turn elicit psychological responses that become enduring and pathological, such as depression and social anxiety.

IMPACT ON THE FAMILY

How the family, both parents and healthy siblings, respond to and cope with a child with a skin disorder is a new area of research. In patients with EB, reactions of family members to the condition have both direct impact on the child and, ultimately, on the family as a whole.[13] Parents of children diagnosed with EB identified distress around themes including their own painful struggle to accept their child as visibly different from others, witnessing their child suffering from pain and sometimes causing the pain while taking care of the wounds, witnessing others' reactions to the child's appearance, feelings of uncertainty, restrictions in employment or leisure time, and guilt at not paying attention to other family members, including siblings.[17] Parents occasionally mention feeling ashamed of their child's appearance—a feeling that in turn engenders enormous guilt. Parental support is crucial and a protective component to improve resilience and lead to more positive psychosocial outcomes for their children.[19,20]

All too often, however, parents feel unprepared, even overwhelmed, with how to manage appearance-related issues.[21] The impact and adjustment on healthy siblings of having a brother or sister with a serious illness and a visible disfigurement are yet not well understood. Although the presence of chronic illness may increase siblings' distress, the adjustment can vary by age, sex, and type of illness.[22] Clinical experience suggests that siblings' reactions are especially complicated when their brother or sister's illness is highly visible or disfiguring in its manifestation.

INTERVENTION

Optimal care for a child's dermatological condition—both medical and psychosocial aspects—ideally includes ongoing and specialized approaches (educational, psychological, and integrative), support for the children and families, and access to an interdisciplinary team. A powerful mediator of adjusting to the impact of a serious skin disorder is effective communication that is open, honest, acknowledges emotions, and actively involves the child, family and the care team.[17] "Psychoeducational" approaches combine the transmission of critical information about the condition and treatment with extreme sensitivity to the impact on the child and family of receiving such information. The team can guide children in adjusting to differences or changes in their appearance while validating their emotional experience throughout the illness.

Early and ongoing psychological guidance for parents—regarding the care of both the patient and the healthy siblings—is invaluable. When available, individual psychotherapy (including play therapy for young children) and expressive therapies (e.g., art and music) permit children to safely explore their extraordinary life circumstances without being overwhelmed by a sense of vulnerability. When children feel validated in their concerns, they are more able to think through their situation and move toward some sense of mastery over the challenges. Family therapy can play a critical integrative role for all members in managing unremitting challenges and stress.

Encouraging and facilitating connections between patients and their peers (with others who are living with a similar condition and with healthy friends) provides a critical opportunity for them to share their experience and gain support.[23] These interactions may be in person or telephone or through various media, including e-mail, texting, and social networking websites.

The care team can recommend and offer integrative modalities to provide relaxation and respite for children, as well as give them a certain sense of control over their symptoms. These include guided imagery, massage, healing touch, hypnosis, acupuncture, and aromatherapy, as well as other mind-body skills. Teaching parents how to implement selected techniques for their child can assuage their sense of helplessness and opens an important avenue of comfort for the child embedded within the family.

Greater attention to understanding the impact and efficacy of interventions for children with skin disease is needed to ease profound suffering and enhance their overall well-being. The integrative palliative team can play an important supportive role in enhancing quality of life for the child and family.

PRURITUS

Pruritus is defined by the International Forum for the Study of Itch (IFSI) as a sensation in the skin that provokes the desire to scratch.[24] Itch can be distressing and sometimes difficult to treat. It may lead to sleep disturbance, difficulty concentrating, anxiety, depression, and agitation. Left inadequately managed, it can have a significantly negative impact on a child and their families quality of life.[25] Itch may impact physical function, impair social relationships and school performance[26,27] and lead to self-consciousness and lower self-esteem.[28] Parents may face financial burdens secondary to the cost of dermatologic care and poor reimbursement for some topical products, struggle with the time commitment for treatment, and experience difficulty meeting the needs of other family members including siblings while taking time to care for a child's skin.[29] The relationship between psychological and dermatological health may be bidirectional, and a comprehensive approach to management is recommended,[27] including multidisciplinary treatment, education, and psychological support.[30,31]

The IFSI identifies six categories for the classification of pruritus based on underlying etiology: dermatological, systemic/neurogenic, neurological, psychological/psychosomatic, mixed, and other.[32] Because the causes of pruritus are numerous, identifying the etiology of pruritus can be helpful when formulating a therapeutic approach. This section of the chapter focuses on common causes of pruritus in seriously ill children. The reader is further directed to the European S2K

Guideline on Chronic Pruritus for additional general and disease specific recommendations.[24]

PATHOPHYSIOLOGY OF PRURITUS

Our understanding of pruritus perception and transmission has progressed over the past decade, with promising treatment targets beginning to emerge while still others are in earlier stages of development.[33] Overall, the neuronal pathways for the transmission of pruritus are thought to be closely related to pain pathways (Figure 26.1).[34]

In chronic pruritus (itch that lasts >6 weeks), peripheral stimulation by a pruritogen has been shown to lead to nonhistaminergic/mechano-sensitive c-fiber and A-delta fiber

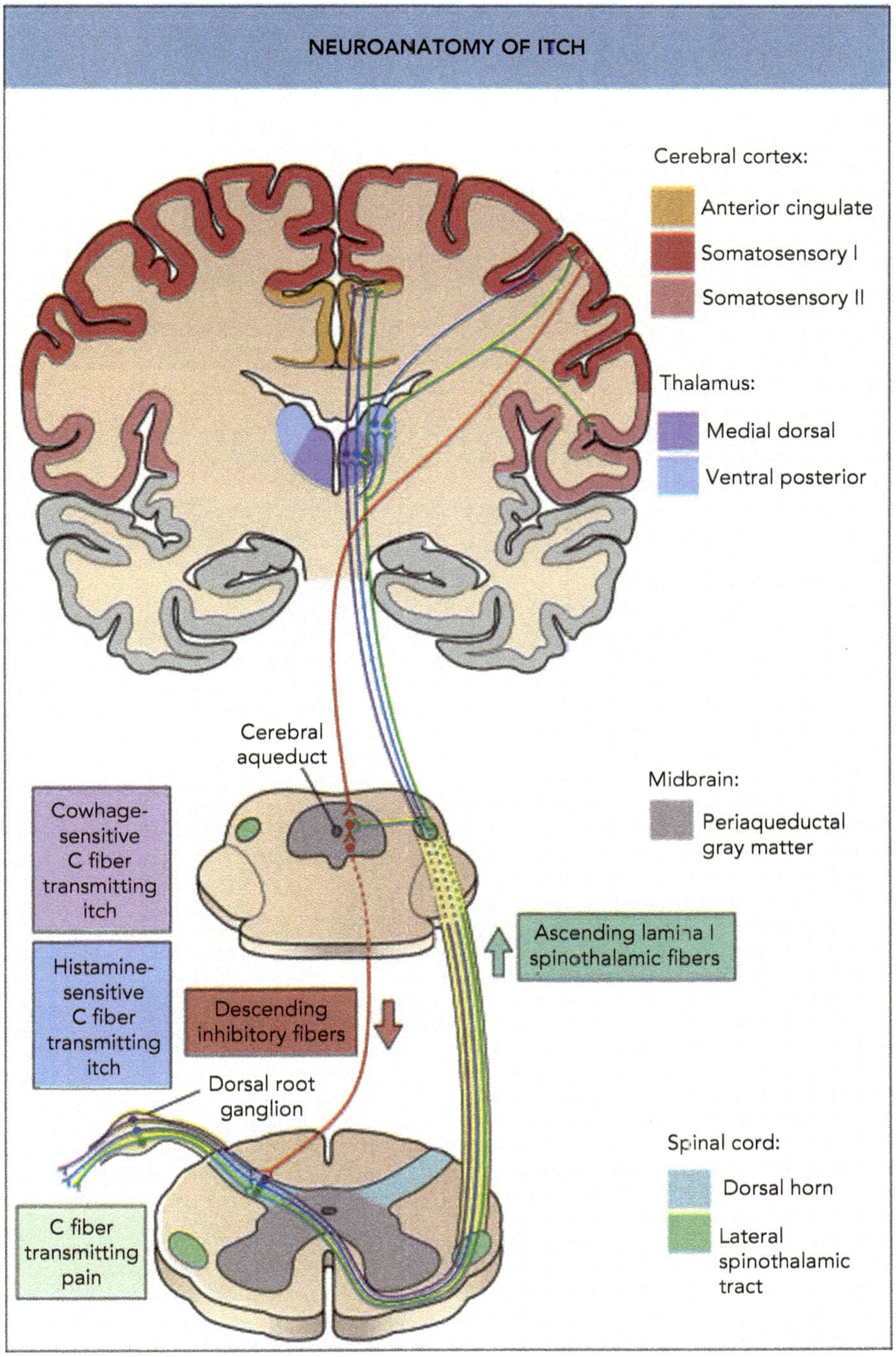

Figure 26.1 Neuroanatomy of itch. Itch and pain transmission occurs via unmyelinated C nerve fibers that excite the lamina I subset of neurons in the dorsal horn of the spinal cord. Two subsets of pruritoceptive C-fiber neurons (which respond to histamine and cowhage, respectively) are conducted through distinct spinothalamic pathways, with projections to the thalamus. Processing of itch through either pathway activates several regions of the brain, which are similar to those involved in pain (see Figure 26.1). Concomitant painful stimuli can reduce the sensation of itch, possibly by a descending inhibitory mechanism resulting from activation of the periaqueductal gray matter. (Adapted from Figure 5.1 Yosipovitch G, Akiyama, T. Pruritus 2018, In Bolognia, Schaffer MD, Cerroni MD editors: Dermatology, 4th ed., Elsevier[34])

pathway activation.[35–37] Meanwhile, histaminergic/mechano-insensitive c-fibers play a lesser role in chronic itch but are still important for acute dermatological conditions like urticaria, insect bites/infestations, and phytodermatoses. These findings help to explain the observation that antihistamines are useful for some itch but are not helpful in others.[38]

Molecules currently known to mediate itch in the periphery include[39–42]

- *Amines*: Histamine, serotonin, proteases (e.g., kallikrein 5 and mucunian), cytokine-interleukins
- *Peptides*: Bradykinin, substance P, calcitonin gene-related peptide, nerve growth factor, endothelin-1, opioid peptides
- *Phospholipid metabolites*: Leukotriene, endocannabinoids

After initial stimulation, G-protein coupled receptors (e.g., transient receptor vallinoid cation channel subfamily V1 [TRPV1], transient receptor potential ankyrin 1 [TRPA1], and voltage-gated sodium channels) depolarize the nerve, leading to sodium influx and potentiation of signal from the periphery to the spinal cord.[43,44]

At the spinal cord level, sensory neurons release gastrin-releasing peptide to activate gastrin-peptide–specific dorsal horn neuron receptors[45] that subsequently carry the itch signal via the spinal cord to the thalamus. Functional magnetic resonance imaging (fMRI) shows activity in multiple areas of the brain which encode sensory location and intensity, emotion, attention regulation, cognitive/evaluative, motor control, and goal-directed movement aspects of itch.[46]

Itch of the neurological classification arises secondary to damage of nerves anywhere along the afferent pathway. Nerve damage can be seen in peripheral neuropathies, nerve compression, or cerebral processes such as tumors, abscess, or thrombosis. Itch caused by psychiatric and/or psychosomatic disease can occur in disorders such as obsessive-compulsive disorder and parasitophobia. It is also believed that both acute and chronic stress can trigger or enhance pruritus.[47]

OVERVIEW OF PROPOSED TREATMENTS

Itch may be inhibited by peripheral, spinal, and/or supraspinal mechanisms. These mechanisms include gamma aminobutyric acid (GABA), glycine, dynorphin, endocannabinoid, norepinephrine, and serotonin and mechanical (scratch) inhibition.[48]

Systemic mediators of itch responses that are under investigation for specific clinical utility in chronic pruritus syndromes [39–41,49–51]include

- Neurokinin 1 (NK-1) antagonists: Aprepitant, serlopitant, tradipitant, orvepitant, fosaprepitant
- Kappa-agonists: Nalfurafine, pentazocine, nalbuphine, difelikefalin
- Mu-opioid receptor antagonists: Naloxone, naltrexone, nalbuphine
- Interleukin antagonists: Cyclosporine, nemolizumab dipilumab, secukinumab, ixekizumab
- IgE blocker: Omalizumab
- Steroids
- Janus kinase (JAK) inhibitors: Tofacitinib, others
- First- and second-generation histamine receptor antagonists: Bilastine, rupatidine, others
- Leukotriene receptor antagonists: Montelukast
- Bile acid transporter inhibitors
- Gabapentinoids

Topical and local therapies under investigation for itch[52] include

- Transient receptor potential vanilloid 1 (TRPV1) inhibitors: Capsaicin, tacrolimus
- Tropomyosin-receptor-kinase A (trka) inhibitors: Pegcantratinib
- Transient receptor potential melastin 8: Menthol creams
- Proteinase-activated receptor 2 (PAR-2) inhibitor: Polidocanol
- Phosphodiesterase-4 (PDE-4) inhibitors: Crisaborole
- Topical analgesics: Ketamine, amitriptyline, lidocaine
- Endocannabinoids: N-palmitoylethanolamine, N-acetyl ethanolamine
- Botulinum toxin type A

ASSESSMENT

Among seriously ill children the most likely etiologies of pruritus include underlying medical disorders, drug therapy, and dry skin. The etiology of pruritus can frequently be determined by history and physical exam. History should include localized versus generalized location, description, temporal profile, provoking factors, effect of medications, current medication list, atopic history, and travel history. Physical exam should include evaluation for dry skin, scabies, icteric conjunctivae, weight loss, and mental status changes. Radiologic and laboratory workup can be considered based on clinical presentation and goals of care.

Validated, universal clinical assessment tools that quantify the severity of pruritus and impact on quality of life are needed in adults and children.[53] The pediatric tools available assess global quality of life (QOL) for children with skin disease[54] or assess itch severity but are designed to be used in specific conditions, such as post-burn pruritus[55] or cholestatic itch.[56] Several existing tools designed to measure disease severity and QOL for children with atopic dermatitis need further validation.[57,58] In children older than 6 years, visual analog scales may be used to evaluate itch intensity.[59] In the research setting, quantitative measures of pruritus can be obtained by devices that assess motor movement at the wrist (actigraphy) or by accelerometers that measure the vibrations of the fingernails in the act of scratching, although relationship between motor movements and subjective experience is influenced by multiple factors.[60]

MANAGEMENT OF SPECIFIC CONDITIONS

The most effective treatment for pruritus is treating the underlying cause of the itch. This is not always possible, and even when it is possible the itch often does not resolve immediately. For this reason it is important to identify treatments specifically aimed at quickly and effectively relieving itch to the extent possible regardless of the state of the patient's underlying condition. In this section, we review management strategies for pruritus that are caused by conditions frequently seen in seriously ill children (Table 26.2).

Practical steps can be taken to prevent, treat, and mitigate pruritus regardless of the etiology.[24] Preventive measures which may help include use of a humidifier if air is dry,

TABLE 26.2 Treatment of pruritus by cause

CAUSE	TREATMENT
General measures for all forms of pruritus (including prevention and management of xerosis)	Insure air is humidified Keep ambient temperature cool and avoid rapid temperature changes in environment Avoid very (thermally) hot, and spicy foods Avoid emotional stressors i.e. extreme excitement, strain Learn relaxation techniques Select coping tools/distracting behaviors to engage in when itch is severe Maintain hydration of body as a whole (enteral, or parenteral if necessary) Wear breathable cotton in layers Bathe in cool/lukewarm bath, add one or more of the following to the bath: sodium bicarbonate, oatmeal, potassium permanganate Select low pH cleaners and moisturizers Use oil-based emollients (avoid- water or alcohol-based) Avoid fragrances, any irritating ingredients specific to your child Keep fingernails short Wear gloves or mittens if scratching is subconscious/occurring at night (remember to allow babies and toddlers time out of gloves to explore sensory world each day)
Opioid-induced	Opioid rotation Add analgesic adjuvants to allow opioid dose to be lowest possible Opioid receptor antagonist Opioid receptor agonist-antagonist Mixed results with: 5-HT_3 receptor antagonists, D_2 receptor antagonists, nonsteroidal anti-inflammatory agents, lidocaine, subhypnotic propofol, midazolam
Cancer-specific	Anticancer therapy H_2 receptor antagonist cimetidine in Hodgkin's lymphoma and polycythemia vera Paroxetine Mirtazapine Possibly: Ondansetron, corticosteroids, H1 antihistamines, gabapentinoids, thalidomide, naloxone, butorphanol
Cholestasis	If extrahepatic: Cholestyramine, bile acids If intrahepatic and obstructed: Phenobarbital Any cause: • Rifampin • Naltrexone • Sertraline • Surgical intervention: Bile duct stenting, external biliary diversion, terminal ileal exclusion, gallbladder to colon diversion depending on location of obstruction • Liver transplantation in severe refractory cases depending on goals of care
Uremia	Enhance dialysis regimen Correct calcium, phosphorus, and magnesium Treat hyperparathyroidism Ultraviolet (UV-B) light therapy Cromolyn sodium Gabapentin Mu-opioid receptor antagonist naltrexone Kappa-opioid receptor agonist nalfurafine (not available in United States at time of publication) Capsaicin cream
HIV/AIDS	Assess for secondary etiology: Infection, peripheral neuropathy, xerosis, primary skin condition, systemic disease, drug reaction, elevated cytokines If HIV is cause: Indomethacin

maintaining a cool ambient temperature, avoiding rapid changes in environmental temperature, limiting the intake of very hot drinks or spicy food, and avoiding emotional stressors including extreme excitement and strain when possible. It can also be beneficial for children to learn relaxation techniques as well as coping strategies to prevent perpetuation of the itch–scratch cycle.

Interventions that maintain or improve skin moisture and integrity are helpful in soothing itch and include: oral rehydration (when dehydration is present); wearing soft, breathable cotton clothing in layers to prevent excessive sweating; restricting time (<20 min) in the bath or shower; bathing in cool or lukewarm water instead of hot water; dabbing skin when wet; and applying emollients to the skin after bathing and on a regular basis (avoiding alcohol- or water-based products in favor of oil-based products). Some children may find adding oatmeal or potassium permanganate to the bath soothing to itchy skin. High skin surface pH has been noted in several skin disorders, including atopic dermatitis, and uremia. Using low pH cleansers and moisturizers, or preparing baths with sodium bicarbonate added to the bath water can address this issue. Attention should also be paid to avoiding skin irritants, including fragrances.

Since it can be quite difficult to keep children from unconsciously scratching areas that itch, it is crucial to keep a child's fingernails cut short to mitigate damage to the skin from scratching. Gloves or mittens can be placed on children's hands, but they are often difficult to keep in place and can limit important developmental exploration of the world early on and impair function in older children.

Additional research is needed to determine treatment efficacy for pharmacologic and nonpharmacologic interventions for chronic pruritus of unknown origin.[61]

OPIOID-INDUCED PRURITUS

Pruritus that may localize to the face and trunk is a common complication of parenteral or neuraxial opioid administration. Pruritus can also be seen with the administration of oral opioids. It is difficult to estimate the incidence of opioids-induced pruritus in children for several reasons including limited data, variation between opioids and routes of administration, and lack of uniformity in methods of evaluation of pruritus. The incidence has been reported to be between 2% and 50% for parenteral administration and between 20% and 100% when neuraxial opioids are administered.[62,63]

The mechanism of opioid-induced pruritus is not fully understood. It is known that orally, intradermally, or parenterally administered codeine, morphine, and meperidine can cause the release of histamine from mast cells, but fentanyl, alfentanil, sufentanil, buprenorphine, and naloxone do not.[64,65] For this reason, histamine cannot play a singular role in opioid-induced pruritus. Furthermore, in studies done in primates, the administration of a histamine antagonist did not attenuate scratch induced by morphine.[66] Some opioid-induced pruritus is known to be mediated centrally through mu-opioid receptors,[67] and additional mechanisms proposed include modulation of serotonin pathways,[68] prostaglandins, the role of an "itch center" in the central nervous system (CNS), medullary dorsal horn activation, antagonism of inhibitory transmitters,[69] and D_2 receptors.[70]

In the initial management of pruritus caused by morphine, it may be helpful to change from morphine to an alternative opioid such as hydromorphone or fentanyl. If this is not effective, an opioid receptor antagonist can be administered in conjunction with the patient's opioid. It is important, however, that the opioid antagonist be used in a low enough dose that it does not reverse the analgesia achieved by the opioid. Both naloxone and naltrexone have been studied. Naloxone can be administered at a starting dose of 0.25 mcg/kg/hr to 1 mcg/kg/hr. Doses of more than 2 mcg/kg/hr are likely to cause an unacceptable degree of reversal of the analgesic effect of the opioid. A pilot study done in children in sickle cell crisis found that patients tolerated co-administration of naloxone and morphine.[71] Two additional small studies of 46 and 59 pediatric postoperative patients, respectively, found that concomitant administration of low-dose naloxone and morphine through patient-controlled analgesia (PCA) significantly reduced opioid-associated pruritus.[72,73]

Opioid agonist-antagonists, including nalbuphine and butorphanol, have also been studied as agents to reduce pruritus. These drugs have conceptual advantages over pure opioid antagonists in that they do not reverse the analgesic effect to the opioid or risk precipitation of opioid withdrawal syndrome. These medications act as antagonists at the mu-receptor and as agonists at the kappa-receptor, which attenuates morphine-induced itch without interfering with analgesia in monkeys.[74] Results of human clinical trials have been mixed, with only limited studies in the pediatric population. One study of 184 pediatric patients found that nalbuphine 50 mcg/kg IV given as a single dose was not effective in the treatment of postoperative opioid-induced pruritus.[75] Nonetheless, a subsequent review found nalbuphine more effective for opioid-induced pruritus when compared to placebo, control, diphenhydramine, naloxone, or propofol in patients receiving neuraxial opioids.[76]

Beyond opioid antagonists and opioid agonist/antagonists, there has not been investigation or consensus specifically in children for other agents to prevent or manage opioid-induced pruritus.[77,78] In adults, and especially laboring women 5-HT_3 receptor antagonists,[68] D_2 receptor antagonists,[70,79] the sodium channel blocker lidocaine[80] and prostaglandin-blocking nonsteroidal anti-inflammatory agents (NSAIDs),[81] have been studied as possible treatments for opioid-induced pruritus, with mixed results. While studies in adults may be promising for some agents (e.g., propofol[82] and midazolam[83]), these studies are in adults exclusively and limit subjects to those receiving intrathecal or epidural opioids. These factors make it difficult to predict the effect that these medications may have in the treatment of opioid-induced pruritus in seriously ill children. It may be that the use of opioid-sparing analgesic strategies that lower the total opioid dose and secondarily mitigate pruritus (e.g., adjuvants such as acetaminophen and NSAIDs, regional techniques, gabapentinoids, etc.) deserve consideration.

CANCER-SPECIFIC PRURITUS

Many children with cancer experience pruritus. Although the incidence of pruritus in children is not known, estimates in adult cancer range from 6% to 50%, with higher prevalence in hematologic malignancies.[24] Children with cancer may experience greater incidence of pruritus than adults with cancer.[84,85] The most common types of cancers that cause pruritus in the pediatric population are cancers of bone, skin, liver, and blood—particularly leukemias and Hodgkin and non-Hodgkin's lymphomas.[84] The exact mechanism by which cancer causes pruritus is unknown, although several factors under investigation include degree of inflammation, presence of eosinophils, role of CD4 helper T cells, and timing of production of IL-31 in the model of cutaneous T-cell lymphoma.[86]

In order to choose the most appropriate treatment, it is important to consider the cause of the symptom. The pruritus may be a direct result of the cancer[84] or a side effect of the child's treatment.[87] Possible etiologies for secondary pruritus include xerosis, radiation desquamation, drug reactions, cholestasis, uremia, side effects from chemotherapy and biologic agents, or graft versus host disease.

The most effective treatment for cancer-related pruritus is anticancer therapy. In advanced illness, however, patients may respond poorly to or are no longer receiving disease-modifying therapies. In these patients, other approaches to the treatment of the pruritus must be identified. There are very limited data on the treatment of pruritus associated with cancer in children, necessitating extrapolation from the adult literature. In Hodgkin's lymphoma[88,89] and polycythemia vera,[90] case reports suggest that the H_2-receptor antagonist, cimetidine, is effective in treating pruritus. A case series[91] that included pediatric patients suggested that pruritus caused by solid tumors may respond to the serotonin selective reuptake inhibitor (SSRI) paroxetine, which was also determined to have moderate evidence of efficacy for pruritus in adults with advanced cancer.[92] While paroxetine's antidepressant effects can take weeks to see, its antipruritic effects may be seen in as little as 24 hours after administration, with the current hypothesis that the more rapid antipruritic effect is serotonin mediated. Mirtazapine has also been shown similarly to improve pruritus related to cancer in three elderly cancer patients[93] in other more recent case reports,[94,95] with recommendation in systematic reviews of the literature to consider paroxetine and mirtazapine as therapeutic options for cancer-related pruritus.[95,96] Anecdotal evidence from small case reports and uncontrolled studies also exist for other medications (e.g., corticosteroids, H_1 antihistamines, gabapentinoids, ondansetron, thalidomide, naloxone, and butorphanol), but too little data exist to support their use over the aforementioned medications. Combined therapy may be needed and efficacious to address multifactorial causes of pruritus from immune, peripheral, and CNS stimulation.[97]

CHOLESTASIS

Cholestasis occurs in children of all ages, but it is particularly common in the neonatal period. The incidence of neonatal cholestasis is estimated to be approximately 1 in 2,500 live births.[98] The mechanism by which cholestasis causes pruritus is unclear; while mechanisms including accumulated bile acids, steroid-derived metabolites, endogenous mu-opioids, and serotonin have been observed, they are also disputed as causative mechanisms.[99,100] The pruritus of cholestasis is not mediated by histamine, and any relief that patients perceive with the administration of antihistamines is likely related to the sedating effects of the medication. It is of interest to note that pruritus often precedes accumulation of bile salts, and it often resolves if patients progress to liver failure.[100]

Therapy for pruritus caused by cholestasis is typically administered in a progressive order until efficacy is achieved, starting with medication directed at decreasing the level of circulating bile acids, including the nonabsorbable anion exchange resin cholestyramine.[101] However, nonabsorbable anion exchange resins are not effective in the case of intrahepatic biliary obstruction because the bile acids must reach the intestine for the medication to be effective; instead, phenobarbital can be used.[102]

If obstruction is partial, and pruritus is refractory to cholestyramine (or cholestyramine is contraindicated), rifampin is considered next. Rifampin appears to act by inhibiting autotaxin expression as its mechanism for reducing cholestatic pruritus.[24,103] The third- and fourth-line agents for cholestatic pruritus are naltrexone then sertraline, respectively.[101,104] Care should be taken when administering mu-opioid antagonists in the seriously ill patient when they are also receiving opioid agonists for pain as there is a risk of loss of analgesia at higher doses of naltrexone.

Although initial studies in adults appeared to show that the 5-HT_3 receptor antagonist ondansetron was effective,[105] subsequent studies[106] failed to show effect. Clinical practice guidelines and systematic reviews consider the use of ondansetron, other medications, and nonsurgical therapies to have insufficient evidence of efficacy and safety.[97,100,101]

Surgical interventions may also be helpful if medical management has not been successful and surgery makes sense within the goals of care. Procedures including partial external biliary diversion,[107,108] terminal ileal exclusion, and gallbladder to colon diversion have shown a trend toward decreased pruritus in some children with intrahepatic cholestasis.[109] In pruritus caused by extrahepatic disease, stenting the bile duct is often the best treatment for pruritus. In extreme cases of pruritus that is refractory to treatment and that is causing significant negative effects on a patient's quality of life, liver transplant may be considered.[101]

UREMIC PRURITUS

Pruritus from uremia is seen in patients with chronic renal failure but rarely in those with acute renal failure. The rate of pruritus is higher in patients receiving dialysis than in those not receiving dialysis, and, in adults, the presence of severe uremic pruritus is a predictive factor for death.[110] The mechanism by which uremia causes pruritus is not fully understood, but, as in other systemic illnesses, it is likely caused by the accumulation of pruritogens in the blood. It is intriguing to note that renal transplantation has been found to reduce, and in some cases relieve chronic pruritus,[111] but the effect is not uniform for all patients.

Limited research has been done in the pediatric population on pruritus secondary to uremia.[112] Therefore, treatments are often based on evidence from the adult literature, which is also lacking in definitive approaches to the condition.[113,114] Initial management in patients on dialysis includes enhancing the dialysis regimen and correcting the patient's calcium, phosphorus, and magnesium. Xerosis, which is very common in uremic patients, should also be treated.[115] If a patient is found to have hyperparathyroidism secondary to renal failure, pruritus can resolve after parathyroidectomy.[116,117] Beyond these steps, ultraviolet light (UV-B) therapy, gabapentin, oral cromolyn sodium, topical capsaicin, the mu-opioid receptor antagonist naltrexone, and the kappa-opioid receptor agonist nalfurafine have shown some promise in adults,[97,118,119] but have yet to be studied systematically in children. As in pruritus caused by most other systemic diseases, antihistamines are not helpful in the treatment of uremic pruritus.

HIV/AIDS

Pruritus is very common in patients with HIV infection. It can be secondary to multiple etiologies, including infection, infestation, peripheral neuropathy, xerosis, a primary skin condition, systemic disease, drug reaction, or elevated levels of cytokines. A thorough evaluation for the most likely causes of the pruritus should be done and should direct treatment. Idiopathic HIV pruritus is uncommon and is diagnosed by the exclusion of other causes. For patients with pruritus associated with HIV infection, a recent Cochrane review in adults concluded that indomethacin may be most effective, but results are tentative and further investigation is necessary to determine ideal therapy.[97]

MUCOSITIS

Oral and gastrointestinal mucositis, referred to collectively as *alimentary tract mucositis*, is very common in children receiving cytotoxic chemotherapy, molecularly targeted agents, hematopoietic stem cell transplantation, and/or radiation to areas encompassing the gastrointestinal tract, including the head and neck. Younger patients develop oral mucositis (OM) more frequently and heal more quickly than older patients receiving similar treatments. This is thought to be secondary to an increased epithelial mitotic rate in children as compared to adults. Mucositis of the oral cavity and esophagus can lead to ulceration, oral pain, dysphagia, and odynophagia while mucositis of the gastrointestinal tract can lead to gastritis, abdominal pain, diarrhea, malabsorption, and bloating. Mucositis can be the dose-limiting factor in administration of chemotherapy, and affected children are at risk of bleeding, local infections, sepsis, and compromised nutritional status. Because mucositis limits treatment, causes serious complications, and leads to significant symptom burden, increasing attention has been paid to understanding its pathogenesis, exploring preventative measures, and investigating treatments. Despite this increased attention, there are few interventions that are supported by a strong evidence base. In 2019, the Multinational Association of Supportive Care in Cancer and the International Society for Oral Oncology (MASCC/ISOO) published their updated evidence-based guidelines for mucositis.[120] These guidelines provide a strong foundation for the evidence-based care of mucositis.

Given that the groups of patients who are likely to develop mucositis is known, it would be ideal to implement a therapy prior to high-risk intervention to reduce the incidence or severity of the symptom. Efforts to prevent OM have traditionally focused on modifying oral microbial load to decrease inflammatory response and subsequently OM severity. The fact that there have been inconsistent results with the use of antimicrobial therapies such as chlorhexidine rinses has led to the exploration of the concept that oral flora dysbiosis observed in patients during cancer therapy is a predisposing factor in the development of OM and achieving oral flora symbiosis rather than sterilization of the oral cavity may be the goal.[121] At this time, though multiple preventative approaches have been studied, the primary recommendation of the MASCC/ISOO is to implement a multiagent combination oral care protocol for the prevention of OM during chemotherapy, head and neck radiation therapy, and hematopoietic stem cell transplantation.[122] These protocols should be formulated by a interdisciplinary team including medical, dental, nursing, and child life/psychosocial professionals. Protocols vary between institutions, but typically include recommendations regarding the timing and frequency of regular assessment of the oral mucosa, tooth brushing, flossing, and the use of a bland mouth rinse such as a saline or sodium bicarbonate rinse. Providing education to patients and families about these protocols and appropriate oral care, though not evidence-based, is generally believed to be helpful. The evidence base reviewed by the MASCC/ISOO was not strong enough to create a guideline around professional oral care, but expert opinion supports dental evaluation and treatment prior to cancer therapy.[122]

Another common preventative measure used to minimize mucositis caused by chemotherapy is cryotherapy. This intervention involves having the child suck on ice for 20–45 minutes while receiving chemotherapy. The ice cools the mucosal tissue and leads to vasoconstriction, decreasing the exposure of the tissue to the chemotherapeutic agent. The MASCC/ISOO guideline supports the use of oral cryotherapy in patients undergoing autologous hematopoietic stem cell transplant (HSCT) with high-dose melphalan conditioning protocols and patients receiving bolus 5-fluorouracil chemotherapy.[123] Growth factors and cytokines have been studied for the prevention and treatment of OM and only keratinocyte growth factor-1 (KGF-1) has been shown to be effective in patients undergoing autologous HSCT conditioned with high-dose chemotherapy and total body irradiation regimens.[124] Laser therapy and other light therapies that have trophic, anti-inflammatory, and analgesic effects have been trialed for both prevention and treatment of OM. In patients receiving HSCT or head and neck radiation this type of therapy may be effective for prevention of OM and related pain.[125]

For the prevention of gastrointestinal mucositis, several therapies are being investigated including palifermin, glutamine, sodium butyrate, and dietary interventions, but the evidence base for these interventions is not strong. The MASCC/ISOO does recommend the use of probiotics containing *Lactobacillus* spp. for prevention of chemotherapy- and radiation-induced diarrhea in patients with pelvic malignancies.[126]

The primary symptom associated with OM that interdisciplinary teams are asked to address is pain. The mainstay of treatment for pain associated with OM remains systemic opioids. In the setting of oral pain and difficulty swallowing, intravenous PCA with a basal rate and a bolus dose may provide the most immediate and effective pain control. Opioids can be very helpful, but they frequently do not completely control the pain and their use may be limited by side effects such as sedation. For this reason many oral rinses have been trialed as adjuvant therapy. Topical agents are often mixed in different combinations and referred to by various colloquial names such as "magic mouthwash." Though these combined rinses are common, the evidence does not support their use. In fact the American Academy of Nursing Choosing Wisely statement recommends against the use of mixed medication mouthwashes to prevent or manage cancer treatment–induced OM. Topical agents that have been tried in the treatment of OM-induced pain include analgesics such as viscous lidocaine, morphine, ketamine, diphenhydramine, capsaicin, doxepin, benzydamine, maltodextrin, and dexamethasone. Mucosal protective agents such as aluminum hydroxide and magnesium hydroxide containing liquid antacids, natural honey, Gelclair, Episil, kaolin/pectin, and propolis have also been tried. The evidence base is not strong enough to recommend the use of any one of these adjuvant treatments over another. Caution needs to be taken when considering the use of topical anesthetics due to the theoretical concern over an increased risk of aspiration secondary to the numbing effects of the drugs and concern over systemic absorption through damaged mucosal surfaces. The MASCC/ISOO guidelines do recommend the use of topical 0.2% morphine mouthwash for the treatment OM pain in head and neck cancer patients treated with radiation and chemotherapy.[127] It is hypothesized that opioid receptors on peripheral nerves could be blocked by topical morphine leading to reduced neuronal excitability of peripheral nociceptors.[127]

One factor that may increase the oral pain associated with OM is secondary infection with fungal organisms, bacteria, or herpes simplex virus. In patients with mucositis, evaluation should be done for any signs of infection, and appropriate treatment should be started based on the results of the evaluation. In immunosuppressed patients, including patients on systemic steroids, topical treatment of oral infections is typically not sufficient and systemic treatment should be considered.

When children have OM, particular care should be taken to make sure they are eating foods that don't increase their pain. Foods that are acidic, salty, dry, or that require a significant amount of chewing should be avoided.

The primary symptom associated with gastrointestinal mucositis that interdisciplinary teams are asked to address is diarrhea. It is important to ensure that adequate hydration is maintained. Diarrhea can be treated with standard antidiarrheal medications including loperamide. If loperamide is not effective, then octreotide can be considered.

DIAPER DERMATITIS

Diaper dermatitis is a broad term used to describe an inflammatory reaction of the skin within the diaper area. Common causes include allergic contact dermatitis (ACD) and irritant contact dermatitis (ICD).

Allergic contact dermatitis can be caused by exposure to an allergen leading to a T-cell–mediated type IV delayed hypersensitivity reaction. The inflammatory response requires sensitization caused by an allergen penetrating the epidermal skin barrier followed by a subsequent exposure to the same allergen.[128] Common allergens include components of topical creams such as lanolin and formaldehyde releasers, preservatives such as benzalkonium chloride used in baby wipes, and topical medications including neomycin, antifungals, and steroids. The clinical presentation in the acute phase typically spares the skin folds and causes erythema, scaling, vesicles, and bullae.[128] Infants and toddlers may be less likely to develop ACD secondary to the immaturity of their immune systems.[129] Treatment includes avoidance of the allergen, regular use of emollients that enhance the barrier function of the skin, and topical corticosteroids. In very severe cases a short course of systemic corticosteroids can be considered.[128]

The most common cause of diaper dermatitis is ICD caused by impairment of the skin's barrier function and subsequent exposure to irritants such as those in urine and stool. Commonly the initial presentation includes erythema, mild maceration, and scaling which spares the inguinal folds. More severe presentations can include papules, pustules, and skin breakdown with open areas[130] (Figure 26.2). Complications of the initial condition can include granuloma gluteal infantum,[131] Jacquet's erosive diaper dermatitis,[132] pseudoverrucous papules,[133] and secondary infection.[134] The incidence of ICD peaks at 9–12 months of age,[129,134,135] but in seriously ill children incontinence and prolonged use of diapers is common and ICD can occur at any age.

The initiating event for ICD is overhydration of the skin from prolonged exposure to urine and stool which is potentiated by the physical occlusion of the diaper.[130,134] Friction from the diaper against the overhydrated skin causes damage to the stratum corneum and epidermis. This increases the skin's permeability to irritants.[130,134] In addition, the pH in the diaper area is increased when fecal ureases catalyze the conversion of urinary urea to ammonia.[130,134] Urease-positive bacteria in feces, which are more common in children who drink

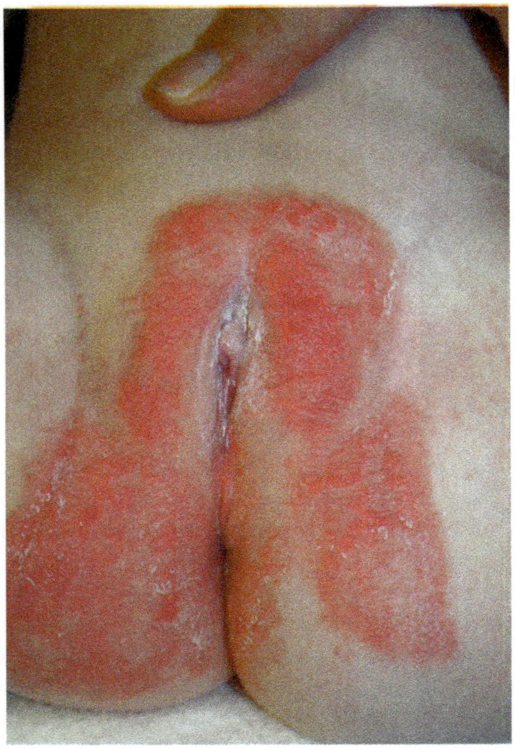

Figure 26.2 Diaper dermatitis.

cow's milk, can also degrade urea and release ammonia.[129] The elevated pH activates fecal proteases and lipases which are considered the most significant irritants leading to ICD.[129] The fecal enzymes further increase the skin's permeability to bile salts and other irritants.[136] It follows that there is a positive correlation between the number of stools per day and the development of ICD.[135] Of note, the faster stool moves through the intestine the higher the proteases and lipases concentration, leading to an even further increased susceptibility to ICD in children having diarrhea.[129] Broad-spectrum antibiotics can play a role by causing diarrhea and increasing the susceptibility to the development of a candida infection.[129] Other factors that may increase the likelihood of ICD are zinc and biotin deficiencies.[129] Additionally, premature infants can take several weeks to develop proper skin pH and full barrier function leading to the need for increased attention to this issue in the neonates.[134] One protective factor against ICD is breastfeeding which results in stools with a lower pH.[136]

The prevention and treatment of ICD starts with trying to keep the skin in the diaper area dry. This can be achieved by ensuring that the diaper is changed as soon as it becomes wet or soiled. An additional helpful approach is exposing the diaper area to air as often as possible,[130] which has the added benefit of decreasing friction on the skin from the diaper. Emollients can be applied to support the skin's barrier function.[137] When the diaper is changed, the skin should be gently cleansed completely removing urine and stool while minimizing friction. Research suggests that there is no significant difference between using a wet washcloth or a baby wipe to clean the skin.[138,139] Traditional soap with an alkaline pH should be avoided and mild cleansers with a slightly acid pH should be used instead.[137] Wipes should not contain alcohol, fragrances, essential oils, soap, or harsh detergents that can lead skin irritation. They should contain well-tolerated preservatives and a pH buffer to maintain slight acidity of the skin.[137] Once the skin is clean, a barrier cream containing zinc oxide or petroleum can be used to reduce the skin's contact with urine and stool. The barrier cream does not need to be fully removed between diaper changes as long as all of the urine and stool has been removed. Modern disposable diaper technology that includes super-absorbent gels, petrolatum-based lotions, breathable outer layers, and a mesh like aperture top sheet has helped in preventing ICD. These modern disposable diapers may be more effective in preventing ICD than cloth diapers.[140–142] If a severe ICD develops that is not responsive to the preceding measures, a short 3–7 day course of low-potency, nonhalogenated topical corticosteroid such as 1% hydrocortisone can be applied twice a day before the barrier cream. High-potency topical steroids and combination antifungal/potent steroid creams should be avoided as there can be systemic absorption leading to adrenal suppression. Topical vitamin A has been studied for treatment and prevention of ICD, but it is unclear whether it is efficacious.[143]

In the setting of diaper dermatitis with skin breakdown and an elevated skin pH that alters the cutaneous microbiome, there is increased risk for developing a secondary fungal or bacterial infection. The most common fungal infection is *Candida albicans*.[136] It commonly involves the deep skin folds and presents as erythematous and scaly plaques with satellite papules and pustules. Microscopic slide examination (KOH) or fungal culture can aid with diagnosis. If diaper dermatitis persists for more than 3 days after initiation of the standard treatments, it is likely that there is a secondary infection with *C. albicans*. Cutaneous infections can usually be easily treated with topical antifungals.[144] Persistent or recurrent infections could be a sign of diabetes mellitus, chronic mucocutaneous candidiasis, or an underlying immune deficiency. Bacterial infections in the diaper area can also occur and often present with vesiculopustular lesions that can be mistaken for fungal infection. The most common bacterial infection is *Staphylococcus aureus*.[136] Bullous impetigo caused by *S. aureus* often presents as large bullae that break down, leaving collarets of scale behind. Newborns are especially prone to development of bullous impetigo. *Staphylococcus* sp., *Escherichia coli*, and *Bacteroides* sp. are common.[145] Appropriate antibiotic therapy can be tailored based on bacterial culture results and organism susceptibility profiles. Typically topical antibiotic treatment is sufficient, but oral antibacterial treatment may be needed for more extensive infections and when topical therapy is not effective.[146] In the event of fever or ill appearance, an evaluation by a healthcare professional is indicated.

For persistent dermatoses that present in the diaper area and are unresponsive to conventional treatment approaches, dermatologic consultation and skin biopsy may be indicated. Skin diseases such as chronic inflammatory dermatoses (atopic dermatitis, seborrheic dermatitis, and psoriasis), infectious diseases (scabies, congenital syphilis, and primary herpes simplex), metabolic diseases (acrodermatitis enteropathica), autoimmune diseases (lichen sclerosis and Kawasaki disease), and neoplasms (Langerhans cell histiocytosis) may present with prominent groin involvement.[129,144]

One study[147] documented parental guilt secondary to a child developing diaper dermatitis, therefore care should be taken not to imply poor parenting when providing education about prevention and treatment of ICD. At the same time child abuse and/or neglect should be listed in the differential diagnosis of severe, recalcitrant, or atypical diaper dermatitis. ICD not responding to treatment may be the result of neglect and the diaper area is a possible site for burns and bruises.

WOUNDS

There are several causes of wounds that occur in seriously ill children. Pressure injuries, malignant wounds, wounds caused by blistering skin conditions, and trauma are the most common. Minimal literature is available regarding treatment of pediatric wounds versus adult wounds due to the fact that a majority of data has focused on the compromised and elderly patient. Lack of scientific data has contributed to ongoing use of modalities that are not optimal in managing wounds in the pediatric population, including saline gauze and leaving wounds open to air so they can breathe.

Unlike wound management in the general population, the first determination that should be made when managing a wound in a seriously ill child is the goal of treatment. Frequently, the goal is to heal the wound. However, in some cases, particularly when the child is near the end of life, there may not be time to heal the wound. The goal then becomes to stabilize the wound and control the symptoms associated with the wound including pain, odor, bleeding, and exudate. Under these circumstances care should be given to managing the periwound area.

TYPES OF WOUNDS

PRESSURE INJURIES

Pressure injuries in the pediatric population, while not as prevalent as in adults, are still a significant dermatologic occurrence that must be appropriately addressed. The incidence of pressure injuries in the pediatric population ranges from 1.4% to 28.8% depending on risk factors, with children in critical care being more likely to develop a pressure injury.[148–150] Minimal data are available on the overall incidence of pediatric pressure injuries, especially in seriously ill children. Data on the incidence and point prevalence of pediatric pressure injuries in different care settings, such as home setting versus hospital, are not available.

Children who are bed- or chair-bound or who have limited ability to reposition themselves are at particularly high risk for developing pressure injuries. Poor nutritional status and conditions leading to moist skin, such as incontinence, are compounding risk factors. It is important to identify patients who are at high risk and take steps to prevent pressure injury formation. If a child is identified as being high risk, his or her skin should be inspected daily so that issues can be identified before they become problematic. A bed-bound patient should be repositioned every 2 hours and a chair-bound patient every hour. An appropriate pressure-reducing mattress is essential to off-load areas of higher pressure.[151] In addition care should be taken to ensure that patients have appropriate cushions for their wheelchairs and other frequently used seating. Donut-type cushions should be avoided because they reduce blood flow to the tissue within the donut. Children should be lifted with the help of a draw sheet or trapeze when repositioned to prevent shearing forces. Pillows, foam wedges, and flotation devices or boots should be used to prevent bony prominences, such as the heels and ankles, from coming into contact with each other and surfaces.

When patients are in a side-lying position, pressure directly on the trochanter should be avoided. When a child is incontinent, an absorbent diaper or brief should be used, and it should be changed as soon as the child becomes wet or soiled. In addition, a barrier cream should be used to protect the skin from moisture. Excessive skin dryness is also a risk factor for skin breakdown. It should be avoided by applying liberal amounts of moisturizer directly to skin that is still damp after bathing (reapply up to 3–4 times daily) and subsequently overlapped with an emollient to serve as an occlusive agent thereby preventing moisture loss. When a child is being cared for at home it is important that parents and other caregivers are educated on how to prevent pressure injuries and how to identify pediatric skin failure at the earliest stage.[152]

Pressure injuries occur in similar locations in both adults and children. The most common locations are the heels, neck, sacrum, and scalp (specifically the occiput), or when any medical device is in contact with skin.[153,154] Whenever possible, avoid adhesives, rotate medical devices, dry skin whenever it is wet, and use appropriate skin barriers.[150] The primary concern, regardless of location of the injury, is addressing and eliminating the source of pressure, shear, friction, and or excess moisture. Examination of pressure sources includes evaluation of support surfaces, splints, braces, clothing, and any other material or device that is in contact with the skin. Unless the underlying etiology is identified, the opportunity to intervene and/or prevent further injury and promote healing is lost and may lead to continued tissue damage and severe injury. Whenever using any product on a child, whether a pressure-reducing surface, device, or other product, it is important to review the information related to age-specific use.

A child's report of pain from a cast, splint, or other supportive device should always be taken seriously pending complete review of the source of the pain. If in doubt, the supportive device should be removed to allow for a full assessment. Medical device–related pressure injuries (MDPIs) most commonly occur with external monitoring, oxygen delivery, and airway maintenance.[153] Sources of pressure that may require removal include but are not limited to casts, other immobilization devices and boards, masks, pressure cuffs, and tubing.

Identification of the underlying pressure injury etiology is critical to optimal outcomes. When treating pressure injuries, it is important to rule out other potential etiologies. These etiologies include fluid extravasation; surgery-related wounds; electrical, thermal, and chemical burns; incontinence-related erosions or lesions; congenital abnormalities; trauma from dressings, adhesives, and clothing; and systemic diseases. Potential abuse should be included in the differential diagnosis based on the presentation and history. Failure to treat underlying pathophysiology will delay or prevent closure of the wound.

Pressure injury staging is the same in adult and pediatric populations. The most commonly accepted system for staging and describing pressure injuries is from the National Pressure Injury Advisory Panel (NPIAP), shown in Box 26.1. The NPIAP updated its name in November 2019 from National Pressure Ulcer Advisory Panel (NPUAP) to reflect a shift to the internationally preferred term "pressure injury" in place of "pressure ulcer" to acknowledge that lesser degrees of skin damage due to pressure may not be associated with skin ulceration. The description and identification for each stage was

BOX 26.1 REVISED NATIONAL PRESSURE INJURY ADVISORY PANEL (NPIAP) PRESSURE INJURY STAGING SYSTEM

Pressure Injury: A pressure injury is localized damage to the skin and underlying soft tissue usually over a bony prominence or related to a medical or other device. The injury can present as intact skin or an open ulcer and may be painful. The injury occurs as a result of intense pressure, prolonged pressure or pressure in combination with shear. The tolerance of soft tissue for pressure and shear may also be affected by microclimate, nutrition, perfusion, comorbid conditions and condition of the soft tissue.

Stage 1 Pressure Injury: Non-blanchable erythema of intact skin. Intact skin with a localized area of nonblanchable erythema, which may appear differently in darkly pigmented skin. Presence of blanchable erythema or changes in sensation, temperature, or firmness may precede visual changes. Color changes do not include purple or maroon discoloration; these may indicate deep tissue pressure injury.

Stage 2 Pressure Injury: Partial- thickness loss of skin with exposed dermis. Partial-thickness loss of skin with exposed dermis. The wound bed is viable, pink or red, moist, and may also present as an intact or ruptured serum-filled blister. Adipose (fat) is not visible and deeper tissues are not visible. Granulation tissue, slough and eschar are not present. These injuries commonly result from adverse microclimate and shear in the skin over the pelvis and shear in the heel. This stage should not be used to describe moisture associated skin damage (MASD) including incontinence associated dermatitis (IAD), intertriginous dermatitis (ITD), medical adhesive related skin injury (MARSI), or traumatic wounds (skin tears, burns, abrasions).

Stage 3 Pressure Injury: Full-thickness skin loss. Full-thickness loss of skin, in which adipose (fat) is visible in the ulcer and granulation tissue and epibole (rolled wound edges) are often present. Slough and/or eschar may be visible. The depth of tissue damage varies by anatomical location; areas of significant adiposity can develop deep wounds. Undermining and tunneling may occur. Fascia, muscle, tendon, ligament, cartilage or bone are not exposed. If slough or eschar obscures the extent of tissue loss this is an unstageable pressure injury.

Stage 4 Pressure Injury: Full-thickness loss of skin and tissue. Full-thickness skin and tissue loss with exposed or directly palpable fascia, muscle, tendon, ligament, cartilage or bone in the ulcer. Slough and/or eschar may be visible. Epibole (rolled edges), undermining and/or tunneling often occur. Depth varies by anatomical location. If slough or eschar obscures the extent of tissue loss this is an unstageable pressure injury.

Unstageable Pressure Injury: Obscured full-thickness skin and tissue loss. Full-thickness skin and tissue loss in which the extent of tissue damage within the ulcer cannot be confirmed because it is obscured by slough or eschar. If slough or eschar is removed, a Stage 3 or Stage 4 pressure injury will be revealed. Stable eschar (i.e. dry, adherent, intact without erythema or fluctuance) on an ischemic limb or the heel(s) should not be softened or removed.

Deep Tissue Pressure Injury: Persistent non-blanchable deep red, maroon or purple discoloration. Intact or non-intact skin with localized area of persistent non- blanchable deep red, maroon, purple discoloration or epidermal separation revealing a dark wound bed or blood filled blister. Pain and temperature change often precede skin color changes. Discoloration may appear differently in darkly pigmented skin. This injury results from intense and/or prolonged pressure and shear forces at the bone-muscle interface. The wound may evolve rapidly to reveal the actual extent of tissue injury, or may resolve without tissue loss. If necrotic tissue, subcutaneous tissue, granulation tissue, fascia, muscle or other underlying structures are visible, this indicates a full thickness pressure injury (Unstageable, Stage 3 or Stage 4). Do not use DTPI to describe vascular, traumatic, neuropathic, or dermatologic conditions.

Additional pressure injury definitions.

Medical Device Related Pressure Injury: This describes an etiology. Medical device related pressure injuries result from the use of devices designed and applied for diagnostic or therapeutic purposes. The resultant pressure injury generally conforms to the pattern or shape of the device. The injury should be staged using the staging system.

Mucosal Membrane Pressure Injury: Mucosal membrane pressure injury is found on mucous membranes with a history of a medical device in use at the location of the injury. These ulcers cannot be staged.

Used with permission of the Prevention and Treatment of Pressure Ulcers/Injuries: Clinical Practice Guideline. The International Guideline 2019. Third edition released November 2019 by the European Pressure Ulcer Advisory Panel, National Pressure Injury Advisor Panel, Pan Pacific Pressure Injury Alliance.

updated to reflect additional mechanisms and areas of injury (e.g., device-related and mucosal pressure injuries).[155,156]

GASTROSTOMY TUBE SITE HYPERGRANULATION TISSUE AND ERYTHEMA

Hypergranulation tissue is common in the first 3 months of gastrostomy tube (G tube) placement and may develop at mature stoma sites due to excess moisture, pressure, or friction caused by tube instability. Hypergranulation tissue may cause discomfort and affect how the device fits in the stoma. It is important to first address proper tube sizing, as a replacement or alternate gauge may be indicated. In addition, some G tubes have a balloon, and it is important to check that the balloon is properly inflated to secure the tube and prevent leakage. Polyurethane foam may be used to reduce friction and absorb leaks. Topical triamcinolone three times daily has been used for the treatment of hypergranulation tissue with good effect.[157] If the problem persists despite these interventions, treatment with silver nitrate may be employed. Before using silver nitrate it is vital to protect the peri-stomal healthy skin with barrier cream to avoid chemical burn of this healthy tissue. The area should then be sprayed with a 20% benzocaine topical anesthetic aerosol spray immediately prior to the procedure since silver nitrate may cause pain. Once the area has been protected and appropriate anesthesia has been achieved, using minimal pressure, quickly touch the silver nitrate stick directly to the hypergranulation tissue, being careful not to allow dripping of fluid onto the surrounding healthy skin. Following the procedure, maintain the skin as clean and dry as possible. Reassess weekly, as reapplication may be necessary to completely eliminate the hypergranulation tissue. If the child is unable to tolerate the treatment (e.g., exhibiting discomfort following the procedure by taking a long time to settle or grabbing at the tube site), stop treatment and consult the surgical team for alternative options.

Erythema around the G tube site is common and typically caused by leakage of gastric content or other factors that cause the skin to become moist. The skin around the G tube site should be gently cleansed and dried daily. It is very important to protect the skin using a barrier cream or ointment. Split gauze is typically not helpful. Candida infections can occur and should be treated with topical antifungal medications. Cellulitis is less common, but should be considered if there is pain at the G tube site. If cellulitis does occur, it is frequently caused by staphylococcal infection, and oral or intravenous antibiotics may be indicated.

MALIGNANT AND FUNGATING WOUNDS

A primary skin cancer, invasion of a primary or metastatic tumor through the skin, or the cutaneous infiltration of a tumor via the bloodstream or lymphatics, may cause malignant wounds. Some of the cancers in adults that commonly cause these types of wounds include melanoma, breast, lung, head and neck, chest, colorectal, cervical, and ovarian.[158,159] In children and young adults sarcomas are more common and can cause fungating malignant wounds.

Malignant wounds alter the perfusion of the involved tissue. There is often significant tumor necrosis. Necrotic tissue can become infected, usually with anaerobic and facultative bacteria, but sometimes also with aerobic bacteria leading to pain and odor.[160] The challenges in the management of a malignant wound are controlling the infection, exudate, odor, bleeding, itching, and denuded periwound skin.[158,159] Signs and symptoms of the wound can impact the child's psychological well-being leading to anxiety, distress, and social isolation.[158] The wound may affect the child's body image, and associated odor may be embarrassing and lead to isolation because family and friends are repulsed.[158]

The principles of management of malignant wounds are the same as those for advanced pressure injuries. In malignant wounds there may be a role for antineoplastic treatments in reducing tumor size and managing symptoms. Radiotherapy, chemotherapy, hormonal therapy, and surgical excision may be incorporated to reduce the size of tumor and control the bleeding, exudate, and pain.[161] Therapies may help slow the progression and severity but rarely heal the wound.[162] The focus of treatment should be on controlling the symptoms associated with the wound.[161]

BLISTERING DERMATOSES

Genetically inherited blistering disorders, such as EB, present a spectrum of disease severity and prognosis depending on type and defect in cell adhesion molecules. EB simplex is due to defects in keratin 5 and 14, and although traditionally it has been described as a more mild form of EB, simplex has a variable phenotype from a mild to severe depending on subtype. Patients with junctional or dystrophic EB have significant morbidity and mortality associated with their disease throughout the life span. The emphasis in children with any form of EB is on adequate nutrition, control of anemia, prevention and treatment of wounds, and infection prophylaxis if indicated.[163] It is important to assess symptom burden in children with EB because pruritus,[164] pain,[165] and other symptoms impacting quality of life are common.[166] For example, nearly all patients with any form of EB report frequent severe pain.[167,168] A Quality of Life EB questionnaire for children and adults 10 years and older is available,[169] while another tool, the EB-specific module of the Infants and Toddlers Dermatology Quality of Life,[170,171] was recently developed. Treatments to improve overall health and specific symptoms while mitigating unwanted side effects are a target of ongoing investigation.[164,172–174]

An attempt to minimize the formation of wounds is important in this group of patients. Minor trauma and shearing forces can cause blistering (Figure 26.3). Using gentle handling techniques is critical. The seams of clothing and elastic on disposable diapers can cause trauma. Loose clothing should be chosen and be turned inside out when worn. Cloth diapers can be used, or the elastic can be cut out of disposable diapers. Fusion of the digits can be a problem in children with EB, and children's fingers and toes can be individually wrapped in an attempt to prevent this from occurring. It is important to avoid adhesives that are frequently used to attach medical

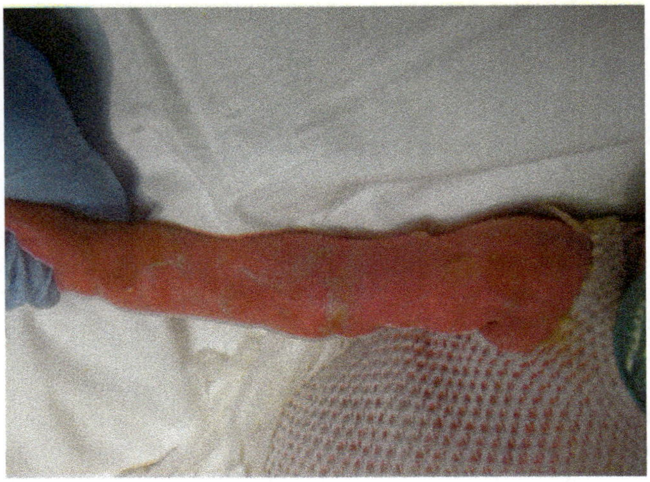

Figure 26.3 Epidermolysis bullosa of the arm.

devices, such as cardiac monitors and pulse oximeters, to the skin. When necessary, children should be bathed in a tub and gently patted dry or allowed to air dry. Breastfeeding and bottle-feeding can cause trauma to the lips. Petroleum should be used to lubricate lips prior to feeding, or syringe or dropper feeds should be considered. Keeping stools soft can minimize trauma to the anal area caused by bowel movements. Controlling the child's environment by avoiding heat and high humidity can be helpful in preventing blister formation.

When large blisters do form, they may need to be gently lanced and drained or aspirated without removal of the roof of the blister, which provides a natural dressing. When there are open wounds the general principles of wound care can be applied (Figure 26.4).[175] Wounds are often treated with an antibiotic cream and covered with a nonadherent dressing. Dressings can be held in place with stretchy tubular gauze netting (Figure 26.3).

DOCUMENTATION AND EDUCATION

An important component for the treatment of problematic pediatric wounds is the documentation of the findings, treatments applied, and family education provided. Documentation in conjunction with family and patient education is an intrinsic component of the care process and is usually more difficult and time-consuming than care of the wound itself. Initial documentation requires measurements, a description including unusual characteristics, photos, staging of pressure injuries, past treatments, and response to treatments. The baseline wound assessment includes location, size, type of tissue, amount and type of exudate, presence of malodor and signs of infection, condition of surrounding skin, and presence of pain.[161,176] A thorough history, including a review of systems, past medical history, and history of past therapies, is a requirement for the development of an appropriate treatment plan. Subsequent documentation should reflect a complete evaluation performed at each examination. Risk assessment is part of the documentation, of which the most commonly used prediction tools are the Norton and Braden scales. It is important to recognize, however, that these risk assessment tools cover a limited range of risk factors, and therefore their use in conjunction with clinical judgment is imperative.

Family education can be challenging when expectations for rapid recovery and optimal outcome are not attainable. Underestimation of time to closure, lack of clarity about expected outcome, and nondisclosure of treatment complications may lead to frustration for the patient and family. A clear, concise, compassionate explanation of the treatment and expected outcome establishes credibility and collaboration.

TREATMENT

Six primary general principles of wound care can be applied when initiating the treatment of any wound.

- Identify and treat underlying pathophysiology if possible
- Debride nonviable tissue
- Provide nutritional support
- Identify and treat infection
- Use appropriate topical therapy
- Consider advanced modalities

When planning wound care with a seriously ill patient, the following principles should be considered as well:[161]

- The wishes of the patient
- The diagnosis and future prognosis
- Psychological impact of the wound on the patient's quality of life, family, and careers
- Availability of social support networks

Along with managing the wound, it is crucial to manage the symptoms that are often associated with wounds including

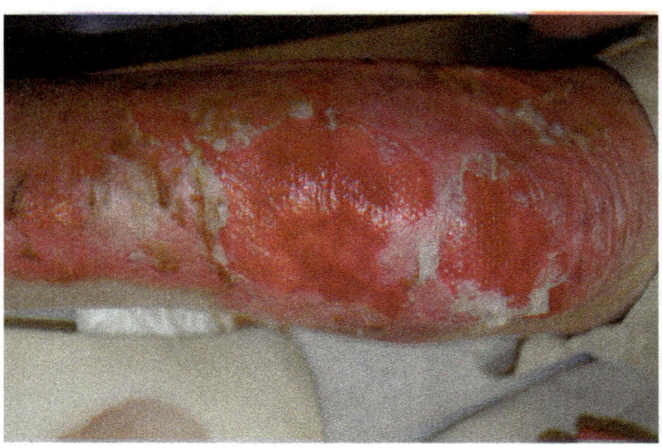

Figure 26.4 Epidermolysis bullosa of the leg.

pain, odor, bleeding, and exudate[161] (Table 26.4). When these symptoms are left untreated there is potential to affect a child's quality of life by leading to anxiety, embarrassment, and social isolation.

When formulating a treatment plan there must be a clear definition about whether the goal is to heal the wound or control the symptoms associated with the wound. For example, when the goal is to heal a wound, debridement is critical to allow wound healing. When the goal is to control symptoms associated with a wound, debridement is important to the extent that it is required to control odor, drainage, or infection. Nutritional support is critical to wound healing, but when a wound won't heal, the child is near the end of life, and the goal is to control the symptoms associated with the wound, then nutrition is not as important. Children who are close to the end of life may have poor appetites. In these cases, there is no need to encourage any more nutritional intake than the child can comfortably tolerate.

DEBRIDEMENT

The evidence-based literature discusses the importance of removing nonviable or infected tissue from a wound bed because it may delay wound closure and contribute to infection.[155,177,178] Unless surgical debridement is necessary due to extensive damage, a conservative approach with debridement outside the operating room is typically successful. Sharp debridement may require premedication or application of a topical anesthetic such as benzocaine spray, EMLA, or sevoflurane.[177] The wound may then be gently debrided by curettage or conservative sharp debridement to remove nonviable tissue. Autolytic, enzymatic, biological, ultrasonic, and mechanical (irrigation, hydrotherapy) debridement have been used successfully in cases where sharp and or more intensive debridement may not be possible or indicated.[178] Wet-to-dry dressings are a nonselective form of mechanical debridement which are no longer recommended for use as they often remove healthy tissues, leading to tissue reinjury, which causes bleeding, pain, and delayed healing.[179] As such, *wet-to-dry* dressings are considered substandard wound care. The primary enzyme available on the US market for *enzymatic debridement* is collagenase, a selective chemical debriding agent indicated in wounds with slough or necrosis. It should be applied after cleansing with normal saline to create an optimal pH environment of 6–8 and should not be used in conjunction with silver, mercury, or certain detergent products as these may inhibit the activity of the collagenase enzyme. As with many products related to wound care, minimal data are available establishing safety and efficacy of enzymes in the pediatric population. Establishing the risk-benefit ratio and reviewing the patient medical history is imperative prior to prescription of any enzyme. No documentation is available regarding the use of this drug category in neonates, therefore, application in this population cannot be recommended.

Autolytic debridement employs the use of occlusion and a moist wound environment. In the presence of normal cell and immune response activity, preventing desiccation of the wound bed allows for a natural debridement accomplished by macrophage activity, endogenous wound bed enzymes (including elastase and collagenase), and subsequent autolytic activity.[178] Medicinal honey is an antimicrobial that promotes autolytic debridement.[180] It has been documented for pediatric use,[181,182] although not in well-designed randomized controlled and adequately powered trials.[181] It appears to be well-tolerated and effective in the limited data available. It is a slower method, but it offers an alternative approach.

NUTRITION

The adverse effects of poor nutritional status on tissue repair, infection rates, morbidity, and mortality are well documented in the literature.[148,150,156,183,184] Understanding the overall nutritional status of the pediatric patient by reviewing markers, including but not limited to albumin and prealbumin levels, is a key component of wound healing. Despite relieving pressure, addressing the underlying wound etiology, and choosing an adequate dressing, tissue repair may not occur in the absence of adequate nutrition. Optimizing nutritional status by including a registered dietician in the interdisciplinary team may be useful.

TOPICAL THERAPY

A myriad of topical dressings, ointments, and treatment modalities is available. The variety of products and manufacturers' claims creates confusion rather than clarity as to which treatment is most appropriate and effective. It is important to explore the information provided with each product, particularly indications and contraindications, before product selection. This overview is intended to categorize each of the primary dressing types. Table 26.3 provides a concise list of product options, their indications, and contraindications, as well as advantages and disadvantages. The data listed are meant as a guideline since individual medical status and goals will vary among patients. Similar products within each category have never been compared with each other in any published Level I or credible trial. Based on the lack of research, it may be justly assumed that the major differences between products within a dressing category are based on cost, qualitative features, patient tolerance, availability, and educational support provided by the industry. Each patient's wound requirements, medical status, tolerance to product components, reaction to adhesives, and other features should be considered before choosing a product in any category. The goal of topical therapy is to collect drainage, protect periwound skin, prevent infection, reduce odor, and promote patient comfort while reducing the frequency of dressing changes.[179,181,185]

Transparent Film

Transparent dressings are primarily polyurethane-based and designed to permit vapor transmission. Their primary purpose is to seal and protect superficial wounds, thus reducing the risk of external contamination or abrasion. This particular category of products are adhesive in nature and, if removed prematurely or less than 48 hours after application, may damage newly formed and periwound tissue. Even when left

TABLE 26.3 Wound dressings

CLASSIFICATION OR DESCRIPTION	INDICATIONS	CONTRAINDICATIONS	ADVANTAGES AND DISADVANTAGES	HELPFUL HINTS
Transparent Films Transparent Polyurethane film Gas permeable Moisture vapor permeable Impermeable to bacteria and liquids Adhesive	Dry to minimally exudating wounds Partial thickness Granular or necrotic, ideal for softening eschar Skin tears May use over absorptive wound fillers or hydrogels on full-thickness wounds	Infected wounds Wounds with heavy exudate Fragile surrounding skin	Advantages: Protection Autolysis, especially eschar Allows visual assessment Waterproof Flexible Pain reducing Moist environment Up to 7-day wear time Disadvantages: Not absorptive Excess drainage may cause maceration of surrounding skin May strip fragile skin upon removal May be difficult to apply	Use a large enough dressing to cover at least 1 inch of surrounding skin. Application of skin sealant to surrounding skin improves seal Change dressing when exudate leaks onto intact skin around the wound to avoid maceration Read package insert and instructions (RPII)
Hydrocolloids Wafer dressing that interacts with wound exudate to form a moist gel on wound bed Impermeable to oxygen (occlusive) Impermeable to bacteria Adhesive	Wounds with low to moderate exudate Partial or full thickness Granular or necrotic Pressure ulcers Venous ulcers May be used over absorptive wound fillers, alginates, or hydrogels depending on amount of drainage	Infected wounds Third-degree burns Diabetic ulcers Arterial ulcers Wounds with heavy exudate Fragile surrounding skin	Advantages: Protection Autolysis Waterproof Flexible Pain reduction Moist environment 3- to 7-day wear time Insulates wound Disadvantages: Odor May strip fragile skin upon removal Excess drainage can cause maceration of surrounding skin Potential for sensitivity to adhesive	Consider patch test to check for allergy to adhesive when using over venous ulcers Cover at least 1 inch of surrounding skin for improved adhesion Change the dressing *before* it leaks Educate families in advance of the odor and drainage associated with this product RPII
Foams Polyurethane foam Varying degrees of thickness and gas permeability Adhesive and nonadhesive forms	Wounds with moderate to high exudate Partial or full thickness Granular or necrotic Pressure ulcers Venous ulcers Diabetic ulcers Arterial ulcers Infected wounds if changed daily Can be used over hydrogels, absorptive wound fillers, or alginates	Stage 1 wounds Dry wounds Fragile surrounding skin	Advantages: Protection Autolysis Conforms to shape Moist environment Insulates wound May decrease excess granulation tissue 4- to 7-day wear time Disadvantages: Some require tape or other securing method Adhesive foams may strip skin upon removal Cavity foams may harm tissue if over-packed	Tape nonadhesive foams across dressing rather than picture-framing with tape; this keeps the foam in contact with the wound Cover at least 1 inch of surrounding skin Most foams should be changed when strike-through of drainage is within 1 inch of the edge. RPII
Absorptive Wound Fillers Sheets, ropes, pastes, granules, or powders that absorb exudate Two main types: *Starch Copolymers* *Alginates:* Naturally occurring polymer of seaweed; gel is formed when fibers interact with wound fluid Some products are fillers, but do not absorb much exudate. Read product insert	Moderate to high exudate Partial or full thickness Granular or necrotic Pressure ulcers Venous ulcers Diabetic ulcers Arterial ulcers Used as a filler with other dressings Infected wounds if changed daily	Dry or low exudating wounds Deep tunneling wounds or deep undermining Alginates not recommended for third-degree burns	Advantages: Autolysis Conforms to shape Moist environment Absorbs exudate Nonadherent Pain reducing No reinjury at removal Up to 7-day wear time Alginates are mildly hemostatic Disadvantages: Requires secondary dressing Alginates may dry out and adhere to wound, requiring saline soak to remove	For very high-draining wounds, cover with gauze or abdominal (ABD) pad and change when drainage strikes through to outside May cover with foam, hydrocolloid, or film, depending on amount of exudate Some starch copolymers should be packed to fill the wound only one-third to one-half full. Absorption capacity varies among fillers. RPII

TABLE 26.3 Continued

CLASSIFICATION OR DESCRIPTION	INDICATIONS	CONTRAINDICATIONS	ADVANTAGES AND DISADVANTAGES	HELPFUL HINTS
Hydrogels Sheets or amorphous gels that have 20–90% water Some have starch copolymers that absorb small amounts of exudate Some products are dehydrated gels that offer more absorption Nonadhesive Gas permeable	Dry to minimally exudating wounds Partial thickness, use sheet gel Full thickness, use amorphous gel Granular or necrotic Pressure ulcers Diabetic ulcers Arterial ulcers, leave dry if there is no healing potential. Amorphous gels may be used on infected wound if changed daily	Wounds with heavy exudate Stage 1 wounds Sheet hydrogels are not recommended on infected wounds	Advantages: Autolysis Conforms to wound bed Moist environment Nonadhesive Pain reduction No trauma upon removal Disadvantages: Potential to macerate surrounding skin May require secondary dressing Some products may dehydrate in wound	Saturate gauze pad with amorphous gel to pack into wounds with depth Change dressing based on amount of drainage. If wound is drying out after one day, change daily; if wound is staying moist longer, change less often if wound not infected Sheet hydrogels work well on skin tears; change only 1–2 times a week RPII
Contact Layers Exudate-permeable sheets that are applied directly over wound to prevent dressing adherence to wound Used commonly under gauze	Wounds in which dressings are adhering Petrolatum-impregnated contact layers may help keep dry wounds moist Used over skin substitutes and extracellular matrices	No major contraindications	Advantages: Provides for atraumatic removal of dressings Disadvantages: Some contact layers may still adhere to wound bed Petrolatum-based contact layers may contribute to periwound maceration in higher draining wounds	Overlap onto surrounding skin by 1–2 cm to protect fragile wound edges RPII
Antimicrobial Dressings Sheets, pastes, foams, films, or gauze dressings with nontoxic antimicrobials that maintain a moist environment, although gauze product may dry out	Indicated to decrease colonization of microbes and reduce the risk of infection in partial- and full-thickness wounds Absorptive capacity varies among products	Sensitivity to ingredients	Advantages: Provides nontoxic alternative to antiseptics in patients at risk for infection Broad-spectrum coverage Reduces wound odor Film dressings provide bacterial barrier Disadvantages: Expensive Some products require secondary dressing	Match dressing to exudate level RPII
Gauze Linen fiber dressing Some are woven, some are nonwoven	Wounds with minimal to heavy exudate Partial or full thickness Granular or necrotic Pressure ulcers Venous ulcers Diabetic ulcers Arterial ulcers May be used on infected wounds Use over topical antibiotics, growth factors, or enzymes	None	Advantages: Universally available Easy to use Ribbon gauze packs deep tunnels Facilitates mechanical debridement Disadvantages: Nonselective debridement, will harm healthy tissue Readily dries out wound Must be kept continually moist with saline to provide moist wound healing Usually requires multiple dressing changes per day Cotton fibers left in wound may cause prolonged inflammation and may interfere with wound healing	Avoid use of wet-to-dry dressings because of pain and tissue damage upon removal For continuously moist dressing, remove secondary dressing and reapply saline to packing q4–6h Use ribbon gauze for packing deep sinus tracts Pack wounds lightly to prevent pressure on tissue RPII

This list is not all-inclusive of every dressing on the market. No inferences should be made regarding the inclusion or exclusion of products on this list.

intact for up to 1 week, they should be removed with the pull and stretch then lift technique. Transparent film dressings are not designed for use with heavily exudating or full-thickness wounds, unless it is being used to secure the primary dressing.[178,179,181,185,186]

Hydrocolloid

Hydrocolloid dressings usually contain guar gum and carboxymethylcellulose in varying degrees and are designed for use on partial and full-thickness wounds that are low to moderately exudating. They may be left intact on clean, noninfected low-exudate wounds for up to a week. Caution must be exerted when removing any adhesive dressings from the skin because continued adhesion may damage the surrounding tissue. Hydrocolloid dressings may allow for limited routine bathing and hygiene because they are water impermeable. This category of products is of particular benefit to the pediatric patient because they conform well to irregular surface areas and are generally well-tolerated. Dressing residue may be present on removal, so this type of dressing should be avoided in very deep wounds with tunneling or sinus tracts where the residue cannot be removed. They should be avoided with high levels of exudate or when friable and fragile tissue is present.[178,179,181,185,186]

Foam Dressings

Foam dressings are minimally traumatic to tissue while being one of the most versatile categories of products on the market. Especially versatile are the configurations without adhesive backings or borders. Other than sensitivity to adhesives or products, there are no major contraindications. Polyurethane foam dressings are designed for heavily exudating wounds. Depending on the level of exudate and bacterial burden, the dressing may be left in place for up to 1 week. Absorption of fluid on low to moderately exudating wounds is good, allowing for the wicking of excess fluid. Foam products are easily applied, well-tolerated by the patient, and painless when removed. Abdominal, back, and scalp wounds, as well as those on relatively flat surfaces, are easily covered with smaller or larger size dressings. When adhesive is not desired, they may be held in place with a burn net or gauze wrap. Modified foams are available for irregularly shaped surfaces, including the buttocks, elbows, and heels. Foams do not provide any significant pressure reduction or relief. Foams are available with a silver antimicrobial component. Avoid using polyurethane foams on no or low exudating wounds to prevent adhesion to granulating tissue and unintentional mechanical debridement.[178,179,181,185,186]

Alginates and Collagen Dressings

Alginates are biodegradable products derived from seaweed and optimal for moderate to heavily exudative wounds with tunneling, undermining, and sinus tracts to which other dressings cannot conform. They are highly absorbent due to the strong hydrophilic gel formation, which simultaneously serves to limit wound secretions and minimize bacterial contamination. Alginates combined with calcium allow for hemostasis in steadily oozing wounds or bleeding friable wounds.[178,179,181,185,186] It is important that these products are "cut to fit" and do not overlap the wound edge as this could lead to maceration of the periwound area. As with all products, caution is needed in deep tracts and cavities to avoid allowing product or residue to remain lodged in areas that cannot be cleansed with gentle irrigation. This category of products usually requires daily dressing changes. Fortunately, removal is painless as they do not adhere to the wound bed in moderate to heavily exuding wounds. The products dissolve and can be removed with gentle rinsing or cleansing as part of normal bathing, and alginate fibers that remain trapped in a wound are readily biodegraded. However, products left on low-exudate wounds for extended periods of time may desiccate and be difficult or painful to remove. Collagen products are an excellent biomaterial for chronic wounds by promoting restoration of tissue structure, regeneration, and functionality.[187] Exogenous collagen (derived from animal sources) is biodegradable and purified to be rendered a weak antigenic. Collagen dressings are available in sheets or powder forms, the latter of which can be easily removed with gentle irrigation between dressing changes. A secondary dressing is typically recommended.

Hydrogel Dressings

These are available in amorphous, sheet, or gauze configurations. They consist of varying degrees of water, polymers, humectants, and preservatives. Their primary use is in maintaining moisture in low-exudate wounds while assisting with debridement through autolysis. They are the standard treatment for clean granulating wounds. Hydrogel dressings and topical hydrogels must be changed daily to keep the wound moist and prevent the hydrogel from evaporating and further drying the wound. Application of hydrogels to moderate to heavily exudating wounds may contribute to maceration of the wound edges. Maceration decreases tissue tensile strength and, in the presence of shear, friction, or ongoing pressure, may contribute to further tissue breakdown. If a moistened normal saline gauze is being applied, consider switching to a hydrogel as it will not cause dessication or tissue trauma.

Silver and Antimicrobial Dressings

Silver and other antimicrobial dressings act on the cell membrane and wall by eliminating existing bacteria, inhibiting bacterial and fungal growth, and promoting wound contraction.[188] They are available in versions of almost all of the preceding products and are also available topically, as in silver sulfadiazine cream. There is no Level I study or other significant data related to antimicrobial dressing use and improved outcomes in pediatric pressure injuries. Patients with heavy colonization of a wound, high risk of wound infection, and/or an immunosuppressive disorder are at risk of developing a clinical infection requiring oral or systemic antibiotic therapy. Reducing or controlling the level of pathogens in a chronic wound to below a critical level in high-risk scenarios may ultimately benefit the patient.[178,179,181,185,186] However, antimicrobial products, while not contraindicated in the presence of infection, are not to be used as the primary treatment for a true clinical infection. Except for an immunocompromised individual, the host immune system may be successful at eradicating bacteria at a local level. Products with high silver content, above 2 parts per million, have not been well studied in the pediatric patient and should be used with caution, particularly in the neonatal population. High concentrations of silver in clean granulating wounds may cause cell stasis and inhibition of migration.

Zinc is another heavy metal with antimicrobial properties. While some benefit has been suggested when applied topically, pediatric data are not available. There is no reason to suspect that limited use of a product with topical zinc on a superficial lesion poses any risk, yet caution is still warranted. Topical antimicrobials are commonly prescribed and available over the counter. Triple antibiotic ointment and similar agents are known to cause sensitizing reactions.[189] Available data suggest they may be of benefit in reducing surface colonization, however, simple daily cleansing with a liquid antimicrobial wound cleanser or normal saline, followed by covering with gauze, is inexpensive and effective.[160,179,186,190–192]

Topical gel with metronidazole offers the benefits of a hydrogel, as listed earlier, while assisting with odor control caused by anaerobes. Other antimicrobial ointments, including mupirocin ointment, address gram-positive organisms in the wound environment. Literature exploring the differences in effectiveness and cytotoxicity levels of different topical antimicrobial agents is available for review.[160,179,186,190–192]

Iodine dressings exert bactericidal action. Two of the most widely used forms are cadexomer iodine (Iodosorb, Iodoform packing strips) and Povidine-iodine (Betadine). Cadexomer iodine is indicated in chronic or heavily colonized wounds as it exhibits dual action with antimicrobial and desloughing properties. It is available in a gel, ointment, powder, or dressing form. For dry ulcers that are not expected to heal or where moist wound healing is contraindicated (e.g., dry stable eschars), providine-iodine is used as an antiseptic for superficial bacteria.

INFECTION CONTROL

Bacteria, fungi, and other infectious agents colonize all wounds. It is not until the infectious agent is present in sufficient quantities that the wound is considered infected. *Staphylococcus epidermis* and *Corynebacterium* are the most common wound colonizers while *Proteus, Klebsiella, Pseudomonas*, and *Candida* are the most common infectious agents. The presence of pathogens at a critically colonized levels are known to delay the tissue repair process.[160,179,186,190–192] They can also lead to purulent exudate, pain, and odor. Clinical and systemic signs of infection must be carefully reviewed to ascertain if the wound and periwound skin condition is consistent with infection. Swabs and wound cultures are most accurate when taken post-debridement or following gentle cleansing with a non-antimicrobial agent use of antimicrobial agents may hinder growth from the fluid retrieved from the culture. Unless superficial debris and contaminants have been removed the swab culture may not be indicative of deep-tissue pathogens. Simple contamination may be addressed through superficial debridement and wound cleansing, thus may not require the use of antibiotic therapy.[160,179,186,190–192] Antimicrobial dressings may be used with caution as previously mentioned. The larger the wound surface area, the greater the need becomes to determine risk of systemic absorption of any agent that may be incorporated into a dressing, including silver, polyhexamethybutylene, iodine, or other antimicrobial. If antibiotic treatment is indicated, selection will be based on numerous factors, including identification of pathogens, spectrum of coverage, and patient tolerance.

ADJUNCTIVE, ADVANCED, AND ANCILLARY TECHNOLOGIES

Modalities that have been developed more recently include the use of growth factors, acellular matrices, cell-based products, topical drugs, and mechanical devices, such as electrical stimulation, moisture vapor therapy, and ultrasound. These technologies are designed to assist with wound closure for the more difficult to heal lesions. Studies related to these products have been conducted on the adult population. Product application, indications, and contraindications must be carefully reviewed to determine if the benefit justifies their risks. There is an abundance of literature on these product categories for the treatment of problematic wounds in the adult population although, except for biological materials, most of the evidence is Level II or usually Level III. Virtually no literature may be found that discusses the same application of any of these products in the pediatric population.

Of the ancillary treatment modalities, negative pressure wound therapy (NPWT) has become one of the most commonly used. NPWT is indicated for full-thickness clean, granulating wounds without slough or necrosis of most etiologies, including pressure injuries. Reading the manufacturer's recommendations for pediatric use and any available literature is a requirement before use of any of the devices. A review of the literature finds no data showing any advantage of using one manufacturer's NPWT product over another's. NPWT is of greatest benefit in larger defects to assist with contraction and granulation for wound closure.[179,185,192,193] The few studies that have been completed investigating the use of NPWT in the pediatric population suggest that NPWT is safe and may assist in rapid granulation and successful wound closure.[193] Limited availability of data does not mean that the products may not be used; rather it strongly suggests that the treating clinician review the evidence for use and contact the manufacturer for any additional information concerning safety and outcomes in the pediatric population (Table 26.3 and Table 26.4).

SYMPTOM CONTROL

Whether or not the goal is to heal a wound, it is critical to assess for and treat the symptoms associated with the wound. Poor control of symptoms may have adverse physical and psychological impacts on children.

TABLE 26.4 Choosing the appropriate dressing

WOUND CHARACTERISTIC	GOAL OF THERAPY	DRESSING EXAMPLES
High exudate	Exudate absorption	Absorptive wound fillers Foams (high MVTR) Gauze
Low to moderate exudate	Maintain moisture Provide some absorption as needed	Hydrocolloids Thin foams or foams with lower MVTR Island dressings (dressings with absorptive island, covered with and surrounded by a transparent film) Gels, creams, ointments, contact layers
Minimal to no exudate	Add moisture	Hydrogels Amorphous for wounds with depth Sheet for superficial wounds Transparent films—add small amount of amorphous hydrogel under film for rapid hydration Hydrocolloids—slower than hydrogels and/or films at hydration
Clinically infected	Systemic treatment of infection Wick away exudate Wound cleansing	Use dressing appropriate for amount of exudate, but change dressing daily Avoid occlusive dressings Antimicrobial dressings may be used Saline irrigation (35 cc syringe/19 g needle)
High infection risk (e.g., immunosuppression, ischemic ulcer, diabetic foot ulcer)	Prevent infection	Use dressing appropriate for amount of exudate, but change dressing every 1–3 days Antimicrobial dressings may be used Utilize occlusive dressings with caution
Wound location	Prevent wound contamination Prevent maceration on plantar foot	Use adhesive dressings, such as films over filler, hydrocolloids, foams, in the sacral area to protect from incontinence Avoid dressings that will compress with ambulation and ooze onto surrounding skin, such as hydrocolloids and paste wound fillers
Skin quality	Fragile skin Risk of contact sensitivity Periwound maceration	Avoid adhesive dressings; use a sheet hydrogel on skin tears secured with gauze wrap or netting Avoid adhesive dressings or products with sensitizing preservatives Use skin sealants on surrounding skin for protection

PAIN

Pain associated with wound care is a complex experience comprising sensory, cognitive, behavioral, and psychological components. Strategies designed to reduce the pain and distress associated with wound care need to combine pharmacologic and nonpharmacologic approaches. Pain intervention often starts with providing the child with developmentally appropriate information about what to expect during the wound care procedure. Other interventions include providing opportunities for emotional expression and establishing trust with the medical team.[194]

Directed medical play in younger children can be beneficial for the child as well as to secondarily ease parental anxiety.[195] Using a distraction technique (e.g., listening to music, watching movies, playing with toys, playing games, talking with another person) is a helpful coping strategy for all ages. Distraction reduces pain by spinal inhibition, as documented on fMRI, which occurs via an opioid inhibitory pathway that can be reversed by naloxone.[196] Recent studies explore using virtual reality (VR) for pain and anxiety in wound care as well. VR was found to help relieve these symptoms and reduced the length of time of the dressing change.[197,198] As a form of distraction, a slower response to the incoming pain signals is likely also occurring.[199] Other nonpharmacological interventions include strategies such as cognitive-behavioral therapy, which can be helpful in targeting negative or unrealistic thoughts and replacing them with positive thoughts and attitudes[200,201] and mind-body therapies including guided imagery, meditation, hypnosis, and biofeedback. These interventions can be helpful but should always be guided by the child's preferences. Children need to be involved in the process since it helps them to feel more secure and to trust their medical team during the wound care.

Pain associated with wounds may be constant or it may occur only with dressing changes. When the pain is constant, an evaluation should be done for treatable factors that may be causing or contributing to the pain, such as wound infection, tissue reaction, or increased pressure, particularly over a bony prominence. Pain associated with wounds can be either nociceptive or neuropathic.[202,203] For constant pain, the principles of pain management discussed in Chapter 23 may be applied. Strategies include treatment with systemic medications including opioids and pain adjuvants. NSAIDs can be particularly helpful in managing wound pain, but if the goal of care is to heal the wound then it should be noted that NSAIDs may interfere with angiogenesis and delay wound healing.[202,203]

Topical treatments can be effective in controlling wound pain. It is known that opioid receptors are not only present in the CNS but also in the periphery.[202,203] Topical opioids can be placed directly on wounds to block these receptors. In case studies, the use of morphine-infused Intrasite gel has been shown to be effective in controlling wound pain.[202,203]

If the patient has pain limited to dressing changes, an evaluation should be made to ensure that the dressing has been carefully selected to minimize tissue adherence. If there is pain related to removal of the dressing, then a 2% to 4% solution of lidocaine may be used to moisten the dressing and wound as the dressing is being removed.[202,203] It typically takes 4 minutes for lidocaine to take effect, and the effect can last anywhere between 30 minutes and 3 hours, depending on the strength.

Finally, sharp and conservative debridement causes acute pain that is present as long as the procedure lasts. If there is slough and debris to be removed, a 20% benzocaine topical anesthetic aerosol spray or dry powder may be applied to the wound immediately prior to debridement, as the onset of action is rapid (less than 1 minute) and the effective duration is up to 10 minutes.[204] Alternatively 2% to 4% lidocaine solution may be applied to the wound. If there is likely to be pain in the tissue surrounding the wound it can be injected with lidocaine before the procedure.[202,203] If local anesthesia is insufficient for pain associated with debridement or dressing changes, a short-acting systemically administered opioid can be used. The patient may also need sedation with a short-acting benzodiazepine, nitrous oxide, or ketamine.[202,203] If there is unstable eschar that requires debridement, the eschar may be scored and EMLA cream applied in a thick layer, then covered with an occlusive dressing and allowed to sit for 30–60 minutes before the procedure.[202,203]

ODOR

Putrefying tissue and infection cause odor associated with wounds. *Pseudomonas* or anaerobic bacteria are the most frequent causes. To minimize odor, the wound should be gently debrided to remove decaying putrefying tissue. If there is a superficial anaerobic infection, treatment with topical metronidazole or silver sulfadiazine may be sufficient to neutralize the odor.[205,206] For deeper infections, systemic metronidazole may be required. If the goal is to control symptoms and not heal the wound, then cytotoxic cleansers such as iodine and diluted Dakin's solution may be used with caution. For *Pseudomonas*, 0.0025% acetic acid may be helpful.[191] Dressings can be placed over the wound to contain the odor. An odor-absorbing dressing, such as charcoal dressings, can also be of benefit.

There are several adjustments that can be made to the child's environment to minimize odor. The child's room should have adequate ventilation. Cat litter or activated charcoal can be placed in a flat container with large surface area, such as a cookie sheet, and placed under the child's bed or close to the child to absorb odor. Using aromatherapy or introducing an alternate odor such as coffee, vanilla, or vinegar may be helpful.[179,185,191] If this approach is used, then it is important to make sure that the aroma is acceptable to the child and does not cause an adverse reaction, such as nausea.

BLEEDING

Bleeding is more common in malignant tumors than in pressure injuries. The surface of malignant tumors is often friable. Dressings should be removed carefully. If the dressing adheres to the wound surface, then it should be moistened with normal saline before the removal to minimize bleeding. If the wound is particularly friable, it may be necessary to apply an inert, nonstick, nonabsorbent synthetic polymer mesh as the primary dressing. This type of dressing does not need to be removed and can be covered with other dressings that can be changed regularly. Alternatively, alginate dressings are hemostatic and may be left in place for several days. They turn to gel when exposed to liquid and can be easily washed off with normal saline with minimal trauma. If there is significant oozing from the wound, then low-dose topical thromboplastin may be sprayed onto the wound.[179] A 0.5% to 1% silver nitrate solution may also be effective. For frank bleeding, silver nitrate sticks, electrocautery, or gentle pressure may be effective.[179,185] A single fraction of radiation directed to the skin will sclerose most vessels and stop bleeding within just a few days. Interventional radiology may be consulted if sclerosing a large vessel is necessary to stop bleeding.

EXUDATE

Exudate can be significant, especially in malignant wounds and Stage 4 pressure injuries. When the amount of exudate is substantial, consideration should be given as to whether edema or infection may be contributing. Both foam and alginate dressings are highly absorptive and can be useful in keeping clothes, intravascular lines, and surrounding healthy skin dry. NPWT has demonstrated effectivity in high-exudate, clean, granulating wounds and dehisced surgical wounds.[179,185,192,193] The goal is to control the exudate without desiccating the wound bed.

REFERENCES

1. LeMone P. Analysis of a human phenomenon: Self-concept. *Nurs Diagn ND Off J North Am Nurs Diagn Assoc.* 1991;2(3):126–130. doi:10.1111/j.1744-618x.1991.tb00347.x
2. Henry M, Ho A, Lambert SD, et al. Looking beyond disfigurement: The experience of patients with head and neck cancer. *J Palliat Care.* 2014;30(1):5–15.
3. Cash TF, Pruzinsky T. *Body Images: Development, Deviance, and Change.* Guilford Press; 1990.
4. Drench ME. Changes in body image secondary to disease and injury. *Rehabil Nurs.* 1994;19(1):31–36. doi:10.1002/j.2048-7940.1994.tb01300.x
5. Teo I, Fronczyk KM, Guindani M, et al. Salient body image concerns of patients with cancer undergoing head and neck reconstruction. *Head Neck.* 2016;38(7):1035–1042. doi:10.1002/hed.24415
6. Hedström M, Haglund K, Skolin I, von Essen L. Distressing events for children and adolescents with cancer: Child, parent, and nurse perceptions. *J Pediatr Oncol Nurs.* 2003;20(3):120–132. doi:10.1053/jpon.2003.76
7. Varni JW, Katz ER, Colegrove R, Dolgin M. Perceived physical appearance and adjustment of children with newly diagnosed cancer: A path analytic model. *J Behav Med.* 1995;18(3):261–278. doi:10.1007/BF01857873
8. Larouche SS, Chin-Peuckert L. Changes in body image experienced by adolescents with cancer. *J Pediatr Oncol Nurs.* 2006;23(4):200–209. doi:10.1177/1043454206289756
9. Bleyer WA. Cancer in older adolescents and young adults: Epidemiology, diagnosis, treatment, survival, and importance of clinical trials. *Med Pediatr Oncol.* 2002;38(1):1–10. doi:10.1002/mpo.1257

10. Eiser C. The impact of treatment: Adolescents' views. In Selby P, Baily C, eds. *Cancer and the Adolescent*. BMJ Publishing; 1996: 264–275.
11. Evan EE, Kaufman M, Cook AB, Zeltzer LK. Sexual health and self-esteem in adolescents and young adults with cancer. *Cancer*. 2006;107(7 Suppl):1672–1679. doi:10.1002/cncr.22101
12. Jain SV, Murrell DF. Psychosocial impact of inherited and autoimmune blistering diseases. *Int J Womens Dermatol*. 2018;4(1):49–53. doi:10.1016/j.ijwd.2017.11.004
13. Margari F, Lecce PA, Santamato W, et al. Psychiatric symptoms and quality of life in patients affected by epidermolysis bullosa. *J Clin Psychol Med Settings*. 2010;17(4):333–339. doi:10.1007/s10880-010-9205-4
14. Van Loey NEE, Van Son MJM. Psychopathology and psychological problems in patients with burn scars: Epidemiology and management. *Am J Clin Dermatol*. 2003;4(4):245–272. doi:10.2165/00128071-200304040-00004
15. Magnan MA. Psychological considerations for patients with acute wounds. *Crit Care Nurs Clin North Am*. 1996;8(2):183–193.
16. Ulmer JF. An exploratory study of pain, coping, and depressed mood following burn injury. *J Pain Symptom Manage*. 1997;13(3): 148–157. doi:10.1016/s0885-3924(96)00301-6
17. van Scheppingen C, Lettinga AT, Duipmans JC, Maathuis KGB, Jonkman MF. The main problems of parents of a child with epidermolysis bullosa. *Qual Health Res*. 2008;18(4):545–556. doi:10.1177/1049732308315110
18. Bernstein NR, Breslau AJ, Graham JA. *Coping Strategies for Burn Survivors and Their Families*. Praeger Publishers; 1988: xiii.
19. Haase JE. The adolescent resilience model as a guide to interventions. *J Pediatr Oncol Nurs*. 2004;21(5):289–299; discussion 300–304. doi:10.1177/1043454204267922
20. Martin K, Geuens S, Asche JK, et al. Psychosocial recommendations for the care of children and adults with epidermolysis bullosa and their family: Evidence-based guidelines. *Orphanet J Rare Dis*. 2019;14(1):133. doi:10.1186/s13023-019-1086-5
21. Williamson H, Harcourt D, Halliwell E, Frith H, Wallace M. Adolescents' and parents' experiences of managing the psychosocial impact of appearance change during cancer treatment. *J Pediatr Oncol Nurs*. 2010;27(3):168–175. doi:10.1177/1043454209357923
22. Drotar D, Crawford P. Psychological adaptation of siblings of chronically ill children: Research and practice implications. *J Dev Behav Pediatr JDBP*. 1985;6(6):355–362.
23. Williams EF, Gannon K, Soon K. The experiences of young people with epidermolysis bullosa simplex: A qualitative study. *J Health Psychol*. 2011;16(5):701–710. doi:10.1177/1359105310387954
24. Weisshaar E, Szepietowski JC, Dalgard F, et al. European S2k guideline on chronic pruritus. *Acta Derm Venereol*. 2019;99(5):469–506. doi:10.2340/00015555-3164
25. Weisshaar E, Diepgen TL, Bruckner T, et al. Itch intensity evaluated in the German Atopic Dermatitis Intervention Study (GADIS): Correlations with quality of life, coping behaviour and SCORAD severity in 823 children. *Acta Derm Venereol*. 2008;88(3):234–239. doi:10.2340/00015555-0432
26. Metz M, Wahn U, Gieler U, Stock P, Schmitt J, Blume-Peytavi U. Chronic pruritus associated with dermatologic disease in infancy and childhood: Update from an interdisciplinary group of dermatologists and pediatricians. *Pediatr Allergy Immunol*. 2013;24(6):527–539. doi:10.1111/pai.12115
27. Na CH, Chung J, Simpson EL. Quality of life and disease impact of atopic dermatitis and psoriasis on children and their families. *Child Basel Switz*. 2019;6(12). doi:10.3390/children6120133
28. Kantor R, Dalal P, Cella D, Silverberg JI. Research letter: Impact of pruritus on quality of life-a systematic review. *J Am Acad Dermatol*. 2016;75(5):885–886.e4. doi:10.1016/j.jaad.2016.07.016
29. Gånemo A. Quality of life in Swedish children with congenital ichthyosis. *Dermatol Rep*. 2010;2(1). doi:10.4081/dr.2010.e7
30. El Hachem M, Di Mauro G, Rotunno R, et al. Pruritus in pediatric patients with atopic dermatitis: A multidisciplinary approach—summary document from an Italian expert group. *Ital J Pediatr*. 2020;46(1):11. doi:10.1186/s13052-020-0777-9
31. Tarikci N, Kocatürk E, Güngör Ş, Topal IO, Can PÜ, Singer R. Pruritus in systemic diseases: A review of etiological factors and new treatment modalities. *SciWorld J*. 2015;2015:803752. doi:10.1155/2015/803752
32. Ständer S. Classification of itch. *Itch Manage Clin Pract*. 2016;50:1–4. doi:10.1159/000446009
33. Yosipovitch G, Rosen JD, Hashimoto T. Itch: From mechanism to (novel) therapeutic approaches. *J Allergy Clin Immunol*. 2018;142(5):1375–1390. doi:10.1016/j.jaci.2018.09.005
34. Yostipovitch, Gil, Akiyama T. Cutaneous neurophysiology. In Bolognia JL, Schaffer JV, Cerroni L, eds. *Dermatology*. Vol 1. 4th ed. Elsevier; 2018: 100–110.
35. Ringkamp M, Schepers RJ, Shimada SG, et al. A role for nociceptive, myelinated nerve fibers in itch sensation. *J Neurosci*. 2011;31(42):14841–14849. doi:10.1523/JNEUROSCI.3005-11.2011
36. LaMotte RH, Dong X, Ringkamp M. Sensory neurons and circuits mediating itch. *Nat Rev Neurosci*. 2014;15(1):19–31. doi:10.1038/nrn3641
37. Jeffry J, Kim S, Chen Z-F. Itch signaling in the nervous system. *Physiology*. 2011;26(4):286–292. doi:10.1152/physiol.00007.2011
38. Namer B, Carr R, Johanek LM, Schmelz M, Handwerker HO, Ringkamp M. Separate peripheral pathways for pruritus in man. *J Neurophysiol*. 2008;100(4):2062–2069. doi:10.1152/jn.90482.2008
39. Song J, Xian D, Yang L, Xiong X, Lai R, Zhong J. Pruritus: Progress toward pathogenesis and treatment. *BioMed Res Int*. 2018;2018(17):1–12. doi:https://doi-org.laneproxy.stanford.edu/10.1155/2018/9625936
40. Rinaldi G. The itch-scratch cycle: A review of the mechanisms. *Dermatol Pract Concept*. 2019;9(2):90–97. doi:10.5826/dpc.0902a03
41. Besner Morin C, Misery L. Emerging treatments and novel pathways in pruritus. *J Cutan Med Surg*. 2019;23(5):528–536. doi:10.1177/1203475419852050
42. Cevikbas F, Lerner EA. Physiology and pathophysiology of itch. *Physiol Rev*. 2020;100(3):945–982. doi:10.1152/physrev.00017.2019
43. Dong X, Dong X. Peripheral and central mechanisms of itch. *Neuron*. 2018;98(3):482–494. doi:10.1016/j.neuron.2018.03.023
44. Carstens E, Follansbee T, Iodi Carstens M. The challenge of basic itch research. *Acta Derm Venereol*. 2020;100(2):2–8. doi:10.2340/00015555-3343
45. Barry DM, Munanairi A, Chen Z-F. Spinal mechanisms of itch transmission. *Neurosci Bull*. 2017;34(1):156–164. doi:10.1007/s12264-017-0125-2
46. Najafi P, Carré J-L, Ben Salem D, Brenaut E, Misery L, Dufor O. Central mechanisms of itch: A systematic literature review and meta-analysis. *J Neuroradiol*. Published online December 3, 2019;47(6):450–457. doi:10.1016/j.neurad.2019.11.005
47. Hunter HJA, Momen SE, Kleyn CE. The impact of psychosocial stress on healthy skin. *Clin Exp Dermatol*. 2015;40(5):540–546. doi:10.1111/ced.12582
48. Carstens E, Akiyama T. Central mechanisms of itch. *Itch Manag Clin Pract*. 2016;50:11–17. doi:10.1159/000446011
49. Tey HL, Yosipovitch G. Targeted treatment of pruritus: A look into the future. *Br J Dermatol*. 2011;165(1):5–17. doi:10.1111/j.1365-2133.2011.10217.x
50. Metz M. Are we facing a change in the treatment of chronic pruritus? *Br J Dermatol*. 2019;181(5):877–878. doi:10.1111/bjd.18298
51. Ständer S, Yosipovitch G. Substance P and neurokinin 1 receptor are new targets for the treatment of chronic pruritus. *Br J Dermatol*. 2019;181(5):932–938. doi:10.1111/bjd.18025
52. McEwen MW, Fite EM, Yosipovitch G, Patel T. Drugs on the Horizon for Chronic Pruritus. *Dermatol Clin*. 2018;36(3):335–344. doi:10.1016/j.det.2018.02.016
53. Ständer S, Zeidler C, Riepe C, et al. European EADV network on assessment of severity and burden of pruritus (PruNet): First meeting on outcome tools. *J Eur Acad Dermatol Venereol*. 2016;30(7):1144–1147. doi:10.1111/jdv.13296

54. Olsen JR, Gallacher J, Finlay AY, Piguet V, Francis NA. Quality of life impact of childhood skin conditions measured using the Children's Dermatology Life Quality Index (CDLQI): A meta-analysis. *Br J Dermatol.* 2016;174(4):853–861. doi:10.1111/bjd.14361
55. Morris V, Murphy LM, Rosenberg M, Rosenberg L, Holzer CE, Meyer WJ. Itch assessment scale for the pediatric burn survivor. *J Burn Care Res.* 2012;33(3):419–424. doi:10.1097/BCR.0b013e3182372bfa
56. Kamath BM, Abetz-Webb L, Kennedy C, et al. Development of a novel tool to assess the impact of itching in pediatric cholestasis. *Patient.* 2018;11(1):69–82. doi:10.1007/s40271-017-0266-4
57. Gabes M, Tischer C, Apfelbacher C. Measurement properties of quality-of-life outcome measures for children and adults with eczema: An updated systematic review. *Pediatr Allergy Immunol.* 2020;31(1):66–77. doi:10.1111/pai.13120
58. Fishbein AB, Silverberg JI, Wilson EJ, Ong PY. Update on atopic dermatitis: Diagnosis, severity assessment, and treatment selection. *J Allergy Clin Immunol Pract.* 2020;8(1):91–101. doi:10.1016/j.jaip.2019.06.044
59. Wahlgren C-F. Children's rating of itch: An experimental study. *Pediatr Dermatol.* 2005;22(2):97–101. doi:10.1111/j.1525-1470.2005.22201.x
60. Pereira MP, Ständer S. Assessment of severity and burden of pruritus. *Allergol Int.* 2017;66(1):3–7. doi:10.1016/j.alit.2016.08.009
61. Andrade A, Kuah CY, Martin-Lopez JE, et al. Interventions for chronic pruritus of unknown origin. *Cochrane Database Syst Rev.* 2020;1:CD013128. doi:10.1002/14651858.CD013128.pub2
62. Ganesh A, Maxwell LG. Pathophysiology and management of opioid-induced pruritus. *Drugs.* 2007;67(16):2323–2333. doi:10.2165/00003495-200767160-00003
63. Reich A, Szepietowski JC. Opioid-induced pruritus: An update. *Clin Exp Dermatol.* 2010;35(1):2–6. doi:10.1111/j.1365-2230.2009.03463.x
64. Flacke JW, Flacke WE, Bloor BC, Van Etten AP, Kripke BJ. Histamine release by four narcotics: A double-blind study in humans. *Anesth Analg.* 1987;66(8):723–730.
65. Blunk JA, Schmelz M, Zeck S, Skov P, Likar R, Koppert W. Opioid-induced mast cell activation and vascular responses is not mediated by mu-opioid receptors: An in vivo microdialysis study in human skin. *Anesth Analg.* 2004;98(2):364–370. doi:10.1213/01.ane.0000097168.32472.0d
66. Ko MCH, Song MS, Edwards T, Lee H, Naughton NN. The role of central mu opioid receptors in opioid-induced itch in primates. *J Pharmacol Exp Ther.* 2004;310(1):169–176. doi:10.1124/jpet.103.061101
67. Golembiewski J. Opioid-Induced Pruritus. *J Perianesth Nurs.* 2013;28(4):247–249. doi:10.1016/j.jopan.2013.05.008
68. Rashid S, Trivedi DD, Al-Shathir M, Moulton M, Baumrucker SJ. Is there a role for 5-HT3 receptor antagonists in the treatment of opioid-induced pruritus? *Am J Hosp Palliat Med.* 2018;35(4):740–744. doi:10.1177/1049909117736062
69. Szarvas S, Harmon D, Murphy D. Neuraxial opioid-induced pruritus: A review. *J Clin Anesth.* 2003;15(3):234–239. doi:10.1016/S0952-8180(02)00501-9
70. Kjellberg F, Tramèr MR. Pharmacological control of opioid-induced pruritus: A quantitative systematic review of randomized trials. *Eur J Anaesthesiol.* 2001;18(6):346–357. doi:10.1046/j.0265-0215.2000.00826.x
71. Koch J, Manworren R, Clark L, Quinn CT, Buchanan GR, Rogers ZR. Pilot study of continuous co-infusion of morphine and naloxone in children with sickle cell pain crisis. *Am J Hematol.* 2008;83(9):728–731. doi:10.1002/ajh.21213
72. Maxwell LG, Kaufmann SC, Bitzer S, et al. The effects of a small-dose naloxone infusion on opioid-induced side effects and analgesia in children and adolescents treated with intravenous patient-controlled analgesia: A double-blind, prospective, randomized, controlled study. *Anesth Analg.* 2005;100(4):953–958. doi:10.1213/01.ANE.0000148618.17736.3C
73. Monitto CL, Kost-Byerly S, White E, et al. The optimal dose of prophylactic intravenous naloxone in ameliorating opioid-induced side effects in children receiving intravenous patient-controlled analgesia morphine for moderate to severe pain: A dose finding study. *Anesth Analg.* 2011;113(4):834–842. doi:10.1213/ANE.0b013e31822c9a44
74. Ko MCH, Lee H, Song MS, et al. Activation of kappa-opioid receptors inhibits pruritus evoked by subcutaneous or intrathecal administration of morphine in monkeys. *J Pharmacol Exp Ther.* 2003;305(1):173–179. doi:10.1124/jpet.102.044909
75. Nakatsuka N, Minogue SC, Lim J, et al. Intravenous nalbuphine 50 microg x kg(-1) is ineffective for opioid-induced pruritus in pediatrics. *Can J Anaesth J Can Anesth.* 2006;53(11):1103–1110.
76. Jannuzzi RG. Nalbuphine for treatment of opioid-induced pruritus: A systematic review of literature. *Clin J Pain.* 2016;32(1):87–93. doi:10.1097/AJP.0000000000000211
77. Jitpakdee T, Mandee S. Strategies for preventing side effects of systemic opioid in postoperative pediatric patients. *Pediatr Anesth.* 2014;24(6):561–568. doi:10.1111/pan.12420
78. Cravero JP, Agarwal R, Berde C, et al. The Society for Pediatric Anesthesia recommendations for the use of opioids in children during the perioperative period. *Paediatr Anaesth.* 2019;29(6):547–571. doi:10.1111/pan.13639
79. Horta ML, Morejon LCL, da Cruz AW, et al. Study of the prophylactic effect of droperidol, alizapride, propofol and promethazine on spinal morphine-induced pruritus. *Br J Anaesth.* 2006;96(6):796–800. doi:10.1093/bja/ael072
80. Waxler B, Dadabhoy ZP, Stojiljkovic L, Rabito SF. Primer of postoperative pruritus for anesthesiologists. *Anesthesiology.* 2005;103(1):168–178. doi:10.1097/00000542-200507000-00025
81. Kumar K, Singh SI. Neuraxial opioid-induced pruritus: An update. *J Anaesthesiol Clin Pharmacol.* 2013;29(3):303. doi:10.4103/0970-9185.117045
82. Kampo S, Afful AP, Mohammed S, Ntim M, Buunaaim ADB, Anabah TW. Sub-hypnotic dose of propofol as antiemetic prophylaxis attenuates intrathecal morphine-induced postoperative nausea and vomiting, and pruritus in parturient undergoing cesarean section: A randomized control trial. *BMC Anesthesiol.* 2019;19(1):177. doi:10.1186/s12871-019-0847-y
83. Makarem J, Mireskandari SM, Jafarzadeh A, Rahbar Nikoukar L, Aghaii S. Intravenous midazolam as more effective than propofol for preventing pruritus after intrathecal sufentanil in surgical patients: A randomized blinded trial. *Anesthesiol Pain Med.* 2017;7(3):e37535. doi:10.5812/aapm.37535
84. Belzberg M, Larson VA, Khanna R, et al. Association between itch and cancer in 3836 pediatric pruritus patients at a tertiary care center. *Medicines.* 2019;6(4). doi:10.3390/medicines6040099
85. Larson VA, Tang O, Ständer S, Kang S, Kwatra SG. Association between itch and cancer in 16,925 patients with pruritus: Experience at a tertiary care center. *J Am Acad Dermatol.* 2019;80(4):931–937. doi:10.1016/j.jaad.2018.08.044
86. Rowe B, Yosipovitch G. Malignancy-associated pruritus. *Eur J Pain.* 2016;20(1):19–23. doi:10.1002/ejp.760
87. Ensslin CJ, Rosen AC, Wu S, Lacouture ME. Pruritus in patients treated with targeted cancer therapies: Systematic review and meta-analysis. *J Am Acad Dermatol.* 2013;69(5):708–720. doi:10.1016/j.jaad.2013.06.038
88. Aymard JP, Lederlin P, Witz F, Colomb JN, Herbeuval R, Weber B. Cimetidine for pruritus in Hodgkin's disease. *Br Med J.* 1980;280(6208):151–152. doi:10.1136/bmj.280.6208.151
89. Stäubli M, Graf W, Straub PW. [Pruritus in Hodgkin's disease responding to cimetidine]. *Schweiz Med Wochenschr.* 1981;111(20):723–724.
90. Tefferi A, Vannucchi AM, Barbui T. Polycythemia vera treatment algorithm 2018. *Blood Cancer J.* 2018;8(1). doi:10.1038/s41408-017-0042-7
91. Zylicz Z, Smits C, Krajnik M. Paroxetine for pruritus in advanced cancer. *J Pain Symptom Manage.* 1998;16(2):121–124. doi:10.1016/s0885-3924(98)00048-7

92. Zylicz Z, Krajnik M, Sorge AA van, Costantini M. Paroxetine in the treatment of severe non-dermatological pruritus: A randomized, controlled trial. *J Pain Symptom Manage.* 2003;26(6):1105–1112. doi:10.1016/j.jpainsymman.2003.05.004
93. Davis MP, Frandsen JL, Walsh D, Andresen S, Taylor S. Mirtazapine for pruritus. *J Pain Symptom Manage.* 2003;25(3):288–291. doi:10.1016/S0885-3924(02)00645-0
94. Bromberg H, Chang Y, Craig D. Pruritic manifestation of peripheral t cell lymphoma effectively managed with mirtazapine: A case report. *J Pain Palliat Care Pharmacother.* Published online March 2, 2020; 34(3):153–154. doi:10.1080/15360288.2020.1734142
95. Khanna R, Boozalis E, Belzberg M, Zampella JG, Kwatra SG. Mirtazapine for the treatment of chronic pruritus. *Medicines.* 2019;6(3). doi:10.3390/medicines6030073
96. Kouwenhoven TA, van de Kerkhof PCM, Kamsteeg M. Use of oral antidepressants in patients with chronic pruritus: A systematic review. *J Am Acad Dermatol.* 2017;77(6):1068–1073.e7. doi:10.1016/j.jaad.2017.08.025
97. Siemens W, Xander C, Meerpohl JJ, et al. Pharmacological interventions for pruritus in adult palliative care patients. *Cochrane Database Syst Rev.* 2016;11:CD008320. doi:10.1002/14651858.CD008320.pub3
98. Fawaz R, Baumann U, Ekong U, et al. Guideline for the evaluation of cholestatic jaundice in infants: Joint recommendations of the North American Society for Pediatric Gastroenterology, Hepatology, and Nutrition and the European Society for Pediatric Gastroenterology, Hepatology, and Nutrition. *J Pediatr Gastroenterol Nutr.* 2017;64(1):154–168. doi:10.1097/MPG.0000000000001334
99. Ben Ameur S, Chabchoub I, Telmoudi J, et al. Management of cholestatic pruritus in children with Alagille syndrome: Case report and literature review. *Arch Pédiatrie.* 2016;23(12):1247–1250. doi:10.1016/j.arcped.2016.09.004
100. Kremer AE, Oude Elferink RPJ, Beuers U. Pathophysiology and current management of pruritus in liver disease. *Clin Res Hepatol Gastroenterol.* 2011;35(2):89–97. doi:10.1016/j.clinre.2010.10.007
101. European Association for the Study of the Liver. EASL Clinical practice guidelines: Management of cholestatic liver diseases. *J Hepatol.* 2009;51(2):237–267. doi:10.1016/j.jhep.2009.04.009
102. Stiehl A, Thaler MM, Admirand WH. The effects of phenobarbital on bile salts and bilirubin in patients with intrahepatic and extrahepatic cholestasis. *N Engl J Med.* 1972;286(16):858–861. doi:10.1056/NEJM197204202861602
103. Kremer AE, Bolier R, Dijk R van, Elferink RPJO, Beuers U. Advances in pathogenesis and management of pruritus in cholestasis. *Dig Dis.* 2014;32(5):637–645. doi:10.1159/000360518
104. Thébaut A, Debray D, Gonzales E. An update on the physiopathology and therapeutic management of cholestatic pruritus in children. *Clin Res Hepatol Gastroenterol.* 2018;42(2):103–109. doi:10.1016/j.clinre.2017.08.007
105. Müller C, Pongratz S, Pidlich J, et al. Treatment of pruritus in chronic liver disease with the 5-hydroxytryptamine receptor type 3 antagonist ondansetron: A randomized, placebo-controlled, double-blind cross-over trial. *Eur J Gastroenterol Hepatol.* 1998;10(10):865–870. doi:10.1097/00042737-199810000-00010
106. O'Donohue JW, Pereira SP, Ashdown AC, Haigh CG, Wilkinson JR, Williams R. A controlled trial of ondansetron in the pruritus of cholestasis. *Aliment Pharmacol Ther.* 2005;21(8):1041–1045. doi:10.1111/j.1365-2036.2005.02430.x
107. Mattei P, von Allmen D, Piccoli D, Rand E. Relief of intractable pruritus in Alagille syndrome by partial external biliary diversion. *J Pediatr Surg.* 2006;41(1):104–107; discussion 104-107. doi:10.1016/j.jpedsurg.2005.10.014
108. Yang H, Porte RJ, Verkade HJ, De Langen ZJ, Hulscher JBF. Partial external biliary diversion in children with progressive familial intrahepatic cholestasis and Alagille disease. *J Pediatr Gastroenterol Nutr.* 2009;49(2):216–221. doi:10.1097/MPG.0b013e31819a4e3d
109. Wang KS, Tiao G, Bass LM, et al. Analysis of surgical interruption of the enterohepatic circulation as a treatment for pediatric cholestasis. *Hepatology.* 2017;65(5):1645–1654. doi:10.1002/hep.29019
110. Wu H-Y, Huang J-W, Tsai W-C, et al. Prognostic importance and determinants of uremic pruritus in patients receiving peritoneal dialysis: A prospective cohort study. *PloS One.* 2018;13(9):e0203474. doi:10.1371/journal.pone.0203474
111. Krajewski PK, Krajewska M, Szepietowski JC. Pruritus in renal transplant recipients: Current state of knowledge. *Adv Clin Exp Med Off Organ Wroclaw Med Univ.* Published online June 23, 2020. doi:10.17219/acem/122174
112. Senturk N, Ozkaya O, Aytekin S, et al. Characteristics of pruritus in children on peritoneal dialysis. *Nephron Clin Pract.* 2008;109(3):c168–172. doi:10.1159/000145461
113. Simonsen E, Komenda P, Lerner B, et al. Treatment of uremic pruritus: A systematic review. *Am J Kidney Dis Off J Natl Kidney Found.* 2017;70(5):638–655. doi:10.1053/j.ajkd.2017.05.018
114. Swarna SS, Aziz K, Zubair T, Qadir N, Khan M. Pruritus associated with chronic kidney disease: A comprehensive literature review. *Cureus.* 2019;11(7):e5256. doi:10.7759/cureus.5256
115. Morton CA, Lafferty M, Hau C, Henderson I, Jones M, Love JG. Pruritus and skin hydration during dialysis. *Nephrol Dial Transplant.* 1996;11(10):2031–2036. doi:10.1093/oxfordjournals.ndt.a027092
116. Neonakis E, Wheeler MH, Krishnan H, Coles GA, Davies F, Woodhead JS. Results of surgical treatment of renal hyperparathyroidism. *Arch Surg.* 1995;130(6):643–648. doi:10.1001/archsurg.1995.01430060081015
117. Chen J, Jia X, Kong X, Wang Z, Cui M, Xu D. Total parathyroidectomy with autotransplantation versus subtotal parathyroidectomy for renal hyperparathyroidism: A systematic review and meta-analysis. *Nephrology.* 2017;22(5):388–396. doi:10.1111/nep.12801
118. Berger TG, Steinhoff M. Pruritus and renal failure. *Semin Cutan Med Surg.* 2011;30(2):99–100. doi:10.1016/j.sder.2011.04.005
119. Pereira MP, Mittal A, Ständer S. Current treatment strategies in refractory chronic pruritus. *Curr Opin Pharmacol.* 2019;46:1–6.
120. Ranna V, Cheng KKF, Castillo DA, et al. Development of the MASCC/ISOO clinical practice guidelines for mucositis: An overview of the methods. *Support Care Cancer.* 2019;27(10):3933–3948. doi:10.1007/s00520-019-04891-1
121. Stringer AM, Logan RM. The role of oral flora in the development of chemotherapy-induced oral mucositis. *J Oral Pathol Med.* 2015;44(2):81–87. doi:10.1111/jop.12152
122. Hong CHL, Gueiros LA, Fulton JS, et al. Systematic review of basic oral care for the management of oral mucositis in cancer patients and clinical practice guidelines. *Support Care Cancer.* 2019;27(10):3949–3967. doi:10.1007/s00520-019-04848-4
123. Correa MEP, Cheng KKF, Chiang K, et al. Systematic review of oral cryotherapy for the management of oral mucositis in cancer patients and clinical practice guidelines. *Support Care Cancer.* 2020;28(5):2449–2456. doi:10.1007/s00520-019-05217-x
124. Logan RM, Al-Azri AR, Bossi P, et al. Systematic review of growth factors and cytokines for the management of oral mucositis in cancer patients and clinical practice guidelines. *Support Care Cancer.* 2020;28(5):2485–2498. doi:10.1007/s00520-019-05170-9
125. Zadik Y, Arany PR, Fregnani ER, et al. Systematic review of photobiomodulation for the management of oral mucositis in cancer patients and clinical practice guidelines. *Support Care Cancer.* 2019;27(10):3969–3983. doi:10.1007/s00520-019-04890-2
126. Bowen JM, Gibson RJ, Coller JK, et al. Systematic review of agents for the management of cancer treatment-related gastrointestinal mucositis and clinical practice guidelines. *Support Care Cancer.* 2019;27(10):4011–4022. doi:10.1007/s00520-019-04892-0
127. Saunders DP, Rouleau T, Cheng K, et al. Systematic review of antimicrobials, mucosal coating agents, anesthetics, and analgesics for the management of oral mucositis in cancer patients and clinical practice guidelines. *Support Care Cancer.* 2020;28(5):2473–2484. doi:10.1007/s00520-019-05181-6
128. Tan C-H, Rasool S, Johnston GA. Contact dermatitis: Allergic and irritant. *Clin Dermatol.* 2014;32(1):116–124. doi:10.1016/j.clindermatol.2013.05.033

129. Tüzün Y, Wolf R, Bağlam S, Engin B. Diaper (napkin) dermatitis: A fold (intertriginous) dermatosis. *Clin Dermatol.* 2015;33(4):477–482. doi 10.1016/j.clindermatol.2015.04.012
130. Merrill L. Prevention, treatment and parent education for diaper dermatitis. *Nurs Womens Health.* 2015;19(4):324–336; quiz 337. doi:10.1111/1751-486X.12218
131. Ingersoll Z, Garza-Chapa JI, Pham R, Malouf P, Susa J, Weis S. Recurrent granuloma gluteale infantum secondary to fecal overflow incontinence. *Case Rep Dermatol.* 2018;10(2):203–207. doi:10.1159/000492270
132. Van L, Harting M, Rosen T. Jacquet erosive diaper dermatitis: A complication of adult urinary incontinence. *Cutis.* 2008;82(1):72–74.
133. Goldberg NS, Esterly NB, Rothman KF, et al. Perianal pseudoverrucous papules and nodules in children. *Arch Dermatol.* 1992;128(2):240–242.
134. Wiesner E, Vassantachart JM, Jacob SE. Art of prevention: The importance of proper diapering practices. *Int J Womens Dermatol.* 2019;5(4):233–234. doi:10.1016/j.ijwd.2019.02.005
135. Shin HT. Diagnosis and management of diaper dermatitis. *Pediatr Clin North Am.* 2014;61(2):367–382. doi:10.1016/j.pcl.2013.11.009
136. Stamatas GN, Tierney NK. Diaper dermatitis: Etiology, manifestations, prevention, and management. *Pediatr Dermatol.* 2014;31(1):1–7. doi:10.1111/pde.12245
137. Blume-Peytavi U, Kanti V. Prevention and treatment of diaper dermatitis. *Pediatr Dermatol.* 2018;35 Suppl 1:s19-s23. doi:10.1111/pde.13495
138. Lavender T, Furber C, Campbell M, et al. Effect on skin hydration of using baby wipes to clean the napkin area of newborn babies: Assessor-blinded randomised controlled equivalence trial. *BMC Pediatr.* 2012;12:59. doi:10.1186/1471-2431-12-59
139. Garcia Bartels N, Massoudy L, Scheufele R, et al. Standardized diaper care regimen: A prospective, randomized pilot study on skin barrier function and epidermal IL-1α in newborns. *Pediatr Dermatol.* 2012;29(3):270–276. doi:10.1111/j.1525-1470.2011.01590.x
140. Odio M, Thaman L. Diapering, diaper technology, and diaper area skin health. *Pediatr Dermatol.* 2014;31 Suppl 1:9–14. doi:10.1111/pde.12501
141. Gustin J, Gibb R, Maltbie D, Roe D, Waimin Siu S. The impact of diaper design on mitigating known causes of diaper dermatitis. *Pediatr Dermatol.* 2018;35(6):792–795. doi:10.1111/pde.13680
142. Burdall O, Willgress L, Goad N. Neonatal skin care: Developments in care to maintain neonatal barrier function and prevention of diaper dermatitis. *Pediatr Dermatol.* 2019;36(1):31–35. doi:10.1111/pde.13714
143. Davies MW, Dore AJ, Perissinotto KL. Topical vitamin A, or its derivatives, for treating and preventing napkin dermatitis in infants. *Cochrane Database Syst Rev.* 2005;(4):CD004300. doi:10.1002/14651858.CD004300.pub2
144. Fölster-Holst R. Differential diagnoses of diaper dermatitis. *Pediatr Dermatol.* 2018;35(Suppl 1):s10–s18. doi:10.1111/pde.13484
145. Brook I. Microbiology of secondarily infected diaper dermatitis. *Int J Dermatol.* 1992;31(10):700–702. doi:10.1111/j.1365-4362.1992.tb01375.x
146. Hartman-Adams H, Banvard C, Juckett G. Impetigo: Diagnosis and treatment. *Am Fam Physician.* 2014;90(4):229–235.
147. Furber C, Bedwell C, Campbell M, et al. The challenges and realities of diaper area cleansing for parents. *J Obstet Gynecol Neonatal Nurs JOGNN.* 2012;41(6):E13–25. doi:10.1111/j.1552-6909.2012.01390.x
148. García-Molina P, Balaguer-López E, García-Fernández FP, Ferrera-Fernández M de LÁ, Blasco JM, Verdú J. Pressure ulcers' incidence, preventive measures, and risk factors in neonatal intensive care and intermediate care units. *Int Wound J.* 2018;15(4):571–579. doi:10.1111/iwj.12900
149. Razmus I, Bergquist-Beringer S. Pressure injury prevalence and the rate of hospital-acquired pressure injury among pediatric patients in acute care. *J Wound Ostomy Cont Nurs.* 2017;44(2):110–117. doi:10.1097/WON.0000000000000306
150. Smith HA, Moore Z, Tan MH. Cohort study to determine the risk of pressure ulcers and developing a care bundle within a paediatric intensive care unit setting. *Intensive Crit Care Nurs.* 2019;53:68-72. doi:10.1016/j.iccn.2019.04.008
151. Delmore B, Deppisch M, Sylvia C, Luna-Anderson C, Nie AM. Pressure injuries in the pediatric population: A national pressure ulcer advisory panel white paper. *Adv Skin Wound Care.* 2019;32(9): 394–408. doi:10.1097/01.ASW.0000577124.58253.66
152. Cohen KE, Scanlon MC, Bemanian A, Schindler CA. Pediatric skin failure. *Am J Crit Care Off Publ Am Assoc Crit-Care Nurses.* 2017;26(4):320–328. doi:10.4037/ajcc2017806
153. Curley MAQ, Hasbani NR, Quigley SM, et al. Predicting Pressure injury risk in pediatric patients: The Braden QD scale. *J Pediatr.* 2018;192:189–195.e2. doi:10.1016/j.jpeds.2017.09.045
154. Sánchez-Lorente MM, Sanchis-Sánchez E, García-Molina P, Balaguer-López E, Blasco J-M. Prevalence of pressure ulcers in the paediatric population and in primary health care: An epidemiological study conducted in Spain. *J Tissue Viability.* 2018;27(4): 221–225. doi:10.1016/j.jtv.2018.07.004
155. Edsberg LE, Black JM, Goldberg M, McNichol L, Moore L, Sieggreen M. Revised National Pressure Ulcer Advisory Panel Pressure Injury Staging System: Revised Pressure Injury Staging System. *J Wound Ostomy Continence Nurs.* 2016;43(6):585–597. doi:10.1097/WON.0000000000000281
156. Kottner J, Cuddigan J, Carville K, et al. Prevention and treatment of pressure ulcers/injuries: The protocol for the second update of the international Clinical Practice Guideline 2019. *J Tissue Viability.* 2019;28(2):51–58. doi:10.1016/j.jtv.2019.01.001
157. Hockenberry, Marilyn J, Wilson, David, eds. The child with gastrointestinal dysfunction. In Hockenberry MJ, Wilson D, eds. *Wong's Nursing Care of Infants and Children.* 9th ed. Elsevier; 2013: 998–1051.
158. Gethin G, McIntosh C, Probst S. Complementary and alternative therapies for management of odor in malignant fungating wounds: A critical review. *Chronic Wound Care Manag Res.* 2016;3:51–57. doi:https://doi.org/10.2147/CWCMR.S85472
159. Neloska L, Damevska K, Kuzmanova A, Pavleska L, Kostov M, Zovic BP. Dermatological diseases in palliative care patients: A prospective study of 271 patients. *JDDG J Dtsch Dermatol Ges.* 2017;15(6):621–627. doi:10.1111/ddg.13236
160. Swanson T, Haesler E, Angel D, Sussman G. IWII wound infection in clinical practice consensus document 2016 update. *Wound Pract Res J Aust Wound Manag Assoc.* 2016;24(4):194.
161. Tandler S, Stephen-Haynes J. Fungating wounds: Management and treatment options. *Br J Nurs Mark Allen Publ.* 2017;26(12 Suppl):S6–S14. doi:10.12968/bjon.2017.26.12.S6
162. National Institute for Health and Care Excellence. Palliative care: Malignant skin ulcer. Published 2017. Accessed January 20, 2020. http://tinyurl.com/yc6gkr2c
163. Bruckner AL, Pope E, Mellerio JE, et al. Supportive care: Bathing, wound care, nutrition, pain and itch management, psychosocial support, palliation. In *Blistering Diseases: Clinical Features, Pathogenesis, Treatment.* Springer Berlin Heidelberg. 2015: 653–666. doi:10.1007/978-3-662-45698-9_70
164. Danial C, Adeduntan R, Gorell ES, et al. Prevalence and characterization of pruritus in epidermolysis bullosa. *Pediatr Dermatol.* 2015;32(1):53–59. doi:10.1111/pde.12391
165. Goldschneider KR, Good J, Harrop E, et al. Pain care for patients with epidermolysis bullosa: Best care practice guidelines. *BMC Med.* 2014;12:178. doi:10.1186/s12916-014-0178-2
166. Togo CCG, Zidorio APC, Gonçalves VSS, Hubbard L, de Carvalho KMB, Dutra ES. Quality of life in people with epidermolysis bullosa: A systematic review. *Qual Life Res.* 2020;29(7):1731–1745. doi:10.1007/s11136-020-02495-5
167. Brun J, Chiaverini C, Devos C, et al. Pain and quality of life evaluation in patients with localized epidermolysis bullosa simplex. *Orphanet J Rare Dis.* 2017;12(1):119. doi:10.1186/s13023-017-0666-5
168. Schräder NHB, Yuen WY, Jonkman MF. Pain quality assessment scale for epidermolysis bullosa. *Acta Derm Venereol.* 2018;98(3): 346–349. doi:10.2340/00015555-2827

169. Frew JW, Martin LK, Nijsten T, Murrell DF. Quality of life evaluation in epidermolysis bullosa (EB) through the development of the QOLEB questionnaire: An EB-specific quality of life instrument. *Br J Dermatol.* 2009;161(6):1323–1330. doi:10.1111/j.1365-2133.2009.09347.x
170. Chernyshov PV, Suru A, Gedeon I, Derevyanko LA, Tiplica GS, Salavastru CM. Epidermolysis bullosa-specific module of the Infants and Toddlers Dermatology Quality of Life (InToDermQoL) questionnaire. *J Eur Acad Dermatol Venereol.* 2019;33(3):612–617. doi:10.1111/jdv.15337
171. Chernyshov PV, Pustišek N, Gedeon I, et al. International pilot tests of the epidermolysis bullosa-specific module of the Infants and Toddlers Dermatology Quality of Life questionnaire. *J Eur Acad Dermatol Venereol.* 2020;34(3):e123–e124. doi:10.1111/jdv.16051
172. Bruckner-Tuderman L. Newer treatment modalities in epidermolysis bullosa. *Indian Dermatol Online J.* 2019;10(3):244. doi:10.4103/idoj.IDOJ_287_18
173. Dwiyana RF, Yogya Y, Gondokaryono SP, et al. Clinical efficacy of biocellulose, carboxymethyl cellulose and normal saline dressing in epidermolysis bullosa. *J Wound Care.* 2019;28(Sup10):S4–S9. doi:10.12968/jowc.2019.28.Sup10.S4
174. Yaşar Ş, Yaşar B, Cebeci F, Bayoğlu D, Nuhoğlu Ç. Topical sucralfate cream treatment for aplasia cutis congenita with dystrophic epidermolysis bullosa: A case study. *J Wound Care.* 2018;27(11):768–771. doi:10.12968/jowc.2018.27.11.768
175. Pope E, Lara-Corrales I, Mellerio J, et al. A consensus approach to wound care in epidermolysis bullosa. *J Am Acad Dermatol.* 2012;67(5):904–917. doi:10.1016/j.jaad.2012.01.016
176. Woo K, Sibbald G, Fogh K, et al. Assessment and management of persistent (chronic) and total wound pain. *Int Wound J.* 2008;5(2):205–215. doi:10.1111/j.1742-481X.2008.00483.x
177. Martínez-Monsalve A, Selva-Sevilla C, Gerónimo-Pardo M. Analgesic effectiveness of topical sevoflurane to perform sharp debridement of painful wounds. *J Vasc Surg.* 2019;69(5):1532–1537. doi:10.1016/j.jvs.2018.08.175
178. Nazarko L. Choosing the correct wound care dressing: An overview. *Br J Community Nurs.* 2018;32(5):43–52.
179. Schultz GS, Sibbald RG, Falanga V, et al. Wound bed preparation: A systematic approach to wound management. *Wound Repair Regen.* 2003;11(s1):S1-S28. doi:10.1046/j.1524-475X.11.s2.1.x
180. Molan P, Rhodes T. Honey: A biologic wound dressing. *Wounds Compend Clin Res Pract.* 2015;27(6):141–151.
181. Mearns ES, Liang M, Limone BL, et al. Economic analysis and budget impact of clostridial collagenase ointment compared with medicinal honey for treatment of pressure ulcers in the US. *Clin Outcomes Res CEOR.* 2017;9:485–494. doi:10.2147/CEOR.S133847
182. Smaropoulos E, Cremers NAJ. Treating severe wounds in pediatrics with medical grade honey: A case series. *Clin Case Rep.* 2020;8(3):469–476. doi:10.1002/ccr3.2691
183. Thomas E, Vinodkumar S, Mathew S, Setia MS. A study of the factors associated with risk for development of pressure ulcers: A longitudinal analysis. *Indian J Dermatol.* 2015;60(6):566. doi:10.4103/0019-5154.169127
184. Saghaleini SH, Dehghan K, Shadvar K, Sanaie S, Mahmoodpoor A, Ostadi Z. Pressure ulcer and nutrition. *Indian J Crit Care Med.* 2018;22(4):283–289. doi:10.4103/ijccm.IJCCM_277_17
185. White R. Wound dressings and other topical modalities in bioburden control. In Cutting K, Percival S, eds. *Microbiology of Wounds.* Taylor & Francis; 2010: 385.
186. Butcher M. Assessment, management and prevention of infected wounds. *J Community Nurs.* 2013;27:25–34.
187. Chattopadhyay S, Raines RT. Collagen-based biomaterials for wound healing. *Biopolymers.* 2014;101(8):821–833. doi:10.1002/bip.22486
188. Nam G, Rangasamy S, Purushothaman B, Song JM. The application of bericidal silver nanoparticles in wound treatment: *Nanomater Nanotechnol.* Published online January 1, 2015;5(23):1–14. doi:10.5772/60918
189. Spring S, Pratt M, Chaplin A. Contact dermatitis to topical medicaments: A retrospective chart review from the Ottawa Hospital Patch Test Clinic. *Dermat Contact Atopic Occup Drug.* 2012;23(5):210–213. doi:10.1097/DER.0b013e31826e443c
190. DaCosta RS, Kulbatski I, Lindvere-Teene L, et al. Point-of-care autofluorescence imaging for real-time sampling and treatment guidance of bioburden in chronic wounds: First-in-human results. *PloS One.* 2015;10(3):e0116623. doi:10.1371/journal.pone.0116623
191. Halstead FD, Rauf M, Moiemen NS, et al. The antibacterial activity of acetic acid against biofilm-producing pathogens of relevance to burns patients. *PloS One.* 2015;10(9):e0136190. doi:10.1371/journal.pone.0136190
192. Li Z, Yu Q, Wang S, et al. Impact of negative-pressure wound therapy on bacterial behaviour and bioburden in a contaminated full-thickness wound. *Int Wound J.* 2019;16(5):1214–1221. doi:10.1111/iwj.13197
193. Baharestani M, Amjad I, Bookout K, et al. V.A.C. Therapy in the management of paediatric wounds: Clinical review and experience. *Int Wound J.* 2009;6:1–26. doi:10.1111/j.1742-481X.2009.00607.x
194. Thompson, RH. *The Handbook of Child Life: A Guide for Pediatric Psychosocial Care.* 2nd ed. Charles C Thomas; 2018. https://web-a-ebscohost-com.laneproxy.stanford.edu/ehost/ebookviewer/ebook?sid=965bd77b-6551-4f3f-b250-49d86fe73812%40session mgr4006&vid=0&format=EB
195. Moore ER, Bennett KL, Dietrich MS, Wells N. The effect of directed medical play on young children's pain and distress during burn wound care. *J Pediatr Health Care.* 2015;29(3):265–273. doi:10.1016/j.pedhc.2014.12.006
196. Sprenger C, Eippert F, Finsterbusch J, Bingel U, Rose M, Büchel C. Attention modulates spinal cord responses to pain. *Curr Biol.* 2012;22(11):1019–1022. doi:10.1016/j.cub.2012.04.006
197. Arane K, Behboudi A, Goldman RD. Virtual reality for pain and anxiety management in children. *Can Fam Physician Med Fam Can.* 2017;63(12):932–934.
198. Hua Y, Qiu R, Yao W-Y, Zhang Q, Chen X-L. The effect of virtual reality distraction on pain relief during dressing changes in children with chronic wounds on lower limbs. *Pain Manag Nurs.* 2015;16(5):685–691. doi:10.1016/j.pmn.2015.03.001
199. Hoffman HG, Chambers GT, Meyer WJ, et al. Virtual reality as an adjunctive non-pharmacologic analgesic for acute burn pain during medical procedures. *Ann Behav Med.* 2011;41(2):183–191. doi:10.1007/s12160-010-9248-7
200. Chester SJ, Tyack Z, De Young A, et al. Efficacy of hypnosis on pain, wound-healing, anxiety, and stress in children with acute burn injuries: A randomized controlled trial. *Pain.* 2018;159(9):1790–1801. doi:10.1097/j.pain.0000000000001276
201. Ali S, McGrath T, Drendel AL. An evidence-based approach to minimizing acute procedural pain in the emergency department and beyond. *Pediatr Emerg Care.* 2016;32(1):36–42; quiz 43-44. doi:10.1097/PEC.0000000000000669
202. Thomas R, Phillips M, Hamilton RJ. Pain management in the pediatric palliative care population. *J Nurs Scholarsh.* 2018;50(4):375–382. doi:10.1111/jnu.12389
203. van der Heijden MJE, de Jong A, Rode H, Martinez R, van Dijk M. Assessing and addressing the problem of pain and distress during wound care procedures in paediatric patients with burns. *Burns.* 2018;44(1):175–182. doi:10.1016/j.burns.2017.07.004
204. Aronson JK, ed. *Meyler's Side Effects of Drugs: The International Encyclopedia of Adverse Drug Reactions and Interactions.* 16th ed. Elsevier Science; 2016: 858–862.
205. Akhmetova A, Saliev T, Allan IU, Illsley MJ, Nurgozhin T, Mikhalovsky S. A comprehensive review of topical odor-controlling treatment options for chronic wounds: *J Wound Ostomy Continence Nurs.* 2016;43(6):598–609. doi:10.1097/WON.0000000000000273
206. Watanabe K, Shimo A, Tsugawa K, et al. Safe and effective deodorization of malodorous fungating tumors using topical metronidazole 0.75% gel (GK567): A multicenter, open-label, phase III study (RDT.07.SRE.27013). *Support Care Cancer.* 2016;24(6):2583–2590. doi:10.1007/s00520-015-3067-0

27 | EASING DISTRESS WHEN DEATH IS NEAR

DEBRA LOTSTEIN AND RACHEL RUSCH

Death is not the opposite of life, but a part of it.

HARUKI MURAKAMI

INTRODUCTION

While in many ways a child's death is always tragic, when inevitable, as palliative care clinicians we aspire to enable a more peaceful death experience for the child and family. Recognizing that what may bring peace will differ across families, this chapter reviews strategies that can address each child and family's unique physical, psychosocial, and spiritual needs at end of life. Care provided in the final days before a child's death can be a profound opportunity to create a strong foundation from which a family may continue to find support in their bereavement.

Importantly, when a child is dying, all care goals may not be uniformly focused on easing suffering. Recent studies affirm the common clinical experience that, even when a child's illness is said to be incurable, parents will hope to extend life, concurrent with ensuring comfort. Family values will differ: While some aspire to focus on a peaceful end-of-life experience for their child, others value continued attempts to sustain a child's life, while others hope for combined considerations of prolonging life and ensuring comfort. As clinicians, it is critical to remember that whatever the primary goals of care and setting of a child's death, treatment should never be at the exclusion of ensuring comfort.

To this end, thoughtfulness surrounding the language clinicians use during such sensitive and vulnerable times builds the foundation for peace at end of life. The ways clinicians describe the shift in goals of care from a focus on disease-directed treatments toward care centering on a child's comfort is significant to families.[1] Terms such as "withdrawal of care," "withdrawal of support," or "allowing natural death" may imply a withholding of attention and services that families may sense as an abandonment of their child or themselves. Alternatively, we can describe how we are partnering with families as they consider and reconsider various medical interventions, including the discontinuation of life-sustaining treatments. As opposed to limiting care, we continue caring deeply for the child and family throughout the dying process and into bereavement. Going further, providing care at the end of a child's life invites clinicians to be present to everything that arises during this most intimate of clinician–family experiences (Figure 27.1).

Of note, studies that assess quality of life at the very end of life in children are limited. Thus, the content of this chapter is guided by clinical experience based on consensus and the existing literature.

INTERDISCIPLINARY CARING

The care of a dying child requires exquisite collaboration among all involved to meet the needs of the child and family. Table 27.1 highlights key roles and activities of the interdisciplinary team. No matter where the child is being cared for, short huddles or meetings among team members may be helpful to maintain open lines of communication.

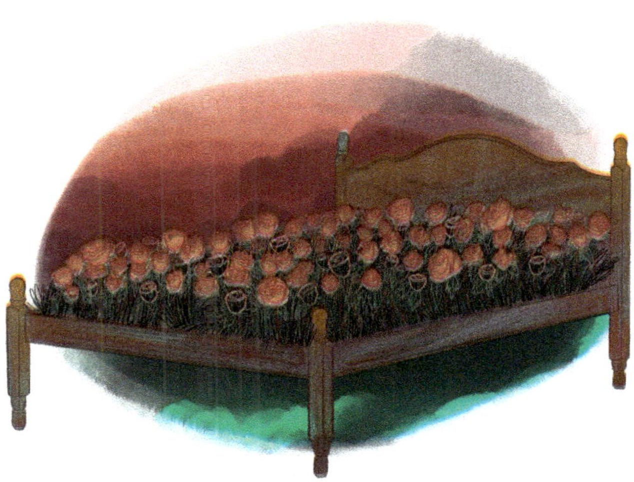

Figure 27.1 *A Bed of Roses [Cradled Vessel], 2020.* Image from an art therapist expressing the vulnerability, pain, strength, and beauty one might encounter when fully present with children and families through a child's death. Artwork by Rebecca Yeretzian-Santana, MA, AMFT, ATR (used with permission).

TABLE 27.1 Interdisciplinary roles in the care of the imminently dying child

CLINICIAN	DISCIPLINE SPECIFIC ROLES	INTERDISCIPLINARY ROLES
Primary physician/Nurse practitioner	Leads discussions related to establishing and re-evaluating goals of care and care plans Therapeutic recommendations to relieve distress Request for organ donation and autopsy	Presence Anticipatory guidance Assessment and relief of child and family distress Respond to questions and/or concerns Perform little acts of kindness
Nurse	Administration of distress relieving interventions Ensure the setting is equipped to meet child's and family's needs with regard to staff, medications and equipment Gatekeeper when requested by family Communicator with larger team regarding bedside experiences of child and family	
Psychosocial clinician	Provide individual or family psychotherapy as a continuation of an ongoing process, or as needed on a crisis basis Facilitate legacy-building opportunities Assist with advanced care planning regarding after-death steps such as wake and/or funeral arrangements Consider larger family and community needs such as siblings and school	
Child life specialist	Play activities to allow legacy-building opportunities Play activities for child if able, siblings and other children to promote expression of feelings regarding child's death Play activities for siblings and other children to create opportunities to escape from the intensity of being with a dying child	
Chaplain	Assess and respond to spiritual needs of child and family Ensure that clinicians are familiar with and respectful of family rituals related to death and dying Meet with community spiritual leader as indicated	
Pharmacist	Advise about distress-relieving medications Ensure adequate supply of distress-relieving medications	

Used with permission from Wolfe J. Easing distress when death is near. In Wolfe J, Hinds P, Sourkes B, eds. *Textbook of Interdisciplinary Pediatric Palliative Care*. Elsevier Saunders; 2011: 368–386.[103]

IN ADVANCE OF CLEAR DECLINE

TOPICS FOR ANTICIPATORY GUIDANCE

Most families will have little prior knowledge of the multiple concerns related to end-of-life care and what happens after a child's death. Notably, anticipatory guidance can help prepare families for the child's end-of-life course and ease the child and family's distress. Each family will have a different comfort level regarding these conversations; for some, knowing more about what lies ahead will increase their sense of control and provide comfort; for others, thinking ahead of the present moment can be overwhelming or generate fear that they are causing or rushing their child's death. Families may be hesitant to openly ask questions, so gently inquiring about their need for information and slowly providing it in manageable quantities is considered a helpful practice.[2] Seeking their permission, as in "Would it be helpful for us to talk now about what the future might look like as your child gets sicker?" can be a way to assess an individual's openness to these conversations. If parents permit it, other close friends or family members can help with logistical information (e.g., funeral arrangements) to alleviate some burden for the family. Box 27.1 provides a guide to important end-of-life topics with suggestions for timing of these discussions and with references to other chapters in this book that cover these topics in more detail.

BOX 27.1 POTENTIAL COMMUNICATION TOPICS IN CHILDREN WITH ADVANCED LIFE-THREATENING ILLNESS, WITH PROPOSED TIMING

Chapters in this book with additional discussion of these topics are listed in parentheses.

- In advance of clear decline:
  - Considerations about resuscitation status and other life-prolonging interventions (Chapter 14)
  - Discussions related to preferred location of care (Chapters 13 and 14)
- During clear decline:
  - Discussion related to preferred location of child's death
  - If dying at home: details for actions at time of death, including who will pronounce the child's death
  - Spiritual and religious practices and legacy activities
- When death appears to be within days:
  - Anticipatory guidance on physical changes at end of life
  - Discussion related to organ and tissue donation and autopsy (Chapter 14)
  - Funeral and commemoration planning
- Following death:
  - Bereavement guidance (Chapter 15)

Timing around these anticipatory conversations can be difficult given the uncertainty in prognosis for children with serious illness. Clinicians may be asked by family members and even the child themselves to share "how much time is left" when these topics are broached. For some children with complex, chronic conditions who have multiple episodes of exacerbations and recoveries, predicting when they are at the point where recovery is not possible and death is near can be especially difficult. Clinicians should use their assessment of the status of the patient and their knowledge of likely disease course to give families an honest time frame stated as a range (i.e., minutes to hours, hours to days, days to weeks, weeks to months). Acknowledging the uncertainty while at the same time preparing families for the likely course ahead helps build and maintain trust, especially for families who have been told many times before that their child is dying. In the following parent reflection, Augustina shares the way the palliative care team used this approach to both prepare and support her through a long period of recoveries and exacerbations prior to her son's eventual death.

Family Reflection

Isai was such an amazing child. Since the day the doctors told me he had hydrocephalus, I said "I'll keep him." I didn't know that he was going to have other health issues. He went to the hospital 2 days after he was born to have a surgery, a shunt put in his head. I was so scared back then not knowing what to expect. We went to the hospital for many years to see a lot of specialists regarding seizures, bone problems, lung disease, GI problems, and for his shunt. Later he was on oxygen because his lungs were just getting so tired. About a year before Isai got sicker, I met with the palliative care team in clinic. We made a care and pain management plan so that he could live a better, more comfortable life.

Isai started getting sicker and was in and out of the intensive care unit (ICU) for the last 3 years of this life. The palliative team came to visit, and we talked about a lot of things, like how to keep him comfortable. They would visit him or come to see how I was doing. I'm so happy they did.

Isai was the strongest boy you could ever meet, and I learned a lot from Isai in the last few days of his life. He graduated high school, and he was healthy for 6 months after that. Then he started going in and out of the ICU, and one day at the end of May, he got very sick and we went to the ICU, not knowing he wouldn't go home anymore. Isai fought for his life like he did many times before, like a warrior, but he was just tired. The palliative care team was there to help him to be as comfortable as he could. They talked to me and gave me moral support.

When Isai passed away the palliative care team helped me a lot. Now they call me and ask how we are doing. I feel so comfortable talking with them, and I'm very grateful for the support they gave me and my son. His legacy will continue to live forever. I'm sure Isai is watching over us and is very happy. He will always be missed.

Augustina Ramos, mother of Isai Carrasco

DISCUSSION OF PREFERRED LOCATION OF CARE AND DEATH

An important consideration as a child is reaching the end of life is the location of care and of death, if that can be arranged. Faced with the reality that their child's death is inevitable, some families hope to spend as much time at home as possible. Others feel more comfortable and supported in the hospital environment, with clinicians close at hand to address symptoms or provide care. Notably, the decision of preferred location of care when time is short may be different from the desired location of death, as some families might hope to be at home and come to the hospital only when it seems that death is very close. In addition to child and family preference, the decision to stay home will depend on other practical matters, including whether support for nursing and symptom needs can be met at home, the availability of hospice care with pediatric expertise, and the resources of the family and home itself. Further issues related to discussion and enrollment in hospice services are discussed in Chapter 4.

WHEN DEATH IS IMMINENT

Dying is a dynamic process that is influenced by many factors. However, it is remarkable how similar the process can be despite very different underlying illnesses. Clinical experience suggests that when approaching death within hours to days, a child is often bedridden, semiconscious, with little or no oral intake. Changes in pulse, respiration, and peripheral circulation may also be apparent. Table 27.2 summarizes changes frequently seen in dying patients which can be indications of timing of death and may also signal the need for specific comfort-focused measures.[3,4]

KEY PRINCIPLES OF CARE

There are several key principles in managing the child's final days. An analytical approach to symptom control continues but usually relies on clinical findings rather than investigation of possible causes. Medication and treatments should be reviewed with regard to how they are contributing to comfort or possibly causing uncomfortable side effects. It is helpful to review of the route of medication administration, as many patients lose the ability to take medications orally. While interdisciplinary team care is always important, perhaps there is no other time where it is quite as essential.[5]

Finally, it is essential that the care team maintains effective communication and ensures that support is in place for the family. A daily visit for inpatients, or for those at home a daily phone call at a planned time or even occasional home visits from either a hospice or hospital-based team, can be very reassuring for families.[6] Importantly, even when the child may be comfortable and symptoms are well-controlled,

TABLE 27.2 Signs of impending death

ORGAN SYSTEM	CHANGE	MANIFESTED BY/SIGNS OF:
Constitutional/ Neurologic	Fatigue	Sleeping more than awake
	Weakness	Inability to get out of bed; inability to lift head off pillow; rarely, there is a burst of energy just before death
	Decreasing level of consciousness	Increasing drowsiness, difficult to arouse; unresponsive to verbal or tactile stimuli
	Decreasing ability to communicate	Difficulty word finding, delayed or inappropriate response, monosyllabic words, verbally unresponsive
	Terminal delirium	Day–night reversal; confusion; agitation/ restlessness; difficult to console; purposeless repetitious movements; moaning, groaning
	Pain	Grimacing; moaning; tension in forehead between eyebrows; difficult to console; agitation
	Loss of ability to close eyes	Whites of eyes showing (with or without pupils visible); conjunctival erythema
	Decreasing appetite/food intake	Refusal of food; emesis; weight loss, wasting; loss of muscle and fat
	Decreasing fluid intake	Dehydration, dry mucous membranes
	Loss of ability to swallow	Dysphagia, coughing, choking, aspiration; loss of gag reflex; buildup of oral and tracheal secretions; gurgling
Skin/Extremities	Peripheral edema	Due to hypoalbuminemia, third spacing
	Cutaneous ischemia	Erythema over boney prominences; skin breakdown, wounds
Cardiac/Renal	Cardiac dysfunction	Tachycardia, weak pulse; hypertension followed by hypotension (not responsive to fluids); mottling and cooling of the skin; dependent venous pooling
	Renal dysfunction	Dark urine; oliguria; anuria
	Loss of sphincter control	Incontinence of urine or bowels; perineal skin maceration and candidiasis
Respiratory	Respiratory dysfunction	Noisy wet-sounding breathing; abnormal breathing patterns (apnea, agonal breaths, and/or Cheyne-Stokes respirations, characterized by oscillation of ventilation between apnea and tachypnea, with a crescendo-decrescendo pattern in the depth of respirations); rarely, aspiration, asphyxiation

Adapted from Bicanovsky L. Comfort care: Symptom control in the dying. In Walsh, D et al. eds, *Palliative medicine*. 1st ed. Saunders; 2009; and Emanuel L, Ferris F, von Gunten C, Hauser J, Von Roenn J. The last hours of living: Practical advice for clinicians. https://www.medscape.com/viewarticle/716463. 2010.

a clinician's presence during the final period can be very comforting to family members. Such a presence reinforces that the dying patient's welfare remains important, and it provides opportunity for support and guidance to the family at a time of extreme stress. It is critical to inform the family that although death may be imminent, the time frame may be hours to days.

LETTING THE FAMILY KNOW WHEN DEATH IS IMMINENT

Parents and other family members are often fearful that if they step away from the bedside, they will not be present at the time of the child's death. As such, it is often helpful to let family and loved ones know about the signs of impending death both to prepare for what to expect and to try to judge when presence at the bedside may be warranted. To introduce this topic, simply ask whether it would be helpful to know more about what to expect as the child is dying. If a parent agrees to be informed, it is important to be clear, provide short pieces of information, and then subsequently check if it is all right to continue.

It is also critical to prepare parents that it may not be possible to know the exact moment when death will occur. Anecdotally, some families may find comfort in knowing that children may choose to die when their parent is not present as a last effort to protect the parent from further suffering, if such a choice is indeed possible.

SETTING THE STAGE

When a child is actively dying and there is consensus that the primary focus of care should be on comfort, there is much that the interdisciplinary team can do to permit a more comfortable death experience with as few medical interruptions as possible. Actions needed to achieve this goal will vary by setting, whether the child is at home or in the hospital.

AT HOME

Families should be informed about the change in their child's status and should be prepared for potential changes in symptoms and signs of impending death (see later discussion). At this time medications and treatments can be reviewed, and those that do not contribute to comfort could be discontinued. The child will need continuous care, and some may require professional in-home care around the clock. If a clinician cannot be present continually, the family must have access to immediate help for symptom management by phone, and it is essential that families have adequate supplies of medications to treat common symptoms in the home, including access to opiates and benzodiazepines. If a child is no longer able to take needed medications orally, alternative forms and methods of giving medications should be explained, including those that can be given by dissolvable forms or rectally. Families should have a signed in-home order for withholding of life-sustaining treatments, especially if emergency medical services may be involved.

In addition to the anticipatory guidance around physical changes immediately before and after death, parents (or a close friend/family member) should be given instruction about what should happen with the body after death. If the family is being cared for by a hospice agency, the family should know to contact the agency at the time of death, and typically a hospice nurse will be available to pronounce the child and contact the funeral home and others who should be informed. If an autopsy or organ donation are being considered, the family should know how to contact the appropriate hospital or organ procurement agency. As families may contact emergency services in a moment of crisis, a call from a clinician ahead of time to the local police department will help them be prepared in case they are called. Providers should help the family determine ahead of time when hospice is not involved who will be called to pronounce the patient and who will be filling out the death certificate, which may need to happen before the funeral home will pick up the body (depending on state and local regulations). Emergency services can be called for pronouncement and presented with an out-of-hospital do-not-resuscitate (DNR) order so they do not need to initiate cardiopulmonary resuscitation or bring the body to a hospital. However emergency services do not necessarily need to be called for expected deaths in the home if one of the child's primary or palliative care physicians may be contacted to pronounce the death. Even in expected deaths, a coroner may be contacted for out-of-hospital deaths, and providers should be familiar with the policies for this in their practice area. The family should have a funeral home chosen ahead of time who will come to remove the body at the appropriate time. Refer to Chapter 4 for further explanation of the role of hospice in out-of-hospital deaths.

IN THE HOSPITAL

Continued medical interventions, including vital sign assessments, pulse oximetry, nonessential medications, and blood work may be disruptive and no longer beneficial to the child's care. However, discussion of discontinuing these procedures is delicate and can be perceived as no longer caring for the child. This is especially true among families who are used to vigilantly monitoring their child. Parents should be made aware that discontinuing these procedures allows them time to be with the child without interference from intermittent procedures, wires and tape, and/or sounds from alarms. Gentle suggestions can be made that discontinuing monitors would enable the family to focus entirely on the child, rather than the surrounding medical equipment. As always, flexibility is essential. Some families may simply not want to forgo what they are used to and will often state that the vital sign assessment and/or the monitor will bring them comfort and help them know when the child's time has come.

Considerations about the physical space within a hospital setting for a child's dying process may be helpful for patient, family, and practitioner alike. When possible, larger and less medicalized rooms may provide feelings of comfort and peace to the child and their family. If such spaces are not available, these intentions can be adapted by bringing in larger beds or doubled beds into standard hospital rooms if it is the wish and hope of a family to be able to lie next to their loved one. If families desire, bringing in photos, blankets, and cherished items from home can bring great meaning and comfort. Some patients and families find support from music, whether it be favorite family songs or important spiritual hymns. Encouragement of playing such music and partnering with music therapists when possible can provide additional meaningful support to the child and their family.[7] Additionally, therapeutic books and tactile interventions such as weighted stuffed animals may be additional appropriate supports for siblings and caretakers when death is imminent.[8,9]

Advocating for families and loved ones to more freely visit a child's bedside throughout the end-of-life period can help them to best support a child. Alongside hospital policy and treatment considerations, PPC practitioners can assist in allowing the patient and family to guide who and what they feel comfortable with having present at bedside during such a deeply personal time. Open communication with bedside nursing and primary medical teams can help ensure compassion for the various ways in which families may navigate this period.[10] For some families, being present at bedside during the death of their loved one may be too difficult, and partnering with supportive services such as social work and spiritual care can facilitate psychological and emotional support for both the child and their family. In cases of psychosocial complexity wherein families may not be allowed to be present within the hospital, additional attention may be needed in supporting bedside nursing and primary care teams in a way that is thoughtful of professional and personal boundaries while continuing to promote compassionate care for a child through the end of their life.[11]

RESPECTING SPIRITUAL AND RELIGIOUS VALUES AT END OF LIFE

Hospital-based spiritual care teams, hospice chaplains, and community clergy can provide expert support and guidance to families for whom religion or spirituality is a part of their adaptive coping.[12] Partnering with these individuals can be particularly supportive of specific traditions that may be important to a child, their family, and their faith community through end-of-life and postmortem care. Remaining present to different forms of spiritual or religious needs within family systems and creating an open forum for communication in this regard can be an additional benefit while partnering with chaplain colleagues.[13] Where spiritual care teams may not be available, it can be beneficial to humbly partner with patients and families directly, as a therapeutic listening presence as opposed to spiritual expert. Seeking guidance and support from community members the family may identify as important in supporting their spiritual needs can be a helpful support of this partnership. Additional guidance on some traditional religious tenets surrounding death and dying is provided in Table 27.3. It is also important to maintain spiritual and cultural humility and not assume that specific religious needs are central for a specific child and/or family.[14]

TABLE 27.3 Examples of religion and care at the time of death

RELIGION	CONCEPTS ABOUT DEATH	RITUALS NEAR AND AT TIME OF DEATH	ROUTINE POSTMORTEM CARE	BODY DISPOSAL	MOURNING RITUALS
Buddhism	Death is seen as a process in the cyclical continuum, which includes birth, sickness, old age, death, rebirth, sickness, old age, death, and so on.	Because death is associated with rebirth, great importance is attributed to the state of mind, which should be calm and clear. This means that serene surroundings are important at the time of death. No formal rituals are customary at the time of death. The family may wish to contact a monk who will pray for the deceased. Prayers do not need to be performed in the presence of the body.	In general, Buddhism does not oppose autopsies. Many Tibetan Buddhists believe that the dead body should not be cut or embalmed until 3 days have passed Routine postmortem care is generally acceptable.	Cremation is typical.	The first 7 days after death are the most important for final and funereal prayer. Prayers are then said weekly, during a 49-day funeral period. It is during this period that the prayers of the mourners are believed to help the deceased during the post-death transformation and awaken their spirit to the true nature of death.
Greek and Eastern Orthodox	Orthodox Christians believe death is a necessary consequence of human life due to original sin. Death is necessary to achieve everlasting life.	When a person nears death, it is customary for the priest of the church to be called. The priest in the family's parish is preferred. If the family does not have its own clergy locally, the chaplain may assist in contacting an Orthodox priest through the local Greek Orthodox Diocese. If the patient is awake, Holy Communion can and should be offered to the dying person. The Orthodox priest may also anoint the ill person on the forehead, cheeks, chest, and hands with holy oil in a ritual of spiritual and bodily healing known as the Sacrament of Holy Unction. There are no Last Rites in the Orthodox Church. When the patient has died, the priest will read special prayers for the dead, as well as provide emotional and spiritual support to the bereaved.	Orthodox persons usually decline autopsies, although they are permitted if there are compelling medical reasons to do so, if the body is treated with dignity and if all the tissues and organs are returned to the body for burial. When a child dies, it is customary to dress him or her in white as a groom or bride of Christ, and great care is taken in the selection of burial clothing.	Burial is preferred by the Orthodox Church; allows cremation if the law of the country requires is.	The Eastern Orthodox hold a special vigil over the dead called the *parastasis* or *panikhida*, as a time of contemplation on death. The funeral service includes hymns, chants, and Bible readings.

TABLE 27.3 Continued

RELIGION	CONCEPTS ABOUT DEATH	RITUALS NEAR AND AT TIME OF DEATH	ROUTINE POSTMORTEM CARE	BODY DISPOSAL	MOURNING RITUALS
Hinduism	Hindus believe that although the physical body dies, the soul of a person has no beginning or end (*Samsara*). Death marks a passage rather than the end of life. At death, the soul may be reborn into another living being. The nature of subsequent rebirth is a consequence of actions taken in this life.	The family may wish to keep vigil at the bedside, and play recordings of sacred Indian music to help the patient detach from pain or other worldly things. While the burning of incense is not permitted in the hospital, special arrangements may be made for the use of incense in the hospital chapel or prayer room. The ashes from the incense are often placed on the forehead of the patient, as a blessing. Hindu clergy is not usually requested; although when present, may tie sacred threads around the wrists or neck of the body. Clinical staff should not remove these threads.	Autopsy is permissible. After death, the family may wish to place drops of holy water and basil leaves in the mouth of the deceased, as well as wash or dress the body. The clinician should wear disposable gloves to show respect in closing the eyes and wrapping the body. The deceased's arms should be straightened.	Cremation is preferred, usually within 24 hours of death. In preparation for cremation, the body is bathed, laid in a coffin, adorned with sandalwood paste and garlands, and wrapped in white cloth. Embalming is not customary.	Survivors may choose to fast until the cremation takes place. If so, families may appreciate advocacy to ensure prompt cremation. Family members sometimes choose to delay the cremation until the arrival of extended family. The remains are usually scattered in the Ganges River in India or another body of water. In the cremation ceremony, the body is carried three times counterclockwise around the pyre, then placed upon it. The chief mourner presses the cremation switch. The days of mourning are considered a time of ritual impurity. Mourners cover all religious pictures in the house and do not attend festivals or visit swamis or take part in marriage ceremonies. Mourning period length varies, though Hindu scriptures caution against excessive mourning. A bereavement ceremony to assist the well-being of the soul takes place in the home between 10 and 30 days after death, often on the 13th day. The first year anniversary and subsequent anniversaries of death are very important to surviving family members and involve sacred religious rites.

(continued)

TABLE 27.3 Continued

RELIGION	CONCEPTS ABOUT DEATH	RITUALS NEAR AND AT TIME OF DEATH	ROUTINE POSTMORTEM CARE	BODY DISPOSAL	MOURNING RITUALS
Islam	Muslims believe that there is another world after death for which believers should prepare during their lives on earth.	The family of a dying Muslim may ask that the patient face the east, with his or her head elevated. At the time of death, the Muslim call to prayer is recited by friends, and a chapter of the Koran is read aloud. An Imam is not customarily present at the time of death, but will come if asked.	The body is considered sacred, thus autopsies are forbidden except in cases of compelling legal or medical reasons. If an autopsy must be done, it should be as noninvasive and minimally disfiguring as possible, such as tissue biopsy, and all body parts and fluids returned to the body for burial. Healthcare providers should speak with the family or the Muslim chaplain before giving postmortem care. Many may prefer that another Muslim of the same sex prepare the body. If no Muslim is present, a non-Muslim should use gloves so as to not touch the body. The body should be draped to ensure privacy at all times. Washing will be done in a ritual way at the funeral home. When doing the postmortem care, the head should be turned to the right, and the arms are laid by the patient's side. No locks of hair should be cut.	Burial is performed as soon as possible because embalming is not customary. Cremation is forbidden. The corpse is bathed and wrapped in a plain cloth called a *kafan*. The deceased is buried in the ground after the funeral service. Only burial in the ground is allowed according to Sharl'ah, Islamic law.	Mourners gather and offer *Janazah*, prayers for the forgiveness of the deceased. Once the body is buried, Muslim mourners offer one final *Janazah* prayer
Judaism	Judaism defines death as occurring when respiration and circulation are irreversibly stopped. Brain death is not generally acknowledged among the most Orthodox, and is a source of debate among Conservatives. Euthanasia and withdrawal of care that hastens death are strictly forbidden. In some cases, extraordinary care may be withheld. There are precise rabbinical guidelines called *Responsa* for such situations, and consultation with the Rabbi around such matters is often sought by the family.	At the time of death, the family may wish to gather at the bedside, read psalms and recite the *vidui*, the last prayer of confession. It is not customary for a rabbi to be present at the time of death, although one may be requested.	Some Orthodox and Conservative Jews do not approve of autopsy, unless required by law or the life of a specific person, such as other family members in the case of a hereditary illness, can be saved by information from the autopsy. If an autopsy is done, the more limited the disfigurement, the better. Needle biopsy, limited autopsy, or in situ examination are preferred. All body parts and fluids need to be returned for burial. Some Orthodox families may request their rabbi to be present to observe the autopsy.	Cremation is forbidden. Burial is required to be done as soon as possible; embalming is not permitted unless legally required. The dead are buried as soon as possible. The body is washed to purify it, dressed in a plain linen shroud. The casket, a plain wooden coffin, remains closed after the body is dressed. The body is watched over from time of death till burial, as a sign of respect. The kaddish, a prayer in honor of the dead, is said.	Jews do not make funeral arrangements on the Sabbath or major holidays. A mourning period follows the funeral for the immediate family (*shiva*). Friends and hospital staff who have come to know the family well are welcome to visit the home in the mourning period. It is customary to make charitable contributions rather than send flowers. There is an intense 7-day mourning period, called *shiva*, following the

TABLE 27.3 Continued

RELIGION	CONCEPTS ABOUT DEATH	RITUALS NEAR AND AT TIME OF DEATH	ROUTINE POSTMORTEM CARE	BODY DISPOSAL	MOURNING RITUALS
	Jews believe death in this life will eventually lead to resurrection in a world to come.		Postmortem care is very important to observant Jews. Medical personnel should consult the family before washing the body. The nurse should provide routine care of the body wearing gloves. The arms are not crossed in postmortem care. Any clothing, dressings, or medical equipment with the patient's blood must be buried with the patient. The Jewish community may use designated individuals to wash the body at a later time and prefer funeral homes that are familiar with Jewish faith and ritual. In the Jewish traditions, the body may not be left alone until the burial. Family may wish to station someone outside the morgue to sit with the body until it is removed from the hospital.		burial. Mourners traditionally rent their garments as a symbol of grief. Today, people often wear a black ribbon instead of tearing their clothes. Mourners also cover mirrors, sit on low stools, and avoid wearing leather. The full mourning period lasts a year, after which mourners observe the dead's *yahrzeit*, or yearly anniversary, of the death.
Protestantism	Conservative Protestants believe that everyone has the gift of eternal life. The body dies, but the soul lives forever. The larger question is where each person will spend eternity. Heaven is a glorious location where there is an absence of pain, disease, sex, depression, etc. and where people exist in the presence of Jesus Christ. Hell is a location where its inmates will be punished without any hope of relief, for eternity. The level of punishment will be the same for everyone.	If a child is critically ill, the nurse may want to ask the family about baptism. If the family wishes to baptize their child in the hospital, the Protestant chaplain can be paged or the church pastor called. The family usually prefers to be present and often finds the pastor to be a reassuring companion at such a time. Providers should inquire if families would like their pastor or chaplain called. There are no essential end-of-life sacraments, although some Episcopalian, Lutheran, and Pentecostal persons may request anointing. Reading of scripture, bedside prayers that are personalized to the particular situation, and singing are common.	There are no special concerns for postmortem care. Organ donation and autopsy are a matter of personal preference.	No restrictions or special concerns.	Funerals, memorial services and burials are scheduled at the family's convenience because embalming and/or creamation are common.

(continued)

TABLE 27.3 Continued

RELIGION	CONCEPTS ABOUT DEATH	RITUALS NEAR AND AT TIME OF DEATH	ROUTINE POSTMORTEM CARE	BODY DISPOSAL	MOURNING RITUALS
	A second major belief is that most humans will be sent to hell after they die. Only those few who have been saved will go to heaven. Salvation requires repentance of sins and trusting Jesus as one's Lord and Savior. Believers who have done many good deeds will be rewarded more in heaven; believers who have led an evil life will be rewarded less.				
Roman Catholicism	The Catholic church has a high regard for the preservation and dignity of life, including the sick, disabled, and unborn. The church does not obligate persons to pursue gravely burdensome or ineffective life-sustaining interventions. Analgesics may be used in sufficient amounts to relieve pain even if life is thereby shortened, so long as death is not the intended effect. Catholics see death as a passage from this life to the new, everlasting life promised by Christ. The soul of the deceased goes on to the afterlife, which includes purgatory as well as heaven and hell. According to Catholic belief, the bodies of the dead will be resurrected at the end of time.	Because the priest is viewed as an intermediary between the believer and God, and one whose prayers have special merit, the priest is often requested at the time of death. Even when all sacramental care has been provided earlier, families may request that the priest be present. Families may request an emergency baptism, or sacrament of the sick before death.	There are no special concerns for postmortem care. Organ donation and autopsy are a matter of personal preference.	No restrictions or special concerns. The Church encourages Catholics to be buried in Catholic cemeteries. In 1963, the Vatican lifted the ban on cremation for Catholics. However, the cremation must be interred, not scattered or kept at home.	The Catholic funeral service is called the Mass of the Resurrection. During it, Jesus Christ's life is remembered and related to that of the deceased. Eulogies are not generally allowed during the funeral Mass, but may be delivered at a wake or other nonreligious ceremony. There is also a final graveside farewell, and additional traditions depending on the region.

This information is an introduction to specific religious traditions and is meant to help clinicians understand variations in religious practice. Providers are cautioned not to overgeneralize or characterize all members of a religious group as being alike. A person's spiritual and religious profile is unique and can only be determined when trust has been established and open-ended assessment questions are asked.

Adapted from Children's Hospital Boston practitioner information pages:

Religious Traditions—Buddhism (1997, revised 2000; Greek (and Eastern) Orthodox (1999); Hinduism (1998); Islam (the faith of Muslims) (1997, revised 2002); Judaism (1998); Protestantism (Christian) (1997); Roman Catholicism (1998).

Clinicians are, at times, asked to pray for a child or to lead a family in prayer. This may be an indication of unmet spiritual needs and further exploration of whether it would be helpful to involve the chaplain, if he or she is not already involved, may be warranted. Regardless, the clinician may feel conflicted about whether to participate in or lead a prayer on behalf of the patient because of considerations of professional–personal boundaries and his or her own religious beliefs or spirituality. Consideration of the following options, which attempt to respect the integrity of the clinician's beliefs and be supportive of the family's needs, may be helpful.[15,16]

1. *Praying for the patient*: If a hospital or community chaplain is involved and available, it may be helpful for the clinician to invite the chaplain to lead those present in prayer. In this way, one is respecting the family's wish to have a prayer led on their behalf while respecting and maintaining therapeutically appropriate boundaries.
2. *Sit with patient and family while the family prays*: A clinician who is uncomfortable praying with the family may choose instead to sit quietly in supportive company while they pray. In this way, clinicians lend support to the patient and family without explicitly endorsing a belief system.
3. *Respectfully decline*: Clinicians may also respectfully decline to pray with the family. To avoid the patient feeling rejected, the clinician may want to say, "Thank you for the invitation. Because of my own beliefs, I am unable to participate; however, please know that you and your child are in my thoughts."

LEGACY AND MEMORY-MAKING ACTIVITIES

Legacy and memory-making activities may feel helpful and important for families to pursue during a child's dying processes and soon after their death.[17,18] When possible, primary social workers, spiritual care providers, and child life specialists should be involved for additional assessment and implementation of such activities. Specific interventions may include creating hand, foot, or thumb prints; saving locks of hair; or recording the child's heartbeat.[19] Obtaining photos or videos, whether by the family or in partnership with community resources, can provide additional activity at bedside and provide comfort in bereavement.

EASING CHILD DISTRESS

SHIFTING THE FOCUS OF MEDICAL CARE

Importantly, when a child is actively dying, comfort can be achieved without a focus on reversing the underlying causes of symptoms (see Table 27.2 for changes seen with impending death). For example, it may no longer be indicated to directly treat severe constipation if the child is not expected to live more than a few days. Rather, abdominal discomfort from constipation could be treated symptomatically with opioids, even though opioids may exacerbate constipation. Similarly, continued dressing changes for bedsores may be more painful and disruptive than opting for a more general approach of titrating symptom-relieving medications. Most importantly, treatment decisions should be guided by the priorities of the child and the parent. Again, these decisions should be individualized and discussed with parents so that they understand that it represents a change in care strategy rather than a decrease in care provided. Guidance for approaching some specific symptoms seen at end of life are described in detail next.

DRAWING INWARD

As they approach death, children may become more withdrawn and less interested in usual activities or in interacting with loved ones. Understandably this can be interpreted as a rejection by family members and so should be explained as a normal aspect of dying. This phase has been described as a "drawing inward."

> The endpoint of the terminal phase is often marked by a turning inward on the part of the child, a decathecting from the external world. Cognitive and emotional horizons narrow, as all energy is needed simply for physical survival. A generalized irritability is not uncommon. The child may talk very little and may even retreat from physical contact. Although such withdrawal is not universal, a certain degree of quietness is almost always evident. The child is pulling into himself or herself, not away from others. (B. Sourkes)[20]

ALTERED CONSCIOUSNESS

Diminished wakefulness is very common during the last days of life[21] and is often desirable for the child and family. However, it is also common for parents and loved ones to want to hold onto every wakeful moment possible. At times this desire for a child's awareness/alertness can hinder titration of pain-relieving medications. The team should continue efforts to try for a careful balance of comfort and an ability to interact, while at the same time encouraging the family to continue their own interactions, such as gentle hugging, touching, talking, or singing, with the hope that the child perceives such gestures. One family reread aloud the first book of the Harry Potter series to their dying child, hoping that the story would bring as much joy to him as it had previously.

ESCALATING PAIN, DYSPNEA, AND AGITATION

Three very common symptoms during the final days of life that may require intensive treatment efforts are escalating pain, dyspnea, and agitation. Further details for management of these distressing symptoms can be found in Chapters 20, 23, 24. There are multiple challenges to successful symptom management at end of life, including lack of knowledge and fear of opioid escalation, communication barriers among team members, and fear of hastening death.[22] Clinicians may need to work at the institutional level to develop guidelines, standard order sets, and policies that will allow greater consistency in medication administration and symptom management outcomes. An example of a standardized order set is provided in Box 27.2. When a patient experiences a refractory symptom that cannot be captured through appropriate titration of symptom-relieving medications, sedation to unconsciousness, or *palliative sedation*, may be indicated. Palliative sedation is discussed in further detail later.

NOISY BREATHING

Due to an inability to handle secretions, breathing can become particularly noisy when death is imminent. This is often described as "the death rattle," a term that should not be used, especially with families, given its harshness. Noisy breathing may be more common in patients with primary lung disease or brain tumors.[23] It is critically important to prepare family members for this possibility. Because this symptom is often present when the child is already unconscious, the child may not experience this as uncomfortable. Deep suctioning should be avoided during this phase due to discomfort and lack of efficacy. However, transdermal scopolamine, L-hyoscyamine drops for smaller patients, and glycopyrrolate may be helpful in drying secretions and diminishing this symptom, although evidence of benefit is limited.[24] Addressing and treating what the family perceives as suffering should be a priority, even if there are differences of opinion within the care team.

EMERGENCIES DURING THE TERMINAL PHASE

Rare circumstances can result in the child experiencing sudden high distress and some are best treated using more invasive strategies. Patients should be assessed for their risk of experiencing these complications so that effective interventions can be readily available.

- *Tension pneumothorax*. Sudden gasping can develop in a child who experiences a tension pneumothorax, which can occur in the setting of pulmonary metastases, for example. It results from a progressive deterioration and worsening of a simple pneumothorax associated with the formation of a one-way valve at the point of a rupture in the lung. Air becomes trapped in the pleural cavity between the chest wall and the lung and builds up, putting pressure on the lung and keeping it from fully inflating. Rapid titration of opioids alone is often insufficient to relieve suffering. Management should involve *needle thoracostomy*, the insertion of a large-bore needle into the second intercostal space on the midclavicular line, thereby releasing the pressure in the pleural cavity and converting the tension pneumothorax to a simple pneumothorax. Hemothorax can result in the same symptoms and can be treated similarly.
- *Upper airway obstruction*. Acute stridor resulting from sudden upper airway obstruction is one of the most feared end-of-life symptoms. Death is near when this occurs, and emergency tracheotomy is not indicated. Instead, rapid initiation of opioids and benzodiazepines, or at times initiation of palliative sedation, is indicated.
- *Urinary retention*. Urinary retention is a known side effect of opioids, and, if time permits, then opioid rotation should be considered. Crede's maneuver, the application of manual pressure over the lower abdomen, can also promote emptying of the bladder. However depending on how imminent death is, or if retention is due to an irreversible cause, such as neurologic compromise or obstruction, then bladder decompression via catheterization can provide tremendous symptomatic relief. In such instances, decisions should be made regarding whether to continue with intermittent straight catheterization or Foley catheter placement depending on child and family preference.
- *Bowel obstruction*. Similarly, there are effective strategies for the medical management of bowel obstruction, as delineated in Chapter 25; however, placement of nasogastric suctioning can provide the most immediate and sustained relief, if doing so will not add to a patient's discomfort.
- *Hemorrhage*. Massive hemorrhage is a catastrophic event If this event is anticipated (e.g., if patient is at risk for gastrointestinal or pulmonary bleeding), the family should be prepared for this, including having dark towels and bedsheets. The only effective medical intervention is rapid initiation of sedation, and medications and orders for this should be prepared ahead of time.
- *Myoclonus and seizure*. Myoclonus is often experienced in association with the use of high-dose opioids and can evolve into overt seizure. Early recognition and treatment with benzodiazepines can effectively treat this symptom. If seizure occurs either as a result of high-dose opioids or other underlying etiologies, it is critical to have antiseizure medications available that can be administered intravenously, such as lorazepam, or rectally, such as diazepam.
- *Delirium and/or hallucinations*. It is common for the child to become less coherent toward the end of life, however, overt hallucinations and agitation can be extremely distressing for both the child and family. Chapter 20 provides an extensive review of assessment and management of delirium. In end-of-life instances,

BOX 27.2 GUIDELINES FOR MANAGEMENT OF ESCALATING PAIN, DYSPNEA, OR AGITATION AT THE END OF LIFE

These guidelines are intended for a patient at the end of life with a do-not-resuscitate order in place, and with escalating pain, dyspnea, or agitation. Palliative sedation may be considered with experienced guidance.

WITH ESCALATING PAIN, DYSPNEA, AGITATION

Identify the doctor or nurse responsible for prescribing for patient.

Care nurse to remain at bedside, and prescriber to remain on unit until symptoms are controlled.

Charge nurse or designated staff member will be available to assist as needed until symptoms are controlled.

Nurse will notify pharmacy of expected need for increased opioid use. A back-up continuous infusion supply will be maintained. Nurse will call for new infusion each time back-up solution is started.

No ceiling dose exists for symptom management at the end of life. The correct dose is the one that relieves the symptoms.

Loading Dose

For patients already on opioids: Administer loading dose of same opioid equal to 10% of total opioid dose from preceding 24 hours.

For patients not already receiving opioids: administer loading dose IV x one as follows:

Morphine 0.1 mg/kg IV
or
Hydromorphone 0.015 mg/kg IV
or
Fentanyl 1 mcg/kg IV

Subsequent Dosing

Doses may be given every 10 minutes as needed for end-of-life symptoms.

Begin intermittent dosing, increasing every third dose, as indicated below:

If pain/dyspnea not relieved:	Example:
Doses given q10min prn	
Dose #1 is starting/loading dose	10 mg
1 × previous dose	10 mg
Increase to 1.5 × previous dose	15 mg
1 × previous dose	15 mg
Increase to 1.5 × previous dose	22.5 mg

If inadequate relief from first dose, give second dose.

If inadequate relief from second dose, notify prescriber of need for additional orders.

If good relief from either dose after 30 minutes, obtain order to begin and/or adjust continuous infusion.

If inadequate relief, continue the same sequence prn: 1×, 1.5×, 1×, 1.5×, 1×, 1.5× previous dose.

Pain assessment may be by pain scale or be descriptive, such as crying, grimacing, moaning when moved.

Continuous Infusion Instructions

Recommended Hourly Rate = total opioid dose administered during rapid titration phase ÷ 6 (which is 2× half-life in hours).

Adjustments for Moderate Increase in Symptoms

If at any time symptoms recur, resume intermittent dosing as recommended above, and then increase hourly continuous infusion dose accordingly.

For a patient who has been stabilized on patient controlled analgesia and then experiences a mild to moderate increase in symptoms, increase continuous infusion and intermittent dose by 1.3–1.5 × current dose.

Always consider use of adjunctive therapy (see guidelines). If morphine equivalent >5 mg/kg/hour, or hydromorphone >0.8 mg/kg/hour, adjunctive therapy is strongly recommended.

(continued)

BOX 27.2 **Continued**

Adjunctive Therapy

For anxiety/agitation (Recommended starting dose):

Intermittent Lorazepam: 0.05 mg/kg IV q4h prn anxiety/agitation

Intermittent Haloperidol: 0.01–0.03 mg/kg/day, IV divided q8h or q12h prn hallucinations/agitation (adult dosing: 0.5–5 mg/dose)

For excess respiratory secretions:

Glycopyrrolate: 4–10 mcg/kg/dose IV q3h prn secretions

Hyoscyamine:

Children 2–12 years: 0.0625–0.125 mg PO/SL q4h as needed; maximum daily dosage 0.75 mg

Children >12 years to adults: 0.125–0.25 mg PO/SL q4h as needed; maximum daily dosage 1.5 mg

Scopolamine:

Children >12 years and adults: Apply 1 disc behind the ear every 3 days as needed

Adapted with permission from Children's Hospital Boston Guidelines for Management of Escalating Pain/Dyspnea/Agitation at the End of Life. Boston, Mass. Revised 9/2000.

the child may respond well to intermittent doses of a neuroleptic such as haloperidol, which can be administered orally or intravenously.

CHILD AND FAMILY DISTRESS

Alongside physical changes and ongoing medical planning, continued assessment of psychosocial concerns is central to meeting the needs of the child and their family at end of life.

WHAT TO SAY TO THE CHILD

A common source of distress for families and clinicians alike is knowing how to talk with a cognitively engaged child about his or her impending death. If welcomed by the patient and their family, PPC interdisciplinary teams can offer guidance around communication as the dying process unfolds. Clinicians should also be respectful of times when parents and caregivers feel able to emotionally care for their loved one without outside support.

The child, regardless of age, is often the best guide to ongoing communication during the end-of-life process. If given the opportunity, many children and adolescents will ask questions or share reflections about their physical, emotional, psychological, or spiritual experience. Allowing the patient to direct these end-of-life conversations may bring a sense of peace for the child and the family. Interdisciplinary teams can model ways to encourage a child's openness to reflect and ask these questions; teams can also share language the family might use to mitigate a child's distress, including expressions of ongoing commitment to the child's comfort and safety.

ADAPTIVE COPING AND LANGUAGE OF HOPE

Some families continue to express hope for recovery and miracles as their child becomes sicker and death becomes more certain. For these families, such talk does not inherently mean that a family is in "denial," but instead reflects how they are coping with their child's illness and may even have benefits for the initial stages of bereavement.[25,26] Clinicians may take the opportunity to both affirm a family's loving and hopeful statements regarding their child's life while also expressing ongoing worry and prognostic education where appropriate. In speaking with primary and bedside clinicians, PPC teams may model compassion toward the family's ability to simultaneously hold their hopes and their worries as their child nears end of life, potentially enhancing empathetic communication and mitigating provider moral distress.[27]

SUPPORT DURING A RESUSCITATIVE EFFORT

Approximately 50% of children who experience cardiac arrest in the hospital and 90% of those who experience an out-of-hospital arrest will die.[28,29] Most hospitals have instituted efforts to preempt unexpected cardiorespiratory arrest by instituting "rapid response teams" and protocols to promote early transfer to the ICU.[30] Despite these efforts, codes continue to occur and efforts should be made to attend to the family's distress. Such efforts include identifying a point person for the family who can serve as a constant presence during the resuscitative effort, provide regular updates, answer questions, and make every effort to meet the family's needs. Families are now regularly invited to be present during resuscitative efforts, and most families report that they want to be given the option. After the event, most report they would choose to be present again.[31–34]

THE CHILD WHO LINGERS

Clinical experience suggests that families may express distress regarding the length of time it is taking for the child to die when active dying lasts for hours or days. It is impossible to imagine the enormity of a family's distress associated with this period; the ambivalence of feelings related to wanting to hold on to every moment versus not being able to bear a moment longer at the child's bedside. Anticipatory guidance aimed at preparing families for this period can be helpful. Furthermore, suggesting ways to be with the child can ease family distress, including encouraging activities that engage the senses, for example through

- Touch, such as lying beside the child, providing gentle massage, or hugging
- Sound, of a family's spoken words, including reading favorite books, reflecting on memories, prayer, or playing music, much of which depends on family background and communication style
- Sight, such as looking at photos and other memorabilia and adjusting the lighting to family preference
- Smell, depending on family culture, incense and other familiar smells may be calming
- Action, continuing to provide care through application of damp cloths to forehead, moistening lips, or gentle suction when helpful

Management of visitors is a key role of the healthcare team. For some families, being surrounded by extended family and friends is critical, for others it is unbearable. Inquiring about what is most comforting is essential.

Clinical staff caring for the patient should also receive anticipatory guidance regarding expected timing of death and guidance and support when the dying process seems prolonged. Staff distress in these instances can be addressed through clear guidance in daily huddles, frequent check-ins by the palliative care team, and additional team meetings to ensure ongoing dialogue and communication.[35] Note that a child may be kept alive through ongoing provision of oxygen via nasal canula or intravenous fluids, and if ongoing survival is perceived as prolonging a child's suffering these interventions could be stopped, with family involvement in decision-making. Throughout this period, attention to the child's comfort remains the top priority and if suffering is apparent to loved ones and clinicians, medications should be further titrated.

ADDRESSING REQUESTS TO HASTEN DEATH

Rarely, a parent will overtly request that the child's death be intentionally hastened,[36] and this is most commonly associated with parental fears about child suffering. A child too might ask about this, or ask about assisted dying, which is legal in some states in the United States (and in some other countries) for those older than 18 with terminal conditions. Voluntary euthanasia is legal in the Netherlands, Belgium, Luxembourg, Colombia, and Canada; in some of these countries the laws include minors who can provide assent.[37,38] There are no legal hastening options for minors in North America. Yet, if the child or parent requests hastening, it is important to respond with more than just a statement about its legal prohibition. Just as other requests should be explored to identify underlying meaning and fears, so should this type of request. Explanation of legal and effective alternatives, such as further titration of symptom-relieving medications and palliative sedation, is helpful, and psychosocial or existential distress can be addressed by members of the interdisciplinary team.

Clinical Vignette

Eddie was 6-year-old boy with advanced metastatic alveolar rhabdomyosarcoma. The primary lesion involved his face and neck, and he also had pulmonary and bone marrow metastases. His parents wanted to be prepared for what to expect for his end-of-life course, and the palliative care team offered the following information. One significant concern was that Eddie's tumor would progress locally faster than in his lungs and bone marrow, and, as a result, he was at high risk for upper airway obstruction and suffocation at the end of life. The family was also told about progressive dyspnea and fatigue, should other sites of disease progress faster. Upon hearing these possibilities, his father, Charlie, asked whether Eddie's life could be intentionally ended when he reached a stage when his life was no longer worth living. Rather than focusing on the illegal nature of such an action, Charlie was asked more about his worries and he described immense concerns about Eddie's experience of suffering. In response, the physician gently informed him that we may not be able to tell when life was not worth living from Eddie's perspective, but that every effort would be made to try to ensure his comfort. Eddie's father was told about strategies for intensive symptom management and palliative sedation, if necessary.

Eddie did not suffer from dyspnea or upper airway obstruction. He simply became less and less responsive and required minimal pain-relieving medications. He died peacefully surrounded by family, friends, and clinical caregivers. Several weeks following his death, Charlie reflected that had Eddie's life been intentionally ended, it would have been treating his own suffering, and not Eddie's.

ENSURING COMFORT DURING SPECIAL CIRCUMSTANCES

There are times at the end of a child's life when the burden of suffering from continuation of life-sustaining medical interventions outweighs their potential benefits in a child who is dying of an irreversible disease process. When these special circumstances arise, expert and compassionate interdisciplinary care is needed to address symptoms and help guide the primary clinical teams, the family, and the child, if he or she is conscious.

WHEN FLUIDS AND NUTRITION ARE DISCONTINUED

Typically, as a child approaches end of life, there is little drive for drinking and eating, and older patients have indicated that this is not experienced as hunger or thirst.[19] It is not uncommon, however, for children to be receiving artificial hydration and nutrition (AHN; i.e., intravenous fluids and/or gastric tube feeding) near the end of life, and this may prolong dying without providing benefit in terms of comfort. In such circumstances, clinicians and parents may opt to discontinue medically administered fluid and nutrition.

The continuation of fluids and nutrition may contribute to significant discomfort in a child at end of life. For example, in a child dying from an advanced brain tumor, fluids can increase cerebral edema and headache. In a child with end-stage lung disease, fluids can increase secretions and, at times, pulmonary edema, both of which can exacerbate dyspnea. Other potential harms from the provision of AHN include risk of emesis and aspiration, abdominal discomfort, compression of lung capacity by abdominal contents, and third spacing of fluids leading to effusions, ascites, and peripheral edema (especially as renal function declines).

Importantly, withholding AHN in dying patients when the harms outweigh the possible benefits is ethical and legal.[39] Despite the acceptability of the withholding of AHN, the potential harms of receiving AHN, and the natural decline in need for nutrition and fluids at end of life, this issue is one of the most difficult and emotionally laden for families and caregivers.[40] Feeding one's child is a primal responsibility of parents and caregivers, and it is distressing to see one's loved one stop eating and drinking. Many (if not most) families can benefit from compassionate guidance about the risks of AHN and can include empathic statements over the distress a caregiver may feel when seeing their loved one decline and an explanation that the dying process includes this natural decline in the need for food and hydration and the ability of the body to digest food, the lack of a normal sense of hunger, and the potential harms of AHN. If a child is alert and shows any interest in eating or drinking, they can take small volumes of whatever food or drink they desire on their own, without external pressure to take more. If complete discontinuation of AHN is not acceptable to the family, a decrease in the volume to minimize risk of harm can often be acceptable.

Moreover, once AHN is discontinued and depending on how long a child is likely to survive, the child's appearance may change over time. Anticipatory guidance is critical to helping the family through this end-of-life period. The following key considerations should be discussed.

DURATION OF SURVIVAL

Before embarking on this conversation, the clinician should assess how long the child is likely to survive without hydration and nutrition. Estimates should be given in terms of hours, days, or weeks, rather than an exact amount of time. The duration that a child may survive depends on multiple factors. One consideration is the condition of internal organs, especially the heart and kidneys. For example, if fluids and nutrition are discontinued in a child in a persistent vegetative state, but without other end-organ damage, the child may live for days to weeks. However, in a child with multisystem organ involvement, the duration is likely to be considerably shorter. One sign that can indicate that death is near is when the child becomes anuric. It is uncommon for a child to live more than a few days once the kidneys have stopped functioning. Importantly, despite the discontinuation of AHN, a child's life expectancy can by impacted by the intravenous fluids received with medications, especially continuous infusions. Estimates in these cases are much more difficult to make.

CHANGE IN APPEARANCE

With discontinuing fluids and nutrition, the child will look increasingly dehydrated and this appearance can be difficult for families to bear. In infants, the fontanel will become sunken. Eye sockets will become sunken in all children. Depending on how malnourished the child was to start, the abdomen may become concave. Mucous membranes become increasingly dry and secretions very thick. The skin will become looser. Though changes are likely, this does not mean the child is feeling uncomfortable. Nonetheless, the physical appearance of the child may invoke images of malnourished children, and although parents may understand that the child is not suffering, emotionally, the changes may be unacceptable to them. As such, it is important to offer parents the opportunity to express their worries, and it may be even helpful to reinstitute some hydration at times.

WAYS TO PROMOTE COMFORT

As noted, most children do not express discomfort when not receiving medically administered fluid and nutrition, especially as consciousness lessens. Nonetheless, simple measures can be helpful to both the child and family. Sips of desired liquid and small bites of any food requested can provide a great deal of comfort. Administration of artificial tears can prevent painful cornea abrasions as the eyes become dryer as dehydration progresses. Gentle moistening of the mouth with water-soaked toothettes or ice chips can also be extremely comforting, as is moistening of the lips with a damp cloth or petroleum hydrolatum. Gentle repositioning to prevent bedsores is also helpful. Finally, opioids should be titrated appropriately in response to any expression of distress.

Clinicians, too, including hospital-based physicians and inpatient and home nurses, may need to be educated about these concerns over the risks of AHN and encouraged to reconsider the routine use of AHN in patients approaching end of life. For example, routinely calculated "maintenance" feeds or fluids are not appropriate in dying patients, who may need little more than the fluids that accompany medications, which even that can be excessive or lead to unintended prolongation of the dying process and should be minimized.

WHEN THE VENTILATOR IS DISCONTINUED

One of the most common ways a child typically dies in the ICU is through the discontinuation of ventilatory support.[41–43] The decision to stop this intervention is typically made when there is consensus that the underlying cause of ventilator dependence is irreversible and continued ventilatory support will not result in a meaningful quality of life. The following considerations are important when the patient, when involved, the family, and the healthcare team reach consensus that ventilator support will be discontinued.

Counseling families[44] is a critical aspect of care for the patient who is to be removed from a ventilator (also known as "compassionate extubation"). Before discontinuing, the following issues should be discussed[45]:

- *Potential outcome of discontinuing the ventilator*: Clinical experience suggests that even when there is clear consensus that the child will not survive for long following discontinuation of ventilator support, at times a child will unexpectedly breathe on his or her own. This is especially possible in the newborn who was initially intubated for apnea. Thus, preparing the family for the possibility that the child may survive is essential. When patients are on maximal respiratory support, and especially if other life-sustaining treatments have been stopped (including vasopressors and/or AHN), death typically occurs within minutes. Patients on lower levels of ventilatory support, with relatively intact neurologic control of breathing may survive for hours or even days. More specific prognostication is often not possible.
- *Assurances about comfort*: It is important to prepare the family for the possibility that breathlessness may occur but that it can be managed. Confirm that medication will be available to manage any discomfort and that the patient will likely need to be kept asleep to control symptoms. It is helpful to further explain that involuntary moving or irregular breathing patterns and gasping do not reflect suffering if the patient is properly sedated or in a coma. Explain that the family can be at the bedside during discontinuation of the ventilator.
- *Reinforce the decision*: Even though a family may make a definite decision for ventilator discontinuation, such a decision is always emotionally difficult. It is helpful to provide reassurance they have made the best decision possible for their child.

OPTIONS FOR VENTILATOR DISCONTINUATION

Two methods have been described for ventilator discontinuation[46,47]: immediate extubation and terminal weaning. The clinician's and patient's comfort, and the family's perceptions, should influence the choice. In *immediate extubation*, the endotracheal tube is removed after appropriate suctioning. Humidified air or oxygen is given to prevent the airway from drying. This is the preferred approach to relieve discomfort if the patient is conscious, the volume of secretions is low, and the airway is unlikely to be compromised after extubation. In other circumstances (e.g., when there is a high risk of significant hemoptysis), patients benefit from a *terminal wean* with the gradual reduction in oxygen and/or ventilator rate at a pace not faster than pharmacologic sedation is administered to treat objective signs of distress from the effects of hypoventilation and hypoxia. Note that increasing levels of carbon dioxide in the blood can be sedating and, as such, can contribute to the patient's comfort. In terminal weaning, the ventilator rate, positive end-expiratory pressure (PEEP), and oxygen levels are decreased while the endotracheal tube is left in place. Terminal weaning may be carried out over a period of as little as 30 minutes, or it can be over a longer period of time. If the patient survives and it is decided to leave the endotracheal tube in place, a Briggs T-piece can be placed.

Each institution and/or critical care unit may want to have a standard protocol or checklist to assure patient, family, and clinician comfort during the process of discontinuing ventilatory support. An example of such a checklist from one institution is provided in Box 27.3. The following are some suggested steps to ensure smooth discontinuation of ventilator support:

- Encourage family members to plan for visits from clergy, special music, or rituals that may be important to them.
- Document clinical findings, discussion with family, and plan of care.
- Turn off all monitors and alarms, when agreed upon by family.
- Remove any unnecessary medical paraphernalia, such as the nasogastric tube.
- Maintain intravenous access for administration of palliative medications.
- Suction patient and set the oxygen to 21%; observe for signs of respiratory distress.
- Adjust medications as needed to relieve distress before proceeding further.

PATIENTS RECEIVING NEUROMUSCULAR BLOCKING AGENTS (NMBA)

Neuromuscular blocking drugs have no sedative or analgesic properties and may mask symptoms of suffering at the end of life. As a general rule, therefore, pharmacologic paralysis should be avoided at the end of life. In most cases, the effect of these agents can be reversed or allowed to wear off within a short period of time, allowing for the discontinuation of mechanical ventilation in the absence of the confounding effects of paralysis. Patients who have been receiving NMBAs chronically for management of their ventilatory failure occasionally can present a more difficult ethical dilemma. In some situations, restoration of neuromuscular function may not be possible for several days or even weeks. When faced with this

BOX 27.3 EXAMPLE OF CLINICAL CHECKLIST FOR COMPASSIONATE EXTUBATION

PRIOR TO EXTUBATION

- Provide patient-specific anticipatory guidance to family regarding time frame, expected symptoms, and terminal manifestations *(reinforce consistency between teams/providers)*
- Inform adjunctive services (social work, chaplaincy, child life)
  - Per hospital policy, liberalize visitation
- Consider limiting or discontinuing
  - Paralytics
  - Restraints/unnecessary medical paraphernalia
  - Inotropes/vasopressors
  - Nutritional support (consider no more than one-third maintenance IVF)
  - Antibiotics
  - Labs/x-rays
  - Monitors in room through covering/silencing (discuss with family first)
- DNR/DNI order signed by attending and ACP note written in chart
- Extubation order in place
- Clarify plan with all providers caring for patient (RN, resident/fellow/APP, RT)

SYMPTOM MANAGEMENT

These are suggested guidelines for starting dosages, please consider on individual basis

- Review orders for symptom management, bolus 15 minutes prior to extubation and have additional PRNs drawn at bedside
  - Dyspnea management:
    - Oxygen-maximum 2 L NC or blow by (avoid face mask)
    - Morphine 0.05 mg/kg IV *or* 0.1 mg/kg PO q15min prn
- Pain management:
  - Consider oral comfort measures if appropriate (sucrose, breast milk)
  - Continue current IV infusion and bolus 15 minutes prior to extubation
    - Morphine beginning doses at 0.05 mg/kg/hr
    - Hydromorphone beginning doses at 0.01 mg/kg/hr
    - Fentanyl beginning doses at 1 mcg/kg/hr
- Agitation:
  - Family presence, low lighting, soothing music
  - Consider lorazepam gtt at 0.02 mg/kg/hr *or* 0.05 mg/kg/dose PO/IV q1–2h
- Secretion management:
  - Glycopyrrolate 0.01–0.02 mg/kg IV q4–6h *or*
  - Atropine 1 drop SL q2h (1% ophthalmic solution)

DURING AND SHORTLY AFTER COMPASSIONATE EXTUBATION

- Provider to stay present at bedside for first 15 minutes after extubation to ensure management relieves symptoms
- Provider to reassess frequently, with input from family and nursing, and increase infusion rates of analgesic and anxiolytic medications as needed
  - Opioids: bolus 1 hour dose equivalent *and* increase infusion rate by 25–50% if moderate and 50–100% if severe dyspnea or pain
  - Lorazepam: increase infusion rate by 25–100% for agitation, later doses may reach or exceed 0.2 mg/kg/hr

FOLLOWING EXTUBATION

- Staff debriefing and support

Abbreviations: IVF, Intravenous fluids; RN, registered nurse; APP, Advanced practice practitioner; RT, respiratory therapist; NC, nasal canula; PRN, as needed.

problem, the clinician must choose between withdrawing the ventilator while the patient is paralyzed versus continuation of life support well beyond the point at which the patient and family have determined that the burdens of such treatments outweigh the probable benefits. In this circumstance, it may be preferable to proceed with discontinuation of life support despite the continued presence of neuromuscular blockade along with the provision of adequate analgesia to mitigated presumed suffering.

SYMPTOM CONTROL

The most common symptoms related to discontinuation of a ventilator are breathlessness and anxiety. Opioids and benzodiazepines are the primary medications used to provide comfort, typically requiring doses that cause sedation to achieve good symptom control. The dose needed to control symptoms will depend on the neurological status of the patient and the amount of similar medication used up to the time of extubation. It should be assumed that even unconscious patients may experience distress, and they should also receive symptom-relieving medications in advance of planned extubation. Patients who are awake at the time of extubation or in whom significant amounts of opioids and benzodiazepines have been used previously will require greater dosages or addition of another agent such as a barbiturate to achieve symptom control.[47,48] Medication titration should proceed according to guidelines discussed in Chapter 23.

Clinical Vignette

Asha was a 6-month-old baby girl born with Trisomy 18. Prenatally diagnosed, Asha's mother, Kamile, traveled from Jamaica to the United States for Asha's birth and for a higher level of medical care that she knew her baby would likely need. For several months, Asha lived locally near the hospital with Kamile and their extended family before she was admitted to the hospital with an aspiration pneumonia. Her respiratory status declined to the point that she needed the support of mechanical ventilation to survive, and Kamile agreed to this intervention. Over the next few weeks, Kamile engaged in thoughtful and extensive discussions with Asha's various primary teams alongside the support of palliative care. Kamile shared her hope that Asha's health could be optimized prior to extubation so that she might be discharged home to live as long as possible, knowing that her time would be short. At the same time Kamile wanted to protect Asha from reintubation or attempted cardiac resuscitation should she not be able to breathe on her own. A do not attempt resuscitation/intubation order was placed, and several days later extubation was attempted. During this time the palliative care team, who had been involved in Asha's care since her admission more than a month prior, provided information, guidance, and supportive reflection surrounding Asha's potential end-of-life experience, sharing their worry that Asha was likely to die shortly following extubation, while also holding hope with Kamile that Asha would be able to breathe on her own. Kamile shared her understanding and appreciation for this guidance, noting her own worry that Asha may not survive extubation alongside her loving hope for her daughter's future. Kamile sought support from the palliative care team in speaking with her husband and extended family in Jamaica and in identifying a local funeral home. Palliative care worked in partnership with the spiritual care team to provide important spiritual rituals at bedside during this time. Child life joined with Kamile in creating handprints and footprints, building a beautiful collage of the prints and photos Kamile had taken of Asha over time. Upon Kamile's request, the minutes prior to extubation were spent quietly with the palliative care social worker at Asha's bedside. During this time Kamile reflected on her love of Asha and sang a quiet prayer. The primary medical team was then invited into the room, providing morphine as needed to assure Asha was comfortable as the endotracheal tube was removed. Cardiopulmonary monitoring was continued due to hospital policy, although alarm settings were decreased and set to "silent" mode. Additional lab tests and medications that did not contribute to comfort were discontinued. Then the endotracheal tube was removed and the bedside nurse swiftly placed Asha in Kamile's arms. Asha breathed for a few moments before dying comfortably within her mother's arms. Following the pronouncement of her death, various medical and supportive care staff members spent time with Kamile at bedside as she bathed Asha and dressed her in a white dressing gown she had brought from home. Kamile remained at Asha's bedside for another 2 hours, calling her family both locally and in her home country. She left the unit to return home, escorted by loved ones and by a known hospital chaplain. The palliative care social worker worked closely with Kamile in the days that followed to ensure continued coordination of funeral planning and to provide additional support. Kamile continually reflected her gratitude for the time, compassion, and supportive care her daughter received throughout her life and in the weeks preceding her death.

BRAIN DEATH

In children, brain death (i.e., "irreversible cessation of all functions of the entire brain, including the brainstem)"[49] most commonly arises from hypoxic brain injury due to cardiac or primary pulmonary arrest, shock, or trauma.[50] It may be difficult for parents and other loved ones to grasp the reality of "death by neurologic criteria" because the typical signs of dying may not be present when a child is brain dead and is still receiving cardiorespiratory support. The clinical neurological examination remains the standard for the determination of brain death and has been adopted by most countries.[51,52] The declaration of brain death requires not only a series of careful neurologic tests but also the establishment of the cause of coma, the ascertainment of irreversibility, the resolution of any misleading clinical neurologic signs, the interpretation of the findings on neuroimaging, and the performance of any confirmatory laboratory tests that are deemed necessary, as outlined in Box 27.4.[51] Despite medical consensus, there continues to be areas of controversy around its definition.[53] Some families may have religious or personal reasons that lead them to not accept the equivalence of brain death and biologic death, and individual team members may have varying degrees of comfort with this concept.[52] Depending on the family's beliefs and those of spiritual or religious advisers, families rarely disagree with this death pronouncement, but when there is conflict, resolution may require ethics consultation and/or judicial involvement. Nonetheless, the use of clear and consistent language in explaining death by neurologic criteria can support a family's understanding and acceptance. Once cardiorespiratory support is discontinued, the typical signs of dying ensue.

ORGAN DONATION

Considerations around potential solid organ donation can impact end-of-life care planning and warrant specific anticipatory guidance to families. Solid organ donation may

BOX 27.4 ALGORITHM TO DIAGNOSE BRAIN DEATH IN INFANTS AND CHILDREN

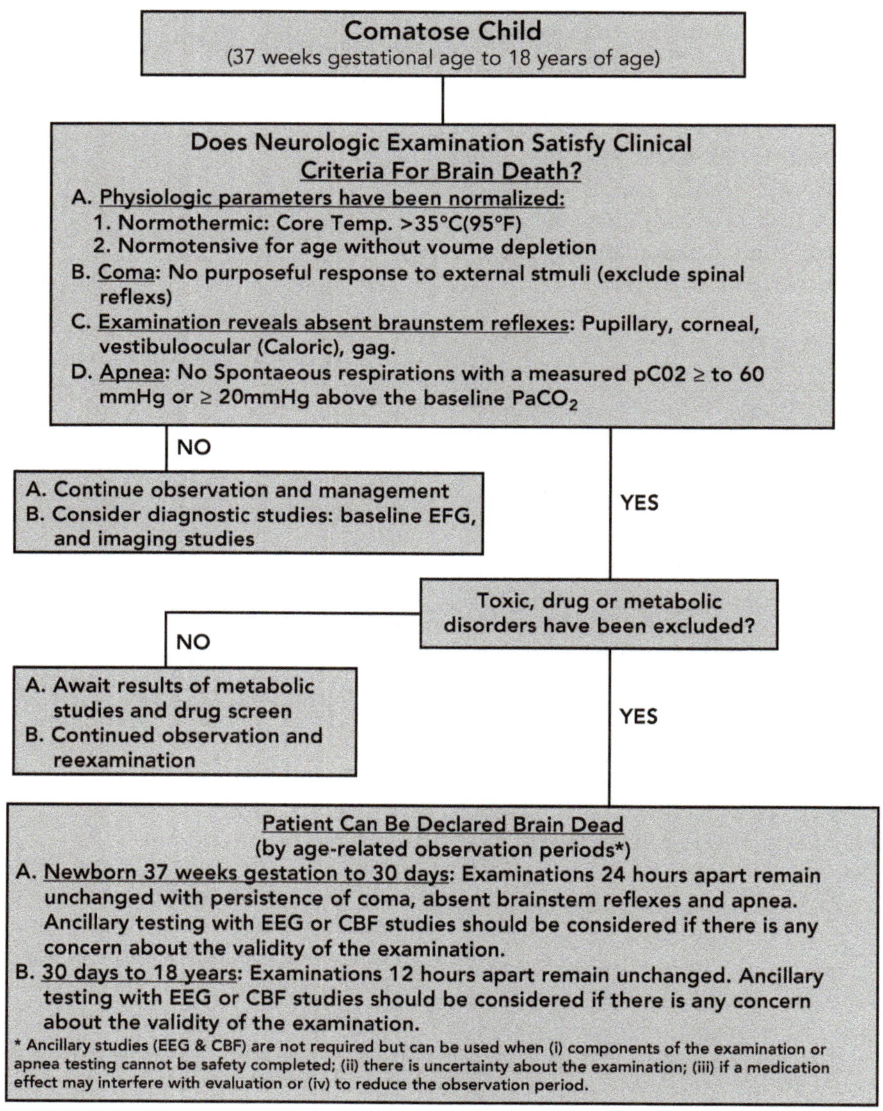

Reprinted with permission from Nakagawa et al. Guidelines for the Determination of Brain Death in Infants and Children: An update of the 1987 Task Force Recommendations. *Pediatrics* 2011; 128;e720.

Abbreviations: CBF, cerebral blood flow, EEG, electroencephalography.

be possible when a child is declared dead by neurologic criteria (i.e., brain dead) or cardiac criteria (i.e., after cardiopulmonary arrest following discontinuation of life-sustaining interventions).[54,55] In the second scenario, the patient has suffered irreversible brain damage, where cortical function is absent, yet the patient has brainstem reflexes so does not meet neurologic criteria for brain death.[55] In either situation, the family should be informed that the patient may require additional interventions to maximize the health of the organs being considered for transplantation. Also, life-sustaining treatment is typically removed in the operating room, such that once cardiac arrest occurs, the organs can be removed as soon as possible. In the case of donation after cardiac death a patient must have cardiac arrest within 60 minutes after removal of ventilatory and circulatory support.[55] Given these requirements, the organ donation process will impact how the child is treated at end of life and where the family will have their final moments with their child. Communication and decision-making concerns related to organ donation are discussed in further detail in Chapter 14.

PALLIATIVE SEDATION THERAPY

On occasion, children with life-threatening illness may suffer from severe or escalating symptoms that are not relieved by the usual palliative interventions. When the overriding goal is comfort for the child, palliative sedation therapy (PST) provides a means to relieve extreme suffering in such rare but critical situations. PST is broadly defined as "the lowering of patient consciousness using medications for the express purpose of limiting patient awareness of suffering that is intractable and intolerable."[56] The addition of "therapy" to the term emphasizes that it is an accepted palliative treatment for symptoms rather than an end in and of itself. PST is usually administered for intractable symptoms at the end of life.

Despite some controversy over the definition and indications for PST, this treatment modality is accepted worldwide as an intervention for patients with refractory suffering at the end of life, and international practice standards for adult care have been published.[57] However, literature regarding the provision of PST in pediatrics is scant.[58-60] In this section we describe situations where PST may be considered in the care of children at end of life, definitions of PST, and details surrounding its implementation. Except where specified in this chapter, evidence presented reflects PST in adults.

INDICATIONS FOR PST

SYMPTOMS PROMPTING CONSIDERATION OF PST

Refractory physical symptoms such as pain, delirium and/or agitation, dyspnea, and nausea and/or vomiting may prompt consideration of PST. The published relative frequencies of physical symptoms invoking PST vary across settings and populations and with the type of sedation studied.[61] Large studies to determine the prevalence of indications for PST in children have not been conducted.

In contrast, the use of PST for refractory distress from nonphysical symptoms (i.e., psychological and existential distress) is more complex.[62] In adults, such distress may involve feelings of meaninglessness and worthlessness; being a burden on others; or death anxiety, fear, a wish to control the time of death. While clinical guidelines for consideration in adults have been published,[56,57,63] PST for nonphysical symptoms in children cannot be recommended and is currently discouraged.[60]

INTOLERABLE SUFFERING

If refractory symptoms escalate to the point of intolerability, the predominant goal of care may shift from extension of life or preservation of function to that of alleviating suffering. As suffering and distress are subjective phenomena, only the individual experiencing such suffering can truly deem his or her condition intolerable.[64] Those who are unable to express themselves verbally rely on proxies (typically parents), in conjunction with the medical team, to decide whether PST should be implemented. When PST is under consideration, distinguishing the child's suffering from that of their parents requires skillful, sensitive discussion.[65,66]

DISTINGUISHING REFRACTORY SYMPTOMS FROM DIFFICULT TO CONTROL SYMPTOMS

Before considering PST, clinicians should assure that symptoms are truly refractory. "Refractory" symptoms are commonly defined as those which cannot be relieved by available measures, within an acceptable time frame, and with acceptable toxicity.[67] Determining if a symptom is refractory then requires that intensive and multidisciplinary efforts to relieve the symptoms have been exhausted.[58,63]

Palliative care consultation, if available, should be a requisite condition whenever PST is considered to help establish that all acceptable interventions to relieve suffering have been considered.[58,60,68] A palliative care team can also ensure that the circumstances are considered from an interdisciplinary perspective and that the physical, emotional, existential, and social dimensions of suffering have been thoroughly explored and addressed. If palliative care consultation is not an option, input from clinicians from different disciplines and with expertise in symptom control, ethics, or the care of seriously ill children should be sought, which may include pain management/anesthesia, psychiatry, psychology, social work, child life, spiritual care, and, potentially, clinical ethics. Hospital policies outlining the appropriate consideration and use of PST are encouraged.[56]

Figure 27.2 provides an algorithm for decision-making on the initiation of PST.[60]

SUBTYPES OF PST

PST may be further described in terms of the level of sedation achieved and its intended duration. Generally, the lowest level of sedation necessary to achieve relief of

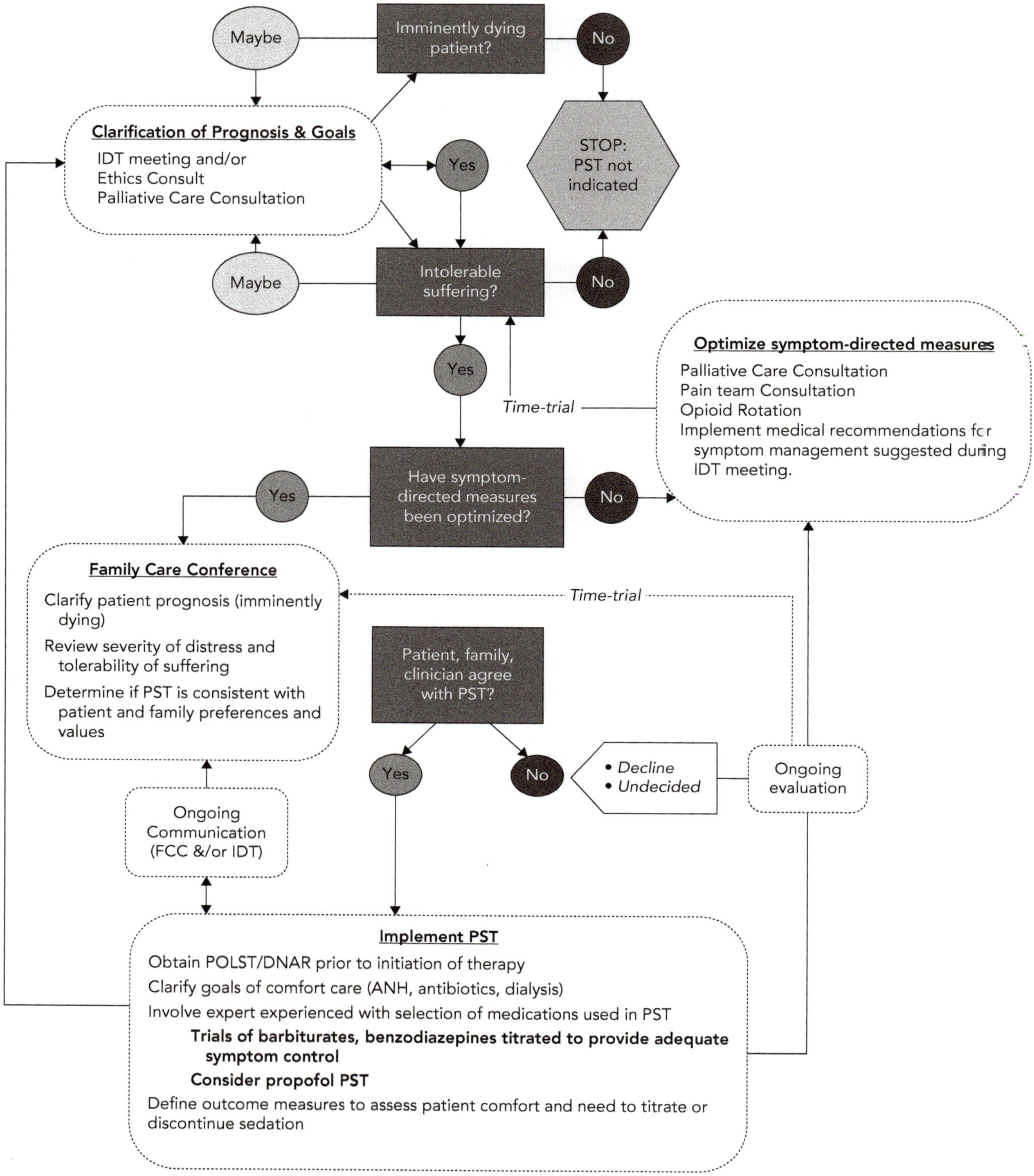

Figure 27.2 *Algorithm for initiation of palliative sedation.*

Abbreviations: IDT, Interdisciplinary Team; PST, Palliative Sedation Therapy; FCC, Family Care Conference; ANH, artificial nutrition/hydration; DNAR, do not attempt resuscitation; POLST, physician orders for life-sustaining treatment. Used with permission from Anghelescu DL, Hamilton H. Faughnan LG, et al. Pediatric palliative sedation therapy with propofol: Recommendations based on experience in children with terminal cancer. *J Palliati Med.* 2012;15:1082–1090.

symptoms is used. *Conscious sedation* describes a state where a patient is receiving sedating medications but is still alert and able to converse, with *deep sedation* being a state that may be indicated in end-of-life situations where comfort cannot be assured without sedation to the point of being noninteractive. *Respite sedation* is a subtype of PST intended to be time-limited for a temporary break from intolerable symptoms, after which time sedation would be decreased with the hope of return to prior level of consciousness.[57] This might be used to support a patient waiting for a procedure intended to alleviate symptoms, while awaiting the arrival of a loved one, or at times prior to the continuation of ongoing disease-directed treatments; further description of the unique considerations for respite sedation are beyond the scope of this chapter. If there is no intention of waking the patient, then continuous sedation is used. Both deep and continuous sedation can be recommended only for patients with an expected prognosis of hours to days without a treatable condition.[63,69]

Emergency sedation is a subtype of PST where sedation to the point of unconsciousness is instituted in the face of a catastrophic event such as massive hemoptysis or acute airway obstruction.[57] Ideally, the potential for emergency sedation is recognized in advance by the care team and discussed with the family before it is needed. If proactive planning has not happened, in a crisis moment, the care team must rapidly evaluate the child's prognosis, goals of care, resuscitation status, and the benefits and burdens of sedation.

ETHICAL CONSIDERATIONS

PST has been criticized as a slow form of euthanasia. *Euthanasia* is the deliberate termination of a patient's life by active intervention, at the request of the patient in otherwise uncontrollable suffering. The aim of PST is the relief of suffering and not the shortening of life.[48,56,65,70] The major distinguishing factor between euthanasia and palliative sedation is the intent of the clinician, patient, and family receiving PST, which is to relieve suffering, not to cause death.[71,72] Another distinguishing factor is the use of the lowest dose of medication in PST to relieve suffering versus the use of lethal doses in euthanasia. The amount of medication, dose, and route for PST needs to be slowly titrated and the patient frequently monitored to establish the minimal level of sedation required to relieve the intolerable suffering. The doctrine of *double effect* is often used to justify PST, but invocation of the doctrine is often unnecessary and overemphasizes an association between PST and hastening death.[71] Ethics consultation is recommended if it would support the patient, family, and/or healthcare team members in the decision-making process or if disagreements exist among those involved.

COMMUNICATION ABOUT PST

COMMUNICATION WITH THE FAMILY

Frequent, open, and honest communication with the family both before and during the provision of PST is crucial.[66] Morita and colleagues have demonstrated that feeling the responsibility for the decision is an independent predictor of high stress in bereaved family members.[73] It is therefore particularly important for the healthcare team to share the responsibility for the decision to administer PST, thus alleviating some of the burden from the family.

Bereaved family members of patients who received PST report having concerns about the patient's distress, whether maximum efforts to control symptoms had been made before initiating PST, having opportunities to say important things to the patients before sedation, to understand their suffering, and for professionals to treat patients with dignity.[66,73] Families also report feeling guilt, helplessness, and exhaustion during the process.

Concern that sedation may shorten life is also common among family members, although several empirical studies have shown no differences in survival when patients who received PST are compared with those who did not receive PST.[61,74] It is therefore important to discuss with families that PST, as with other forms of sedation, is generally very safe although rarely patients experience complications that may shorten life. The degree of focus on risks should also be influenced by the clinical context. For example, presentation of the risks and plans to reduce them, such as monitoring vital signs, may be different depending on whether there is a plan to reverse sedation and awaken the patient after a certain amount of time. In any event, discussion of the risks should never leave families feeling as though they must choose between their child's life and comfort.

Opportunities, both initially and every 24–48 hours while PST is in place, are needed to address these concerns and feelings, which may compound the suffering that families endure during their loved one's last days.[66,75] All discussions should be documented in the medical record as they occur to maximize clear and consistent communication between staff members and the family; specific elements that should be included are described in Box 27.5.

Special attention to regular interdisciplinary communication with families may be needed if PST is administered in the home. Such communication is important not only for the family, but also for staff providing direct care in the home. PST places higher demands on home-care staff.[76,77]

COMMUNICATION WITH THE CHILD

The ability to communicate is diminished in most patients who receive PST. This is one of the more challenging aspects of PST for families, who deeply miss the ability to communicate with their loved one, and, once the patient is comfortable and sedated, they often wish for opportunities to reawaken and communicate with their loved one.[78] Such longing may lead to feelings of anger, frustration, and disappointment. Families should be encouraged to continue to talk to their child and participate in their care if desired. Some family members may be hesitant to touch their child. To the extent that they are comfortable doing so, family members should be encouraged to do certain things for their child, such as washing and dressing or holding or massaging the child. The use of respite sedation may be another strategy for permitting meaningful interactions with their loved one, if interrupted sedation does not evoke a crisis of uncontrolled suffering.

During PST, families are also acutely aware of the way the care team interacts with their loved one. Even small gestures, such as talking to the child and attending to the environment, conveys compassion for the child as well as the message that the child will continue to receive the same attentive care

BOX 27.5 DOCUMENTATION OF COMMUNICATION ABOUT PALLIATIVE SEDATION THERAPY

When beginning palliative sedation therapy (PST), the physician should be responsible for documenting the following:

- The nature of the child's life-threatening illness and their limited prognosis, death anticipated in hours to days
- The patient's and/or family's goals of care. For PST to be considered, the overriding goal must be comfort as opposed to function or preservation of consciousness
- The nature of the distressing and intolerable symptom
- Refractoriness of symptom
- Outcomes of interdisciplinary assessment
- Findings of relevant consultants
- Limitations of the available techniques
- The option of PST
- Intended outcome of sedation, the degree and duration of sedation, its goals, and expected outcomes
- Risks have been discussed (including aspiration, paradoxical agitation, respiratory suppression) and treatment alternatives
- Indications for titrating the sedative upward or downward
- Plans for monitoring the child with vital signs, laboratory tests, if indicated
- Discussion of plans for continuing or withholding artificial nutrition and hydration
- Resuscitation status and life-sustaining treatments, such as dialysis
- If the child is involved in the decision, the child's ability to make decisions about their ongoing care should be specified
- Any specific goals that the patient or family may have, such as a visit from a family member before initiating sedation

Adapted with permission from Naipaul AD, Ullrich C. Palliative sedation. In Wolfe J, Hinds P, Sourkes B, eds. *Textbook of Interdisciplinary Pediatric Palliative Care*. Philadelphia, PA: Elsevier Saunders; 2011: 204–214.

received before sedation. A respectful manner that preserves the individual's dignity and individuality is needed from all members of the care team, as its absence can deeply impact families and their subsequent bereavement.[73,78]

INTERDISCIPLINARY TEAM COMMUNICATION

Caring for a patient with intractable suffering can strain every member of a care team physically, emotionally, and morally. Although PST is a widely accepted therapy for otherwise intractable suffering at the end of life in many countries,[56,63,65] support for PST may not necessarily be unanimous, particularly so when PST is administered for nonphysical suffering. It is imperative that all members have the freedom to share their views with others on the team in a nonjudgmental and respectful environment. Those who object or who are significantly distressed by providing palliative sedation should be given the opportunity to change patient assignments without concern for repercussions. Frequent opportunities for staff to debrief are essential.

Psychosocial team members (e.g., social work, child life, spiritual care) can support opportunities for the family to participate in meaningful activities regardless of whether a decision is made for palliative sedation. Furthermore, bereavement support should consider the fact that PST was used. Uncontrolled symptom distress, a prerequisite for PST, and PST itself may place surviving loved ones at increased risk for complicated grief. As a complex and multifaceted palliative care intervention for proportionally serious distress, skilled interdisciplinary bereavement support is essential, preferably from the same team that followed the patient and family during PST.

ADDITIONAL CONSIDERATIONS PRIOR TO INITIATING PST

LOCATION OF CARE

The location of the child's care should also be determined before initiating discussion of PST, because this is likely to affect whether PST will be an option. As in most clinical situations, determining the range of treatment options prior to presenting the idea of PST to the family is recommended. Offering to relieve a child's suffering through sedation when this is not a realistic option can leave a family feeling abandoned and the care team demoralized and guilty.[79]

PROVISION OF ARTIFICIAL HYDRATION AND NUTRITION

Although provision of AHN may be continued during PST, it is unlikely to contribute to the patient's comfort. It may actually detract from the goal of maximizing comfort by contributing to fluid overload or gastrointestinal discomfort.[80] Discontinuation of AHN when PST is implemented has not been associated with shorter survival times,[74] perhaps because patients with severely distressing and uncontrolled symptoms are unlikely to sustain themselves with oral intake for extended periods of time. In some cases where respite sedation is intended, ongoing provision of AHN may be consistent with the family's primary goals.

RESUSCITATION STATUS

Given the premises of PST, implementation of a DNR order is required if there are no intentions to lift sedation. Even if sedation is intended to be temporary (i.e., respite sedation), it is possible that the child will not regain consciousness. To prevent undue suffering, it is recommended that a DNR order be in place for respite sedation in patients with advanced illness and a limited prognosis.

DOCUMENTATION

The importance of documentation whenever PST is considered cannot be overstated. Outcomes of interdisciplinary assessments in determination of a symptom's refractoriness, discussions with families regarding the PST option and ongoing assessments of clinicians caring for a child receiving PST must all be thoroughly and routinely documented. Such documentation should be readily accessible by all members of the child's care team. Documentation is particularly important for caregivers who may not have participated in discussions but are involved in providing sedation.

MEDICAL CONSIDERATIONS

DEPTH OF SEDATION

In general, the targeted level of sedation should be the lowest that relieves distress. Conscious sedation, where the patient is calm and able to respond to verbal commands, is often considered the ideal level of sedation for PST. This mild degree of sedation should be attempted first because it preserves interactive function. If the patient experiences persistent distress, deeper sedation should be pursued. Once symptoms are controlled, the sedative dose may be titrated downward to potentially reestablish consciousness after a specified interval to allow for planned family interactions and to reevaluate the child's condition and the family's preferences for sedation. In other instances, such as intense distress, severely refractory symptoms, or anticipated death within hours to a few days, continuous deep sedation may be indicated.

CHOICE OF SEDATIVE

In the absence of controlled trials evaluating sedatives for PST, the choice of sedative is often driven by the clinical scenario, including the nature of the refractory symptoms, location of care, and duration and depth of sedation desired. Medications with rapid onset and short duration of action are most useful in delivering PST; commonly used medications for PST are summarized in Table 27.4. Most commonly, benzodiazepines, neuroleptics, or barbiturates are used in PST, and use of other anesthetic agents such as propofol and ketamine have been described. [60,81,82]

Midazolam and barbiturates such as pentobarbital were some of the first agents reported to be used for PST.[81,83] In the absence of delirium, midazolam is the agent of choice and is the most commonly used agent for PST. It has a rapid onset and short duration of action, facilitating titration. Pentobarbital also has a short onset of action and may alternatively be used, but it has a long half-life and is not readily reversed. Because of these properties, pentobarbital is not ideal for respite sedation.

If available, propofol is frequently an excellent choice for use in PST because its rapid onset and duration of action (5–10 minutes) allow for close control of sedation in response to symptoms and for variable depths of sedation.[60,82,84] Propofol also has many other beneficial properties, including anxiolytic, antiemetic, antipruritic, anticonvulsant, and antimyoclonic effects. Use of propofol may be limited by inability to use this agent outside of an ICU setting and concerns over propofol-related infusion syndrome with longer term use.[82,84]

Dexmedetomidine holds promise as another potential agent for use in PST. Dexmedetomidine acts in the descending pain modulating system on postsynaptic alpha-2 receptors.[85] It is associated with less delirium than midazolam in intubated ICU patients, has analgesic effects, and frequently allows patients to be sedated but communicative and cooperative.[86]

Other medications commonly used at end of life are best used in conjunction with the medications just described during PST. For example, opioids do not effectively produce reliable, prolonged sedation. Furthermore, escalating opioids may have neuroexcitatory side effects such as delirium, hyperalgesia, or myoclonus. However, opioids should be continued in children already receiving opioids for ongoing analgesia and to avoid withdrawal symptoms. Although ketamine has sedative and analgesic properties, it may cause unpleasant dysphoric or dissociative reactions, particularly in older children, and is not recommended as monotherapy for PST. Neuroleptics such as haloperidol and chlorpromazine do not reliably induce unconsciousness on their own, though they may be a good choice in conjunction with another agent (such as a benzodiazepine) in terminal agitated delirium.[81]

ADMINISTRATION OF PST

Suggested guidelines for the initial and ongoing administration of medications for PST are described in Box 27.6. Once sedation has been titrated to relieve symptoms, the physician should ensure that clear parameters for sedative titration and physician notification are documented and discussed, including initial infusion rate, rate of continuous infusion, and dose and time interval for bolus doses, as well as indications for infusion rate increases or bolus dose administration.

As in other situations where comfort is the primary focus of care in a dying child, the physician should also discontinue all orders not contributing to the patient's comfort or goals of care. For example, routine cardiopulmonary monitoring (e.g., heart rate, blood pressure) is typically not necessary during continuous sedation when there is no intent to awaken the patient and a DNR order is in place.[65] Observational assessments and physical exam can be used to adjust therapy to the desired effects.

During the initiation of PST, continuous nursing care will be required with a nurse/patient ratio of 1:1 preferred until the desired treatment effects are reached and may then be reconsidered. A patient may experience diminished or loss of protective reflexes such as blinking, gagging, and coughing. Routine eye and mouth care, as well as skin protection to prevent breakdown, will be necessary and important to maximize comfort. Families may be provided with the opportunity to participate in the patient's hygiene.

MONITORING COMFORT AND SEDATION

Optimal tools to quantitatively measure comfort are not yet established. Monitoring comfort level will vary among each patient and family's perspective.[87] Due to this individualized approach, when communicating with the family, clinicians should avoid ambiguous terms such as "comfort care" and focus on the specific indicators of comfort established for a particular child and family. During the initiation and titration of therapy, the level of sedation is monitored frequently. The level of sedation may be documented using a tool such as the Ramsay Scale,[88] as consistent monitoring of comfort and

TABLE 27.4 Medications commonly used for palliative sedation therapy

	DOSE	TITRATION	SYMPTOM CONTROL	COMMENTS
Benzodiazepines			Anxiolytic, amnestic, and anticonvulsant properties; synergistic sedativeeffect with opioids and neuroleptics	Monotherapy with benzodiazepines occasionally fails to provide adequate sedation. May cause paradoxical agitation, especially in those with impaired liver function.
Midazolam	Loading dose 0.03–0.05 mg/kg slow push IV/SC; may repeat loading dose every 5 min to achieve desired effect (to maximum of 2 mg). Continuous infusion: hourly dose 25–33% of the cumulative loading dose.	Additional bolus doses equal to the hourly infusion dose may be given up to every 5–15 min. If >3 boluses are required within an hour, the continuous infusion may be increased by 30%. Tolerance may develop.		One of the most commonly used drugs for PST. Short-acting benzodiazepine; because of rapid redistribution, administer by continuous infusion. Maintain continuous infusion because of short duration of action. Compatible with many other IV medications, including opioids. Midazolam infusions are stable for 24 hrs after preparation by pharmacy.
Lorazepam	Loading dose 2–3 mg/kg IV over 30 min (no faster than 50 mg/min). If inadequate sedation after 30 min, a second loading dose of 1–2 mg/kg should be administered over 30 min. At the time of initial loading dose, begin continuous infusion at 1–2 mg/kg/hr			Peak effect 30 min after IV administration. Because of slower pharmacokinetics, less amenable to titration than midazolam
Other anesthetics Pentobarbital	Loading dose 2–3 mg/kg IV over 30 min (no faster than 50 mg/min). If inadequate sedation after 30 min, a second loading dose of 1–2 mg/kg should be administered over 30 min. At the time of initial loading dose, begin continuous infusion at 1–2 mg/kg/hr	For escalating symptoms, a bolus dose of 1 mg/kg IV over 30 min may be given. Tolerance may develop quickly, prompting increases in infusion rate. Titrate continuous infusion every 30–60 min.	Anticonvulsant, antipruritic, antiemetic properties; no analgesic properties	Pentobarbital infusions are stable for 7 days after preparation by pharmacy.
Dexmedetomidine	Initial loading infusion of 1 mcg/kg IV over 10 min; continuous infusion of 0.1–1 mcg/kg/hr). Dosing guidelines are undetermined in pediatrics and warrant further investigation	Titrate infusion up to 1 mcg/kg/hr every 10 min to reach desired effect. Maximum dosing in pediatrics requires further investigation	Analgesic, sympatholytic, and anxiolytic effects	Alpha-2 agonist; May cause sedation without respiratory depression; may cause bradycardia and hypotension; has a rapid distribution phase with a distribution half-life (t1/2) of approximately 6 minutes. Consider close monitoring of heart rate and blood pressure during initiation and with increases in dose. However, gradual changes in blood pressure and heart rate unrelated to dose changes should not be attributed to dexmedetomidine and are more likely to be a reflection of the dying process.

TABLE 27.4 Continued

	DOSE	TITRATION	SYMPTOM CONTROL	COMMENTS
Propofol	Start at 1 mg/kg/hr/ IV	Titrate dose in steps of 0.5 mg/kg/hr every 30 min. For acute management of severe symptoms, may give bolus dose every 10 min. With prolonged use tolerance may develop–dose range usually 1–4 mg/kg/hr Most respond to 1–2 mg/kg/hr. Avoid exceeding 3 mg/kg/hr long-term.	Anxiolytic, antiemetic, antipruritic, anticonvulsant, antimyoclonic bronchodilation. No analgesic effects	Widely used for general anesthesia and sedation of ICU patients. *Cannot* be given SC. May be used for PST if midazolam fails. Incompatible with other IV meds commonly given at end of life, therefore requiring a dedicated line. Onset of action 30 sec, allowing for rapid titration Change tubing every 12 hrs and discard vial and any unused drug if not infused after 12 hrs. Duration of action 5–10 min, do not interrupt infusion for >60 sec when changing tubing. Useful for renal or hepatic insufficiency; metabolites not thought to have biologic activity. Mechanism of action includes inhibition of GABA uptake Negative inotrope; high doses may cause hypotension, bradycardia, respiratory depression May cause pain on infusion into small peripheral veins Risk of infection due to high lipid content; change tubing every 12 hrs and discard any unused drug not infused after 12 hrs Synergistic with midazolam in causing sedation

Reproduced with permission from Naipaul AD, Ullrich C. Palliative sedation. In Wolfe J, Hinds P, Sourkes B, eds. *Textbook of Interdisciplinary Pediatric Palliative Care.* Philadelphia: Elsevier Saunders; 2011:204–214.[104]

sedation may guide subsequent sedative dosing, as outlined in Box 27.7. Once sedation has been achieved, the level of sedation and comfort should be regularly evaluated and documented.

CARE AT THE TIME OF DEATH

Several activities will need to be carried out at the time of death, ideally happening as sensitively and smoothly as possible. If a child is at home with hospice, the hospice agency should be contacted if staff are not present. If hospice is not involved in the case of an expected death, the plans made earlier (described earlier) should be enacted, and a hospital-based provider, if not able to pronounce the patient themselves, may help a family navigate the phone calls to emergency services/paramedics and the funeral home, which can assist with completion of the death certificate (according to local regulations). When a child dies in the hospital, typically a member of the house staff is called for the pronouncement.

THE PRONOUNCEMENT

There is no one standard for declaring that a patient has died. Having a nurse, social worker, or chaplain accompany the clinician who is doing the pronouncement can be helpful for introductions and to provide support to the clinician and family. The clinician should introduce themselves, including their role, to each person present and explain his or her purpose at this time. Empathetic statements, such as "I am sorry for your loss," can ease the distress, as can telling the family that they are welcome to stay while their loved one is examined. Additional testing such as electrocardiograms or electroencephalograms are not required for pronouncing that a child has died, and carrying out these tests could interfere with the family's very emotional and private time with their

BOX 27.6 GUIDELINES FOR ADMINISTRATION OF PALLIATIVE SEDATION THERAPY

- Prior to initiation:
  - The pharmacy should be notified well in advance of the anticipated need for ongoing supply of medication, to assure adequate supply.
  - Drug solutions should be inspected visually for evidence of precipitation prior to administration. If precipitation is present, the solution should not be used.
- Initiation:
  - The patient's nurse and prescribing physician should remain with the patient during the initiation and initial titration of sedative to achieve relief from suffering.
  - The physician should administer the loading dose.
  - An initial bolus (loading) dose should be accompanied by the start of a continuous infusion. Continuous infusions must be administered via an infusion pump and should be interrupted or discontinued only upon a physician's order.
- Titration:
  - Additional boluses may be delivered to capture uncontrolled symptoms. A nurse or physician should remain at the bedside to observe the effect, about 5 minutes for propofol, 10 minutes for midazolam, and 15 minutes for pentobarbital.
  - The infusion rate may also be increased until sedation and comfort are achieved, or until the patient exhibits evidence of distress or other undesired effects of the medications. Lowered blood pressure and gradual changes in respiratory rate or oxygen saturation are expected in a dying patient and should not, by themselves, lead to reduction of the infusion rate. However, abrupt onset of apnea or snoring may indicate oversedation, and should prompt consideration of decreasing sedative infusion rate.
  - Once the desired level of symptom control is achieved, the infusion should be maintained at the lowest rate that supports this desired level of symptom control. Further dose adjustments require documentation of the adjustment and the level of comfort before and after the adjustment.

Adapted with permission from Naipaul AD, Ullrich C. Palliative sedation. In Wolfe J, Hinds P, Sourkes B, eds. *Textbook of Interdisciplinary Pediatric Palliative Care*. Elsevier Saunders; 2011: 204–214.

child. (Special considerations in the event of death by neurologic criteria were described earlier.) Consider the following steps to pronounce the death[89]:

1. Identify the patient by the hospital ID tag (if in the hospital).
2. Note the general appearance of the body; ensure that the patient is not overtly hypothermic at the time of this assessment.
3. Ascertain that the patient does not rouse to verbal or tactile stimuli. Avoid overtly painful stimuli such as deep sternal pressure.

BOX 27.7 MONITORING RECOMMENDATIONS

Patient monitoring recommendations during the initiation and titration of palliative sedation therapy in the hospital or home environment are noted here.

Degree of comfort, level of consciousness (using scale below), and potential adverse effects of sedation (e.g., agitation) should be evaluated regularly:

- Every 15 minutes × 1 hour
- Then, every 30 minutes × 1 hour
- Then every 2 hours × 6 hours
- Then may increase interval to every 4 hours

Note: Cardiac monitors, oxygen monitors, and other monitors are generally not used or discontinued, except in the case of respite sedation.

A scale such as the modified Ramsay Scale[a] should be used to consistently rate degree of sedation:

1. Patient is anxious and agitated or restless, or both
2. Patient is cooperative, oriented, and tranquil
3. Patient responds to commands only
4. Patient exhibits brisk response to light glabellar tap or equivalent, or auditory stimulus
5. Patient exhibits a sluggish response to light glabellar tap or equivalent, or auditory stimulus
6. Patient exhibits no response

[a]Reproduced with permission from Ramsay MA, Savege TM, Simpson BR, Goodwin R: Controlled sedation with alphaxalone-alphadolone. *Br Med J*. 1974;2:656–659.

Reproduced with permission from Naipaul AD, Ullrich C. Palliative sedation. In Wolfe J, Hinds P, Sourkes B, eds. *Textbook of Interdisciplinary Pediatric Palliative Care*. Philadelphia: Elsevier Saunders; 2011:204–214.

4. Listen for the absence of heart sounds; feel for the absence of carotid pulse.
5. Look and listen for the absence of spontaneous respirations. Note that there is no standard amount of time for steps 4 and 5; at some hospitals it is recommended to observe for at least 60 seconds.
6. Record the position of the pupils and the absence of pupillary light reflex.
7. Record the time at which assessment is completed.
8. Once completed, it is considerate to again make an empathetic statement acknowledging the family's loss.

DOCUMENTATION IN THE MEDICAL RECORD

A simple statement in the medical record is all that is required, "Called to pronounce (name); there were absent heart sounds and respirations (and other pertinent physical examination findings if present). Time and date of death was (include)." The following additional items should also be noted[89]:

- If the attending physician and family, if not present, were notified

- If the organ bank was notified, which is required in the United States
- If the coroner or medical examiner was notified, which is required in some states for a child death regardless of cause

DEATH CERTIFICATE COMPLETION

There is tremendous variability in diagnoses used for completion of the death certificate; however, experience suggests that what is written can hold great importance for family members and is important for accurate epidemiologic recordkeeping. In the United States, guidance is available from various sources, including the Centers for Disease Control and Prevention and the National Association of Medical Examiners and includes the following[90,91]:

1. Make every effort to report a specific underlying etiology that is the cause of death. A modifier like "probable" can be used if there is diagnostic uncertainty.
2. Use a Sequential Part I Format, if possible, meaning:
   a. The first diagnosis listed is the most immediate cause of death
   b. The condition after that is the cause of the condition above
   c. This can be continued to the most specific diagnosis
3. Fill out Part II with other significant conditions that may have contributed to the patient's death but did not directly lead to the cause of death
4. Example:

   Part I.

   1. Acute exacerbation of chronic lung disease
   2. Neuromuscular scoliosis
   3. Spastic quadriparesis
   4. Hypoxic ischemic encephalopathy

   Part II.

   Seizure disorder
5. Err on the side of reporting too much rather than too little.
6. Do not report mechanistic terminal events such as:
   - Cardiac arrest
   - Asystole
   - Cardiopulmonary arrest
   - Respiratory arrest
   - Electromechanical dissociation
   - Ventricular fibrillation
7. Do not report symptoms or signs.
8. Do not report a condition if its existence in the patient is obviously based on another reported condition (e.g., hyperglycemia and diabetes).
9. Do not use abbreviations.

AFTER-DEATH CARE

ACUTE BEREAVEMENT SUPPORT TO THE FAMILY

Even alongside the most exquisite planning, preparation, and guidance surrounding the death of a child, supporting families through this moment and the initial experience of grief must be met with a spirit of family-centered compassion.[92] Suggestions for helpful phrases and actions after a child dies, and those that should be avoided, are provided in Table 27.5.

In the hospital and at home if available, clinicians should ensure appropriate supportive staff such as social work, spiritual care, and child life are available to families, if such services have been previously beneficial. Families may find comfort in having trusted clinicians to bear witness in this moment. They may seek a hand to hold or a shoulder to quite literally cry on. With respect to one's own professional assessment and personal comfort, such human gestures of care may be sincerely appreciated by some families. When a family has decided that it is time to leave the hospital, the accompaniment of supportive staff provides assurance of continued care and availability.

Some families may have religious or personal practices that require a child who has died in the hospital to be directly transferred to a mortuary or funeral home, thus bypassing the hospital's morgue. Such requests require prior communication and planning in partnership with the family's chosen funeral home, the hospital's morgue staff, and the primary medical team. Such special circumstances are a reminder that early assessment of any unique supportive needs to be respected at end of life can be beneficial in ensuring comfort to a family when appropriate.

TABLE 27.5 Helpful and unhelpful things to say and do when caring for a family whose child has died

	HELPFUL	NOT HELPFUL
Words	• "I'm sorry" • "This is so hard" • "What are you remembering about your child today?" • Say the child's name • Talk about your memories of the child	• "I know how you feel" • "She's/he's happy now" • "It was probably for the best" • "It is God's will" • "You are strong enough to deal with this"
Actions	• Be present • Be silent • Get support from others • Take care of yourself	• Avoiding the family • Comparing with other losses • Pressuring positivity • Locating their "stage of grief"

In the hours and days after a child's death, newly bereaved families may have logistical questions that they may or may not have desired to discuss prior to their loved one's death. They may seek guidance regarding funeral arrangements, working with mortuaries, or protocol surrounding a hospital's morgue should the death occur in the hospital. Ongoing communication between the family and the PPC team or other hospital-based providers in the days following a child's death can provide a sense of orientation and a modicum of solace to families during this acute initial period of grief.

PREPARING THE BODY

The most important message to relay to parents is that nothing needs to be done in a hurry when their child dies. This is very much a private time for family to say their individual goodbyes. Saying goodbyes and performing rituals are important because they enable parents, siblings, and other family members to express their love, sorrow, relief, and regrets, and share precious memories. Washing the child for the last time, dressing the child in special clothes, taking photos, playing favorite music, praying together, touching and cuddling the child, talking to the child, taking foot- and handprints, cutting a lock of hair, and writing a message or poem for the child are all examples of rituals that families have found helpful. Some families may be guided by religious practices after death,[14] which can vary considerably, some of which are summarized in Table 27.2. This refers to the religion table 27.2

When death occurs in the hospital, preparation of the body will vary depending on religious and cultural preference, hospital policy, and whether the body will be examined by the medical examiner and/or an autopsy will be performed.[14] When the body is formally examined in these situations, all indwelling lines and tubes must remain intact. Appropriate pads should be placed over puncture or wound sites and under the perineum to contain body fluids if necessary. The autopsy consent form may be modified if parents object to any aspects of this practice.

If formal postmortem exam is not anticipated, the body should be bathed, and attempts made to restore as normal an appearance as possible. Families may request special handling or positioning, and they should be offered to participate in the bathing and dressing of their child along with nursing staff. The body should be dressed in a hospital gown or clothing designated by family. Chaplain assistance may be helpful and requested if indicated.

Hospital policy will dictate how long a family may stay in a hospital room with their child's body. If there is an amount of time specified in the policy, consideration should be made as to how this time frame is communicated with the family. For some parents being told they can be there for 4 hours (for example) can lead to a sense the family is obligated to stay longer than perhaps they felt necessary. Likewise stating a time frame can feel to families as if we are pressuring them to leave.

Once the family has left the hospital, nurses typically perform any additional postmortem care by two staff members who can support one another. Taking the body to the morgue should be done as a team, using discrete means of transport.

PHYSICAL CHANGES AFTER DEATH

If the family plans to be with the child's body for a prolonged period, it may be helpful to gently prepare them for how the body will change over time. "Cuddle cots" have been used for infant deaths; these keep the body cool, slowing deterioration and allowing loved ones to spend longer periods of time with the child.[93]

LIVOR MORTIS

One of the early changes that can be observed is *livor mortis*, also referred to as *lividity*, *postmortem hypostasis*, *vibices*, and *suggilations*.[94] This is a physical process. While the individual is alive, the heart circulates the blood. When death occurs, circulation stops and the blood begins to settle, by gravity, to the lowest portions of the body. This results in a discoloration of those lower, dependent parts of the body. Although beginning immediately, the first signs of livor mortis are typically seen about 1 hour following death, with full development being observed 2–4 hours following death.[94]

RIGOR MORTIS

Rigor mortis is a chemical change resulting in a stiffening of the body's muscles following death, resulting from changes in the myofribrils of the muscle tissues. Immediately following death, the body becomes limp and is easily flexed.[94] As adenosine triphosphate (ATP) is converted to adenosine diphosphate (ADP) and lactic acid is produced lowering the cellular pH, locking chemical bridges are formed between actin and myosin resulting in formation of rigor. Typically, the onset of rigor is first observed 2–6 hours following death and develops over the first 12 hours. The onset begins with the muscles of the face and then spreads to all the muscles during the next 4–6 hours. Rigor typically lasts from 24 to 36 hours, after which the muscles begin once again to relax.

HOSPITAL STAFF SUPPORT

PPC clinicians may play an important role in the support of staff after a patient's death. Whether after an acute change in status or following a prolonged illness, staff members may need additional support following a child's death. Such support can occur both in acute follow-up and in more formalized debriefing, wherein the processing of the end of a patient's life may be discussed and reviewed in a supportive setting. Some settings may additionally elect to build community rituals, memorials, or gatherings to acknowledge the process of caring for children who have died. These types of activities have the potential to support community, deepen sustainability, and promote resilience for clinical staff.[95]

DEBRIEFING STAFF

No matter how common or rare it is for staff to care for a child through death, it is always helpful to create a safe and nonjudgmental forum for staff to reflect on the experience.[96] Such forums can be gathered formally by a unit or informally by support staff in response to an unexpected death. Encouragement of interdisciplinary engagement and participation from senior staff can be beneficial toward ensuring participation and supporting strengthened communities.

Helpful guideposts in structuring such debriefs may include[96]

1. Reflecting upon the care delivered to the child and family regarding what went well and what could be improved upon
2. Discussing the initial bereavement experience of the family to ensure that their support needs are being met
3. Taking time to remember and celebrate the life of the child

COMMEMORATION OF THE CHILD BY STAFF

Regardless of how long a child has been cared for by staff, following a child's death clinicians may appreciate the opportunity to commemorate the child.[97,98] In a study of more than 200 pediatric critical care specialists,[99] 79% contacted families following the child's death at least sometimes, 72% attended funerals, and only 2.5% thought that it was inappropriate for clinicians to attend funerals. A total of 76% agreed that follow-up contact helps the family, whereas 47% agreed that follow-up contact helps the physicians.

The condolence letter or card is one of the simplest gestures that can be made by a clinician and is typically highly valued by family members. Personal experience suggests that these notes are kept indefinitely and become a part of the child's legacy. A helpful condolence letter may contain both a personal reflection regarding the deceased and can contain guidance surrounding ongoing bereavement support. One of the greatest hurdles to writing these letters is simply finding the right words.[100,101] One can begin the letter with a direct expression of sorrow about the death, such as "I am writing to send you my condolences on the death of your son/daughter." Typical themes to include in the letter are

- A personal memory of the patient and family
- Specific references to qualities of the child, such as courage, humor, and kindness, can bring life to the letter
- An acknowledgment of all the family did for the child
- A statement that it was a privilege to have participated in the child's care
- Let the family know that it is fine to contact caregivers with questions or concerns
- Conclude with a statement that the child will be remembered, which can also be very comforting

Even the simplest and most succinct message from clinicians in a store-bought sympathy card can mean a great deal to families. If an in-depth card feels daunting, uncomplicated language such as "you are in my thoughts" or "I will always remember your child" communicates the sentiment of warmth and care.

Clinician's acts of kindness and commemoration following a child's death should not be taken lightly. In a qualitative study[102] of bereaved parents whose child was in the care of the ICU, three critical themes were identified:

1. Parents place great importance on the hospital's memorial service and on staff presence at such a service.
2. Parents often find it difficult to return to the hospital after the child's death, but attending the memorial service is common and helps with their bereavement.
3. Parents greatly appreciate receiving cards, clinician efforts to telephone, visit, and attend the funeral, and these little acts of kindness are recalled months, even years, later. Conversely, parents express disappointment when clinicians did not engage in these activities.

It is increasingly common for palliative care programs to offer longer term bereavement support to families, and these efforts are described in detail in Chapter 15.

CONCLUSION

Caring for a dying child is a truly intimate experience and a privilege that brings with it great sadness but also enormous gifts, especially when clinicians are prepared to participate in this process and are given the opportunity to provide unhurried, compassionate care. The following case exemplifies such an experience.

Clinical Vignette

Mary was a 16-year-old girl with an advanced brain tumor and spinal metastases. Together with her family, her goals were to continue to strive for cancer control, but at the same time enjoy as much time at home in her community, which was several hours away from the hospital. She was passionate about attending school, being with family and friends, and painting (Figure 27.3).[103] Comprehensive support was put into place at home, and Mary's many symptoms were managed proactively. Her medication regimen was extensive, including the following:

Dexamethasone 2 mg QID	Cerebral edema
Omeprazole 20 mg BID	Gastric prophylaxis
Bisacodyl 2 tabs BID	Constipation
Ondansetron 8 mg TID	Nausea
Metoclopramide 10 mg TID	Nausea
Methadone 15 mg TID	Pain

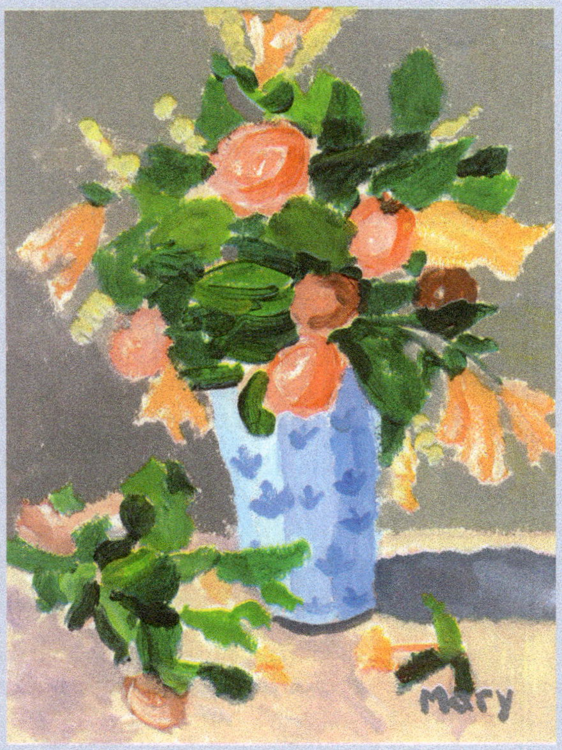

Figure 27.3 *Painting by Mary in the last year of her life.*

Oral medication	Indication
Methylphenidate 15 mg every am, 15 mg every noon	Daytime drowsiness
Celecoxib 100 mg BID	Antiangiogenic agent
Nortriptyline 20 mg qhs	Neuropathic pain
Gabapentin 300 mg TID	Neuropathic pain
Baclofen 15 mg TID	Muscle spasm
Sertraline 100 mg qhs	Depression, anxiety
Trazodone 25 mg qhs	Depression, insomnia

Unfortunately, 1 month before death, Mary was admitted to the hospital in pain crisis, and it took 3 days before her distress could be eased. The team was concerned that the only way to achieve comfort would be through palliative sedation, and Mary's family was prepared for this possibility. But, in true Mary fashion, despite substantial escalation of symptom-relieving medications, she woke up and was comfortable. The next phase of conversation related to whether it would be possible to transition Mary back home. Unfortunately, her home hospice team believed that they could not manage her complex regimen. Instead, she resided in the hospital's homelike suite, "The Comfort Care Room," for the final weeks of life. Fortunately, her community came to her. Mary continued to be involved in decision-making. One such decision was related to her continuing to take food by mouth. Despite many hours of being asleep a day, Mary would regularly wake up in the morning and asked to be wheeled down to the cafeteria for a breakfast of bacon, eggs, and potatoes. However, her ability to swallow effectively was diminishing, and she was at high risk for aspiration. Nonetheless, she chose to continue her passion for eating breakfast. Comfort was achieved through a modified medication regimen.

Intravenous medication	Indication
Dexamethasone 4 mg QID	Cerebral edema
Ondansetron 8 mg TID	Nausea
Methadone 10 mg QID	Pain
Fentanyl 225 mcg/h PCA with 180 mcg bolus q6min	Pain
Ativan 1.75 mg IV q4h, 1 mg IV q1h prn	Anxiety
Haldol 1 mg IV q6h	Anxiety, agitation, hallucinations
Scopolamine patch	Excess secretions

Three days before death, Mary experienced an aspiration event and progressive respiratory distress. Opioids were further titrated to comfort. She died surrounded by family, friends, and the care team. As stated by Mary's mother, "To me, the comfort corner room was beyond words in our last days with Mary. To have the safety of the hospital (doctors, nurses, all caregivers, Father Nee) and for all of us to be with her until the end was the ultimate blessing."

Consistent with her passion for education and generous spirit, Mary's family agreed to an autopsy. In her usual manner, the neuropathologist, Dr. Hannah Kinney, extensively reviewed Mary's record and spoke with many clinicians in advance of performing the autopsy. Her discoveries inspired the following poem.

In Honor of Mary by Hannah Kinney

What does courage look like
Under the microscope?
I want to know,
Me, the disease detective
Who entrusts in the power
Of the microscope
To reveal the truth.
Here is tumor
Deep in the eye's pathways
That transmit the faces we love;
Here is tumor
Deep in the hypothalamus
That generates the daily rhythms
Of vitality;
And here is tumor
Destroying the spinal cord
Beyond recognition,
No chance ever to stand again.
But looking down the microscope
I see the young woman
Who refused to sit in a wheelchair
At the special class picture
As she was losing strength in both legs

Forever.
I see the young woman
Who painted pink-tipped flowers
On brilliant blue water
With a background
Of life's greenery
Just before dying.
The pathologist's job
Is to integrate
Microscopic findings
With clinical history:
Looking down the microscope,
I correlate the devastation
Of the spinal cord
With the joyful spirit
Of the doomed woman
To stand anyway,
And I see courage.

May 1, 2003

ACKNOWLEDGMENT

D.L. and R.R. gratefully acknowledge Joanne Wolfe, Amitra D. Naipual, and Christina Ullrich, authors of the original sections of the first edition of this textbook from which this chapter is adapted.[103,104]

REFERENCES

1. McGinley JM, Waldrop DP. Navigating the transition from advanced illness to bereavement: How provider communication informs family-related roles and needs. *J Soc Work End Life Palliat Care.* 2020:1-24.
2. Pease K, McMillin SE. Practice concepts and innovations for pediatric end-of-life care by the interdisciplinary care team. *J Soc Work End Life Palliat Care.* 2018;14(2-3):143–152.
3. Emanuel L, Ferris F, von Gunten C, Hauser J, Von Roenn J. The last hours of living: Practical advice for clinicians. 2010. https://www.medscape.com/viewarticle/716463
4. Bicanovsky L. Comfort care: Symptom control in the dying. *In* Walsh D, Caraceni AT, Fainsinger R, et al., eds. Palliative Medicine. Saunders; 2009:997–1000.
5. Ferrell BR, Twaddle ML, Melnick A, Meier DE. National consensus project clinical practice guidelines for quality palliative care guidelines. *J Palliat Med.* 2018;21(12):1684–1689.
6. Cherin DA, Enguidanos SM, Jamison P. Physicians as medical center "extenders" in end-of-life care: Physician home visits as the lynch pin in creating an end-of-life care system. *Home Health Care Serv Q.* 2004;23(2):41–53.
7. Duda LJ. Integrating music therapy into pediatric palliative care. *Prog Palliat Care.* 2013;21(2):65–77.
8. Rusch R, Greenman J, Scanlon C, Horne K, Jonas DF. Bibliotherapy and bereavement: Harnessing the power of reading to enhance family coping in pediatric palliative care. *J Soc Work End Life Palliat Care.* 2020:1–14.
9. Arruda-Colli MNF, Weaver MS, Wiener L. Communication about dying, death, and bereavement: A systematic review of children's literature. *J Palliat Med.* 2017;20(5):548–559.
10. Butler AE, Hall H, Copnell B. Becoming a team: The nature of the parent-healthcare provider relationship when a child is dying in the pediatric intensive care unit. *J Pediatr Nurs.* 2018;40:e26–e32.
11. Browning ED, Cruz JS. Reflective debriefing: A social work intervention addressing moral distress among ICU nurses. *J Soc Work End-of-Life Palliat Care.* 2018;14(1):44–72.
12. Fitchett G, Lyndes KA, Cadge W, Berlinger N, Flanagan E, Misasi J. The role of professional chaplains on pediatric palliative care teams: Perspectives from physicians and chaplains. *J Palliat Med.* 2011;14(6):704–707.
13. Lo B, Ruston D, Kates LW, et al. Discussing religious and spiritual issues at the end of life: A practical guide for physicians. *JAMA.* 2002;287(6):749–754.
14. Wiener L, McConnell DG, Latella L, Ludi E. Cultural and religious considerations in pediatric palliative care. *Palliat Support Care.* 2013;11(1):47.
15. Cooper RS, Ferguson A, Bodurtha JN, Smith TJ. AMEN in challenging conversations: Bridging the gaps between faith, hope, and medicine. *J Oncol Pract.* 2014;10(4):e191–e195.
16. Orr RD. Responding to patient beliefs in miracles: Spirituality/medicine interface project. *South Med J.* 2007;100(12):1263–1267.
17. Foster TL, Dietrich MS, Friedman DL, Gordon JE, Gilmer MJ. National survey of children's hospitals on legacy-making activities. *J Palliat Med.* 2012;15(5):573–578.
18. Johnson LM, Snaman JM, Cupit MC, Baker JN. End-of-life care for hospitalized children. *Pediatr Clin North Am.* 2014;61(4): 835–854.
19. Schreck B, Economos A. Perinatal music therapy: Using Doppler recordings to connect and create. *Music Med.* 2018;10(1):22–25.
20. Sourkes BM. *Armfuls of Time: The Psychological Experience of the Child with a Life-Threatening Illness.* University of Pittsburgh Press; 1995.
21. Drake R, Frost J, Collins JJ. The symptoms of dying children. *J Pain Symptom Manage.* 2003;26(1):594–603.
22. Greenfield K, Holley S, Schoth DE, et al. A mixed-methods systematic review and meta-analysis of barriers and facilitators to paediatric symptom management at end of life. *Palliat Med.* 2020:0269216320907065.
23. Twomey S, Dowling M. Management of death rattle at end of life. *Br J Nurs.* 2013;22(2):81–85.
24. Lokker ME, van Zuylen L, van der Rijt CCD, van der Heide A. Prevalence, impact, and treatment of death rattle: A systematic review. *J Pain Symptom Manage.* 2014;47(1):105–122.
25. Kaye EC, Kiefer A, Blazin L, Spraker-Perlman H, Clark L, Baker JN. Bereaved parents, hope, and realism. *Pediatrics.* 2020;145(5).
26. van der Geest IMM, van den Heuvel-Eibrink MM, Falkenburg N, et al. Parents' faith and hope during the pediatric palliative phase and the association with long-term parental adjustment. *J Palliat Med.* 2015;18(5):402–407.
27. October TW, Dizon ZB, Arnold RM, Rosenberg AR. Characteristics of physician empathetic statements during pediatric intensive care conferences with family members: A qualitative study. *JAMA Network Open.* 2018;1(3):e180351–e180351.
28. Naim MY, Burke RV, McNally BF, et al. Association of bystander cardiopulmonary resuscitation with overall and neurologically favorable survival after pediatric out-of-hospital cardiac arrest in the United States: A report from the Cardiac Arrest Registry to Enhance Survival Surveillance Registry. *JAMA Pediatr.* 2017;171(2):133–141.
29. Knudson JD, Neish SR, Cabrera AG, et al. Prevalence and outcomes of pediatric in-hospital cardiopulmonary resuscitation in the United States: An analysis of the Kids' Inpatient Database. *Crit Care Med.* 2012;40(11):2940–2944.
30. Chan PS, Jain R, Nallmothu BK, Berg RA, Sasson C. Rapid response teams: A systematic review and meta-analysis. *Arch Intern Med.* 2010;170(1):18–26.
31. Tinsley C, Hill JB, Shah J, et al. Experience of families during cardiopulmonary resuscitation in a pediatric intensive care unit. *Pediatrics.* 2008;122(4):e799–e804.

32. Shaw K, Ritchie D, Adams G. Does witnessing resuscitation help parents come to terms with the death of their child? A review of the literature. *Intensive Crit Care Nurs.* 2011;27(5):253–262.
33. Pasek TA, Licata J. Parent advocacy group for events of resuscitation. *Crit Care Nurse.* 2016;36(3):58–64.
34. Nishisaki A, Diekema DS. Mind the gap and narrowing it: Family presence during pediatric resuscitation and invasive procedures. *Resuscitation.* 2011;82(6):655–656.
35. Jonas DF, Bogetz JF. Identifying the deliberate prevention and intervention strategies of pediatric palliative care teams supporting providers during times of staff distress. *J Palliat Med.* 2016;19(6):679–683.
36. Dussel V, Joffe S, Hilden JM, Watterson-Schaeffer J, Weeks JC, Wolfe J. Considerations about hastening death among parents of children who die of cancer. *Arch Pediatr Adolesc Med.* 2010;164(3):231–237.
37. Procon.org. Euthanasia & physician-assisted suicide (PAS) around the world. 2020. https://euthanasia.procon.org/euthanasia-physician-assisted-suicide-pas-around-the-world/
38. End of Life Law and Policy in Canada: Euthanasia. http://eol.law.dal.ca/?page_id=238. Accessed June 27, 2021.
39. Diekema DS, Botkin JR. Forgoing medically provided nutrition and hydration in children. *Pediatrics.* 2009;124(2):813.
40. Rapoport A, Shaheed J, Newman C, Rugg M, Steele R. Parental perceptions of forgoing artificial nutrition and hydration during end-of-life care. *Pediatrics.* 2013;131(5):861–869.
41. Dupont-Thibodeau A, Langevin R, Janvier A. Later rather than sooner: The impact of clinical management on timing and modes of death in the last decade. *Acta Paediatrica.* 2014;103(11):1148–1152.
42. Burns JP, Sellers DE, Meyer EC, Lewis-Newby M, Truog RD. Epidemiology of death in the pediatric intensive care unit at five US teaching hospitals. *Crit Care Med.* 2014;42(9):2101.
43. Trowbridge A, Walter JK, McConathey E, Morrison W, Feudtner C. Modes of death within a children's hospital. *Pediatrics.* 2018;142(4).
44. Weise KL, Okun AL, Carter BS, Christian CW. Guidance on forgoing life-sustaining medical treatment. *Pediatrics.* 2017;140(3):e20171905.
45. Truog RD, Campbell ML, Curtis JR, et al. Recommendations for end-of-life care in the intensive care unit: A consensus statement by the American College of Critical Care Medicine. *Crit Care Med.* 2008;36(3):953–963.
46. Robert R, Le Gouge A, Kentish-Barnes N, et al. Terminal weaning or immediate extubation for withdrawing mechanical ventilation in critically ill patients (the ARREVE observational study). *Intensive Care Med.* 2017;43(12):1793.
47. Downar J, Delaney JW, Hawryluck L, Kenny L. Guidelines for the withdrawal of life-sustaining measures. *Intensive Care Med.* 2016;42(6):1003–1017.
48. Truog RD, Berde CB, Mitchell C, Grier HE. Barbiturates in the care of the terminally ill. *N Engl J Med.* 1992;327(23):1678–1682.
49. American Academy of Pediatrice. Guidelines for the determination of brain death in children. *Pediatrics.* 1987;80(2):298–300.
50. Kirschen MP, Francoeur C, Murphy M, et al. Epidemiology of brain death in pediatric intensive care units in the United States. *JAMA Pediatrics.* 2019;173(5):469–476.
51. Nakagawa TA, Ashwal S, Mathur M, Mysore M, Society of Critical Care M. Guidelines for the determination of brain death in infants and children: An update of the 1987 Task Force recommendations. *Am Acad Pediatr.* 2011.
52. Russell JA, Epstein LG, Greer DM, Kirschen M, Rubin MA, Lewis A. Brain death, the determination of brain death, and member guidance for brain death accommodation requests: AAN position statement. *Neurology.* 2019;92(5):228–232.
53. Truog RD, Paquette ET, Tasker RC. Understanding brain death. *JAMA.* 2020.
54. Eichner JM, Chitkara MB, Lye PS, et al. Policy statement-pediatric organ donation and transplantation. *Pediatrics.* 2010;125(4):822–828.
55. Nakagawa TA, Shemie SD, Dryden-Palmer K, Parshuram CS, Brierley J. Organ donation following neurologic and circulatory determination of death. *Pediatr Crit Care Med.* 2018;19(8S):S26–S32.
56. Kirk TW, Mahon MM, Palliative Sedation Task Force of the NHPCO Ethics Committee. National Hospice and Palliative Care Organization (NHPCO) position statement and commentary on the use of palliative sedation in imminently dying terminally ill patients. *J Pain Symptom Manage.* 2010;39(5):914–923.
57. Cherny NI, ESMO Guidelines Working Group. ESMO Clinical Practice Guidelines for the management of refractory symptoms at the end of life and the use of palliative sedation. *Ann Oncol.* 2014;25(3):143–152.
58. Kiman R, Wuiloud AC, Requena ML. End of life care sedation for children. *Curr Opin Support Palliat Care.* 2011;5(3):285–290.
59. Kenny NP, Frager G. Refractory symptoms and terminal sedation of children: Ethical issues and practical management. *J Palliat Care.* 1996;12(3):40–45.
60. Anghelescu DL, Hamilton H, Faughnan LG, Johnson L-M, Baker JN. Pediatric palliative sedation therapy with propofol: Recommendations based on experience in children with terminal cancer. *J Palliat Med.* 2012;15(10):1082–1090.
61. Beller EM, Van Driel ML, McGregor L, Truong S, Mitchell G. Palliative pharmacological sedation for terminally ill adults. *Cochrane Database Syst Rev.* 2015;(1):1–38.
62. Rodrigues P, Crokaert J, Gastmans C. Palliative sedation for existential suffering: A systematic review of argument-based ethics literature. *J Pain Symptom Manage.* 2018;55(6):1577–1590.
63. Schildmann E, Schildmann J. Palliative sedation therapy: A systematic literature review and critical appraisal of available guidance on indication and decision making. *J Palliat Med.* 2014;17(5):601–611.
64. Cassell EJ. Diagnosing suffering: A perspective. *Ann Intern Med.* 1999;131(7):531–534.
65. Cherny NI. ESMO Clinical Practice Guidelines for the management of refractory symptoms at the end of life and the use of palliative sedation. *Ann Oncol.* 2014;25(suppl 3):iii143–iii152.
66. Tursunov O, Cherny NI, Ganz FD. Experiences of family members of dying patients receiving palliative sedation. *Oncol Nurs Forum.* 2016;43(6):E226–E232.
67. Cherny NI, Portenoy RK. Sedation in the management of refractory symptoms: Guidelines for evaluation and treatment. *J Palliat Care.* 1994;10(2):31–38.
68. Twycross R. Reflections on palliative sedation. *Palliat Care.* 2019;12:1178224218823511.
69. Graeff AD, Dean M. Palliative sedation therapy in the last weeks of life: A literature review and recommendations for standards. *J Palliat Med.* 2007;10(1):67–85.
70. Abarshi E, Rietjens J, Robijn L, et al. International variations in clinical practice guidelines for palliative sedation: A systematic review. *BMJ Support Palliat Care.* 2017;7(3):223–229.
71. Hahn MP. Review of palliative sedation and its distinction from euthanasia and lethal injection. *J Pain Palliat Care Pharmacother.* 2012;26(1):30–39.
72. Olsen ML, Swetz KM, Mueller PS. Ethical decision making with end-of-life care: Palliative sedation and withholding or withdrawing life-sustaining treatments. *Mayo Clin Proc.* 2010;85(10):949–954.
73. Morita T, Ikenaga M, Adachi I, et al. Concerns of family members of patients receiving palliative sedation therapy. *Support Care Cancer.* 2004;12(12):885–889.
74. Maltoni M, Scarpi E, Rosati M, et al. Palliative sedation in end-of-life care and survival: A systematic review. *J Clin Oncol.* 2012;30(12):1378–1383.
75. Eun Y, Hong I-W, Bruera E, Kang JH. Qualitative study on the perceptions of terminally ill cancer patients and their family members regarding end-of-life experiences focusing on palliative sedation. *J Pain Symptom Manage.* 2017;53(6):1010–1016.
76. Rosengarten OS, Lamed Y, Zisling T, Feigin A, Jacobs JM. Palliative sedation at home. *J Palliat Care.* 2009;25(1):5–11.
77. Mercadante S, Porzio G, Valle A, Fusco F, Aielli F, Costanzo V. Palliative sedation in patients with advanced cancer followed at home: A systematic review. *J Pain Symptom Manage.* 2011;41(4):754–760.

78. Brajtman S. The impact on the family of terminal restlessness and its management. *Palliat Med.* 2003;17(5):454–460.
79. Quill TE, Lo B, Brock DW, Meisel A. Last-resort options for palliative sedation. *Ann Intern Med.* 2009;151(6):421–424.
80. Siden H, Tucker T, Derman S, et al. Pediatric enteral feeding intolerance: A new prognosticator for children with life-limiting illness? *J Palliat Care.* 2009;25(3):213–217.
81. Bodnar J. A review of agents for palliative sedation/continuous deep sedation: Pharmacology and practical applications. *J Pain Palliat Care Pharmacother.* 2017;31(1):16–37.
82. McWilliams K, Keeley PW, Waterhouse ET. Propofol for terminal sedation in palliative care: A systematic review. *J Palliat Med.* 2010;13(1):73–76.
83. Quill TE. Barbiturates in the care of the terminally ill. *N Engl J Med.* 1993;328(18):1350–1351.
84. Mele E, Mastronuzzi A, Cefalo MG, et al. Propofol-based palliative sedation in terminally ill children with solid tumors: A case series. *Medicine (Baltimore).* 2019;98(21):e15615.
85. Burns J, Jackson K, Sheehy KA, Finkel JC, Quezado ZM. The use of dexmedetomidine in pediatric palliative care: A preliminary study. *J Palliat Med.* 2017;20(7):779–783.
86. Soares LGL, Naylor C, Martins MIA, Peixoto G. Dexmedetomidine: A new option for intractable distress in the dying. *J Pain Symptom Manage.* 2002;24(1):6–8.
87. Brinkkemper T, van Norel AM, Szadek KM, Loer SA, Zuurmond WWA, Perez RSGM. The use of observational scales to monitor symptom control and depth of sedation in patients requiring palliative sedation: A systematic review. *Palliat Med.* 2013;27(1):54–67.
88. Sessler CN, Gosnell MS, Grap MJ, et al. The Richmond Agitation–Sedation Scale: Validity and reliability in adult intensive care unit patients. *Am J Respirat Crit Care Med.* 2002;166(10):1338–1344.
89. Weissman D, Heidenreich C. Fast Facts and Concepts #004. Death pronouncement in the hospital. 2015. https://www.mypcnow.org
90. US Department of Health and Human Services, Center for Disease Control and Prevention, National Center for Health Statistics. Instructions for completing the cause-of-death section of the certificate. https://www.cdc.gov/nchs/data/dvs/blue_form.pdf. Issued August 2004.
91. National Association of Medical Examiners. Writing cause of death statements-basic principles. 2005. https://name.memberclicks.net/assets/docs/76bc59b3-9464-4ca8-8b2a-1f0624b22f99.pdf
92. October T, Dryden-Palmer K, Copnell B, Meert KL. Caring for parents after the death of a child. *Pediatr Crit Care Med.* 2018;19(8S Suppl 2):S61–S68.
93. Smith P, Vasileiou K, Jordan A. Healthcare professionals' perceptions and experiences of using a cold cot following the loss of a baby: A qualitative study in maternity and neonatal units in the UK. *BMC Pregnancy Childbirth.* 2020;20(1):1–9.
94. Goff ML. Early post-mortem changes and stages of decomposition in exposed cadavers. *Exp Appl Acarol.* 2009;49(1-2):21–36.
95. Kearney MK, Weininger RB, Vachon MLS, Harrison RL, Mount BM. Self-care of physicians caring for patients at the end of life: "Being connected . . . a key to my survival." *JAMA.* 2009;301(11):1155–1164.
96. Leff V, Klement A, Galanos A. A successful debrief program for house staff. *J Soc Work End-of-Life Palliat Care.* 2017;13(2-3):87–90.
97. Lichtenthal WG, Sweeney CR, Roberts KE, et al. Bereavement follow-up after the death of a child as a standard of care in pediatric oncology. *Pediatr Blood Cancer.* 2015;62(S5):S834–S869.
98. Kim K, Churilov L, Huang A, Weinberg L. Bereavement practices employed by hospitals and medical practitioners toward attending funeral of patients: A systematic review. *Medicine (Baltimore).* 2019;98(36):e16692.
99. Borasino S, Morrison W, Silberman J, Nelson RM, Feudtner C. Physicians' contact with families after the death of pediatric patients: A survey of pediatric critical care practitioners' beliefs and self-reported practices. *Pediatrics.* 2008;122(6):e1174.
100. Bedell SE, Cadenhead K, Graboys TB. The doctor's letter of condolence. *N Engl J Med.* 2001;344(15):1162–1164.
101. Weaver MS, Lichtenthal WG, Larson K, Wiener L. How I approach expressing condolences and longitudinal remembering to a family after the death of a child. *Pediatr Blood Cancer.* 2019;66(2):e27489.
102. Macdonald ME, Liben S, Carnevale FA, et al. Parental perspectives on hospital staff members' acts of kindness and commemoration after a child's death. *Pediatrics.* 2005;116(4):884.
103. Wolfe J. Easing distress when death is near. In Wolfe J, Hinds P, Sourkes B, eds. *Textbook of Interdisciplinary Pediatric Palliative Care.* Elsevier Saunders; 2011: 368–386.
104. Naipaul AD, Ullrich C. Palliative sedation. In Wolfe J, Hinds P, Sourkes B, eds. *Textbook of Interdisciplinary Pediatric Palliative Care.* Elsevier Saunders; 2011: 204–214.

SECTION IV | ILLNESS AND TREATMENT EXPERIENCE

Enough
When they came to take you
in that dark night, their hands
gathering up what was left of you
as you lay in your mother's arms,
the blood going to your brain
without sufficient oxygen to keep you,
we said: If she can live . . .

A mother whose 11-month-old child had lived with dilated cardiomyopathy and then underwent heart transplant wrote these lines. As her poem continues, it articulates the experience of so many parents of seriously ill children: times of hope intermixed with times of despair, and a course all too unpredictable.

The first chapter in this book, on the language of interdisciplinary pediatric palliative care, distinguished between the illness experience and the underlying disease or condition. The aim of this section is to describe selected life-threatening *diseases and conditions*, how the child's experience transforms them into *illnesses*, and how pediatric palliative care emerges as the overarching framework for clinical intervention. The very nature of the interdisciplinary team is ideally suited to address these complex disorders as they are *lived* by a broad diversity of children and their families.

The chapters in this section introduce the reader to serious illnesses in childhood, from their epidemiology and disease-specific characteristics and treatments to illness-specific guidance and communication. The knowledge of—and appreciation for—the unique qualities of each clinical entity (or grouping) are an essential foundation for the pediatric palliative care team, as they contribute their language and skills to the optimal care of the child and family.

And when they carried you
to the airplane and lifted
their tiny cargo up
into the sky, we said: If they
can carry her safely.
And when they opened
your delicate rib cage to reveal
the overgrown bird struggling
inside to be free of you, we said:
If she can lose her worn heart.

And when the child, your secret brother,
gave up his heart when it entered the cave
of your body, we pledged: We will always
remember your secret brother.

But the new heart rested
like a hibernating creature, barely
fluttering within you, and you grew
cold, first your feet and then
your legs. We promised:
Whatever it takes.

And when the heart began
to awaken, to send the blood strongly
along all its channels like a great engine
dreaming of air, we said:
She must live.

When that heart
pumped oxygen hungrily
through the great vessels
of your body when you saw us with
your eyes and your hands,
when you asked your father
if it was night and he carried you
to the window, we said: Now there are
mornings and evenings.

And when the world began
to breathe again, we said all
those things you might say
when a child is born
and you are planning
the long life ahead of her.
It is never enough.

MYRA SKLAREW[1]

REFERENCE

1. Cross SN, Berlin R, Jo Blank D, et al. Illness: A collection of poems. *J Med Humanit.* (2010) 31:176–178. With kind permission of Springer Science and Business Media.

28 | PRENATAL AND NEONATAL PALLIATIVE CARE

CHRISTY CUMMINGS, ANNE SULLIVAN, LAUREN CRAMER, AND RENEE BOSS

Having the baby was a surreal experience; it was entering a world of unknowns and uncertainties. Would he be born alive? Would he live for minutes, hours, days or months?

A MOTHER

INTRODUCTION

For most, pregnancy is a time filled with joyful anticipation of welcoming a new life into the family. Technological advances provide early confirmation of pregnancy, thus allowing parents to share their news with others, often just weeks after conception. Technology also permits clinicians to detect life-threatening fetal complications and potentially even intervene via fetal surgeries or genetic therapies.[1] Each year in the United States, more than 1 million pregnancies will end in fetal death, many due to genetic abnormalities. More than 23,000 babies between 20 and 40 weeks gestation will be stillborn, and nearly 16,000 neonates will die within the first 28 days of life, with nearly half of these deaths due to congenital diseases and/or prematurity.[2] Gestational risk factors such as a family history of genetic diseases or maternal chronic illness can result in repeated losses. Concurrently, there are increasing numbers of infants born who survive with medical complexity. Factors that may impact survivorship include the advancement of medical technology, specific institutional practices of hospitals, and range of accessibility to outpatient and home-based supports to care for these medically fragile children.

Families may learn that their baby has a life-threatening diagnosis early in pregnancy, in the prenatal period just prior to delivery, or in the neonatal period after birth. As parents learn of a life-threatening fetal condition, they bear the difficult task of shifting from joyful welcoming of a healthy newborn to comprehending the ramifications of their baby's diagnosis. Palliative care in each scenario is targeted to families' unique needs after diagnosis, when families begin to grieve the loss of a "normal" pregnancy or infant.[3] Fetal-neonatal conditions which would benefit from the interventions and support of palliative care can include rare syndromes such as anencephaly and Potter's syndrome, all extremely premature infants, infants with severe birth injuries, and complex neonatal conditions when no diagnosis can be identified. We describe how interdisciplinary team (IDT) clinicians can deliver integrated, compassionate, and evidence-based services for these infants and families.

In this chapter, we discuss prenatal-neonatal palliative and end-of-life care. Often the phrase "perinatal" is used to describe care around the time of birth; we will use "prenatal" and "neonatal" to be more precise. We will highlight the unique contributions of IDT clinicians as related to four distinct periods as demonstrated in Figure 28.1.

- *Early Prenatal Period*: The life-threatening fetal diagnosis is made weeks to months before birth
- *Late Prenatal Period*: The life-threatening fetal diagnosis is made hours to days before birth
- *Early Neonatal Period*: The neonatal diagnosis and palliative care intervention occurs in the first hours to days of life
- *Late Neonatal Period*: The neonate's or infant's diagnosis and palliative care intervention occurs in the first weeks to months of life

A general overview of concepts and issues common to all periods will be presented first, followed by more specific information pertinent to each of the four periods. In this chapter, we conclude with information specific to end-of-life care and bereavement. Whenever available, data from relevant clinical research across disciplines are referenced. Because of the ethical and logistical limitations to research with pregnant women, women in labor, and parents of critically ill newborns, data are sometimes limited or absent. Where data

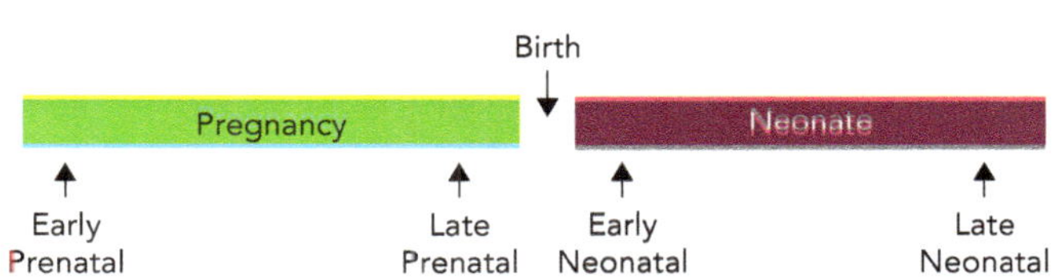

Figure 28.1 *Periods of prenatal and neonatal palliative care.*

are lacking, our recommendations are drawn from historical and current texts and from the clinical experience of interdisciplinary experts.

EPIDEMIOLOGY OF LIFE-THREATENING NEONATAL CONDITIONS

The landscape for decision-making for infants with potentially life-limiting conditions continues to evolve as advances in therapies and new outcomes data are published. For example, for infants born extremely preterm, near the limit of viability, defined broadly as birth between 20 and 25 weeks' gestation, there remains substantial infant morbidity and mortality, with wide variation among hospitals and continuously evolving outcomes.[4–6] Some centers do not offer resuscitation at less than 24 weeks' gestation while others offer active resuscitation and antenatal corticosteroids to all infants as early as 22 weeks with survival rates at 22–23 weeks gestation of 25–50% across the United States.[6,7] Decisions surrounding antenatal interventions and postnatal resuscitation for these infants should be made in conjunction with the family using a shared decision-making approach.

Similarly, for infants diagnosed with Trisomy 13 or 18, there remains high neonatal and infant mortality, and surviving children may have significant impairments. After such a diagnosis, many parents choose termination of pregnancy or to focus on the comfort of their child at birth, though many others wish for treatment to attempt to prolong the lives of their children. However, in the past decade, studies have revealed these conditions are heterogeneous, with increasing numbers of centers providing life-prolonging interventions for these children with survival reported as high as 15 and 16 years for Trisomy 13 and 18, respectively, after receiving interventions for congenital heart disease.[8,9]

Given the wide range of possible outcomes for some infants, it is important to elicit families' understanding, hopes, and worries and determine what's most important to them, as well as support them along with the rest of the IDT in delineating an approach to their child's care.[10] Parental preferences often fall into one of three categories: support the child in living as long as possible (leave no stone unturned in pursuit of possible life-sustaining interventions, may impact quality of life), support the child in living as well and as long as possible (most common—blended approach), or support the child in living as well as possible (prioritizing quality of life, even if for moments, hours, or days). A shared decision-making approach regarding options for termination/continuation of the pregnancy, interventions to prolong life, and choices about potential procedures should be practiced.[10]

INTERDISCIPLINARY TEAM CLINICIANS AND ROLES

The diagnosis and management of a life-threatening condition for an infant can potentially span the prenatal and neonatal periods and beyond and may require the involvement of unique IDT clinicians not found in other areas of pediatric palliative care (PPC) as shown in Figure 28.2. Palliative care in these scenarios may be delivered by palliative care specialists who work alongside the infant's primary team or by clinicians without subspecialty palliative care training who care for children with serious illness, referred to as primary, or generalist palliative care.[11] Not uncommonly, IDT clinicians work in different clinics, hospitals, or even cities due to the nature of regionalized neonatal care. For example, a life-threatening fetal diagnosis may be made by a community obstetrician, with subsequent management of both the pregnant woman and baby by multiple subspecialists at a large referral center. Particular effort must be made to communicate well and provide seamless care to families throughout this trajectory of care.

SUPPORTING FAMILIES' PRACTICAL NEEDS

Women with a high-risk pregnancy are often hospitalized for a prolonged period before birth. The pregnant woman's hospitalization can profoundly disrupt the life of the family, and these women often worry about this burden on their loved ones.[12] Distance from home to the regional hospital may be

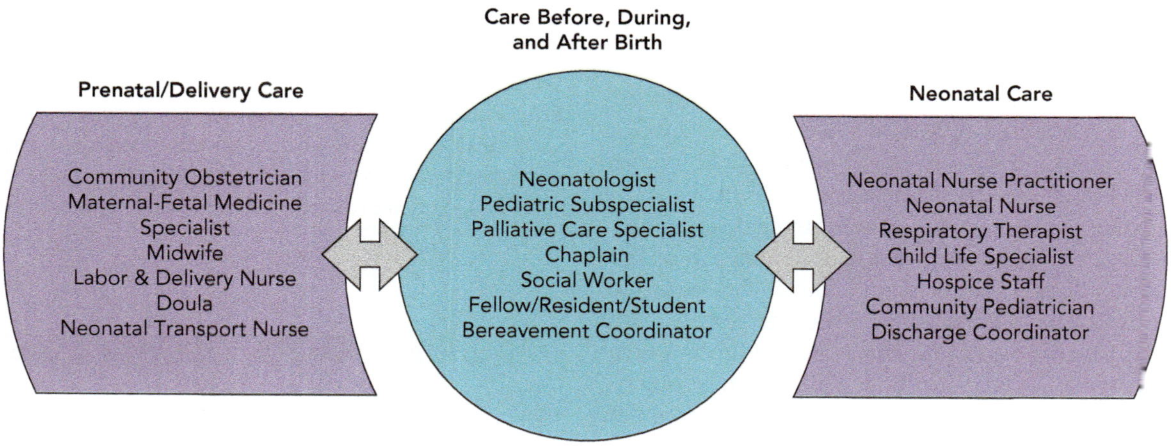

Figure 28.2 Potential interdisciplinary team members.

100 miles or more, with the associated costs of traveling including lodging, meals, and parking. Families with a limited income may be forced to restrict visits or visit in the evening after completing a full workday, which can impact communication with daytime clinicians.

Environments that are conducive to and promote family presence are essential. Privacy and lenient visitation hours are important to women hospitalized prenatally.[12] When private rooms are not available, strategies are needed to maintain confidentiality during parent–clinician discussions. Parents are very cognizant of and appreciative for those clinicians who "go out of their way" to enable family members to be present with them at their time of distress.[13–15]

Parents may need to balance multiple demands to be physically present at the hospital, care for other children, and work to provide for the family. Grandparents may not know how to support their children through something that they themselves have never experienced. Staff can help families with simple gestures like obtaining a food tray for the visiting father or informing the family about hospital specific and locally based resources to ensure that families' most basic needs are being addressed. There has been a focused effort in many neonatal intensive care unit (NICU) settings to introduce technology that complies with the Health Insurance Portability and Accountability Act (HIPAA) to keep parents informed about the status of the child when they are not able to be immediately at the bedside. This has been implemented in the form of cameras focused on the infant, videoconferencing and videophone, all with positive results and reduced anxiety and stress among parents.[16] Such technologies also allow other family members, such as elderly grandparents and young siblings who would not otherwise be able to visit the NICU, to see the infant, and this has been reported as valuable.[16]

Siblings may be aware of a baby's expected arrival before a potential life-threatening fetal diagnosis is made. Siblings have their own unique feelings of anticipation, excitement, sadness, or ambivalence. IDT clinicians may need to provide families with strategies to allow siblings to maintain closeness with their mother during her hospitalization while maintaining as normal a home and school routine as possible. Parents may need suggestions about how to include their children in the events surrounding the baby's birth, life, and possible death.[17] Child life specialists can offer creative avenues of art, play, and interactive therapies to assist these children in coping with their sibling's medical complexity and uncertainty about outcome as well as how to say good-bye to their baby brother or sister in the case of the death of that sibling.

COMMUNICATION

When families learn of a life-threatening fetal or neonatal condition, clinicians may feel an urgency to communicate essential information quickly, without careful attention to the way it is presented. Whenever possible, clinicians should anticipate the impact of information on a family already under significant stress. Priority should be placed on asking parents who else should be present for discussions regarding treatment decisions. Meeting times should not be restricted to routine morning or evening rounds and should allow for extended family presence. Family members often assist the parent to recall information given during these meetings. If a discussion must occur with the mother or father alone, a nurse or other clinician should be assigned the role of helping the parent to interpret the information. Sequential discussions are often needed. Parents should be encouraged to write down information and questions and should be provided with a means to do so.

The importance of clear, honest, and compassionate communication is central to prenatal and neonatal palliative care.[18–21] Clinicians can convey empathy through careful listening and anticipation of the family's needs. Respect is apparent when clinicians refer to the baby by his or her given name, if known. Respect extends to colleagues when conflicting opinions, which often arise in prenatal and neonatal decision-making, are approached in a professional manner. A family's confidence and trust in the healthcare team are eroded if they witness disrespectful behavior among members of the team. An example of disrespectful behavior is when clinicians are openly critical of the competency of their colleagues because of a disagreement with a medical diagnosis and/or a management decision. These conversations should never occur in the family's presence or in close proximity to family members where the conversations could be overheard. A family needs to know that clinicians work collaboratively as a team and with the family to identify a plan of care.

DECISION-MAKING

Families who receive a diagnosis of a potentially lethal fetal or neonatal condition face decisions that are unparalleled in other areas of pediatrics and range from pregnancy termination to fetal surgery, including experimental fetal therapies such as in utero gene therapy and stem cell transplantation.[1] The level of uncertainty is also unparalleled, as decisions are often necessary before birth when diagnosis and prognosis are rarely definite. This can create emotional distress and moral dilemmas for clinicians and parents alike as they consider management options.[22]

Internationally, there is significant variation in the process of decision-making for these infants. In countries with paternalistic models of medical care, physicians decide which infants will receive life-sustaining therapies, without family input.[23] In the United States, parent–clinician collaboration in shared decision-making has become increasingly important.[24] Neonatologists acknowledge that, at times, parental authority in decision-making may even surpass the authority of the medical team.[25–28] For instance, a neonatologist may not feel comfortable limiting delivery room resuscitation for an infant born at 22 weeks' gestation if the family requests that "everything be done," even when the likelihood of survival is low.

Best practices for engaging in shared decision-making before, during, and after birth are not clear. Ideally, multiple interdisciplinary discussions would occur with families over time while minimizing the stressors of maternal illness, pain, and home-life disruption. But this rarely occurs. While data about these interactions are limited, retrospective data suggest that parent–clinician collaboration in these scenarios is incomplete. For example, Zupancic et al. interviewed parents and neonatologists within 24 hours of counseling; there was only 59% agreement that a management plan had been formulated.[29]

Parents and clinicians may come to these conversations with very different priorities. Neonatologists often emphasize predictions of morbidities and mortality[30–32] based on large population aggregate data, yet families often focus on emotions, hope, and religious and spiritual beliefs, with their specific child in mind (e.g., "*n* of 1 mindset").[24,33–35] Families who have become pregnant through assisted reproduction or who have suffered repeated losses may be particularly committed to continuing a pregnancy, regardless of predictions of illness or death.[36] Families may also possess unrealistic expectations for their infant based on media portrayal of "miracle babies."

As with older children, parents have the right to act as surrogate decision-makers for their infants. But surrogate decision-making for infants is unique in several ways. The concept of "prior preferences" does not apply to newborns. Parents and clinicians may differ significantly in their perceptions of a "good" quality of life for infants; in one study, parents were more likely than clinicians to believe that attempts should be made to save all infants, regardless of projected outcomes.[37] New parents already expecting to bring home a totally dependent infant may underestimate the consequences of decisions which may extend this dependence indefinitely.

Shared decision-making requires IDT clinicians to assist families in expressing their values and goals while focusing on the infant's best interest and minimizing harm. Families should be asked about what the pregnancy or the infant means to them, and what they believe is a good quality of life. They should be encouraged to talk with important extended family members and religious leaders. They should be asked about their preferred decision-making role and reminded that the IDT is there to support them regardless of the decision.[24]

Families must be cautioned that, once a decision is made, diagnostic and prognostic uncertainty may translate into unexpected outcomes. The family who makes a carefully detailed birth plan involving out-of-state family members and religious rituals may suffer a fetal death before birth. Families who opt for nonresuscitation of an extremely premature infant to prevent infant suffering may deliver a vigorous baby weighing 200 grams more than predicted. Clinicians and families alike should prepare for the possibility that management decisions may need to be altered quickly based on new information.[4,38,39] Finally, it should be noted that not all management options are equally available to families. Hospital policies and state policies can impact clinician willingness to offer the options of pregnancy termination, noninitiation of resuscitation, and withdrawal of therapy.[40] Availability of resources in the hospital or community setting may also limit options, such as home hospice and visiting nurse or IDT clinician support.

HOPE

Redefining hope is critical during prenatal and neonatal palliative care. Families are often unprepared for the diagnosis of a potentially lethal fetal or neonatal condition. Physicians may worry that talking about hope will create unrealistic expectations, yet parents who have gone through this have emphasized that, regardless of the infant's prognosis, parents need clinicians to give them hope for something.[33,34,41] One study found that physicians who provided more hope to families were not necessarily more likely to predict survival, but they did express emotion and showed parents that they were touched by the tragedy of the situation.[33] Adult patients with a terminal diagnosis describe that clinicians can provide hope by shifting the focus to what can be realistically achieved versus what can only be wished for but never achieved.[42] For the IDT that is counseling a family, this might mean openly acknowledging the grief and pain of the situation, reassuring the family that the team will join in their hope that the infant's outcome will be a good one, and helping them to imagine how they might want events to proceed if the outcome is death or severe disability.

It is helpful to talk with families about what is meaningful to them, such as the possibility of holding a baby who is alive or without any medical equipment or technology for the first time or making sure that the infant does not experience pain. Hope for a "good outcome" may need to be redefined repeatedly over time, in a way that helps families to cherish what is possible with their infant. For parents expecting multiple babies, parental hope for each of the developing fetuses in utero may hang in a delicate balance, especially if one is diagnosed with a life-threatening condition. When the death of a multiple occurs, parents must simultaneously maintain hope for the surviving babies while experiencing grief for their loss.[43]

CULTURAL, RELIGIOUS, AND SPIRITUAL ISSUES

Families often struggle to make meaning of a child's death in the context of their cultural, religious, spiritual, or existential beliefs. This struggle may inform the decisions families make regarding their infant. Kenner and Boykova[44] provide an excellent reference for neonatal end-of-life care issues as related to variety of religious traditions. Several unique aspects of religion and prenatal/neonatal end-of-life care should be noted. In some traditions, a fetus is not recognized as a person until it is born alive. Parents from these traditions who experience a miscarriage or stillbirth may feel abandoned by their communities and may need additional resources from the IDT. In other traditions, families may struggle to reconcile pregnancy termination or withdrawal of life-supporting technology with church doctrine. Talking with their own religious leader and/or a hospital chaplain can be invaluable, both by alleviating family guilt and by helping the medical team to better understand the parents' values. While religious leaders can provide invaluable support for families, the medical team should be sure such leaders are aware of the medical possibilities to guide the family appropriately. Obstetrical and neonatal wards often limit visitors; when possible, accommodations need to be made for families' cultural or religious end-of-life rituals. One advantage of home hospice for infants is the opportunity for families to participate in religious and cultural rituals more freely.

Studies of adults who face end-of-life decisions for themselves or their family members suggest that race and ethnicity impact choices about life-sustaining therapies. While this issue has not yet been evaluated for prenatal-neonatal end-of-life care, IDT clinicians should be prepared to assess the role that race, or ethnicity may play in parents' decisions.

PROFESSIONAL CAREGIVER SUFFERING AND MORAL DISTRESS

As in other areas of PPC, being with families throughout their baby's dying can be deeply rewarding but can also lead to professional caregiver suffering. Suffering is intensified in situations involving moral distress, which often characterizes the uncertainty of prenatal and neonatal prognosis.[45] Tragic infant deaths and cumulative losses can make it difficult for a clinician to create meaning in their profession. Clinicians who themselves are childbearing or childrearing may closely identify with families, particularly when clinicians have a long-term relationship with the family. Though such sensitivity can promote empathy, it can also lead to intense feelings of anxiety and grief in the clinician, who then may benefit from personal therapeutic supports to cope and process these experiences. A dual-process model of clinician's grief has been described: clinicians may simultaneously experience grief reactions by focusing on the loss and avoid grief reactions by focusing on other aspects of a patient's care.[46]

Infant deaths often occur in environments that do not support clinicians' needs. Prenatal deaths may occur in birth centers, where care is focused on healthy births, often evidenced by names such as the "New Life Center." Clinicians in birth centers may struggle to care for bereaved families while simultaneously caring for parents who are birthing healthy infants.[47] Neonatal deaths often occur in ICUs which rarely emphasize the sacredness of the end-of-life experience. Though clinicians may join in annual rituals to honor deceased patients and process their own grief, support during acute losses may not be available.

IDT clinicians from varying disciplines have unique experiences with families at the end of life. For example, while neonatal nurses rarely feel involved in decision-making, neonatal physicians feel very responsible for end-of-life decision-making.[48] These differences may make it difficult for clinicians to fully support each other. IDT clinicians with expertise in addressing suffering, such as palliative care team members, chaplaincy, or specially trained nurses,[49] could facilitate self-care for others.

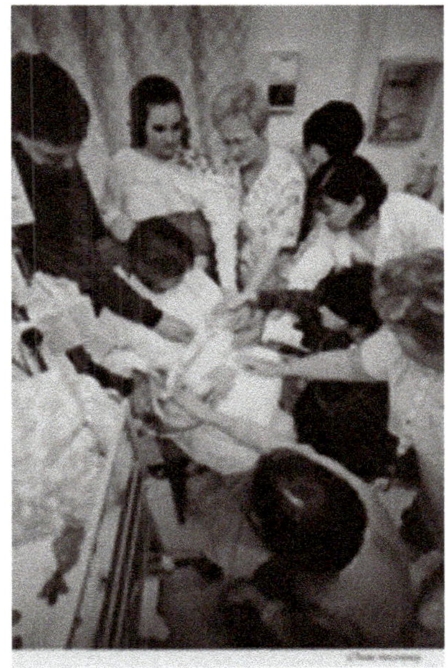

Figure 28.3 Interdisciplinary team (IDT) clinicians join parents in a ritual of thanksgiving and blessing for baby Logan before his death. Photograph provided courtesy of Todd Hochberg.

Strategies for minimizing professional caregiver suffering must also take place at the organizational level. An educational intervention in end-of-life care, which included content on prevention of compassion fatigue, has been shown to increase the comfort of neonatal nurses with the care of the dying infant.[50] Other strategies might include a core group of clinicians to serve as a resource on all shifts, case reviews of each death for all disciplines, engaging mental health liaisons for debriefing, and providing meaningful gestures to clinicians, such as meditation or massages. Co-creation of ritual may provide clinicians with unique opportunities to both support bereaved families and facilitate their own grief work, as demonstrated in Figure 28.3.[46]

THE FOUR PERIODS OF PRENATAL AND NEONATAL PALLIATIVE CARE

In this next section, we discuss considerations for patients and families in each of four periods: early prenatal period, late prenatal period, early neonatal period, and late neonatal period. Clinical Vignettes are followed by recommendations for specific interventions for each unique patient population.

EARLY PRENATAL PALLIATIVE CARE

Clinical Vignette

Early Prenatal Palliative Care

Mr. and Mrs. Chang are expecting their fourth baby, with prenatal care from a community obstetrician who speaks the family's primary language, Korean. A routine ultrasound at 18 weeks gestation reveals the baby has probable cardiac, renal, and neural tube defects. The obstetrician recommends further testing at an urban medical center 60 miles away.

Hesitantly, the Changs travel to the medical center, where further testing reveals a diagnosis of Trisomy 18 and multiple anomalies. Without an interpreter, the medical center team shares the diagnosis, offering Mrs. Chang the option to terminate her pregnancy. Upon hearing this news, Mr. and Mrs. Chang decline discussing other options for their baby's care and return home. No further communication occurs between the medical center staff, the community obstetrician, or the family.

At 37 weeks' gestation, Mrs. Chang presents at the local community hospital in active labor. As she is admitted to labor and delivery, her 12-year-old daughter translates, telling the nurse, "My mother is very scared because my father is at work right now and they think the baby may be sick."

Before a thorough history can be obtained, the baby is born. He requires immediate intubation, chest compressions, umbilical line placement, and medications. Within 30 minutes of birth, the baby is stabilized, and transport is arranged for the baby to a Level 3 NICU at a regional medical center. Mrs. Chang briefly views her son prior to signing consents for the transfer of his care. Mr. Chang arrives at the community hospital just minutes after the ambulance's departure with his son.

Upon arrival at the NICU, the neonatologist suspects a chromosomal disorder and orders genetic testing. Intensive intervention is provided to sustain the baby until a diagnosis can be confirmed. With aid of an interpreter, the baby's current condition and suspected diagnosis is shared with Mr. and Mrs. Chang over the phone. Mr. Chang tells the staff to "do everything" for their baby.

Twelve hours later, Baby Chang's condition deteriorates. He does not respond to resuscitative efforts and dies. His parents receive a phone call in Mrs. Chang's postpartum room, notifying them of their son's death.

The delivery of palliative care in the early prenatal period presents the unique challenge of planning for a patient who is not yet born. As a life-threatening condition is identified in-utero, both parents and clinicians must integrate their care goals in preparation for the uncertainty surrounding the baby's prognosis after birth. The provision of palliative care subsequently unfolds during three distinct phases: in the prenatal period, during labor and delivery, and eventually throughout the baby's living and dying.

SETTING

As illustrated in the clinical vignette, early prenatal period advanced care planning may initially begin in the obstetrician's office. Further evaluation may involve specialist consultations at a regional hospital far from the family's home. In some instances, diagnosis of a specific prenatal condition, such as twin-to-twin transfusion or monoamniotic twins, may require the parents to travel out of state for specialized prenatal care. The emergence of hospital-based fetal care programs affords each IDT clinician the opportunity to integrate palliative care throughout the trajectory of care.[51] Some families may opt for home birth, with care provided by a hospice and midwife team.

INTERDISCIPLINARY TEAM CLINICIANS

Parents who receive a life-threatening fetal diagnosis may interact with numerous IDT clinicians at multiple sites of care. In fact, each discipline represented in Figure 28.2 could potentially interact with the family throughout pregnancy, delivery, and the baby's birth and potential death. Therefore, it is of utmost importance that a key point person be identified who can facilitate continuity throughout the trajectory of care.

COMMUNICATION

In addition to the principles of communication discussed in this chapter's introduction, there are particular considerations during the early prenatal period. IDT clinicians should establish and maintain a relationship with the family as the pregnancy continues, supporting the family and facilitating bonding with the baby. Clinicians can help parents anticipate questions from acquaintances, such as work colleagues or neighbors, about the pregnancy. It may be helpful to schedule prenatal visits before or after regular office hours. Some sites may offer separate childbirth education sessions separate from classes for families expecting healthy babies.[52]

Throughout the early prenatal period, clinicians may find themselves reviewing test results and other prognostic information with parents on multiple occasions. Patience and empathetic listening skills are important. Clinicians should explore with parents how best to provide updates on the baby's status before, during, and after birth. Parents may worry about how their baby will tolerate labor. Clear expectations should be established about the management plan should fetal distress during labor occur. When the plan is for noninitiation of delivery room resuscitation, good communication between the obstetrical, neonatal, and pediatric teams can help to make this experience the least obtrusive as possible for families, so that they can cherish the time that they have with their infant. As shown in Box 28.1, an end-of-life care order set protocol can be a helpful communication tool and should specify orders for vital signs, medications, fluids and/or nutrition, and who should be called to declare death and complete postmortem documentation. Staff training and preparation is important, as obstetrical and newborn nursery staff who typically care for healthy infants may be unfamiliar with and uncomfortable with neonatal end-of-life care.

CREATION OF BIRTH PLAN AND ADVANCE DIRECTIVE

The use of a written birth plan and advance directive can facilitate communication during the early prenatal period.[21,52–55] The co-creation of a birth plan between parents and clinicians

BOX 28.1 SAMPLE END-OF-LIFE CARE ORDER SET FOR NEONATE FOLLOWING DELIVERY

1. Admiss on Diagnosis: ______________________
2. Birth Weight __________ kg
3. Do Not Resuscitate (Refer to DNR Order Form)
4. Admit to ___NICU ___Newborn Nursery for comfort care
5. Infant to stay in mother's postpartum room at all times. If respite care needed, may transfer to NICU per parents' request
6. No cardiorespiratory monitoring. Assess for breathing/heart beat prn, per patient status changes
8. Nutrition/Hydration: Per family's request (e.g., breastfeeding prn as tolerated. No formula supplementation.)
9. Provide nonpharmacological measures prn for irritability or mild pain:
   - Swaddle in warm blankets
   - Holding
   - Pacifier
   - Sucrose
10. For moderate pain and/or dyspnea control: __________ (e.g., morphine)
11. With cessation of breathing/heart rate, page __________ for death pronouncement.
12. Expiration paperwork to be initiated by ____________.

provides a unique opportunity for parents to be actively involved in their baby's care while also preparing the parents for a variety of possible outcomes. Clinicians can help prepare families by acknowledging and naming the uncertainty while still emphasizing the goals and values of the parents regardless of the outcome.

A well-crafted planning tool should effectively communicate parents' wishes for care of the mother during labor and delivery and should be partnered with advance directives outlining appropriate interventions for the baby. Box 28.2 highlights possible components of a birth plan and advance directives. It is important to note that this tool is effective only if it is shared, discussed, and readily accessible to all IDT clinicians prior to the baby's birth.

DECISION-MAKING

The process of decision-making in the early prenatal period begins at the time of diagnosis. As reflected in the clinical vignette, parents may be offered the option to terminate the pregnancy. Prior to discussing these options, the clinician should explore family values and considerations around termination as many families find this conversation distressing, and it has the potential to be perceived as disrespectful and devaluing their child.[56,57] Clinicians presenting such options should be clear about any institutional policies related to terminations such as family counseling, ethical review, or committee approval. Terminations may not be permitted at a religiously affiliated hospital. Decisions about termination often reflect parents' moral, ethical and religious views. Current data are limited regarding pregnancy outcome following a potentially life-limiting fetal diagnosis, with two programs reporting 60% of parents opting to terminate the pregnancy.[51,58] Termination decisions may be complicated if the family has experienced infertility or with the diagnosis of a life-threatening condition with one fetus of a multiple pregnancy.

For those parents who choose to continue the pregnancy, subsequent decision-making is guided by the certainty of diagnosis, the certainty of prognosis, and the meaning of that prognosis to the parents.[54] Together, IDT clinicians and parents work to determine those interventions which are of best interest for the baby, weighing treatment benefits and burdens. The American Academy of Pediatrics (AAP)[39] and the Neonatal Resuscitation Program[59] confirm that resuscitation may be forgone in any scenario if infant survival is unlikely. It is important to note that the number of conditions for which there are clear recommendations for nonresuscitation has decreased steadily over time as medicine and technology diminish the chance that a disease will be "lethal."[60] For example, for infants with Trisomy 13 or 18, previously referred to as "lethal" conditions due to the high mortality and severe disability among survivors, there has been a shift toward a shared decision-making approach to help better understand families' values and goals in the context of current medical facts in order to weigh the benefits and burdens of any potential intervention for their child.[61,62]

Clinicians should be aware that death at very early gestational ages may present unique issues regarding hospital practices and disposition options. In most states, pregnancies ending prior to 20 weeks completed gestation do not require reporting or generation of a fetal death certificate. Therefore, parents experiencing an early pregnancy loss are not legally bound to make any disposition choice, and most states do not require clinicians to notify parents that they have a choice in the disposition of their tiny baby's body. If and when a fetal death occurs, IDT clinicians should be mindful of hospital, local, and state ordinances and practices regarding options for disposition and communicate these to parents in an appropriate, considerate, and consistent manner.

For infants who survive birth, decision-making is an ongoing process guided by the infant's status during critical transition points including the immediate postpartum period and the time around maternal hospital discharge. Together, IDT clinicians work to promote maximum comfort for the family and infant while accommodating evolving needs and preferences. If a mother requests hospital discharge soon after birth and prior to the baby's death, staff may have little time to adequately provide information and address all of the parents' needs. Routine follow-up after hospital discharge is essential as decision-making unfolds. Many families will choose to support the child in living as long as possible with support of medical technology; the IDT can provide support throughout this decision-making process through the post-discharge period.

REDEFINING HOPE

Families in the early prenatal period face the daunting task of understanding their unborn child's poor prognosis while

BOX 28.2 COMPONENTS OF A PRENATAL PALLIATIVE BIRTH PLAN AND NEONATAL ADVANCE DIRECTIVE

OPENING STATEMENT

Summarizes parents' overall goal for their baby

Example: *We would like to honor our son's life and prolong it if able while minimizing his suffering, and share as many meaningful moments with him as possible*

CARE OF MOTHER AND BABY DURING LABOR AND DELIVERY

- Timing, route and location of the baby's delivery
- Management of mother's pain during labor
- Extent of monitoring baby's heart beat during labor
- If parents have strong desire to meet the baby alive, possible interventions for fetal distress
- Presence of family members or friends
- Faith traditions, prayers, or rituals to be initiated soon after baby's birth

INITIAL CARE MANAGEMENT OF THE BABY

- Extent of desired resuscitation measures or clear DNR/limitation of emergency treatment orders
- Drying baby thoroughly after birth and placing on warm, clean blankets
- Use of warmth to maximize comfort and minimize unwanted symptoms
- Use of suctioning and free flow oxygen
- Management of pain, dyspnea, seizures or other symptoms

CARE FOR THE FAMILY FOLLOWING DELIVERY

- Opportunities to maximize family's time together including: sibling presence, memory-making and keepsake activities, ritual, photographs.
- Plan for communicating baby's status to family and friends not at hospital

ONGOING CARE MANAGEMENT FOR THE BABY

- Comfort measures including warmth, mouth and lip care, kangaroo care, skin care
- Potential initiation of nutrition: breast/bottle feeding, formula via dropper, gavage feedings
- Use of suctioning and free flow oxygen
- Management of pain, dyspnea, seizures, or other symptoms
- Plan for extent of diagnostic testing, such as no x-rays, ultrasounds, blood draws
- Plan for if baby will stay in mother's postpartum room, newborn nursery, or NICU

DISCHARGE PLAN FOR INFANTS WHO SURVIVE THE POSTPARTUM PERIOD

- Anticipatory plan for baby's care when mother is ready to be discharged from the hospital
- Care of the baby in the NICU, home palliative and/or hospice care, community hospice

END-OF-LIFE CARE NEEDS

(Some families may not want to address these issues prior to baby's death)

- Location of death
- Family's preferred funeral director
- Autopsy, postmortem biopsy, and/or special genetic testing
- Organ or tissue donation plans if appropriate

CONTACT INFORMATION

For the following as needed: Palliative care coordinator or primary IDT contact, consulting physicians, family's clergy or pastor, photographer, local prenatal/PPC, or hospice program simultaneously waiting to meet their baby face to face. IDT clinicians must always be mindful that some parents may maintain seemingly unrealistic hope that the diagnosis will be proven false upon the baby's birth. Facilitating choices in care for both mother and child can nurture a sense of control, provide meaning, and foster hope for the family in the midst of chaos and heartbreak.[63] Parental hopes may shift throughout the early prenatal period care trajectory, and IDT clinicians should be prepared to address these preferences accordingly.

MANAGEMENT OF INFANT SUFFERING

IDT clinicians should anticipate and prepare for potential symptoms of infant suffering after birth. Table 28.1 presents pharmacological and nonpharmacological options for pain and symptom management. Table 28.2 presents medication dosing appropriate for term newborns and infants.

TABLE 28.1 Strategies to minimize infant suffering

SITE OF CARE	PHARMACOLOGIC	NONPHARMACOLOGIC
In the delivery room	Oral or rectal • Acetaminophen • Midazolam • Morphine • Sucrose	Warmth Minimal stimulation Swaddling Kangaroo care Non-nutritive sucking
NICU care	IV bolus/IM** • Midazolam • Lorazepam (no IM dosing) • Morphine • Fentanyl • Acetaminophen IV continuous infusion • Midazolam • Morphine • Fentanyl Oral or rectal • Acetaminophen • Sucrose • Midazolam • Morphine • Furosemide • Midazolam • Glycopyrrolate Topical • Fentanyl (patch) • EMLA	Warmth Minimal stimulation Minimal painful procedures Swaddling Non-nutritive sucking Noise reduction Light reduction Nesting Kangaroo care Massage Music
Home care	Oral or rectal • Acetaminophen • Sucrose • Midazolam • Morphine • Furosemide • Midazolam • Glycopyrrolate Topical • Fentanyl (patch) • EMLA	Warmth Swaddling Nutritive or Non-nutritive sucking Kangaroo care Massage Music

Adapted with permission from IBM Micromedex Neofax. Available at http://neofax.micromedexsolutions.com

**minimize intramuscular (IM) dosing when able

Also see Chapter 21 "Prevention and Treatment of Pain in Children with Serious Illness."

Clinical Vignette #1 Revisited

Care for the Chang family could have been improved by the following palliative care measures:

- Establish what is most important to this family, their understanding of the diagnosis, and what it means to them. Also identify the family's wishes and preferences for the baby's care and work to honor those wishes.
- Identify cultural needs that may impact the Changs' understanding of their baby's condition.
- Learn how the Changs prefer to receive information and prepare family for a life-threatening diagnosis.
- Use a professional medical interpreter throughout the trajectory of care.
- Establish clear lines of communication between the community hospital and regional medical center.
- Create a birth plan.
- Provide opportunities for the parents and siblings to connect with the baby and make memories, including honoring cultural and religious traditions and/or rituals

LATE PRENATAL PALLIATIVE CARE

Clinical Vignette #2

Mrs. Reynolds is admitted at 23 1/7 weeks of gestation with bulging membranes and preterm labor. She had been monitored closely during prenatal care because of bleeding in the first trimester. A cerclage was placed early on in her pregnancy because of a history of preterm labor 3 years prior. For that prior pregnancy, she selected a rescue cerclage at 20 weeks of gestation over termination and gave birth to a premature infant at 36 weeks gestation who suffered no major complications.

For the current pregnancy, Mrs. Reynolds's membranes ruptured shortly after admission. It seemed as if many different doctors gave her information, but none supported her in decision-making. Mr. Reynolds was not able to be present for any of these discussions. Within 2 days of hospital admission, she delivered a stillborn infant girl who weighed 525 grams.

Mrs. Reynolds had not expected her infant to be born so soon and thought she would be able to "hold on to this baby like her first one." She and her husband selected hospital burial because of financial reasons and were given pictures of their baby. At her request, Mrs. Reynolds was discharged the same day as the birth, before their families could come to the hospital to see her and the infant. Mrs. Reynolds was instructed to call her obstetrician and schedule a postpartum visit for 6 weeks post-discharge.

Palliative care in the late prenatal period is focused on those families who face an acute delivery of an infant with a life-threatening condition. Examples include mothers with a previously uncomplicated pregnancy who suddenly develop extremely premature labor, or mothers who develop

TABLE 28.2 Dosing for term neonates and infants

	ROUTE					
	ORAL	RECTAL	INTRANASAL	IV BOLUS	IM[a]	IV DRIP
Medication						
Acetaminophen	12–15 mg/kg q6h	12–18 mg/kg q6h	X	12.5 mg/kg/dose q6 hr	X	X
Fentanyl	X	X	1.5–2 mcg/kg divided between each nostril q30–60min PRN	0.5–4 mcg/kg q2–4h	X	1–5 mcg/kg/hr
Furosemide	1–6 mg/kg q12h	X	X	1–2 mg/kg q12h	1 mg/kg q12h	X
Glycopyrrolate	0.04–0.1 mg/kg q4–8h			0.004–0.01 mg/kg q4–8h	0.004–0.01 mg/kg q4–8h	
Lorazepam	X	X	X	0.05–0.1 mg/kg/dose	X	X
Midazolam	0.25 mg/kg q2–4h	X	0.2–0.3 mg/kg q2–4h	0.05–0.15 mg/kg q2–4h	0.05–0.15 mg/kg q2–4h	0.01–0.06 mg/kg/hr
Morphine	3–5× the IV dose	X	X	0.05–0.2 mg/kg q4h	0.05–0.2 mg/kg q4h	0.1–0.2 mg/kg/hr
Sucrose 24%	Max 2 mL/dose via pacifier	X	X	X	X	X

[a]Minimize intramuscular (IM) dosing when possible.

Please refer to original source for dosing in premature infants.

Adapted with permission from IBM Micromedex Neofax. Available at http://neofax.micromedexsolutions.com

their own life-threatening condition, such as pre-eclampsia, so that delivery of the infant must occur emergently. Other families who may benefit from palliative care in the late prenatal period are those who have known about a potential fetal complication for weeks but who have not developed close relationships with clinicians and have not made any decisions for their infant's care.

SETTING

A pregnant woman's medical complications may be diagnosed during a routine prenatal visit, or she may present to a local hospital. Women are not always aware of the signs of preterm labor and premature rupture of membranes[13] and may delay seeking care. Pregnant women who present with urgent medical conditions to local hospitals that lack expertise in high-risk pregnancies may receive inaccurate prognostic information or outdated medical management. If the woman can be stabilized, she may be quickly transferred to a regional medical center far from home. If she cannot be transferred, she may deliver at the local hospital.

Typically, the antepartum unit or the labor and delivery unit do not routinely integrate palliative care as the focus of care on these units is the birth of a healthy infant. Families who deliver a critically ill infant may have a heightened sensitivity to the sights and sounds of the unit, such as cries of other healthy babies or jingles that play over the hospital intercom each time a baby is born. If the family chooses a comfort-focused approach to their infant, clinicians need to modify environments to promote privacy and family togetherness and support grief. One such strategy is to use door markings which signify the special care that the mother and her family need.

INTERDISCIPLINARY TEAM CLINICIANS

The IDT varies depending on the presence of a subspecialty palliative care team and the institutional practice of including neonatal clinicians in prenatal decision-making. Figure 28.2 highlights typical IDT clinicians in the late prenatal period, which can include obstetricians, nurse midwives, labor room and/or triage nurses, antepartum nurses, neonatal physicians, nurse practitioners, social workers, and chaplains. If the woman was transported, a transport nurse may be the person to spend the most amount of time with the woman and may best get to know her and her family. IDTs that do not include neonatal clinicians in the late prenatal period can lead to distress and frustration among obstetrical and neonatal nurses.

COMMUNICATION

Communication during the late prenatal period is often rushed and easily fragmented. Multiple clinicians speak with the family about the mother's and infant's condition. A maternal-fetal medicine specialist may be the first to meet a woman after she has been transferred to a regional medical center with imminent delivery. If involved, neonatologists or neonatal nurse practitioners typically provide prognostic information to the parents regarding infant survival and morbidity. Regardless of the discipline involved, the clinicians must be knowledgeable about local and national data for infant outcome. This is especially critical because treatment decisions made by physicians have been shown to be influenced by their knowledge of outcomes and the type of information that is available.[64]

Data suggest that women may experience a profound sense of responsibility for preventing preterm birth.[65] Clinicians should choose their words carefully to avoid enhancing mothers' guilt. For example, phrases such as "hold on for 2 more weeks" should be avoided. Mothers may also fault themselves for somehow "causing" premature birth. Providing accurate information is critical to reassure mothers who did nothing wrong to cause the events.

The benefits of a prenatal tour to the NICU during a high-risk pregnancy have been documented.[66] However, the practice of giving a prenatal tour is not consistent and may be dependent on the institution's philosophy of care regarding involvement of neonatal clinicians. For pregnant women restricted to bedrest, information about the NICU can be presented in a variety of innovative ways, including photo albums and/or digital recordings.

Parents who rely on other sources, such as the internet, to supplement healthcare information may feel hampered by limited availability or access to these external resources in the hospital setting. Families who do access the internet may develop unrealistic expectations for their infant's outcome. Parents who access chat rooms with other parents can become frustrated with limited options offered at their site of care if they hear of other possible care practices. Clinicians must listen carefully to the families to understand their ongoing need for information and care options as well as provide support throughout each family's individual decision-making process.

DECISION-MAKING

For diagnoses made in the late prenatal period, termination is generally not an option. Instead, decisions include

- Tocolysis versus induction of labor
- Whether to monitor for fetal well-being
- The use of antenatal steroids
- Whether to perform a cesarean section for fetal distress
- Whether to initiate resuscitation in the delivery room
- How many neonatal interventions and treatments should be undertaken at birth and in the first days of life
- Discontinuation of neonatal therapies

Decisions for life-threatening fetal conditions diagnosed in the late prenatal period are often rushed and chaotic, with inadequate time to explore parents' authentic values and goals. The role of the IDT and palliative care clinicians here is to provide a sense of calmness amid the chaos and a focus on family goals.

Despite an attempt to account for prognostic indicators beyond gestational age,[4,6,67] the ability to give an accurate prognosis in the late prenatal period is limited.[38] Therefore, the AAP recommends that clinicians guide families through a process of deciding whether to initiate life-sustaining therapies in the delivery room.[4,39] A clinician skilled in the care of newborns should be present at delivery to evaluate the infant. Ideally, this clinician will have been a part of the management plan. The World Health Organization (WHO) definition of "live born" should be used to document infant condition at birth.[68] Parents will notice any signs of life in the infant at birth and may need help to understand that a weak cry or reflexive movement do not change the infant's prognosis. If the infant's condition is the same as anticipated, then the plan of care can be followed. If the condition is different or if the parent requests, then treatment decisions might change from the earlier plan.

REDEFINING HOPE

There may not be an opportunity for hope to be redefined by parents in the late prenatal period because of the short time between diagnosis and birth. Clinicians may feel reluctant to even begin a preliminary discussion about hope with parents because of the high probability of infant death.[41,69] Clinicians can mistakenly equate hope with intact survival of an infant. In an attempt to avoid giving false hope, clinicians overemphasize poor prognostic data to try to "convince" parents of the gravity of the condition. Discussions about hope are most easily started by asking families what they value and then reframing hope within those parameters, such as hoping that the baby can live until a grandmother arrives. This "breadth of hopes" allows families to cope with the retreat of a particular hope while their other hopes emerge into the forefront.[70]

MANAGEMENT OF INFANT SUFFERING

In the delivery room, drying and warming the infant are key methods for minimizing infant suffering. Additional measures to reduce infant suffering are listed in Tables 28.1 and 28.2.

Clinical Vignette #2 Revisited

Several interventions might have improved care for the Reynolds family:

- Learning about the parents' past experiences, hopes, and preferred role in decision-making.
- Making sure the father was involved in communication with the physicians.
- Creating a birth plan.
- Suggesting ways for the Reynolds to create meaningful memories in the short time they have with their infant.
- Providing comprehensive information about burial or cremation options.
- Providing follow-up after the death, including a phone call within 2 weeks, a chance for the Reynolds to meet with clinicians to review the death, and assistance with coordinating follow-up appointments including bereavement counseling referral. Staff involved in the care of the infant may also outreach the family with a bereavement call or collectively sign and mail a bereavement card.

Clinical Vignette #3

Ms. Jones is 20 years old and pregnant for the first time. She is no longer involved with the baby's father and plans to raise the infant alone. She has an uneventful pregnancy and goes into labor on her due date. During labor at a local hospital, fetal bradycardia occurs. A stat cesarean section reveals total placental abruption. The infant is pale, limp, and apneic at birth. A neonatal nurse practitioner begins resuscitation, and first detects the infant's heart rate at 12 minutes of life. He is brought to the special care nursery and placed on a ventilator. He is profoundly acidotic, and within 1 hour he has a seizure. He is transferred by helicopter at 3 hours of life to a regional NICU 100 miles away.

The infant is encephalopathic and hypotensive. An electroencephalogram (EEG) is consistent with hypoxic ischemic encephalopathy and seizures. Ms. Jones is recovering from her surgery at the community hospital, and the NICU team speaks with her by telephone. They tell her the infant's condition is very serious.

When Ms. Jones arrives at the NICU on hospital day 2, the on-call resident reports that her son is "doing OK." She tells Ms. Jones that the day team will meet with her in the morning. When Ms. Jones asks the nurse for information, the nurse states this is the first time she has cared for her son. She tells Ms. Jones that the baby has "had a good evening."

The attending physician meets alone with Ms. Jones the next day. He discusses the infant's diagnosis and his current treatments. Ms. Jones is told that should the infant survive, he is very likely to have profound disability. She is also told that, in scenarios like this, some parents do not want their baby to be supported by machines, and they decide to take the baby off the ventilator. "Ms. Jones, do you want us to take your son off the machines?"

Palliative care in the early neonatal period targets those families who experience a normal pregnancy, but whose neonate develops a life-threatening condition during birth or in the first few hours of life. Common neonatal diagnoses in this period include birth traumas, overwhelming infections, and previously undiagnosed congenital conditions. These families are generally stunned by the abrupt onset of their infant's condition. The primary surrogate decision-maker, the mother, has just given birth. Palliative care is appropriate for all of these families from birth, even as acute care and diagnostic evaluation proceeds. A palliative approach, either by the NICU team or a subspecialty team, should elicit family goals and support them in achieving these goals whether focused on life extension, comfort, or a blended approach.

SETTING

Care for critically ill infants in the early neonatal period nearly always occurs in the NICU. Intensive care for newborns was regionalized in the 1970s in an attempt to maximize neonatal outcomes by designating hospitals with special technologies and expertise. Critically ill newborns born at community hospitals are often transferred to regional NICUs. When a neonatal life-threatening diagnosis is certain at birth, and the infant is likely to die during transport or soon after, clinician should consider whether end-of-life care should be provided by the local clinician in lieu of neonatal transport, if this approach aligns with the family's values.

Providing end-of-life care in the NICU can be challenging. NICUs are fast-paced and loud, with many staff members. There is often little privacy for families and restrictions on visits by siblings and extended family members. Successful models for NICU palliative care rooms have included drapes, a bed and a refrigerator for the family, music, disposable cameras, and video cameras for parent use.

For many newborns with life-threatening conditions in the early neonatal period, hospital discharge may be possible ranging from hospice care to home care with extended hour nursing care for technology-dependent infants, if resources are available, with palliative care integrated throughout. Inpatient hospice is rarely available for newborns, particularly in rural areas. Home hospice is available to some, though not all, families. In one study of 62 infants who died at home, only 20 received home hospice.[55] Although little research has examined parent preferences for place of death for newborns, clinical experience suggests that important family–infant bonding can occur when newborns are allowed to go home. Families often treasure the memories of a newborn sleeping in her own crib, wearing her own clothes, being held by family members. Bonding between extended family members and the newborn has been found to improve the support of parents by the extended family during the bereavement period.[71]

INTERDISCIPLINARY TEAM CLINICIANS

IDT clinicians in the early neonatal period include many prenatal and neonatal clinicians involved in the late prenatal period as well as pediatric subspecialists, child life clinicians, and community neonatal clinicians including pediatricians and the home-hospice team. Figure 28.2 highlights some of the common roles for these clinicians. As with other intensive care environments, many NICUs do not integrate subspecialty palliative care early in medical management. In one study, the median time between NICU palliative care consult and infant death was 2.5 days.[72] However, a primary palliative care IDT member who is fully integrated into the NICU team can increase opportunities for integrating palliative care earlier into neonatal care. Within a given NICU, it is recommended there be a "champion" for neonatal palliative care who will collaborate with unit-specific interdisciplinary staff and partner with subspecialist palliative care clinicians to address unit needs and incorporate palliative care strategies into everyday care.[73]

COMMUNICATION

When diagnosis of a life-threatening neonatal condition is made in the early neonatal period, clinician coordination and communication must be established quickly. For infants who must be transferred, arrangements should be made for the mother to be transferred as well so that the family can be closer to the infant and communication can improve.

In the early neonatal period, the first hours to days after birth are often filled with tests and subspecialist evaluations. Clear and timely communication among IDT clinicians and the family can be challenging. A central IDT member should be designated as the primary person to deliver information and recommendations to the family. The goal is to integrate information into a "big picture" and to formulate goals of care. Clinicians should avoid the temptation to tell families that their infant is "doing OK" or "having a good day" when the overall status is uncertain. This provides families with false hope and does not allow them time to prepare for the grave reality of their infant's condition. Instead, families may benefit from clinicians sharing if their baby looks comfortable in the moment or that the medical teams are continuing to work hard to help them feel comfortable and maintain clinical stability.

For infants who are discharged to home, communication between hospital and community clinicians can be facilitated by the involvement of specialty palliative care or home hospice. Where these options are not available, hospital clinicians must confirm that the community pediatrician is comfortable with caring for the dying infant, including managing seizures, dyspnea, secretion management, and pain, and can access resources for the family. When appropriate, documentation of resuscitation status should be completed as required by the state and provided to the family before discharge from the hospital.

DECISION-MAKING

There are several decisions particular to the early neonatal period, which should be noted. Because the neonatal diagnosis was not made prenatally, intensive delivery room resuscitation is typical in these scenarios. In the first hours and days of life, as the prognosis becomes grim, decisions arise regarding whether additional therapies such as extracorporeal membranous oxygenation, are indicated or if current life-sustaining therapies, such as mechanical ventilation, should be discontinued. The withholding of fluid and nutrition is particularly controversial in neonates. Some clinicians have concerns about withholding nutrition in light of the Baby Doe regulations.[74] The 2014 report of the AAP Committee on Bioethics reaffirms that nutrition may be withheld from newborns and infants when their benefit to the infant is outweighed by the burden.[75]

These discussions must center on the parents' values and goals and on the infant's best interest. Although parents should be encouraged to share in decision-making, clinicians can ease guilt and regret by framing these discussions not in terms of "do you want us to stop the ventilator?" but instead focusing on what might be of greatest benefit to the infant in the short- and long-term and make recommendations for care based on family values.

When discontinuation of life-sustaining therapies occurs, clinicians should prepare families for what they will see, hear, and feel as their infant dies. Sensitive introduction of the concept of autopsy may be necessary before removing central lines or thoracostomy tubes in some hospitals; hospital regulations may require that medical devices remain in place. In the case of a suspected congenital syndrome which could impact future pregnancies, genetic specialists should advise about neonatal testing needed before death. Many genetic tests can be performed on a postmortem skin biopsy.

Families should be prepared that, while neonatal death typically occurs within hours of extubation, some infants may survive for days. Gasping respirations often occur and an anticipatory symptom management plan should be in place to ease the baby's distress. The neonatal heart rate may persist for hours after breathing stops. Dying may be prolonged if the infant is not bundled closely and kept warm. IDT clinicians may hear parents questioning their decisions and the plan of care for the baby when the dying process seems to be prolonged, and they should be prepared to answer questions and provide support accordingly

REDEFINING HOPE

Families in the early neonatal period are understandably overwhelmed by the need to assimilate complicated medical information, understand the prognosis, articulate goals of care, and focus on maximizing the time they have with their infant. Clinicians can help families focus on what can be realistically achieved in hours or days and make meaning from those goals. For instance, limiting painful procedures, being able to deliver kangaroo (skin-to-skin) care, or seeing their baby open her eyes have been important to some families.

MANAGEMENT OF INFANT SUFFERING

Nearly all sick newborns in the early neonatal period are exposed to painful intravenous access, phlebotomy, intubation, and ventilation. Newborns are often agitated by concomitant exposure to cold, noise, and light. Assessing and managing neonatal pain is a skill that differs from pain assessment of older children.[76] While the motor response to pain evolves and becomes more pronounced near term, perception of pain is present as early as 16–18 weeks' gestation. Several scales have been developed to assess pain in infants.[77–81] Only a subset of these scales is appropriate for use with premature infants.[77–79] Facial grimacing is central to most of these scales; brow furrowing, nasolabial bulge, and squeezing the eyes shut also indicate pain. When facial movements are decreased by sedation, then heart rate variability can be a reliable indicator of pain.

There may be reluctance to treat sick newborns with medications that depress the central nervous system because the neurologic exam is often a critical component of accurate diagnosis and prognosis. There may also be concern that the infant's tenuous cardiorespiratory status will be irrevocably depressed before a clear diagnosis is made. Nevertheless, clinicians should strive to minimize pain and discomfort with pharmacologic and nonpharmacologic therapies as appropriate, as referenced in Tables 28.1 and 28.2.

Clinical Vignette #3 Revisited

Several interventions might have improved care for Ms. Jones and her son.

- Concurrent with the infant's transfer, the NICU clinicians could have facilitated transfer of Ms. Jones' obstetrical care to the regional hospital.
- A single IDT member could have been designated to speak with Ms. Jones.
- Ms. Jones could have been encouraged to have a support person present for discussions regarding withdrawing life-sustaining therapies.
- Clinicians could have avoided using euphemisms to describe her son's status to Ms. Jones.
- Clinicians could have initiated a discussion about Ms. Jones's values and the infant's best interest and avoided asking her if she wanted the staff to discontinue the ventilator.

LATE NEONATAL PALLIATIVE CARE

Clinical Vignette #4

Anna is born at 24 weeks' gestation. She is very sick from birth with severe lung disease. On day of life 3, she is diagnosed with large, bilateral intraventricular hemorrhages. The family is told that Anna could die and that if she survives she may have neurological impairment or cerebral palsy. The family is religious and asks the neonatologist to do everything possible for Anna. They pray for a miracle.

Over the coming weeks, Anna remains critically ill and mechanically ventilated. She has one surgery for a persistent ductus arteriosus and another surgery to place a ventricular shunt. She develops repeated infections related to her immature immune system. She does not tolerate enteral feeding. The family visits infrequently; they live 90 miles away and have had to return to work. With each crisis, they are told that Anna may die. The parents remain hopeful. Privately, Anna's father is becoming more anxious about his daughter's condition and wonders what they should do.

At 10 weeks of age, Anna remains partially dependent on parenteral feeding, and multiple attempts at extubation have been unsuccessful. She develops seizures, which are poorly controlled; twice she has needed cardiopulmonary resuscitation (CPR) during a seizure. She has bradycardia in response to routine cares or being held by her parents.

Because it is an academic hospital, the clinical staff rotates frequently, and no one develops a rapport with the parents. The team worries that Anna is suffering, and several clinicians wonder about the option of discussing discontinuation of life-sustaining therapies. A consulting physician who has not previously been involved in her care tells the parents it would be wrong to stop treating Anna. The father has a hard time trusting the medical team and argues with the mother about what should be done.

One night Anna has a prolonged seizure and goes into cardiac arrest; she dies before her parents arrive at the hospital.

Palliative care in the late neonatal period targets families whose infant develops a life-threatening condition in the first weeks to months of life. Common neonatal diagnoses in this period include surgical complications, such as diaphragmatic hernia repair; profound neurologic diseases; and severe sequelae of prematurity, including cor pulmonale. These diseases often manifest as a roller coaster of improvements and decompensations; families endure multiple crises over time. Many of these infants have long-term dependence on life-sustaining technology and multiorgan involvement, representing a population of chronically critically ill patients.[82] Palliative care is appropriate throughout the disease trajectory.

SETTING

Care for critically ill infants in the late neonatal period nearly always occurs in the hospital. In periods of relative stability, the infant may be transferred to a non-acute hospital ward, facility, or home. The infant is then often transferred back to a neonatal or pediatric acute-care setting for worsening disease.

As noted previously, providing end-of-life care in the neonatal or pediatric ICU can be challenging. Both inpatient and home-based hospice is more available for older infants than for newborns but remains a scarce resource in the late neonatal period.

INTERDISCIPLINARY TEAM CLINICIANS

Many of the IDT clinicians in the early neonatal period maintain important roles in the late neonatal period. Figure 28.2 highlights some of these roles.

COMMUNICATION

Continuity of communication with families easily breaks down when infants are hospitalized for weeks to months. Families who live far away may only be able to visit infrequently. Parents may be forced to return to work soon after birth, so that parental leave can be saved until the infant is discharged. Parent–infant bonding can be disrupted because of the infant's prolonged illness, and parents may feel a loss of their role as parent. For mothers, postpartum depression can increase feelings of sadness and detachment. Regular meetings with the family throughout the hospitalization can assess their evolving needs.

Poor communication between IDT clinicians, resulting in a loss of focus on the goals of care, can occur. Multiple strategies are needed to improve communication. Regular IDT meetings, with minutes distributed to missing clinicians, are helpful. This is particularly true when multiple subspecialists have recommendations that must be placed in the context of the infant's overall condition. Family satisfaction is improved when IDT clinicians deliver consistent information.[34] In settings with regularly rotating clinicians, a nonrotating IDT member, such as a social worker, may best serve as the primary contact person for the family.

As noted earlier, hospital clinicians must ensure clear communication with community clinicians for infants who are discharged to home with or without home hospice. Explicit discussions about pain and symptom control, resuscitation status, and family resources are needed.

DECISION-MAKING

There are several decisions particular to the late neonatal period that should be noted. When infants have been critically ill for weeks to months, families have often been asked to make repeated decisions about life-sustaining therapies. Some families become immune to the gravity of these discussions. They find it difficult to trust clinicians' judgment of a new crisis as life-threatening when the infant has already survived similar crises in the past. Families may develop conflicting goals at different points during the hospitalization. One parent may wish to pursue all therapies regardless of the outcome, while the other wishes to focus on their child's comfort. Clinicians encourage families to talk about their disagreements. Clinicians should anticipate that parents' goals often evolve over time, and decisions to not discontinue therapies early in the infant's hospitalization may change as parents develop a greater understanding of the prognosis. It is particularly important to elicit the parents' values regarding quality of life, as these may differ from clinicians'.[37]

REDEFINING HOPE

Parents and clinicians who pursued life-prolonging interventions during earlier medical crises may have difficulty recognizing that an infant's death is near. It can be helpful to reframe the choice of limiting or discontinuing therapies as not giving up, but instead as an active choice to limit suffering and enhance comfort. Working toward discharge with home hospice, organizing a religious ritual with extended family members, or spending some time in a private room with the infant before extubation may all be goals for which parents can hope.

MANAGEMENT OF INFANT SUFFERING

Infants who have had repeated painful experiences may manifest hyperalgesia in response to minor procedures such as heel sticks or immunizations.[83] These older infants may tolerate a wider variety of pharmacologic formulations of analgesia and anxiolytics than newborns, such as patches and sublingual and rectal applications. Older infants may also benefit from help with secretions, gastroesophageal reflux, and anemia. Pharmacologic and nonpharmacologic strategies that reduce infant suffering are listed in Tables 28.1 and 28.2.

Clinical Vignette #4 Revisited

A number of strategies could have improved care for Anna and her family.

- Family meetings should have been scheduled regularly from early in the Anna's hospitalization.
- IDT meetings should be scheduled regularly to review the goals of care.
- Early discussions should have been held with Anna's family to help them anticipate a prolonged hospitalization.
- Creative methods for enhancing parents' bond with their infant could have been developed, such as encouraging them to leave a camera for staff to take pictures of Anna when the parents cannot visit.
- The family should have been informed that the social worker should be their primary contact person throughout the hospitalization, as he or she can always identify the clinicians responsible for their infant's care.
- Staff should have inquired about disagreement between Anna's parents regarding the goals of care.
- Staff should ask the family about their religious beliefs, and involve chaplain support.

TRANSITIONING PALLIATIVE CARE FROM THE NICU TO OTHER SETTINGS

Clinical Vignette #5

Jasper is a 6-month-old infant, born at 23 weeks' gestation with a history of necrotizing enterocolitis, severe bronchopulmonary dysplasia, and feeding intolerance. He has had a prolonged NICU stay and recently had a tracheostomy and gastrostomy (G) tube placed to help facilitate transfer to home with his family.

Due to his medical complexity, the NICU team recommends transfer to a rehabilitation facility prior to discharge home, to achieve further medical stability before discharge, foster development, and work on teaching for home care.

Jasper's parents do not own a car, and it will be a 60-minute commute to the facility. They are very anxious about the transfer as they have become quite attached to the NICU staff and worry that the care will not be same. Jasper's mother plans to stop working to take care of Jasper full time but they are worried how they will make this work financially.

Families who care for chronic critically ill children who survive the NICU face many challenges in transitioning their child to another unit, another facility, or home. Many of these remain dependent on mechanical ventilation and feeding tubes, with some requiring parenteral nutrition. For these infants and their families, palliative care remains important for interdisciplinary team and psychosocial support while emphasizing pain and symptom management for the infant.

Care for chronic critically ill infants with evolving complex needs usually starts in a NICU, with eventual transfer out of the NICU to home, home hospice or a hospice house, a rehabilitation facility, a pediatric floor, or pediatric ICU.

In these settings, subspecialty palliative care plays an important role for continuity of care throughout these transitions as it is unlikely that the primary clinicians will be able remain a reliable source of support once the infant has transitioned out of the NICU.

TRANSITIONAL SUPPORT AND COMMUNICATION

Families of infants with complex chronic serious illness are often overwhelmed by the prospect of their child leaving a unit they have called home for the past few months. Many families feel attached to their care team in the NICU, and, if they are being transferred to another unit or facility, they may feel abandoned by this primary team and uncertain about what their new team will bring. Tours of the new unit or facility can help facilitate this transition, including introduction to the new team.

The coordination of transitional care from the NICU to home, inpatient hospice house, or rehabilitation facility should include the primary care pediatrician, specialty clinicians, and the subspecialty palliative care team as an extra layer of support and continuity for patient families.[73] Child life services can play an important role in supporting families during this transition as well, specifically surrounding explanations of G tubes and tracheostomies, what these might look like at home and why a new sibling may be different from others.

There are also a unique set of challenges for families transitioning their medically complex child to home. Many caregivers may question their parenting self-efficacy in their developing role as a parent.[84] Even experienced parents will be navigating a new path of parenthood with their child's differing healthcare needs. Many parents appreciate resources for parent support groups to connect with families in similar situations. In addition, as families prepare to bring their medically complex child into a fragmented healthcare system with limits on home nursing support, the IDT can help facilitate care coordination; provide referrals to national, state, or local financial resources; and empower parents to participate in their child's healthcare needs by teaching them to manage oxygen and monitors and replace gastric and tracheostomy tubes.[85] Such tailored support for each family can help them navigate the emotional and systemic stressors that may be involved in the care of a medically complex child.

Clinical Vignette #5 Revisited

Several interventions might have improved care for Jasper and his family.

- Early consultation with a palliative care subspecialist may have helped facilitate the challenges of transitioning out of the NICU and provided an extra layer of support for the family.
- Early connection with social work could have addressed financial concerns and facilitated identification of financial assistance programs.
- Staff could have provided resources for support systems and parent support groups in the community or online.

END-OF-LIFE AND BEREAVEMENT CARE

Though caring for families during their child's dying and throughout bereavement have been described by several other authors in this book, several issues unique to prenatal and neonatal loss should be recognized.

MEMORY-MAKING

For families whose infant dies around the time of birth, an entire lifetime of meeting, treasuring, and loving their babies may be wrapped up in mere minutes, hours, or days. Parents value the choice to interact and make memories with their baby during this brief time.[18,20,86] Rituals to acknowledge the baby's living and dying can provide meaning and nurture relationships among the parents, siblings, and baby.[87,88] All IDT clinicians can play an integral role in facilitating such moments between parent and child.

Some families willingly accept opportunities to interact with their baby and make memories. Others may hesitate initially, but may appreciate time to consider the options. Opportunities for memory-making and ritual are highlighted in Box 28.3. Families should be encouraged to interact with their baby at a pace and in ways that are most meaningful to them, even if their choices differ from how clinicians believe memories should be made, as demonstrated in Figure 28.4.[89,90]

CARE OF THE FAMILY DURING THE DYING PROCESS

IDT clinicians should ascertain how much information parents wish to know about what death may be like, including anticipated changes in the baby's breathing, level of consciousness, color, and heart rate. Parents should be encouraged to be with their baby during death in ways that are meaningful and comfortable to them. Child life specialists and nurses may help to prepare siblings for what they will see and experience prior to meeting their dying sibling, keeping in mind that this may be their first time actually seeing and interacting with their baby brother or sister.

Special cultural or religious actions, including proper care of the body, should be determined before the baby's death and implemented accordingly. A safe, private location should be established, providing families the opportunity to be with their baby's body after death if desired. A time limit should

BOX 28.3 CREATING MEANINGFUL MEMORIES

Photographs and Video

Both serve as touchstones to the family's moments of interacting with their baby.

Photography Considerations

- Prenatal photography with pregnancy or family portraits
- Photographs of multiples together, including, if needed, photographing baby who has died with surviving multiples (Pector EA. Views of bereaved multiple-birth parents on life support decisions, the dying process, and discussions surrounding death. *J Perinatol* 2004;24:4–10).
- Parents encouraged to bring their own cameras to the hospital
- Digital or disposable cameras available on the units for both staff and family use
- Method of providing digital images to family including CD-ROM or SD card
- Method of storing digital images should parents decide not to receive the photographs at discharge

Photography Resources

- Now I Lay Me Down to Sleep: A national organization that links volunteer photographers to families experiencing the death of a baby: www.nilmdts.org
- Todd Hochberg Bereavement Photography: Todd Hochberg is a pioneer in the field of photojournalistic style bereavement photography. His website is a resource for clinicians in utilizing this style of photography: www.toddhochberg.com
- RTS Bereavement Services Guidelines for photographing babies at end-of-life (Daley M, Limbo R, eds. *Creating memories. RTS bereavement training in early pregnancy loss, stillbirth, and newborn death.* La Crosse, WI: Gundersen Lutheran Medical Foundation, Inc.; 2008).

Plaster Molds

Molds can be created of a baby's hands and feet using a variety of products

- 3D mold kits such as Precious Hands or Wedding Hands
- Modeling compound used to make an impression such as Crayola's Model Magic or dental resins

Ink Prints and Other Memories

Prints can be created of baby's hands and feet on the following:

- Complimentary hospital birth certificate, card stock, or in a baby book
- Hats, t-shirts, or other items of clothing for the parents or siblings
- Child life specialists can often facilitate the creation of an art piece that includes fingerprints of the child, family, and medical team members providing care.
- Heart Doppler reading and/or an audio recording of an infant's heartbeat incorporated into a soundtrack of songs families played for their infant.

Locks of Hair

- Can be carefully collected and placed in a small sealable plastic bag for safe-keeping

Scrapbooking

- Can be done during the prenatal period or after the baby's birth. Some antenatal and neonatal units provide scrapbooking opportunities for parents as a way to connect for support while creating memory pages (Schwarz B, Fatzinger D, Meier PP. Rush SpecialKare Keepsakes. *MCN Am J Maternal Child Nurs.* 2004;29:354–361).

Personal Items

- Can be brought by the family or offered by IDT clinicians. Hospital auxiliary members, church, or community service groups may provide donations. Patterns for very small size gowns and blankets can be found online. Examples of personal items include:
  Baptismal gowns and baby clothing in a variety of sizes
  Hand-knit caps and blanket
  Small toys
  Tape recorders of parents' voices talking, reading, or singing
  Baby rings (Figure 28.4) available from www.bereavementservices.org

(continued)

BOX 28.3 CONTINUED

Memory Boxes

- Plain boxes can be purchased inexpensively at local craft stores or online and then decorated by siblings

Opportunities to Interact with the Baby

Touching and holding the baby, including kangaroo care
Rituals of blessing, naming, dedication, recognition of life, or baptism
Bathing and caring for the baby's body both while living and after death
Rocking, cuddling, or lying down with the baby in a bed
Reading special books or singing to the baby
Taking the baby outdoors or allowing the baby to experience sunshine

not be imposed, as parental contact with their deceased baby's body poses little risk for infection and also does not impact potential postmortem testing.[91] In addition, IDT clinicians should ensure processes are in place should a mother hospitalized on a postpartum unit wish to be with her baby's body again before discharge.[91]

Recognizing that many young parents have never before made arrangements for the care of a loved one's body after death, IDT clinicians should be prepared to provide both verbal and written information on choosing a funeral director. An appropriate IDT member should be knowledgeable of the hospital's process for release of remains, as well as local choices for burial or cremation. It is also helpful for IDT clinicians to explore the availability of hospital- and community-based resources (e.g., local funeral homes) that may provide financial assistance to families' hoping to pursue various cremation or burial practices to honor their child. In addition, the options for autopsy and organ or tissue donation should be discussed with the parents as appropriate. IDT clinicians may choose to develop a process to notify staff members of a baby's death, thus allowing staff who were not working at the time of the baby's death the opportunity to say good-bye to their tiny patient.

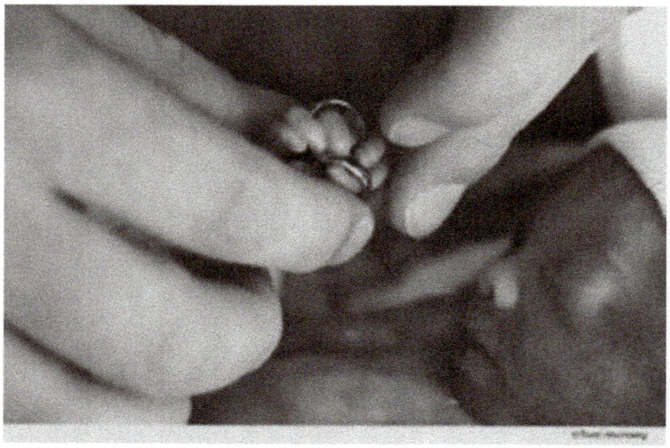

Figure 28.4 A father gently places baby rings on the hands of his twin babies. Photograph provided courtesy of Todd Hochberg.

BEREAVEMENT SUPPORT

Grief support begins with the diagnosis of the life-limiting condition and continues months after the baby's death.[3] Follow-up with these families is essential. Parents' recollections of events surrounding birth and death may differ from the reality, specifically concerning the infant's condition at birth and the type of treatment that was given. The IDT can review the information with the family, even when there are no autopsy findings to review. The meeting should include IDT clinicians who can review the events around the death, provide recommendations for a subsequent pregnancy, and assess how the parents are working through their grief.

Parents face ongoing challenges when they are back in their community, where the infant's death may not be known or the details misunderstood. When others do not know about the birth and death of the infant, they may approach the mother as if she is still pregnant, thereby creating an uncomfortable situation. Also, it is not uncommon for this type of a loss to be perceived as and called a miscarriage by the lay public. IDT clinicians can help families anticipate the heartbreaking task of returning home to a waiting nursery without their baby. Parents may appreciate the opportunity to consider how they will share the news of the baby's death with their children, other family members, friends, colleagues, and strangers. A packet of supportive literature written specifically for parents experiencing the death of a baby should be provided prior to discharge from the hospital.

IDT clinicians should create avenues for bereavement follow-up tailored to their particular population. Such follow-up may occur through phone calls, bereavement mailings, hospital memorial services, or anniversary acknowledgments. Some parents may find comfort from a bereavement support group or may access similar programs for their surviving children. A full discussion of prenatal and neonatal grief is outside the scope of this chapter. Readers are encouraged to access the following resources for further information:

- Resolve Through Sharing (RTS): www.bereavementservices.org
- National Pregnancy Loss and Infant Death Alliance: www.plida.org

- SHARE Pregnancy and Infant Loss Support: www.nationalshare.org
- MISS Foundation: www.missfoundation.org
- Centering Corporation: www.centering.org
- Perinatal Hospice and Palliative Care: www.perinatalhospice.org
- Center for Loss in Multiple Birth: www.climb-support.org
- The Compassionate Friends: www.compassionatefriends.org
- Support Organization for Trisomy 18, 13, and related disorders (SoFT): www.trisomy.org

CONCLUSION

The needs of families anticipating the birth of a baby with a life-threatening condition offer unique opportunities to implement palliative care measures throughout the prenatal and neonatal periods. IDT clinicians who participate in the provision of such care have the privilege of welcoming new life, creating meaningful moments, and facilitating good-byes while honoring family's hopes, beliefs, and preferences.

Family Reflection

When our beautiful baby was born it started as a normal labor, but then I was rushed into an emergency c-section when doctors couldn't find her heartbeat. Cindy Sue was resuscitated and rushed to the children's hospital where she was put on life support.

What followed was a series of events, tests, meetings, and decisions for which there is no handbook for parents. We relied on the information and advice that we were given; we had to trust that the people who were caring for her, knew exactly what she needed. We asked endless questions, even though the answers were hard to hear. We were given the information, and then also given the space to process and the support to make difficult decisions.

We connected with the PPC team. They helped us navigate conversations with our 2-year-old son, to help him understand, to the best of his toddler ability, what was going on with our family. We had intimate, middle of the night conversations with nurses, and bedside talks with the NICU doctors. Somehow, the human element rose high above the medical jargon and the machines, and that was what kept us moving forward.

We made a promise to our daughter that we would be stronger, better because of her and that we would find the joy that comes with the birth of a new baby. We are so grateful to everyone who surrounded us during those difficult times, and we are forever grateful for the 13 days with our sweet Cindy Sue.

Please see Figure 28.5 for a photograph of Cindy Sue and her family (provided by her parents).

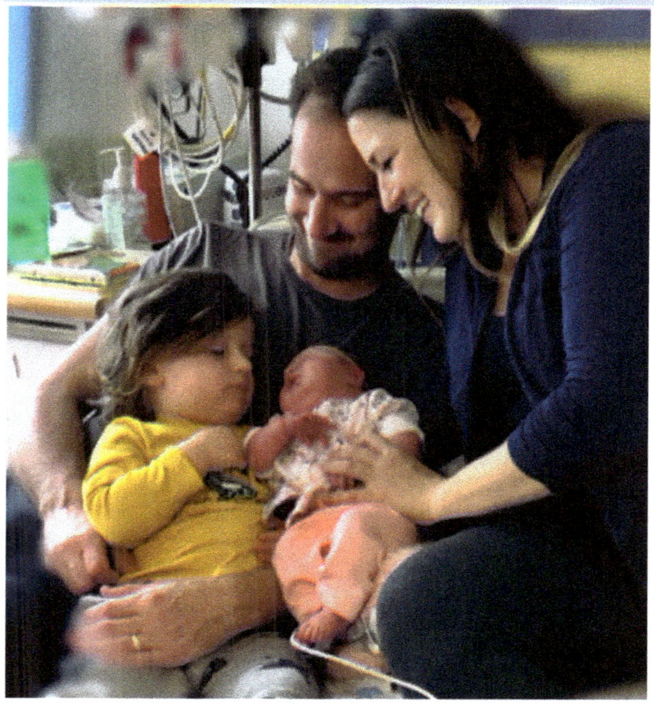

Figure 28.5 Cindy Sue and her family. Photograph courtesy of Tim, Amy, and Ray Deihl-Butterworth.

REFERENCES

1. Witt R, MacKenzie TC, Paranteau WH. Fetal stem cell and gene therapy. *Sem Fetal Neonatal Med.* 2017;22:410–414.
2. MacDorman MF, Gregory ECW. Fetal and perinatal mortality: United States, 2013. *Nat Vital Stat Rep.* 2015;64(8):1–24.
3. Milstein JM. Introducing spirituality in medical care: Transition from hopelessness to wholeness. *JAMA.* 2018;299:2440–2441.
4. Cummings J. Antenatal counseling regarding resuscitation and intensive care before 25 weeks of gestation. *Pediatrics.* 2015;136(3):588–595.
5. Raju TNK, Mercer BM, Burchfield DJ, Joseph GF. Periviable birth: Executive summary of a joint workshop by the Eunice Kennedy Shriver National Institute of Child Health and Human Development, Society for Maternal-Fetal Medicine, American Academy of Pediatrics, and American College of Obstetricians. *J Perinatol.* 2014;34(5):333–342.
6. Rysavy MA, Horbar JD, Bell EF, et al. Assessment of an updated neonatal research network extremely preterm birth outcome model in the Vermont Oxford network. *JAMA Pediatr.* Published online 2020;174(5):e196294.
7. Watkins PL, Dagle JM, Bell EF, Colaizy TT. Outcomes at 18 to 22 months of corrected age for infants born at 22 to 25 weeks of gestation in a center practicing active management. *J Pediatr.* 2020;217:52–58.e1.
8. Peterson JK, Kochilas LK, Catton KG, Moller JH, Setty SP. Long-term outcomes of children with trisomy 13 and 18 after congenital heart disease interventions. *Ann Thorac Surg.* 2017;103(6):1941–1949.
9. Janvier A, Farlow B, Barrington K. Cardiac surgery for children with trisomies 13 and 18: Where are we now? *Semin Perinatol.* 2016;40(4):254–260.
10. Haug S, Goldstein M, Cummins D, Fayard E, Merritt TA. Using patient-centered care after a prenatal diagnosis of trisomy 18 or trisomy 13: A review. *JAMA Pediatr.* 2017;171(4):382–387.

11. Quill TE, Abernethy AP. Generalist plus specialist palliative care—creating a more sustainable model. *N Engl J Med.* 2013;368(13):1173–1175.
12. Richter, M. S., C. Parkes, and J. Chaw-Kant. Listening to the voices of hospitalized high-risk antepartum patients. *J Obstet Gynecol Neonatal Nurs.* 2007;36:313–318.
13. Kavanaugh K. Parents' experience surrounding the death of a newborn whose birth is at the margin of viability. *J Obstet Gynecol Neonatal Nurs.* 1997;26:43–51.
14. Richardson B, Dol J, Rutledge K, et al. Evaluation of mobile apps targeted to parents of infants in the neonatal intensive care unit: A systematic app review. *JMIR Mhealth Uhealth.* 2019;7(4):e11620.
15. Makkar A, McCoy M, Hallford G, et al. Evaluation of neonatal services provided in a level II NICU utilizing hybrid telemedicine: A prospective study. *Telemed J E Health.* 2020;26(2):176–183.
16. Epstein EG, Arechiga J, Dancy M, Simon J, Wilson D, Alhusen JL. Integrative review of technology to support communication with parents of infants in the NICU. *J Obstet Gynecol Neonatal Nurs.* 2017;46(3):357–366.
17. Limbo R, Kobler K. "Will our baby be alive again?" Supporting parents of young children when a baby dies. *Nurs Women's Health* 2009;13:302–311.
18. Widger K, Picot C. Parents' perceptions of the quality of pediatric and perinatal end-of-life care. *Pediatr Nurs.* 2008;34:53–58.
19. Williams C, Munson D, Zupancic J, Kirpalani H. Supporting bereaved parents: Practical steps in providing compassionate perinatal and neonatal end-of-life care. a North American perspective. *Semin Fetal Neonat Med.* 2008;13:335–340.
20. Gold KJ. Navigating care after a baby dies: A systematic review of parent experiences with health providers. *J Perinatol.* 2007;27:230–237.
21. Moro T, Kavanaugh K, Okuno-Jones S, Vankleef JA. Neonatal end-of-life care: A review of the research literature. *J Perinat Neonatal Nurs.* 2006;20:262–73.
22. Knapp B, Decker C, Lantos JD. Neonatologists' attitudes about diagnostic whole-genome sequencing in the NICU. *Pediatrics.* 2019;143:S54–S57.
23. Carnevale FA, Canoui P, Cremer R, et al. Parental involvement in treatment decisions regarding their critically ill child: A comparative study of France and Quebec. *Pediatr Crit Care Med.* 2007;8:337–342.
24. Lantos JD. Ethical problems in decision making in the neonatal ICU. *N Engl J Med.* 2018;379(19):1851–1860.
25. Doron MW, Veness-Meehan KA, Margolis LH, Holoman EM, Stiles AD. Delivery room resuscitation decisions for extremely premature infants, *Pediatrics.* 1998;102:574–582.
26. Peerzada JM, Richardson DK, Burns JP. Delivery room decision-making at the threshold of viability. *J Pediatr.* 2004;145:492–498.
27. van der Heide A, van der Maas PJ, van der Wal G, Kollée LA, de Leeuw R, Holl RA. The role of parents in end-of-life decisions in neonatology: Physicians' views and practices. *Pediatrics.* 1998;101:413–418.
28. Morrison W, Clark JD, Lewis-Newby M, Kon AA Titrating clinician directiveness in serious pediatric illness. *Pediatrics.* 2018;142(S2):S178–S186.
29. Zupancic JA, Kirpalani H, Barrett J, et al. Characterising doctor-parent communication in counselling for impending preterm delivery. *Arch Dis Child Fetal Neonatal Ed.* 2002;87:F113–117.
30. Bastek TK, Richardson DK, Zupancic JA, Burns JP. Prenatal consultation practices at the border of viability: A regional survey. *Pediatrics.* 2005;116:407–413.
31. Martinez AM, Partridge JC, Yu V, et al. Physician counselling practices and decision-making for extremely preterm infants in the Pacific Rim. *J Paediatr Child Health.* 2005;41:209–214.
32. Partridge JC, Martinez AM, Nishida H, et al. International comparison of care for very low birth weight infants: Parents' perceptions of counseling and decision-making. *Pediatrics.* 2005;116:e263–271.
33. Boss RD, Hutton N, Sulpar LJ, West AM, Donohue PK. Values parents apply to decision-making regarding delivery room resuscitation for high-risk newborns. *Pediatrics.* 2008;122:583–589.
34. Miquel-Verges F, Woods L, Aucott SA, Boss RD, Donohue PK. Prenatal consultation for congenital anomalies: Parental expectations and perceptions. *Pediatrics.* 2009;124(4):e573–e579.
35. Carter BS, Lantos JD. Disclosing adverse events and near misses to parents of neonates. *Semin Perinatol.* 2019;43(8):151182.
36. Freda MC, Devine KS, Semelsberger C. The lived experience of miscarriage after infertility. *MCN Am J Matern Child Nurs.* 2003;28:16–23.
37. Streiner DL, Saigal S, Burrows E, Stoskopf B, Rosenbaum P. Attitudes of parents and health care professionals toward active treatment of extremely premature infants. *Pediatrics.* 2001;108:152–157.
38. Chiswick M. Infants of borderline viability: Ethical and clinical considerations. *Sem Fetal Neonat Med.* 2008;13:8–15.
39. American Academy of Pediatrics Committee on Fetus and Newborn, Bell EF. Noninitiation or withdrawal of intensive care for high-risk newborns. *Pediatrics.* 2007; reaffirmed 2015;119:401–403.
40. Hurst I. The legal landscape at the threshold of viability for extremely premature infants: A nursing perspective, part I. *J Perinat Neonatal Nurs.* 2005;19:155–166; quiz 167–168.
b. Hurst I. The legal landscape at the threshold of viability for extremely premature infants: A nursing perspective, Part II. *J Perinat Neonatal Nurs.* 2005;19:253–262; quiz 263–264.
41. Kavanaugh K, Savage T, Kilpatrick S, Kimura R, Hershberger P. Life support decisions for extremely premature infants: Report of a pilot study. *J Pediatr Nurs.* 2005;20:347–359.
42. Evans WG, Tulsky JA, Back AL, Arnold RM. Communication at times of transitions: How to help patients cope with loss and re-define hope. *Cancer J.* 2006;12:417–424.
43. Pector EA. Views of bereaved multiple-birth parents on life support decisions, the dying process, and discussions surrounding death. *J Perinatol.* 2004;24:4–10.
44. Kenner C, Boykova M. Palliative care in the neonatal intensive care unit. In B Ferrell, N Coyle, eds. *Textbook of Palliative Nursing.* 3rd ed. Oxford University Press; 2010: 1065–1080.
45. Kain VJ. Moral distress and providing care to dying babies in neonatal nursing. *Int J Palliat Nurs.* 2007;13:243–248.
46. Papadatou D. A proposed model of health professionals' grieving process. *Omega.* 2000;41:59–77.
47. Roehrs C, Masterson A, Alles R, Witt C, Rutt P. Caring for families coping with perinatal loss. *J Obstet Gynecol Neonatal Nurs.* 2008;37:631–639.
48. Epstein EG. End-of-life experiences of nurses and physicians in the newborn intensive care unit. *J Perinatol.* 2008;28:771–778.
49. Pavlish C, Brown-Saltzman K, So L, Wong J. SUPPORT: An evidence-based model for leaders addressing moral distress. *J Nurs Admin.* 2016;46(6):313–320.
50. Rogers S, Babgi A, Gomez C. Educational interventions in end-of-life care: Part I: An educational intervention responding to the moral distress of NICU nurses provided by an ethics consultation team. *Adv Neonatal Care.* 2008;8:56–65.
51. Leuthner S, Jones EL. Fetal concerns program: A model for perinatal palliative care. *MCN Am J Matern Child Nurs.* 2007;2:272–278.
52. Sumner LH, Kavanaugh K, Moro T. Extending palliative care into pregnancy and the immediate newborn period: State of the practice of perinatal palliative care. *J Perinat Neonatal Nurs.* 2006;20:113–116.
53. Munson D, Leuthner SR. Palliative care for the family carrying a fetus with a life-limiting diagnosis. *Pediatr Clin North Am.* 2007;54:787–798.
54. Leuthner SR. Palliative care of the infant with lethal anomalies. *Pediatr Clin North Am.* 2004;51:747–759.
55. Leuthner SR, Boldt AM, Kirby RS. Where infants die: Examination of place of death and hospice/home health care options in the state of Wisconsin. *J Palliat Med.* 2004;7:269–277.
56. Coleman PK, Coyle CT, Rue VM. Late-term elective abortion and susceptibility to posttraumatic stress symptoms. *J Pregnancy.* 2010;2010:130519.
57. Langford K, Maxwell D. Late termination for fetal abnormality: Providing essential information for parents. *J Obstet Gynaecol (Lahore).* 2001;21(2):171–172.

58. Breeze AC, Lees CC, Kumar A, Missfelder-Lobos HH, Murdoch EM. Palliative care for prenatally diagnosed lethal fetal abnormality. *Arch Dis Child Fetal Neonatal Ed*. 2007;92:F56–58.
59. Weiner GM, Zaichkin J, eds. *Textbook of Neonatal Resuscitation (NRP)*. 7th ed. American Academy of Pediatrics; 2016.
60. Koogler TK, Wilfond BS, Ross LF. Lethal language, lethal decisions. *Hastings Center Rep*. 2003;33:37–41.
61. Andrews SE, Downey AG, Showalter DS, et al. Shared decision making and the pathways approach in the prenatal and postnatal management of the trisomy 13 and trisomy 18 syndromes. *Am J Med Genet Part C Semin Med Genet.* 2016;172C:257–263.
62. Nelson KE, Janvier A, Nathanson PG, Feudtner C. Ethics and the importance of good clinical practices. *Am J Bioeth*. 2020;20(1):67–70.
63. Milstein, J. A paradigm of integrative care: Healing with curing throughout life, "being with" and "doing to." *J Perinatol*. 2005;25:563–568.
64. Janvier A, Lantos J, Deschênes M, Couture E, Nadeau S, Barrington KJ. Caregivers attitudes for very premature infants: What if they knew? *Acta Paediatrica* 2008;97:276–279.
65. MacKinnon K. Living with the threat of preterm labor: Women's work of keeping the baby in. *J Obstet Gynecol Neonatal Nurs*. 2006;35:700–708.
66. Griffin T, Kavanaugh K, Soto CF, White M. Parental evaluation of a tour of the neonatal intensive care unit during a high-risk pregnancy. *J Obstet Gynecol Neonatal Nurs*. 1997;26:59–65.
67. Tyson JE, Parikh NA, Langer J, Green C, Higgins RD, National Institute of Child Health and Human Development Neonatal Research Network. Intensive care for extreme prematurity: Moving beyond gestational age. *N Engl J Med*. 2008;358:1672–1681.
68. World Health Organization. *International Statistical Classification Of Diseases And Related Health Problems.* World Health Organization; 1993.
69. Reder EA, Serwint JR. Until the last breath: Exploring the concept of hope for parents and health care professionals during a child's serious illness, *Arch Pediatr Adolesc Med*. 2009;163:653–657.
70. Feudtner C. The breadth of hopes. *N Engl J Med.* 2009;361:2306–2307.
71. Lauer ME, Mulhern RK, Schell MJ, Camitta BM. Long-term follow-up of parental adjustment following a child's death at home or hospital. *Cancer*. 1989;63:988–994.
72. Pierucci RL, Kirby RS, Leuthner SR. End-of-life care for neonates and infants: The experience and effects of a palliative care consultation service. *Pediatrics*. 2001;108:653–660.
73. Carter BS. Pediatric palliative care in infants and neonates. *Children (Basel).* 2018;5(2):21.
74. Child Abuse and Prevention Act, 42 U.S.C. 1994. US Department of Health and Human Services.
75. Diekema DS, Botkin JR, and the Committee on Bioethics American Academy of Pediatrics. Clinical report--forgoing medically provided nutrition and hydration in children, reaffirmed. *Pediatrics*. 2014;124:813–822.
76. Batton DG, Barrington KJ, Wallman C. 2006. Prevention and management of pain in the neonate: An update. *Pediatrics*. 118:2231–2241.
77. Stevens B, Johnston C, Petryshen P, Taddio A. Premature infant pain profile: Development and initial validation. *Clin J Pain*. 1996;12:13–22.
78. Grunau RV, Johnston CC, Craig KD. Neonatal facial and cry responses to invasive and non-invasive procedures. *Pain*. 1990;42:295–305.
79. Krechel SW, Bildner J. CRIES: A new neonatal postoperative pain measurement score. Initial testing of validity and reliability. *Paediatr Anaesth*. 1995;5:53–61.
80. van Dijk M, de Boer JB, Koot HM, Tibboel D, Passchier J, Duivenvoorden HJ. The reliability and validity of the COMFORT scale as a postoperative pain instrument in 0 to 3-year-old infants. *Pain*. 1000;84:367–377.
81. Lawrence J, Alcock D, McGrath P, Kay J, MacMurray SB, Dulberg C. The development of a tool to assess neonatal pain. *Neonatal Netw*. 1993;12:59–66.
82. Shapiro MC, Henderson CM, Hutton N, Boss RD. Defining pediatric chronic critical illness for clinical care, research, and policy. *Hosp Pediatr*. 2017;7(4):236–244.
83. Taddio A, Shah V, Gilbert-MacLeod C, Katz J. Conditioning and hyperalgesia in newborns exposed to repeated heel lances. *JAMA*. 2002;288:857–861.
84. Lakshmanan A, Kubicek K, Williams R, et al. Viewpoints from families for improving transition from NICU-to-home for infants with medical complexity at a safety net hospital: A qualitative study. *BMC Pediatr* 2019;19,223.
85. Allshouse C, Comeau M, Rodgers R, Wells N. Families of children with medical complexity: A view from the front lines. *Pediatrics*. 2018;141(Supplement 3):S195 LP–S201.
86. Meert KL, Thurston CS, Briller SH. The spiritual needs of parents at the time of their child's death in the pediatric intensive care unit and during bereavement: A qualitative study. *Pediatr Crit Care Med*. 2005;6:420–427.
87. Kobler K, Limbo R, Kavanaugh K. Meaningful moments: The use of ritual in perinatal and pediatric death. *MCN Am J Matern Child Nurs*. 2007;32:288–295.
88. Fanos JH, Little GA, Edwards WH. Candles in the snow: Ritual and memory for siblings of infants who died in the intensive care nursery. *J Pediatr*. 2009;154:849–853.
89. Daley M, Limbo R, eds. *Creating Memories. RTS Bereavement Training in Early Pregnancy Loss, Stillbirth, and Newborn Death.* Gundersen Lutheran Medical Foundation; 2008.
90. Schwarz B, Fatzinger C, Meier PP. Rush SpecialKare Keepsakes. *MCN Am J Matern Child Nurs*. 2004;29:354–361; quiz 62–63.
91. Pregnancy Loss and Infant Death Alliance. PLIDA position statements: Delaying postmortem pathology studies; infection risks are insignificant when parents have contact with their baby after death. 2016. Online https://www.plida.org/position-statements_non-members

29 | CHILDREN WITH COMPLEX CHRONIC CONDITIONS

JORI BOGETZ, CHRISTOPHER A. COLLURA, AND CHRISTY TORKILDSON

Family Reflection

A Parent's Perspective

The COVID-19 pandemic has impacted our lives in many ways. As the family of a child with many complex chronic conditions, we have always managed to normalize our very abnormal life. In some ways, I believe families of disabled and chronically ill children may find this time in history a little less disturbing than normal families. We are accustomed to social isolation. We have mastered handwashing and keeping our homes safe and clean. We frequently have to prohibit visitors and activities we deem unsafe. On the other hand, our feelings of vulnerability are heightened. We absolutely must not risk endangering our children. If our son gets this virus it would have a potentially devastating outcome for him. We have stopped home nursing. No family or friends are allowed to come into our home. Last month, we had the difficult conversation with him about what our plan would be if he began to show symptoms. We have decided to keep him home, no hospitalization, start hospice immediately, and care for him ourselves until his death. A local hospice doctor would coordinate his care and end-of-life needs. I've made myself an isolation gown and a face shield. Just as in the past when we have had to worry about the unthinkable, we have to deal with such abnormal subjects and plan for the pandemic. Despite all of this, we still focus on finding joy in every day and follow our son's motto of "Love Life."

Mother of a 21-year-old son
with complex chronic conditions

When God is going to do something wonderful, He or She always starts with a hardship; when God is going to do something amazing, He or She starts with an impossibility.

Anne Lamott

INTRODUCTION TO CHILDREN WITH COMPLEX CHRONIC CONDITIONS

In the United States, advances in pediatric healthcare continue to reduce childhood mortality while allowing children with complex illness to live longer. Many of these children have special healthcare needs (CSHCN)—defined as those "at risk for a chronic physical, developmental, behavioral, or emotional condition requiring health related services beyond that required by children generally."[1] A subset of CSHCN with medically complex illness account for an increasing trend in healthcare utilization including hospital admissions, readmissions, prolonged length of stay, pediatric healthcare expenditure, and death.[2–5]

To better account for healthcare use by medically complex children and identify those at risk of death, Feudtner et al. defined complex chronic conditions (CCCs) as "any medical condition that can be reasonably expected to last at least 12 months (unless death intervenes) and to involve either several different organ systems or one organ system severely enough to require specialty pediatric care and probably some period of hospitalization in a tertiary care center."[6] This definition is widely accepted to best account for those children who commonly and recurrently receive care in intensive inpatient settings. To better delineate children with the most intensive healthcare needs among those with CCCs, the term "children with medical complexity (CMC)" is often used. While this terminology may best describe children with substantial caregiver needs, functional limitations, and healthcare service utilization, this chapter will use the umbrella term CCCs to describe the overarching population of CMC.

Children with CCCs and their families live with the lifelong joys of having a child with special needs and also the challenge of life-threatening and life-limiting illness. Specialty pediatric palliative care (PPC) teams partner with the child, family, and primary and subspecialty care teams to navigate a child's chronic illness trajectory while balancing medical interventions intended to prolong life and restore function while helping the child and family thrive amid life-threatening illness. Increasingly, this includes interdisciplinary complex care teams that provide primary palliative care for patients and families. By centering values-based goals of care, treating physical and emotional pain, and supporting the psychosocial well-being of the child and family, PPC is an essential resource in the care for children with CCCs.[7] Throughout the chapter, PPC will refer to the added layer of support provided by specialty pediatric palliative care teams.

Clinical Vignette (Part 1)

Charlie is 2-year-old boy with complex medical needs. He was born extremely premature at 23 weeks of gestation due to preterm labor. He experienced a very complicated neonatal intensive care course, including severe intraventricular hemorrhage, retinopathy of prematurity, and severe bronchopulmonary dysplasia requiring long-term ventilation via tracheostomy. He is assisted by a gastrostomy tube for enteral nutrition and had a ventriculoperitoneal shunt placed due to posthemorrhagic hydrocephalus. He was hospitalized at the children's hospital for 6-months with the last several months of long-term inpatient care for chronic lung disease, while home nursing was secured to provide necessary support in the family's house to optimize safe care of a child with chronic technology needs.

His parents, Sarah and Neal, understand that Charlie will likely have significant neurologic and physical disability from complications related to extreme prematurity. They remain hopeful that, with growth and development, he will not require lifelong invasive chronic mechanical ventilation. His family's goals are to provide medical interventions that help Charlie experience joy and loving relationships with his family.

ILLNESS TRAJECTORIES

Palliative care has used illness trajectory frameworks to help map prognostic time frames and anticipated needs of patients in order to best aid healthcare and social service support.[3] The trajectory most commonly associated with children with CCCs is "long-term limitations with intermittent serious illness." This trajectory, developed for adults with chronic conditions like heart failure and chronic obstructive pulmonary disease, details gradual functional decline with sudden and severe periods of deterioration and recovery toward a return to a diminished functional outcome. Acute episodes within this trajectory are often life-threatening and may result in death. For children with CCCs, multiple hospital admissions are strongly associated with decreased survival, yet uncertainty remains.[9] Such data support the "long-term limitations with intermittent serious illness trajectory" for children with CCCs because recurrent acute episodes may eventually progress to a life-limiting outcome. Intensive care unit (ICU) admissions for children with CCCs are significantly associated with prolonged length of stay and mortality in the ICU.[5] One cross-sectional survey of bereaved parents demonstrated that nearly two-thirds of children with life-threatening CCCs died in the hospital, with more than half dying in the ICU.[10] Children with static encephalopathy, congenital and chromosomal disorders, and pulmonary disorders are at highest risk of in-hospital death.[10]

Using such illness trajectories may be helpful in understanding mortality risk for children with CCCs when recurrent hospitalizations for acute illness occur, but its application to the individual patient with CCCs likely oversimplifies an unpredictable and complicated course. Often recurrent admissions, especially to the ICU, involve multiple diagnostic and therapeutic interventions administered with restorative intent. In addition, for children with CCCs, their functional baseline may be unknown as the illness trajectory does not necessarily begin at the peak of function with subsequent gradual decline. Rather, for many children with CCCs with primarily neurologic, metabolic, congenital, or chromosomal disorders, or complications from premature birth, the "starting point" of the child's disease—the neonatal ICU (NICU)—may encompass the sickest the patient will be for several years of life. Subsequent neurologic and physical development with multiple medical interventions with restorative intent may facilitate a new, higher functioning baseline (Figure 29.1).

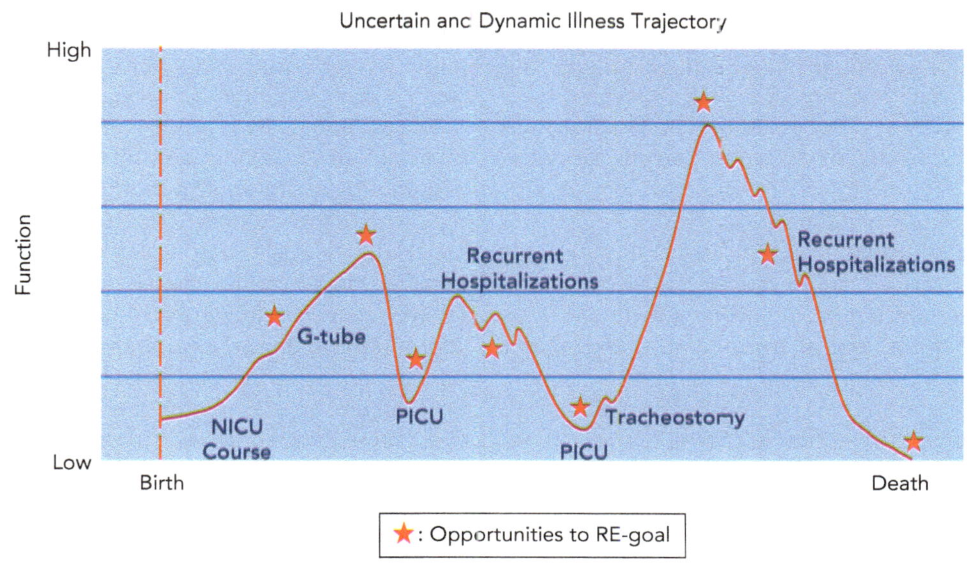

Figure 29.1 Dynamic goals of care.

Unlike an adult patient with chronic illness who may follow an anticipated trajectory of gradual functional decline compounded by acute exacerbations toward eventual end of life, children with rare CCCs may not follow such a predictable course. Figure 29.1 illustrates that goals of care consultation (denoted by the red stars) by perinatal PPC teams may be indicated prior to birth if congenital or chromosomal disease is anticipated. The NICU course often presents a life-threatening hospitalization, and shared decision-making is indicated toward long-term medical interventions that may or may not allow for improved functional status, development, and growth for the infant. Following NICU discharge, acute life-threatening hospitalizations including intensive care utilization may pose greater need for PPC consultation over the age continuum, outlining family-centered and values-driven recommendations regarding further complex medicalization and technology needs. Again, such interventions may or may not have profound restorative effects that allow the child and family to thrive and are balanced against an unpredictable time frame that often leads to an eventual recurrent pattern of hospitalizations, functional decline, and end of life. The dynamic nature of the clinical course for children with CCCs illustrates the need for the close partnership with families that PPC can foster to support the assessment of benefits and burdens of proposed interventions. The long-term relationship between PPC and children with CCCs and their families recognizes the need to "re-goal" or reassess goals of care as the benefit-burden calculus changes over the course of a child's illness trajectory—meaning what is weighed as beneficial at one point in time may be considered burdensome at another depending on the holistic consideration of the child's life.[11]

HEALTH SERVICES RECEIVED BY CCCS

Hospital data support a growing proportion of admissions in children with CCCs, and though these patients make-up only 10–22% of hospital admissions,[2,3] such admissions account for a far greater proportion of intensive care utilization, total hospital days, and nearly half of all pediatric hospital charges.[3,12] These data are driven most significantly by children with CCCs related to cardiovascular, congenital, neuromuscular, respiratory, and malignant disease. Readmissions for children with CCCs are influenced by polypharmacy and technology use.

Like hospital admissions for children with CCCs, technology use, including feeding tubes and tracheostomy along with long-term invasive and noninvasive mechanical ventilation, has increased in recent years. Children with CCCs account for the vast majority of gastrostomy tube placements, tracheostomies, and cerebral spinal fluid shunts in children.[3,13] Such interventions present high resource utilization and need for hospitalization often occurring in the last year of life.[14] Again, such findings speak to the uncertain nature of illness trajectories for children with CCCs. With declining functional status, it is paramount to identify that such decline may predict higher rates of hospitalization, intensive care utilization, and procedural and surgical interventions toward impending end of life and should be a trigger for PPC consultation.

PPC has been demonstrated to increase the frequency of establishing goals of care and advance care planning for children with life-threatening and life-limiting illness. This includes addressing resuscitation status and hospice involvement compared with patients who did not receive PPC consults.[15]

Clinical Vignette (Part 2)

Charlie has been hospitalized nine times since his initial discharge from the NICU for viral lower respiratory tract infections, new onset of seizures, ventriculoperitoneal shunt revision, and routine airway interventions. He has been diagnosed with epilepsy with multiple seizure types including infantile spasms and is maintained on three antiepileptic medications. He has a new diagnosis of spastic diplegia and is enrolled in the pediatric complex care clinic which specializes in the care of children with complex medical conditions and provides care coordination across the seven subspecialty providers who care for Charlie in the children's medical center.

Mary and Neal worry that Charlie's complex medical needs are causing pain and suffering. PPC is consulted to consider goals of care, symptom management, and support the family during this challenging course.

THE IMPACT OF CCCS ON THE FAMILY

Long-standing research has consistently demonstrated the psychosocial impact that CCCs may have on children and families. Studies on the psychological adjustment of parents of children with CCCs have demonstrated increased rates of mental health treatment, depression, and other affective disorders, including disparate coping processes between mothers and fathers.[16] Role conflicts significantly impact families of CCCs as parents and often siblings balance their family duties with also being an expert caregiver. Families must accommodate the technically challenging and substantial responsibilities of caring for a medically complex child, including teaching in-home and in-hospital healthcare professionals how best to care for their child while maintaining identities as a mother and father.[17] Siblings of children with CCCs may also experience impaired psychological functioning including depression and anxiety and even impaired cognitive development—although they may also experience tremendous growth, responsibility, and pride.[8] In addition to psychosocial challenges, families of children with CCCs often experience financial hardship. Many families report changes to employment, financial burdens related to the child's healthcare costs, and difficulty in paying mortgages or utilities.[19] Despite these challenges, families also find strength, resilience, joy, and love as a result of parenting a child with CCCs, and more research is needed to understand these from both parent and sibling perspectives.

As such, the care of children with CCCs must consider family-based outcomes through a comprehensive scope. This should not only consider the health and quality of life of the child, but also the function and resilience of the entire family.[7] The role of PPC in the care of the family is consistently cited as an essential standard of care.[20,21] Parental and family support from PPC over the trajectory of the child's illness offers essential critical partnership in decision-making, coping, and identifying mechanisms to address financial stressors, access to mental health services, spiritual support, and counseling.

TRANSITION TO ADULTHOOD

As children with CCCs live longer, there are mounting challenges in the transition into adulthood. Often children with CCCs continue living with genetic or congenital, neurologic, or childhood multisystem diseases traditionally cared for by pediatric experts. For many, chronological age alone drives a transition into adult care, and families may be asked to leave a long-standing supportive care structure for a new adult healthcare setting. Such a transition risks imparting a sense of abandonment, loss, and even fear with the loss of care coordination and family support integral in pediatric care.[22] PPC can play a valuable role in facilitating a holistic transition by outlining the family's goals of care with new providers while reviewing advance care planning. Depending on the child's cognitive capacity, such a transition should support psychosocial development as much as clinical care with careful steps to empower the child to gradually gain ownership of her or his complex medical management when possible. Given the expertise by which PPC builds a trusted clinical relationship with families, PPC is essential to ensure a successful goals-driven transition.

In addition to the clinical and psychosocial transition into adulthood, there are additional legal considerations to ensure a seamless transition across the care continuum. For young adults with significant neurologic or psychomotor impairment who are dependent on their caregivers for medical decision-making and delivery of complex technology-assisted home care, legally appointed guardianship for parents is necessary to ensure the family maintains parental authority for medical and social decision-making for their child. Pediatric complex care programs in partnership with PPC should anticipate the need to legally secure guardianship at the age of 18 for the majority of young adults with severe cognitive disabilities. This planning should begin in early adolescence and requires integral knowledge of a community's social and legal resources, potential out-of-home placement options, and advance care planning.

UNIQUE NEEDS OF PATIENTS WITH CCCS AND THEIR FAMILIES

This section explores the needs, challenges, and opportunities of caring for children with CCCs and their families. As previously noted, the population of children with CCCs has been increasing steadily with advances in technology and medical care. However, the ability to meet the varied needs of this vulnerable population has lagged behind.[23] A 2016 National Academies Press Workshop that focused on quality and accessible care for children with disabilities and complex health needs summarized the challenges many of these children and their families face

> Uneven public and professional awareness of their conditions and a research base marked by significant gaps have led to programs, practices, and policies that are inconsistent in quality and coverage. Parents often have to navigate and coordinate, largely on their own, a variety of social, medical, and educational support services, adding to the already daunting financial, logistical, and emotional challenges of raising children with special needs. The unmet needs of children with disabilities and complex medical and educational needs can cause great suffering for these children and for those who love and care for them.[24]

HOME CARE AND NURSING CHALLENGES

Children with CCCs typically require 24-hour care. Most of these children are dependent on two or more technologies, such as tube feeding and ventilatory support.[25,26] Most, if not all, of this care falls to the family caregiver, most often the mother.[26,27] Home nursing care is often prescribed to assist the children and families, offer some respite, and allow parents to attend to other children and other needs. Additionally, home nursing can provide education and support for the family to learn how to care for the varied needs of their child.

Home care can be provided in the home with a physicians' order and third-party payer authorization, most commonly Medicaid.[4] Home care can be visit or shift-based care. The care coordination and networks of care needed to support children with CCCs at home can be extensive, and community coalitions can help to strength collaborative ties between organizations.[28] Challenges to home care include variability in available services across and within states. Additionally, home care agencies often face significant staffing shortages which impact the number of patients that can be served and the number of shifts that can be covered for any child.

Parents may need to be better prepared for some of these challenges, including the difficulty in filling home nursing hours and the potential for fluctuating levels of support at home over time. For nurses working in home care, there can be significant professional satisfaction, providing autonomy in practice, the opportunity to establish a close relationship with patient and family, and the ability to advocate for the patients' needs. However, home care can also be challenging for a nurse who is used to working within a structured environment such as a hospital, where the professional providers are in the positions of authority. For many nurses, home care may be a completely new experience. Nurses in home care are guests in their patients' home; they are not in charge. Add to this the needs of a child with CCCs, sibling support, parents/

guardian needs, and the needs of other family members. There are additional challenges in providing care in a patients' home such as isolation, boundary issues, limited resources, differences in socioeconomic status, and differences in living conditions (such as the number of members in a household). Additionally, practical needs include space for all the equipment, medications, and supplies needed for the care of the child, which can be significant.

The addition of community-based PPC services also increases opportunities for healthcare providers and services for children and their families. Unfortunately, community-based PPC is often not available, and access to services can be difficult. With the Affordable Care Act, children with CCCs nearing end of life can be supported by home hospice in addition to home nursing through the *concurrent care* provision—although there is substantial variability state to state, and access to services must be determined on a local level. Palliative and hospice care in the home is visit-based: it is different from home visit or shift-nursing care. This is a common source of misunderstanding when a family is first introduced to PPC or hospice care at home, as many expect shift-nursing care similar to what they received in the hospital. PPC is always provided by an interdisciplinary team, whereas home care can be provided by an interdisciplinary team if the physician orders discipline-specific therapies for the care of the patient. Unfortunately, all these factors contribute to more confusion and disconnects for the family.

IT TAKES A COMMUNITY: SCHOOL AND DEVELOPMENTAL SERVICE PROVISIONS

The primary goal for most families with children with CCCs is to provide as normal a lived experience as possible for their child; for many that includes going to school. School programs for children with special needs are not uncommon; however, the services provided may range from simply custodial to full integration with needed services such as physical therapy, occupational therapy, or speech therapy integrated into the special needs programs.

Grouped services are much more common for younger children in schools than they are for older children and adolescents, and families may have to try to maneuver between school and several different appointments and settings to get the services their child needs.[29] A useful tool is *care mapping*. Antonelli and Lind define care mapping as, "a process which guides and supports the ability of families and care professionals to work together to achieve the best possible health outcomes."[30] This tool helps facilitate the many needs between "home care, healthcare, school and community." There are "how-to" PDFs available for families and professionals; family information about care mapping can be found at http://www.childrenshospital.org/~/media/care-coordination/caremappingforfamilies21813.ashx?la=en&hash=DF739259501C48A1B099375D79D944F2D5478E2A. For professionals, information can be found at https://www.childrenshospital.org/~/media/care-coordination/caremappingforprofessionals21813.ashx?la=en

ISOLATION AND THE LOSS OF "NORMAL"

Despite the many appointments a child with CCCs has and the number of individuals needed to provide care for each child, having a child with significant medical needs can be isolating.[31] Often the parenting role is focused on the medical needs of their child, determining signs of imminent decline or pain and discomfort. As noted previously, these children require around-the-clock care and technology to help them survive, which means several pieces of equipment to provide that technology. The practical challenge of trying to go anywhere, in addition to the multiple healthcare appointments, can be daunting and so going out of the home is often avoided. Added to that are the risk of infection for children who are often immunocompromised, which often also results in parents avoiding family gatherings or other social events, thus complicating an already isolating existence.[32–34]

Often with the birth of a child with CCCs or a diagnosis later on in childhood or adolescence, there is a sense of loss and grief.[31,35,36] This loss includes thoughts of what might have been and the grief that comes with that loss. Amber Conn writes on her blog about the grief she feels since she heard of her daughters' condition. With more than 1.7 million subscribers, her words hit home for many.

> The moment we heard the words "Alexander disease" and "three-to-five-year life expectancy," I began grieving. . . . I grieve for my child, who was at one point healthy, vibrant, and full of life. I grieve for the life we dreamed of having—watching our child play sports and having play dates like typical kids. (Conn, 2018, https://themighty.com/2018/09/grief-parenting-medically-complex-child/)

MULTIDISCIPLINARY CARE

There is a growing body of literature focused on the many needs of a child with CCCs, including the need for specialized equipment, multidisciplinary specialty care, the fragmentation of care, and the challenges of navigating that care.[36] Box 29.1 is a list of providers who can support CCCs and their families; it also demonstrates the number of providers that families often interact with for the care of their child. This list is not exhaustive; it is not unusual, for example, for one child to have multiple subspecialty physicians involved with their care such as pulmonary, gastroenterology, neurology, orthopedics, and rehabilitation medicine.

The *medical home model* is often cited as preferred to provide comprehensive care to a child with CCCs. The medical home provides the advantage of limiting the number of appointments at different clinics or providers, decreasing fragmentation of care, increasing the ability for comprehensive care coordination, and enhancing communication between providers. Unfortunately, although the medical home model is growing, most families find their care fragmented between the tertiary medical center for subspecialty care and their community providers with limited ability to coordinate appointments.[23,27] An example of the complexity of

BOX 29.1 PROVIDERS WHO CAN SUPPORT CHILDREN WITH COMPLEX CHRONIC CONDITIONS AND THEIR FAMILIES

- Social worker
- Clinical nurse
- Child psychologist/Psychiatrist
- Child life specialist
- Chaplain
- Art therapist
- Music therapist
- Physical therapist
- Occupational therapist
- Speech therapist
- Subspecialty physicians
- Hospice providers
- Grief specialist/Therapist
- Pediatrician
- School counselor/Principal
- Camp/Camp staff

multidisciplinary needs for a family with a child with CCCs is shown in Figure 29.2.

Clinical Vignette (Part 3)

In partnership with complex care, PPC outlines goals of care that align with prioritizing home care for Charlie in lieu of hospitalization whenever possible. Mary and Neal hope that by doing so, this will allow Charlie to engage with his family as much as possible and avoid long-term hospitalizations that significantly burden him and his family physically, emotionally, and financially. Multispecialty clinic visits are streamlined, and action plans regarding mechanical ventilation support, antibiotic prescribing, breakthrough seizure control, and pain management are created to assist Mary and Neal along with home nursing to address clinical concerns in the home with the goal of preventing hospitalization.

THE ROLE OF PEDIATRIC PALLIATIVE CARE TEAMS

This section explores the different roles of the PPC team and how they support children with CCCs and their families.

COLLABORATION WITH CHILDREN AND PARENTS

PPC teams often form partnerships with families to provide the best care possible for children with CCCs.[37,38] Children with CCCs may be able share what makes them happy and what gives their life meaning with PPC teams.[39] For younger children or those with severe cognitive disabilities, parents and families are often experts in understanding what brings their child joy and when their child is well. This can be understood through facial expression, vocalization, energy level, excitement, and posturing. Similarly, for parents who are unable to interpret these details about their child for whatever reason, PPC teams can ask questions to elucidate these aspects of quality of life. "All About Me" posters and signs can be created to share more about specific likes and dislikes of an individual child as well as what brings them comfort (Figure 29.3). The PPC team's ability to astutely listen for this information is essential to formulating care plans with the child's joy, comfort, and quality of life in mind.

PPC teams can also support children with CCCs and parents through ongoing psychosocial support as they adjust to the roller coaster of the ups and downs associated with complex chronic disease. Whether adapting to an unexpected genetic diagnosis prenatally or a traumatic injury resulting in a new baseline health status, PPC teams know that grief is a part of the journey.[40] They also know that "new norms" are created and that there is tremendous growth that comes along with the hardships of caring for a chronically ill child.[37] PPC teams can stay attuned to this as it happens naturally and at its own pace—while knowing that sometimes this peace may not be reached at all or is only achieved many years after a child's death.

COLLABORATION WITH OTHER HEALTHCARE PROVIDERS AND CLINICAL TEAMS

PPC teams can also help to meet the needs of children with CCCs and their families through collaborative care with other clinical teams.[37] Increasingly, children with CCCs are cared for by a myriad of subspecialists or in complex care programs.[41] These programs are designed to help families through care coordination and access to community services.[42] These programs often have dedicated resources for coordinating appointments, streamlining communication with medical teams, and accessing home nursing care and developmental therapies. All of these aspects of care are essential for children with CCCs.

What these programs may be less attuned to is the need to tease apart the nuances of tradeoffs in medical decision-making with families. Often, parents of children with CCCs live in constant uncertainty about the future. Given our limited ability to prognosticate, they typically do not know what to expect in terms of life expectancy and/or further decline in their child's health. Children may also go without a unifying diagnosis. Although healthcare providers have become increasingly comfortable with a "wait and see" approach, parents can be left feeling isolated and alone with little to no answers as a scaffold for their child's care plan. Although uncertainty is the norm, PPC teams can listen to these concerns, normalize, and provide an illness trajectory framework to limit uncertainty and anticipate future decision points.[43] Having walked with other families on similar journeys, PPC teams can meet families where they are, help them to anticipate both good days and bad days as part of their child's health trajectory, and provide psychosocial support.[44]

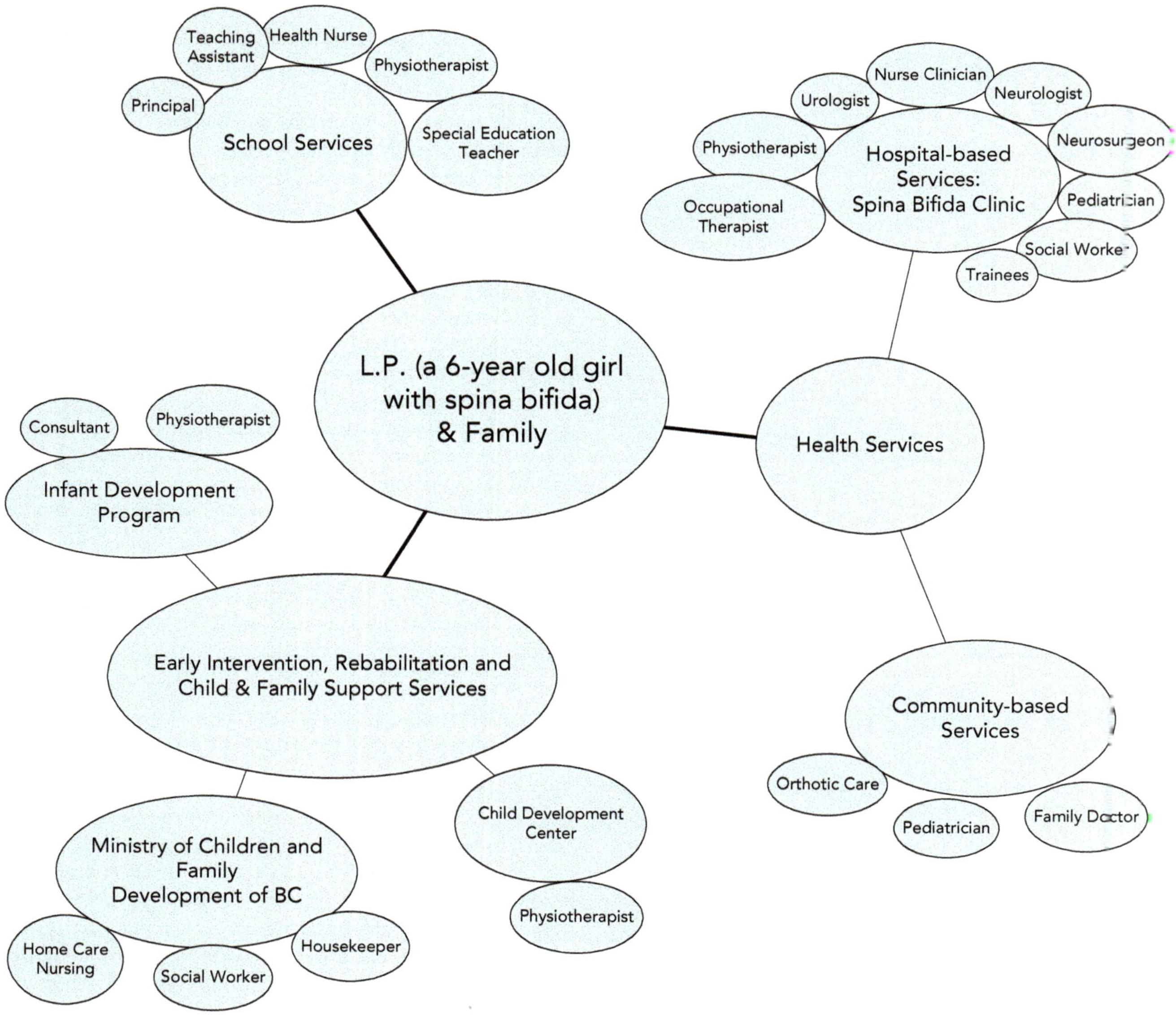

Figure 29.2 *Service network diagram.*

This is particularly important in times of stress, such as during a hospitalization or acute decline. Parents of children with CCCs can be better served by anticipating care decisions beforehand in less urgent or emergent circumstances.[45] This can be accomplished through gentle and compassionate conversations with the PPC team about concerns that may arise in the future. The PPC team can also determine if other healthcare providers, such as the child's long-term pulmonologist or pediatrician, is the best person to have these discussions. If so, the PPC team can encourage these conversations, provide recommendations or training on how to proceed in a way that is supportive to families, and help to complete any documentation needed to support family decisions.[45] Many healthcare providers are not aware of advance care planning tools such as Voicing My Choices, Five Wishes, or Physician Orders for Life-Sustaining Treatment (POLST, https://polst.org/national-form/) forms, and PPC teams can share these resources.[46] PPC teams can also provide direct communication training and education to healthcare providers in their community or help providers identify national/international resources on palliative care for children, including the American Academy of Pediatrics (AAP), VitalTalk (vitaltalk.org), the End of Life Nursing Education Consortium (ELNEC; aacnnursing.org/ELNEC), and the National Consensus Project (https://www.nationalcoalitionhpc.org/ncp/).

PPC teams also can help to determine when further testing and medical evaluations including imaging or laboratory testing are unlikely to reveal new or actionable information.[43] This can be hard for other healthcare providers to adapt to because it is far from the norm when it comes to medical care, especially when there are ongoing intractable medical issues. PPC teams can offer recommendations regarding time-limited trials of interventions or "testing" interventions, such as feeding, through the "lens of comfort" for the child.[43] For example, for a child with severe cognitive disability, a decision

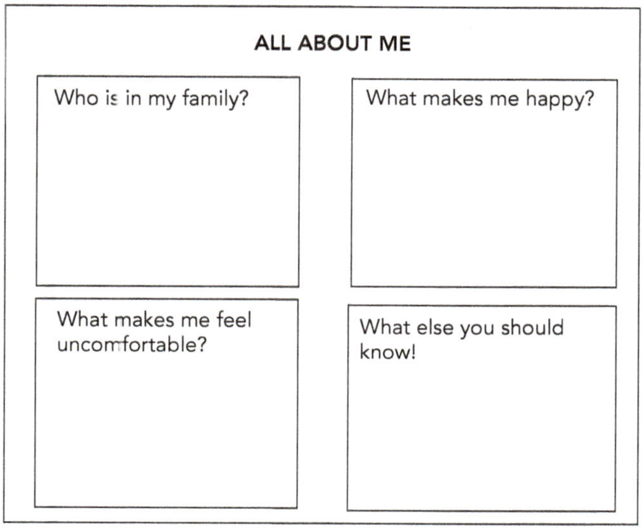

Figure 29.3 All about me.

might be made to determine what level of feeding is comfortable for the child and use that as the "test" to determine what is optimal.[47] In contrast, a family with a child with Trisomy 18 with abdominal discomfort might feel that their concerns are being brushed aside because of their child's underlying condition, and PPC teams can help advocate for more testing and evaluation when needed and if consistent with family values.

ADDRESSING SYMPTOMS

PPC teams can also support children with CCCs by paying attention to their symptoms and having a symptom-focused approach to treatment. Other healthcare providers may be more focused on fixing the underlying medical problem, such as addressing poor ventilation with increased respiratory support. PPC teams can complement this by simultaneously addressing dyspnea and also how the increased use of ventilatory support is affecting quality of life.[48] For children with CCCs, both of these perspectives about care are essential.

PPC teams are also expert in thinking through how symptoms are impacting daily routines and activities that are important to the child and family. PPC teams can help negotiate medication and treatment schedules so that they also take these issues into account.[49] For example, a young adult who is struggling to come to dialysis may not be giving signs that they are ready for a more comfort-focused approach to care, but instead may need additional psychosocial support and a reassessment of how to fit dialysis into the life they want to live. Attention to timing, schedules, and how chronic care fits into quality of life are often important roles for PPC teams.

PPC teams can also address symptoms through active symptom assessment over time and medication management. Increasingly, there are validated measures for symptom assessment and tracking.[50,51] For children with severe cognitive disabilities, the individualized numeric rating scale can give parents more control in helping healthcare providers and other caregivers to recognize their child's symptoms, such as pain or discomfort.[50] PPC teams can also notice drug-drug interactions and assess for side effects from medications. Similarly, they also know that many symptoms are interrelated—such as pain and sleep—and can assess for these simultaneously.[49,51]

For children with CCCs, another essential aspect of symptom management is nonpharmacologic. Children and their parents want a holistic approach to symptoms through the use of techniques such as positioning, massage, acupuncture, and aromatherapy.[52] This is particularly important for children with severe cognitive disabilities.[52] Many of these children have sensitivities and particular needs to support their comfort. This can include positioning, vibration, light/dark, noise, and music. Each child is different and talking to parents about what makes their child special and how the environment and play can be adapted for them is essential to honoring them as children and supporting parents. Other healthcare providers that may work in conjunction with the PPC team, such as child life specialists, are essential.

In addition, PPC teams often are comfortable with a "trial and error" approach and can counsel families about this, particularly when symptoms are expected to be difficult to treat or get rid of completely.[49] PPC teams can set these expectations ahead of time with children with CCCs and their families, along with the promise of non-abandonment and a willingness to keep trying and to use a multimodal approach.[49] (For further details about specific management of common neurological symptoms in children with CCCs please see Chapter 19.)

RELATIONSHIPS

Children with CCCs and their families often require frequent medical care that necessitates coming in and out of the medical system. Unfortunately, our medical system is still struggling to meet the needs of medically complex patients. PPC teams can offset this by being a consistent presence for families through various siloed outpatient clinics and during inpatient care. Having a small team that knows you and your child is often the antidote families need when facing complex systems, when they need additional advocacy, and during times of crisis.[53] To provide continuity of care, sign-out between PPC team members is important so that everyone knows the child and family. Hospital-based PPC teams can also partner with home-based PPC and hospice teams in the community to streamline services and continuity of care.[54,55] Often community teams know best about how care is being provided in the home and what would make things easier for the child and family.[56] They are often creative problem-solvers who find resources and help create joyful experiences in the home. Hospital-based teams can be in close contact with home-based teams to get updates on children and their families. In this way, when families are in subspecialty clinics or hospitalized, the hospital based PPC team is up to date and ready to address issues in real-time. Hospital-based teams may also have more dedicated PPC expertise and can provide back-up and training for more adult-focused home-based palliative care and hospice teams so that children and families can receive care in the home if that is what is important to them.[55]

These relationships are also essential to making decisions about goals of care and about advance care planning.[44] It often takes healthcare providers who have known the child and family long-term to be able to point out how quality of life has changed and to be a "safe" person for parents to talk to about regret, challenges, and how care goals may have shifted. PPC teams can use their communication skills and listening presence to have these conversations to tease out what is most important and create care plans that honor children and family's values.[20]

GRIEF AND LOSS SUPPORT

Children with CCCs and their families face ongoing losses and grief throughout their child's life. This may start perinatally with decisions about how to move forward when a child is expected to be born with multiple medical problems, such as severe complex congenital heart disease. It may occur following a traumatic brain injury in an otherwise healthy child. It can also be more insidious, as children with CCCs become frailer or need to compromise/change their lifestyle over time due to their health. These losses often go unaddressed and underappreciated by healthcare providers. Even very young children may struggle with how their bodies are changing and what limitations they have in comparison to their peers. The feelings of loss that go along with these issues can be isolating—particularly when popular culture denies opportunities to share sadness, guilt, and loneliness and when people are supposed to present themselves as strong and self-sufficient. PPC teams know that children and parents need outlets to express themselves. They can provide that outlet and/or help families explore what gives them strength and purpose.

Another significant aspect of chronic disease is anticipatory grief. Young adults with CCCs may think about the future, including their own death, and they need outlets to express these concerns. Similarly, parents of children with CCCs may be grieving not only the loss of having a "normal," healthy child, but also worry about expected changes in their child's health and their child's eventual death. Even when issues such as worsening lung function or changes in mobility are not predicted for many years, children and parents can grieve their eventual loss even if the timeline is uncertain. Similarly, death can be very present for families even from the start of a CCC, and typically healthcare providers are not equipped to address these ongoing or taboo concerns. PPC teams who build relationships may be the most able to speak directly to these fears in a gentle and compassionate manner that feels welcoming and supportive.[40]

PPC teams also know that support needs to be ongoing throughout chronic illness and also after a child's death. There is no expiration date on grief, and parents can continue to grieve and grow following the death of their child for the rest of their lives.[40] PCC teams can provide opportunities to talk about ongoing grief, offer support groups, and tailor resources to meet individual family needs. PPC teams who participate in research can also give parents the opportunity to be a part of ongoing studies aimed at improving care for children with CCCs.[57,58] This may not be right for every family, but many parents welcome the opportunity to "give back" and help make the struggles they and their child faced "mean something larger than themselves."[57,58] Regardless, many families want their child's life to extend beyond their death, and PPC teams can find opportunities to support this for parents. Other important resources include those created by other parents who have had children with CCCs and have also experienced grief/loss. Courageous Parents Network (https://courageousparentsnetwork.org/) can help parents navigate many of these experiences.

Clinical Vignette (Part 4)

Over the course of the next several years, with intensive concurrent complex and palliative supportive care, Charlie is able to "finally thrive and be happy for the first time in his life," according to Mary. Charlie remains relatively healthy, avoiding respiratory infections and only rarely requiring hospitalization for acute illness or seizures. Neal identifies that complications related to polypharmacy or medical interventions are very infrequent and credits expert care coordination and goals-driven care plans for the significant improvement in Charlie's quality of life. "Charlie is the core of our family and brings joy to us and his sisters every day."

With marked pulmonary improvement and lung development, Charlie's tracheostomy is removed, and he is liberated from chronic mechanical ventilation. He is nonambulatory, but social work support from PPC has been instrumental in identifying local- and state-level resources to support assisted equipment to aid his mobility. The family is well-connected with Charlie's interdisciplinary team and navigates most acute clinical concerns as an outpatient.

REFERENCES

1. Newacheck PW, Strickland B, Shonkoff JP, et al. An epidemiologic profile of children with special health care needs. *Pediatrics.* 1998;102(1 Pt 1):117–123. doi:10.1542/peds.102.1.117
2. Bucholz EM, Toomey SL, Schuster MA. Trends in pediatric hospitalizations and readmissions: 2010–2016. *Pediatrics.* 2019;143(2):e20181958–12. doi:10.1542/peds.2018-1958
3. Simon TD, Berry J, Feudtner C, et al. Children with complex chronic conditions in inpatient hospital settings in the United States. *Pediatrics.* 2010;126(4):647–655. doi:10.1542/peds.2009-3266
4. Agrawal R, Smith T, Li Y, Cartland J. Rate of spending on chronic conditions among Medicaid and CHIP recipients. *Pediatrics.* 2014;134(1):e80–e87. doi:10.1542/peds.2013-2947
5. Edwards JD, Houtrow AJ, Vasilevskis EE, et al. Chronic conditions among children admitted to U.S. pediatric intensive care units: Their prevalence and impact on risk for mortality and prolonged

length of stay. *Crit Care Med.* 2012;40(7):2196–2203. doi:10.1097/CCM.0bC13e31824e68cf
6. Feudtner C, Hays RM, Haynes G, Geyer JR, Neff JM, Koepsell TD. Deaths attributed to pediatric complex chronic conditions: National trends and implications for supportive care services. *Pediatrics.* 2001;107(6):e99–e99. doi:10.1542/peds.107.6.e99
7. Cohen E, Kuo DZ, Agrawal R, et al. Children with medical complexity: An emerging population for clinical and research initiatives. *Pediatrics.* 2011;127(3):529–538. doi:10.1542/peds.2010-0910
8. Murray SA, Kendall M, Boyd K, Sheikh A. Illness trajectories and palliative care. *BMJ.* 2005;330(7498):1007.
9. Kalzén H, Larsson B, Eksborg S, Lindberg L, Edberg KE, Frostell C. Survival after PICU admission: The impact of multiple admissions and complex chronic conditions. *PLoS One.* 2018;13(4):e0193294–14. doi:10.1371/journal.pone.0193294
10. DeCourcey D, Silverman M, Oladunjoye A, Balkin E, Wolfe J. Patterns of care at the end of life for children and young adults with life-threatening complex chronic conditions. *J Pediatrics.* 2018;193:196–203.e2. doi:10.1016/j.jpeds.2017.09.078
11. Klick JC, Ballantine A. Providing care in chronic disease: The ever-changing balance of integrating palliative and restorative medicine. *Pediatr Clin N Am.* 2007;54(5):799–812. doi:10.1016/j.pcl.2007.07.003
12. Silber JH, Rosenbaum PR, Pimentel SD, et al. Comparing resource use in medical admissions of children with complex chronic conditions. *Med Care.* 2019;57(8):615–624. doi:10.1097/MLR.0000000000001149
13. McDougall CM, Adderley RJ, Wensley DF, Seear MD. Long-term ventilation in children: Longitudinal trends and outcomes. *Arch Dis Child.* 2013;98(9):660–665. doi:10.1136/archdischild-2012-303062
14. Ananth P, Melvin P, Feudtner C, Wolfe J, Berry JG. Hospital use in the last year of fife for children with life-threatening complex chronic conditions. *Pediatrics.* 2015;136(5):938–946. doi:10.1542/peds.2015-0260
15. Harmoney K, Mobley EM, Gilbertson-White S, Brogden NK, Benson RJ. Differences in advance care planning and circumstances of death for pediatric patients who do and do not receive palliative care consults: A single-center retrospective review of all pediatric deaths from 2012 to 2016. *J Palliat Med.* 2019;22(12):1506–1514. doi:10.1089/jpm.2019.0111
16. Wallander JL, Varni JW. Effects of pediatric chronic physical disorders on child and family adjustment. *J Child Psychol Psychiatry.* 1998;39(1):29–46.
17. Ratliffe CE, Harrigan RC, Haley J, Tse A, Olson T. Stress in families with medically fragile children. *Issues Compr Pediatr Nurs.* 2002 25(3):167–188. doi:10.1080/01460860290042558
18. Sharpe D, Rossiter L. Siblings of children with a chronic illness: A meta-analysis. *J Pediatr Psychol.* 2002;27(8):699–710. doi:10.1093/jpepsy/27.8.699
19. Thomson J, Shah SS, Simmons JM, et al. Financial and social hardships in families of children with medical complexity. *J Pediatr.* 2016;172:187–193.e1. doi:10.1016/j.jpeds.2016.01.049
20. Section on Hospice and Palliative Medicine and Committee on Hospital Care. Pediatric palliative care and hospice care commitments, guidelines, and recommendations. *Pediatrics.* 2013;132(5):966–972. doi:10.1542/peds.2013-2731
21. Kearney JA, Salley CG, Muriel AC. Standards of Psychosocial Care for Parents of Children with Cancer. *Pediatr Blood Cancer.* 2015;62:S632–S683. https://doi.org/10.1002/pbc.25761
22. Davies H, Rennick J, Majnemer A. Transition from pediatric to adult health care for young adults with neurological disorders: Parental perspectives. *Can J Neurosci Nurs.* 2011;33(2):32–39.
23. Cohen E, Berry JG, Sanders L, Schor EL, Wise PH. Status complexicus? The emergence of pediatric complex care. *Pediatrics.* 2018;141(Suppl 3):S202–S211. doi:10.1542/peds.2017-1284E
24. Planning Committee for the Workshop on Funding Opportunities for Evidence-Based Prevention and Interventions to Promote Children's Cognitive, Affective, and Behavioral Health, Forum on Promoting Children's Cognitive, Affective, and Behavioral Health, Board on Children, Youth, and Families, Division of Behavioral and Social Sciences and Education, National Academies of Sciences, Engineering, and Medicine. Ensuring quality and accessible care for children with disabilities and complex health and educational needs: Workshop in brief. June 2016. doi:10.17226/23544.
25. Feudtner C, Villareale N, Morray B, Sharp V, Hays RM, Neff JM. Technology-dependency among patients discharged from a children's hospital: A retrospective cohort study. *BMC Pediatr.* 2005;5(1):8. doi:10.1186/1471-2431-5-8
26. Lazzarin P, Schiavon B, Brugnaro L, Benini F. Parents spend an average of nine hours a day providing palliative care for children at home and need to maintain an average of five life-saving devices. *Acta Paediatr.* 2017;107(2):289–293. doi:10.1111/apa.14098
27. Cordeiro A, Davis RK, Antonelli R, et al. Care coordination for children and youth with special health care needs: National survey results. *Clin Pediatr.* 2018;57(12):1398–1408. doi:10.1177/0009922818783501
28. Nageswaran S, Golden SL, Easterling D, O'Shea TM, Hansen WB, Ip EH. Factors associated with collaboration among agencies serving children with complex chronic conditions. *Matern Child Health J.* 2013;17(9):1533–1540. doi:10.1007/s10995-012-1032-9
29. Bailey S, O'Connell B, Pearce J. The transition from paediatric to adult health care services for young adults with a disability: An ethical perspective. *Aust Health Review.* 2003;26(1):64–67. doi:10.1071/AH030064
30. Antonelli R, Lind C. Care Mapping: A how-to guide for patients and families. 2020. www.childrenshospital.org
31. Collins A, Hennessy-Anderson N, Hosking S, Hynson J, Remedios C, Thomas K. Lived experiences of parents caring for a child with a life-limiting condition in Australia: A qualitative study. *Palliat Med.* 2016;30(10):950–959. doi:10.1177/0269216316634245
32. Mesman GR, Kuo D, Carroll JL, Ward WL. The impact of technology dependence on children and their families. *J Pediatr Health Care.* 2013;27(6):451–459. doi:10.1016/j.pedhc.2012.05.003
33. Alfonso M, Walker A, Gupta A, Telfair J, Colquit G. "It all goes back to the services": A rural/urban comparison of service providers' perceptions of challenges and facilitators to disability services. *OJPM.* 2015;05(10):434–440. doi:10.4236/ojpm.2015.510048
34. Yantzi NM, Rosenberg MW, McKeever P. Getting out of the house: The challenges mothers face when their children have long-term care needs. *Health Social Care Commun.* 2006;15(1):45–55. doi:10.1111/j.1365-2524.2006.00663.x
35. Miller AR, Condin CJ, McKellin WH, Shaw N, Klassen AF, Sheps S. Continuity of care for children with complex chronic health conditions: Parents' perspectives. *BMC Health Serv Res.* 2009;9(1):242. doi:10.1186/1472-6963-9-242
36. Currie G, Szabo J. "It is like a jungle gym, and everything is under construction": The parent's perspective of caring for a child with a rare disease. *Child Care Health Dev.* 2019;45(1):96–103. doi:10.1111/cch.12628
37. Carosella A, Snyder A, Ward E. What parents of children with complex medical conditions want their child's physicians to understand. *JAMA Pediatr.* 2018;172(4):315–316. doi:10.1001/jamapediatrics.2017.3931
38. Walter JK, DeCamp LR, Warrier KS, Murphy TP, Keefer PM. Care of the complex chronically ill child by generalist pediatricians: Lessons learned from pediatric palliative care. *Hosp Pediatr.* 2013;3(2):129–138.
39. Vuillerot C, Hodgkinson I, Bissery A, et al. Self-perception of quality of life by adolescents with neuromuscular diseases. *J Adolesc Health.* 2010;46(1):70–76. doi:10.1016/j.jadohealth.2009.05.005
40. Snaman JM, Kaye EC, Torres C, Gibson DV, Baker JN. Helping parents live with the hole in their heart: The role of health care providers and institutions in the bereaved parents' grief journeys. *Cancer.* May 2016. doi:10.1002/cncr.30087

41. Pordes E, Gordon J, Sanders LM, Cohen E. Models of care delivery for children with medical complexity. *Pediatrics.* 2018;141(Suppl 3):S212–S223. doi:10.1542/peds.2017-1284F
42. Cohen E, Lacombe-Duncan A, Spalding K, et al. Integrated complex care coordination for children with medical complexity: A mixed-methods evaluation of tertiary care-community collaboration. *BMC Health Serv Res*. 2012;12(1):1–11.
43. Bogetz JF, Hauer J. Certainty of decisions: A process-based model for decision making for children with severe neurological impairment. *Clin Pediatr.* 2018;57(10):1227–1231. doi:10.1177/0009922817740668
44. Levetown M, American Academy of Pediatrics Committee on Bioethics. Communicating with children and families: From everyday interactions to skill in conveying distressing information. *Pediatrics.* 2008;121(5):e1441–e1460. doi:10.1542/peds.2008-0565
45. Orkin J, Beaune L, Moore C, et al. Toward an understanding of advance care planning in children with medical complexity. *Pediatrics.* 2020;145(3):e20192241. doi:10.1542/peds.2019-2241
46. Fraser J, Harris N, Berringer AJ, Prescott H, Finlay F. Advanced care planning in children with life-limiting conditions: The Wishes Document. *Arch Dis Childh.* 2010;95(2):79–82. doi:10.1136/adc.2009.160051
47. Hauer J. Feeding intolerance in children with severe impairment of the central nervous system: Strategies for treatment and prevention. *Children*. 2018;5(1):1. doi:10.1136/adc.2004.061440
48. Hauer JM. Respiratory symptom management in a child with severe neurologic impairment. *J Palliat Med.* 2007;10(5):1201–1207. doi:10.1089/jpm.2007.9907
49. Hauer J. *Caring for Children Who Have Severe Neurological Impairment*. Johns Hopkins University Press; 2013.
50. Solodiuk JC, Scott-Sutherland J, Meyers M, et al. Validation of the Individualized Numeric Rating Scale (INRS): A pain assessment tool for nonverbal children with intellectual disability. *Pain*. 2010;150(2):231–236. doi:10.1016/j.pain.2010.03.016
51. Hauer J, Houtrow AJ, Section on Hospice and Palliative Medicine, Council on Children with Disabilities. Pain assessment and treatment in children with significant impairment of the central nervous system. *Pediatrics.* 2017;139(6):e20171002–e20171002. doi:10.1542/peds.2017-1002
52. Friedrichsdorf SJ, Kang TI. The management of pain in children with life-limiting illnesses. *Pediatr Clin N Am*. 2007;54(5):645–672. doi:10.1016/j.pcl.2007.07.007
53. Weaver M, Wichman C, Darnall C, Bace S, Vail C, Macfadyen A. Proxy-Reported Quality Of Life And Family Impact For Children Followed Longitudinally By A Pediatric Palliative Care Team. *J Palliat Med*. 2018;21(2):241–244. doi:10.1089/jpm.2017.0092
54. Foster CC, Agrawal RK, Davis MM. Home health care for children with medical complexity: Workforce gaps, policy, and future directions. *Health Affairs (Project Hope)*. 2019;38(6):987–993. doi:10.1377/hlthaff.2018.05531
55. Kaye E, Gattas M, Kiefer A, et al. Provision of palliative and hospice care to children in the community: A population study of hospice nurses. *J Pain Symptom Manage*. December 2018:1-10. doi:10.1016/j.jpainsymman.2018.10.509
56. Carroll JM, Torkildson C, Winsness JS. Issues related to providing quality pediatric palliative care in the community. *Pediatr Clin N Am*. 2007;54(5):813–827. doi:10.1016/j.pcl.2007.06.002
57. Steele R, Cadell S, Siden H, Andrews G, Smit Quosai T, Feichtinger L. Impact of research participation on parents of seriously ill children. *J Palliat Med*. 2014;17(7):788–796. doi:10.1089/jpm.2013.0529
58. Weaver MS, Mooney-Doyle K, Kelly KP, et al. The benefits and burdens of pediatric palliative care and end-of-life research: A systematic review. *J Palliat Med.* March 2019:jpm.2018.0483–12. doi:10.1089/jpm.2018.0483

30 | ADVANCED HEART DISEASE

MELISSA K. COUSINO, CHELSEA HENEGHAN, AND ELIZABETH D. BLUME

> She looks *good* today. . . . I actually said that to a visitor today. My daughter just came off ECMO, is on continuous dialysis and has tubes coming out of nearly every part of her. She is no longer an ECMO candidate, and we aren't sure if her (transplanted) heart will recover . . . and I said that . . . *she looks good today.* How desensitized am I? She said she wants this still. And I want this still. But, I worry about her future . . . our future.

INTRODUCTION

In contrast to adults, advanced heart disease (AHD) is a rare condition in children, with approximately 11,000–14,000 heart failure-related pediatric hospitalizations occurring annually in the United States.[1] There are two primary etiologies of pediatric AHD: cardiomyopathy and congenital heart disease (CHD). The overall incidence of CHD is approximately 8–10 per 1,000 live births,[2] and the incidence of cardiomyopathy is estimated at 1 per 100,000 children.[3,4] Only a fraction of children diagnosed with either form of pediatric heart disease eventually progress to AHD[5] (Box 30.1), necessitating long-term intensive medical management and/or recurrent hospitalization. Those who do are at high risk for developing end-stage heart disease,[5,6] a clinical syndrome characterized by marked reduction in quality of life, functional status, nutritional deficiency, and respiratory distress. Similar to adults, the high mortality associated with pediatric AHD stems from its sequelae, including low cardiac output, respiratory failure, malignant arrhythmias, stroke, thromboembolism, multiorgan dysfunction, and infection.[5] As such, children with AHD represent a diverse group ranging from those cared for at home by their parents while still participating in childhood activities to those in hospice care at the end of life. For some, advanced therapies, such as transplantation, ventricular assist device, or other high-risk interventions may be indicated. For others, therapies may be limited. Across this diverse patient population, there is increasing evidence that pediatric AHD impacts the physical and psychosocial health of affected children as well as their families. Palliative care provides an opportunity to proactively intervene across physical, psychosocial, and spiritual domains in order to maximize the quality of life and symptom management of children living with AHD and their families, as well as prepare families for complex treatment decision-making and end-of-life care.

BOX 30.1 ADVANCED HEART DISEASE DEFINITION

PANEL 1: CRITERIA FOR DEFINITION OF AHD

- Lesions with higher risk of morbidity and mortality
- Single ventricle physiology
- Congenital heart disease with associated genetic syndrome
- Pulmonary vein stenosis
- Pulmonary hypertension
- Evaluation or listing for heart transplantation
- Need for mechanical circulatory support
- Hospital admission length >30 days
- Multiple cardiac surgeries or catheterizations (>3 times in 1 year)
- Mechanical ventilator support >14 days
- Hospital admission more than 3 per year for cardiac cause (i.e., arrhythmia management and heart failure)

Reprinted with permission from Morrell E, Moynihan K, Wolfe J, and Blume E. Palliative care and paediatric cardiology: current evidence and future directions. *Lancet Child Adolesc Health.* 2019;3:502–510.

INCIDENCE AND EPIDEMIOLOGY OF ADVANCED HEART DISEASE

The reported prevalence of CHD varies widely depending on the method of diagnosis and whether the data reflect prenatally detected CHD or live births of children with CHD. In general, the prevalence of CHD is approximately 3 per 1,000 for clinically severe defects (those requiring an intervention in the first year of life), 6 per 1,000 when including the more moderate defects, and 9–20 per 1,000 when including smaller septal defects and mild valve stenosis. Between 1940 and 2002, approximately 2 million infants were born with CHD in the United States.[7] Over this same period, tremendous achievements in surgical and medical care led to improvements in long-term survival of children with CHD. Surgical procedures have been developed to treat most congenital heart defects, including those that were historically uniformly fatal, such as hypoplastic left heart syndrome. Major advances have also been achieved in intensive care management, ventilatory support, mechanical support, intraoperative management, long-term medical management, and diagnostic imaging.[8,9] Prenatal detection of CHD has led to more controlled perinatal transitions and earlier surgical repairs. As a result, the number of young people living with severe CHD has increased. In 1985, the median age of all patients living with severe CHD was 11 years. In 2000, the median age was 17 years, with 49% of the CHD population being adults.[10] There are currently more than 2.4 million people (1 million children and 1.4 million adults) living with CHD.[11]

Despite dramatically improved short- and long-term outcomes, CHD is the leading cause of infant deaths owing to congenital anomalies worldwide, and palliated heart disease remains one of the leading causes of nonaccidental death in childhood in the United States.[2,7] Although only a small number of children with CHD will progress to AHD, morbidity and mortality among this group is high. Approximately 14,000 children experience heart failure related hospitalizations annually in the United States, and 7% die during their hospitalization. This mortality rate is nearly 20 times greater than hospitalized children without heart failure and approximately double that seen in adult heart failure.[1] For those with end-stage disease, ventricular assist device therapies and heart transplantation offer the potential for extended survival. However, almost 20% of children listed for transplant will die waiting for an organ, and an additional 1 in 10 heart transplant recipients will die within the first year post-transplant.[12]

PALLIATIVE CARE IN PEDIATRIC ADVANCED HEART DISEASE

To improve quality of life, reduce suffering, and support patient and family medical decision-making, there is growing attention being paid to the role of palliative care within pediatric AHD. However, the evolution of palliative care in children with AHD has occurred slowly. The slow progress is likely due to the growing perception of heart disease as highly treatable via surgical and mechanical interventions and the variable disease course with periods of both stability and acute-on-chronic decompensation (Figure 30.1).[13–15]

Involvement of palliative care services for pediatric patients with AHD is considerably less when compared to other critical pediatric illnesses, although trends suggest this is changing.[16] In a large, multisite study, only 8% of pediatric palliative care consults were for patients with underlying cardiac disease.[17] Among pediatric patients who died of AHD at a single institution, 16% received a palliative care consult.[13] In a recent study of circumstances surrounding death in pediatric heart transplant recipients, 30% had received a palliative care consult.[18] There is emerging evidence highlighting the benefits of palliative care involvement for pediatric patients with critical heart disease and their families. In a randomized controlled trial of early palliative care referral for infants prenatally diagnosed with single-ventricle heart disease, maternal anxiety of surviving infants was less with improved family communication and relationships reported among those receiving early consultation.[19]

Despite high morbidity and mortality, along with increasing evidence for the important role of palliative care within pediatric[19,20] and adult AHD,[21] pediatric cardiologists endorse barriers to requesting palliative care consultations. The most notable barriers include undermining parental hope and worry that parents would perceive the referral as their cardiology team giving up.[22] In a recent study of communication about difficult topics in pediatric end-stage organ disease (e.g., advance care planning), multidisciplinary pediatric healthcare clinicians endorsed a number of communication challenges, including parents not wanting difficult conversations to occur with their child.[23] Despite many perceived barriers, it is encouraging to note that the majority (85%) of cardiologists find palliative care involvement to be helpful,[24] and many cardiologists feel comfortable providing care at end of life.[22] The role of the specialty palliative care team in continuing to collaborate with and educate pediatric cardiologists and cardiothoracic surgeons to overcome barriers to move forward palliative care in pediatric cardiology cannot be underestimated.

Although there are no clinical practice guidelines specific to palliative care involvement within pediatric cardiology or AHD, the small but growing literature highlights diagnoses and patient populations that may especially benefit from specialty palliative care, including single ventricle anatomy, CHD associated with genetic disorders, pulmonary vein stenosis, and/or heart transplant/mechanical circulatory support (Figure 30.2).[25,26] A national survey of pediatric cardiologists found that palliative care referrals most commonly occurred for patients with pulmonary vein stenosis or those needing heart transplantation or mechanical circulatory support.[22] Palliative care involvement specific to psychosocial support and goals of care discussions has been most common.[27] Symptom management of thirst may also be an area where palliative care can be particularly helpful.[22] Looking forward, the establishment of "automatic" consults for specific triggers may help augment and systematize specialty palliative care consults.

While there has been considerable uptake of palliative care clinical services and research within pediatric cardiology, there remains additional opportunity for improvements. Figure 30.3 depicts the collaborative contributions of disciplines across palliative care and cardiology teams to the care of pediatric patients with AHD and their families. The interdisciplinary nature of palliative care, in partnership with cardiology teams, is helpful for promoting quality of life through reducing physical and psychosocial symptom burden and facilitating communication and decision-making.

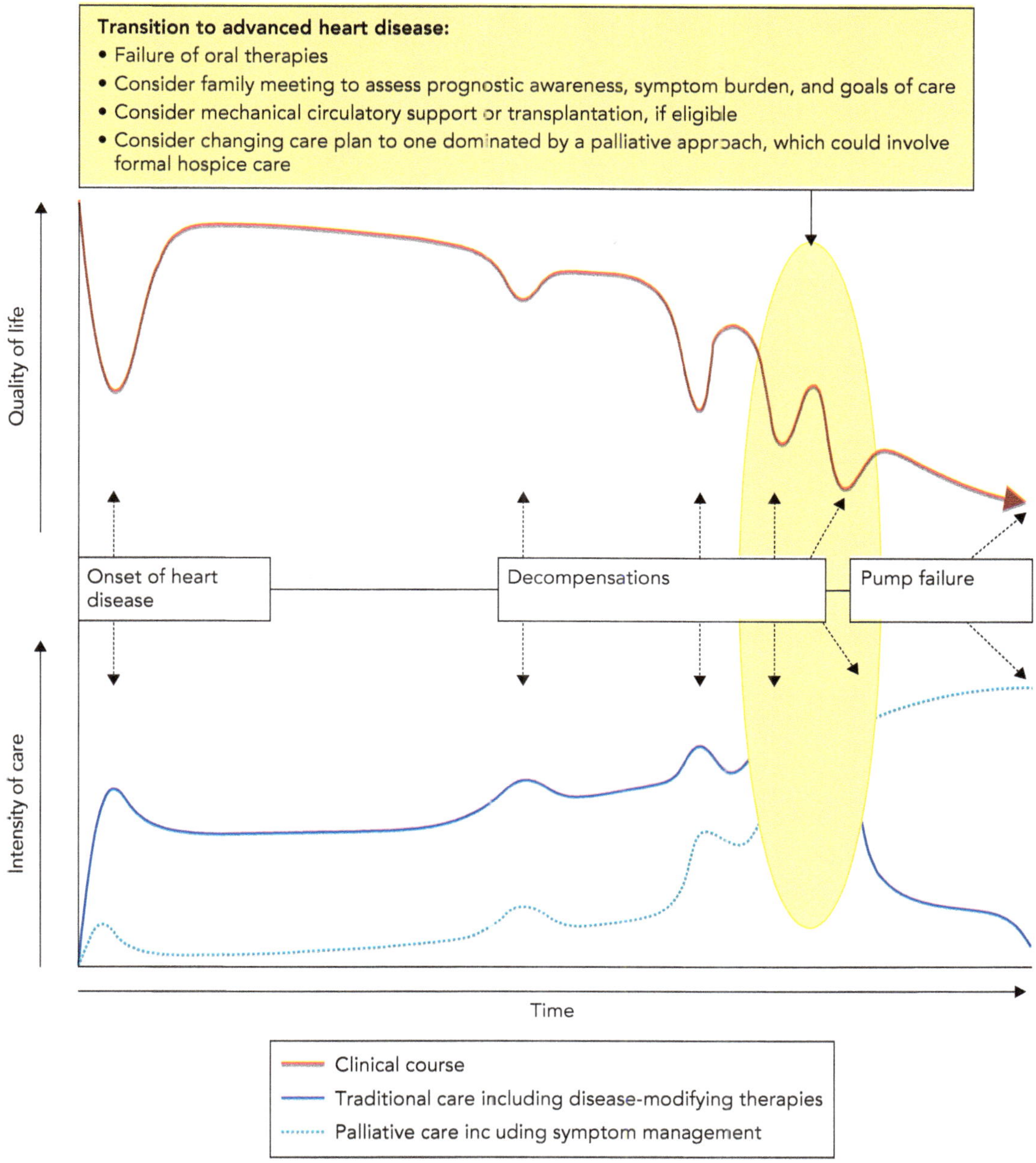

Figure 30.1 Clinical course of pediatric heart disease with integration of palliative care. Reprinted with permission from Morrell E, Moynihan K, Wolfe J, Blume ED. Palliative care and paediatric cardiology: Current evidence and future directions. *Lancet Child Adolesc Health*. 2019;*3*(7):E10–E10.

PROMOTING QUALITY OF LIFE FOR CHILDREN WITH ADVANCED HEART DISEASE AND THEIR FAMILIES

Although the past decade has shown an increase in studies evaluating the quality of life in children with AHD, this continues to be an underresearched field.[28–32] Early research described abnormalities in both the physical and psychosocial domains of quality of life, with 20% of children with mild to moderate CHD reporting significantly impaired quality of life. Parents and healthcare providers of children and adolescents with CHD more frequently identified physical dimensions, most often physical limitations, as quality-of-life concerns.[33] Physical limitations are a critically important element to quality of life in the subset of children with AHD who lack the physical stamina to participate in many developmentally appropriate activities. Scarring, medication regimens, receiving special treatment, school issues, and social issues were identified by school aged children and/or their parents as negatively affecting the children's quality of life. Adolescents also noted the negative impact of feeling different from peers and recognition of their own mortality as contributing to lower quality of life.[33]

In one of the first studies to explore parental perspectives on suffering and quality of life at the end of life in children with AHD, almost half of bereaved parents perceived their child experienced suffering at end of life. Furthermore, more than two-thirds of parents perceived their child's quality of

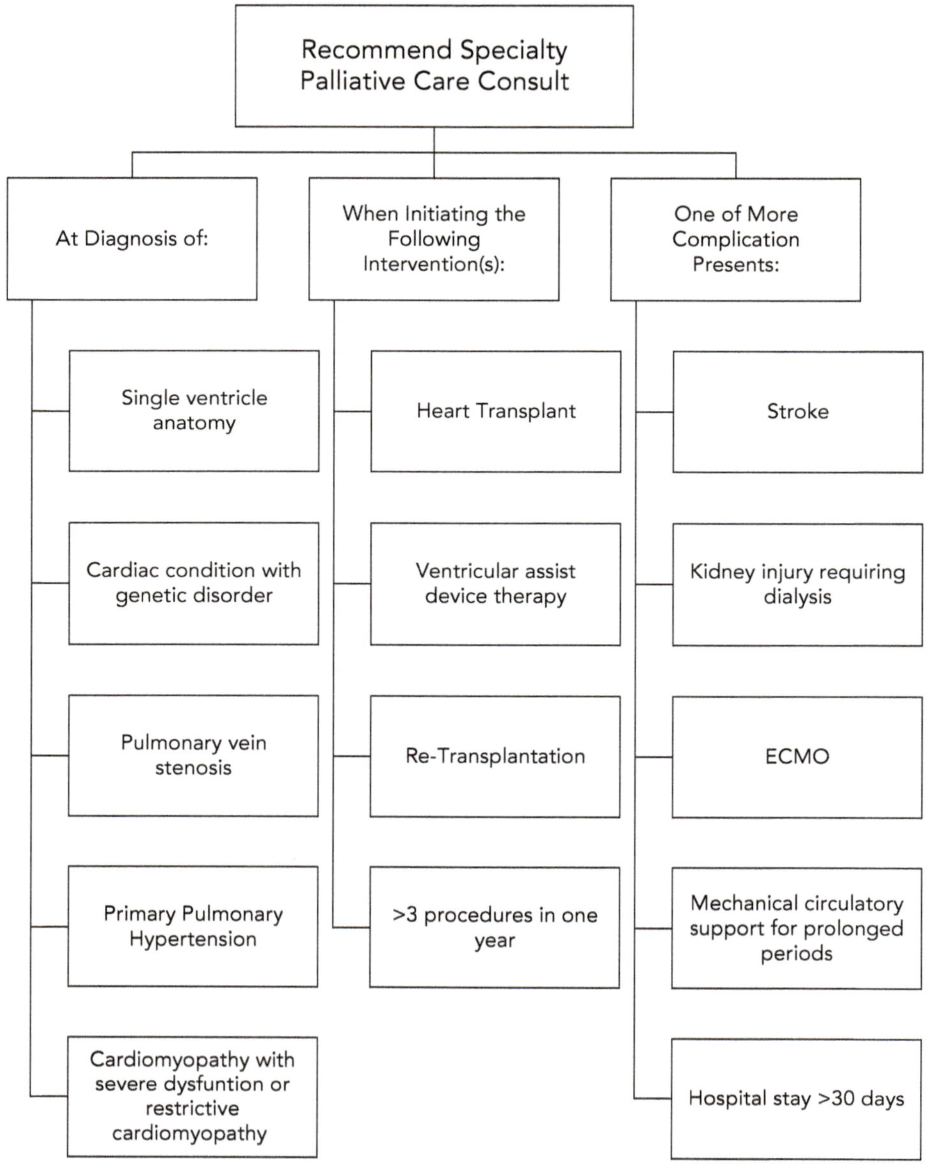

Figure 30.2 *Triggers for specialty palliative care involvement in pediatric advanced heart disease.*

life in the last month of life as poor or fair. These parents specifically noted that symptoms contributed to suffering. Parents of children younger than 2 years perceived breathing difficulties, feeding difficulties, and pain to be associated with a great deal of suffering. Parents with children older than 2 years reported fatigue, sleep disturbances, breathing difficulties, poor appetite, and chest pain as contributing to significant suffering.[15] Further research supports pain, fatigue, breathing difficulties, and feeding difficulties as contributing to suffering in children with AHD.[34] These studies highlight an opportunity for improvement in quality of life by specifically addressing symptoms.

Understanding the medical context, including prognostic indicators of a child's AHD, can be helpful to identify the need for consulting specialty palliative care. As described earlier, many children with AHD would accept a consult to specialty palliative care at any time within the disease course. Additionally, earlier conversations about prognosis may help families make decisions that fit within their personal values. Continued conversations with the child and family may shed light and offer opportunities to optimize quality of life through symptom management according to patient and family priorities. Interventions and symptom management recommendations must be tailored to the needs of the patient and family. If the family's stated goals are to have every opportunity to pursue disease-directed therapies and interventions, medications with side-effect profiles that may risk those goals would likely not be appropriate interventions. On the other hand, many patients and families make the loving decision to focus on comfort and symptom management, forgoing future interventions. Specialty palliative care may be particularly beneficial in clarifying and delineating some of these hopes to further align the teams' approach with the goals of the child and family. We will note particular branch points

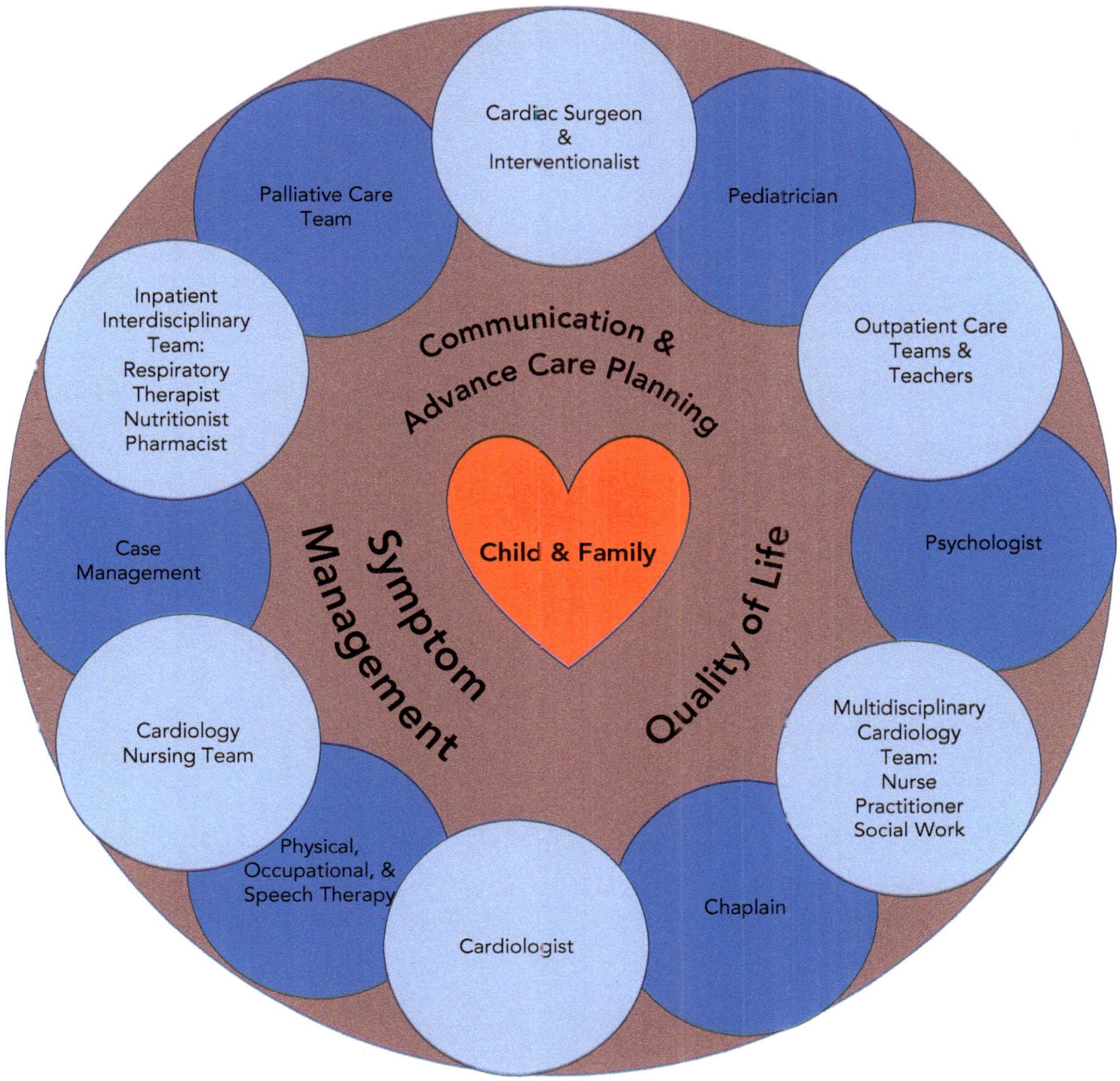

Figure 30.3 Interdisciplinary collaboration between palliative care and pediatric cardiology.

in symptom management recommendations later based on stated goals while also acknowledging that, for many pediatric patients and their families, goals may continue to remain blended and become clearer throughout the illness course.

SYMPTOM MANAGEMENT FOR CHILDREN WITH ADVANCED HEART DISEASE

Symptom management includes a variety of complex medical and psychosocial interventions to optimize quality of life. As cardiac function deteriorates, traditional symptoms of heart failure can ensue. Symptom management can be complex, and side effects of drugs can worsen these symptoms. The first strategy to good symptom management in children with AHD is good heart failure management. Improved cardiac output will improve symptoms. Some guidelines are offered in Table 30.1.

PAIN

To best understand pain in children with AHD, it is important to first review and understand the pain etiology (see Chapter 23). From recent research we know that parents of children with AHD report almost 80% of children hospitalized with AHD suffered considerably due to pain.[34] The most commonly experienced types of pain in patients with AHD are abdominal pain from fluid overload and/or ischemia as well as procedural pain. Furthermore, as with all symptoms, it is important to obtain a full understanding of the pain a child is experiencing, how they are experiencing it, and what interventions (both pharmacologic and nonpharmacologic) have been most helpful.

Much of the pain experienced in both the ambulatory and inpatient setting in children with AHD is procedural pain, particularly needle-stick pain. For outpatient procedures, it may be helpful to provide a written prescription for topical anesthetic cream and instructions for application for

TABLE 30.1 Symptom management medication guidelines

MEDICATION	INDICATION FOR USE	DOSING	SIDE EFFECTS/ CONTRAINDICATIONS	COMMENTS
Dopamine	Increase cardiac output, blood pressure, and urine output	Renal and mesenteric: 2–5 mcg/kg/min (beta) effect: 5–10 mcg/kg/min IV infusion	Tachydysrhythmia, vasoconstriction at higher doses. Anginal pain, and palpitations	Volume depletion should be corrected before starting. No hypersensitivity to sulfites. Extravasation can cause severe tissue damage
Dobutamine	Increase cardiac output and manage short-term cardiac decompensation	2–20 mcg/kg/min IV infusion Transient hypotension	Ectopic heart beats, increased heart rate, chest pain, headache, nausea and vomiting, dyspnea	Volume depletion should be corrected before starting. No hypersensitivity to sulfite and idiopathic hypertrophic subaortic stenosis
Milrinone	Treat low cardiac output syndrome and congestive heart failure	0.2–1 mcg/kg	Headache, ventricular dysrhythmias, hypotension, and chest pain	Do not use in patients with severe pulmonary or aortic obstructive disease
Furosemide	Loop diuretic Reduce preload	0.05 mg/kg/hour (titrated as infusion) 1–2 mg/kg/dose q6–12h 2 mg/kg PO TID	Hypotension, dizziness, urticaria, electrolyte imbalances, potential ototoxicity with high doses, jaundice	Indomethacin decreases the effect
Bumetanide	Loop directed Reduce preload	0.015–0.1 mg/kg/dose q6–24h IV/PO	Hypotension, chest pain, dizziness, rash, hyperglycemia, electrolyte imbalance, elevated liver enzymes, ototoxicity, elevated serum creatinine	Do not use if hypersensitivity to bumetanide and anuria or increasing azotemia
Spironolactone	Potassium-sparing diuretic acting on distal collecting duct of the nephron Treat congestive heart failure	1–2 mg/kg/day orally daily or divided into BID dosing	Dysrhythmias, lethargy, confusion, ataxia, rash, electrolyte imbalance, dehydration, decreased renal function	Indicated for CHF, can be used in conjunction with Lasix and digoxin
Prostaglandin E_1	Maintain patency of the ductus arteriosus, used in severe coarctation of the aorta, critical pulmonary stenosis, TGA	0.05 mcg/kg/min, can be doubled every 15–30 min to max 0.2 mcg/kg/min	Apnea, hypotension, seizures, flushing, elevated temperature	
Gabapentin	Neuropathic pain Visceral pain	2 mg/kg/dose TID Increase 2 mg/kg/dose every 3–4 days Goal: 30–45 mg/kg/day	Sedation	Monitor renal function

the parents. Additionally, managing inpatient needle sticks with pain prevention protocols, including distraction techniques and topical anesthetic creams, may reduce trauma. Optimizing nonpharmacologic strategies, such as a cold compress, applying pressure or vibration, and repositioning can also help to lower levels of anxiety, distress, and pain.[35] In a focus group of parents of children on ventricular assist devices, dressing changes were the most distressing reason for perceived pain (Cousino, May, and Blume, 2019, direct communication). Collaborating with child life specialists to develop patient unique coping strategies (e.g., iPad distraction, diaphragmatic breathing) around procedural pain can be incredibly beneficial.

Abdominal pain can be challenging to diagnose and treat, particularly in children with AHD. The later section on gastrointestinal (GI) disturbances offers differentials for nausea/vomiting that may contribute to abdominal discomfort. Visceral pain, which is diffuse in character, can be a symptom in children with CHD. Pain is initiated when visceral receptors, located on smooth tissue membranes, within intestinal muscle, and in the mucosa of hollow organs, are stimulated by excessive contraction, stretching, tension, or ischemia. Visceral pain in children with AHD may result from vasoconstriction and/or ventricular injury causing decreased skeletal perfusion and ischemia to the organs and gut. Some studies and anecdotal evidence suggest gabanoids (gabapentin/pregabalin) can be successful in treating this type of pain.[36] Consultation to specialty palliative care may offer further expertise in titration of gabanoids and use of amitriptyline/nortriptyline for visceral hyperalgesia, as well as possible recommendations for methadone (see Chapter 23).

Specific considerations for methadone initiation in patients with AHD include potential risk of QTC prolongation, and increased risk of torsades de pointes. Research of the side effect profile of methadone in children with cardiac disease is limited. Most research comes from the adult literature and pediatric oncology patients and excludes patients with cardiac disease. Adult literature has identified individuals with cardiac disease are at significant risk for QTC prolongation on methadone.[37,38] The APS guidelines, in adult patients, recommend reconsideration of methadone use with a QTC interval between 450 and 500 ms and avoidance of methadone with a QTC above 500 ms.[39] There are no recommendations on guidelines for ECG monitoring for methadone addition in pediatric patients with AHD. Thus, when adding any potential QTC prolonging medication, careful and thoughtful evaluation of the child's and family's goals for treating the symptom, as well as weighing the child's potential risk for that symptom is necessary. Close collaboration with specialty palliative care and cardiology teams can be particularly helpful in this instance.

Pain may also result from excessive fluid overload and edema of neck, abdomen, back, and extremities. Diuretics can provide symptom relief caused by peripheral edema, and postural changes can help with back pain related to edema in the sacral area. Although chest pain is rare, it is very frightening for children and families. Opioids can improve coronary perfusion and may have a primary cardiac role in patients with ischemic disease. Discussions about pain management should occur early on. Many families and caretakers worry about the cardiac and respiratory effects of opioids. Understanding a family's specific worries about opioids will strengthen the therapeutic relationship between patient/family and provider and allow the provider to address those concerns. Most cardiac ICUs are comfortable with opioids in the postoperative period. Providing education about opioid use to cardiology staff outside of the postoperative period may improve provider comfort. Recognizing symptoms which might benefit from opioids and creating a trial period with opioids for these symptoms can be a helpful approach. Pain management is critical to improve suffering throughout the disease course while continuing life-extending measures in children with AHD.

FATIGUE

The activation of both the renin-angiotensin system and the sympathetic nervous system results in vasoconstriction and poor skeletal muscle perfusion. This often leads to overwhelming fatigue, sometimes out of proportion to the cardiac dysfunction. For patients in the early phases of AHD, fatigue can be particularly difficult to sort out, as it can often be confused with laziness or depression. Modified physical therapy and cardiac rehabilitation programs can be useful to avoid deconditioning and maintain muscle tone. In addition, modified exercise programs have been shown to be beneficial to outlook and endurance in patients with CHD.[40,41] Fatigue may be a marker of overall symptom burden (Molloy, personal communication). If fatigue is the most prominent symptom, it is useful to do a comprehensive symptom history. For those AHD patients whose fatigue is secondary to poor muscle perfusion, systemic vasodilators, such as milrinone, can help lower systemic vascular resistance and result in temporary improvement of fatigue. Many children and young adults describe "something lifting off my chest" after a few hours of a milrinone infusion. There is some anecdotal evidence that a short infusion holiday of 3–5 days can have an improved effect lasting for several weeks. Some patients may benefit from this therapy either intermittently or as a continuous infusion.

SLEEP DISTURBANCES

Poor sleep in children with AHD may be a variable that contributes to overall fatigue as well exacerbates other symptoms. Understanding a child's sleep routine will provide valuable insight into guiding management. Parents of children with AHD reported that sleep disturbance contributed to their child's suffering.[15] Sleep disturbances may be caused from a number of different reasons including obstructive apnea, environmental factors (hospital setting, timing of medications), dyspnea, pain, depression, and anxiety. Trialing nonpharmacologic management (as described in Chapter 22) by optimizing the environment to support circadian rhythm throughout the day and nighttime is typically a good first step. In addition, timing of diuretics is critical in maintaining good sleep hygiene because diuretics before bedtime will interrupt sleep. Diuretics should not be given within 4 hours of bedtime. We recommend twice-daily diuretics be retimed to 8 AM and 4 PM to allow for minimal sleep disturbances secondary to need to void. Pharmacologic therapy can start with melatonin. Though ramelteon, olanzapine, trazodone, and clonidine are all medications that have been used with good effect in children for insomnia, each of these medications has potential cardiac side effects. Special care in understanding insomnia as well as goals of care must be made prior to initiation of any of these medications. Olanzapine and trazodone both have QTC prolongation side effects. Clonidine reduces sympathetic outflow from the central nervous system, thus special attention to blood pressure must be noted prior to initiation. Furthermore, trials of methylphenidate may be trialed in patients experiencing extreme fatigue who have not benefited from methods discussed earlier (both pharmacologic and nonpharmacologic). However, methylphenidate may increase the risk of arrhythmia and should be thought about carefully with primary cardiology team.

BREATHING DIFFICULTIES

Breathing difficulties in children may be a result of a variety of different reasons. In a study of parental perspectives, while almost all children hospitalized with AHD who reported breathing difficulties were treated for this symptom, only about 40% of parents felt their child was treated successfully.[34] One common reason for breathing difficulties in children, adolescents, and young adults with AHD is fluid overload. Although many children do not present with the traditional adult heart failure congestion with rales, respiratory distress, and shortness of breath, some children do present with these symptoms. Discussions around what interventions make the most sense for the patient physiologically should be considered.

Children with end-stage disease may experience dyspnea, the subjective feeling of breathlessness. Dyspnea may be managed through nonpharmacologic techniques as well as pharmacologic (see Chapter 24). A fan near the face is very effective for relief of the breathlessness of dyspnea in this population. Children as young as 3 or 4 years can ask for and control the use of a small handheld fan effectively. Oxygen can be added if the patient feels relief from it, though some children are bothered more by the cannula and the dryness versus the relief from oxygen itself. It is important to have specific conversations with families, as many families believe that oxygen will prolong life or improve symptoms, when the cannula themselves are causing more distress.

GASTROINTESTINAL DISTURBANCES, FEEDING DIFFICULTIES, AND THIRST

Children with congestion and heart failure often have GI symptoms such as nausea, vomiting, anorexia, and extreme thirst. Diuretics and fluid management are the key therapy for congestive symptoms in heart failure in children and can improve GI symptoms rapidly. Many loop diuretics, such as furosemide, have a threshold effect, and if patients with normal renal function are not responding, then doses can be doubled. Ascites can present as pain or feeding intolerance. This is often accompanied by edema of the bowel wall and poor GI absorption of diuretics, requiring intravenous diuretics.

Fluid restriction for these patients is critical in maintaining homeostasis and decreasing hospital admissions. However, fluid restriction can be very difficult as the body's response to lower output is secretion of anti-diuretic hormone (ADH) and subsequent thirst. Discussion about the utility of fluid restriction and the understanding that the thirst response is counter-regulatory may help some patients and families. The maintenance of fluid restriction for many families is endless and futile, and increasing diuretics may be the simplest action. Some children find that sour candies and hot sauce in small amounts seem to satiate the thirst response. Frozen fruits such as grapes and watermelon can help with thirst as well. Working with child life to set up a chart for fluid allowance throughout the day is helpful. Additionally, collaborating with a team nutritionist can be beneficial in thinking about how to modify diet to best aid in fluid restriction. Many children with AHD have a nasogastric or gastrostomy tube to assist with feeding. Modifying feeding regimens to deliver feeds continuously rather than bolus feeds may also improve abdominal discomfort.

DIZZINESS AND/OR SYNCOPE

Syncope can be a result of primary ventricular arrhythmia secondary to myocyte fibrosis and can be very frightening for families and patients. It may be worsened by electrolyte abnormalities such as hypomagnesemia and hypokalemia, which should be monitored closely. Dizziness can also be very disturbing for patients as it may remind them of the presyncopal state. It may be due to low cardiac output More often, however, it is a symptom related to side effects of the cardiac medications and can limit quality of life. The use of multiple antihypertensives together in the morning can often lead to dizziness and headache. Awareness of the total medical picture can help improve timing of medications for patient comfort. Vasodilating medications given at bedtime may reduce dizziness during the day.

PSYCHOSOCIAL FUNCTIONING

Similar to other serious pediatric illnesses, children and young adults with AHD experience increased rates of emotional and behavioral challenges. In a sample of adolescents with single ventricle anatomy, lifetime prevalence of a psychiatric diagnosis was 65%, with nearly half of the participants meeting criteria for a diagnosis at time of study assessment.[42] Moreover, the sample had an approximately five times increased rate of lifetime anxiety disorders (35%) and attention deficit hyperactivity disorder (ADHD) when compared to healthy controls. In a recent study of children and adolescents pre-heart transplantation, 14% presented with a psychiatric admission during their hospitalization.[43] Of those 8 years or older with a ventricular assist device (VAD) in place, 40% met criteria for a psychiatric diagnosis, with adjustment (20%) and anxiety (17%) disorders being most common. For those with AHD who go on to receive heart transplantation, psychosocial risks persist. Approximately 20–50% of pediatric heart or heart-lung transplant recipients have been found to have impaired psychological functioning many years post-transplant.[44–46]

Notably, psychological symptoms and advancing heart disease symptoms often overlap. For example, fatigue and anhedonia may be due to worsening depression, heart failure or a combination of both. Thus, thoughtful and frequent assessment of psychological health throughout the heart disease course is important.[44] Antidepressant therapy, specifically the use of selective serotonin reuptake inhibitors (SSRIs) for anxiety and/or depression, are used in a subset of patients with AHD requiring heart transplantation (7%), with more common use seen among those on VAD therapies (25%).[43] In addition, psychological support is recommended utilizing evidence-based interventions, including cognitive-behavioral therapy and relaxation skills training, to address psychological symptoms commonly experienced among this population. Both psychology intervention and child life support services can be utilized for patients with significant procedural distress (e.g., needle-based procedures, dressing changes) to enhance coping and improve quality of life.

FAMILY IMPACT

It is important to recognize that AHD impacts the entire family system. Parents of children with CHD have higher rates of psychosocial morbidity than do parents of either healthy children or those with other chronic medical conditions.[33] Sources of stress include medical and surgical procedures, activity restrictions, uncertainty, the child's prognosis, the child's behavior, decisions about disclosing medical details to the child, transitioning older children to self-management, and perceptions that their child is different.[34–38] Parents also experience significant rates of psychiatric comorbidities, including depression, anxiety, and somatization, and there is evidence that these are chronic in nature.[39] Approximately 9% of parents of children post-heart transplantation endorsed symptoms of posttraumatic stress,[40] further underscoring that the impact of pediatric heart disease on parents is long-lasting.

Although less is known about the psychosocial impact of AHD on siblings, one study found that 30% of parents reported adverse sequelae of CHD on healthy siblings, including anxiety, depression, anger, jealousy, feeling left out, and perceptions that the child with CHD lived under different rules.[43] Given the impact of pediatric AHD on the psychosocial well-being of the affected child and his or her parents and siblings, palliative care for this population involves attention to the psychosocial health of the entire family.

COMMUNICATION AND ADVANCED CARE PLANNING

Although it is widely recommended that adults with AHD participate in advance care planning,[47,48] minimal prognostic, advance care planning, and end-of-life care focused communication occurs across adult heart failure populations. Among adults with CHD, only 1% recalled discussing advance care planning with their medical team even though 78% of the participants believed their healthcare providers should initiate end-of-life decision-making discussions early in the disease course.[49] Advance care planning and end-of-life care communication occurs even less frequently in pediatric AHD populations.

In a recent pilot study of adolescents and young adults with AHD undergoing heart transplant evaluation,[20] the majority of participants (83%) indicated that they wanted to discuss their prognosis, while 67% stated that they would want to discuss their end-of-life care preferences if very sick. Although few had engaged in formal advanced care planning discussions, study participants expressed preferences for how such conversations should occur. The majority expressed a preference for family involvement in end-of-life decision-making. There was wide-ranging variability in terms of when young people would want to start such a discussion, thus highlighting the importance of tailoring advance care planning discussions to the individual needs and preferences of patients and families. It is also important to recognize that although parents understood their child's desire to be involved in medical treatment decision-making (e.g., decision to be listed for heart transplant), only 58% of parents perceived that their child would want to be involved in end-of-life decision-making.[20]

Findings align with research in other pediatric illness groups suggesting that young people desire prognostic information and want to be made aware of their options and engage in shared decision-making with caregivers.[50,51] Randomized controlled intervention research in both pediatric cancer and HIV populations has demonstrated that family-centered advance care planning with young people results in increased awareness of adolescents' and young adults' end-of-life wishes, reductions in invasive interventions at end of life, reduced decisional burden, and increased likelihood of home deaths.[51–54] Advanced care planning should begin with the primary cardiology team. Research from pediatric oncology patients and their families endorsed preferring to have these discussions with trusted and established care providers.[55] Specialty palliative care can further support the primary team as well as the patient and family.

Taken together, advance care planning for children with AHD should be tailored to the individual needs and preferences of patients and families with specific attention paid to clear communication about possible interventions and their limitations, such as extracorporeal membrane oxygenation (ECMO), transplant, and VAD, as well as less invasive interventions, such blood draws and cardiac catherizations. Providers can establish consistent time points for when preferences for end-of-life decision-making are assessed and revisited. Honest and systematic conversations that occur throughout the disease trajectory decrease unexpected decision-making discussions during highly stressful times.[56]

DECISION-MAKING

Shared decision-making in pediatric cardiology is critical yet challenging amid the changing landscape of improved long-term outcomes, more children living into adolescence and adulthood, and the rapid emergence of highly technologic therapies. Decision-making specific to life-prolonging interventions is complicated by the highly variable trajectory of AHD, with many patients experiencing acute exacerbations followed by periods of stability. Furthermore, risk stratification depends on large numbers of randomized studies which are not possible in this field. Many parents have been told their child's anatomy is unique and that options and outcomes for each child are uncertain and unknown. In addition, many families of infants with complex CHD have already made significant important decisions about goals of care by continuing the pregnancy. It is imperative that pediatric cardiologists review with new families their previous experience and their prior decisions. Understanding this will encourage this important connection between primary cardiac subspecialist and parents. Specialty palliative care support and consultation to assist with understanding decision-making can be especially helpful to support primary care teams, patients, and their families—who are likely to encounter a number of high-stakes decisions, such as decisions regarding surgical interventions, transplant listing, use of technology and/or mechanical support, and end-of-life care.

FETAL COUNSELING

For many families, challenging decision-making occurs at the time of prenatal diagnosis of severe CHD. Although staged reconstruction is often the most common path and provider recommendation for hypoplastic left heart syndrome,[57] a single-center retrospective study found that 11% of families chose to terminate the pregnancy and 7% opted to proceed with comfort care only at birth.[58] Specialty palliative care consultation in the prenatal period, especially for complicated CHD,[59] provides an opportunity for cardiology and palliative care teams to work together to guide families through their decision-making. Furthermore, in a randomized controlled trial, Hancock et al. showed a decrease in maternal stress in the postpartum period among patients born to families who had a specialty palliative care consult in the fetal period.[19] For many families where palliative resources are not available, primary palliative care skills for the fetal cardiologist are critical. Starting the encounter with questions about what the parents understand about their child's condition and whether there are any care plan decisions already made will help this first encounter move more successfully. For example, for parents who are not considering termination to hear about termination as an option for the first 10 minutes of the encounter can derail the relationship from the start.

TECHNOLOGY, VENTRICULAR ASSIST DEVICES, AND MECHANICAL CIRCULATORY SUPPORT

Decisions regarding technological devices are another important component to decision-making in pediatric cardiology. The wider acceptance of mechanical support in the form of VAD and ECMO support bring another level of complexity to the decision-making process. The acceptance of technology must not be seen as working in contrast with palliative care. These technologies must be incorporated into the spectrum of therapy for AHD. Families and caregivers can hold on to the hope of recovery or transplant while supported by a device, while also making preparations and plans for symptom relief and minimizing suffering. This balance often feels more delicate to the provider than to the family. Most families can hold both if the presentation is clear and direct. Pediatric cardiologists should set aside time to discuss the "what ifs" with parents away from the bedside, in a conversation that does not include a medical update or plan for the week. Interdisciplinary team huddles to enhance coordination of roles during family meetings may increase family involvement in these important discussions.[60]

Consultation with specialty palliative care prior to initiation of these therapies can be particularly helpful for enhancing the longitudinal relationship with the patient, family, and care teams. Reliance on mechanical support strategies will provide an important new area for understanding palliative care needs in all AHD patients and in children in particular. Because of the advanced nature of the heart disease of children who require ECMO or VAD support, there may be instances when discontinuing mechanical support is a consideration. Although complications such as stroke with VAD are decreasing, discussing end-of-life care process prior to implantation is critical. The difficulties for families of patients with a VAD often revolve around the patient who may be cognitively aware and neurologically healthy, with the heart beating, but with severe end-organ dysfunction, and thus no longer a transplant candidate. This type of discontinuation by terminating the pump function may feel different to medical providers and families than discontinuation of an endotracheal tube. Specialty palliative care involvement for VAD patients has been shown to be valuable, with early involvement leading to increased discussions about goals of care and advanced directives.[60]

Moreover, the development of a deactivation checklist for providers and families has been offered as a starting point to be sure the goals are reviewed and that pertinent people are present.[61] It is important to note that recommendations about premedications and symptom management for these situations vary between institutions. General guidance advises avoiding neuromuscular blocking agents and titrating sedatives and analgesia to treat objective signs of discomfort that evolve with the discontinuation of life-sustaining therapies. Providers continue to have diverse views about the process of deactivation of VAD in children, and knowledge gaps are notable.[62,63]

In addition to ECMO and VAD, many children who progress to AHD already have an implantable defibrillator (ICD). Again, this technology provides some safety from sudden death but at the expense of pain and anxiety from defibrillation if the device fires, as well as the possibility of continued firing at end of life. Turning off the defibrillator is a difficult decision for families and patients, and plans should be set in place before end of life. Many families cannot bear to turn it off until the end stage, which can sometimes be disturbing at end of life. Formal institutional policies for end-of-life care for pediatric patients with ECMO, VAD, and/or ICD may help reduce medical provider and family decisional stress, burden, and regret.

Clinical Vignette

AB was diagnosed with cardiomyopathy at 1 year of age and underwent cardiac transplantation without complication. His course was uncomplicated for the first 5 years post-transplant, and he was managed as an outpatient by the multidisciplinary team. At 5 years of age, he presented to clinic because his mother observed that he "did not look right," had poor appetite, and was uninterested in play. On echocardiogram, his cardiac function was very poor, and he had evidence of acute rejection and cardiac allograft vasculopathy. He was admitted to the ICU for intravenous inotropes to maintain cardiac output. Because of progressive cardiac allograft vasculopathy, persistent poor cardiac function, and continued need for high-dose inotropes, he was relisted for transplant. Workup revealed exposure to parvovirus, a likely cause of his acute decompensation. His mother, who was pregnant, was also exposed to parvovirus and delivered at 33 weeks' gestation. The infant died in the newborn period of viral sepsis and cardiomyopathy. AB's physical condition stabilized on IV inotropes, and symptoms were manageable medically. Specialty palliative care was consulted to provide additional decision-making and bereavement support to AB's family. Palliative care social work provided primary bereavement support to the family, while transplant social work focused on supporting AB and his family through with his worsened health status. In addition, transplant psychology worked one-on-one with AB with interventions targeting his new-onset medical anxieties and procedural distress. Although the family wanted to "do everything" for AB, decision-making about retransplant was more complicated than their first experience with transplant listing. They very much trusted their transplant team but benefited from discussions with the specialty palliative care team with whom they could comfortably discuss all options, including not moving forward with retransplantation. Together with their primary transplant team and palliative care team, the family decided on relisting.

AB underwent his second cardiac transplantation, requiring the need for ECMO for 6 days postoperatively for graft failure. Once more, psychosocial support was provided by both the transplant and palliative care teams as they worked to manage the uncertainty of AB's condition in the context of the recent loss of his parents' newborn. He required intensive rehabilitative physical and occupational therapy to restore function after his lengthy critical illness.

Other than a short hospitalization for cytomegalovirus pneumonia, he enjoyed his relatively normal life. About 3 years post-transplant, he again developed signs of heart failure and evaluation revealed accelerated cardiac allograft vasculopathy, which once again progressed rapidly. When he required IV inotropes for his decompensated heart failure, treatment options, including ECMO and VAD, were considered. Because he had developed cardiac allograft vasculopathy with both his first and second transplant, he was not a candidate for a third transplant. Although the family had not actively followed with the palliative care team for some time, they welcomed reconsultation and some familiar supports. AB did not have a long-term option, and, as such, the family and team elected to forego mechanical support and concentrate on supportive care. AB had a wish to see the Disney princesses, therefore the team and family focused on transitioning AB to oral medications to manage his heart failure. The palliative care team worked with the primary transplant team to discharge AB home with hospice care. He went to Disney World with his family. He rode all the rides and saw all the Disney princesses. On the last day of the trip, he was laughing on the water ride with his mom and sister, "fell asleep," and died. His mother continues to participate in the bereavement program organized by the palliative care team.

FUTURE DIRECTIONS

The role of palliative care for children with AHD is expanding. Although many issues are like other serious illness in children, continued examination of the unique and specific needs and barriers is needed to maximize the impact of palliative care for children with AHD and their families. A necessary first step is gaining understanding of and identifying clear prognostic indicators for children with AHD. This will help to inform timing of palliative care involvement and decision-making support provided to families.

Second, descriptive studies have provided a framework for understanding current practices, needs, and targets for intervention. However, palliative care interventions in pediatric cardiology are needed. Randomized controlled clinical trials targeting physical and psychological symptoms, along with communication and quality of life, are critical to move this field forward and gain key stakeholders for increasing the provision of palliative care within cardiology. Defining protocols, decisional support aids, and communication templates for high-risk surgical interventions and mechanical support will further align cardiology and palliative care teams to support the physical, psychosocial, and spiritual needs of patients and families. Third, bereavement research among this population is an important area of study to improve the care provided to patients and their families across the entirety of the disease course.

Last, education initiatives targeting both cardiologists and palliative care specialists will be important. There is a role for both primary palliative care and specialty palliative care in pediatric AHD. Determining when, how, and why each of those are most appropriate will be an important next step, especially as the demand and need for palliative care in pediatric cardiology grows with changes in the field and disease course.

Family Perspective

As mom to a heart angel, a heart transplant recipient, and a heart-healthy 4-year-old daughter, my identity as a mother is a unique one, spanning through a wide range of experiences and related emotions. My journey as a "heart mom" began in May 2007, with the birth and subsequent cardiomyopathy diagnosis of my firstborn child, Joseph, and it has followed a path of enlightenment, heartbreak, and hope. Six-year-old Joseph very suddenly passed away in 2013, just 1 month after his brother, Jack, was born with the same condition. With the support of our boys' medical team, our family was able to take on the herculean task of grieving one child while regaining the confidence to care for his brother who had a shared diagnosis. Through it all, our path to transplant was our beacon of hope giving Jack the opportunity to live his best life.

In September 2014, after an extensive multidisciplinary evaluation process, Jack was found to be a good candidate for a heart transplant and was officially listed. On

Friday February 16, 2018 we received an early morning call informing us a heart was available. This began a brand new journey for Jack and our entire family. A new path.

Although filled with great appreciation for this gift of life, the time immediately following the transplant was extremely challenging for me as a mother. I had come to be an expert on my son's heart condition. I had years of experience in watching for specific warning signs, understanding the significance of physical changes, and caring for his poorly functioning heart. I knew my son better than anyone and was his best advocate. All of this changed the night his sick heart was removed and a healthy one was put into his body. With this beautiful gift of life came a huge learning curve with new information and care practices. Essentially, I had to relearn how to care for my child, all the while supporting him through the intense postoperative period. This was incredibly overwhelming for me, and, once again, I leaned on Jack's medical team for support. Knowing they had walked parents through this post-transplant process hundreds of times brought me great comfort.

The next 2 weeks were filled with countless learning experiences as different team members stepped in to provide the support and education my husband and I needed to bridge the gaps in our understanding. Social workers and chaplains helped us sort through a multitude of intense emotions, various medical specialists trained us in each transplant-related discipline, and cardiologists and nursing staff provided ongoing care while empowering us as parents. It was collaboration at its best, highlighted by the gradual transfer of responsibility from staff to parent, with careful assessment and scaffolding of new knowledge. By the time Jack was medically ready to be discharged from the hospital, my husband and I were once again feeling competent in our role as primary caregivers and ready to let our beautiful boy experience this new chapter in his life outside of the hospital walls. Our transformation during Jack's 2-week post-transplant stay was nothing short of amazing and all due to the comprehensive care our family received.

As I reflect on my history as a "heart mom" and revisit each unique phase including prenatal diagnosis, introduction to hospital life, medical management, bereavement, and the transplant process, one thing is abundantly clear: the relationship my husband and I had with our sons' primary cardiologist was the cornerstone of our entire care experience. In times of both heartbreak and joy, this relationship, built on trust, shared decision-making, and effective communication, was absolutely essential to our survival as a family unit. I firmly believe the time our cardiologist invested in understanding our needs, values, and goals as a family not only served as a guide for medical intervention but was the most critical component of our positive care experience. My family is forever grateful for the exceptional care we received. We are thriving as a family because of this and have great hope for the future.

REFERENCES

1. Rossano JW, Kim JJ, Decker JA, et al. Prevalence, morbidity, and mortality of heart failure-related hospitalizations in children in the United States: A population-based study. *J Card Fail.* 2012;18(6):459–470. doi:10.1016/j.cardfail.2012.03.001
2. Hoffman JIE, Kaplan S. The incidence of congenital heart disease. *J Am Coll Cardiol.* 2002;39(12):1890–1900. doi:10.1016/S0735-1097(02)01886-7
3. Nugent AW, Daubeney PEF, Chondros P, et al. The epidemiology of childhood cardiomyopathy in Australia. *N Engl J Med.* 2003;348(17):1639–1646. doi:10.1056/NEJMoa021737
4. Wilkinson JD, Sleeper LA, Alvarez JA, Bublik N, Lipshultz SE, Group PCS. The pediatric cardiomyopathy registry: 1995–2007. *Prog Pediatr Cardiol.* 2008;25(1):31–36.
5. Rosenthal D, Chrisant MRK, Edens E, et al. International Society for Heart and Lung Transplantation: Practice guidelines for management of heart failure in children. *J Heart Lung Transplant.* 2004;23(12):1313–1333.
6. Canter CE, Shaddy RE, Bernstein D, et al. Indications for heart transplantation in pediatric heart disease: A scientific statement from the American Heart Association Council on Cardiovascular Disease in the Young. *Circulation.* 2007;115(5):658–676. doi:10.1161/CIRCULATIONAHA.106.180449
7. Lock JE, Keane JF, Mandell VS, Perry SB. *Nadas' Pediatric Cardiology.* Published online 2006.
8. Noonan JA. A history of pediatric specialties: The development of pediatric cardiology. *Pediatr Res.* 2004;56(2):298–306.
9. Freedom RM, Lock J, Bricker JT. Pediatric cardiology and cardiovascular surgery: 1950–2000. *Circulation.* 2000;102(suppl_4):Iv-58.
10. Marelli AJ, Mackie AS, Ionescu-Ittu R, Rahme E, Pilote L. Congenital heart disease in the general population. *Circulation.* 2007;115(2):163 LP—172. http://circ.ahajournals.org/content/115/2/163.abstract
11. Gilboa SM, Devine OJ, Kucik JE, et al. Congenital heart defects in the United States: Estimating the magnitude of the affected population in 2010. *Circulation.* July 5, 2016. http://circ.ahajournals.org/content/early/2016/06/30/CIRCULATIONAHA.115.019307.abstract
12. Dipchand AI, Rossano JW, Edwards LB, et al. The Registry of the International Society for Heart and Lung Transplantation: Eighteenth official pediatric lung and heart-lung transplantation report—2015; Focus theme: Early graft failure. *J Heart Lung Transplant.* 2015;34(10):1255–1263. doi:10.1016/j.healun.2015.08.005
13. Morrell E, Moynihan K, Wolfe J, Blume ED. Palliative care and paediatric cardiology: Current evidence and future directions. *Lancet Child Adolesc Health.* 2019;3(7):E10–E10.
14. Morell E, Wolfe J, Scheurer M, et al. Patterns of care at end of life in children with advanced heart disease. *Arch Pediatr Adolesc Med.* 2012;166(8):745–748. doi:10.1001/archpediatrics.2011.1829
15. Blume ED, Balkin EM, Aiyagari R, et al. Parental perspectives on suffering and quality of life at end-of-life in children with advanced heart disease. *Pediatr Crit Care Med.* 2014;15(4):336–342. doi:10.1097/PCC.0000000000000072
16. Moynihan K, Kaye E, Bailey V, Wolfe J, Thiagarajan R, Snaman J 41 Palliative Care Integration in Pediatric Cardiac Intensive Care Units: A Novel Champion-Based Model. *Crit Care Med.* 2019;47:189. doi:10.1097/01.ccm.0000551170.37983.db
17. Feudtner C, Kang TI, Hexem KR, et al. Pediatric palliative care patients: A prospective multicenter cohort study. *Pediatrics.* 2011;127(6):1094–1101. doi:10.1542/peds.2010-3225
18. Hollander SA, Dykes JC, Chen S, et al. The end-of-life experience of pediatric heart transplant recipients. *J Pain Symptom Manage.* 2017;53(5):927–931.
19. Hancock HS, Pituch K, Uzark K, et al. A randomised trial of early palliative care for maternal stress in infants prenatally diagnosed with single-ventricle heart disease. *Cardiol Young.* 2018;28(4):561–570.
20. Cousino MK, Miller VA, Smith C, et al. Medical and end-of-life decision making in adolescents' pre-heart transplant: A descriptive pilot study. *Palliat Med.* Published online 2019;34(3):272–280.

21. Rogers JG, Patel CB, Mentz RJ, et al. Palliative care in heart failure: The PAL-HF randomized, controlled clinical trial. *J Am Coll Cardiol.* 2017;70(3):331–341. doi:10.1016/j.jacc.2017.05.030
22. Balkin EM, Kirkpatrick JN, Kaufman B, et al. Pediatric cardiology provider attitudes about palliative care: A multicenter survey study. *Pediatr Cardiol.* 2017;38(7):1324–1331.
23. Cousino MK, Schumacher K, Magee J, et al. Communication about prognosis and end-of-life in pediatric organ failure and transplantation. *Pediatr Transplant.* Published online 2019:e13373. doi:10.1111/petr.13373
24. Balkin EM, Sleeper LA, Kirkpatrick JN, et al. Physician perspectives on palliative care for children with advanced heart disease: A comparison between pediatric cardiology and palliative care physicians. *J Palliat Med.* 2018;21(6):773–779.
25. Marwi ML, Henner N, Kirsch R. The role of palliative care in critical congenital heart disease. In *Seminars in Perinatology*. Vol 41.2017: 128–132.
26. Goloff N, Joy BF. A part of the team: The changing role of palliative care in congenital heart disease. *Prog Pediatr Cardiol.* 2018;48:59–62.
27. Marcus KL, Balkin EM, Al-Sayegh H, et al. Patterns and outcomes of care in children with advanced heart disease receiving palliative care consultation. *J Pain Symptom Manage.* 2018;55(2):351–358.
28. Uzark K, Jones K, Burwinkle TM, Varni JW. The Pediatric Quality of Life Inventory in children with heart disease. *Prog Pediatr Cardiol.* 2003;18(2):141–149. doi:https://doi.org/10.1016/S1058-9813(03)00087-0
29. Uzark K, Griffin L, Rodriguez R, et al. Quality of life in pediatric heart transplant recipients: A comparison with children with and without heart disease. *J Heart Lung Transplant.* 2012;31(6):571–578.
30. Uzark K, Zak V, Shrader P, et al. Assessment of quality of life in young patients with single ventricle after the Fontan operation. *J Pediatr.* 2016;170(Suppl C):166–172.e1. doi:https://doi.org/10.1016/j.jpeds.2015.11.016
31. Werner H, Latal B, Buechel EV, Beck I, Landolt MA. Health-related quality of life after open-heart surgery. *J Pediatr.* 2014;164(2):254–258.
32. Latal B, Helfricht S, Fischer JE, Bauersfeld U, Landolt MA. Psychological adjustment and quality of life in children and adolescents following open-heart surgery for congenital heart disease: A systematic review. *BMC Pediatr.* 2009;9(1):6.
33. Marino BS, Tomlinson RS, Drotar D, et al. Quality-of-life concerns differ among patients, parents, and medical providers in children and adolescents with congenital and acquired heart disease. *Pediatrics.* 2009;123(4):e708–e715.
34. DeWitt ES, Balkin EM, Reichman JR, et al. Parent-reported symptoms and effectiveness of treatment in children hospitalized with advanced heart disease. *J Heart Lung Transplant.* 2019;38(4):S464.
35. Wong C, Lau E, Palozzi L, Campbell F. Pain management in children: Part 1: Pain assessment tools and a brief review of nonpharmacological and pharmacological treatment options. *Can Pharm Journal.* 2012;145(5):222–225.
36. Sikandar S, Dickenson AH. Visceral pain–the ins and outs, the ups and downs. *Curr Opin Support Palliat Care.* 2012;6(1):17.
37. Madden K, Jo E, Williams JL, Liu D, Bruera E. Corrected QT interval prolongation in pediatric and young adult patients on methadone for cancer-related pain. *J Pain Symptom Manage.* 2019;58(4):678–684. doi:10.1016/j.jpainsymman.2019.05.021
38. McPherson ML, Walker KA, Davis MP, et al. Safe and appropriate use of methadone in hospice and palliative care: Expert consensus white paper. *J Pain Symptom Manage.* 2019;57(3):635–645.e4. doi:10.1016/j.jpainsymman.2018.12.001
39. Chou R, Cruciani RA, Fiellin DA, et al. Methadone safety: A clinical practice guideline from the American pain society and college on problems of drug dependence, in collaboration with the heart rhythm society. *J Pain.* 2014;15(4):321–337. doi:10.1016/j.jpain.2014.01.494
40. Rhodes J, Curran TJ, Camil L, et al. Impact of cardiac rehabilitation on the exercise function of children with serious congenital heart disease. *Pediatrics.* 2005;116(6):1339–1345.
41. Rhodes J, Curran TJ, Camil L, et al. Sustained effects of cardiac rehabilitation in children with serious congenital heart disease. *Pediatrics.* 2006;118(3):e586–e593.
42. DeMaso DR, Calderon J, Taylor GA, et al. Psychiatric disorders in adolescents with single ventricle congenital heart disease. *Pediatrics.* 2017;139(3):e20162241.
43. Diaz I, Thurm C, Hall M, et al. Disorders of adjustment, mood, and anxiety in children and adolescents undergoing heart transplantation and the association of ventricular assist device support. *J Pediatr.* Published online 2019;217:20–24. doi:10.1016/j.jpeds.2019.10.022
44. Cousino MK, Schumacher KR, Rea KE, et al. Psychosocial functioning in pediatric heart transplant recipients and their families. *Pediatr Transplant.* Published online 2018;2(2):e13110.
45. DeMaso DR, Kelley SD, Bastardi H, O'Brien P, Blume ED. The longitudinal impact of psychological functioning, medical severity, and family functioning in pediatric heart transplantation. *J Heart Lung Transplant.* 2004;23(4):473–480.
46. McCormick AD, Schumacher KR, Zamberlan M, et al. Illness Specific Anxiety Following Pediatric Heart Transplant. *J Heart Lung Transplant.* 2019;38(4):S94.
47. Goodlin SJ, Hauptman PJ, Arnold R, et al. Consensus statement: Palliative and supportive care in advanced heart failure. *J Card Fail.* 2004;10(3):200–209. doi:10.1016/j.cardfail.2003.09.006
48. Warnes CA, Williams RG, Bashore TM, et al. ACC/AHA 2008 Guidelines for the management of adults with congenital heart disease. *J Am Coll Cardiol.* 2008;52(23):1890–1947. doi:10.1016/j.jacc.2008.10.002
49. Tobler D, Greutmann M, Colman JM, Greutmann-Yantiri M, Librach LS, Kovacs AH. End-of-life in adults with congenital heart disease: A call for early communication. *Int J Cardiol.* 2012;155(3):383–387. doi:10.1016/j.ijcard.2010.10.050
50. Lyon ME, McCabe MA, Patel KM, D'angelo LJ. What do adolescents want? An exploratory study regarding end-of-life decision-making. *J Adolesc Health.* 2004;35(6):529. e1–529.e6. doi:https://doi.org/10.1016/j.jadohealth.2004.02.009
51. Lotz JD, Jox RJ, Borasio GD, Fuhrer M. Pediatric advance care planning: A systematic review. *Pediatrics.* 2013;131(3):e873–e880. doi:10.1542/peds.2012-2394
52. Lyon ME, Jacobs S, Briggs L, Cheng Y, Wang J. Family-centered advance care planning for teens with cancer. *JAMA Pediatr.* 2013;167(5):460–467. http://dx.doi.org/10.1001/jamapediatrics.2013.943
53. Lyon ME, Garvie PA, Briggs L, He J, McCarter R, D'Angelo LJ. Development, Feasibility, and Acceptability of the Family/Adolescent-Centered (FACE) advance care planning intervention for adolescents with HIV. *J Palliat Med.* 2009;12(4):363–372. doi:10.1089/jpm.2008.0261
54. Lyon ME, Garvie PA, McCarter R, Briggs L, He J, Angelo LJ. Who will speak for me? Improving end-of-life decision-making for adolescents with HIV and their families. *Pediatrics.* 2009;123(2):e199 LP-e206. http://pediatrics.aappublications.org/content/123/2/e199.abstract
55. Teno JM, Clarridge BR, Casey V, et al. Family perspectives on end-of-life care at the last place of care. *J Am Med Assoc.* 2004;291(1):88–93. doi:10.1001/jama.291.1.88
56. Rosenberg AR, Wolfe J, Wiener L, Lyon M, Feudtner C. Ethics, emotions, and the skills of talking about progressing disease with terminally ill adolescents a review. *JAMA Pediatr.* 2016;170(12). doi:10.1001/jamapediatrics.2016.2142
57. Yates AR, Hoffman TM, Boettner B, Feltes TF, Cua CL. Initial counseling prior to palliation for hypoplastic left heart syndrome. *Congenit Heart Dis.* 2011;6(4):347–358.
58. Rychik J, Szwast A, Natarajan S, et al. Perinatal and early surgical outcome for the fetus with hypoplastic left heart syndrome: A 5-year single institutional experience. *Ultrasound Obstet Gynecol.* 2010;36(4):465–470.
59. Rychik J. What does palliative care mean in prenatal diagnosis of congenital heart disease? *World J Pediatr Congenit Hear Surg.* 2013;4(1):80–84.

60. Knoll C, Kaufman B, Chen S, et al. Palliative care engagement for pediatric ventricular assist device patients. *ASAIO J*. Published online November 2019;66(8):929–932.
61. Machado DS, Hollander SA, Murray J, Philip J, Bleiweis M, Kittelson S. Ventricular assist device deactivation in children: Preparedness planning and procedural checklist. *J Heart Lung Transplant*. 2019;38(10):1116–1118.
62. Hollander SA, Axelrod DM, Bernstein D, et al. Compassionate deactivation of ventricular assist devices in pediatric patients. *J Heart Lung Transplant*. 2016;35(5):564–567. doi:10.1016/j.healun.2016.03.020
63. Hollander SA, McElhinney DB, Almond CS, et al. Rehospitalization after pediatric heart transplantation: Incidence, indications, and outcomes. *Pediatr Transplant*. 2017;21(1). doi:10.1111/petr.12857

31 | CYSTIC FIBROSIS AND OTHER CHILDHOOD LUNG DISEASES

ELISABETH POTTS DELLON, JESSICA GOGGIN, AND ELLIOT RABINOWITZ

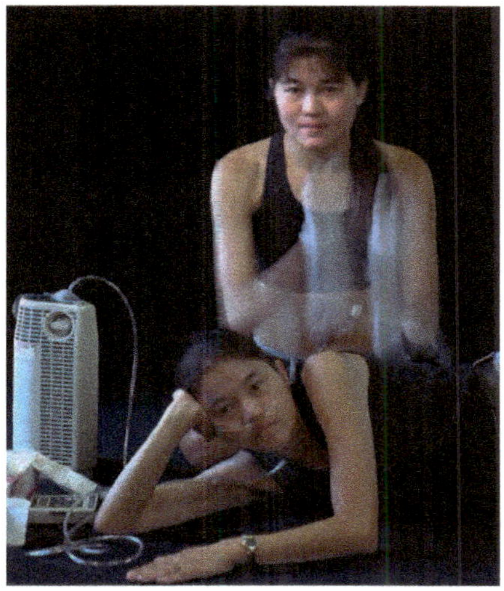

Photo by David Myers

Therapy
An endless rhythmic beat
A sort of faint knocking in the distance.
The hands of a mutual therapist
Pounding hard on the delicate chest
Beating delicately on the hard chest.
A cruel and merciless treatment
Scuenching our precious time on this earth.
Depleting such valuable energy from our souls
As the timer ticks away – anyway.
Faster! Faster!
Harder! Harder!
Day in, day out
A mindless routine sets in.

The anxiety of every breath grows stronger
With each cupped pound.
The aching back, sore muscles.
The bleeding hands gloved for protection
The cup overflows.
What meaning gives this bizarre and undignified practice
To the core of our existence?

"I love you!"
says the beating rhythm.
With each beat a reminder that you are no burden
A cherished moment of togetherness
Of deep connection between you and me.
A synchronicity of beating arms
Is a synchronicity of love and affection.

Isabel Stenzel Byrnes
(with permission from Isabel Stenzel Byrnes)

INTRODUCTION

Cystic fibrosis (CF) is a well-known disease to many pediatricians and pediatric palliative care (PPC) clinicians. PPC teams may encounter other life-threatening childhood lung diseases, but these are less common than CF. The focus of this chapter is on CF, with a brief overview of other childhood lung diseases. At the same time, readers will find much of the content also applies to these less familiar illnesses. Given the degree of familiarity with CF for the readers of this chapter, this chapter intertwines two goals: to provide an updated view of the rapidly evolving landscape of CF in the past decade and to present a model of primary and specialty palliative care delivery for children and families affected by CF. The typical patterns of care for individuals with CF have historically presented predictable barriers to successful integration of palliative care. Understanding the natural history, changing epidemiology and cultural understanding, and the perceived and actual physical and psychosocial burden of the disease will help palliative care specialists better understand how to integrate their clinical expertise into the established and successful CF model of clinical care. Furthermore, integration of palliative care does not need to disrupt the typically well-established relationships between children and their families with the CF care team.

OVERVIEW

CF is a life-limiting genetic disorder with an incidence of 1 in 3,200 live births in the United States. CF affects approximately 30,000 in North America and more than 70,000 individuals and their families worldwide.[1] CF is a multisystem disease resulting from mutations in the CF transmembrane regulator (CFTR) gene, causing abnormal chloride ion transport across epithelial cells lining the airways, pancreatic ducts, gastrointestinal (GI) tract, and reproductive organs. This abnormal transport leads to dehydrated and viscous secretions. Clinical manifestations of this defect include recurrent respiratory infections, nutritional deficiencies related to malabsorption from pancreatic exocrine insufficiency, intestinal obstruction, hepatobiliary disease, diabetes, and male azoospermia.[2] The natural history of CF is a progressive decline in lung function due to recurrent infection, inflammation, and bronchial obstruction leading to bronchiectasis and subsequent ongoing inflammation, infection, and airway damage. Chronic inflammation and infection of the airways accounts for most morbidity in CF, and the vast majority of people eventually die from respiratory failure.[3]

Once known as a pediatric illness due to short life expectancy, therapeutic advances have transformed CF into a chronic disease, with adults comprising more than half of those with CF in the United States and the United Kingdom.[4,5] Despite increased life expectancy, CF remains life-limiting, and people still die quite young, with a median age at death of approximately 31–32 years in 2018.[4,5] Unfortunately, children with CF and their families still endure the challenges associated with chronic illness, including the burden of numerous therapies and disease exacerbations, the knowledge of a limited life span, the responsibility of complex decision-making regarding lung transplant and other intensive treatments, and the stigma and reproductive choices associated with a genetic disease.

MODEL OF CYSTIC FIBROSIS CARE DELIVERY

The care of individuals with CF involves multiple interdisciplinary clinicians collaborating with parents and caregivers, often following guidelines and recommendations from the Cystic Fibrosis Foundation. While this model provides structure and guidance, the specific care delivered is tailored to each individual's needs and accessibility of available resources.

ACCREDITED CYSTIC FIBROSIS CARE CENTERS

Due to its complexity, clinical CF care in the United States is usually received at accredited CF care centers.[6] Part of a comprehensive network of clinical care, research, support, and quality improvement, accredited care centers were established in 1961 by the Cystic Fibrosis Foundation. There are about 130 accredited care centers across the United States, and people are encouraged to be seen at least quarterly.[7] Accredited CF care centers must adhere to established guidelines; however, variation may exist related to differences in location, institution, or health systems. For example, children who live a long distance from their closest center may receive primarily consultative care, with much of their day-to-day care provided by a local primary physician. Additionally, children without health insurance may have limited or no access to a CF center at all, especially if the institution does not provide charity care or the child does not have documented status as a US citizen or resident.

INTERDISCIPLINARY TEAMS

An interdisciplinary approach to care is essential to manage this complex illness. Specialized care is provided through interdisciplinary teams with physicians, nurses, social workers, dietitians, and respiratory therapists; disciplines required for CF care center accreditation.[6] Some teams also include other specialists like pharmacists, gastroenterologists, endocrinologists, psychologists, psychiatrists, physical therapists, or child life specialists. Close relationships often form between children, their families, and CF teams after working together for years and sometimes decades. With outcomes in CF closely linked with adherence to the daily treatment regimen, parents and other caregivers are essential partners in the CF care delivery model.

PALLIATIVE CARE IN CYSTIC FIBROSIS

There are no accreditation requirements or standards for integration of specialty palliative care within CF care in the United States; however, the Cystic Fibrosis Foundation that states palliative care may be useful in symptom management.[8–10] Similarly, the European Cystic Fibrosis Society Guidelines call for "attention to communication, symptom control and a multi-disciplinary approach to care, including expertise in palliative care."[11] Access to specialty palliative care varies by institution due to differences in size, scope, and availability of palliative care. For example, some CF centers are in an institution that only provides inpatient palliative care, limiting access for those with CF who could benefit from palliative care but are not hospitalized. Institutions that offer outpatient palliative care may have variable scope of services.

IMPORTANT THINGS TO KNOW ABOUT CYSTIC FIBROSIS CARE

Routine care in CF aims primarily to control and/or improve symptoms, prevent or treat respiratory infection, and optimize nutrition.[10,12] This treatment, including airway clearance and medications for respiratory symptoms, pancreatic enzymes to improve GI symptoms and weight, and sometimes other medications to treat complications such as diabetes, forms the foundation of the treatment regimen in CF.

TREATMENT BURDEN

Treatment regimens in CF can be time-consuming, sometimes requiring 2–4 hours of therapy daily.[13] Children with CF require close supervision from caregivers, and even adults often need assistance from caregivers to carry out respiratory therapies and other treatments.[14] Adolescents may be particularly vulnerable if, as they strive to assert independence as part of usual growth and development, they decrease adherence to their CF treatment regimen. The time required is most always burdensome and challenging for both children and their families to maintain. Care should be nonjudgmental, with emphasis on partnering with children and families to focus on making the best decisions they can today and in the future, without blame or guilt related to past decisions.

INFECTION CONTROL

As more evidence has become available over the past several decades, infection control has become a significant component of treatment. Over time, the lungs become colonized with various organisms, and people with CF risk exposing each other to dangerous respiratory pathogens. Current infection control and prevention guidelines call for people with CF to avoid close proximity to others with CF, staying a minimum of 6 feet apart at all times.[15] An unfortunate consequence of the guidelines is the potential for decreased interaction and social support between people with CF.[16]

MENTAL HEALTH

In addition to physical symptoms, people with CF, including children and adolescents, experience a high rate of depression and anxiety, and an association has also been found with effective management of CF.[17,18] Mental health care in CF has been emphasized through recent requirements for anxiety and depression screening and efforts to facilitate social support for people with CF and their families.[18]

CARE DURING ADVANCED ILLNESS

CF is a lifelong illness that necessitates frequent and never-ending therapies. While intensive therapies aimed at maintaining airway clearance and nutrition may stave off exacerbations, individuals with CF will invariably experience progressive loss of function; live with the unpredictable risk of exacerbations, worsening lung function, and frequent hospitalizations; and, ultimately, suffer a premature death. Unfortunately, even the most experienced CF clinician is unable to predict when these episodes of acute illness and loss may occur, and the disease carries a large degree of uncertainty.[19] Many individuals with CF experience acute decompensations in health, recoveries, and periods of relative stability, usually superimposed on a gradual downward trajectory in lung function (Figure 31.1). An individual's functional capacity over time often mirrors this course. Most people will have periodic setbacks, and while some of these setbacks will be followed by complete recovery, others may result in a decline of overall function. Lung transplant is a choice for some people with advanced illness but is not curative and comes with a host of burdens and uncertainties along with the potential for life extension and improved quality of life.

INNOVATIVE THERAPIES

When the CF gene was initially described in 1989, many believed a cure was imminent.[20] This hope led to great optimism, followed by disappointment when a cure did not readily arrive.[21] While there is still no cure at this time, new and improved therapies, as well as the possibility of lung transplant, offer hope to many people living with CF.[22] Recent development of cystic fibrosis transmembrane conductance regulator (CFTR) modulator medications have led to many in the CF community feeling that the future, long-anticipated following identification of the CFTR gene, is happening now.[23] CFTR modulators address the underlying cause of CF, restoring function to the defective CFTR protein and potentially altering the natural course of the illness.[23] The first CFTR modulator, ivacaftor (Kalydeco), was approved in the United States in 2012, but only about 8–10% of people with CF were eligible to take it. Recent studies report improved clinical outcomes and quality of life in people with CF taking ivacaftor.[24,25] After interim progress with additional modulators, elexacaftor/ivacaftor/tezacaftor (Trikafta) was approved in the United States in late 2019. Close to 90% of adults are now eligible for a CFTR modulator, with hope that approval for children will soon follow. Long-term safety, tolerability, and effectiveness are under study and much has been written about the high cost of these new medications. Ongoing research is already seeking the next generations of CFTR modulators and other innovative therapies.

This is an unprecedented and exciting time, but people with CF, especially those who are ineligible or cannot tolerate CFTR modulators because of drug interactions, hepatic insult, or adverse mental health outcomes, and those with accumulated damage to lungs and other organs will continue to

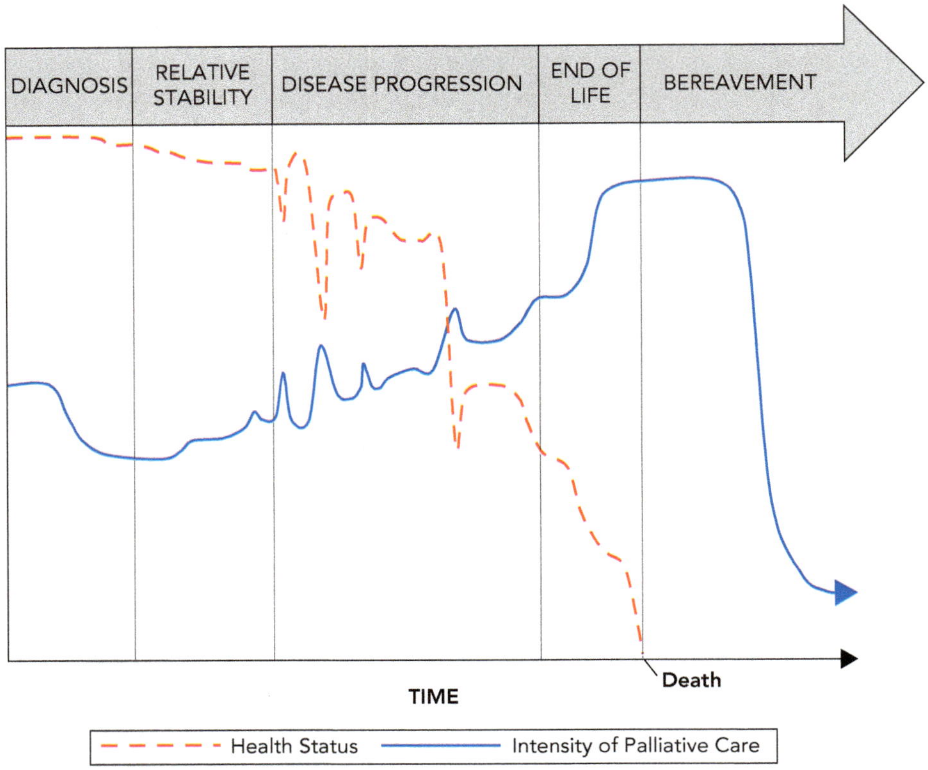

Figure 31.1 *Anticipated trajectory of illness in cystic fibrosis.*

need comprehensive care, including primary and specialty palliative care for years to come.[26–30] It can be difficult to balance hope and optimism when seeing progress made in CF while at the same time confronted by the reality of disease progression and disappointment when a long-awaited therapy is not available or cannot reverse years of damage and other sequelae of CF.

HOPE

For individuals with CF and those who care for them, hope and despair are inextricably intertwined. Widespread and consistent application of chronic treatments has led to increasing life expectancy, and new and improved treatments have shown more promise than ever. Understandably, most individuals with CF, family caregivers, and clinicians maintain an attitude of vigorous optimism. Experience suggests that CF teams generally adopt an enthusiastic approach, emphasizing optimistic increases in life expectancy and encouraging hope for improved survival and quality of life. This attitude is in part a response to the outdated image of CF among the general public as a killer of children, in part a strategy to encourage adherence to a time-consuming daily regimen, and in part an antidote to the unpredictable course of the illness.

Despite increasing life expectancy, people with CF still experience significant suffering.[17,31–33] In some circumstances, hopeful enthusiasm of CF care team members and parents may crowd out concerns of the child regarding what he or she has heard about limited life expectancy in CF. At other times, optimism may inhibit frank discussion of the reality of life with CF. The same enthusiasm may discourage reporting of bothersome symptoms or concerns about burdens of treatment. In these instances, a CF team's enthusiastic optimism may worsen the child's or family's anxiety, when a quiet but hopeful discussion might have alleviated their concerns. An overly optimistic approach may also prevent the CF care team from recognizing benefits of collaboration with the palliative care team. A rejection of the either/or attitude toward hope and despair encourages recognition that hope can flourish even in the face of the difficult truth of symptom burden and limited life expectancy of CF.

CYSTIC FIBROSIS ILLNESS TRAJECTORY

CF is a lifelong, multisystem, progressive illness characterized by gradual decline in lung function and GI/nutritional difficulties, with worsening symptom and treatment burden over time. In considering when and how to incorporate palliative care into CF care, it is helpful to consider both disease milestones and stage of illness across the life span of individuals with CF, including (1) diagnosis, (2) relative stability, (3) disease progression, and (4) end of life.

DIAGNOSIS

CF is an autosomal recessive genetic disorder. Although many older children and adults were diagnosed following onset of symptoms or diagnosis of a sibling, most new diagnoses are now made through newborn screening, resulting in a population of asymptomatic infants diagnosed in the first month of life.[5,33–35] Earlier diagnosis has led to some improved clinical outcomes, but does carry some risks for families, including emotional impact of indeterminate testing results with diagnostic uncertainty and implications of diagnosis of a genetic disease.[36–39] Because of their experience with discussing difficult news and helping families manage grief, palliative care teams are in a good position to help CF teams develop a compassionate approach to revealing the diagnosis.[40]

Families must process not only shock of the diagnosis, but also begin a complex care regimen to be followed every day if the benefit of earlier diagnosis via newborn screening is to be realized. CF care teams are accomplished at helping families with this news, but advent of newborn screening brings a new group to light: the largely asymptomatic child with a genetic diagnosis. The change in the experience of diagnosis may offer an opportunity for palliative care teams to approach the CF care team with an offer to help them do the best possible job supporting families affected by CF.

RELATIVE STABILITY

Two events may provide room for palliative care teams to partner with CF care teams. The first is preparing the team to respond to children and families when they bring up limited life expectancy with CF. Many CF clinicians prefer to minimize this issue by focusing on the progress in CF so far, while many individuals with CF, especially by adolescence, are aware of limited life expectancy and should be offered the opportunity to talk about it.[41–43] CF care team members do not want to be surprised when an adolescent asks about mortality, and the palliative care team may be able to help develop an educational approach which explores a range of developmentally appropriate responses to a child's questions.

Second, palliative care teams may have a window of opportunity to assist CF care teams during the first hospitalization for a pulmonary exacerbation. The first pulmonary exacerbation can be a time of substantial stress for the whole family as they are confronted with the reality of worsening illness.[44] Habituating the family to a routine of careful surveillance and vigorous treatment of any drop from "baseline" is an important goal. CF care teams may not recognize the increased symbolic meaning of this first exacerbation in an era of newborn screening and highly effective modulator therapy. Although pulmonary exacerbations and their treatment remain routine for CF teams, they are new to people with CF and their families.

DISEASE PROGRESSION AND END OF LIFE

There are many opportunities for integration of specialty palliative care within CF as the disease progresses: expert assessment and management of CF-related physical and emotional symptoms; communication augmentation, including assistance with goals of care, advance care planning (ACP), and complex treatment decision-making; caregiver support with shifting burdens and needs; and care coordination. These topics will be addressed in the next section.

With progress in therapies, some of the burden of symptoms and therapies may be lessening for children and adolescents. However, many young people currently living with CF face the challenges of progressive disease and end of life. As such, palliative care specialists should be familiar with the unique needs of children with CF and their caregivers.

DELIVERING PALLIATIVE CARE TO CHILDREN WITH CYSTIC FIBROSIS

Palliative care is ideally a partnership, whereby CF care team members provide continuous monitoring and support for palliative needs, or primary palliative care, while palliative care specialists support the CF care team with expert management of complex or severe concerns.[45,46] Long-term, trusting relationships often exist between CF care teams and individuals with CF and their caregivers, thus facilitating CF care teams in addressing primary palliative care needs. CF care team members endorse the need for focused training in primary palliative care skills, including basic pain and symptom management, communication about goals of care, prognosis, and treatment decisions.[8,46–48] Palliative care specialists can offer expert management of complex or intractable distress that is beyond the scope or skill set of the CF care team (i.e., specialty palliative care) and can provide training and support around primary palliative care skills.

Historically, there has been no standard for incorporating specialty palliative care within CF care. Not unlike the general public and even some healthcare clinicians, many CF care teams inappropriately regard specialty palliative care as associated only with end of life. As a result, specific palliative interventions, including therapies directed at managing symptoms in those with mild to moderate disease, are often not introduced until the person is clearly dying—often too late to derive the benefits of specialty palliative care. A palliative care approach, clearly differentiated from end-of-life care and integrated with disease-directed and restorative measures from the time of diagnosis, may limit the burden of disease, maximize quality of life at all stages of illness, and provide effective support to individuals with CF and their families.[45] The intensity of palliative care should match the unique needs of each individual, including but not limited to physical and emotional symptom management, addressing existential and spiritual suffering, communicating about prognosis and treatment options, eliciting goals of care, engaging children with CF and caregivers in ACP, and, when relevant, offering support during lung transplant evaluation and following transplantation.

The remainder of this section will emphasize the role of the palliative care specialist in caring for individuals with CF, complementing primary palliative care offered by the CF care team. While consultation is more likely to occur in later stages of disease, it is important to recognize the value that specialty palliative care could bring throughout the life

BOX 31.1 HOW CAN THE PEDIATRIC PALLIATIVE CARE TEAM HELP THE CYSTIC FIBROSIS (CF) TEAM CARE FOR CHILDREN, ADOLESCENTS AND FAMILIES WITH CF THROUGHOUT THE LIFE SPAN?

At the time of diagnosis

- Help the care CF team develop strategies to reveal the diagnosis in a compassionate manner and to mitigate the impact of parental grief.

During routine care

- Help the CF care team anticipate and prepare for emotional reactions to setbacks and especially the first hospitalization, which can trigger parental anxiety about disease progression and mortality.
- Help the CF care team become comfortable with discussions of mortality throughout the life span of the child and adolescent, so that the team is prepared for inevitable questions and discussion with children and families and prioritizes communication about prognosis as a part of routine care.

As the disease progresses

- Help the CF care team gain expertise in the assessment and treatment of symptoms throughout the life span, including expertise in pain management and assessment of nonpulmonary, non-GI symptoms such as fatigue and anxiety.
- Provide advice and approaches to raising and discussing complex issues like advance care planning, facing prognostic uncertainty.
- Help the CF care team plan a comprehensive roadmap for the decisions which will be faced by individuals with CF, caregivers, and clinicians, including anticipatory guidance about the use of intensive technologies like mechanical ventilation and extracorporeal life support (ECLS).
- Offer the CF care team and transplant team assistance with planning and carrying out the process of transplant decision-making.

At end of life

- Offer expertise and experience with managing symptoms and end-of-life care in different settings, including accessing pediatric hospice services if available.

After the death of the child or adolescent

- Offer direct bereavement services (or referral to community bereavement services) for caregivers and siblings.
- Offer grief and bereavement support to CF care team and transplant team members.

---

span. For examples of how palliative care teams can partner with CF care teams in providing palliative care to children with CF throughout the life span, please refer to Box 31.1 and the Family Reflection at the end of this chapter. Table 31.1 highlights examples of primary and specialty palliative care within the domains of palliative care.

SYMPTOM ASSESSMENT AND MANAGEMENT

Distressing physical and emotional symptoms are common in individuals with CF throughout the life span.[49–53] While clinicians typically expect both physical and emotional symptoms to worsen as lung disease progresses, they are not as clearly associated as one might expect.[10,51–55] Little research describes the impact of symptoms on quality of life or on the end-of-life experience for individuals with CF, but existing literature and clinical practice suggest much room for improvement in both care delivery and support for CF team members in managing symptoms.[47,56] General principles of symptom management can be applied in CF, and the multidisciplinary nature of CF care should allow for regular attention to symptoms with input from palliative care specialists for complex and/or severe symptoms and spiritual/existential distress. Because other chapters focus on assessment and management of symptoms, this section covers issues specific to symptom management in CF.

RESPIRATORY SYMPTOMS

Respiratory symptoms such as cough and dyspnea may be only minimal or intermittent in younger people, but worsen as lung disease progresses, with periods of increased cough and dyspnea occurring during respiratory exacerbations. Basic CF respiratory care, directed at reducing respiratory symptoms, involves a combination of airway clearance techniques, aerosolized therapies, antimicrobials, anti-inflammatory medications, and exercise.[57] Devices like percussive vests are used several times daily to help loosen and dislodge thick, sticky mucus. Daily airway clearance therapies are essential to maintain lung health and quality of life in CF. Respiratory exacerbations of CF manifest in many ways, with symptoms including increased cough and sputum production, dyspnea, fatigue, fever, chest pain, hemoptysis, sleep disturbance, and weight loss.

Cough is necessary for clearance of thick respiratory secretions, but excessive cough may be distressing and disruptive. Aerosolized therapies and airway clearance techniques facilitate cough and are routinely recommended for maintenance of health and are intensified during respiratory exacerbations. While these treatments are intended to reduce chronic respiratory symptoms, they are also burdensome due in part to the extensive amount of time required for treatments, but also the discomforts associated with respiratory therapies, such as pain, dyspnea, sleep disturbance, and urinary incontinence.[58,59] Treatment of increased cough includes aerosols and airway clearance therapies, antibiotics for infection, and specific treatments for other common causes of cough in CF, including gastroesophageal reflux disease, sinus disease, asthma, and allergies. Antitussives are typically avoided due to their negative impact on airway clearance. For severe exacerbations, hospitalization may be necessary. Intravenous antibiotics are commonly used, often in combination given the challenges of combating virulent and often drug-resistant respiratory pathogens, along with intensified airway clearance therapies.[3]

TABLE 31.1 Primary versus specialty palliative care for individuals with cystic fibrosis and their families

PALLIATIVE CARE DOMAIN	PRIMARY PALLIATIVE CARE (PPC) PALLIATIVE CARE CONCERNS ADDRESSED BY CF CARE TEAM[a]	SPECIALTY PALLIATIVE CARE (SPC) REASONS TO CONSIDER CONSULTING A PALLIATIVE CARE SPECIALIST
Symptom management	Basic physical symptoms like pain, cough, dyspnea, anorexia (MD/NP; dietitian; RT; PT) Basic management of emotional symptoms like anxiety and depression (MD/NP, psychologist, SW)	Assist with managing physical symptoms refractory to PPC interventions Assist with managing emotional symptoms refractory to PPC interventions Address existential/spiritual distress
Communication: Goals of care, advance care planning, and decision-making	Educate about CF as a chronic, progressive condition (MD/NP, RN) Discuss prognostic uncertainty (MD/NP, RN, SW, psychologist) Communicate distressing news related to CF (MD/NP, RN, SW) Engage patient and caregivers in discussions about goals of care (MD/NP, RN, SW, psychologist) Describe options for life-sustaining treatments for respiratory failure (MD/NP) Identify surrogate decision maker (MD/NP) Guide documentation of legal, actionable advance directives (MD/NP, SW) Educate and support around transplantation, including medical indications, processes, and outcomes (MD/NP)	Address resuscitation status, advance directives when there are misunderstandings of options and prognosis Navigate discordance among patients, caregivers, and healthcare providers Address concerns about misalignment of goals and treatment decisions Address fears about future illness and preferences for communication (e.g., family vs. patient-centered, amount of information desired about illness, and benefits versus burdens of treatment options) Act as third party for conversations about lung transplantation Additional exploration of wishes around end-of-life care
Caregiver support	Supportive listening (all team members) Screen for caregiver anxiety and depression (SW, psychologist) Identify resources for emotional support (SW, psychologist) Address financial needs and identify resources (SW)	Address needs that exceed expertise of CF care team, particularly if conflict exists Address existential/spiritual distress of caregivers Explore grief and bereavement needs and assist with community referrals
Care coordination	Communicate with other relevant healthcare providers (all team members) Referral to community resources (RN, SW)	Communicate with CF care team and other relevant healthcare providers Introduce and assist with referrals to hospice and community palliative care resources; hospice eligibility review

[a] CF care team members' contributions to primary palliative care of individuals with CF by discipline are noted in parenthesis. Abbreviations: Physician (MD), nurse practitioner (NP), CF nurse (RN), social worker (SW), respiratory therapist (RT), physical therapist (PT).

Hemoptysis may occur in association with cough, particularly in the setting of lower respiratory infections. Small volume hemoptysis is generally managed with antibiotics, correction of bleeding disorders, and cautious use of or temporary suspension of aerosols and airway clearance therapies. Massive hemoptysis (more than 240 milliliters in 24 hours or recurrent bleeding of more than 100 milliliters per day) occurs in approximately 1% of children with CF and is unrelated to severity of lung disease, is associated with other respiratory complications, and has a high likelihood of recurrence.[60] Bronchial artery embolization is utilized for acute treatment, but recurrent and unremitting end-stage hemoptysis may require sedation and measures such as the use of dark towels and linens to reduce visualization of bright red blood and help lessen anxiety.

Dyspnea is commonly reported as CF lung disease progresses.[10,59–61] This complex symptom is related to increased ventilatory demand due to increased dead space in abnormal CF lungs, increased respiratory effort to move air through dilated and obstructed airways, and increased muscle force required for maintenance of normal ventilation because of abnormal airway resistance and flattening of the diaphragm by hyperinflated lungs.[62] Notably, the interplay between dyspnea and anxiety can be complicated.[63,64] Enhanced airway clearance and treatment of infection and inflammation with standard CF therapies may reduce acute or subacute dyspnea. With disease progression, dyspnea may become less responsive to such treatments.

For those with chronic dyspnea and more advanced lung disease, physical therapy to improve conditioning may be helpful. The use of oxygen to support gas exchange with exertion, during sleep, and on a continual basis later in the course of disease may reduce the sensation of dyspnea. Oxygen is usually administered by nasal cannula, although some people prefer to use face masks during periods of acute illness. Noninvasive positive pressure ventilation for management of dyspnea, hypoxemia, and hypercapnia was often avoided in the past because of concern for applying positive pressure to airways which are abnormally dilated and impacted with thick mucus, making airway clearance more difficult, but it has gained favor over time for those with sleep disturbance and daytime fatigue and as a bridging therapy for those with respiratory insufficiency awaiting lung transplantation.[65,66] Intubation with mechanical ventilation, and even extracorporeal life support (ECLS), may also be considered for some people with "reversible" causes of respiratory failure and for lung transplant candidates.[67,68] Ventilator modes and settings that combat hypercapnia in advanced CF lung disease are uncomfortable and typically necessitate the use of sedative medications which interfere with the ability to communicate. ECLS as a bridge to lung transplantation is intended to be provided to people who are awake and ambulatory, but the risk for complications is not insignificant.[68,69] The decision to use these interventions must be made with the knowledge that, while they may provide relief of severe dyspnea and possibly prolong life, their use has many associated risks which must be understood by individuals with CF and caregivers, along with continued exploration of goals of care.

Decreasing the sensation of dyspnea using opioids and benzodiazepines may be considered for use in advanced CF lung disease.[70,71] However, despite evidence that these medications can be used safely in people with respiratory diseases, concerns about respiratory depression in advanced CF lung disease have been described and may act as barriers to effective palliation of dyspnea.[9,55,67,70,72,73] Aerosolized opioids have not been found to be efficacious.[74] Concerns about the use of opioids to relieve dyspnea may be alleviated by starting with very low doses and titrating to effect, monitoring closely for undesirable secondary effects and managing constipation proactively. This strategy also allows everyone the time to become more comfortable with the use of opioids to treat dyspnea. Other supportive and adjunctive therapies, including blowing cool air with fans, maintaining cooler ambient temperatures, positioning, relaxation techniques, and psychotherapy may be beneficial for some people. Clusters of symptoms like dyspnea and anxiety require thoughtful management.

PAIN

Pain, including headache and sinus, chest, back, abdominal, and joint pain, is common in individuals with CF throughout the life span and negatively affects adherence, emotional symptoms, quality of life, and survival.[33,52,75] Headache may be due to cough, sinus disease, or hypercapnia in addition to the numerous other causes of headache in people without CF, and treatment should reflect the cause. Sinus pain may respond to treatment for infection with systemic or nasally instilled antibiotics or use of intranasal steroids and saline to facilitate drainage of secretions. Surgical intervention by an otolaryngologist for severe or persistent pain may be warranted.[76] Chest pain that originates from the lung may be due to infection, mucus plugging, hemoptysis, or pneumothorax; it is often localized and may be pleuritic and/or associated with symptoms like cough and dyspnea. Musculoskeletal chest pain may result from frequent cough and increased thoracic volume.[77] Individuals with CF may also be at increased risk of rib and vertebral compression fractures in the setting of osteoporosis related to chronic vitamin D deficiency and/or systemic steroid use.[78,79] Physical therapy, pharmacologic agents, and orthopedic referral can be considered depending on the etiology of the pain. Joint pain may be due to typical injuries or causes of arthritis in the non-CF population and to fluoroquinolone antibiotic use, but *CF arthropathy*, a diagnosis of exclusion, affects a small proportion of people with CF.[80] Symptoms are typically episodic and present at times of illness and stress. Treatment may involve analgesics and anti-inflammatory medications, sometimes including disease-modifying anti-rheumatic drugs.[81] Caution should be given to concurrent use of nonsteroidal anti-inflammatory drugs (NSAIDs) in patients who are treated with nephrotoxic antibiotics for pulmonary exacerbations or with known comorbid kidney or liver disease; acetaminophen should be used carefully in those with CF-associated liver disease.

Distressing and/or debilitating pain from any source warrants careful evaluation. Appropriate management involves identifying and, if possible, eliminating underlying causes. Establishing goals of treatment and selection of medications and other treatments, and monitoring response to therapies and treatment side effects, should follow standard approaches to pain management addressed in previous chapters. Concerns about opioid use are often amplified in CF due to concerns about respiratory depression and severe constipation in addition to the societal concerns about misuse, abuse, and addiction. Additionally, lung transplant eligibility may affect opioid prescribing given concerns from transplant centers about perioperative management and long-term outcomes. There is not enough evidence to either support or refute withholding opioids from individuals with CF who have appropriate indications, including moderate to severe acute or chronic pain, painful therapies, dyspnea in severe lung disease, or pain/dyspnea at end of life.[82,83] As such, consideration around opioid prescribing must be individualized, with lung transplant not being an absolute contraindication.

GASTROINTESTINAL SYMPTOMS

Gastrointestinal manifestations of CF are numerous and include steatorrhea and malnutrition related to pancreatic exocrine insufficiency (present in approximately 85% of individuals with CF), gastroesophageal reflux, and obstructive biliary tract disease.[5] Symptoms related to these problems include abdominal pain, constipation, anorexia, and, for a small percentage of people, symptoms of progressive hepatobiliary disease.[84] Abdominal pain associated with an increase in bowel movements, urgency, or distension should prompt optimization of pancreatic enzyme replacement. Constipation may be acute or chronic in nature and may be treated with oral electrolyte solutions and/or stimulant laxatives. Distal intestinal obstruction syndrome may occur when excessively viscid intestinal contents become impacted in the distal small intestine and proximal colon and should be suspected when pain and obstipation occur concomitantly. Treatment involves intestinal lavage and close monitoring for progression to frank bowel obstruction, which warrants surgical intervention.[85] Gastroesophageal reflux is managed with standard therapies, including histamine receptor antagonists and proton pump inhibitors. Surgical treatment of reflux does not appear to confer benefit but is considered in some cases.[86] Other causes of GI symptoms which are not specific to or more common in CF must not be overlooked.

Because of malabsorption and increased metabolic demands, individuals with CF require greater caloric intake to achieve and maintain adequate nutritional status. As lung disease progresses, cough and increased work of breathing may make eating laborious and maintenance of weight difficult or impossible without medical intervention. Behavioral interventions around feeding, calorie-dense oral supplements, and appetite stimulants are typically offered in a stepwise fashion as other causes of and contributors to anorexia, including gastroesophageal reflux disease, sinus disease, depression, and anxiety are addressed.[87,88] For those who are unable to maintain acceptable nutritional status, feeding tubes may be recommended.[88] Individuals with advanced disease who choose to pursue lung transplantation may be required to pursue intensive nutritional interventions in order to reduce operative and recovery-related risks. Those for whom transplantation is not desired or not an option may be offered more choices about the ongoing use of nutritional interventions.

PSYCHOLOGICAL SYMPTOMS

Depression and anxiety are known to be more prevalent in CF compared to the general population.[89] They may adversely impact health outcomes and quality of life. Screening for depression and anxiety and guiding those affected to appropriate interventions and support are recommended as a routine part of CF care.[18] For patients and families affected by any chronic illness, disease-specific social support plays a vital role in coping with stress and managing depression and anxiety. In contrast to past extensive social support available through cohorting of children with CF on hospital wards and summer camps, strict guidelines for infection control have led to physical isolation of individuals with CF and thus often their families. This has led to social networking and support via the internet and other media which allow for indirect contact.[90] For some, this is extremely effective, but for others this isolation leads to loneliness which may theoretically impact disease-related coping.[91,92]

Treatment of depression in CF does not differ from standard treatment, apart from the recognition of chronic illness as a provocative factor.[18] Anxiety about disease progression is common, suggesting the need for ongoing attention to this symptom throughout the life span. Symptom clusters may occur, such that anxiety may be perpetuated by dyspnea, cough, pain, and fatigue; thus, addressing these symptoms may reduce and indirectly treat anxiety. Medications commonly used to treat CF, such as beta-agonists and steroids, may also contribute to anxiety symptoms. Treatment of anxiety may involve cognitive-behavioral therapy, psychotherapy, and complementary techniques such as biofeedback and relaxation. Pharmacologic agents may be added in select cases, with favor given to selective serotonin reuptake inhibitors (SSRIs) and selective-norepinephrine reuptake inhibitors (SNRIs), noting potential for drug interactions in those using CFTR modulators or antimicrobial drugs with shared hepatic metabolism; this is most commonly the case with SSRIs.[93] Oral benzodiazepines are considered for short-term treatment of acute anxiety but otherwise reserved for those with severe and unremitting symptoms or advanced lung disease as per Cystic Fibrosis Foundation guidelines.[18,83]

FATIGUE

Fatigue is a highly prevalent but often underappreciated symptom in childhood chronic disease and is a common symptom in CF.[49,64,94] Fatigue is reported to impact adherence to treatment and quality of life.[94–96] This complex symptom is often unresponsive to rest, limits functioning, and affects physical, cognitive, and emotional stamina.[64] The interaction between fatigue and other symptoms such as cough, dyspnea, pain, and depression may be substantial.[95] Treatment for fatigue is also complex and not well studied in CF, but interventions including exercise, psychotherapy and disease-specific support networks, complementary and alternative therapies, improving sleep hygiene, and the use of stimulants are possible options.[64,97] Management of sleep disturbance, either on its own or as a contributor to fatigue, centers on improving nocturnal hypoxemia or sleep-disordered breathing. If present, treatment with supplemental oxygen or noninvasive positive pressure ventilation and avoiding use of hypnotics in favor of nonpharmacological strategies may be beneficial, with melatonin felt to be safe and efficacious for children with CF.[98,99]

ROLE OF THE PALLIATIVE CARE TEAM IN SYMPTOM MANAGEMENT

While CF clinicians and other care team members are aware of the high symptom burden in CF, many lack specific training in thorough assessment and management of symptoms. Additionally, the focus of routine CF care is often on preservation of "baseline" health and lung function rather than on chronic management of symptoms, even for those symptoms which are more likely to progress than to remit. Concerns about medication side effects and long-term implications of certain symptom-specific treatments, as well as a lack of clinical decision support, may lead to under-prescribing of medications and other symptom-specific treatments, particularly in the late stages of CF lung disease. Palliative care clinicians may use their expertise to bring attention to and offer relief from distressing symptoms experienced by individuals with CF as their disease progresses.

COMMUNICATION: GOALS OF CARE, ADVANCE CARE PLANNING, AND DECISION-MAKING

Most individuals with CF will live into their adult years, necessitating a transition of decision-making from surrogates to autonomous decisions. Often, in this transition, adults with CF may defer decision-making to the parent who has carried that responsibility all their lives.[13] For this reason, special care should be taken to assess the role of each individual in the decision-making process, and effort should be made to actively include the adolescent and young adult.[100]

While few people give no thought at all to the life-threatening nature of their disease, some adolescents and young adults develop certain fantasies or beliefs about their life span and may develop symbolic meaning to living past a certain age.[43,101,102] These expectations and perceptions may directly influence planning for the future, adherence to the therapeutic regimens, and quality of life. Prognostic uncertainty and discussions about life expectancy lead to anticipatory grief in children with CF. This grief may intensify during hospitalization and when health declines, as well as through observation of serious illness and death in CF peers. Children, caregivers, and clinicians should be encouraged to see grief as an expected part of life with CF. Much like other children with chronic life-threatening illnesses, children with CF are often aware they are dying even if never told directly, and they have concerns about impending death and separation from caregivers, family, and friends.[103] They may also grieve the loss of function, lack of interaction with family and peers, and changes in body image. Palliative care specialists and others with expertise in psychosocial support can help children communicate these concerns and find meaning and control as illness progresses. They can also be helpful in educating caregivers and members of the CF care team in how to provide appropriate supports to the child and how best to involve children in planning and decision-making, which could help mitigate anxiety and grief around serious illness and disease progression.

While ACP for children does not carry legal weight, the American Academy of Pediatrics recommends that children, adolescents, and young adults with a life-limiting illness be involved in ACP.[104] As such, children with CF should be included in medical decision-making in a culturally and developmentally appropriate way with an effort of transition from assent to autonomy.[41,105,106] Information about ACP in CF is limited, especially in children. A study of adults with CF revealed that most recognized the life-threatening nature of their disease and have considered the type of care they would want to have if unable to decide for themselves, and many even developed specific plans about end-of-life care.[107] While these adults discussed their plans with family members and said they would be comfortable discussing them with the CF care team, only one-third had in fact discussed ACP with any member of the team. Subsequent studies suggest greater rates of ACP, but this is not universal among adults with this known life-limiting illness.[48,105,108] Reasons for lack of communication include perceptions that these discussions will hinder hope, optimistic expectations of treatment outcomes, denial of disease severity, delaying conversations until patients themselves are too ill to participate, and beliefs that they only need to occur when death is imminent.[109,110]

Existing ACP tools may not fit the clinical characteristics of CF given the unique aspects of the CF illness trajectory and disease-specific therapies. In an attempt to improve ACP, some CF care centers have developed CF-specific tools or have adapted programs such as Voicing My Choices and Five Wishes for use in CF clinical care.[111] Do not attempt resuscitation (DNAR) and do not attempt intubation (DNAI) orders appear to be perceived as having limited practical use in ACP in CF in the United States because a DNAR order is not in place for most people with CF until very late in the course of illness.[112] In practice, DNAR and DNAI orders should not be used as the sole document regarding appropriate interventions near the end of life, particularly as the roles and outcomes of advanced therapies like extracorporeal membrane oxygenation (ECMO) to support respiratory failure evolve.[68] Instead, these orders should be used as part of meeting the goals of care of the individual and family and should be consistent with the anticipated outcome of the intervention.

LUNG TRANSPLANTATION FOR ADVANCED CF LUNG DISEASE: SPECIAL CONSIDERATIONS

Lung transplantation is the most intensive treatment available for advanced CF lung disease and is considered when one's functional status and quality of life are significantly impaired, with listing occurring when anticipated survival with a transplant is greater than without.[113] Transplant may improve survival and quality of life for selected patients. Length of survival after transplant is unpredictable for an individual, and shorter on average in children than adults: median survival is currently 9.9 years for adults with CF versus 5.6 years for children.[114] While some people have relatively benign operative and post-transplant courses, complications are unfortunately difficult to predict and count as the second leading cause of death among people with CF.[5] Quality-of-life outcomes are variable throughout the transplant course, often affected by medical complications, and accompanied by anxiety and depression.[115,116] With advances in therapies, the time frame for transplant consideration may be shifted away from childhood, but, at this time, many children and adolescents/young adults with CF still face this decision.

The pursuit of lung transplantation may inherently change the focus of care from restorative and palliative to "curative" in the eyes of individuals with CF, caregivers, and medical providers.[9,117] It is important to recognize that the additional stress of waiting for a transplant may have great emotional impact, with candidacy for transplant always at risk because of development of disease complications that might preclude it and the risk of dying before transplant.[118] Discussions about transplant provide a natural opportunity to address wishes for ongoing medical care, including hopes for survival, goals and expectations for palliation of symptoms, and desired roles of caregivers. While meeting new clinicians and teams may be an additional stressor, palliative care consultation during the transplant decision-making process and after transplant—ideally with continuity throughout—may have many benefits.

It is important that individuals with CF and their caregivers fully understand the risks and benefits of transplant as well as alternative treatment options. Earlier referral for transplant evaluation is recommended to allow people time to process information and make a truly informed decision in the context of their goals and values.[113] Discussions about transplant often take place with various clinicians, including members of the CF care team, lung transplant team, and palliative care team. Input from different parties may help individuals with CF and caregivers decide whether transplant falls within the context of their goals and values. Open communication among clinicians and teams is essential so that decisions can be supported.[119] In addition, offering peer decision-support by means of support groups and mentoring programs may be helpful. Issues of caregiver stress and fatigue should be acknowledged and addressed.[120]

For those considering or awaiting lung transplantation, decisions to limit life-sustaining treatments can be particularly complex. Challenges exist in simultaneously managing end-of-life care/ACP and candidacy for lung transplantation. As previously discussed, transplant eligibility may limit or preclude use of opioids and benzodiazepines for severe symptoms or when end of life may be near but hope for transplant remains. This is primarily because of perceptions, despite lack of evidence, that perioperative management and long-term outcomes might be negatively affected by use of these classes of medications.[73,82,83] CF and transplant care clinicians are encouraged to engage people in honest conversations about implications and anticipated outcomes of treatments like mechanical ventilation and/or ECLS as a bridge to lung transplantation and decisions to forego or limit symptom-relieving medications in the face of this uncertainty. Palliative care specialists can be helpful to individuals with CF, their families, and CF clinicians as they balance these often conflicting choices. Regardless of transplant eligibility or candidacy, preferences may change as one's condition changes, and clinicians should invite ongoing conversations about ACP.

Individuals with CF who pursue lung transplant but are deemed ineligible for transplant because of medical or psychosocial contraindications deserve thoughtful discussion of their goals for ongoing medical care, which may include continuation of standard CF therapies, incorporation of palliative treatments, and/or transition to hospice care. Palliative care consultation for discussion of treatment options and further planning may be beneficial for individuals with CF, caregivers, and the CF care team.

Family Reflection

My name is Alyssa. I am 35 years old, and I have CF. My brother Danny, also had CF. We were both diagnosed in 1990, I was 5 years old, and he was 3 years old.

When Danny was 17 years old, his disease had progressed and transplant was considered a very risky option. He made the choice that he would rather go home and be with his family than attempt a transplant and pass away on his own in an operating room. When the decision was made our CF care team connected us with a palliative care nurse. Being in the care of a palliative care nurse made it possible for Danny to continue his treatments and IV antibiotics at home with his family. Palliative care made it possible for us to be able to spend time with him and take care of him with the added support of our nurse and our CF team. The ability to keep in contact and even have our CF team visit our home meant so much to us. Our CF team had been part of our lives for 10 years and were a huge source of support for us.

Danny was in palliative care for about a year. Our nurse was not only a care giver for Danny, but she was also a support system for us as his family. My mom became good friends with our nurse, as did I, and we still have a relationship to this day. End-of-life care and accepting end-of-life care is a very emotional and exhausting experience, and I believe that our time with palliative care is what helped us get through caring for Danny and saying goodbye to him.

Palliative care was the best thing for myself and my family. Knowing that we had the support of our CF care team as well as a highly skilled nurse who facilitated communication between us made all the difference in how we spent time with Danny toward the end of his life.

Alyssa Doyle

CAREGIVER SUPPORT

Caregivers are central to CF care from diagnosis to death, with needs and roles changing with patient age and disease progression.[14,121] Healthy siblings who frequently receive less attention than their brothers or sisters with CF may experience feelings of guilt and may struggle to understand their roles within the family and their relationships with their parents. Additionally, families may experience multiple losses through the death of more than one child with CF, with each loss perhaps impacting family members in different ways. Siblings who also have CF must face both their own mortality and that of their sibling(s). Each affected sibling may experience anticipatory grief surrounding their own disease progression and mortality as well as grief around the potential loss of a sibling. Offering support and identification of resources for grieving and bereaved family members can be helpful.

Caregivers of individuals with CF may experience emotional distress, mental health challenges, and financial strain.[89,122] It is well-characterized that certain individuals with CF and their families are disproportionately impacted in these areas as well as in many others, with the existence of multiple healthcare disparities and inequalities largely based on social determinants of health.[123–125] CF care team members are accustomed to addressing the burden of caring for individuals with CF throughout the life span and should be able to offer a range of supports, including empathic listening, education around caregiving, screening for anxiety and depression, assistance with referrals for emotional support and mental health interventions, and addressing financial and insurance concerns.[93] When needs exceed the expertise of the CF care team, or when individuals with CF, caregivers, or CF care team members feel that third-party support is indicated, palliative care teams have much to offer. When existential or spiritual distress related to caregiving is identified, or when grief and bereavement needs arise, palliative care specialists can be especially helpful in direct support or assistance with appropriate referrals. Screening caregivers for caregiver burden and support needs will allow for better care coordination and resource allocation.

CF care team members may have ongoing involvement with bereaved families in the period following death. In an unpublished study, bereaved caregivers expressed gratitude toward members of the CF care team who sent cards, attended funerals or memorial services, and welcomed the family back to the care center for a visit after a period of grieving. Many described the CF care team as "extended family" and the care centers as a "second home," making communication with team members during the grieving process seem natural. It is important to recognize that there are no standards for bereavement care of CF caregivers, and it is likely that practices vary from one care center to another. Palliative care consultants may be able to provide valuable education to CF care teams regarding bereavement care.

CARE COORDINATION

Palliative care teams are expert at navigating partnerships between and among individuals with CF, caregivers, and other medical providers and teams and in helping with transitions as care needs change throughout the course of serious illness. The current model of CF care allows for multidisciplinary expertise that can meet many, but not all of the needs of individuals with CF. Palliative care specialists can provide complementary care to the "primary" teams, including CF care teams and transplant teams, filling in gaps and offering third-party presence and input around symptom management, ACP, and decision-making. Involvement of palliative care specialists may begin at any time in the illness course, and engagement is likely to wax and wane along with changing needs. Role delineation can be challenging at times but establishing open communication among all parties with the goal of seamless communication encourages reengagement with palliative care specialists anytime an individual with CF, caregiver, or clinician feels it's appropriate. Box 31.1 offers examples of care coordination and support of primary teams throughout the life span.

The time of transition from pediatric to adult clinicians and care teams can be complicated under the best of circumstances. Many CF care centers offer formal transition programs with an aim to enhance both satisfaction and health outcomes.[126,127] For children with more advanced disease and greater palliative needs, this time is especially critical and must be tailored to the unique needs of child and family. Consideration of transition from pediatric to adult palliative care clinicians/teams and also the timing of transition may be driven by institutional practices and resources but should ideally be individualized.

Transition to end-of-life care is another particularly challenging time. Palliative care specialists can offer education about symptom management, consultation about continuation of therapies, investigation of hospice services, and communication with hospice teams about the intricacies of CF care at end of life. Palliative care specialists can help foster collaborative care between hospice teams and CF care teams, highlighting the importance of involving CF care experts in end-of-life care, both for assistance with symptom management and for emotional support of the individual with CF and their family who have established long-term relationships with their CF care teams and/or transplant teams.

NON-CYSTIC FIBROSIS CHILDHOOD LUNG DISEASES

While the primary focus of this chapter is palliative care for children with CF, children living with a variety of other pulmonary diseases may also benefit from palliative care. Some of these diseases are primary pulmonary disorders, such as bronchopulmonary dysplasia in premature infants or forms of childhood interstitial lung disease. Others are secondary pulmonary disorders in which the lung disease is a manifestation of their underlying illness, such as restrictive lung disease in the setting of muscular dystrophies. However, there is little published research on palliative care integration in these non-CF forms of lung disease. Therefore, much of the practice of palliative care for children with these diseases is informed from the literature in CF and other nonpulmonary conditions, clinical expertise, and core principles that guide palliative care more broadly.

The same general palliative care domains apply to children living with non-CF pulmonary diseases, including symptom management, communication and ACP, caregiver support, and care coordination. Clinicians on the pulmonary team likely assume similar roles in providing primary palliative care within these domains, as outlined in Table 31.1. Notably, many of these lung diseases are relatively rare and face financial and logistical barriers to robust, large, research studies to understand the disease pathophysiology, develop therapeutic options, and guide clinical practice. These challenges, along with prognostic uncertainty in many circumstances, highlight the benefit of specialty-level palliative care consultation. Specialty palliative care experts may serve many similar roles as they do for children living with CF, as outlined in Table 31.1. Furthermore, Table 31.2 summarizes some of these other forms of lung disease and describes how palliative care may provide benefit throughout the lives of children living with these diseases.

CONCLUSION

CF is a complex and burdensome genetic condition with implications on quality of life for the child and family. Advances in care are leading to better outcomes, including both survival and quality of life, but CF remains incurable and each individual's course is unique and unpredictable. People with CF and their caregivers stand to benefit from both primary and specialty palliative care throughout the life span, and while more work is needed to inform optimal integration of palliative care into routine CF care, advances are

TABLE 31.2 Palliative care opportunities for individuals with pediatric lung diseases other than cystic fibrosis

DISEASE	DESCRIPTION	ILLNESS TRAJECTORY	HIGHLIGHTED PALLIATIVE CARE NEEDS
Pulmonary hypertension	High blood pressure in the arteries of the lungs. May be seen in conjunction with other congenital heart or lung disease or be idiopathic. Patients may be cared for primarily by cardiologists and/or pulmonologists, depending on the care center.	In severe forms, may develop right ventricular failure, poor weight gain, syncope, and progress to lung transplantation evaluation.	Psychosocial support is crucial, especially in certain familial phenotypes that run in families, leading to multiple family members affected across generations. Associated with significant morbidity and mortality. Complex decision-making especially should lung transplantation be considered.
Childhood interstitial lung disease (ILD) or diffuse lung disease (DLD)	Heterogeneous group of rare lung diseases that impact neonates, infants, children, and teenagers by impacting the pulmonary parenchyma and/or impairing gas exchange. May be characterized as a primary pulmonary process, associated with a known systemic disorder, or classified histopathologically, each of which may inform the prognosis and guide potential treatment.	Depending on the form, may lead to tachypnea, hypoxemia, poor weight gain, cough, and dyspnea. Prognosis can range depending on the specific form of ILD, from improvement over time to lung transplantation and death.	Proper diagnosis can be challenging given nonspecific symptoms, and timely referrals are crucial in providing opportunities for treatment in certain severe forms. Families may benefit from support around complex decision-making in the setting of significant prognostic uncertainty.
Bronchopulmonary dysplasia	Chronic lung disease in premature infants related to disrupted pulmonary development. Varying definitions often involve a combination of gestational age and degree of supplemental oxygen use and characterize extent of disease as mild, moderate, or severe.	At increased risk of pulmonary infections, wheezing, persistent abnormalities in pulmonary function, prolonged mechanical ventilation, growth restriction, and neurodevelopmental impairment. Severe form has an increased risk of pulmonary artery hypertension, which significantly increases the risk of morbidity and mortality.	Premature birth is often associated with caregiver psychosocial challenges, including potentially unpredicted prolonged hospitalizations. Families may benefit from longitudinal psychosocial support to assist with decision-making and goals of care over time.
Neurologic impairment	Heterogeneous group of disorders characterized by alterations to neurologic function and muscle strength. This can manifest as hypotonia, weakness, dystonia, spasticity, seizures, sleep disordered breathing, cognitive impairment, and with other neurologic changes depending on the specific etiology. There are multiple potential causes, including but not limited to genetic syndromes, inborn errors of metabolism, endocrinopathies, trauma, neonatal infections, primary neuromuscular disorders, and cerebral palsy.	Specific symptoms are highly variable depending on the specific disorder or disease. Often characterized as either progressive or nonprogressive neurologic impairment.	In the setting of severe neurologic impairment and/or progressive neurologic disease, recurring complex decision-making may arise in regards to technological interventions aimed toward providing nutrition/hydration and to assisting with ventilation. These decisions often involve multiple care teams to fully anticipate an individual person's illness trajectory, explore patient and family goals, and decide treatment options aligned with those goals.
Sickle cell disease	Group of hemoglobinopathies leading to vaso-occlusive complications and red cell hemolysis. This genetic change can lead to a number of pulmonary manifestations over time, including dyspnea, decreased pulmonary function, acute chest syndrome, venous thromboembolic disease, pulmonary hypertension, pulmonary fibrosis, asthma, and recurrent wheezing.	At risk of a number of complications to multiple organ systems, largely related to the vaso-occlusive episodes in the chest, bone, brain, liver, kidney, and other organs. Some children may be eligible for bone marrow transplantation.	It is a chronic disease which benefits from life-long collaboration with clinical teams focusing on prevention of infectious and vaso-occlusive episodes. Comprehensive pain management, often involving opioids, is typically necessary during severe vaso-occlusive crises. Recurrent acute chest syndrome can lead to chronic dyspnea and other pulmonary complications over time.
Anatomic airway abnormalities	Various congenital airway anomalies can impact the structure of the trachea and bronchi of the lungs, leading to chronic respiratory stridor or wheeze, impaired ventilation, and increased risk of aspiration. This can include malformations such as tracheal stenosis, tracheoesophageal fistula, and tracheobronchomalacia.	Highly dependent on the specific anatomic changes to the airway, severity of symptoms, and associated comorbidities. Some of these anatomic malformations may be approached surgically for repair, while others may be monitored conservatively.	When these airway malformations are severe, surgical interventions may be carefully considered depending on the patient's airway anatomy and age. Help with complex decision-making may be important, especially if other complicating comorbidities exist that impact the patient's quality of life and the family's decision-making.

(continued)

TABLE 31.2 Continued

DISEASE	DESCRIPTION	ILLNESS TRAJECTORY	HIGHLIGHTED PALLIATIVE CARE NEEDS
Congenital diaphragmatic hernia	A defect prenatally in the development of the diaphragm which allows herniated abdominal organs into the chest, which impairs lung development and can lead to lung hypoplasia and pulmonary hypertension.	Often attempt to first stabilize pulmonary and cardiac function via intubation with mechanical ventilation, placement of nasogastric tube to decompress the stomach and intestine, and extracorporeal membrane oxygenation (ECMO) for infants in distress despite medical management. Prognosis and interventions pursued are highly dependent on the degree of lung hypoplasia and pulmonary hypertension, with increased risk of mortality in settings of comorbid prematurity or cardiac abnormalities.	May be prenatally diagnosed, and thus families may benefit from prenatal palliative care consultation to help understand the family's goals and discuss advance care planning in thinking about the delivery and potential intensive interventions in the immediate postnatal period.

also being made in this area with the development of clinical practice guidelines and investment in palliative care research by the Cystic Fibrosis Foundation. The interdisciplinary models of both CF care and palliative care afford opportunities for collaboration to improve quality of life and other health outcomes. While the care of children with non-CF lung diseases may include unique differences from CF care, models and principles of palliative care in CF can be applied to other disease populations.

Team Reflection

Kylie

Kylie's newborn screen was positive for CF, and a sweat chloride test confirmed the diagnosis. Kylie's parents couldn't help but search the internet before going to the CF clinic. There was some good news—much progress had been made in CF, but also bad news—memorials for so many, including children. With the confirmation of CF came a flood of new information. A thousand questions all at once. It's in our genes: Is it our fault? Are we good enough parents to handle this? What about having more children? How will we pay for everything? Will one of us have to quit work? Will she be normal? When will the cure come?

Kylie's parents learned quickly and settled into a routine of regular visits with the CF team. She was thriving and got through the usual daycare colds without too much difficulty. Her parents found comfort in blogging about their experiences and fundraising for CF research. They welcomed a son, Charlie. They decided against prenatal genetic testing because they couldn't imagine what to do with the results. They were relieved to learn Charlie did not have CF.

When Kylie started kindergarten, her coughs lingered and she began to lose weight. Each clinic visit brought new concerns: decreased lung function, respiratory infections, and poor weight gain. Kylie's doctor always had something new to try and focused on returning to her previous "baseline." If the doctor was optimistic, Kylie's parents could be optimistic, too. Particularly excited about a new CFTR modulator drug approved for older people with CF, they were delighted to get in a clinical trial for her age group. Kylie's health improved after starting the modulator—she had more energy, coughed less, and gained weight. But unfortunately, abnormal liver function necessitated stopping the drug. Her parents were reassured that more new therapies were coming, and something would be available in a few years.

Kylie was hospitalized for a pulmonary exacerbation at 8 years of age. Anxious about everything, she wouldn't let her mother leave. For her parents, the hospital was a harsh reminder that Kylie really was sick. She improved, but never back to baseline. The hospital became the "new normal." Finding it impossible to support a frightened Kylie through hospitalizations while caring for another child and working full time, her mother took time off to focus on Kylie's health and the family's well-being. She administered IV antibiotics at home, provided airway clearance therapies, and tube feedings through Kylie's new gastrostomy tube, something previously perceived as a "last resort" but now essential. The tube made it easier to get her enough calories and to end the constant fights about eating.

Around her twelfth birthday, Kylie had a severe coughing fit, chest pain, and couldn't catch her breath. They rushed to the emergency room, where her oxygen saturation was 85%. Her chest x-ray showed a pneumothorax, something they had never heard of. A surgeon placed a chest tube; she was terrified but afraid to ask for medication to calm her down. In the ICU, the doctor told her parents, "We need to do everything to avoid putting her on the ventilator. CF patients don't make it off the ventilator." Kylie overheard but was afraid to ask what he meant. After a few days with BiPAP, Kylie started weaning from oxygen, her chest tube was removed, and she moved to a regular room, relieved to be in a familiar place with nurses she had known for years.

But things were different now. Her lung function was much lower, and she needed oxygen for exercise and sleep. Kylie struggled with the CF care routine and lost interest in eating. Afraid to go back to school, she argued about doing schoolwork at home. Her cough was constant, and her chest and head hurt most of the time. She seemed unable to go more than a few days without antibiotics, and they always gave her nausea and diarrhea. She dreaded CF clinic and the reactions of her parents and doctor to her declining weight and lung function. The social worker was concerned about her mood, and screening led to referrals to a therapist and psychiatrist. She agreed to go only to please her parents—it felt like a waste of time to her.

At her next clinic visit, Kylie and her family heard the words they never said out loud: lung transplant. Kylie didn't think she wanted one—she knew it meant more tubes, more ICUs, and probably lots of pain. But her parents were interested, and she agreed to hear what the transplant team had to say. They were told that transplant was like trading one disease for another. There would still be pills, appointments, and procedures. But her parents felt encouraged by the transplant team's optimistic views of outcomes. Kylie read about others' experiences with transplant. She still felt uncertain, but worried about what would happen to her family if she died. And she wanted to know what it was like to run and laugh without coughing. She couldn't remember ever being able to do those things.

Kylie waited for new lungs for nearly a year and finally had her transplant. After a smooth surgery and easier than expected recovery, Kylie went home 3 weeks later without oxygen, delighted to shout her goodbyes as she left.

The next 2 years brought ups and downs, with periods of good health interrupted by infections and episodes of rejection. Kylie eventually returned to school. Her mother returned to work and encouraged Kylie to take more responsibility with her medications. Kylie, now 15, disliked some of the side effects and began taking them sporadically. Over time, she noticed it was harder to carry her backpack at school, especially up the stairs. She started to cough again, which she tried to hide. A big drop in lung function led to a lung biopsy, with bad news: chronic rejection. Kylie reluctantly admitted that she often skipped her anti-rejection medications. Her parents felt angry, worried, sad, and desperate, all at the same time.

Kylie's graft rejection progressed rapidly. She needed continuous oxygen again, lost weight, and stopped attending school. After signing a contract to take her medications, Kylie was listed for a second lung transplant. Now short of breath all the time, she began to feel anxious about another transplant and the possibility of dying. Her parents worried about her fragile condition and asked the transplant team to talk with her about the future. Once again, everyone was worried about the same thing, but just didn't know how to talk about it. The transplant team enlisted the social worker to address Kylie's fears, but the team didn't directly discuss what might happen in the future. Taking this as a signal not to talk about it, Kylie's parents did not ask questions.

One afternoon, Kylie's mother found her on the floor, unconscious. The ambulance team intubated her and rushed her to the hospital. Throughout the week, her lungs worsened and her kidneys began to fail. The transplant doctor said he had to remove Kylie from the wait list. The ICU doctor said she did not think Kylie was going to make it and recommended withdrawal of life support. But Kylie's parents shared that she had pulled through many times before and asked her transplant team, "Didn't you always tell us to be optimistic?"

In the days that followed, Kylie's parents watched her struggle and prayed for a miracle. They felt comforted seeing familiar faces from the transplant and CF teams, but were uncertain who to ask for help about what to do next. Conversations with the medical team grew shorter. They spent time talking and praying with the hospital chaplain. When they felt ready to withdraw life support, they were relieved to be offered help for their family to grieve. After all they had been through, they would have to find a way to go home without Kylie.

REFERENCES

1. Cystic Fibrosis Foundation. About cystic fibrosis. n.d. https://www.cff.org/What-is-CF/About-Cystic-Fibrosis/
2. Knowles MR, Durie PR. What is cystic fibrosis? *N Engl J Med.* 2002;347(6):439–442.
3. Flume PA. Pulmonary complications of cystic fibrosis. *Respir Care.* 2009;54(5):618–627.
4. Cystic Fibrosis Trust. *UK Cystic Fibrosis Registry Annual Data Report 2018.* Cystic Fibrosis Trust; 2019.
5. Cystic Fibrosis Foundation. *Cystic Fibrosis Foundation 2018 Patient Registry Annual Data Report.* Cystic Fibrosis Foundation; 2019.
6. Mogayzel PJ, Dunitz J, Marrow LC, Hazle LA. Improving chronic care delivery and outcomes: The impact of the cystic fibrosis care center network. *BMJ Quality & Safety.* 2014;23(Suppl 1):i3.
7. Cystic Fibrosis Foundation Patient Registry Annual Data Report to the Center Directors 2013. http://www.cff.org/UploadedFiles/research/ClinicalResearch/PatientRegistryReport/2013_CFF_Annual_Data_Report_to_the_Center_Directors.pdf. Cystic Fibrosis Foundation, Bethesda, MD USA 2013.
8. Linnemann RW, O'Malley PJ, Friedman D, et al. Development and evaluation of a palliative care curriculum for cystic fibrosis healthcare providers. *J Cyst Fibros.* 2016;15(1):90–95.
9. Robinson W. Palliative care in cystic fibrosis. *J Palliat Med.* 2000;3(2):187–192.
10. Yankaskas JR, Marshall BC, Sufian B, Simon RH, Rodman D. Cystic fibrosis adult care: Consensus conference report. *Chest.* 2004;125(1 Suppl):1S.
11. Castellani C, Duff AJA, Bell SC, et al. ECFS best practice guidelines: The 2018 revision. *J Cyst Fibros.* 2018;17(2):153–178.

12. Davis PB. Cystic fibrosis since 1938. *Am J Respirat Crit Care Med.* 2006;173(5):475–482.
13. Sawicki GS, Sellers DE, Robinson WM. High treatment burden in adults with cystic fibrosis: Challenges to disease self-management. *J Cyst Fibros.* 2009;8(2):91–96.
14. McGuffie K, Sellers DE, Sawicki GS, Robinson WM. Self-reported involvement of family members in the care of adults with CF. *J Cyst Fibros.* 2008;7(2):95–101.
15. Saiman L, Siegel JD, LiPuma JJ, et al. Cystic Fibrosis Foundation Guideline: Infection prevention and control guideline for cystic fibrosis: 2013 update. *Infect Control Hosp Epidemiol.* 2014;35:S1–S67.
16. Flewelling KD, Sellers DE, Sawicki GS, Robinson WM, Dill EJ. Social support is associated with fewer reported symptoms and decreased treatment burden in adults with cystic fibrosis. *J Cyst Fibros.* 2019;18(4):572–576.
17. Moraru E, Diaconu R, Anton E, et al. Understanding the relevance of pain, depression and anxiety-like manifestations in the management of cystic fibrosis. *Arch Biol Sci.* 2015;67(3):1067–1070.
18. Quittner AL, Abbott J, Georgiopoulos AM, et al. International Committee on Mental Health in Cystic Fibrosis: Cystic Fibrosis Foundation and European Cystic Fibrosis Society consensus statements for screening and treating depression and anxiety. *Thorax.* 2016;71(1):26.
19. Konstan MW, Wagener JS, VanDevanter DR. Characterizing aggressiveness and predicting future progression of CF lung disease. *J Cyst Fibros.* 2009;8 Suppl 1:S15–19.
20. Koshland DE, Jr. The cystic fibrosis gene story. *Science.* 1989;245(4922):1029.
21. Couzin-Frankel J. Genetics. The promise of a cure: 20 years and counting. *Science.* 2009;324(5934):1504–1507.
22. Edmondson C, Davies JC. Current and future treatment options for cystic fibrosis lung disease: Latest evidence and clinical implications. *Ther Adv Chronic Dis.* 2016;7:170–183.
23. Bell SC, Mall MA, Gutierrez H, et al. The future of cystic fibrosis care: A global perspective. *Lancet Respir Med.* 2020;8(1):65–124.
24. Bell SC, Mainz JG, MacGregor G, et al. Patient-reported outcomes in patients with cystic fibrosis with a G551D mutation on ivacaftor treatment: Results from a cross-sectional study. *BMC Pulm Med.* 2019;19(1):146.
25. Higgins M, Volkova N, Moy K, Marshall B, Bilton D. Real-world outcomes among patients with cystic fibrosis treated with ivacaftor: 2012-2016 experience. *Pulm Ther.* 2020;6(1):141–149.
26. Keating D, Marigowda G, Burr L, et al. VX-445-tezacaftor-ivacaftor in patients with cystic fibrosis and one or two phe508del alleles. *N Engl J Med.* 2018;379(17):1612–1620.
27. McKinzie CJ, Goralski JL, Noah TL, Retsch-Bogart GZ, Prieur MB. Worsening anxiety and depression after initiation of lumacaftor/ivacaftor combination therapy in adolescent females with cystic fibrosis. *J Cyst Fibros.* 2017;16(4):525–527.
28. Shteinberg M, Taylor-Cousar JL. Impact of CFTR modulator use on outcomes in people with severe cystic fibrosis lung disease. *Eur Respir Rev.* 2020;29(155).
29. Taylor-Cousar JL, Munck A, McKone EF, et al. Tezacaftor-ivacaftor in patients with cystic fibrosis homozygous for phe508del. *N Engl J Med.* 2017;377(21):2013–2023.
30. Middleton PG, Mall MA, Drevinek P, et al. Elexacaftor-tezacaftor-ivacaftor for cystic fibrosis with a single phe508del allele. *N Engl J Med.* 2019;381(19):1809–1819.
31. Havermans T, Colpaert K, De Boeck K, Dupont L, Abbott J. Pain in CF: Review of the literature. *J Cyst Fibros.* 2013;12(5):423–430.
32. Lee AL, Rawlings S, Bennett KA, Armstrong D. Pain and its clinical associations in individuals with cystic fibrosis: A systematic review. *Chron Respir Dis.* 2016;13(2):102–117.
33. Allgood SJ, Kozachik S, Alexander KA, Thaxton A, Vera M, Lechtzin N. Descriptions of the pain experience in adults and adolescents with cystic fibrosis. *Pain Manage Nurs.* 2018;19(4):340–347.
34. Farrell PM, White TB, Howenstine MS, et al. Diagnosis of cystic fibrosis in screened populations. *J Pediatr.* 2017;181S:S33–S44 e32.
35. Farrell PM, White TB, Ren CL, et al. Diagnosis of cystic fibrosis: Consensus guidelines from the Cystic Fibrosis Foundation. *J Pediatr.* 2017;181S:S4–S15 e11.
36. Coffey MJ, Whitaker V, Gentin N, et al. Differences in outcomes between early and late diagnosis of cystic fibrosis in the newborn screening era. *J Pediatr.* 2017;181:137–145.e131.
37. Rock MJ. Newborn screening for cystic fibrosis. *Clin Chest Med.* 2007;28(2):297–305.
38. Course CW, Hanks R. Newborn screening for cystic fibrosis Is there benefit for everyone? *Paediatr Respir Rev.* 2019;31:3–5.
39. Lewis S, Curnow L, Ross M, Massie J. Parental attitudes to the identification of their infants as carriers of cystic fibrosis by newborn screening. *J Paediatr Child Health.* 2006;42(9):533–537.
40. Grob R. Is my sick child healthy? Is my healthy child sick?: Changing parental experiences of cystic fibrosis in the age of expanded newborn screening. *Social Sci Med (1982).* 2008;67(7):1056–1064.
41. Kazmerski TM, Weiner DJ, Matisko J, et al. Advance care planning in adolescents with cystic fibrosis: A quality improvement project. *Pediatr Pulmonol.* 2016;51(12):1304–1310.
42. Christian BJ, D'Auria JP, Moore CB. Playing for time: Adolescent perspectives of lung transplantation for cystic fibrosis. *J Pediatr Health Care.* 1999;13(3 Pt 1):120–125.
43. Farber JG, Prieur MG, Roach C, et al. Difficult conversations: Discussing prognosis with children with cystic fibrosis. *Pediatr Pulmonol.* 2018;53(5):592–598.
44. Bluebond-Langner M. *The Private Worlds of Dying Children.* Princeton University Press; 1978.
45. Bourke SJ, Doe SJ, Gascoigne AD, et al. An integrated model of provision of palliative care to patients with cystic fibrosis. *Palliat Med.* 2009;23(6):512–517.
46. Quill T, Abernathy A. Generalist plus specialist palliative care: Creating a more sustainable model. *N Engl J Med.* 2013;368(13):1173–1175. doi:1110.1056/NEJMp1215620. Epub 1212013 Mar 1215626.
47. Goggin J, Cohen R. CF healthcare workers feel unprepared in providing suitable end of life care and desire more education: Results of a nationwide survey. *J Cyst Fibros.* 2016;15(1):85–89.
48. Chen E, Killeen KM, Peterson SJ, Saulitis AK, Balk RA. Evaluation of pain, dyspnea, and goals of care among adults with cystic fibrosis: A comprehensive palliative care survey. *Am J Hospice Palliat Med.* 2017;34(4):347–352.
49. Sawicki GS, Sellers DE, Robinson WM. Self-reported physical and psychological symptom burden in adults with cystic fibrosis. *J Pain Symptom Manage.* 2008;35(4):372–380.
50. Dellon EP, Shores MD, Nelson KI, Wolfe J, Noah TL, Hanson LC. Caregiver perspectives on discussions about the use of intensive treatments in cystic fibrosis. *J Pain Symptom Manage.* 2010;40(6):821–828.
51. Friedman D, Linnemann RW, Altstein LL, et al. The CF-CARES primary palliative care model: A CF-specific structured assessment of symptoms, distress, and coping. *J Cyst Fibros.* 2018;17(1):71–77.
52. Lechtzin N, Allgood SJ, Hong G, et al. The association between pain and clinical outcomes in adolescents with cystic fibrosis. *J Pain Symptom Manage.* 2016;52(5):681–687.
53. Hayes M, Yaster M, Haythornthwaite JA, et al. Pain is a common problem affecting clinical outcomes in adults with cystic fibrosis. *Chest.* 2011;140(6):1598–1603.
54. Ravilly S, Robinson W, Suresh S, Wohl ME, Berde CB. Chronic pain in cystic fibrosis. *Pediatrics.* 1996;98(4):741–747.
55. Robinson WM, Ravilly S, Berde C, Wohl ME. End-of-life care in cystic fibrosis. *Pediatrics.* 1997;100(2 Pt 1):205–209.
56. Friedman D, Linnemann RW, Altstein LL, et al. Effects of a primary palliative care intervention on quality of life and mental health in cystic fibrosis. *Pediatr Pulmonol.* 2019;54(7):984–992.
57. O'Sullivan BP, Freedman SD. Cystic fibrosis. *Lancet.* 2009;373(9678):1891–1904.
58. Sawicki GS, Sellers DE, Robinson WM. High treatment burden in adults with cystic fibrosis: Challenges to disease self-management. *J Cyst Fibros.* 2009;8(2):91–96.

59. Dill EJ, Dawson R, Sellers DE, Robinson WM, Sawicki GS. Longitudinal trends in health-related quality of life in adults with cystic fibrosis. *Chest.* 2013;144(3):981–989. doi:910.1378/chest.1312-1404.
60. Garcia B, Flume PA. Pulmonary complications of cystic fibrosis. *Semin Respir Crit Care Med.* 2019;40(6):804–809.
61. Dhingra L, Walker P, Berdella M, et al. Addressing the burden of illness in adults with cystic fibrosis with screening and triage: An early intervention model of palliative care. *J Cyst Fibros.* 2019.
62. Orenstein DM, Rosenstein BJ, Stern RC. *Cystic Fibrosis Medical Care.* Lippincott Williams & Williams; 2000.
63. Luce JM, Luce JA. Perspectives on care at the close of life. Management of dyspnea in patients with far-advanced lung disease: "Once I lose it it's kind of hard to catch it. . . ." *JAMA.* 2001;285(10):1331–1337.
64. Ullrich CK, Mayer OH. Assessment and management of fatigue and dyspnea in pediatric palliative care. *Pediatr Clin North Am.* 2007;54(5):735–756, xi.
65. Noone PG. Non-invasive ventilation for the treatment of hypercapnic respiratory failure in cystic fibrosis. *Thorax.* 2008;63(1):5–7.
66. Moran F, Bradley JM, Piper AJ. Non-invasive ventilation for cystic fibrosis. *Cochrane Database Syst Rev.* 2017;2:Cd002769.
67. Kremer TM, Zwerdling RG, Michelson PH, O'Sullivan P. Intensive care management of the patient with cystic fibrosis. *J Intensive Care Med.* 2008;23(3):159–177.
68. King CS, Brown AW, Aryal S, Ahmad K, Donaldson S. Critical care of the adult patient with cystic fibrosis. *Chest.* 2019;155(1):202–214.
69. Hayes D, Jr., Kopp BT, Preston TJ, et al. Survival of patients with cystic fibrosis on ECMO: Analysis of the Extracorporeal Life Support Organization Registry. *Int J Clin Exp Med.* 2014 7(5):1370–1372.
70. Lanken PN, Terry PB, Delisser HM, et al. An official American Thoracic Society clinical policy statement: Palliative care for patients with respiratory diseases and critical illnesses. *Am J Respir Crit Care Med.* 2008;177(8):912–927.
71. Ambrosino N, Fracchia C. Strategies to relieve dyspnoea in patients with advanced chronic respiratory diseases. A narrative review. *Pulmonology.* 2019;25(5):289–298.
72. Ekstrom MP, Bornefalk-Hermansson A, Abernethy AP, Currow DC. Safety of benzodiazepines and opioids in very severe respiratory disease: National prospective study. *BMJ.* 2014;348:g445.
73. Colman R, Singer LG, Barua R, Downar J. Outcomes of lung transplant candidates referred for co-management by palliative care: A retrospective case series. *Palliat Med.* 2015;29(5):429–435.
74. Currow DC, Ward AM, Abernethy AP. Advances in the pharmacological management of breathlessness. *Curr Opin Support Palliat Care.* 2009;3(2):103–106.
75. Blackwell LS, Quittner AL. Daily pain in adolescents with CF: Effects on adherence, psychological symptoms, and health-related quality of life. *Pediatr Pulmonol.* 2015;50(3):244–251.
76. Chang MT, Patel ZM. Update on long-term outcomes for chronic rhinosinusitis in cystic fibrosis. *Curr Opin Otolaryngol Head Neck Surg.* 2020;28(1):46–51.
77. Ross J, Gamble J, Schultz A, Lewiston N. Back pain and spinal deformity in cystic fibrosis. *Am J Dis Child (1960).* 1987;141(12):1313–1316.
78. Jones AM, Dodd ME, Webb AK, Selby PL. Acute rib fracture pain in CF. *Thorax.* 2001;56(10):819.
79. Schendel A, Mai J, Espinosa R, Tomcyzk CT, Laguna TA. Unexpected height loss in an adolescent with cystic fibrosis. *Global Pediatr Health.* 2018;5:2333794x18773662.
80. Sendzik J, Lode H, Stahlmann R. Quinolone-induced arthropathy: An update focusing on new mechanistic and clinical data. *Int J Antimicrob Agents.* 2009;33(3):194–200.
81. Roehmel JF, Kallinich T, Staab D, Schwarz C. Clinical manifestations and risk factors of arthropathy in cystic fibrosis. *Respir Med.* 2019;147:66–71.
82. Drees D, Tumin D, Miller R, et al. Chronic opioid use and clinical outcomes in lung transplant recipients: A single-center cohort study. *Clin Respir J.* 2018;12(9):2446–2453.
83. Kapnadak SG, Dimango E, Hadjiliadis D, et al. Cystic Fibrosis Foundation consensus guidelines for the care of individuals with advanced cystic fibrosis lung disease. *J Cyst Fibros.* 2020;19(3):344–354.
84. Lusman SS, Grand R. Approach to chronic abdominal pain in cystic fibrosis. *J Cyst Fibros.* 2017;16 Suppl 2:S24–S31.
85. Abraham JM, Taylor CJ. Cystic fibrosis and disorders of the large intestine: DIOS, constipation, and colorectal cancer. *J Cyst Fibros.* 2017;16 Suppl 2:S40–S49.
86. Maqbool A, Pauwels A. Cystic fibrosis and gastroesophageal reflux disease. *J Cyst Fibros.* 2017;16 Suppl 2:S2–S13.
87. Stallings VA, Stark LJ, Robinson KA, Feranchak AP, Quinton H. Evidence-based practice recommendations for nutrition-related management of children and adults with cystic fibrosis and pancreatic insufficiency: Results of a systematic review. *J Am Diet Assoc.* 2008;108(5):832–839.
88. Schwarzenberg SJ, Hempstead SE, McDonald CM, et al. Enteral tube feeding for individuals with cystic fibrosis: Cystic Fibrosis Foundation evidence-informed guidelines. *J Cyst Fibros.* 2016;15(6):724–735.
89. Quittner AL, Goldbeck L, Abbott J, et al. Prevalence of depression and anxiety in patients with cystic fibrosis and parent caregivers: Results of the International Depression Epidemiological Study across nine countries. *Thorax.* 2014;69(12):1090–1097.
90. Bowmer G, Latchford G, Duff A, et al. Adherence to infection prevention and control guidelines: A vignette-based study of decision-making and risk-taking in young adults with cystic fibrosis. *J Cyst Fibros.* 2017;16(1):146–150.
91. Moola F. The complexities of contagion: The experience of social isolation among children and youth living with cystic fibrosis in Canada. *J Child Health Care.* 2018:1367493518767784.
92. Jamieson N, Fitzgerald D, Singh-Grewal D, Hanson CS, Craig JC, Tong A. Children's experiences of cystic fibrosis: A systematic review of qualitative studies. *Pediatrics.* 2014;133(6):e1683–1697.
93. Quittner AL, Abbott J, Georgiopoulos AM, et al. International Committee on Mental Health in Cystic Fibrosis: Cystic Fibrosis Foundation and European Cystic Fibrosis Society consensus statements for screening and treating depression and anxiety. *Thorax.* 2016;71(1):26–34. doi:10.1136/thoraxjnl-2015-207488. Epub 202015 Oct 207489.
94. Nap-van der Vlist MM, Dalmeijer GW, Grootenhuis MA, et al. Fatigue in childhood chronic disease. *Arch Dis Child.* 2019;104(11):1090–1095.
95. Nap-van der Vlist MM, Burghard M, Hulzebos HJ, et al. Prevalence of severe fatigue among adults with cystic fibrosis: A single center study. *J Cyst Fibros.* 2018;17(3):368–374.
96. Prasad SA, Cerny FJ. Factors that influence adherence to exercise and their effectiveness: Application to cystic fibrosis. *Pediatr Pulmonol.* 2002;34(1):66–72.
97. Gruet M. Fatigue in chronic respiratory diseases: Theoretical framework and implications for real-life performance and rehabilitation. *Front Physiol.* 2018;9:1285.
98. de Castro-Silva C, de Bruin VM, Cunha GM, Nunes DM, Medeiros CA, de Bruin PF. Melatonin improves sleep and reduces nitrite in the exhaled breath condensate in cystic fibrosis: A randomized, double-blind placebo-controlled study. *J Pineal Res.* 2010;48(1):65–71.
99. Shakkottai A, O'Brien LM, Nasr SZ, Chervin RD. Sleep disturbances and their impact in pediatric cystic fibrosis. *Sleep Med Rev.* 2018;42:100–110.
100. Malone H, Biggar S, Javadpour S, Edworthy Z, Sheaf G, Coyne I. Interventions for promoting participation in shared decision-making for children and adolescents with cystic fibrosis. *Cochrane Database Syst Rev.* 2019;5:Cd012578.
101. Kazmerski TM, Borrero S, Tuchman LK, et al. Provider and patient attitudes regarding sexual health in young women with cystic fibrosis. *Pediatrics.* 2016;137(6).
102. Freyer DR. Care of the dying adolescent: Special considerations. *Pediatrics.* 2004;113(2):381–388.
103. Poltorak DY, Glazer JP. The development of children's understanding of death: Cognitive and psychodynamic considerations. *Child Adolesc Psychiatric Clin N Am.* 2006;15(3):567–573.

104. American Academy of Pediatrics. Committee on Bioethics and Committee on Hospital Care. Palliative care for children. *Pediatrics.* 2000;106(2 Pt 1):351–357.
105. Linnemann RW, Friedman D, Altstein LL, et al. Advance care planning experiences and preferences among people with cystic fibrosis. *J Palliat Med.* 2019;22(2):138–144.
106. Wiener L, Ballard E, Brennan T, Battles H, Martinez P, Pao M. How I wish to be remembered: The use of an advance care planning document in adolescent and young adult populations. *J Palliat Med.* 2008;11(10):1309–1313.
107. Sawicki GS, Sellers DE, McGuffie K, Robinson W. Adults with cystic fibrosis report important and unmet needs for disease information. *J Cyst Fibros.* 2007;6(6):411–416.
108. Dellon EP, Chen E, Goggin J, et al. Advance care planning in cystic fibrosis: Current practices, challenges, and opportunities. *J Cyst Fibros.* 2016;15(1):96–101.
109. Dellon EP, Sawicki GS, Shores MD, Wolfe J, Hanson LC. Physician practices for communicating with patients with cystic fibrosis about the use of noninvasive and invasive mechanical ventilation. *Chest.* 2012;141(4):1010–1017.
110. Dellon EP, Basile M, Hobler MR, et al. Palliative care needs of individuals with cystic fibrosis: Perspectives of multiple stakeholders. *J Palliat Med.* 2020.
111. Aging With Dignity. Five Wishes. 2020. https://fivewishes.org
112. Dellon EP, Leigh MW, Yankaskas JR, Noah TL. Effects of lung transplantation on inpatient end of life care in cystic fibrosis. *J Cyst Fibros.* 2007;6(6):396–402.
113. Ramos KJ, Smith PJ, McKone EF, et al. Lung transplant referral for individuals with cystic fibrosis: Cystic Fibrosis Foundation consensus guidelines. *J Cyst Fibros.* 2019;18(3):321–333.
114. ISHLT Registry. 2019. https://ishltregistries.org/registries/slides.asp.
115. Vermuelen KM, van der Bij W, Erasmus ME, TenVergert EM. Long-term health-related quality of life after lung transplantation: Different predictors for different dimensions. *J Heart Lung Transplant.* 2007;26(2):188–193.
116. Kugler C, Fischer S, Gottlieb J, et al. Symptom experience after lung transplantation: Impact on quality of life and adherence. *Clin Transplant.* 2007;21(5):590–596.
117. Dellon EP, Leigh MW, Yankaskas JR, Noah TL. Effects of lung transplantation on inpatient end of life care in cystic fibrosis. *J Cyst Fibros.* 2007;6(6):396–402.
118. Vermeulen KM, Bosma OH, Bij W, Koeter GH, Tenvergert EM. Stress, psychological distress, and coping in patients on the waiting list for lung transplantation: An exploratory study. *Transplant Int.* 2005;18(8):954–959.
119. Wentlandt K, Weiss A, O'Connor E, Kaya E. Palliative and end of life care in solid organ transplantation. *Am J Transplant.* 2017;17(12):3008–3019.
120. Rosenberger EM, Dew MA, DiMartini AF, De Vito Dabbs AJ, Yusen RD. Psychosocial issues facing lung transplant candidates, recipients and family caregivers. *Thorac Surg Clin.* 2012;22(4):517–529. doi:510.1016/j.thorsurg.2012.1008.1001.
121. Ernst MM, Johnson MC, Stark LJ. Developmental and psychosocial issues in cystic fibrosis. *Pediatr Clin North Am.* 2011;58(4):865–885, x.
122. Orenstein DM, Abood RN. Cost(s) of caring for patients with cystic fibrosis. *Curr Opin Pediatr.* 2018;30(3):393–398.
123. Kerem E, Cohen-Cymberknoh M. Disparities in cystic fibrosis care and outcome: Socioeconomic status and beyond. *Chest.* 2016;149(2):298–300.
124. Rho J, Ahn C, Gao A, Sawicki GS, Keller A, Jain R. Disparities in mortality of Hispanic patients with cystic fibrosis in the United States: A national and regional cohort study. *Am J Respir Crit Care Med.* 2018;198(8):1055–1063.
125. McGarry ME, Williams WA, 2nd, McColley SA. The demographics of adverse outcomes in cystic fibrosis. *Pediatr Pulmonol.* 2019;54 Suppl 3:S74–S83.
126. Tuchman L, Schwartz M. Health outcomes associated with transition from pediatric to adult cystic fibrosis care. *Pediatrics.* 2013;132(5):847–853.
127. Chaudhry SR, Keaton M, Nasr SZ. Evaluation of a cystic fibrosis transition program from pediatric to adult care. *Pediatr Pulmonol.* 2013;48(7):658–665.

32 | SOLID ORGAN TRANSPLANT

TIMOTHY KLOUDA, DEBRA BOYER, LYNNE HELFAND, MICHAEL MCCOWN, NICHOLAS PUROL, AND DAWN FREIBERGER

Every obstacle I have overcome
Has made me stronger in some way
And to get the best out of life
I must live it day by day.
So this bump I've now stumbled upon
Is no different from the rest
I must smile, hope, and fight
And try my very best.
As my hair may all fall out
My diabetes out of whack
I will continue to get better
And my hair will grow back
So accept me as I am
While I go around this bend
Cause I'm going to get through this
I'm fighting till the end.

CYSTIC FIBROSIS PATIENT

Providing palliative care to patients pursuing an intensive, life-extending treatment such as organ transplantation may seem paradoxical. However, the presence of severe end-stage disease, insufficient organ availability, and significant morbidity and mortality associated with transplantation requires the application of palliative care concepts through every step of the transplant process. The disparity between the number of patients listed for solid organ transplant and donors is significant. Finding a viable organ for a recipient leaves listed patients with unpredictable waiting times, potentially lasting years. This can leave both patients and care givers experiencing a wide array of emotions due to their uncertain future. During this period, the patient's medical status may worsen and his or her care needs could change dramatically. Patients and caregivers may also no longer wish to pursue transplantation for medical or personal reasons. Therefore, transplant medicine is focused on providing life-extending treatments but must always recognize the medical realities, symptom management challenges, and emotional needs of the patients and families involved.

The frequency of organ transplantation has grown dramatically over the past 30 years and has increasingly become a part of patient care. In 2017, there were 34,770 solid organ transplants in the United States, with 1,899, roughly 5%, of these procedures occurring in patients less than 18 years of age (Table 32.1).[1] The number of total solid organ transplants has gradually increased for 6 consecutive years, and this trend is likely to continue due to greater experience with surgical techniques and improved treatment and therapies for end-stage disease. These advanced therapies, such as ambulatory extracorporeal membrane oxygenation (ECMO), have led to increased patient survival, thus increasing the number of

TABLE 32.1 Distribution of pediatric solid organ transplants in 2018

ORGAN	NUMBER OF PEDIATRIC TRANSPLANTS N (%)	5-YEAR SURVIVAL RATES (%)
Kidney	756 (40.5)	98.4
Liver	563 (30.1)	88.4
Heart	473 (25.3)	81.5
Intestine	37 (2.0)	76.4
Lung	40 (2.1)	60.6

Data compiled from United Network for Organ Sharing 2018 and https://srtr.transplant.hrsa.gov/annual_reports/2018_ADR_Preview.aspx

recipients listed for organ transplant and prolonging the lives of those waiting for transplantation.

The specific criteria to be listed for organ transplantation vary depending on which organ is involved, but generally patients are referred when the morbidity and mortality associated with their underlying disease is greater than that associated with transplant. Mortality rates reflect a variety of factors, including the impact of the patient's underlying disease and the technical and medical difficulties associated with the transplant procedure and post-transplant complications. Morbidity rates are more difficult to quantify, and the impact of transplantation on a patient's quality of life is similarly challenging. Reported morbidity associated with transplant includes complications from the surgery, chronic organ dysfunction due to ischemic injury or rejection, infection, and side effects associated with long-term immunosuppressive therapy (Table 32.1). Ultimately, all transplants require a patient and caregiver commitment to continued medical care and frequent follow-up. Transplantation should not be viewed as a complete cure of the underlying disease process, but rather a transition to a different chronic medical condition. Recipients of solid organ transplants may struggle with increased anxiety after transplantation resulting from trauma often associated with waiting for an organ offer and terminating treatments for their previous chronic illness as well as learning new therapies and complications associated with transplant.

Solid organ transplantation is offered in many but not all countries, generally in more developed and financially sound environments. However, patients often must travel great distances to obtain needed services, adding an emotional and potential financial burden to patients and their caregivers. In addition, patients do come to the United States from abroad seeking organ transplantation, adding further complexity to their clinical and psychosocial situations.

Family Reflection

Thankfully many parents don't have to "live" in a hospital with their child. They visit, have short or long stays, but they go home. Being in the hospital is like living in a fishbowl; there's no privacy, your autonomy as a parent is gone *but* you have a wonderful support system if you're lucky.

My son lived for a month after I was told he wouldn't be coming, home and there was nothing more the hospital could do except keep him comfortable? I grieved even before he died. I grieved for his future, for the things he would never do, people he would never meet, fall in love with, fall out of love with. Even after virtually living in the hospital for 16 years with cystic fibrosis, I always expected to leave with him. It was a daze. The first day I walked around in pain, anger, resignation. I pleaded to all of the deities, wished I could go back in time and find out where I lost the ability to impact his life. How do you parent a child who is dying? He was justifiably ANGRY; at the doctors, nurses and at me, mostly at me. It's my job as a mom to care for him, and I failed at it. He acted out and if he was disciplined, his response was "so what? I'm gonna die anyway." At that point, all you can do is love them soak in every moment, experience, word. You stay up late and talk, play games, cry together. You bust your butt trying to make wishes come true quickly in such a short period of time because you don't know when his last breath will come. You lean on the nurses like they're your brothers and sisters, you hide your soul-ripping grief behind smiles and laughs to keep from screaming at the top of your lungs. You cry in the shower, so your child doesn't see you break down because you've always been the strong one. You wake up and wonder if that day is going to be the day your baby leaves you forever, and you hope for just one more day to love them. And one more day is never enough. Life shifts when you're in the hospital with a dying child. Problems don't seem as insurmountable or difficult anymore and it all becomes background noise.

I was angry, unjustifiably, at the doctors because they're the ones who you trust to heal your child. They had done everything they could, I knew that, but as my son focused his anger at me, I focused mine at them. We had fought his disease for 17 years and now were stuck "waiting to die," a situation that no parent should have to endure. It's unnatural. We hold the hands of our elders as they pass, celebrate the life they lived, but what's to celebrate about a teenager dying?

TRANSPLANT EVALUATION

Transplantation is an extraordinarily stressful time from every perspective. Careful patient selection is required due to the physical demands involved with the actual procedure, the psychosocial upheaval involved throughout the process, and the extensive financial and social support required after a transplant. Transplant evaluation includes a comprehensive review of the patient's medical history, current physical condition, psychological and/or emotional status, and available financial resources. Evaluation is also a time when the family and patient are introduced to the entire transplant team and the process of transplantation. The development of relationships with the care team during this process can have a lasting impact on patient care throughout the transplant process.

It is essential that the family learn about all aspects of transplantation, including anticipated time on wait lists, potential risks associated with the procedure, and what level of care and lifestyle they can expect post-transplant. In addition to their medical/psycho/social assessments, often the teams that are consulted as part of the evaluation are educating the patient and family about post-transplant care. The transplant consent process generally occurs during the transplant evaluation. At the end of the evaluation, the patient may be actively listed for transplant, placed on deferred status until they meet criteria, or be declined for a specific reason. Occasionally, the patient and/or family may elect to not pursue transplantation, may choose to visit other centers, or decide to postpone listing.

The medical evaluation includes an assessment of the underlying disease process for which the patient was referred, as well as a comprehensive assessment to identify comorbid conditions that may complicate or preclude transplantation. The substantial risks involved with transplantation and the relative scarcity of available organs mandates an intensive evaluation of the patient's current and past medical history to ensure the best possible outcome. Each transplant team will have specific requirements for further testing, but, in general, patients undergo a variety of physical exams, laboratory tests, radiographic procedures, and consultations. Patients are frequently referred to a transplant program from remote locations with little or no preceding contact with the transplant center. Referral may follow a dramatic decline in the patients' medical condition and can be at a particular time of crisis for the family. Because of this, it is not uncommon for transplant centers to repeat testing that has already been completed at the referring institution to confirm results and evaluate for disease progression. The tests and studies that are repeated vary between individual transplant centers, along with the criteria they use to determine transplant candidacy.

Each patient being referred for solid organ transplantation will be evaluated by an interdisciplinary team including various medical and surgical providers, social workers, financial planners, mental health professionals, and pharmacists. Social workers will assess a family's ability to handle post-transplant care and identify their practical and emotional means of support. There are numerous psychosocial stressors present throughout the transplant process, including living with chronic disease, frequent medical evaluation and treatment, the uncertainty of when the transplant will occur, and the substantial requirements for ongoing care throughout the transplant process. In addition to the impact of these stressors on the patient's and family's psyche, there are significant associated financial expenses involved in the process. These include the need for frequent admissions, clinic visits, and procedures that are commonly at centers remote from their home. Families may miss work and have travel and food expenses that they would not normally have. Depending on the patient's insurance, uncovered medical expenses can be overwhelming. A social worker will evaluate the family's strengths and ability to cope with these stressors as well as identify potential areas of concern that may impact the care of the transplanted patient. The social worker will also assist the family in locating and developing the resources and supports they will need to successfully navigate this process. A mental health professional will assess the readiness of the patient and family for transplant and evaluate the level of understanding regarding the child's health and prognosis. There are times when a family and medical team are ready to list for transplant, but the child is not ready. A child may be fearful of the surgery itself or its associated pain and potential complications. Some children may doubt the necessity of the transplant. In these instances, the psychosocial support team can be very helpful in preparing the child and navigating issues of assent in these young patients.

Prior adherence to medical regimens must also be considered, as well as a patient and family's understanding of pre- and post-transplant care needs. It is not uncommon for patients and families to be presented with patient/caregiver agreements, with the goal of setting clear expectations around what is expected while on the wait list and after transplant. Such agreements may also help identify barriers to a successful care plan and allow the interdisciplinary care team to help support the family in reaching expectations. Examples of areas for agreement could include maintaining fluid restrictions or meeting enteral nutrition goals, which may involve assessment and concrete support planning from a transplant nutritionist, psychologist, and/or social worker. As the inability to meet these expectations puts the patient at risk of being inactivated on the transplant list, clearly identifying these expectations and addressing specific challenges to them becomes crucially important in meeting the shared goal of a successful transplant.

At the conclusion of the evaluation process, the patient's disposition regarding transplant will be determined. Patients are formally presented to the transplant team for discussion and all factors—medical, psychosocial, financial, developmental, and family resources—are taken into consideration. Therefore, both medical and psychosocial factors play a large role in the ultimate decision about whether to list a patient for transplantation.

A decision to list a patient will occur when the benefits of a transplant are greater than the predicted morbidity and mortality of the patient's current disease. There are no clear criteria as to when this threshold is met, and therefore listing can be a complicated decision. Importantly, the patient's quality of life is a vital factor in deciding when to proceed with transplantation. Application of this standard must be tempered by a thorough understanding of the overall health of the patient, and care must be taken to not wait too long when comorbid conditions and overall poor health may adversely affect the post-transplant prognosis. Consideration of a subspecialty palliative care team consult is often made during the evaluation phase of transplant. The decision if or when to list is not always straightforward. Palliative care teams can help families sort out goals of care, quality of life, and treatment burden as it relates to the medical teams listing recommendations.

Ethical issues arise when transplant teams are faced with a family with psychosocial limitations. The team must ensure that resources are available to allow the family to overcome obstacles so that they do not compromise the child's care. It is well-documented that proper post-transplant care is essential to ensure a good outcome. Therefore, in some instances, patients are declined for transplant due to insurmountable psychosocial limitations. On rare occasions, support from child protective services is sought out to provide a safe environment for the child post-transplant (Table 32.2).

While many transplant clinicians practice and effectively utilize strong communication and symptom management skills as part of their regular practice, there may also be times to consult a separate subspecialty palliative care service. This referral can assist the primary team with managing complex

TABLE 32.2 Transplant team and their roles

TRANSPLANT TEAM MEMBER	ROLE
Surgeon	Performs transplant surgery and post-transplant care
Physician	Provides medical care both pre- and post-transplant
Nurse coordinator	Responsible for pre- and post-transplant care from a nursing perspective, coordination of care, evaluations and patient and/or family education
Social worker	Provides assessment and care around psychosocial needs of family during all phases of transplant process
Psychologist	Performs pre-transplant evaluation to identify any contraindications to transplant. Identifies need for continued therapy pre- and post-transplant
Registered dietitian	Performs nutritional assessment and evaluation during pre- and post-transplant process
Physical therapist	Provides pre- and post-transplant care to encourage recovery and ambulation
Administrative team	Centralized team consisting of clinical and administrative staff focused on outcomes and patient care experiences
Infectious disease	Responsible for infection-related pre- and post- transplant care for immunocompromised organ recipients
Child life specialist	Provides support before and after medical procedures, aids with patients and families adjustment and understanding of the transplant process
Transplant pharmacist	Provides education and medication management of immunosuppression medications pre- and post-transplant
Financial coordinator	Aids families with the financial aspect of transplant care
Chaplaincy	Works with families and patients alongside the medical team to prove psych-social-spiritual services
Palliative care team	Assists the medical team, family, and patient by providing an additional layer of support and focusing on advanced care planning, quality of life, and symptom burden

symptom burden, ethical considerations with exceptionally high-risk transplant cases, and clarity when there may be competing or deeply unclear goals in the family. At these times, introducing the idea of a separate yet collaborative palliative care team may ultimately provide an added layer of focused symptom management and goals of care decision-making conversations that enhances the already complex evaluation process. In addition, the palliative care team can aid the patient and family with many of these competing and conflicting aspects of their care.

TRANSPLANT PREPARATIONS

Once the determination has been made to list a patient for transplantation, the child is placed on the national wait list, thus beginning a new period of uncertainty. The waitlist process varies by organ type, with some organs using allocation scores based on disease severity to determine the place on the list. Some organs use pure time on the list, with some preference given to children and adolescents. For some organs, allocation may depend on where the donor hospital is located. When this system is used, it is a combination of distance and medical urgency that determines to which patients the organs are offered. The goal of this allocation process is to ideally transplant the sickest patients with the highest likelihood of a wait list death.

Waiting for a transplant can be very stressful for the patient and family. Families are aware that in hoping for a transplant for their child, they are often waiting for a tragic event to happen to another family. Understandably, this can be very difficult for older children and families to process. It is explained that, for a donor family, organ donation enables them to see some benefit come from their tragic situation. While no religion outright forbids the donation or receipt of solid organs, some may discourage donation in certain scenarios. For example, in Japan, the national Shinto religion states that the integrity of a dead body should be preserved, and the injuring of one is a serious crime.[2] Other religions share similar beliefs, making solid organ transplantation less common. A chaplain can help provide spiritual guidance and counseling to patients and families, emphasizing their religious beliefs and helping facilitate communication between the patient and transplant team to provide the best possible care.

Waiting times on the list vary from a day to years. Families are required to be easily reached and remain available to come quickly to the transplant center when an organ becomes available. Arrangements need to be made in advance for other family responsibilities such as sibling childcare. Not uncommonly, patients are called in for a transplant only to be sent home without the surgery when complications with the donor arise. Patients can also be listed in more than one region, which may mean twice the clinic visits and added travel expenses. Certainly, this compounds the time and financial investment for the family.

It can feel as if life is put on hold while a patient is listed for transplant. With the need to be near the transplant center, vacations generally need to be close to home or require a period of inactivation on the list. Activities that have a high exposure to potentially sick contacts should be curtailed. The uncertainty that the patient may not survive to transplant leads to an extraordinarily stressful time in many patients' and families' lives.

It is during this pre-transplant phase that applying palliative care strategies can be extremely helpful. The patient will frequently be receiving intensive medical care to optimize his or her overall health for when the transplant occurs. Regardless if a patient is hospitalized or waiting at home for a transplant, keeping up with the medical regime is important. This includes optimizing nutrition, physical therapy, and mental health. Patients waiting for transplant often struggle with nutrition, commonly due to the severity of their underlying illness and associated comorbidities. Patients may undergo gastrostomy (G) tube placement to provide adequate nutrition during this time period and after the transplant. This decision can lead to complications itself and may provide additional stress, especially in adolescents and young adults. Optimizing medical care when a patient is ill is not always consistent with quality-of-life goals. Balancing the benefits of intensive continued disease-directed therapy with an acceptable quality of life needs to be continually considered and assessed. Open and frank discussions with the patient and family regarding their goals and wishes should occur regularly between the patient and transplant team. There could come a time when a patient decides that continuing therapies is too difficult and severely interfering with their quality of life. In these instances, patients and their families should talk with their transplant teams to see if it is possible to alter treatments and still stay active on the transplant list. If it is not, some patients may decide they no longer wish to be listed for transplant. Clearer understanding of a patient and family's goals and priorities for treatment may help avoid or ameliorate potential conflicts or tensions when addressing pain or symptom management as it relates to recovery from transplant. Similarly, palliative care teams can be very helpful in working with the patient's primary physicians and the transplant teams to ensure that the goals and wishes of the patient and family are continually respected.

While waiting for transplantation, patients may experience chronic pain, discomfort, and dyspnea. Patients may have suffered from chronic pain for years and, as a result, been prescribed analgesics such as opioids and benzodiazepines. While these medications can improve quality of life, evidence concerning the effects of opioid use on transplant outcomes remains limited. Some studies have shown that pre-transplant opioid use is associated with an increased risk of graft loss, readmissions, and higher mortality rates, while others have demonstrated no association between pre-transplant opioid use and retransplant-free survival.[3,4] Other possible side effects include decreased gastrointestinal motility; suppression of respiratory drive, making it more difficult to wean from ventilator support; and increased tolerance, making pain control in the postoperative period more complex. While there are no national guidelines across specific organ systems, some centers consider the chronic use of these medications in the pre-transplant period a contraindication to listing. If the use of opioids is accepted by the transplant team, being on the smallest effective dose possible is preferable. The palliative care team can provide specialty guidance and recommendations around the safe use of opioids and other medications while supporting an underlying goal for transplant eligibility and success.[5] To this end, the palliative care teams can also assist in identifying and supporting integrative, nonpharmacological strategies for symptoms while also providing education to families around risks and benefits of opioids when indicated.

It is important to acknowledge that some patients become too ill and no longer remain transplant candidates, meaning they no longer are predicted to survive a transplant. When facing the decision to inactivate a patient on the transplant list, providers are wrestling with the concern that the patient would not survive the transplant as well as consideration of the allocation of a scarce resource. Many families are conflicted over this, because some believe that if their child is going to die regardless, they ought to be given a chance with transplant. It is advised that the possibility of this happening be addressed with families at the time of transplant listing, especially for organs that have a higher waitlist mortality. This allows the family to mentally prepare for the possibility of their child no longer being a transplant candidate. Often, a palliative care specialist can help to facilitate these conversations and better prepare patients and families for these potential events.

There are also a number of waitlist deaths each year, where the appropriate organ is not found in time to save the child. Transplant caregivers can find themselves in the situation of concurrently managing and maintaining end-stage diseases while simultaneously navigating the dying process. This can feel contradictory to the requirements of staying active on a transplant list. It is not uncommon for members of the medical teams to have differing opinions on how to handle these situations. Families are also conflicted with their desire to not give up and yet spare their child any unnecessary pain or discomfort. Discussions about whether a patient can have a do not attempt resuscitation (DNAR) order in place and still be active on the transplant list are not infrequent. An example might be a patient with cystic fibrosis who faces potential intubation for progressive end-stage lung disease yet still hopes to reach transplantation. In this situation, some patients and/or families elect to proceed with intubation in the hope that an organ will be located in time. Others will choose to pursue medical management while maintaining firm limitations around specific interventions such as ventilatory support. This decision-making can become even more salient and challenging in situations where a ventricular assist device (VAD) or ECMO may need to be considered. While this level of mechanical support is not uncommon in patients waiting for heart or lung transplantation, for instance, it may represent varying degrees of quality or suffering to different patients and their families. The palliative care team can be instrumental in guiding the patient, family, and caregivers through these difficult decisions (Figure 32.1).

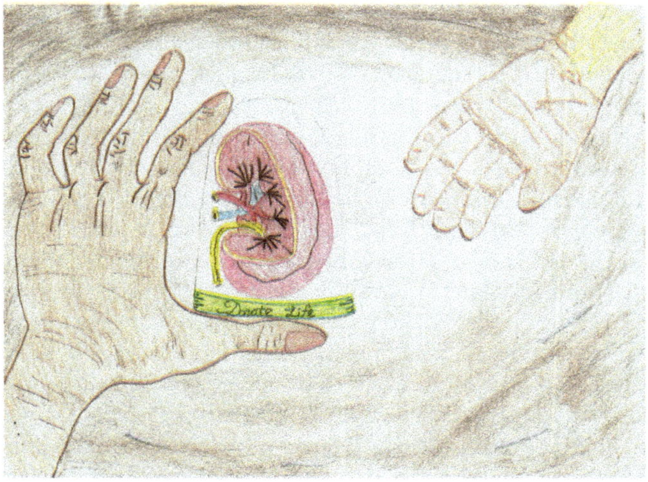

Figure 32.1 Drawing by a child awaiting an organ transplant at Children's Hospital Boston.

TRANSPLANT

The actual transplant procedure is the start of a new experience for the patient and his or her family. While many of these patients have lived their lives with a chronic disease, they are now facing procedures, medications, and complications that are vastly different. Each organ transplant has its own set of immediate surgical risks and subsequent recovery period. Patients are at increased risk for specific organ-related complications during and after surgery along with the general risks associated with surgery. Postoperatively, patients may require varying periods of ventilatory support and intensive care unit interventions. Hospitalizations vary in length, with discharge occurring within 1 week after transplantation to lasting multiple months should complications arise.

In general, patients undergoing transplant will receive immunosuppressive therapy to minimize the chances of rejection. Many solid organ transplant patients will receive induction therapy, which provides intensive and immediate immunosuppression in the postoperative period. Depending on the organ and transplant center, this may consist of a few doses of a medication or months of intermittent therapy. Patients will then receive maintenance immunosuppression, which is generally lifelong. Most solid organ transplant patients are at risk for both acute and chronic rejection. While acute rejection most often occurs in the first few years post-transplant and chronic rejection most often after 1 year, these distinctions are not absolute. Each transplant team will have individualized plans on how to monitor patients for rejection. Secondary to immunosuppressive medications, patients are at risk for long-term complications. While the degree of immunosuppression differs with each organ system and patient, each patient receiving immunosuppressive therapy is at increased risk for infection. For some organs, this risk decreases over time as immunosuppression is lowered; however, for others, it is significant and lifelong. Other common complications include hypertension, renal insufficiency, fluid retention, diabetes, dyslipidemias, seizures, and malignancy. While each patient will have a variable medication regimen, common side effects experienced by this patient population include gastrointestinal upset, thrush, tremors, headaches, hirsutism, and mood changes, all of which can cause increased morbidity and discomfort to patients (Table 32.3).

A second important consideration after transplant is adequate pain control, both in the immediate post-transplant period and afterward. Patients may have multiple lines for intravenous access, chest tubes, and other drains, as well as incisions related to their transplant surgery. While most transplant surgeons, physicians, and nurses are well-versed in adequate pain control, a palliative care service can be vital at this time to ensure that the patient is receiving the appropriate degree of analgesia. Delirium and withdrawal may also be experienced by patients undergoing prolonged hospital courses and medications. Furthermore, if the palliative care service has a long-standing relationship with the patient and family, they may be aware of differing mechanisms both pharmacologic and nonpharmacologic to help individualize the patient's treatment plan.

After transplant, patients and families are often adjusting to a new care team with physicians, surgeons, nurses, and hospitals. This period of adjustment can be stressful and having the continuity of their palliative care team can be very beneficial.

POST-TRANSPLANT PERIOD

In the period immediately following transplant, patients and families are adjusting to new medical issues, trauma experienced while waiting for transplant, and a new lifestyle. Many families have experienced years of coping with the illness that brought them to transplant, and they have developed a level of comfort with the way they feel and how they care for themselves or their child. Post-transplant patients are now relearning about their care. Patients' bodies feel different as they incorporate the new organ and begin to feel that it is truly theirs. Despite education around post-transplant complications, patients and families are often anxious when complications do occur and may worry that the graft could fail.

Patients and families may feel that they have been given a second chance. When the transplant was received from a cadaveric donation, they are aware of this gift being the result of a tragedy. This can lead to feelings of guilt as patients and families try to reconcile their joy with the tragedy that another family has experienced. Patients often wonder about the identity of the donor and may wish to write a letter to the donor family and have difficulty expressing their gratitude along with their sympathy. All communication is organized through the specific transplant center and organ procurement organization (OPO). While each transplant center has a different procedure for contacting donor families or recipients, the United Network for Organ Sharing (UNOS) has universal guidelines on what information can and cannot be

TABLE 32.3 Transplant immunosuppressive therapies

MEDICATION	MECHANISM	ADVERSE EFFECTS
INDUCTION AGENTS		
Rabbit anti-thymocyte globulin (Thymoglobulin)	Polyclonal antibody decreases CD4 lymphocytes	Persistent lymphopenia
Horse anti-thymocyte globulin (Atgam)	Polyclonal antibody against T lymphocytes	Persistent lymphopenia Severe thrombocytopenia
Basiliximab (Simulect)	Monoclonal antibody to IL-2 receptor complex	Anaphylactoid and hypersensitivity reactions
Alemtuzumab (Campath)	Monoclonal antibody to CD52	Severe cytopenia Hypersensitivity with infusion
Maintenance medications		
Tacrolimus (Prograf)	Calcineurin inhibitor	Nephrotoxicity Diabetes mellitus Hyperkalemia Hypertension Hepatic toxicity
Cyclosporine (Neoral/ Sandimmune)	Inhibition of T-cell activation	Nephrotoxicity Hypertension
Mycophenolate mofetil (CellCept)	Inhibition of inosine monophosphate dehydrogenase (IMPDH) with decreased T- and B-cell proliferation	GI disturbance Bone marrow suppression
Mycophenolic acid (Myfortic)	IMPDH inhibition with decreased T- and B-cell proliferation	GI disturbance Bone marrow suppression
Azathioprine (Imuran)	Purine metabolism antagonist	GI toxicity Dose-related hematologic toxicity Hepatotoxicity Mutagenic effects
Sirolimus (Rapamune) or everolimus (Afinitor)	Suppresses cytokine mediated T-cell proliferation	Anaphylaxis and/or angioedema Interstitial lung disease Lymphocele Proteinuria and/or nephro toxicity Impaired wound healing
Prednisone	Inhibits leukocyte migrations and decreases inflammatory response	Hypertension Hyperglycemia Cataracts Osteoporosis Cushing disease

included in correspondences to protect the privacy of both parties.

The literature describes increased incidence of mental health symptoms including depression, anxiety, and post-traumatic stress disorder for parents and/or patients after transplant.[6] Mental health concerns and poor health outcomes are associated with higher rates of nonadherence.

Patients and their families have heard from the medical team that transplant essentially trades one disease process for another. Post-transplant, patients face a new set of medical issues and may realize they must adapt to a new normal. Adjusting to these changes can be a challenging process that varies with the patient's developmental level. Young children tend to incorporate their new medical regime into their life and continue to work with their parents to manage their medications and medical appointments. Some adults may adjust easily, while others may find their new medical regime difficult to adapt to. However, as they become more comfortable with their post-transplant care, they may become less adherent or feel frustrated when their care needs interfere with school, work, or other activities. Families and older patients may wonder how long their new organ will remain viable and feel they are "living on borrowed time." In time, recipients become more comfortable with their changed bodies, and the organ becomes a part of their sense of self. For some this level of comfort is challenged with any medical complication.

Adolescent patients pose a different set of concerns to the transplant professionals. During this stage of development, children feel invincible and are struggling to assert themselves as autonomous individuals. "Risk-taking behaviors function to fulfill developmental needs for independence, autonomy and self-competence."[7] This is the most difficult developmental period for parents and medical professionals. A healthy teen would be given increasing autonomy and responsibility. For the teen with a transplant, however, parents need to walk a fine line between helping their child learn to manage their own care while they remain involved to ensure that their child is adhering to the medical regime. Their goal is to prepare their child to become an independent adult, able to manage his or her own medical care. The foremost concern certainly is that the adolescent will not adhere to the medication regime. In a transplant patient, this can have life-threatening consequences. Teens often want to test the limits of their bodies and may not fully believe that they need the medications. They may purposefully or subconsciously forget to take their medication for a day or longer. When they realize their error, they may not bring this to the attention of their parents. Additionally, teenagers generally have a strong desire to be like their peers and feel normal. "During adolescence, a sense of identity and self-understanding is created through social relationships with peers."[8] They may want to feel that they can have days without medications, like their healthy friends. Patients whose friends do not know about their transplant may prefer the risk of missing a dose of medication rather than the risk of having a peer ask them about their treatments. All these challenges for the adolescent patient lead to higher risk for rejection in a variety of solid organ transplant populations.[9,10]

An additional stressor for the adolescent transplant patient is the eventual transfer of care to an adult center. This is a difficult transition period both medically and psychosocially for the transplant patient. Patients may struggle transitioning from the pediatric center and care team where they have received care their entire life. Furthermore, adjusting to a new mode of care delivery in an adult center can be challenging to emerging adult patients. From a medical standpoint, studies have shown an increased incidence of organ rejection during adolescence, with further risk during the period of transfer to an adult center.[11]

Before transfer to an adult center, adolescents need to gain independence in their care. This is a gradual process that should happen over years. It is important that pediatric centers have a formal process to help adolescents achieve this goal. Parents learn when to have confidence in allowing their child to be independent and when to continue to oversee their child's medical regime. This may or may not correlate with their chronological age or when their peers may be ready for more independence. Additionally, adolescents and adults often have questions regarding pregnancy post-transplant. Depending on the health of the transplant patient and the particular organ that they received, the risk of pregnancy is variable. For some organ groups, such as a lung transplant patient, the risk of experiencing significant and potentially life-threatening rejection after pregnancy is quite high.[12] For other patients, such as kidney transplant recipients, the risk is far less.[13] For all transplant patients, they must be aware of the potential risks to a fetus of all medications they are taking. As patients think about their future, it can be distressing to learn this information.

For a child undergoing transplantation, there are many social stressors. These include extended absences from school, work, or other activities, as well as restricted exposures to ill contacts. Physical changes can follow from prolonged immunosuppressive therapy such as hair growth or loss, weight gain, and cushingoid like features. The potential for organ rejection, infection, and the overall uncertain future of the transplant course can add stress to the recipient and their family.

As mentioned previously, there are significant financial stressors for families that continue to accumulate over the post-transplant period, including lost work time and costs inherent in hospital admissions. For siblings, there can be a sense of deprivation and anger, as more attention must be paid to the patient, thus fostering the perception that the sick sibling is more important. They may also harbor feelings of guilt or fear that they have caused or contributed to their sibling's illness. The patient may also feel guilty because he or she is aware that time spent with them is time away from the sibling.

Patients and their families may be faced with transitioning from end-of-life disease to post-transplant recovery and, in some instances, to morbidity from post-transplant complications. Patients can feel well and be more active and then experience complications that quickly reverse these gains. In other instances, there may be gradual post-transplant complications such as living with chronic rejection. One complication in particular, post-transplant lymphoproliferative disorder (PTLD) can cause significant anxiety and stress for families. PTLD is most commonly due to uncontrolled proliferation of B cells infected with Epstein Barr virus (EBV). Rates of PTLD vary between solid organ transplant groups, ranging from 1% to 30%, with roughly 80% of cases occurring within the first year post-transplant.[14] The main risk factor among all solid organ transplant groups is the degree of immunosuppression and the EBV status of the donor organ and recipient. Therapeutic strategies primarily consist of reduction, alteration, or cessation of immunosuppressive medications, however more aggressive therapies such as monoclonal CD20 antibodies (rituximab) or chemotherapy may be necessary.

When complications occur, patients and their families may need to shift their mindsets from one of recovery to, once again, facing loss and possibly death.[15] Both children and their parents may be surprised when a transplant does not go as planned. Even when education is done prior to listing about potential post-transplant complications, it can be hard to comprehend the significance of these complications. Families may question if they made the right decision for their child to move forward with transplant at all, particularly if complications happen soon after the transplant surgery. Other families feel that any extra time the child received was valuable and worth the burden inherent in the transplant process. This is typically true for children who have a good post-transplant outcome and lead normal lives for a period.

END OF LIFE

When a transplanted organ begins to fail, many of the issues surrounding end-stage disease and end-of-life care are again a reality for a patient and their family. This will certainly vary by organ, with various salvage therapies available to each.

For example, renal transplant recipients may be faced with considering restarting dialysis. When a transplanted organ has failed, an organ recipient and his or her caregivers must consider whether re-transplantation is an option. This decision is generally quite difficult for patients and the transplant team for a variety of reasons. One main consideration is outcomes following re-transplant. In some cases, outcomes of re-transplant are worse compared to the primary transplant, although this varies significantly with the organ involved.[16–18] Additionally, medications and therapies may have caused complications with other organ systems, such as the kidneys or liver. In some cases, these consequences have resulted in situations in which re-transplantation is of higher risk or not possible. Furthermore, it is essential to continue to assess psychological and social factors that could make re-transplantation more difficult. Examples include issues with nonadherence, changes in caregiver circumstances, illicit drug use, and poor medical follow-up. Because each individual transplant center will have its own criteria for re-transplant, it is not uncommon for a patient to be referred to a new program for consideration. In some cases, this program may be at quite a distance from the patient's home.

Families themselves may be ambivalent about re-transplant. If the first transplant went well, then a family is generally more interested in relisting than if there were significant complications. Some ethicists would argue that with all the waitlist deaths that occur each year, it is unfair to list someone for a re-transplant when so many have been waiting long periods of time for their first transplant.

When a patient is relisted for transplant and the organ continues to fail, all the same issue and feelings return that existed while waiting for the first transplant. Medical providers and families once again face a parallel process of addressing end-of-life issues and optimizing medical care to maintain the patient as a re-transplant candidate. Just as in the initial pre-transplant period, these goals can seem contradictory both for patients and caregivers alike. For example, pain medication meant to enhance comfort and potentially allow for engagement in activities of daily living can sometimes result in initial drowsiness or a lessened ability to be ambulatory. In this and other scenarios, the palliative care team can be helpful by offering a perspective that is informed by both the medical and psychosocial realities and the goals of a patient and family, while existing outside of a specific transplant assessment paradigm. Involvement of the subspecialty palliative care team, therefore, ultimately allows an opportunity for a potentially more balanced and holistic approach to care.

Multiple factors, including the patient's age, insurance, and place of residence, can influence the services offered to a patient in the advanced stages of their disease course. Families and patients are sometimes faced with difficult decisions regarding the resources that can be provided to them, including home nursing services, hospice care teams, and medications. In these cases, involvement of palliative care services in the hospital and community may be beneficial to help assess patient needs and support them with symptom management, advance care planning, and anticipatory counseling regarding the status of individual therapies and medication even should re-transplantation not be sought.

Transplant patients may also face particular and unique challenges around anticipatory grief—the grief and mourning experienced prior to or in anticipation of a death.[19,20] Patients may have worries around their own mortality in the stages prior to a transplant and experience complex feelings and ambivalence around the circumstances of acquiring and living with their transplant and the medical care to follow. Due to the resources and circumstances of organ donation and transplantation, patients may worry that expression of complex emotions and grief reactions may be tantamount to lack of gratitude for the medical marvel of a transplant. While the transplant team is best suited to awareness of these potential issues, a palliative care team or provider may also serve to help assess and address these challenges given their unique clinical role situated outside of the primary team.

Because the goal of transplant is giving life, death in transplant patients requires a different focus of care that can be exceedingly difficult on the healthcare team itself. Transplant teams often cultivate close, lasting, and intense bonds with families in pursuit of a shared goal. Healthcare professionals may therefore benefit from continued education and support when helping patients and families through the dying process and into bereavement. Having a member of the palliative care team at family meetings and rounds assures that all aspects of care are considered for the patient and family and also provides an added layer of support for the transplant and medical teams. Medical professionals, especially nursing and direct-care staff, need both the emotional tools and the educational resources to care for the dying patient. In both end-of-life and bereavement care, palliative care providers may therefore help provide guidance, resources, and potential structure for desired follow-up with patient families in collaboration and support of the transplant team to help maintain connections.

Clinical Vignette

CK was a 22-year-old man who was diagnosed with cystic fibrosis as a toddler. At age 12, he was referred to the transplant center for evaluation because of declining pulmonary function and was listed for a double lung transplant. CK waited for 2 years before lungs became available. After transplant CK had several admissions for treatment of infection but was healthy overall.

During this period CK returned to school and, for the first time, had peers who did not know of his medical background. Initially, CK took his medications on time, monitored his pulmonary function by home spirometry, exercised, and was followed closely in transplant clinic. He was independent with most of his care because his father worked full-time. Several years after transplant, CK missed several doses of his anti-rejection medications and stopped doing his home spirometry when his friends were around as he struggled to "live like a normal teenager." Three years after his transplant, CK was diagnosed with chronic rejection. He was again evaluated for a double lung transplant. During the re-evaluation period, CK's medical status was reviewed, and significant concerns were expressed regarding his previous nonadherence. Ultimately, the transplant team believed that this was an isolated event of adolescence and were confident that CK could continue to adhere to the challenging medical regimen required of him with a re-transplant.

CK's lung function continued to decline rapidly. CK and his father questioned if he would survive long enough to receive a second transplant. His parents were able to discuss procedures and choices around his care with their son but had an increasingly difficult time staying at the hospital during his lengthy admissions. In light of the complexities around the possibility of a second transplant, CK worked closely with the palliative care team and mental health providers at the transplant center and began to clarify his goals for treatment and for his quality of life, which included doing everything possible to receive a transplant but focusing on comfort and de-medicalization of his life if transplant would no longer be an option.

Fortunately, CK did receive a second double lung transplant. Unfortunately, this transplant led to additional complications, ultimately resulting in a return to chronic rejection. Building from previous conversations with his care team, psychosocial providers, and the palliative care team, CK made the difficult decision to not pursue evaluation for a third transplant, wishing instead to maximize the time he had left with his family and friends and focus on comfort while maintaining dedicated medical management of his disease. Based on his goals, CK pursued interventions to extend his quality of life outside of transplant that would allow for spending time with friends and his dog, go to church, and participate in various art projects. CK continued to work closely with the transplant team to manage his medical regimen while also increasing his involvement with the palliative care team to manage worsening dyspnea and cope with gradual declines in his functional status. During this period, CK began to refine his advance care planning documentation to better express his wishes. Through collaborative interventions between palliative care and the primary transplant team, CK received ongoing monitoring, psychosocial support, and medical management until the time of his death.

CONCLUSION

Outcomes from organ transplantation have improved dramatically since the first organ transplant was performed in 1954. However, as with all patients with complex medical conditions, it remains a process with variable outcomes. Through every step of the transplant process from referral and evaluation, to listing, the transplant procedure, and the post-transplant period, numerous challenges are faced by patients and caregivers. Palliative care has a role in all these stages and can help to improve the quality of life for patients in these very challenging situations as well as support the providers caring for these complex patients.

REFERENCES

1. Scientific Registry of Transplant Recipients. OPTN/SRTR 2018 Annual Data Report. https://srtr.transplant.hrsa.gov/annual_reports/Default.aspx
2. Eshraghian A. Religion, tradition, culture and solid organ transplantation. *Crit Care Med.* 2013;41(7):134.
3. Bruschwein H, Andersonm V, Patel H, Fleming J, Shahane A, Weder M. Opioid and benzodiazepine use in lung transplant candidates: A national survey of polices and practices. *AM J Transplant.* 2019; 19(3):395–396.
4. Vahidy S, Li D, Hirji A, Kapasi A, Weinkauf J, Laing B, Lien D, Halloran K. Pretransplant opioid use and survival after lung transplantation. *Transplantation.* 2020 Aug;104(8):1720–1725
5. Colman R, Singer LG, Barua R, Downar J. Outcomes of lung transplant candidates referred for co-management by palliative care: A retrospective case series. *Palliat Med.* 2015;29(5):429–435.
6. Cousino MK, Rea KE, Schumacher KR, Magee JC, Fredericks EM. A systematic review of parent and family functioning in pediatric solid organ transplant populations. *Pediatr Transplant.* 2017;21(3):e12900.
7. Millstein SG, Ingra V. Theoretical models of adolescent risk-taking behavior. In Wallander JL, Siegel LJ, eds. *Adolescent Health Problems.* Guilford; 1995: 52–71.
8. Sroufe LA, Cooper RG, Dehart G. *Child Development: Its Nature and Course.* 3rd ed. McGraw Hill; 1996.
9. Boyer D. Poor outcomes in adolescent lung transplant patients: Why the gap? *J Heart Lung Transplant.* 2019;37(3):315–316.
10. Paraskeva MA, Edwards LB, Levvey B, et al. Outcomes of adolescent recipients after lung transplantation: An analysis of the International Society for Heart and Lung Transplantation Registry. *J Heart Lung Transplant.* 2018;37:323–331.
11. Bell LE, Bartosh SM, Davis CL, et al. Adolescent transition to adult care in solid organ transplantation: A consensus conference report. *Am J Transplant.* 2008;8:2230–2242.
12. Armenti VT, Radomski JS, Moritz MJ, Gaughan WJ, McGrory CH, Coscia LA. Report from the National Transplantation Pregnancy Registry (NTPR): Outcomes of pregnancy after transplantation. *Clin Transpl.* 2003:131–41.
13. Zachariah MS, Tornatore KM, Venuto RC. Kidney transplantation and pregnancy. *Curr Opin Organ Transplant.* 2009;14:386–391.
14. Hussein K, Tiede C, Maecker-Kolhoff B, Kreipe H. Posttransplant lymphoproliferative disorder in pediatric patients. *Pathobiology.* 2013;80:289–296.
15. Berzoff J, Silverman PR, eds. *Living with Dying. A Handbook for End-of-Life Healthcare Practitioners.* Columbia University Press; 2004.
16. Aurora P, Edwards LB, Christie JD, et al. 2009 Registry of the International Society for Heart and Lung Transplantation: Twelfth Official Pediatric Lung and Heart/Lung Transplantation Report, 2009. *J Heart Lung Transplant.* 2009;28:1023–1030.
17. Kanter KR, Vincent RN, Berg AM, Mahle WTM, Forbess JM, Kirshbom PM. Cardiac retransplantation in children. *Ann Thoracic Surg.* 2004;78:644–649.
18. Shen ZY, Zhu ZJ, Deng YL, et al. Liver retransplantation: Report of 80 cases and review of the literature. *Hepatobiliary Pancreat Dis Int.* 2006;5(2):180–184.
19. Poole J, Ward JW, DeLuca E, Shildrick M, Abbey S, Mauthner O, Ross H. Grief and loss for patients before and after heart transplant. *Heart Lung.* 2016;45:193–198.
20. Gill P, Lowes L. Renal transplant failure and disenfranchised grief: Participants' experiences in the first year post-graft failure: A qualitative longitudinal study. *Int J Nurs Studies.* 2014;51(9):1271–1280.

33 | ONCOLOGICAL ILLNESSES

SARAH MCCARTHY, KIMBERLY A. PYKE-GRIMM, AND ANGELA M. FERACO

I have loved [Catullus poem 101] since the first time I read it in high school Latin class and I have tried to translate it a number of times. Nothing in English can capture the passionate, slow surface of a Roman elegy. No one (even in Latin) can approximate Catullan diction, which at its most sorrowful has an air of deep festivity, like one of those trees that turns all its leaves over, silver, in the wind. I never arrived at the translation I would have liked to do of poem 101. But over the years of working at it, I came to think of translating as a room, not exactly an unknown room, where one gropes for the light switch. I guess it never ends. A brother never ends. I prowl him. He does not end.

ANNE CARSON, excerpt from *Nox*

Vignette

Lawrence, a 15-year-old boy active on his school's soccer team, collides with another player on the field during practice and feels his right leg go out from under him. When he tries to get up, his pain is severe, and he struggles to stand. His coach calls his mother, Diana, who is at work. Diana picks Lawrence up and brings him to the emergency room at the small hospital that serves his town. The emergency room physician suspects a tibial fracture and obtains radiographs. These confirm a fracture, but also show an abnormal mass that appears to arise from the bone. The emergency room physician contacts the on-call orthopedist who reviews the images, calls a colleague who specializes in orthopedic oncology at the closest children's hospital, and then comes to the emergency room. He tells Lawrence and Diana that Lawrence needs a cast, which he applies, and he prescribes oral medication for pain. The orthopedist explains to Diana and Lawrence that they can go home tonight but that Lawrence needs to go to the children's hospital 60 miles away later that week for additional imaging because "the bone around the area of the break looks abnormal." When Lawrence asks if he will get to play again this season, he notices that the orthopedist looks uncomfortable. "I think that's hard to say right now," the orthopedist replies. "You'll like Dr. Jensen at Children's, though. She'll talk to you about the next steps."

Lawrence and Diana meet Dr. Jensen later that week, after Lawrence undergoes a magnetic resonance imaging (MRI) scan of his painful right leg. Lawrence has had to miss school and Diana has had to miss work and to arrange for her sister to pick up Maya, her youngest, from school. The MRI confirms a mass lesion suspicious for osteosarcoma. After asking Diana and Lawrence to tell her what they know and getting permission to share the results of the MRI with them, Dr. Jensen discloses this news and recommends a biopsy. The biopsy is scheduled for early the following week. On the long drive home, Lawrence is very quiet and Diana's tries to imagine what this means for their family. Her only experience with cancer so far has been in her 75-year-old uncle who has lung cancer.

The biopsy confirms that Lawrence has osteosarcoma, a malignant bone tumor, and Diana and Lawrence return to the children's hospital for more imaging scans and a visit with another physician, Dr. Wilson. Diana has had to miss several days of work already, and her co-workers are starting to grumble about covering her shifts. She explains to Lawrence's guidance counselor at school what is going on. Lawrence's grandmother comes to stay with them so that Maya will have someone to focus on her and so Diana can worry less about household issues.

Dr. Wilson explains that he is a pediatric oncologist and that he will work with Dr. Jensen, the orthopedic oncologist, to treat Lawrence's cancer. He recommends chemotherapy, an operation to remove the cancer, and then more chemotherapy. Dr. Wilson explains that the entire treatment course will take several months and that Lawrence and Diana will have to work with Dr. Jensen to decide what kind of an operation he will have. Lawrence learns that the bone that helps to form his right knee will have to removed and that the possibilities are either an internal metal prosthesis or a rotationplasty, a procedure where his ankle will be "turned around" to become a new knee. This second procedure would enable him to learn to play soccer again, while the first procedure will lead to less function but more typical looks. Lawrence cannot believe that his leg will never be as it was before. Dr. Jensen and his mother, Diana, urge him to consider rotationplasty and suggest that he talk to his coach. Dr. Jensen puts him in touch with a college student who had the same cancer that he has. Three days later, Lawrence and Diana drive back to the children's hospital for his first chemotherapy treatment. Maya has not been sleeping well, and they are all exhausted.

A BRIEF HISTORY OF CHILDHOOD CANCER

Cancer arising in childhood is rare. It encompasses a diverse collection of diseases that can affect every organ system. The most common childhood cancers include leukemias, brain tumors, lymphomas, and extracranial solid tumors arising from the kidney, neuroendocrine tissues, and bone.[1] Over the past 45 years, the overall survival rate for children with cancer has increased dramatically, from approximately 45% in 1975 to more than 80% in recent years.[2] This substantial increase in survival is driven largely by successes in treating acute lymphoblastic leukemia, the most common cancer of childhood.[3] At the end of 2013, approximately 420,000 pediatric cancer survivors were currently living in the United States,[4] and 1 of every 530 young adults aged 20–39 years had been treated for childhood cancer.[5] Yet while gains made in pediatric cancer survival over this period are among the most dramatic success stories of modern medicine, pediatric cancer remains a leading cause of death in children living in the United States. More than 15,000 children ages 0–19 are diagnosed with cancer each year, and approximately 1,700 die from their disease.[1] Childhood cancer is a profoundly life-altering experience for the affected child, the child's family, and the surrounding community.[6] Children treated for cancer experience immediate and late effects of malignancy and treatment that can affect physical health, cognition, and psychosocial functioning.[4] Importantly, children, their siblings, and their parents also report substantial psychological growth and resiliency.[7]

PALLIATIVE CARE AS A STANDARD OF CARE IN PEDIATRIC ONCOLOGY

The integration of palliative care into the care of children and adolescents with cancer is supported as best practice by numerous professional organizations.[8] Palliative care is useful for and intended to be an enhancement to the care of patients with oncological disease at any time during the disease trajectory, from diagnosis to end-of-life[9,10] (Figure 33.1). The role of the interdisciplinary palliative care team may vary with regard to the child with cancer, the child's family caregivers, and the child's pediatric oncology team.[9] For example, the interdisciplinary palliative care team may act as a consultative resource to the interdisciplinary pediatric oncology team, may provide direct care to children and their family caregivers, and, in some circumstances, may assume the role of primary team.[11,12] Patient and family/caregiver distress related to the child's symptoms, psychosocial distress, and poor communication can occur at any time and can benefit from

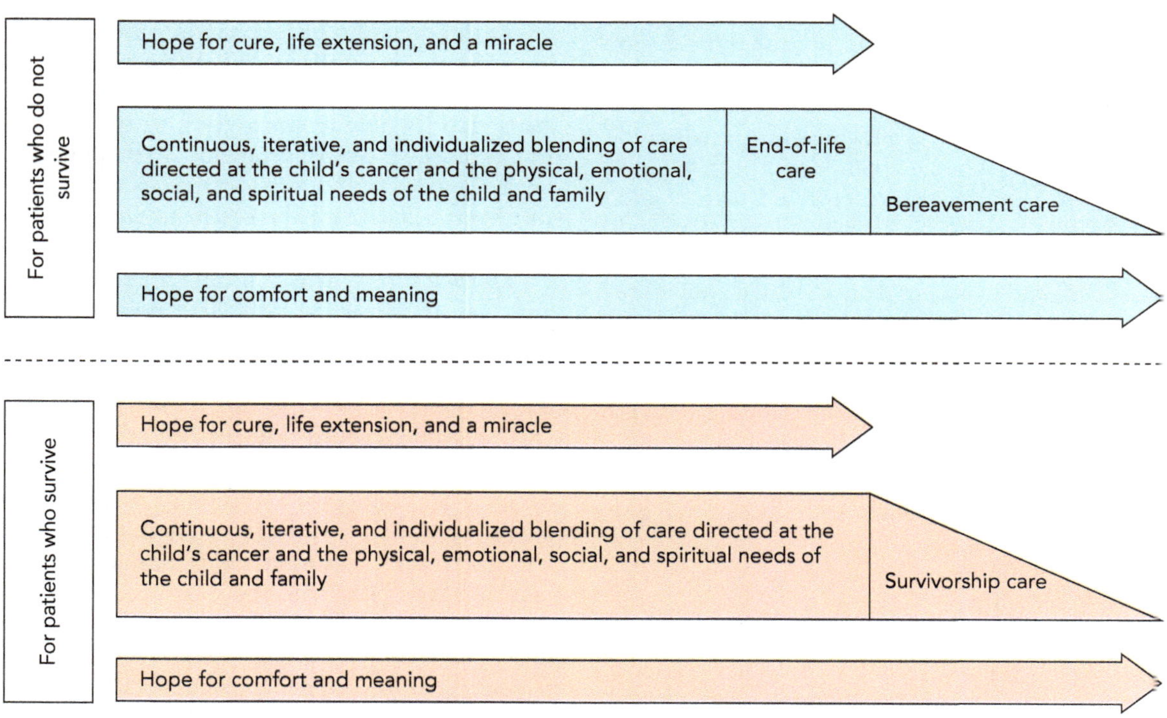

Figure 33.1 *Conceptual model of palliative care integration across the continuum for patients who do not or do survive.* Reprinted with permission from Rosenberg AR, Wolfe J. Approaching the third decade of paediatric palliative oncology investigation: Historical progress and future directions. *Lancet Child Adolesc Health.* 2017 Sep;1(1):56–67. doi: 10.1016/S2352-4642(17)30014-7. Epub 2017 Jul 24. PMID: 29333484; PMCID: PMC5764167

palliative care therapies provided alongside cancer-directed therapy.[9,11,13] Furthermore, patients and families have reported receptivity to early integration of palliative care principles and personnel.[14]

In a landmark paper, Wolfe and colleagues made visible the suffering children with cancer experienced at the end of their lives.[15] At that time, few pediatric oncologists had received formal training in managing symptoms and suffering at the end of life, and few seemed to understand the scope of the problem.[16] Beyond demonstrating the high-intensity care that many children receive at end-of-life, these studies highlighted the need for training in palliative care principles among interdisciplinary clinicians who constitute the pediatric oncology team ("primary" palliative care) as well as the need for specialty pediatric palliative care (PPC) in more complex scenarios. Since that time, the American Academy of Pediatrics has recognized the essential roles that primary and specialty PPC play in the care of seriously ill children.[17] The American Board of Medical Specialties began offering subspecialty certification for Hospice and Palliative Medicine in 2008. The early integration of primary palliative care for all children diagnosed with cancer has been proposed as a standard of care within pediatric oncology.[18] The core tenets of PPC within oncology include systematic symptom assessment and intervention (see Section III), facilitation of family-centered communication (see Chapter 13) including prioritization of the patient's voice (see Chapters 3 and 9), and developmentally informed advance care planning (see Chapter 14).[18] The provision of psychosocial care for patients and families is a key element of palliative care for pediatric oncology patients; see also Chapter 3, "Children's Voices" and Chapter 17, "Psychological Symptoms."[19] PPC teams often include social workers, some of whom have specific training in the field, and may also offer access to assessment and intervention through psychology and psychiatry services. In addition, professionals with expertise in child life, expressive therapies, and chaplaincy can be extremely helpful in promoting coping and augmenting quality of life. Current clinical standards of care[20,21] emphasize the importance of early psychosocial assessment and the development of an individualized psychosocial care plan for the child and the family for all pediatric oncology patients, including those receiving palliative care services.

Research has demonstrated that pediatric oncology patients and their families who receive specialty palliative care experience improvements in psychological and physical symptoms,[22] report better quality of life,[23] are more likely to engage in end-of-life discussions and to enroll in hospice,[24] and are less likely to die in an intensive care unit (ICU) and/or to receive mechanical ventilation immediately prior to death.[25] In addition, specialty palliative care has been associated with improved outcomes for parents before[23] and after their child's death.[26] However, despite the call for early integration of services and the documented positive impact of palliative care involvement, a recent systematic review found that only 54% of children with cancer who subsequently died received any specialty palliative care services prior to their death, and, for the majority, services were not initiated until near the time of death.[27] Of note, this literature examines the role of specialty PPC. Primary palliative care efforts are more difficult to identify and study retrospectively.

LANGUAGE, COMMUNICATION, AND UNCERTAINTY IN CHILDHOOD CANCER

Communication is fundamental to PPC. This includes communication with the child and family as well as among all members of the interdisciplinary team.[28] As highlighted in Chapter 13 and throughout this book, effective patient- and family-centered communication stems from foundational knowledge and attitudes and requires deliberate practice.[29–32] Within pediatric oncology, the practice of compassionate and honest communication throughout the disease trajectory has been shown to enhance patient, parent, and provider outcomes.[12,33] Because pediatric cancer occurs throughout childhood and adolescence, each child's developmental context shapes the care that is needed.[34]

As noted in the first chapter, language is powerful, and language and narrative are important drivers of how children and their families experience childhood cancer.[35] Clinicians frequently use the term "cure" when discussing the goal of treatment for cancer arising in childhood.[3,36] The word "cure" is meant to imply lifelong disease eradication. Despite the incredible progress made in treating childhood cancers, many children face lifelong changes in health due to consequences of their underlying cancer or the treatment they receive.[37–40] The life-threatening nature of cancer, the possibility of cancer progression or recurrence, and the possibility of future health conditions resulting from cancer treatment all contribute to a future that may feel profoundly uncertain.[41] Likewise, clinicians who care for children with cancer over the course of a career see that illness trajectories are frequently uncertain. Children expected to live a long life after completing treatment sometimes die suddenly from infection or from unintended effects of that very treatment, while children with advanced cancer may live far longer than anticipated. This should not discourage clinicians from sharing their best understanding of what a child and family are likely to experience immediately and in the long-term.[42,43] We encourage clinicians to describe the goal of proposed cancer treatments, whether that goal is to live a long life with disease eradication, life extension without expectation that the cancer can be eradicated, or to reduce symptoms arising from active cancer, perhaps without an expectation that this will extend life.

Parents of children with cancer have reported wanting detailed prognostic information, opportunities to revisit initial discussions, and time to consider treatment decisions.[44,45] The time around diagnosis has also been identified to be important for influencing patterns of communication.[46] Open communication between the team and the patient/family all along the illness trajectory can enhance the therapeutic relationship, improve quality of life, and facilitate shared decision-making (Figure 33.2).[47] Other benefits include reducing decisional regret,[48] optimizing medical treatment, and ensuring that

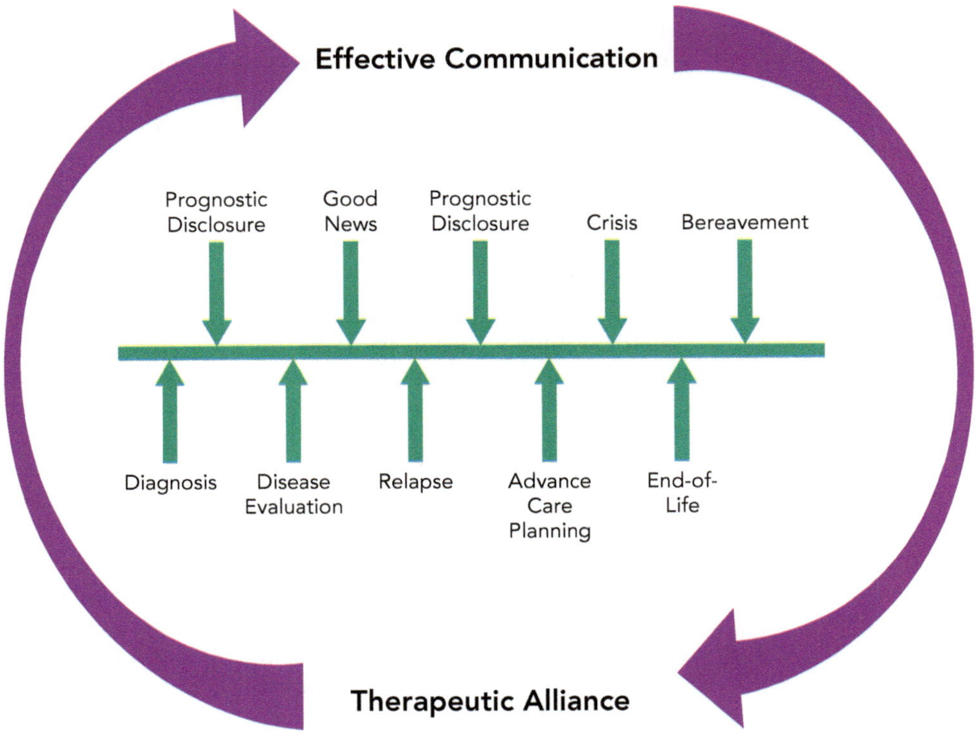

Figure 33.2 *A note on communicating with children and members of the child's extended family.* Reprinted with permission from Blazin LJ, Cecchini C, Habashy C, Kaye EC, Baker JN. Communicating effectively in pediatric cancer care: Translating evidence into practice. *Children (Basel).* 2018 Mar 11;5(3):40. doi: 10.3390/children5030040. PMID: 29534479; PMCID: PMC5867499

treatment is aligned with the goals of care desired by the patient and family. High-quality communication ideally begins with the initial visits[49] and continues throughout the relationship with the interdisciplinary team.[20,50–52] Importantly, communication takes place between the patient/family and multiple individuals from different disciplines who may bring complementary perspectives. These interactions may focus on different aspects of care reflecting the expertise of each discipline (e.g., medicine, nursing, social work, psychology, chaplaincy, child life, rehabilitative therapists). To ensure a clear message and that everyone is "working in the same direction" it is critical that there is also clear communication and mutual exchange among these professionals.[51]

A developmentally sensitive approach to communicating with children is critical in establishing a relationship with them. Table 33.1 highlights the typical cognitive development of children and recommendations for communication matched to developmental level. Increasingly, children who survived cancer and their families believe that the diagnosis and management should be discussed with the child starting early at diagnosis if possible.[34,53–55] Learning how the parents have approached scary or difficult situations with their child prior to the child's diagnosis can begin a conversation about how to involve the child or adolescent in discussions of the child's health. Attending to families' approaches to communication and decision-making and eliciting the cultural, ethnic, or religious basis of these preferences demonstrates respect for the family's norms, rules, and cohesiveness.[56] When there is news to share with the child, such as a diagnosis of cancer, questions to consider discussing with the parents might include: Do they want or need additional time before involving the child? And Do they want to talk with the child privately or with a professional present for support? Eliciting and respecting parents' preferences for how and when to share news with children reinforces the parental role and shows the healthcare team's commitment to aligning with the family.[57,58] Once parents have indicated their readiness, involvement of the child in these conversations should be with the participation of the parents and carefully orchestrated to address concerns and issues in an age-appropriate manner.[34] For many children and most adolescents, the question isn't if they should participate but how, when, and to what extent.[34,59,60] For adolescents, there is also the consideration of their evolving sense of themselves apart from their parents, siblings, and extended family members. Adolescents might want to meet privately with the team. Participation in these conversations serves not only to impart information but also to enhance feelings of control and to establish trust with clinicians.[18]

Communicating with siblings and extended family members[57,61] is very important. Prior to meeting with extended family, it is important to discuss with the parents and, if developmentally appropriate, the child, to determine what and with whom the team can communicate. Direct communication by the healthcare team with siblings and other family members can improve family adjustment, enhance sibling understanding, and help siblings adjust to new life circumstances.[57] When desired by parents, communicating

TABLE 33.1 Developmental considerations and interplay with cancer care

AGE GROUP	PSYCHOSOCIAL CHALLENGES	COGNITIVE CHALLENGES	POTENTIAL BEHAVIORAL MANIFESTATIONS	COMMUNICATION STRATEGIES
Infant/Toddlers (0–2 years)	Difficulties with regular feeding, comfort, and cares in can lead to caregiver mistrust and attachment disruptions.	Developing sensory and motor curiosities can be particularly disrupted by pain, nausea, and discomfort of treatment.	Decreasing abilities to self-soothe and be soothed. Increased irritability with touch or aversion to it.	Engage in play-based interactions with child and parent/trusted caregiver present.
Preschool (3–5 years)	Failure to develop sense of personal control over environment and physical tasks such as toileting, feeding self, walking can lead to fearfulness, anxiety, doubt, frustration, and guilt.	Imagination and magical thinking develop. Fantasy and fears can be complex around physical and environmental difficulties of treatment. Complex abstract thought about death is still limited.	Temper tantrums and procedural resistance can develop when unable to have control, experiencing inconsistent limits/messages, and changing routines.	Use curiosity to gently understand the child's sense of how her world is ordered. Examples: Ask "How does this work/what does this do?" of common things in the child's environment
School-age (6–11 years)	Disruptions in school, sports, and activities valued by family units can lead to sense of inferiority and guilt/shame.	More concrete understanding of treatment including length, number of treatments, and developing understanding of death.	Frequent aversion to medicine, nutrition, and other differences compared to family members due to sense of unfairness and disruption of normalcy.	Engage children around activities that bring them pleasure and a sense of accomplishment. Ask how things are different now and how they explain what is going on to others. Gently probe fears and worries.
Adolescence (12–18 years)	Inability to find acceptance in peer groups and explore different roles can lead to frustration and confusion. Profound loneliness and isolation can develop without intimate peer relationships.	Abstract reasoning and theoretical concepts of death develop. Concepts learned in one context can be applied to others. Critical thinking, planning, and agency in care are possible.	Risk-taking and nonadherence due to sense of invincibility or active denial. Behavior often for the benefit of social/peer values. May seem less influenced by family preferences or values	Strategies such as "Ask-Tell-Ask," are equally useful with adolescents and adults. Expect and acknowledge that adolescents may vary in how, and to what extent, they wish to engage. Provide privacy for at least some portion of clinical visits.

Adapted with permission from Brand et al. The impact of cancer and its treatment on the growth and development of the pediatric patient. *Curr Pediatr Rev.* 2017;13(1):24–33. doi:10.2174/1573396313666161116094916

directly with key extended family members may reduce the burden on them to remember to inform and interpret complicated concepts and issues. Developing relationships between members of the healthcare team, siblings, and other family members may contribute to the overall coping of the family.

IMPACT OF CANCER AND CANCER TREATMENT ON QUALITY OF LIFE

Quality of life encompasses all facets of life, including physical, emotional, social, and spiritual domains.[62] Children with cancer are at high risk for poor quality of life,[63] and efforts to promote well-being should include all these domains. Important symptoms that result from cancer and its treatment (e.g., pain, nausea/vomiting, insomnia, bodily changes, cognitive dysfunction, and psychological symptoms) all impact quality of life. Changes in daily life that may contribute to social isolation also have enormous implications. Much of the empiric evidence and available interventions focus on the role of physical symptoms. Efforts to promote standardization of symptom detection and management include patient-report symptom tools[64] and consensus- and evidence-based guidelines.[65,66] Interdisciplinary palliative care teams facilitate detection and amelioration of poor quality of life related to physical and psychological suffering, social isolation, or spiritual suffering.[67] Supportive discussion characterized by deeply attentive listening and sensitive questioning may at times be the most powerful intervention for children and families experiencing sudden, progressive, or severe changes to the quality of their lives.

IMPACT OF CHILDHOOD CANCER ON THE CHILD'S FAMILY

The diagnosis and treatment of pediatric cancer stresses the psychosocial functioning of the family, including health-related quality of life and marital adjustment.[68–70] Milestones in the cancer trajectory, including initial diagnosis, relapses, and even the positive step of moving to "off-treatment" status place additional stress on caregivers and family relationships.[70,71]

Intensive treatment schedules frequently remove the child from the rhythms of daily family life[72] because of prolonged hospitalizations or long-distance travel to receive cancer care. In two-parent families, frequently one parent will accompany the child to outpatient appointments or stay with the child in the hospital, while the other parent cares for the siblings, while continuing to work and maintain the household. Posttraumatic stress symptoms have been reported in siblings; fortunately, there is some awareness of these problems among parents and growing awareness among professionals.[73]

Interventions such as dedicated programs for siblings may be a useful preventive approach, while group interventions can be useful[74] to treat symptoms of depression in siblings.

Grandparents may become important caregivers for the child with cancer and siblings and provide support to the parents.[75–77] Families frequently experience financial disruption, including high out-of-pocket medical expenses and loss of income due to missed work and job loss.[78–80] There is profound economic loss and material hardship among families of children with cancer, which is associated with psychological distress[78,81] and reduced marital adjustment. Those with preexisting stressors, such as underemployment, poverty, inadequate transportation, lack of legal protections, caregiver mental illness, or poor family functioning, are in particular need of support.[68] This may take the form of concrete resources, legal advocacy, caregiver or family counseling, and spiritual support. Interdisciplinary palliative care teams may be particularly helpful in eliciting sources of stress and identifying supports within the healthcare system or in the surrounding community.[12] When there are psychologists and psychiatrists with expertise in pediatric psycho-oncology, collaboration between interdisciplinary palliative care teams and these clinicians will ensure optimal comprehensive care.[51,82] Spiritual assessment and support from hospital chaplaincy or their own clergy may be particularly important for some families as the experience of receiving a life-threatening diagnosis may change individuals' sense of the world and how it is ordered.[67,83] If a chaplain is not available, another clinician on the interdisciplinary team may at least open the conversation.

PARTICIPATING IN THE CARE OF CHILDREN WITH CANCER: IMPACT ON CLINICIANS

Pediatric oncology, especially, attracts clinicians who wish to help children and families who are at special risk. Caring for children with cancer and their families can be fulfilling and inspiring. Yet this setting can be both personally and professionally demanding (see also Chapter 12).[84–86] Participating in the care of children with cancer can lead to burnout.[84,87,88] Long-term relationships, incurable diseases, unanticipated complications, suffering, loss, grief, and ethical dilemmas—each characteristic of pediatric oncology practice—increase the risk of clinicians developing burnout.[85] Manifestations of burnout can include disengagement from or depersonalization of needy patients and families, poor communication with patients, increased medical errors, physician job dissatisfaction, guilt, and reduced feelings of accomplishment and work effort.[89–91]

Clinicians caring for children with cancer and their families are also at risk for compassion fatigue, moral distress, and moral injury.[92] These forms of work-associated distress may arise when clinicians feel unable to meet the needs of a child or their family due to barriers that may stem from personal, financial, cultural, institutional, ethical, or other sources. When this perception is repeated or prolonged, the clinician's resources are ultimately depleted, and they may retreat to harmful (or at least unhelpful) coping strategies. Use of education and self-care activities reduces compassion fatigue in inpatient pediatric oncology nurses.

All clinical care providers are at risk including nurses, physicians, social workers, psychologists and other clinicians. Rates of burnout among oncology healthcare professionals are reported to be elevated.[93] Burnout among female physicians has been reported to be higher compared to males in various healthcare settings.[88,94]

Barriers to providing optimal care for families might include suboptimal clinical team dynamics[94] and structural barriers such as excessive workload or work hours.[94–96] Institution level barriers include demands for excessive documentation and order entry requirements caused by the electronic health record which might lead to a higher risk for burnout[97] and lack of institutional support.[87,96]

When clinicians experience these barriers infrequently, their ability to cope is likely to remain intact. However continuous exposure can deplete coping reserves and lead to problematic coping mechanisms. Efforts to reduce these barriers, such as increasing work hour flexibility, lightening the schedule, organizational support, improved team communication, and self-care interventions, all may help to mitigate the risk of burnout.[98] Interdisciplinary palliative care teams frequently possess expertise in facilitating reflection and meaning-making. This expertise can be a support to professionals at risk for burnout due to the stresses associated with caring for children with cancer and their families.[99]

Palliative Care Throughout the Continuum of Childhood Cancer Care Palliative care should be offered throughout the continuum of the child's care beginning at diagnosis through to survivorship care or bereavement care if the child does not survive. Palliative care may be delivered by cancer care teams (primary palliative care) or by specialty palliative care teams. Ideally, all children with cancer would receive primary palliative care from skilled clinicians and some children would receive specialty palliative care. Specialty palliative consultation is particularly appropriate when advanced expertise would enhance the child's quality of life and/or family's experience of their child's interest.

PALLIATIVE CARE NEEDS OF CHILDREN AND FAMILIES AT THE TIME OF DIAGNOSIS

Children and families experience high degrees of distress at the time of diagnosis, particularly around symptoms related to the underlying disease, learning the diagnosis, hearing about cancer treatments and participating in treatment decisions, and trying to make sense of how the diagnosis will affect their lives immediately and in the future.[100,101]

How a family learns that their child has cancer has implications for their subsequent expectations and experiences of their child's care. For many, the period of time between suspecting that their child is very ill and learning that their child has cancer is characterized by repeated medical visits in which the suspicion for cancer slowly increases.[46] In most situations, the patient is referred to the oncology team once cancer is thought to be highly likely. Initial visits, which may include diagnostic disclosure and discussions of treatment recommendations, sometimes referred to as the "Day One talk,"[49] may set the tone for many aspects of the long-term relationship between oncology team members and the patient and their family. However, parents and children may be highly distressed during these conversations.[100] As such, there has been recent focus on the importance of deepening these initial discussions to ensure that each family's hopes, worries, and unique context are elicited to enable family-centered care.[100,102]

Patients and families bring with them as many backgrounds as there are human beings when they come to the "Day One Talk."[49] They may have suspected cancer and feel that they are finally receiving the answers they sought, or the possibility of cancer may be completely unexpected and learning the diagnosis will be akin to "shell shock." They may have experience with friends or family members that may influence their perceptions of cancer.[103] Family members may have backgrounds in the health sciences or hospital services and may have encountered people with cancer in their workplace, as a volunteer, or in their faith communities. In preparation for the "Day One talk," team members may seek advice or insight from the medical record or from clinicians who have already interacted with the family. However, much of this information may not be available. It is important that team members be sensitive and flexible in their approach. During this talk, they must continually assess the family for their understanding of the material, ability to hear and entertain new material, emotional responses, and priorities. Rarely can the team share all the information and provide anticipatory guidance in a single visit—nor is it a realistic goal. "Telling" is never a one-time occurrence: it is a process over time. Clinicians may have to modify their approaches based on the family's cultural, scientific, and cognitive background and abilities. Interdisciplinary participation in discussions during the early treatment period, such as the "Day Two Talk"[102] and the "Day 100 Talk,"[104] amplifies the family's voice in the child's care. Engaging in ongoing assessment and taking a flexible approach are critical to developing successful long-term relationships with the child and family and facilitate their eventual participation in truly shared decision-making.

PROGNOSIS AND HOPE

In disclosing the diagnosis and prognosis, the clinician must begin by learning what the family already knows and then seek permission to proceed.[105] By continually assessing the patient and family's reaction and ability to continue the conversation, the clinician will maximize the likelihood of matching the pace and content of the discussion to the family's needs. Techniques such as assessing understanding, providing succinct information, and then reassessing ("ask-tell-ask") can be very useful.[32] Assessing what information is desired and matching this with what is told can prevent families from becoming overwhelmed by information and demonstrates sensitivity and respect.

With the diagnosis of cancer, families—including some children—may wonder (either silently or aloud) "What does this mean for me/us?" or even more explicitly, "How long does he/she/I have?" Disclosing prognosis may be anxiety-provoking for clinicians because they are concerned that families may become overwhelmed and excessively distressed[42] and lose hope. Multiple studies show that patients and families want to hear prognostic information even if the prognosis is poor.[42,106] Most want as much detail as possible.[107] In the face of the unknown, some people prefer to receive even negative information as a way to reduce uncertainty and anxiety.[108]

There is evidence that receiving more information about prognosis (even when poor) is associated with increased hope.[109] The commitment of the healthcare team to provide information is beneficial and may reduce decisional regret.[48] In a study of parental hope for children with advanced cancer, Kamihara and colleagues found that while the vast majority (88%) of parents recognized their child's poor condition, they still maintained hope for a cure and most (66%) continue to hope for a long life.[110] Prognostic knowledge allows parents to adjust their goals and expectations[111] and may result in prioritizing quality time with their children.[112] For some parents of children with advanced cancer, the act of seeking cancer-directed therapy may become part of the parental role.[113]

OVERVIEW OF CANCER-DIRECTED TREATMENTS

Childhood cancers are treated with chemotherapy, radiation, surgery, immune-based therapies, and/or cellular therapies. The following sections provide an overview of these treatment strategies, as well as of the child and family experiences engendered by them. The child's developmental stage, the body systems affected by the cancer and treatment, the family's previous experiences of cancer, cultural depictions of cancer,[114] and significant stressors[115] all contribute to the patient's and family's experience.

LEUKEMIAS AND LYMPHOMAS

These entities are treated mainly with chemotherapy and sometimes radiation therapy. Treatment durations range from a few months for low-stage Hodgkin lymphoma[116] to 2–3 years for acute lymphoblastic leukemia.[117] Children with leukemia frequently require blood and platelet transfusions throughout the initial months of treatment due to replacement of the healthy blood-forming elements by leukemic cells as well as the myelosuppressive effects of leukemia treatment.[66] Though once universally employed in the treatment of acute lymphoblastic leukemia, radiation therapy is now typically reserved only for patients who have frank central nervous system (CNS) involvement by leukemia at diagnosis. Radiation therapy is still commonly employed in the treatment of pediatric Hodgkin lymphoma. Leukemias with certain high-risk features and relapsed leukemias and lymphomas may be treated with immunotherapies or cellular therapies, such as stem cell transplant and chimeric antigen receptor (CAR) T cells, bispecific antibodies, tumor-specific antibodies, or immune checkpoint inhibitors.[118,119] Treatment of select leukemias, such as chronic myelogenous leukemia and Philadelphia-positive acute lymphoblastic leukemias, utilizes tyrosine kinase inhibitors, which have distinct side-effect profiles.[120] Children with high-risk acute myeloid leukemia, relapsed acute lymphoblastic or myeloid leukemia, or relapsed Hodgkin lymphoma cancer may receive infusions of stem cells as a component of cancer-directed treatment. Stem cell transplantation is a particularly intensive treatment as children typically must undergo "conditioning" with high doses of myeloablative chemotherapy and/or immunosuppressive medications prior to infusion of the cellular product. Whole-body irradiation may be a component of some conditioning regimens.

CENTRAL NERVOUS SYSTEM TUMORS

The concept of "local control" stipulates that the primary mass of cancer cells in the brain and/or spinal cord must be surgically removed and/or irradiated in order to prevent additional growth or, for some CNS tumors, metastatic spread. For some children with brain tumors, an operation may completely remove the cancer and may be the definitive treatment. Radiation therapy is a mainstay of treatment for many CNS tumors. Radiation treatment doses for most common childhood CNS cancers range from 18 Gy to 55 Gy. Radiation therapy is typically delivered in daily fractions of approximately 150–180 cGy. Thus, treatment may require daily visits for a period of a few days up to 6 weeks for the highest total doses. Increasingly, adjuvant (postsurgical or post-radiation) chemotherapy, including high-dose chemotherapy with autologous stem cell rescue or targeted therapies, are also employed in the initial treatment of CNS tumors. Tumors such as medulloblastoma in children younger than 3 years are treated exclusively with high-dose chemotherapy with autologous stem cell rescue due to the devastating neurologic consequences of high doses of radiation to the developing brain and spinal cord.[121] Even among older children, tradeoffs between neurologic function (including long-term cognitive outcomes) and disease control may require complex decision-making on the part of the families and treating clinicians. Thus, expert interprofessional support, such as that available from an interdisciplinary palliative care team, may be particularly helpful to families of children with CNS tumors. Finally, targeted therapies are increasingly important in the treatment of cancers of the brain and spinal cord. Identification of BRAF mutations in low-grade gliomas, which were previously treated with months or years of cytotoxic chemotherapy, is altering the treatment paradigm for this disease, enabling some children to receive oral medications and avoid chemotherapy.

EXTRACRANIAL SOLID TUMORS

As for CNS tumors, treatment for extracranial solid tumors emphasizes "local control" through surgical resection and/or radiation therapy.[122] For some children with extracranial solid tumors, an operation may completely remove the cancer and may be the definitive treatment. Neoadjuvant (pr-surgical or pre-radiation) and/or adjuvant (postsurgical or post-radiation) chemotherapy is also used for many of the most common extracranial solid tumors, even if the cancer is confined to a single location or organ at the time of diagnosis. Osteosarcoma, a malignant tumor of bone, is treated with both neoadjuvant and adjuvant chemotherapy in addition to surgical removal of the tumor.[123] For children and adolescents with bone tumors, local control decisions may involve tradeoffs between the appearance of an intact limb and limb function. These decisions require complex decision-making by families and treating clinicians, and patients and families may particularly benefit from skilled communication that can elicit goals and values to enable the best possible treatment decision. In addition to chemotherapy, surgical resection, radiation, and immunotherapy, children with high-risk neuroblastoma receive high-dose chemotherapy and infusions of autologous stem cells. At the time of this writing, treatment for high-risk neuroblastoma is among the most intensive due to the prolonged nature of treatment (~18 months) and the use of multiple modalities, each with the potential for severe side effects during and after treatment.[124] Finally, as is true for leukemia, lymphomas, and brain and spinal cord tumors, treatment of extracranial solid tumors increasingly includes so-called *targeted therapies* that act on a biochemical pathway important to the growth or survival of the cancerous cells.

GENOMICS, PRECISION MEDICINE, AND TUMOR PROFILING

Profiling the genome and mutations of the tumor is a relatively new field of precision cancer treatment that allows the oncologist to select therapies based on the individual patient's tumor biology.[125] In this way, it is hoped to improve the success of therapy and decrease toxicity by avoiding medications that are unlikely to be successful.[126]

Increasingly, the fields of cancer genomics and so-called *precision medicine* are being incorporated into clinical research studies of children with cancer. The Children's Oncology Group, St. Jude Children's Research Hospital, and other national and international childhood cancer research consortia are studying whether gathering information about the specific genomes and epigenomes of advanced childhood cancers can enable "rationally targeted" treatments.[127] Gathering information about the biology of a cancer arising in individual persons is sometimes referred to as "tumor profiling." This strategy has significantly altered the landscape of adult oncology, where the approach to advanced lung cancer, colon cancer, and breast cancers now incorporates genomic information to help determine recommended treatments.[128–130] In childhood cancer, tumor profiling is contributing to changes in recommended treatments, particularly among cancers viewed as "high risk" or "advanced."[131,132] "Advanced cancer" is a term used to describe cancer that is either metastatic at the time of diagnosis, relapsed, or that progresses during treatment.[133]

In pediatric cancer, leukemia has been the area of the most rapid progression in this field. The Children's Oncology Group (COG)/National Cancer Institute Pediatric Molecular Analysis for Therapy Choice (MATCH) trial opened in 2017 and is still under way. Other, disease-specific trials taking place include profiling mutations in leukemia and lymphoma and newly diagnosed medulloblastoma patients.[126] Other areas of rapid progress are in immune modulation (checkpoint inhibitor) and genetically engineered CAR-T cells. This field is rapidly developing and the value and limitations of this technology are still emerging.

EXPERIENCES OF RECEIVING CANCER THERAPEUTICS

Vignette Continued

During his first two cycles of chemotherapy, Lawrence experiences acute and delayed nausea and vomiting and begins to lose his hair. He meets with Jana, a child life specialist, and Richard, a social worker. He attends a social event where he meets other teens who are getting cancer treatment. The pain that has been awakening him at night begins to ease a bit. Over FaceTime, he meets Michael, a college student who was previously treated for osteosarcoma. Lawrence is impressed with all Michael can do with the rotationplasty. He's also relieved to see that Michael has hair. Listening to Michael talk about his classes and his friends, Lawrence begins to believe that he will get through this.

Lawrence struggles with the decision about his upcoming operation. He talks with a social worker, his coach, friends, and his family. He ultimately decides that he wants the internal metal prosthesis. Diana and Dr. Jensen respect his decision, agreeing that it is his body and that he is old enough to guide this decision. Thinking back to the soccer practice when he collided with his teammate, Lawrence realizes it was his last.

His teammates come to visit him in the hospital while he is recovering from his operation. He begins working with a physical therapist and restarts chemotherapy soon after. Dr. Jensen tells him the operation went very well, and Dr. Wilson, the oncologist, tells him that the cancer responded well to chemotherapy. He continues to struggle with nausea, despite receiving medications for nausea. Dr. Wilson consults with Dr. Hanford, a PPC specialist, to discuss additional pharmacologic and integrative approaches. Dr. Hanford consults and suggests that the interdisciplinary palliative care team meet with Lawrence and Diana. Lawrence expresses interest in acupressure and aromatherapy and reveals that he is not always taking the prescribed antiemetics or the antibiotic intended to prevent *Pneumocystis* pneumonia because he dislikes taking pills. Lawrence, Diana, and Nancy, a nurse on the PPC team, collaborate to design a regimen for Lawrence.

Individual experiences of receiving cancer therapeutics will vary widely and will be influenced by the child's developmental stage, underlying health, comorbidities, the family's history of experiences with illness and healthcare systems, and the child's and family's additional stressors, supports, and strengths. Knowledge of common experiences and side effects will enable the clinician to be most helpful to a child or family experiencing symptom distress or poor quality of life. The following sections provide an introduction to facets of cancer care most likely to have a significant impact on quality of life.

CENTRAL VENOUS ACCESS DEVICES

Children receiving treatment for cancer typically require central venous access, either an implanted port or a central venous catheter that communicates with the external environment.[66] For children with implanted ports, the port is accessed via a Huber needle that penetrates the skin and enters the subcutaneous reservoir that connects to the internal central venous catheter. For many families, particularly those whose children are toddlers, acclimating to Huber needle placement can be challenging. Children frequently develop procedural anxiety around placement of the Huber needle. Integrative strategies such as preparatory medical play distraction and self-hypnosis may reduce distress around Huber needle placement.[134] Topical anesthetics may reduce the physical discomfort associated with the Huber needle penetrating the skin.

Children who require more than one lumen of central venous access may have a Hickman or Broviac central venous line (CVL) placed surgically. Others may have a nonsurgical peripherally inserted central catheter (PICC). Both CVLs and PICCs require instillation of anticoagulants at regular intervals to maintain patency of the lumens. Families are frequently expected to learn to perform this "line care," as well as learn how to prevent microbial contamination of the CVL/PICC. Line care contributes to the burden of medical caregiving families face during the period of active treatment for childhood cancer.[135]

CYTOTOXIC CHEMOTHERAPY

CHEMOTHERAPY-INDUCED NAUSEA AND VOMITING

Children who receive cytotoxic chemotherapy are at risk for experiencing chemotherapy-induced nausea and vomiting (CINV). Emetogenicity of chemotherapeutics and chemotherapeutic combinations vary widely. The chemoreceptor trigger zone, an area of the medulla characterized by serotonergic ($5HT_3$), dopaminergic (DA_2), and neurokinin (NK_1) receptors, receives afferent input from the gut and communicates with the vomiting center. See Chapter 25 for a more in-depth discussion of the neurophysiology of vomiting. The Children's Oncology Group, a consortium of pediatric cancer centers largely based in North America, has published evidence-based guidelines for use of pharmacologic antiemetics and integrative strategies to reduce acute, delayed, refractory, and anticipatory CINV.[65,66] In the current era, the $5HT_3$ class of antiemetics, of which ondansetron is a prototypical agent, is a mainstay of pharmacologic treatment for acute CINV. Dexamethasone is also highly effective, particularly in regimens that contain anthracyclines and for prevention of delayed CINV such as that classically associated with platinum compounds.[66] Dexamethasone may be contraindicated in certain populations, such as those with lymphoid malignancies and those where CNS penetration of chemotherapy is of particular concern.[66] Aprepitant, an agent that prevents signaling through NK_1 receptors, is increasingly utilized in children receiving highly emetogenic chemotherapy but alters blood concentrations of common chemotherapeutic agents due to its interaction with the cytochrome p450 isoforms 3A4 and 2C9.[136,137] Olanzapine is also increasingly used for enhanced control of acute CINV in children, though sedative effects may be dose-limiting.[138,139] Multiagent antiemetic regimens that incorporate multiple mechanisms of action are associated with enhanced prevention of CINV, and prevention of acute CINV is associated with prevention of delayed CINV.[140] Thus, pharmacologic antiemetic regimens should be constructed with attention to the child's overall treatment plan, active symptoms, and with the goal of minimizing bothersome side effects. Integrative therapies such as aromatherapy and acupressure may be helpful for preventing and treating CINV, and specialty palliative care teams are encouraged to master these strategies and/or to serve as liaisons to hospital- or community-based practitioners.[134]

ALOPECIA

Alopecia is a common, highly visible, and distressing side-effect of many cytotoxic chemotherapies and cranial radiation.[141,142] Alopecia is the sign that is perhaps most culturally symbolic of cancer and cancer treatment. Prevention of alopecia has been explored through cooling the skin during chemotherapy administration.[143] This strategy is not commonly integrated into current pediatric oncology practice but may be considered for patients for whom alopecia is particularly distressing. Promotion of a positive self-image among children, adolescents, and young adults experiencing alopecia may take the form of adornment through use of wigs, hats, headscarves, makeup, and/or jewelry. Family caregivers of children with cancer and children themselves may benefit from supportive listening to enable them to voice feelings of overall loss and fear related to hair loss.

MYELOSUPPRESSION

Consequences of myelosuppression include fatigue and pallor from anemia, easy bruising and abnormal bleeding from thrombocytopenia, and mucosal ulceration and risk from infection from granulocytopenia. Although anemia and abnormal bleeding are typically managed with transfusions of erythrocytes and platelets, mucosal ulceration and infection present much greater challenges. Strategies under study to prevent mucosal ulceration include light therapy. Treatment of the pain associated with mucosal ulceration (mucositis) may include use of topical anesthetics and systemic analgesics including acetaminophen and opioid medications. If mucosal ulceration interferes with the provision of oral medications, the intravenous route is preferred. Integrative strategies such as self-hypnosis, guided imagery, and Reiki may all be useful in mitigating the pain of mucositis and may have the added benefit of promoting a sense of empowerment among children and families since some of these strategies can be learned and subsequently used without requiring the input of a healthcare professional.[144] The risk of infection is mitigated in part through cleansing the body and teeth regularly, sterilizing the point of entry of CVLs and implanted ports prior to use, prophylactic antibiotics, and, in some cases, use of granulocyte colony-stimulating factors to reduce the duration of neutropenia. Of note, lifestyle and behavioral recommendations for individuals with myelosuppression vary widely, and patients and families may receive conflicting information about what to eat, how to dress (e.g., whether to don a mask), whether school attendance is permitted, and whether intimate contact such as sexual intercourse should be avoided. These recommendations may have profound impacts on patients' and families' experience of the illness and quality of life. Interdisciplinary palliative care teams may be ideally positioned to elicit what is most important to the patient and family, identify the rationale for the recommendation or restriction, and facilitate negotiation toward shared understanding on how to proceed.

UNIQUE SYMPTOMS AND SIDE-EFFECTS ASSOCIATED WITH INDIVIDUAL CHEMOTHERAPEUTIC AGENTS

Several commonly used chemotherapeutic medications have distinct side effects that require preventive medication administration and familiarity with the phenomenon. Examples of these include irinotecan-associated diarrhea, cutaneous reactions to tyrosine kinase inhibitors (e.g., sorafenib), and hemorrhagic cystitis associated with cyclophosphamide administration.[66] While pediatric oncologists and pediatric oncology nurses are typically highly knowledgeable about these side effects and their prevention, identification, and treatment, interdisciplinary palliative care teams should also develop familiarity with these symptoms and side effects to enable collaborative symptom management efforts.

RADIATION THERAPY

Though treatment sessions are typically brief, radiation therapy requires precise positioning to ensure that the dose is delivered to the intended body tissues. For young children, this may require sedation, which carries with it the burden of refraining from eating and drinking in the hours before radiation. In addition to the experience of traveling to and from the treatment center and remaining still for treatments, children receiving radiation frequently experience fatigue and may experience acute symptoms resulting from damage to healthy tissue in the radiation field, such as radiation-induced dermatitis, esophagitis, pneumonitis, or colitis. If hematopoietic marrow is in the radiation field, children may experience myelosuppression requiring transfusions. Children who receive chemotherapy after receiving radiation therapy may experience an inflammatory phenomenon known as "radiation recall," which frequently manifests as dermatitis in the skin overlying previously irradiated areas. Radiation recall reactions can present in other tissues as well, including the lungs, gastrointestinal tract, and muscles.

STEM CELL TRANSPLANTATION, IMMUNOTHERAPIES, AND CELLULAR THERAPIES

The experience of stem cell transplantation is marked by prolonged hospitalization and relative isolation as well as high symptom burdens from mucositis, fevers, and other cutaneous and gastrointestinal symptoms.[66] Interprofessional palliative care consultation may be particularly helpful for patients who are undergoing stem cell transplantation.

Complications of immune-based therapies include *cytokine release syndrome*, which has been well-characterized in recipients of CAR-T cell therapy and can produce severe neurologic symptoms.[145] Aberrant inflammation such as pneumonitis, hepatitis, and hypophysitis has been characterized in patients receiving immune checkpoint inhibitors such as the anti-programmed death-1 agents nivolumab and pembrolizumab and the anti-cytotoxic T-lymphocyte-associated protein 4 (anti-CTLA 4) agent ipilimumab. As these and other novel, immune-based treatments become more common in the treatment of pediatric cancers, knowledge of immune-related complications will be important for members of interdisciplinary palliative care teams.

TARGETED THERAPIES

Use of targeted therapies is likely to increase substantially over the next 5–10 years, especially as tumor profiling becomes more common.[126] Knowledge of the unique symptom profiles associated with each of these agents will become increasingly important to promote quality of life among children receiving these treatments. Rash is a particularly common side effect of many tyrosine kinase inhibitors, the most common class of targeted therapies used today in treating childhood cancers.[1–6]

SURGERY

Undergoing surgery for cancer may lead to marked, permanent body changes. For example, treatment of bone tumors may require either amputation of a limb or replacement of the limb with an internal prosthesis or allograft that renders the limb less functional.[147] Treatment of Wilms tumor typically requires complete removal of a kidney.[131,148] As noted earlier, operative management of CNS tumors may lead to compromised neurologic function. In the immediate postoperative period, acute pain is common and may require systemic and regional analgesic strategies. Amputation may lead to phantom limb pain, which may require multiple treatment modalities, such as pharmacologic treatments for neuropathic pain and integrative strategies such as mirror therapy.[149–152] Diagnosing and managing phantom limb pain may be particularly challenging in younger children, who may not be able to express their symptoms verbally. All children who undergo operations to treat cancer may be at risk for dysesthesia at the site of surgical incision. Careful assessment and provision of multimodal strategies, including medical play, Reiki, and healing touch or massage may be helpful to alleviate distress associated with undergoing a surgical operation.[153–155]

SPECIAL CONSIDERATIONS FOR CHILDREN WITH ADVANCED CANCER AND RARE CANCERS

While cancers are inherently life-threatening entities, advanced cancer tends to be associated with much higher risks of death.[156] An important role for interdisciplinary PPC teams is to facilitate communication that enables true understanding among the child with advanced cancer, the parent(s) or other important family figures in the child's life, and the treating clinicians.[12] How families approach their child's medical care in these circumstances will be shaped in part by what is communicated to them and in part by their own appraisal of the possibilities and tradeoffs.[113] Importantly, parents and children may hold many hopes and expectations that may reflect complicated prognostic understanding: a hope for a long life and yet an expectation that death from progressive cancer is near.[157] Increasingly, the fields of pediatric oncology and PPC recognize that hopes for a long, healthy life and expectations for death from progressive cancer may coexist. Engaging in shared decision-making requires eliciting these frames of reference and making recommendations that reflect what is most important to the child and family.[110,157]

For children facing advanced cancer and those with rare cancers, there may be no agreed upon standard treatment. In this setting, it is increasingly common for families to consider traveling to receive treatment at a highly specialized center that offers experimental treatments.[113] Experimental treatments are sometimes referred to as "Phase I" or "Phase II" clinical trials.[118] Phase I clinical trials are typically dose-finding studies in small numbers of individuals. The safety of the treatment under study may not be known, or there may be preliminary information about the safety of the treatment in adults.[158] Phase II clinical trials are slightly larger studies that are typically studying the apparent effect of the treatment as well as evaluating side effects of the treatment. Several groups have studied decision-making around participation in Phase I trials[159–161] and tumor profiling studies.[162,163] Among children enrolling in Phase I oncology clinical trials, median life expectancy is frequently 6 months or fewer.[164–166] As such, children enrolled on early-phase clinical trials are likely to be at particular risk for symptom distress related to progressive cancer and may benefit from discussions that allow for sharing of illness understanding, goals, and values. Collaboration between early therapeutics programs and interdisciplinary PPC teams can increase the likelihood of providing "total care" for children, particularly if trial participation requires travel away from the child's home and community. Interdisciplinary PPC teams may be able to engage the child and family in discussions of what may lie ahead and provide anticipatory guidance based on discussions of the family's goals and values.[167] Involvement in a Phase I trial should not preclude involvement with and care by palliative care clinicians. Palliative care clinicians/teams can manage symptoms and address distress felt by the child and the family.[113,168,169] There is evolving evidence that involvement in Phase I trials may be associated with delayed utilization of palliative care.[170] At the same time, interdisciplinary PPC teams may enhance the care of children with advanced cancer through collaboration with experimental therapeutics programs.[9,12,168] As such palliative care professionals should redouble their efforts to be involved at this stage in the disease care continuum.

PALLIATIVE CARE AT END OF LIFE

Palliative care at end of life should be available to all children with cancer, but this goal has not yet been achieved in the United States. Certain areas of the United States and larger hospitals are more likely to provide palliative care.[171,172] Multiple professional organizations support an interdisciplinary approach to care for children at end of life that ensures attention to physical, psychosocial, and spiritual distress.[17,173]

Acknowledging that a child is nearing the end of his or her life may be very difficult for parents, clinicians who may have cared for the child for prolonged periods, and for the children themselves.[167,174] If an interdisciplinary PPC team and/or primary palliative care delivered by an interdisciplinary pediatric oncology team has been a routine part of the care of the patient from diagnosis, with careful attention to symptom management and communication through all phases of the illness, then there is less likely to be a sense that palliative care stands in conflict with disease-directed care.[14,102] However, lack of provision of primary or specialty palliative care in early stages of cancer care means there are many patients for whom palliative care is introduced only near end of life.[175,176] Concurrent palliative care and disease-directed care is sometimes conceptualized as "blended" care. The role of palliative care may become more prominent as issues such as pain, existential distress, and consideration of the child's legacy emerge more near the end of life. Ideally, open communication enables recognition that goals and values may evolve in step with changes in the child's health.[167,177–179]

In the United States, "hospice" typically refers to an insurance benefit, and hospice services are typically delivered in the home of the seriously ill individual, whether that individual is an adult or a child. Hospice houses do exist in North America, though the number of free-standing children's hospice houses is small.[180] For children and young adults with serious illness, laws vary at the state level with regard to whether concurrent disease-directed care and hospice benefits can be received.[181] Many children may live in communities where access to hospice services with pediatric expertise is limited.[182] Hospice benefits also typically exclude certain treatments, such as the transfusion of blood products.[183] This may have implications for children with advanced cancer, and decision-making around the location of end-of-life care and whether to involve hospice services should be individualized to promote the child's comfort and the family's peace of mind and to enable care provision by clinicians with the skills to meet the child's and family's needs.[180]

ADDRESSING SYMPTOMS AMONG CHILDREN WITH CANCER AT END OF LIFE

Children with cancer at end of life are at risk for distress from symptoms related to progressive cancer, such as bone pain, bowel obstruction, paralysis, dyspnea, and hemoptysis from metastatic lesions to the skeleton, abdomen, spinal cord, and chest.[184] Poly-symptomatology is common.[15,184] Bone pain is frequently encountered in children with metastatic cancer. Treatments for bone pain from metastatic disease include dexamethasone, hypofractionated radiation therapy, systemic opioids, nonsteroidal anti-inflammatory drugs, regional analgesia, and intravenous bisphosphonates.[185,186] Observable and predictably distressing end-of-life symptoms include altered breathing and handling of secretions, loss of neurologic function, and bleeding.[15,184,187,188] Ideally, the approach to assessing and treating symptom distress in children at the end of their lives is holistic, incorporating both the best evidence for what helps as well as child and family preferences. Relevant preferences might include the location of care, the route by which a medication is administered, or the ability to engage in a treasured activity. For example, a celiac plexus block for pain arising from tumor infiltration into the liver or other upper abdominal viscera may enable a child to be relatively comfortable while reducing the need for systemic opioids that may be contributing to unwanted fatigue.[186] However, this may not be the optimal approach for a child whose family prefers not to travel to a tertiary care center that offers regional analgesia/anesthesia. Integrative treatments and attention to the child's and family's environment may be particularly helpful at end of life. Beyond treating symptom distress as it arises, anticipatory guidance to the child and family about the end-of-life period[189] and efforts to honor the child's life and role in the family and community[11] are key components of palliative care. See Table 33.2 for descriptions of end-of-life symptoms and multimodal approaches to addressing symptom distress.

Facilitating a comfortable death for children with cancer has been identified as an important measure of quality care.[8,173,188] This planning can include development of specific symptom management plans, contingency plans if new or severe symptoms develop, indications for return to hospital or escalation of care, availability of other resources that may be necessary later in the process of dying, etc. These plans should be developed in partnership with all involved participants, including the family and the patient, and should be continually updated. Age-appropriate involvement by the ill child and siblings is beneficial to both patient and family.[190–192] Discussions with ill children or siblings might incorporate children's books that introduce death and dying.[193]

TABLE 33.2 Addressing symptoms[a] at end-of-life among children, adolescents and young adults with advanced cancer[b]

SYMPTOM	CONTEXTUAL CONSIDERATIONS	MEDICATIONS AND PROCEDURAL TREATMENTS	INTEGRATIVE THERAPIES AND ENVIRONMENTAL ADAPTATIONS
Anorexia and cachexia	Anorexia may be adaptive as death nears—approach to this should be guided by whether the child appears distressed by lack of appetite; assessment includes appraisal and treatment of any contributory nausea	Promotility agents such as cyproheptadine may enhance appetite if this is desired Cannabinoids may enhance appetite	Aromatherapy, acupressure, healing touch (particularly if nausea is contributing to anorexia) Tastes or sips of food may still be pleasing to the child and family, even as appetite wanes; consider eliminating dietary restrictions, reduce portions sizes and more frequent meals, avoid undesirable food odors Anticipatory guidance that feeling less hungry is part of the dying process
Anxiety	Source informs approach to treatment; e.g., anxiety due to dyspnea or unrelieved pain versus anxiety related to leaving behind loved ones; consider other contributions, e.g. sleep disturbance	Serotonin reuptake inhibitors are mainstay medications and should be started early to allow for sufficient benefit If anxiety is predominantly related to dyspnea and/or pain, target dyspnea and pain Cannabinoids may enhance sleep Benzodiazepines such as lorazepam or clonazepam should be avoided though may be helpful near end of life	Aromatherapy, acupressure, healing touch, massage therapy, music therapy, animal-assisted therapy, distraction, legacy work Younger children: play therapy, art therapy, storytelling Older children and adolescents: talk therapy, writing, bibliotherapy, self-hypnosis; directed therapy (e.g., dignity therapy) Family therapy may be particularly successful at treating anxiety related to existential distress Changes to room lighting, sound level, and the number of clinical and family visitors may reduce generalized anxiety To minimize sleep disturbance, maintain pattern of day and night
Bleeding	• Care location, source of bleeding, rapidity/chronicity of bleeding and degree of distress influence management • Airway bleeding, especially massive hemoptysis, can be particularly scary to experience and witness; developing plans for how to appraise and address bleeding before it begins is advised to facilitate timely response and minimize patient, family, and staff distress	• Risks and benefits of blood products, such as platelets, packed red cells, and fresh frozen plasma, should be weighed carefully. Ideally, recommendations for or against blood products are grounded in an understanding of the child's overall clinical condition and the family's goals and priorities Mucosal bleeding: • Antifibrinolytic agents (e.g., aminocaproic acid, tranexamic acid) Airway bleeding: • For hemoptysis, interventional strategies such as bronchial artery embolization may be helpful in select cases • Radiation therapy may reduce the likelihood of recurrent hemoptysis • Suctioning may be indicated to relieve upper airway obstruction by blood, particularly if the child is sputtering • Palliative sedation (see also Chapter 27) may be indicated to relieve distress in the setting of large volume, rapid arterial bleeding Intracranial bleeding: • Surgical interventions such as craniectomy may be considered. Ideally, recommendations for or against surgical intervention are grounded in an understanding of the child's overall clinical condition and the family's goals and priorities • Systemic opioids and benzodiazepines to reduce agitation and treat pain	Because bleeding can be highly anxiety-provoking, integrative treatments for anxiety may be indicated (see above) If hemorrhage or bleeding are anticipated, choosing dark bed sheets, pillowcases, and clothing before significant bleeding occurs may reduce visibility of blood; keeping dark towels close at hand allows for rapid response to the bleeding, which may reduce the distress of loved ones looking on

(*continued*)

TABLE 33.2 Continued

SYMPTOM	CONTEXTUAL CONSIDERATIONS	MEDICATIONS AND PROCEDURAL TREATMENTS	INTEGRATIVE THERAPIES AND ENVIRONMENTAL ADAPTATIONS
Bone pain	Types and severity of pain experienced varies. Consideration of the mechanism of pain is helpful throughout the illness trajectory, including at end-of-life. See Chapter 23 for discussion of treating other forms of pain (e.g., neuropathic pain) Measure pain as part of pain assessment: self-report, behavioral/physiologic observation measures, proxy (caregiver) report	Reducing tumor-associated osteolysis: • Hypofractionated radiation therapy to metastatic bony sites • Bisphosphonates (intravenous) Analgesia: • Dexamethasone (oral or intravenous) • Systemic opioids (oral or intravenous, including patient-controlled analgesic setups) • Nonsteroidal anti-inflammatory drugs (oral or intravenous) • If localized bony pain, regional analgesia/anesthesia may be indicated (e.g., epidural or intrathecal catheter-directed treatment)	Aromatherapy, acupressure, healing touch, guided imagery Older children and adolescents: self-hypnosis
Bowel obstruction	Bowel obstruction may not mean that a child must cease eating and drinking; careful attention to the child's and family's questions around food and drink will assist in making a recommendation that maximizes the child's comfort	• Nasogastric sump to decompress the abdomen • Systemic opioids (to treat pain and reduce peristalsis) • Octreotide (subcutaneous or intravenous infusion) • Dexamethasone (reduce tumoral edema, which may decrease degree of obstruction, and antiemetic) • Consider regional analgesia/ anesthesia	Careful positioning of the child may facilitate comfort, particularly if there is abdominal distention
Delirium/ Agitation	• Address contributory symptoms such as dyspnea and pain • Consider the role of polypharmacy	• Haloperidol (oral, subcutaneous, rectal, intravenous, or sublingual) • Phenobarbital (oral, subcutaneous, or intravenous) • Trial of medication omission if polypharmacy suspected	Provide consistent cues for day and night Orient child/adolescent to features of the environments, such as calendars, clocks, toys/ games and photographs or wall artwork Minimize noise and light at night. Organize care to minimize disruption to sleep Promote relaxation through massage and music therapy Talk to the child prior to all care activities narrating what is happening and why using developmentally tailored language and familiar terms Consider need for augmented communication strategies, such as through picture boards
Dyspnea/ Air hunger	There are many respiratory symptoms the child might experience Dyspnea is very common in children with advanced cancer and may be due to: • Erosion of pulmonary parenchyma or airways by metastatic cancer leading to hemorrhage • Airway obstruction directly by metastatic cancer, indirectly due to neurologic injury, or due to upper airway edema, mucus, or salivary secretions • Pleural effusion or hemothorax compressing the lung and impairing gas exchange • Pneumonitis related to radiation treatment or immunotherapies • Tension pneumothorax	• Systemic opioids with rapid titration (see Chapter 27) • Intravenous or intranasal midazolam may relieve agitation related to air hunger • Procedures that evacuate liquid or air from the airway or thorax (see also "airway bleeding," above). Ideally, recommendations for or against procedures are grounded in an understanding of the child's overall clinical condition and the family's goals and priorities • oral suctioning • thoracentesis • thoracostomy • needle thoracostomy (for tension pneumothorax)	Guided imagery Placement of a fan gently blowing air onto the face

TABLE 33.2 Continued

SYMPTOM	CONTEXTUAL CONSIDERATIONS	MEDICATIONS AND PROCEDURAL TREATMENTS	INTEGRATIVE THERAPIES AND ENVIRONMENTAL ADAPTATIONS
Seizures	Seizures may result from disruption of the brain parenchyma by cancer or from metabolic derangements due to organ dysfunction	Prophylaxis: • Long-acting benzodiazepines (e.g., clonazepam) Rapid treatment for active seizures: • Benzodiazepines (oral, rectal, or intranasal route) • Barbiturates, especially phenobarbital	Position child for comfort, using positioning aids; if concern for overstimulation triggering seizures, consider ways to reduce over-handling of the child Music therapy, massage therapy
Spinal cord compression	Progressive loss of function may result from compression/ infiltration of the spinal cord by metastatic tumor	If early presentation, surgery presents the best option to regain function Slowing the process: • Hypofractionated radiation therapy • Dexamethasone (oral or intravenous) Analgesia: • Dexamethasone (oral or intravenous) • Systemic opioids (oral or intravenous) • Nonsteroidal anti-inflammatory drugs (oral or intravenous) Facilitating elimination in setting of altered bowel and bladder function: • Urinary catheterization • Diapering, laxatives versus tolerance of constipation	• Routine skin assessment • Specialized mattresses and careful rotation of the child who has reduced mobility protect against skin and soft tissue injury

[a] Other symptoms might include nausea and vomiting (Chapter 25); difficulty urinating (Chapter 27); constipation or diarrhea (Chapter 25); itching; headache (Chapter 19); lack of energy, drowsiness, or fatigue; (Chapter 21); irritability (Chapter 19); difficulty sleeping (Chapter 30); sadness and worry (Chapter 18, Chapter 27).

[b] See also Pediatric Palliative Care Approach to Pain and Symptom Management, available from https://pinkbook.dfci.org/assets/docs/blueBook.pdf, revised May 2020

Conversation guides such as "Voicing My Choices," which is specifically targeted to adolescents and young adults, can be very useful to assist these discussions.[194] Adolescents with cancer and children younger than 5 years tend to receive more intensive care than school-aged children with cancer near end of life, and the reasons for this are likely complex.[171] Chronically ill adolescents are strongly supportive of being part of their own end-of-life decision-making.[195] End-of-life planning aids, such as videos or questionnaires, and involvement by palliative care services have been shown to be helpful and useful to adolescents with cancer and may decrease the use of high-intensity interventions at end of life,[25,196,197] though adolescents may be more interested in advance care planning discussions to engage on how they would like to be treated and remembered, rather than focusing heavily on medical decision-making.[198]

Bereaved parents advocate that children with cancer should continue to receive the care they received prior to the end-of-life phase and maintain long-term relationships with healthcare providers that have developed over time. Abandonment by well-known healthcare providers is a common concern voiced by families.[159] When a child dies, the surviving parents and siblings have ongoing needs.[26,192,199,200] Members of an interdisciplinary palliative care team or pediatric oncology team who maintain contact with bereaved families can provide important guidance. Useful programmatic interventions include an annual "Day of Remembrance," referral to bereavement programs and community agencies for counseling or psychotherapy, participation in family support groups, and regular follow-up telephone calls from the healthcare team.[201–204] Refer to Chapter 15.

LOCATION OF DEATH

Where a child dies may be influenced by many factors. More than a third of the children who die of cancer die in a hospital.[205–207] When death is anticipated, many children and families prefer death to occur at home, though clinicians are more likely than parents to report that home is the preferred location for a child's death.[180] However, beyond the actual location of death, what may be most important is engaging the family in considering the circumstances of their child's death.[208] There are many factors that are associated with death in the hospital. In addition to the adolescent age group, being of Hispanic ethnicity or "other race," living in a low-income neighborhood, being female, having public insurance, and living farther than 5 miles from a specialty center are predictive of death in hospital.[205] If an interdisciplinary PPC team is involved, rates of hospital and ICU admission at the time of death are lower and end-of-life care is less intensive.[25]

Palliative care involvement should be planned well in advance of expected death. When palliative care teams are involved more than 1 month before death, the likelihood of hospital admission, ICU admission, and high-intensity technology involvement in the dying process is reduced by up to fivefold.[209] When a home death is feasible and consistent with the family's goals and values, the healthcare team may turn to the specialty palliative care team and community home care/hospice service that would make it possible for families to care for their dying child at home. This may allow for the family's control of their environment, encourage more sibling participation, and facilitate responsiveness to the needs of the extended family.

Whether a child's location of death is anticipated to be at home or in a clinical setting, education is required for the family (and for less experienced professional caregivers) about what to expect: changes in clinical condition; symptoms such as air hunger, anxiety, or dehydration; and appropriate management and use of appropriate resources, medications, and devices.[210] Siblings should be asked if they wish to be included in the patient's end-of-life care and allowed to participate at a developmentally appropriate level. At this point, gently providing an outline of the issues involved in declaring death, autopsy options and processes, selecting a funeral home, and planning arrangements should be part of the care plan. A written plan such as a Physicians Order for Life-Sustaining Treatment (POLST) form that delineates the content of advance care planning discussions can be helpful, particularly if a child's anticipated location of death is at home and emergency response personnel may be involved.

Families' wishes and clinicians' recommendations may be dynamic, particularly in the setting of fluctuating symptoms and family stressors. As such, children may spend time at home and in a hospital during the end-of-life period.[180,211] Indications for hospitalization could include refractory or rapidly escalating symptoms, complicated treatment regimens, or need for respite.[212] If the patient is admitted to die in hospital, consideration about any intervention should be concordant with the goals of care. These might include physical exams, routine blood work, and routine vital signs. However, recommendations should be guided by an understanding of the role these activities hold in the life of the child and the family. While vital signs may be bothersome for one child, for another they may form part of a reassuring routine. Visitation policies should aim to promote contact with important loved ones, including a favorite pet when possible. When the child dies, time should be allowed for friends and family to pay their respects and be with the child's body. Clinicians should be available to explain and assist the family throughout the period of active dying. Rituals of preparing the body may be performed by the hospital staff or in collaboration with the family members, as preferred by the family.

DIFFERENCES VERSUS DISPARITIES IN PATTERNS OF END-OF-LIFE CARE

As discussed in the "location of death" section of this chapter, there are socioeconomic and geographic variations in patterns of palliative and end-of-life care experienced by children with cancer. An important ongoing area of research seeks to understand when differences are due to disparities—namely, when care received is not consistent with care desired and when this care is systematically delivered to certain groups of people.[213] Where differences do represent disparities, there are several hypothesized mechanisms by which such disparities may arise. As death approaches, admissions may occur in nonspecialty centers, possibly due to geographic distance to the specialty center.[172] Other factors found to influence the intensity of care (defined as cardiopulmonary resuscitation [CPR], intubation, ICU admission, or hemodialysis) within 30 days of dying include living closer to the hospital, being an underrepresented minority, and receiving care in a nonspecialty center.[171]

Kaye et al. found that African American children with cancer were more likely to receive CPR at the end of life compared to white children, though the reasons for this are unclear.[214] Though this was a single site study, African American children may be more likely to receive care at institutions that provide higher intensity care at the end of life, as has been demonstrated for adults.[215] Observed differences may also be attributable to patient/parent preferences or systematic differences in communication.[216,217] Further investigation is needed to determine to what degree observed patterns of end-of-life care reflect differences versus disparities.[217,218] Hospital-level interventions as well as greater efforts to enhance communication may promote goal-concordant care and mitigate existing care disparities.[172,219,220]

PALLIATIVE CARE DURING SURVIVORSHIP

Vignette Continued

Lawrence runs into Nancy, the PPC nurse, in the hall at the children's hospital. He is 19 years old. He finished his treatment 3 years ago and is now attending community college. He is there for a survivorship visit, including scans of his right leg and lungs, an echocardiogram, and lab work. He confesses to Nancy that although he is glad to see her, these visits fill him with anxiety and remind him of his treatment, which he describes as "a very rough time" in his life. Lawrence thanks Nancy for helping him through his treatment. His college coursework is going fairly well. He notes that he has started to have trouble hearing people when there is a great deal of background noise and is guessing his hearing test today is going to be abnormal. He brightens when he talks about his girlfriend and his new car.

A few months later, Nancy attends a talk about long-term health concerns of adults treated for cancer as children and reaches out to a colleague who works in the outpatient palliative care practice. She learns that there is no formal relationship between the adult outpatient palliative care practice and the childhood cancer survivorship clinic. Since the childhood cancer survivorship clinic frequently sees patients well into adulthood, Nancy suggests to the survivorship clinic director that they form a connection with the adult palliative care practice.

Children and adults who have received treatment for cancer are frequently referred to as "survivors."[221] This term's connections to such phrases as "only the strong survive" can contribute to notions that those who die from cancer or adverse effects of treatment are somehow weak.[222] However, the term is firmly rooted in the lexicon of childhood cancer and has been important for raising awareness that "late effects" of childhood cancer are common and require ongoing care from clinicians with expertise in the special health concerns that may arise.[223] Long-term psychological and physical late effects of childhood cancer and its treatment are increasingly known as the population of childhood cancer survivors increases and as some survivors enter older adulthood.[221,224–227] Though adults who were treated for childhood cancer are resilient, chronic conditions are common.[228] Though studies of long-term survivors reflect risks of previous treatment paradigms, issues experienced by survivors include higher rates of risk behaviors, such as smoking, than age-matched peers, psychological distress, financial hardship, and subfertility or infertility.[37,38,229–234] Adults who received cranial radiation as a component of childhood leukemia treatment are less likely to be employed, are employed in lower status occupations than siblings, and are less likely to be married,[226,235,236] while adults treated for extremity sarcomas have chronic orthopedic needs but were equally likely to be married and employed as their peers.[237] The transition from active treatment to survivorship and the transition from pediatric to adult care are areas of research. Adolescent and young adult cancer survivors have been reported to have poor knowledge of their risk of late effects.[238] Overall health may be diminished by poorly controlled physical, emotional, and/or spiritual distress experienced by the patient and family at any stage in the evolution of the illness.[14,235,236,239] Early engagement by palliative care clinicians and research on these topics are important to identify potential benefits of palliative care and high-impact interventions that could improve the quality of life for these patients and families immediately and long-term.

CURRENT AND FUTURE RESEARCH

Since the early 2000s, pediatric palliative oncology research has grown dramatically. As outlined by Rosenberg and Wolfe,[240] the first decade of research focused on the end-of-life experience of children and their families, highlighting the extraordinary symptom burden and the need for bereavement services after the death of the child. Research during this time developed tools to measure symptoms and quality of life in children with cancer[64,241,242] and identified obstacles to communication about prognosis[106] and goals and tradeoffs that parents considered when making decisions about care at the end of life.[113] In the past 10 years, areas of research have expanded, moving from a focus on the end-of-life period to the whole disease trajectory,[22] broadening symptom burden to include emotional functioning and quality of life[243] and investigating the impact of cancer on the entire family.[81,244] Household material hardship has emerged as an important consequence of childhood cancer care.[80,245] In addition, there has been increasing focus on potential disparities in access to PPC[171] and differences in end-of-life care and outcomes experienced by persons who belong to groups that have been subject to structural discrimination[214] as well as the role of PPC within the global oncology community.[246] Finally, interventions have been developed and tested within pediatric palliative oncology.[240]

As we look toward the next decade of pediatric palliative oncology research, a number of investigative priorities have emerged, all of which build on the important work conducted over the past 20 years. To decrease the suffering of seriously ill children and their families, it is imperative that we first be able to measure and track symptoms over time. This will require longitudinal studies incorporating measures that span the pediatric age spectrum and allow for both child and parent report.[247] The second step to improving symptom management and decreasing suffering is the continued development and testing of interventions that are readily amenable to implementation within clinical practice.[248] Finally, work to enhance advance care planning, decision-making, and systems of care must continue. As PPC research continues to grow, it is important to acknowledge the challenges inherent in designing and producing high-quality research within this area. A recent report from the Pediatric Palliative Care Research Network State of the Science Workshop highlighted five common challenges: small and heterogeneous populations; interdynamic interactions between children, their family members, and the disease process over time; lack of consistent measurement instruments; workforce and infrastructure limitations and the presumed burden of palliative care research on participants.[248] The next phase of research must tackle these challenges through development and refinement of additional clinically meaningful measures, use of innovative methodologies,[247] and the leveraging of research cooperatives.

AUTHORS' NOTE

A note on authorship: Dr. McCarthy and Dr. Pyke-Grimm contributed equally to the chapter and share first authorship. Dr. Feraco is the third and senior co-author. Kimberly A. Pyke-Grimm received partial funding from the Stanford Nurse Alumnae during her Postdoctoral Fellowship in Palliative Care, which occurred during the chapter development.

REFERENCES

1. Siegel RL, Miller KD, Jemal A. Cancer statistics, 2019. *CA Cancer J Clin.* 2019;69(1):7–34.
2. Howlader N, Noone A, Krapcho M, et al. Cancer epidemiology in older adolescents and young adults 15 to 29 years of age, including SEER incidence and survival: 1975–2000. *Institute NC, editor NIH Pub.* 2013(06-5767):1975–2010.
3. Silverman LB. Balancing cure and long-term risks in acute lymphoblastic leukemia. *Hematology Am Soc Hematol Educ Program.* 2014;2014(1):190–197.
4. Robison LL, Hudson MM. Survivors of childhood and adolescent cancer: Life-long risks and responsibilities. *Nat Rev Cancer.* 2014;14(1):61–70.
5. Ward E, DeSantis C, Robbins A, Kohler B, Jemal A. Childhood and adolescent cancer statistics, 2014. *CA Cancer J Clin.* 2014;64(2): 83–103.

6. Clarke-Steffen L. Reconstructing reality: Family strategies for managing childhood cancer. *J Pediatr Nurs.* 1997;12(5):278–287.
7. Rosenberg AR, Baker KS, Syrjala KL, Back AL, Wolfe J. Promoting resilience among parents and caregivers of children with cancer. *J Palliat Med.* 2013;16(6):645–652.
8. Kirch R, Reaman G, Feudtner C, et al. Advancing a comprehensive cancer care agenda for children and their families: Institute of Medicine Workshop highlights and next steps. *CA: Cancer J Clin.* 2016.
9. Brock KE, Snaman JM, Kaye EC, et al. Models of pediatric palliative oncology outpatient care-benefits, challenges, and opportunities. *J Oncol Pract.* 2019;15(9):476–487.
10. Mack JW, Wolfe J. Early integration of pediatric palliative care: For some children, palliative care starts at diagnosis. *Curr Opin Pediatr.* 2006;18(1):10–14.
11. Foster TL, Lafond DA, Reggio C, Hinds PS. Pediatric palliative care in childhood cancer nursing: From diagnosis to cure or end of life. *Semin Oncol Nurs.* 2010;26(4):205–221.
12. Snaman J, McCarthy S, Wiener L, Wolfe J. Pediatric palliative care in oncology. *J Clin Oncol.* 2020;38(9):954–962.
13. Snaman JM, Kaye EC, Baker JN, Wolfe J. Pediatric palliative oncology: the state of the science and art of caring for children with cancer. *Curr Opin Pediatric.* 2018:30(1):40–48.
14. Levine DR, Mandrell BN, Sykes A, et al. Patients' and parents' needs, attitudes, and perceptions about early palliative care integration in pediatric oncology. *JAMA Oncol.* 2017.
15. Wolfe J, Grier HE, Klar N, et al. Symptoms and suffering at the end of life in children with cancer. *N Engl J Med.* 2000;342(5):326–333.
16. Hilden JM, Emanuel EJ, Fairclough DL, et al. Attitudes and practices among pediatric oncologists regarding end-of-life care: Results of the 1998 American Society of Clinical Oncology survey. *J Clin Oncol.* 2001;19(1):205–212.
17. Section On H, Palliative M, Committee On Hospital C. Pediatric palliative care and hospice care commitments, guidelines, and recommendations. *Pediatrics.* 2013;132(5):966–972.
18. Weaver MS, Heinze KE, Kelly KP, et al. Palliative care as a standard of care in pediatric oncology. *Pediatr Blood Cancer.* 2015;62 Suppl 5:S829–833.
19. Waldman E, Wolfe J. Palliative care for children with cancer. *Nat Rev Clin Oncol.* 2013;10(2):100–107.
20. Kazak AE, Abrams AN, Banks J, et al. Psychosocial assessment as a standard of care in pediatric cancer. *Pediatr Blood Cancer.* 2015;62 Suppl 5:426.
21. Weaver MS, Heinze KE, Bell CJ, et al. Establishing psychosocial palliative care standards for children and adolescents with cancer and their families: An integrative review. *Palliat Med.* 2016;30(3):212–223.
22. Kaye EC, Friebert S, Baker JN. Early integration of palliative care for children with high-risk cancer and their families. *Pediatr Blood Cancer.* 2016;63(4):593–597.
23. Groh G, Vyhnalek B, Feddersen B, Fuhrer M, Borasio GD. Effectiveness of a specialized outpatient palliative care service as experienced by patients and caregivers. *J Palliat Med.* 2013;16(8):848–856.
24. Vern-Gross TZ, Lam CG, Graff Z, et al. Patterns of end-of-life care in children with advanced solid tumor malignancies enrolled on a palliative care service. *J Pain Symptom Manage.* 2015;50(3):305–312.
25. Snaman JM, Kaye EC, Lu JJ, Sykes A, Baker JN. Palliative care involvement is associated with less intensive end-of-life care in adolescent and young adult oncology patients. *J Palliat Med.* 2017;20(5):509–516.
26. Snaman JM, Kaye EC, Torres C, Gibson DV, Baker JN. Helping parents live with the hole in their heart: The role of health care providers and institutions in the bereaved parents' grief journeys. *Cancer.* 2016;122(17):2757–2765.
27. Cheng BT, Rost M, De Clercq E, Arnold L, Elger BS, Wangmo T. Palliative care initiation in pediatric oncology patients: A systematic review. *Cancer Med.* 2019;8(1):3–12.
28. Dahlin C. Palliative care nursing an emerging specialty. *Imprint.* 2000;47(2):38–39.
29. Feraco AM, Brand SR, Mack JW, Kesselheim JC, Block SD, Wolfe J. Communication skills training in pediatric oncology: Moving beyond role modeling. *Pediatr Blood Cancer.* 2016;63(6):966–972.
30. Ericsson KA. Deliberate practice and acquisition of expert performance: A general overview. *Acad Emerg Med.* 2008;15(11):988–994.
31. Fryer-Edwards K, Arnold RM, Baile W, Tulsky JA, Petracca F, Back A. Reflective teaching practices: An approach to teaching communication skills in a small-group setting. *Acad Med.* 2006;81(7):638–644.
32. Back AL, Arnold RM, Baile WF, Tulsky JA, Fryer-Edwards K. Approaching difficult communication tasks in oncology. *CA Cancer J Clin.* 2005;55(3):164–177.
33. Blazin LJ, Cecchini C, Habashy C, Kaye EC, Baker JN. Communicating effectively in pediatric cancer care: Translating evidence into practice. *Children (Basel).* 2018;5(3).
34. Brand SR, Fasciano K, Mack JW. Communication preferences of pediatric cancer patients: Talking about prognosis and their future life. *Support Care Cancer.* 2017;25(3):769–774.
35. Rallison L, Limacher LH, Clinton M. Future echoes in pediatric palliative care: Becoming sensitive to language. *J Palliat Care.* 2006;22(2):99–104.
36. Rubnitz JE, Inaba H, Leung WH, et al. Definition of cure in childhood acute myeloid leukemia. *Cancer.* 2014;120(16):2490–2496.
37. Cheung YT, Brinkman TM, Li C, et al. Chronic health conditions and neurocognitive function in aging survivors of childhood cancer: A report from the childhood cancer survivor study. *J Natl Cancer Inst.* 2018;110(4):411–419.
38. Edelmann MN, Daryani VM, Bishop MW, et al. Neurocognitive and patient-reported outcomes in adult survivors of childhood osteosarcoma. *JAMA Oncol.* 2016;2(2):201–208.
39. Bhatia S, Yasui Y, Robison LL, et al. High risk of subsequent neoplasms continues with extended follow-up of childhood Hodgkin's disease: Report from the Late Effects Study Group. *J Clin Oncol.* 2003;21(23):4386–4394.
40. Gurney JG, Krull KR, Kadan-Lottick N, et al. Social outcomes in the Childhood Cancer Survivor Study cohort. *J Clin Oncol.* 2009;27(14):2390–2395.
41. Bishop G. The arc of therapy: From cure to humbling legacy. *J Clin Oncol.* 2019;37(34):3320–3322.
42. Mack JW, Smith TJ. Reasons why physicians do not have discussions about poor prognosis, why it matters, and what can be improved. *J Clin Oncol.* 2012;30(22):2715–2717.
43. Mack JW, Joffe S. Communicating about prognosis: Ethical responsibilities of pediatricians and parents. *Pediatrics.* 2014;133 Suppl 1:S24–30.
44. Sisk BA, Greenzang KA, Kang TI, Mack JW. Longitudinal parental preferences for late effects communication during cancer treatment. *Pediatr Blood Cancer.* 2018;65(1).
45. Levi RB, Marsick R, Drotar D, Kodish ED. Diagnosis, disclosure, and informed consent: Learning from parents of children with cancer. *J Pediatr Hematol Oncol.* 2000;22(1):3–12.
46. Dixon-Woods M, Findlay M, Young B, Cox H, Heney D. Parents' accounts of obtaining a diagnosis of childhood cancer. *Lancet.* 2001;357(9257):670–674.
47. Mack JW, Wolfe J, Cook EF, Grier HE, Cleary PD, Weeks JC. Parents' roles in decision making for children with cancer in the first year of cancer treatment. *J Clin Oncol.* 2011;29(15):2085–2090.
48. Mack JW, Cronin AM, Kang TI. Decisional regret among parents of children with cancer. *J Clin Oncol.* 2016;34(33):4023–4029.
49. Mack JW, Grier HE. The day one talk. *J Clin Oncol.* 2004;22(3):563–566.
50. Sisk BA, Kang TI, Mack JW. Prognostic disclosures over time: Parental preferences and physician practices. *Cancer.* 2017;123(20):4031–4038.
51. Wiener L, Kazak AE, Noll RB, Patenaude AF, Kupst MJ. Interdisciplinary collaboration in standards of psychosocial care. *Pediatr Blood Cancer.* 2015;62 Suppl 5:S425.
52. Steele AC, Mullins LL, Mullins AJ, Muriel AC. Psychosocial interventions and therapeutic support as a standard of care in pediatric oncology. *Pediatric blood & cancer.* 2015;62 Suppl 5:S585.

53. Slavin LA, O'Malley JE, Koocher GP, Foster DJ. Communication of the cancer diagnosis to pediatric patients: Impact on long-term adjustment. *Am J Psychiatry.* 1982;139(2):179–183.
54. Chesler MA, Paris J, Barbarin OA. "Telling" the child with cancer: Parental choices to share information with ill children. *J Pediatr Psychol.* 1986;11(4):497–516.
55. Weaver MS, Baker JN, Gattuso JS, Gibson DV, Sykes AD, Hinds PS. Adolescents' preferences for treatment decisional involvement during their cancer. *Cancer.* 2015;121(24):4416–4424.
56. Wiener L, McConnell DG, Latella L, Ludi E. Cultural and religious considerations in pediatric palliative care. *Palliat Support Care.* 2013;11(1):47–67.
57. Levetown M, American Academy of Pediatrics Committee on B. Communicating with children and families: From everyday interactions to skill in conveying distressing information. *Pediatrics.* 2008;121(5):e1441–1460.
58. Landier W, Ahern J, Barakat LP, et al. Patient/family education for newly diagnosed pediatric oncology patients. *J Pediatr Oncol Nurs.* 2016;33(6):422–431.
59. Hinds PS, Drew D, Oakes LL, et al. End-of-life care preferences of pediatric patients with cancer. *J Clin Oncol.* 2005;23(36):9146–9154.
60. Zwaanswijk M, Tates K, van Dulmen S, et al. Communicating with child patients in pediatric oncology consultations: A vignette study on child patients', parents', and survivors' communication preferences. *Psychooncology.* 2011;20(3):269–277.
61. Gaab EM, Owens GR, MacLeod RD. Siblings caring for and about pediatric palliative care patients. *J Palliat Med.* 2014;17(1):62–67.
62. Anthony SJ, Selkirk E, Sung L, et al. Considering quality of life for children with cancer: A systematic review of patient-reported outcome measures and the development of a conceptual model. *Qual Life Res.* 2014;23(3):771–789.
63. Sung L, Klaassen RJ, Dix D, et al. Identification of paediatric cancer patients with poor quality of life. *Br J Cancer.* 2009;100(1):82–88.
64. Collins JJ, Devine TD, Dick GS, et al. The measurement of symptoms in young children with cancer: The validation of the Memorial Symptom Assessment Scale in children aged 7-12. *J Pain Symptom Manage.* 2002;23(1):10–16.
65. Dupuis LL, Robinson PD, Boodhan S, et al. Guideline for the prevention and treatment of anticipatory nausea and vomiting due to chemotherapy in pediatric cancer patients. *Pediatr Blood Cancer.* 2014;61(8):1506–1512.
66. Altman AJ, Children's Oncology Group. *Supportive Care of Children with Cancer: Current Therapy and Guidelines from the Children's Oncology Group.* 3rd ed. Johns Hopkins University Press; 2004.
67. Robert R, Stavinoha P, Jones BL, et al. Spiritual assessment and spiritual care offerings as a standard of care in pediatric oncology: A recommendation informed by a systematic review of the literature. *Pediatr Blood Cancer.* 2019;66(9):e27764.
68. Lavi I, Fladeboe K, King K, et al. Stress and marital adjustment in families of children with cancer. *Psychooncology.* 2018;27(4):1244–1250.
69. Wiener L, Battles H, Zadeh S, Pelletier W, Arruda-Colli MNF, Muriel AC. The perceived influence of childhood cancer on the parents' relationship. *Psychooncology.* 2017;26(12):2109–2117.
70. Rensen N, Steur LM, Schepers SA, et al. Gender-specific differences in parental health-related quality of life in childhood cancer. *Pediatr Blood Cancer.* 2019;66(7):e27728.
71. Wilford JG, Hopfer S, Wenzel L. Perceptions of changes in clinical, informational, and supportive relationships after end of treatment among parents of young childhood cancer survivors. *Psychooncology.* 2019;28(4):913–919.
72. Brand S, Wolfe J, Samsel C. The impact of cancer and its treatment on the growth and development of the pediatric patient. *Curr Pediatr Rev.* 2017;13(1):24–33.
73. Long KA, Lehmann V, Gerhardt CA, Carpenter AL, Marsland AL, Alderfer MA. Psychosocial functioning and risk factors among siblings of children with cancer: An updated systematic review. *Psychooncology.* 2018;27(6):1467–1479.
74. Barrera M, Atenafu E, Nathan PC, Schulte F, Hancock K. Depression and quality of life in siblings of children with cancer after group intervention participation: A randomized control trial. *J Pediatr Psychol.* 2018;43(10):1093–1103.
75. Kelada L, Wakefield CE, Doolan EL, et al. Grandparents of children with cancer: A controlled comparison of perceived family functioning. *Support Care Cancer.* 2019;27(6):2087–2094.
76. Wakefield CE, Drew D, Ellis SJ, Doolan EL, McLoone JK, Cohn RJ. Grandparents of children with cancer: A controlled study of distress, support, and barriers to care. *Psychooncology.* 2014;23(8):855–861.
77. Moules NJ, McCaffrey G, Laing CM, Tapp DM, Strother D. Grandparents' experiences of childhood cancer, part 2: The need for support. *J Pediatr Oncol Nurs.* 2012;29(3):133–140.
78. Bona K, Dussel V Orellana L, et al. Economic impact of advanced pediatric cancer on families. *J Pain Symptom Manage.* 2014;47(3):594–603.
79. Bona K, London WB, Guo D, Abel G, Lehmann L, Wolfe J. Prevalence and impact of financial hardship among New England pediatric stem cell transplantation families. *Biol Blood Marrow Transplant.* 2015;21(2):312–318.
80. Bilodeau M, Ma C, Al-Sayegh H, Wolfe J, Bona K. Household material hardship in families of children post-chemotherapy. *Pediatr Blood Cancer.* 2018;65(1).
81. Ilowite MF, Al-Sayegh H, Ma C, et al. The relationship between household income and patient-reported symptom distress and quality of life in children with advanced cancer: A report from the pediquest study. *Cancer.* 2018;124(19):3934–3941.
82. Kasl-Godley JE, King DA, Quill TE. Opportunities for psychologists in palliative care: Working with patients and families across the disease continuum. *Am Psychol.* 2014;69(4):364–376.
83. Woodgate RL, Degner LF. A substantive theory of Keeping the Spirit Alive: The Spirit Within children with cancer and their families. *J Pediatr Oncol Nurs.* 2003;20(3):103–119.
84. Whitford B, Nadel AL, Fish JD. Burnout in pediatric hematology/oncology-time to address the elephant by name. *Pediatr Blood Cancer.* 2018;65(10):e27244.
85. Zander M, Hutton A, King L. Coping and resilience factors in pediatric oncology nurses. *J Pediatr Oncol Nurs.* 2010;27(2):94–108.
86. Rasmussen V, Turnell A, Butow P, et al. Burnout among psychosocial oncologists: An application and extension of the effort-reward imbalance model. *Psychooncology.* 2016;25(2):194–202.
87. Mukherjee S, Beresford B, Glaser A, Sloper P. Burnout, psychiatric morbidity, and work-related sources of stress in paediatric oncology staff: A review of the literature. *Psychooncology.* 2009;18(10):1019–1028.
88. Roth M, Morrone K, Moody K, et al. Career burnout among pediatric oncologists. *Pediatr Blood Cancer.* 2011;57(7):1168–1173.
89. Ramirez AJ, Graham J, Richards MA, et al. Burnout and psychiatric disorder among cancer clinicians. *Br J Cancer.* 1995;71(6):1263–1269.
90. Stenmarker M, Hallberg U, Palmerus K, Marky I. Being a messenger of life-threatening conditions: Experiences of pediatric oncologists. *Pediatr Blood Cancer.* 2010;55(3):478–484.
91. Baer TE, Feraco AM, Tuysuzoglu Sagalowsky S, Williams D, Litman HJ, Vinci RJ. Pediatric resident burnout and attitudes toward patients. *Pediatrics.* 2017;139(3):2163.
92. Feudtner C. Holding the tension. *Hastings Cent Rep.* 2016;46(3):inside back cover.
93. Trufelli DC, Bensi CG, Garcia JB, et al. Burnout in cancer professionals: A systematic review and meta-analysis. *Eur J Cancer Care (Engl).* 2008;17(6):524–531.
94. Embriaco N, Azoulay E, Barrau K, et al. High level of burnout in intensivists: Prevalence and associated factors. *Am J Respir Crit Care Med.* 2007;175(7):686–692.
95. Shirom A, Nirel N, Vinokur AD. Work hours and caseload as predictors of physician burnout: The mediating effects by perceived workload and by autonomy. *Applied Psychology.* 2010;59(4):539–565.
96. Dougherty E, Pierce B, Ma C, Panzarella T, Rodin G, Zimmermann C. Factors associated with work stress and professional satisfaction in oncology staff. *Am J Hosp Palliat Care.* 2009;26(2):105–111.

97. Shanafelt TD, Dyrbye LN, Sinsky C, et al. Relationship between clerical burden and characteristics of the electronic environment with physician burnout and professional satisfaction. *Mayo Clin Proc.* 2016;91(7):836–848.
98. Sands SA, Stanley P, Charon R. Pediatric narrative oncology: Interprofessional training to promote empathy, build teams, and prevent burnout. *J Support Oncol.* 2008;6(7):307–312.
99. Imes RS, Omilion-Hodges LM, Hester JDB. *Communication and Care Coordination for the Palliative Care Team: A Handbook for Building and Maintaining Optimal Teams.* Springer; 2021.
100. Feraco AM, Brand SR, Gagne J, Sullivan A, Block SD, Wolfe J. Development of the "Day 100 Talk": Addressing existing communication gaps during the early cancer treatment period in childhood cancer. *Pediatr Blood Cancer.* 2018;65(6):e26972.
101. Greenzang KA, Dauti A, Mack JW. Parent perspectives on information about late effects of childhood cancer treatment and their role in initial treatment decision making. *Pediatr Blood Cancer.* 2018;65(6):e26978.
102. Waldman ED, Levine JM. The day two talk: Early integration of palliative care principles in pediatric oncology. *J Clin Oncol.* 2016;34(34):4068–4070.
103. Kazak AE, Barakat LP, Ditaranto S, et al. Screening for psychosocial risk at pediatric cancer diagnosis: The psychosocial assessment tool. *J Pediatr Hematol Oncol.* 2011;33(4):289–294.
104. Feraco AM, McCarthy, SR, Revette AC, Stevens SE, Das PJ, Al-Sayegh H, Ma C, Tulsky JA, Wolfe J. Feasibility and acceptability of the "day 100 talk": An interdisciplinary communication intervention during the first six months of childhood cancer treatment. *Cancer.* 2020;127(7):1134–1145.
105. Baile WF, Buckman R, Lenzi R, Glober G, Beale EA, Kudelka AP. SPIKES-A six-step protocol for delivering bad news: Application to the patient with cancer. *Oncologist.* 2000;5(4):302–311.
106. Mack JW, Cook EF, Wolfe J, Grier HE, Cleary PD, Weeks JC. Understanding of prognosis among parents of children with cancer: Parental optimism and the parent-physician interaction. *J Clin Oncol.* 2007;25(11):1357–1362.
107. Mack JW, Wolfe J, Grier HE, Cleary PD, Weeks JC. Communication about prognosis between parents and physicians of children with cancer: Parent preferences and the impact of prognostic information. *J Clin Oncol.* 2006;24(33):5265–5270.
108. Wolfe J, Klar N, Grier HE, et al. Understanding of prognosis among parents of children who died of cancer: Impact on treatment goals and integration of palliative care. *JAMA.* 2000;284(19):2469–2475.
109. Mack JW, Wolfe J, Cook EF, Grier HE, Cleary PD, Weeks JC. Hope and prognostic disclosure. *J Clin Oncol.* 2007;25(35):5636–5642.
110. Kamihara J, Nyborn JA, Olcese ME, Nickerson T, Mack JW. Parental hope for children with advanced cancer. *Pediatrics.* 2015;135(5):868–874.
111. Feudtner C. Collaborative communication in pediatric palliative care: A foundation for problem-solving and decision-making. *Pediatr Clin North Am.* 2007;54(5):583–607, ix.
112. Nyborn JA, Olcese M, Nickerson T, Mack JW. "Don't try to cover the sky with your hands": Parents' experiences with prognosis communication about their children with advanced cancer. *J Palliat Med.* 2016;19(6):626–631.
113. Bluebond-Langner M, Belasco JB, Goldman A, Belasco C. Understanding parents' approaches to care and treatment of children with cancer when standard therapy has failed. *J Clin Oncol.* 2007;25(17):2414–2419.
114. Pavisic J, Chilton J, Walter G, Soh NL, Martin A. Childhood cancer in the cinema: How the celluloid mirror reflects psychosocial care. *J Pediatr Hematol Oncol.* 2014;36(6):430–437.
115. Patterson JM, Holm KE, Gurney JG. The impact of childhood cancer on the family: A qualitative analysis of strains, resources, and coping behaviors. *Psychooncology.* 2004;13(6):390–407.
116. Tebbi CK, Mendenhall NP, London WB, et al. Response-dependent and reduced treatment in lower risk Hodgkin lymphoma in children and adolescents, results of P9426: A report from the Children's Oncology Group. *Pediatr Blood Cancer.* 2012;59(7):1259–1265.
117. Larsen EC, Devidas M, Chen S, et al. Dexamethasone and high-dose methotrexate improve outcome for children and young adults with high-risk b-acute lymphoblastic leukemia: A report from Children's Oncology Group Study AALL0232. *J Clin Oncol.* 2016;34(20):2380–2388.
118. von Stackelberg A, Locatelli F, Zugmaier G, et al. Phase I/Phase II study of blinatumomab in pediatric patients with relapsed/refractory acute lymphoblastic leukemia. *J Clin Oncol.* 2016;34(36):4381–4389.
119. Grupp SA, Kalos M, Barrett D, et al. Chimeric antigen receptor-modified T cells for acute lymphoid leukemia. *N Engl J Med.* 2013;368(16):1509–1518.
120. Slayton WB, Schultz KR, Kairalla JA, et al. Dasatinib plus intensive chemotherapy in children, adolescents, and young adults with Philadelphia chromosome-positive acute lymphoblastic leukemia: Results of Children's Oncology Group Trial AALL0622. *J Clin Oncol.* 2018;36(22):2306–2314.
121. Dhall G, Grodman H, Ji L, et al. Outcome of children less than three years old at diagnosis with non-metastatic medulloblastoma treated with chemotherapy on the "Head Start" I and II protocols. *Pediatr Blood Cancer.* 2008;50(6):1169–1175.
122. DuBois SG, Krailo MD, Gebhardt MC, et al. Comparative evaluation of local control strategies in localized Ewing sarcoma of bone: A report from the Children's Oncology Group. *Cancer.* 2015;121(3):467–475.
123. Bielack SS, Smeland S, Whelan JS, et al. Methotrexate, doxorubicin, and cisplatin (MAP) plus maintenance pegylated interferon alfa-2b versus MAP alone in patients with resectable high-grade osteosarcoma and good histologic response to preoperative MAP: First results of the EURAMOS-1 good response randomized controlled trial. *J Clin Oncol.* 2015;33(20):2279–2287.
124. Yu AL, Gilman AL, Ozkaynak MF, et al. Anti-GD2 antibody with GM-CSF, interleukin-2, and isotretinoin for neuroblastoma. *N Engl J Med.* 2010;363(14):1324–1334.
125. Ahmed AA, Vundamati DS, Farooqi MS, Guest E. Precision medicine in pediatric cancer: Current applications and future prospects. *High Throughput.* 2018;7(4).
126. Forrest SJ, Geoerger B, Janeway KA. Precision medicine in pediatric oncology. *Curr Opin Pediatr.* 2018;30(1):17–24.
127. Allen CE, Laetsch TW, Mody R, et al. Target and agent prioritization for the Children's Oncology Group-National Cancer Institute Pediatric MATCH Trial. *J Natl Cancer Inst.* 2017;109(5).
128. Solomon BJ, Mok T, Kim DW, et al. First-line crizotinib versus chemotherapy in ALK-positive lung cancer. *N Engl J Med.* 2014;371(23):2167–2177.
129. Turner NC, Ro J, Andre F, et al. Palbociclib in hormone-receptor-positive advanced breast cancer. *N Engl J Med.* 2015;373(3):209–219.
130. Innocenti F, Ou FS, Qu X, et al. Mutational analysis of patients with colorectal cancer in CALGB/SWOG 80405 identifies new roles of microsatellite instability and tumor mutational burden for patient outcome. *J Clin Oncol.* 2019;37(14):1217–1227.
131. Fernandez CV, Mullen EA, Chi YY, et al. Outcome and prognostic factors in stage III favorable-histology Wilms tumor: A report from the Children's Oncology Group Study AREN0532. *J Clin Oncol.* 2018;36(3):254–261.
132. Vrooman LM, Blonquist TM, Harris MH, et al. Refining risk classification in childhood B acute lymphoblastic leukemia: Results of DFCI ALL Consortium Protocol 05-001. *Blood Adv.* 2018;2(12):1449–1458.
133. Dussel V, Orellana L, Soto N, et al. Feasibility of conducting a palliative care randomized controlled trial in children with advanced cancer: Assessment of the Pediquest study. *J Pain Symptom Manage.* 2015;49(6):1059–1069.
134. Friedrichsdorf SJ. Four steps to eliminate or reduce pain in children caused by needles (part 1). *Pain Manag.* 2017;7(2):89–94.

135. Klassen AF, Klaassen R, Dix D, et al. Impact of caring for a child with cancer on parents' health-related quality of life. *J Clin Oncol.* 2008;26(36):5884–5889.
136. Navari RM. Aprepitant: A neurokinin-1 receptor antagonist for the treatment of chemotherapy-induced nausea and vomiting. *Expert Rev Anticancer Ther.* 2004;4(5):715–724.
137. Patel P, Leeder JS, Piquette-Miller M, Dupuis LL. Aprepitant and fosaprepitant drug interactions: A systematic review. *Br J Clin Pharmacol.* 2017;83(10):2148–2162.
138. Samsel C, Kearney J, Meadows AL, Abrams A, Hirst JM, Muriel AC. Olanzapine for chemotherapy-induced nausea: Lessons learned from child and adolescent psychiatry. *Pediatr Blood Cancer.* 2018;65(10):e27289.
139. Flank J, Schechter T, Gibson P, et al. Olanzapine for prevention of chemotherapy-induced nausea and vomiting in children and adolescents: A multi-center, feasibility study. *Support Care Cancer.* 2018;26(2):549–555.
140. Dupuis LL, Tomlinson GA, Pong A, Sung L, Bickham K. Factors associated with chemotherapy-induced vomiting control in pediatric patients receiving moderately or highly emetogenic chemotherapy: A pooled analysis. *J Clin Oncol.* 2020:JCO2000134.
141. Kinahan KE, Sharp LK, Seidel K, et al. Scarring, disfigurement, and quality of life in long-term survivors of childhood cancer: A report from the Childhood Cancer Survivor study. *J Clin Oncol.* 2012;30(20):2466–2474.
142. Heffron WA, Bommelaere K, Masters R. Group discussions with the parents of leukemic children. *Pediatrics.* 1973;52(6):831–840.
143. Munzone E, Bagnardi V, Campenni G, et al. Preventing chemotherapy-induced alopecia: A prospective clinical trial on the efficacy and safety of a scalp-cooling system in early breast cancer patients treated with anthracyclines. *Br J Cancer.* 2019;121(4):325–331.
144. Liossi C, White P, Hatira P. A randomized clinical trial of a brief hypnosis intervention to control venepuncture-related pain of paediatric cancer patients. *Pain.* 2009;142(3):255–263.
145. Fitzgerald JC, Weiss SL, Maude SL, et al. Cytokine release syndrome after chimeric antigen receptor T cell therapy for acute lymphoblastic leukemia. *Crit Care Med.* 2017;45(2):e124–e131.
146. Belum VR, Washington C, Pratilas CA, Sibaud V, Boralevi F, Lacouture ME. Dermatologic adverse events in pediatric patients receiving targeted anticancer therapies: A pooled analysis. *Pediatr Blood Cancer* 2015;62(5):798–806.
147. Mankin HJ, Gebhardt MC, Jennings LC, Springfield DS, Tomford WW. Long-term results of allograft replacement in the management of bone tumors. *Clin Orthop Relat Res.* 1996(324):86–97.
148. Dix DB, Seibel NL, Chi YY, et al. Treatment of Stage IV favorable histology Wilms tumor with lung metastases: A report from the Children's Oncology Group AREN0533 Study. *J Clin Oncol.* 2018 36(16):1564–1570.
149. Ramsey LH, Karlson CW, Collier AB. Mirror therapy for phantom limb pain in a 7-year-old male with osteosarcoma. *J Pain Symptom Manage.* 2017;53(6):e5–e7.
150. Wong SS, Svingos AM, Heaton SC. Behavioral therapy for acute post-surgical phantom limb pain in a young adult with osteosarcoma. *Pain Pract.* 2019;19(5):571–572.
151. Friedrichsdorf SJ, Nugent AP. Management of neuropathic pain in children with cancer. *Curr Opin Support Palliat Care.* 2013;7(2):131–138.
152. Loucas CA, Brand SR, Bedoya SZ, Muriel AC, Wiener L. Preparing youth with cancer for amputation: A systematic review. *J Psychosoc Oncol.* 2017;35(4):483–493.
153. Lopes-Júnior LC, Bomfim EO, Nascimento LC, Nunes MD, Pereira-da-Silva G, Lima RA. Non-pharmacological interventions to manage fatigue and psychological stress in children and adolescents with cancer: An integrative review. *Eur J Cancer Care (Engl).* 2016;25(6):921–935.
154. Kazak AE, Noll RB. The integration of psychology in pediatric oncology research and practice: Collaboration to improve care and outcomes for children and families. *Am Psychol.* 2015;70(2):146–158.
155. American Academy of Pediatrics Child Life C, Committee on Hospital C, Wilson JM. Child life services. *Pediatrics.* 2006;118(4):1757–1763.
156. Rosenberg AR, Orellana L, Kang TI, et al. Differences in parent-provider concordance regarding prognosis and goals of care among children with advanced cancer. *J Clin Oncol.* 2014;32(27):3005–3011.
157. Feudtner C. The breadth of hopes. *N Engl J Med.* 2009;361(24):2306–2307.
158. Dubois SG, Shusterman S, Ingle AM, et al. Phase I and pharmacokinetic study of sunitinib in pediatric patients with refractory solid tumors: A children's oncology group study. *Clin Cancer Res.* 2011;17(15):5113–5122.
159. Maurer SH, Hinds PS, Spunt SL, Furman WL, Kane JR, Baker JN. Decision making by parents of children with incurable cancer who opt for enrollment on a phase I trial compared with choosing a do not resuscitate/terminal care option. *J Clin Oncol.* 2010;28(20):3292–3298.
160. Hinds PS, Oakes LL, Hicks J, et al. "Trying to be a good parent" as defined by interviews with parents who made phase I, terminal care, and resuscitation decisions for their children. *J Clin Oncol.* 2009;27(35):5979–5985.
161. Johnson LM, Leek AC, Drotar D, et al. Practical communication guidance to improve phase 1 informed consent conversations and decision-making in pediatric oncology. *Cancer.* 2015;121(14):2439–2448.
162. Marron JM, Cronin AM, DuBois SG, et al. Duality of purpose: Participant and parent understanding of the purpose of genomic tumor profiling research among children and young adults with solid tumors. *JCO Precis Oncol.* 2019;3.
163. Marron JM, DuBois SG, Glade Bender J, et al. Patient/parent perspectives on genomic tumor profiling of pediatric solid tumors: The Individualized Cancer Therapy (ICAT) experience. *Pediatr Blood Cancer.* 2016;63(11):1974–1982.
164. Morgenstern DA, Hargrave D, Marshall LV, et al. Toxicity and outcome of children and adolescents participating in phase I/II trials of novel anticancer drugs: The Royal Marsden experience. *J Pediatr Hematol Oncol.* 2014;36(3):218–223.
165. Kim A, Fox E, Warren K, et al. Characteristics and outcome of pediatric patients enrolled in phase I oncology trials. *Oncologist.* 2008;13(6):679–689.
166. Bautista F, Di Giannatale A, Dias-Gastellier N, et al. Patients in pediatric phase I and early phase II clinical oncology trials at Gustave Roussy: A 13-year center experience. *J Pediatr Hematol Oncol.* 2015;37(2):e102–110.
167. Hurwitz CA, Duncan J, Wolfe J. Caring for the child with cancer at the close of life: "There are people who make it, and I'm hoping I'm one of them." *JAMA.* 2004;292(17):2141–2149.
168. Meyers FJ, Linder J, Beckett L, Christensen S, Blais J, Gandara DR. Simultaneous care: A model approach to the perceived conflict between investigational therapy and palliative care. *J Pain Symptom Manage.* 2004;28(6):548–556.
169. Cassel JB, Del Fabbro E, Arkenau T, et al. Phase I cancer trials and palliative care: Antagonism, irrelevance, or synergy? *J Pain Symptom Manage.* 2016;52(3):437–445.
170. Ananth P, Monsereenusorn C, Ma C, Al-Sayegh H, Wolfe J, Rodriguez-Galindo C. Influence of early phase clinical trial enrollment on patterns of end-of-life care for children with advanced cancer. *Pediatr Blood Cancer.* 2018;65(1).
171. Johnston EE, Alvarez E, Saynina O, Sanders L, Bhatia S, Chamberlain LJ. Disparities in the intensity of end-of-life care for children with cancer. *Pediatrics.* 2017;140(4).
172. Johnston EE, Alvarez E, Saynina O, Sanders LM, Bhatia S, Chamberlain LJ. Inpatient utilization and disparities: The last year of life of adolescent and young adult oncology patients in California. *Cancer.* 2018;124(8):1819–1827.

173. National Institutes of Health. NIH State-of-the-Science Conference Statement on improving end-of-life care. *NIH Consens State Sci Statements.* 2004;21(3):1–26.
174. Crane S, Haase JE, Hickman SE. Parental experiences of child participation in a Phase I pediatric oncology clinical trial: "We don't have time to waste." *Qual Health Res.* 2019;29(5):632–644.
175. Kaye EC, Jerkins J, Gushue CA, et al. Predictors of late palliative care referral in children with cancer. *J Pain Symptom Manage.* 2018;55(6):1550–1556.
176. Ulrich CM, Grady C, Wendler D. Palliative care: A supportive adjunct to pediatric phase I clinical trials for anticancer agents? *Pediatrics.* 2004;114(3):852–855.
177. Hill DL, Miller V, Walter JK, et al. Regoaling: A conceptual model of how parents of children with serious illness change medical care goals. *BMC Palliat Care.* 2014;13(1):9.
178. Akard TF, Dietrich MS, Friedman DL, et al. Digital storytelling: An innovative legacy-making intervention for children with cancer. *Pediatr Blood Cancer.* 2015;62(4):658–665.
179. Akard TF, Dietrich MS, Friedman DL, et al. Randomized clinical trial of a legacy intervention for quality of life in children with advanced cancer. *J Palliat Med.* 2020;24(5):680–688.
180. Kassam A, Skiadaresis J, Alexander S, Wolfe J. Parent and clinician preferences for location of end-of-life care: Home, hospital or freestanding hospice? *Pediatr Blood Cancer.* 2014;61(5):859–864.
181. Miller EG, Laragione G, Kang TI, Feudtner C. Concurrent care for the medically complex child: Lessons of implementation. *J Palliat Med.* 2012;15(11):1281–1283.
182. Kaye EC, Gattas M, Kiefer A, et al. Provision of palliative and hospice care to children in the community: A population study of hospice nurses. *J Pain Symptom Manage.* 2019;57(2):241–250.
183. Odejide OO, Steensma DP. Patients with haematological malignancies should not have to choose between transfusions and hospice care. *Lancet Haematol.* 2020;7(5):e418–e424.
184. Goldman A, Hewitt M, Collins GS, Childs M, Hain R, United Kingdom Children's Cancer Study Group/Paediatric Oncology Nurses' Forum Palliative Care Working G. Symptoms in children/young people with progressive malignant disease: United Kingdom Children's Cancer Study Group/Paediatric Oncology Nurses Forum survey. *Pediatrics.* 2006;117(6):e1179–1186.
185. Varma S, Friedman DL, Stavas MJ. The role of radiation therapy in palliative care of children with advanced cancer: Clinical outcomes and patterns of care. *Pediatr Blood Cancer.* 2017;64(5).
186. Rork JF, Berde CB, Goldstein RD. Regional anesthesia approaches to pain management in pediatric palliative care: A review of current knowledge. *J Pain Symptom Manage.* 2013;46(6):859–873.
187. Schmidt P, Otto M, Hechler T, Metzing S, Wolfe J, Zernikow B. Did increased availability of pediatric palliative care lead to improved palliative care outcomes in children with cancer? *J Palliat Med.* 2013;16(9):1034–1039.
188. Wolfe J, Hammel JF, Edwards KE, et al. Easing of suffering in children with cancer at the end of life: Is care changing? *J Clin Oncol.* 2008;26(10):1717–1723.
189. Kassam A, Skiadaresis J, Alexander S, Wolfe J. Differences in end-of-life communication for children with advanced cancer who were referred to a palliative care team. *Pediatr Blood Cancer.* 2015;62(8):1409–1413.
190. Lyon ME, Jacobs S, Briggs L, Cheng YI, Wang J. A longitudinal, randomized, controlled trial of advance care planning for teens with cancer: Anxiety, depression, quality of life, advance directives, spirituality. *J Adolesc Health.* 2014;54(6):710–717.
191. Kreicbergs U, Valdimarsdottir U, Onelov E, Henter JI, Steineck G. Talking about death with children who have severe malignant disease. *N Engl J Med.* 2004;351(12):1175–1186.
192. Lovgren M, Jalmsell L, Eilegard Wallin A, Steineck G, Kreicbergs U. Siblings' experiences of their brother's or sister's cancer death: A nationwide follow-up 2-9 years later. *Psychooncology.* 2016;25(4):435–440.
193. Arruda-Colli MNF, Weaver MS, Wiener L. Communication about dying, death, and bereavement: A systematic review of children's literature. *J Palliat Med.* 2017;20(5):548–559.
194. Wiener L, Zadeh S, Battles H, et al. Allowing adolescents and young adults to plan their end-of-life care. *Pediatrics.* 2012;130(5):897–905.
195. Jacobs S, Perez J, Cheng YI, Sill A, Wang J, Lyon ME. Adolescent end of life preferences and congruence with their parents' preferences: Results of a survey of adolescents with cancer. *Pediatr Blood Cancer.* 2015;62(4):710–714.
196. Lyon ME, McCabe MA, Patel KM, D'Angelo LJ. What do adolescents want? An exploratory study regarding end-of-life decision-making. *J Adolesc Health.* 2004;35(6):529 e521–526.
197. Lyon ME, Garvie PA, Briggs L, He J, McCarter R, D'Angelo LJ. Development, feasibility, and acceptability of the Family/Adolescent-Centered (FACE) Advance Care Planning intervention for adolescents with HIV. *J Palliat Med.* 2009;12(4):363–372.
198. Wiener L, Ballard E, Brennan T, Battles H, Martinez P, Pao M. How I wish to be remembered: The use of an advance care planning document in adolescent and young adult populations. *J Palliat Med.* 2008;11(10):1309–1313.
199. Rosenberg AR, Postier A, Osenga K, et al. Long-term psychosocial outcomes among bereaved siblings of children with cancer. *J Pain Symptom Manage.* 2014;49(1):55–65.
200. Kreicbergs UC, Lannen P, Onelov E, Wolfe J. Parental grief after losing a child to cancer: Impact of professional and social support on long-term outcomes. *J Clin Oncol.* 2007;25(22):3307–3312.
201. Donovan LA, Wakefield CE, Russell V, Cohn RJ. Hospital-based bereavement services following the death of a child: A mixed study review. *Palliat Med.* 2015;29(3):193–210.
202. Heiney SP, Wells L, Ruffin J. A memorial service for families of children who died from cancer and blood disorders. *J Pediatr Oncol Nurs.* 1996;13(2):72–79; discussion 80.
203. Macdonald ME, Liben S, Carnevale FA, et al. Parental perspectives on hospital staff members' acts of kindness and commemoration after a child's death. *Pediatrics.* 2005;116(4):884–890.
204. Lichtenthal WG, Corner GW, Sweeney CR, et al. Mental health services for parents who lost a child to cancer: If we build them, will they come? *J Clin Oncol.* 2015;33(20):2246–2253.
205. Johnston EE, Bogetz J, Saynina O, Chamberlain LJ, Bhatia S, Sanders L. Disparities in inpatient intensity of end-of-life care for complex chronic conditions. *Pediatrics.* 2019 May;143(5):e20182228. doi: 10.1542/peds.2018-2228. Epub 2019 Apr 10.
206. Kaye EC, DeMarsh S, Gushue CA, et al. Predictors of location of death for children with cancer enrolled on a palliative care service. *Oncologist.* 2018;23(12):1525–1532.
207. Bradshaw G, Hinds PS, Lensing S, Gattuso JS, Razzouk BI. Cancer-related deaths in children and adolescents. *J Palliat Med.* 2005;8(1):86–95.
208. Dussel V, Kreicbergs U, Hilden JM, et al. Looking beyond where children die: Determinants and effects of planning a child's location of death. *J Pain Symptom Manage.* 2009;37(1):33–43
209. Widger K, Sutradhar R, Rapoport A, et al. Predictors of specialized pediatric palliative care involvement and impact on patterns of end-of-life care in children with cancer. *J Clin Oncol.* 2018;36(3):801–807.
210. Hinds PS, Schum L, Baker JN, Wolfe J. Key factors affecting dying children and their families. *J Palliat Med.* 2005;8 Suppl 1:70.
211. Kreicbergs U, Valdimarsdottir U, Onelov E, Bjork O, Steineck G, Henter JI. Care-related distress: A nationwide study of parents who lost their child to cancer. *J Clin Oncol.* 2005;23(36):9162–9171.
212. Johnston EE, Martinez I, Currie E, Brock KE, Wolfe J. Hospital or home? Where should children die and how do we make that a reality? *J Pain Symptom Manage.* 2019;60(1):106–115.
213. Currie ER, McPeters SL, Mack JW. Closing the gap on pediatric palliative oncology disparities. *Semin Oncol Nurs.* 2018;34(3):294–302.
214. Kaye EC, Gushue CA, DeMarsh S, et al. Impact of race and ethnicity on end-of-life experiences for children with cancer. *Am J Hosp Palliat Care.* 2019;36(9):767–774.
215. Barnato AE, Berhane Z, Weissfeld LA, et al. Racial variation in end-of-life intensive care use: A race or hospital effect? *Health Serv Res.* 2006;41(6):2219–2237.

216. Elliott AM, Alexander SC, Mescher CA, Mohan D, Barnato AE. Differences in physicians' verbal and nonverbal communication with black and white patients at the end of life. *J Pain Symptom Manage.* 2016;51(1):1–8.
217. Wright AA, Mack JW, Kritek PA, et al. Influence of patients' preferences and treatment site on cancer patients' end-of-life care. *Cancer.* 2010;116(19):4656–4663.
218. Johnston EE, Rosenberg AR, Kamal AH. Pediatric-specific end-of-life care quality measures: An unmet need of a vulnerable population. *J Oncol Pract.* 2017;13(10):e874–e880.
219. Ilowite MF, Cronin AM, Kang TI, Mack JW. Disparities in prognosis communication among parents of children with cancer: The impact of race and ethnicity. *Cancer.* 2017;123(20):3995–4003.
220. Eggly S, Tkatch R, Penner LA, et al. Development of a question prompt list as a communication intervention to reduce racial disparities in cancer treatment. *J Cancer Educ.* 2013;28(2):282–289.
221. Hudson MM, Mertens AC, Yasui Y, et al. Health status of adult long-term survivors of childhood cancer: A report from the Childhood Cancer Survivor Study. *JAMA.* 2003;290(12):1583–1592.
222. Ehrenreich B. Welcome to Cancerland. (criticism of "cult of the survivor" which has grown up around breast cancer fear that disease is being presented as a positive even normal experience and its causes ignored). *Harper's.* 2001;303(1818):43.
223. Parikh RB, Kirch RA, Brawley OW. Advancing a quality-of-life agenda in cancer advocacy: Beyond the war metaphor. *JAMA Oncol.* 2015;1(4):423–424.
224. Bishop G. Seeking the proper tense. *J Gen Intern Med.* 2009;24 Suppl 2:S436–437.
225. Zebrack BJ, Zeltzer LK, Whitton J, et al. Psychological outcomes in long-term survivors of childhood leukemia, Hodgkin's disease, and non-Hodgkin's lymphoma: A report from the Childhood Cancer Survivor Study. *Pediatrics.* 2002;110(1 Pt 1):42–52.
226. Pui CH, Cheng C, Leung W, et al. Extended follow-up of long-term survivors of childhood acute lymphoblastic leukemia. *N Engl J Med.* 2003;349(7):640–649.
227. Mariotto AB, Rowland JH, Yabroff KR, et al. Long-term survivors of childhood cancers in the United States. *Cancer Epidemiol Biomarkers Prev.* 2009;18(4):1033–1040.
228. Oeffinger KC, Mertens AC, Sklar CA, et al. Chronic health conditions in adult survivors of childhood cancer. *N Engl J Med.* 2006;355(15):1572–1582.
229. Anestin AS, Lippe S, Robaey P, et al. Psychological risk in long-term survivors of childhood acute lymphoblastic leukemia and its association with functional health status: A PETALE cohort study. *Pediatr Blood Cancer.* 2018;65(11):e27356.
230. Lehmann V, Chemaitilly W, Lu L, et al. Gonadal functioning and perceptions of infertility risk among adult survivors of childhood cancer: A report from the St Jude Lifetime Cohort Study. *J Clin Oncol.* 2019;37(11):893–902.
231. Fisher RS, Rausch JR, Ferrante AC, et al. Trajectories of health behaviors across early childhood cancer survivorship. *Psychooncology.* 2019;28(1):68–75.
232. Huang IC, Brinkman TM, Mullins L, et al. Child symptoms, parent behaviors, and family strain in long-term survivors of childhood acute lymphoblastic leukemia. *Psychooncology.* 2018;27(8):2031–2038.
233. Brinkman TM, Li C, Vannatta K, et al. Behavioral, social, and emotional symptom comorbidities and profiles in adolescent survivors of childhood cancer: A report from the Childhood Cancer Survivor Study. *J Clin Oncol.* 2016;34(28):3417–3425.
234. Huang IC, Bhakta N, Brinkman TM, et al. Determinants and consequences of financial hardship among adult survivors of childhood cancer: A report from the St. Jude Lifetime Cohort Study. *J Natl Cancer Inst.* 2019;111(2):189–200.
235. Mody R, Li S, Dover DC, et al. Twenty-five-year follow-up among survivors of childhood acute lymphoblastic leukemia: A report from the Childhood Cancer Survivor Study. *Blood.* 2008;111(12):5515–5523.
236. Seitzman RL, Glover DA, Meadows AT, et al. Self-concept in adult survivors of childhood acute lymphoblastic leukemia: A cooperative Children's Cancer Group and National Institutes of Health study. *Pediatr Blood Cancer.* 2004;42(3):230–240.
237. Fernandez-Pineda I, Hudson MM, Pappo AS, et al. Long-term functional outcomes and quality of life in adult survivors of childhood extremity sarcomas: A report from the St. Jude Lifetime Cohort Study. *J Cancer Surviv.* 2017;11(1):1–12.
238. Lee JL, Gutierrez-Colina A, Williamson Lewis R, et al. Knowledge of late effects risks and healthcare responsibility in adolescents and young adults treated for childhood cancer. *J Pediatr Psychol.* 2019;44(5):557–566.
239. Mitchell HR, Lu X, Myers RM, et al. Prospective, longitudinal assessment of quality of life in children from diagnosis to 3 months off treatment for standard risk acute lymphoblastic leukemia: Results of Children's Oncology Group study AALL0331. *Int J Cancer.* 2016;138(2):332–339.
240. Rosenberg AR, Wolfe J. Approaching the third decade of paediatric palliative oncology investigation: Historical progress and future directions. *Lancet Child Adolesc Health.* 2017;1(1):56–67.
241. Collins JJ, Byrnes ME, Dunkel IJ, et al. The measurement of symptoms in children with cancer. *J Pain Symptom Manage.* 2000;19(5):363–377.
242. Varni JW, Burwinkle TM, Katz ER, Meeske K, Dickinson P. The pedsql in pediatric cancer: Reliability and validity of the Pediatric Quality of Life Inventory Generic Core Scales, Multidimensional Fatigue Scale, and Cancer Module. *Cancer.* 2002;94(7):2090–2106.
243. Rosenberg AR, Orellana L, Ullrich C, et al. Quality of life in children with advanced cancer: A report from the Pediquest study. *J Pain Symptom Manage.* 2016;52(2):243–253.
244. Bona K, Dussel V, Orellana L, et al. Economic impact of advanced pediatric cancer on families. *J Pain Symptom Manage.* 2014;47(3):594–603.
245. Pelletier W, Bona K. Assessment of financial burden as a standard of care in pediatric oncology. *Pediatr Blood Cancer.* 2015;62 Suppl 5:S619–631.
246. Esmaili BE, Stewart KA, Masalu NA, Schroeder KM. Qualitative analysis of palliative care for pediatric patients with cancer at Bugando Medical Center: An evaluation of barriers to providing end-of-life care in a resource-limited setting. *J Glob Oncol.* 2018;4:1–10.
247. Nelson KE, Feinstein JA, Gerhardt CA, et al. Emerging methodologies in pediatric palliative care research: Six case studies. *Children (Basel).* 2018;5(3).
248. Feudtner C, Rosenberg AR, Boss RD, et al. Challenges and priorities for pediatric palliative care research in the US and similar practice settings: Report from a Pediatric Palliative Care Research Network Workshop. *J Pain Symptom Manage.* 2019;58(5):909–917 e903.

34 | HEMATOLOGIC SYMPTOMS

BARBARA SPELLER-BROWN, JILLIAN CAMPBELL, ALLISTAIR ABRAHAM, PRIYAL PATEL, LISA HUMPHREY, AND JENNIFER WEBB

Overnight medication for these yellow eyes, tired of Sickle Cell taking people from their lives, Fam keep stressin' about this pain in my system, doctors ask me to rate them, list em. Trapped in my dreams, slaying all my demons, IV needles pokin 'while I'm screamin.' How high I fly the life is my expression. Overnight, the hospitals is my depression. I feel caught in this internal fight; People don't understand my blood, my height. Pain coming out of nowhere, & when it hurts, don't share. When I feel it coming, I know it's another absence in the running.

Sickle Cell Teens Raising Awareness, Initiating Change, Voicing Thoughts, and Empowering Themselves (STRIVE) DC Participants, 2016–2017

Many patients develop hematologic symptoms requiring medical intervention. As suggested in the poem, the manner in which we go about attending to these symptoms can be as important as relief of the symptoms. In this chapter, we address hereditary anemias focusing on sickle cell disease (SCD); platelet disorders, including thrombocytopenia; bleeding disorders; and thrombosis. In each section, the critical roles of an interdisciplinary team will be highlighted (see Figure 34.1).

PALLIATIVE DOMAINS AND HEMATOLOGIC CONDITIONS

Modern medical advancements have improved the survival rates of several hematologic illnesses that were once considered fatal. The treatments discussed throughout this chapter have helped many patients live well into adulthood. While these advancements have improved the quantity of life for many, these patients are still faced with enormous challenges that impact quality of life. Therefore, the potential role of palliative care for these patients is immeasurable.

Palliative care encompasses the following domains of care: (1) structure and process, (2) physical health, (3) psychological and psychiatric health, (4) social health, (5) spirituality and religion, (6) culture, (7) end-of-life care, and (8) ethics and legality.[1–3] Depending on the underlying condition, children with hematologic conditions experience significant symptomatic and psychosocial burdens that are impacted by chronic pain, treatment side effects, multiple hospitalizations, and missed days from school/work. For example, the authors of the aforementioned poem depict perfectly the internal and external struggles associated with living with SCD. Such people are faced with sudden-onset, intense pain episodes referred to as "pain crises," infections, and disease complications that lead to multiple hospitalizations, missed days from school, social separation from their healthy peers, mood dysfunction, and existential hardships. In addition, some people express feeling isolation from the medical community who may not always recognize the severity of their pain and other symptoms, which can add to their overall distress. The burdens of living with such chronic illnesses also extend to caretakers in the form of financial, emotional, and social stress. Healthy siblings also feel the impact as they often grapple with their own emotions around "survivor" guilt, redefinition of their role in the family, hidden grief, and unintended benign neglect from their parents.

Unfortunately, specialty palliative care is often overlooked in these patients as there may be a misconception that palliative care should be reserved for patients with a terminal illness. Hospice care, which is defined as end-of-life management for people who have an estimated survival of fewer than 6 months, is only a small part of specialty palliative care.[4] This distinction is crucial to define when considering specialty palliative care for patients with chronic hematologic conditions. In fact, pediatric palliative care offers much more than end-of-life care and should be considered for any patients who have a life-limiting or life-altering illness. The World Health Organization defines palliative care as care (1) that is providing pain and symptom management; (2) does not postpone or hasten death; (3) starts at diagnosis and is continued regardless of what treatment is offered; (4) encompasses a holistic mind, body, and spirit approach; (5) includes family support and coping; (6) can be provided in the inpatient, outpatient, and/or home settings; (7) includes a broad multidisciplinary approach;

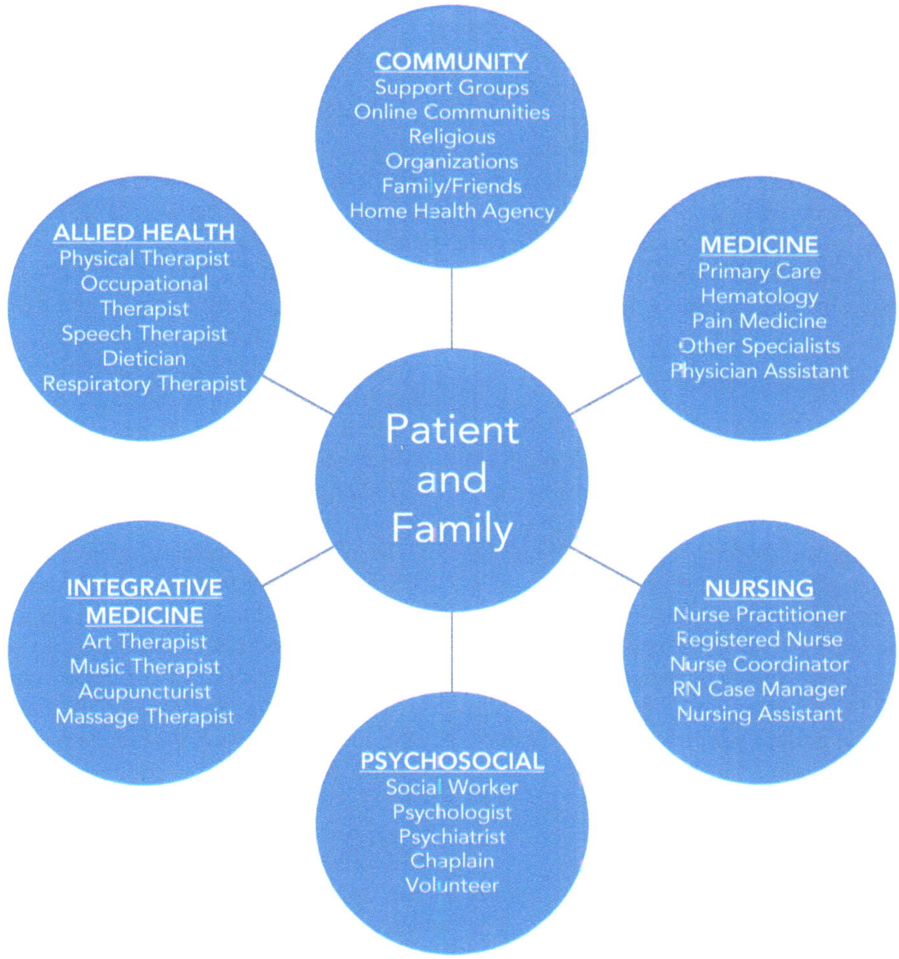
COMMUNITY
Support Groups
Online Communities
Religious
Organizations
Family/Friends
Home Health Agency
ALLIED HEALTH
Physical Therapist
Occupational
Therapist
Speech Therapist
Dietician
Respiratory Therapist
MEDICINE
Primary Care
Hematology
Pain Medicine
Other Specialists
Physician Assistant
Patient
and
Family
INTEGRATIVE
MEDICINE
Art Therapist
Music Therapist
Acupuncturist
Massage Therapist
NURSING
Nurse Practitioner
Registered Nurse
Nurse Coordinator
RN Case Manager
Nursing Assistant
PSYCHOSOCIAL
Social Worker
Psychologist
Psychiatrist
Chaplain
Volunteer

Figure 34.1 *Model of the interdisciplinary roles necessary for the comprehensive care of pediatric patients with hematologic disorders.*

and (8) includes physical, psychological, and social health.[5] Under this definition, palliative care offers a comprehensive approach to taking care of children with serious hematologic conditions.

SICKLE CELL DISEASE

SCD is a group of autosomal recessive hemolytic anemias characterized by erythrocytes that have a propensity to change into "sickle" or crescent shapes.[6] It is a multisystem disease that is associated with episodes of acute illness, vaso-occlusive crisis, chronic inflammation, and progressive multisystem organ damage.[7]

BACKGROUND

SCD affects millions of people around the world and is the most common genetic condition identified via newborn screen in the United States.[8] It affects approximately 1 out of every 365 black or African American births and 1 out of every 16,300 Hispanic American births.[9] Approximately 100,000 people are living with SCD in the United States.

SCD previously was considered a childhood disease since many patients did not survive into adulthood.[8] The introduction of vaccines that protect against invasive pneumococcal disease led to a 42% decrease in sickle cell–related deaths in children younger than 4 years.[9] Today, more than 95% of children with SCD survive to adulthood. However, the average life expectancy for people with SCD is just 40 years.[8]

The most common form of SCD, hemoglobin SS (sickle cell anemia), is caused by the inheritance of two sickle beta-globin genes, one from each parent.[10] Other forms of the disease are caused by inheritance of one sickle beta-globin gene plus another beta-globin chain defect[10]; the most common heterozygous forms of SCD are hemoglobin SC disease, hemoglobin S/beta+ thalassemia, and hemoglobin S/beta0 thalassemia. People with hemoglobin SS and hemoglobin S/beta0 thalassemia have no normal beta-globin production. They generally have a more severe clinical course compared to people with hemoglobin SC disease and hemoglobin S/beta+ thalassemia. However, phenotypic severity can vary significantly among patients.[11]

Acute vaso-occlusive (VOC) pain is the hallmark of SCD, which is caused by entrapment of rigid, deformed erythrocytes in the microcirculation causing tissue injury.[7] The process of sickling and unsickling continues until the erythrocyte membrane is no longer flexible, and irreversibly sickled cells undergo hemolysis.[6]

The shift in mortality from childhood to adulthood has led to an increase in serious morbidity among teens and young adults.[8] Chronic inflammation and vascular damage lead to progressive vasculopathy, which is characterized by systemic and pulmonary hypertension, endothelial dysfunction, and proliferative changes in the blood vessels. Parenchymal damage develops in nearly every organ system of the body, including the brain, eyes, lungs, heart, kidneys, and bones.

SYMPTOMS AND MANAGEMENT

Medical management of SCD generally focuses on detection and prevention of severe complications, as well as alleviating acute and chronic symptoms. Early in life, prophylactic antibiotics, supplemental vaccines, and hydroxyurea (HU) may avoid long-term complications of SCD. Folic acid may be supplemented to support red cell production. Complications can be acute (have a rapid onset and are immediately obvious) or chronic (occurring over time with more subtle symptoms), but both can lead to organ damage and failure. Many symptoms of SCD can be managed through periodic outpatient clinic visits and patient education. However, hospitalization may still be indicated.

PAIN

Patients with SCD are impacted by unpredictable amounts of intermittent and constant pain, known as VOC, that is often poorly managed over their lifetime.[11] Pain is often the hallmark feature of SCD, and unrelieved pain contributes to life-threatening complications, such as acute chest syndrome (ACS). Pain in SCD can be acute, chronic, or mixed, and can be related to tissue injury (nociceptive), nerve injury (neuropathic), or causes unknown (idiopathic). It is often not possible to differentiate between different types of pain.[11]

Acute pain is the most common reason for emergency room visits and admission to hospital for both children and adults. A VOC can present as excruciating pain, most common in the extremities, back, and chest; however, it can occur anywhere throughout the body. Onset can be sudden or gradual and can last from hours to days to weeks. Common triggers for VOC include dehydration, infection, exposure to extreme temperatures (hot or cold), and stress. Frequent episodes of acute pain are associated with disease severity, low fetal hemoglobin concentrations, high hematocrit, and nocturnal hypoxemia.[12]

The management of acute pain is paramount in caring for patients with SCD. Often, the goal of treatment is to minimize the frequency and duration of hospitalizations and emergency room visits and facilitate home management of pain. Treatment of VOC often requires medication. Mild to moderate pain may be treated with nonsteroidal anti-inflammatory medications (NSAIDs), while moderate to severe pain may require oral opioid analgesia in addition to NSAIDs. For severe pain, parenteral (IV) opioids may be needed.

Opioids are the standard treatment for acute and chronic sickle cell pain. There is significant variability in analgesic effect of opioids among patients with SCD.[13] Some of this variability can be attributed to genetic variations in opioid receptors and differences in drug metabolism. Therefore, treatment plans need to be individualized for each patient.

Intermittent injection of IV opioids versus patient-controlled analgesia (PCA) may be considered for a patient hospitalized with acute pain. Studies have shown variable outcomes comparing intermittent injection to PCA; subsequently, the choice of intermittent opioids versus PCA should be individualized to the patient. PCA initiation in the emergency room compared to PCA initiation after hospitalization is associated with fewer opioid boluses and less time without analgesic treatment.[14]

Patients with SCD often face stigma surrounding opioid use and potential for addiction. However, there is no evidence to support increased rates of addictions or association with the US opioid epidemic. Although adults with SCD have high opioid use, total opioid use across insurance payers has remained constant over time. In comparison, reported opioid use in a broader US population has increased to epidemic levels.[15] Patients with SCD on opioids can and do develop tolerance, which is often confused with addiction, and is more common in SCD patients than opioid addiction. One study found that approximately 50% of emergency department providers have concerns about addiction when treating sickle cell patients.[16] Inadequately treated pain can precipitate other SCD complications, and higher VOC rates correlate with early mortality in patients with SCD.[17]

Among sickle cell patients and healthcare providers, there is increasing interest in and acceptance of effective alternative treatments for sickle cell pain. Adjunctive, nonpharmacologic pain management approaches have been shown to be useful, including distraction, heat application, acupuncture, aromatherapy, and healing touch. Acupuncture is a well-tolerated intervention that is associated with improved pain scores in inpatient and outpatient settings.[18] One study found that more than 90% of patients with SCD used some form of complementary and alternative medicine (CAM) to treat pain.[19] Prayer, spiritual and energy healing, relaxation techniques, exercise, imagery, diet, and herbal medicines were among those alternatives. However, further studies are needed to measure their effectiveness.

It is important to collaborate with families when managing frequent and chronic pain, which can become a significant source of stress. Patients and their caregivers may have feelings of hopelessness and despair. Cognitive-behavioral therapy (CBT) should be considered for all patients with chronic pain and is associated with decreased admissions and hospital days.[20] A psychologist who is familiar with SCD can be especially helpful. Unanticipated emergency room visits, hospitalizations, and frequent office visits can lead to many missed work and school days. Loss of employment can occur, and children can be penalized for truancy. Many children fall behind in school due to frequent absences. Social workers can help to ensure all appropriate accommodations are in place at school through implementation of Individualized Education Plans (IEP) and that parents have appropriate accommodations at work, such as access to Family and Medical Leave (FMLA). Families may need the help of an education specialist to navigate complex school issues related to SCD.

NEUROLOGIC COMPLICATIONS

Among the most debilitating effects of SCD are neurological complications, which occur in as many as one-third of patients with SCD. There is a peak of ischemic stroke during the first decade of life. Symptoms of ischemic stroke include aphasia, hemiparesis, facial droop, and sometimes seizures. Transcranial Doppler ultrasound (TCD) is a noninvasive means of identifying patients in childhood who are at highest risk of stroke. In the Stroke Prevention in Sickle Cell Anemia (STOP) study, chronic transfusion to keep Hb S below 30% reduced the risk of stroke by 90% in patients with increased TCD velocities.[21] Adults with SCD more commonly experience hemorrhagic stroke which may present with severe headache, altered level of consciousness, speech impairments, and/or paralysis. By the age of 20, approximately 7–17% of children and adolescents with sickle cell anemia will have sustained a stroke.[21,22] Neuroimaging is used to confirm acute stroke, and, if present, exchange transfusion should be performed (see the section "Transfusion Support"). Care for patients with stroke requires a multidisciplinary approach that includes neurologists, neurosurgeons, interventional radiologists, critical care physicians, and hematologists working collaboratively to optimize patient outcomes.[23] Unfortunately, children and adolescents with SCD who suffer a stroke are at high risk for subsequent strokes.

Silent cerebral infarcts (SCI), which are cerebral infarctions that occur without focal neurologic deficit by exam or history,[23] typically involve watershed areas of the frontal lobes of the brain. They reflect microvascular accidents that are detectable on radiography. Approximately 20% of children with hemoglobin SS disease have SCI, which are linked to neurocognitive problems, poorer educational attainment,[24] and greater risk of further brain injury.[25] Cognitive impairment also occurs without brain infarction and may be partially attributed to chronic anemia and brain hypoxia.[26]

INFECTION

Patients with sickle cell are at increased risk for life-threatening bacterial infections, which are a major cause of morbidity and mortality. The increased susceptibility results from several causes: impaired splenic function, tissue ischemia, defects in complement activation, and micronutrient deficiencies. Several organisms are of particular risk to patients including *S. pneumoniae*, *H influenza*, non-typhi *Salmonella* species, and *Escherichia coli*.[27] The mortality rate among children with SCD who develop *S. pneumoniae* septicemia or meningitis is 11–24%.[28] Early intervention with prophylactic penicillin has become the standard of care. Patients with SCD who have a fever should be encouraged to seek prompt medical attention. Evaluation for infection should include a complete blood count (CBC), reticulocyte count, blood culture due to risk of bacteremia, chest x-ray if respiratory symptoms are present, and urine culture when urinary tract infection is suspected. Treatment includes broad-spectrum antibiotics.

ACUTE CHEST SYNDROME

The second most common cause of hospitalization in patients with SCD is ACS. It resembles pneumonia and is characterized by a new pulmonary infiltrate and signs of lower respiratory tract disease.[29] ACS is caused by a combination of infection, fat embolism, and vaso-occlusion of the pulmonary vasculature.

Evaluation of ACS should include chest x-ray, oxygen saturation measurements, CBC, reticulocyte count, and blood culture. Treatment includes broad-spectrum antibiotics and supplemental oxygen to maintain greater than 95% oxygen saturation. In some cases, bronchodilators and inhaled corticosteroids may also be appropriate. Severity of ACS varies, but about 13% of patients require mechanical ventilation, resulting in approximately 3% mortality.[30] ACS is the most common cause of death in adults with SCD. Blood transfusions or exchange transfusions may be utilized for severe cases with rapid deterioration in clinical status.[30] Deep breathing exercises and use of incentive spirometry can improve lung expansion in hospitalized patients.

Other complications of SCD are reviewed in Table 34.1.

Family Reflection

I've had SCA my whole life, but as I became a teenager, the pain started to be chronic. I continue to take medications such as HU daily to treat pain and recently started taking methadone in hopes of alleviating more pain. Living with chronic pain will never be simple, but throughout my life, I've learned how to cope with my pain in various ways that are suitable to my everyday life. I've developed many skills such as being able to give my pain a score, which helps me know when to take medicine, or use other mechanisms such as hot water bottles, distraction, and simply relaxing. Although I have pain, I push myself in order to get things done because I don't want to allow sickle cell to stand in the way of anything I wish to accomplish. Having a big support system makes living easier for anyone, chronic pain or not. I am fortunate enough to go to a good school with teachers that understand sickle cell. My teachers work with me to ensure that I put my health needs first and my work in school second. Even though I have the opportunity to turn work in late if need be, I always try my best to stay on top of my work when I can. My family is another support system that continues to be very helpful. I can always count on them to distract me from the pain. Some days being 16 with sickle cell is a challenge but I have learned how to deal with the pain in order to continue to do things I love. In the future hopefully there will be more efficient and healthy ways to cope with chronic pain.

Zion Thompson, age 16

TABLE 34.1 Complications of sickle cell disease

COMPLICATION	SYMPTOMS	MANAGEMENT
Splenic sequestration	Sudden enlargement of the spleen Sudden decrease in hemoglobin concentration by at least 2 gm/dL below baseline value Sudden decrease in platelets, pallor, lethargy, ill appearing	Partial correction of anemia.[35] Excessive transfusion over 8 g/dL should be avoided since sequestered erythrocytes in the enlarged spleen reenter the circulation after sequestration resolves; hyperviscosity due to a large transfusion could lead to cerebral infarction Referral to surgery for splenectomy in patients with frequent sequestration, life-threatening sequestration, or chronic splenic sequestration There is no evidence that chronic blood transfusions are effective for the management of recurrent splenic sequestration
Priapism	Sickling in the sinusoids of the penis Painful erection that may last for hours or days or become chronic Sustained, unwanted erection that is often extremely painful Can be a medical emergency if it lasts more than 2 hours Delayed diagnosis and treatment can result in impotence or erectile dysfunction	Pain management[35] Home management: voiding, hydration, warm shower or bath For erection more than 2 hours: IV hydration in emergency setting, oral or IV analgesia, consider urology consult Chronic transfusions may be considered for recurrent priapism
Retinopathy	Most common in Hb SC disease Aggregation of abnormal hemoglobin in the red blood cells in the retinal microcirculation Leads to reduced deformability of the red blood cells, decrease blood flow in the retinal precapillary arterioles, thrombosis, and ischemia Paracentral middle maculopathy or sequelae of proliferative retinopathy, such as vitreous hemorrhage and retinal detachment Precipitated by hypoxia, acidosis, and hyperosmolarity Asymptomatic in the early stages Can lead to blindness if left untreated	There is lack of evidence regarding the optimal management of sickle retinopathy[35] Annual screening by an ophthalmologist starting at 10 years of age Appropriate use of laser surgery may reduce the severity of complications
Avascular necrosis (AVN)	A form of ischemic bone injury that leads to degenerative joint disease Most commonly affects the femoral head (often bilaterally, with asymmetric clinical and radiographic progression) Can have multifocal joint involvement Can cause significant chronic pain and decrease quality of life	All patients with SCD should be evaluated for AVN with x-ray and/or MRI if they present with intermittent or chronic hip pain[35] Treat pain with analgesics and physical therapy Refer to an orthopedic surgeon for evaluation and possible hip core decompression or arthroplasty for advanced stages of avascular necrosis
Pulmonary hypertension (PH)	Progressive, chronic disease that results in a decrease in nitric oxide and prostacyclin production resulting in vasoconstriction Multifactorial etiology: hemolysis, hypercoagulability, hypoxemia, ischemic-reperfusion injury and oxidative stress A mean pulmonary arterial pressure >25 mm Hg with a pulmonary capillary wedge pressure < 15 mm Hg at rest Increased pulmonary vascular resistance Tricuspid regurgitant velocity (TRV) ≥2.5 m/sec Dyspnea, especially on exertion, dizziness, fatigue. High mortality risk Increased in patients with lower levels of fetal hemoglobin and lower systolic blood pressure Increases in prevalence with age	An echocardiogram (ECHO) should be performed to assess for PH, as it provides an estimation of right ventricular systolic pressure (RVSP) and information about the heart's overall size and function There is currently no cure for PH Management of adults with sickle-related PH is based on anticoagulation for those with thromboembolism; oxygen therapy for those with low oxygen saturation; treatment of left ventricular failure in those with postcapillary pulmonary hypertension; and hydroxyurea or transfusions to raise the hemoglobin concentration, reduce hemolysis, and prevent vaso-occlusive events that cause additional increases in pulmonary pressure[135] Refer to PH specialists May need supplemental oxygen when traveling on commercial flights or visiting areas of high altitudes because of the possibility of hypoxemia causing pulmonary vasoconstriction.[136] Randomized trials have not identified drugs to lower PH in SCD patients with precapillary PH[135] Prevention of PH should start early in childhood.

TABLE 34.1 Continued

COMPLICATION	SYMPTOMS	MANAGEMENT
Nephropathy	Repeated vaso-occlusive episodes leading to ischemic injury to glomeruli and the medullary vasa recta Decreased urinary concentrating ability, renal tubular acidosis and glomerular ischemia with secondary hyperfiltration Microalbuminuria (early manifestation); random urine albumin to creatinine ratio (ACR) of 30–300 mg/g creatinine Proteinuria; ACR >300 mg/g creatinine Associated with older age, hemolysis, higher absolute reticulocyte count, cardiovascular disease (i.e., high systolic BP)	Identifying patients most at risk of sickle cell nephropathy is paramount for delivering effective care to prevent progression to end stage renal disease[35] Few options are available for the treatment of SCD nephropathy. Angiotensin-converting enzyme inhibitors (ACE) may reduce overt proteinuria Multiple case studies have suggested that hydroxyurea may have short-term benefits in reducing proteinuria[137,138]
Hepatobiliary complications	Biliary tract abnormalities occur due to increased hemolysis, which leads to increased unconjugated bilirubin that leads to gallstones and sludge[35] Abnormalities include cholelithiasis, cholecystitis, choledocholilithiasis, hepatic sequestration, and acute intrahepatic cholestasis Gallstones may be asymptomatic Symptomatic gallstones often present as colicky pain in the right upper quadrant Cholecystitis can present as severe colicky pain in the right upper quadrant with tenderness, fever, leukocytosis, nausea, and vomiting Hepatic sequestration presents with marked hepatic enlargement and hemoglobin decrease of 2 g/dL or greater Intrahepatic cholestasis presents with sudden RUQ pain, increasing jaundice, enlarging liver, light-colored stools, and extreme hyperbilirubinemia (>50 mg/dL)	Patients with asymptomatic gallstones may be treated with a watch and wait approach[35] Patients with symptomatic cholelithiasis should be treated with cholecystectomy Acute cholecystitis should be treated with antibiotics and referred to surgery for cholecystectomy Acute hepatic sequestration and acute intrahepatic cholestasis are rare complications with high mortality rates; these patients often require exchange transfusion
Leg ulcers	More common in males and older people, although among those with active leg ulcers approximately 22% were between the ages of 10 and 20[35] Occur most frequently on the medial or lateral surfaces of the ankle Range from mild and small to large and severe May be complicated by osteomyelitis Leg ulcers are often chronic	Prevention is key. Seek prompt medical attention for wounds or open sores. Treat with standard wound therapy Monitor for signs of infection

PSYCHOLOGICAL AND SOCIAL STRESSORS

Chronic illnesses like SCD can have a profound impact on patient and family psychosocial and social functions. Painful episodes, frequent emergency visits, and hospitalizations can negatively impact physical function, sleep, academic achievement, and overall quality of life.[31] Patients are at greater risk for poor academic functioning, frequent school absences, social withdrawal, increased anxiety, and depression as compared to their healthy peers.[32] This can have an impact on siblings and other family members as well.

Physical factors that place patients at risk for low-self-esteem, anxiety, depression, and social isolation include delayed puberty (patients are usually smaller than their peers), scleral icterus (due to constant breakdown of red blood cells), physical limitations (due to chronic anemia), and learning difficulties (due to silent and overt strokes).

Patients and families are best supported by comprehensive care that addresses both medical and psychosocial needs to better control the disease and ultimately maximize function.

Patient and caregiver education has been identified as an important part of comprehensive care. Improved parental knowledge for at-risk groups like SCD has been associated with increased treatment adherence, reduced frequency of complications, and alleviation of fears associated with SCD diagnosis.[33] This leads to improved disease management and outcomes.

Prevention, education, and management are important factors to consider when caring for a patient with a chronic illness like SCD. Routine screening for stressors and for internalizing symptoms may be particularly important for these patients, and interventions focused on identifying and treating psychological symptoms are essential. Interventions should be culturally sensitive and should focus on decreasing internalizing symptoms through supportive counseling, including CBT.

TRANSFUSION SUPPORT

Blood transfusions are a critical disease-modifying therapy for patients with SCD. In general, leukoreduced, ABO, and RhD blood group–appropriate and cross-matched red blood cells (RBCs) are used to treat patients with symptomatic anemia. Leukoreduction removes a significant number of contaminating white blood cells, thus decreasing rates of cytomegalovirus (CMV) transmission, human leukocyte antigen (HLA) sensitization, and febrile nonhemolytic transfusion reactions.[34] For patients with SCD, transfusions carry an increased risk of alloimmunization, or antibody formation, to additional minor RBC antigens. This is thought to be due to their intact immune system and chronic inflammation, as well as to ethnic differences in the prevalence of minor RBC antigens. It is generally recommended to match a priori at ABO, RhD, RhCE, and Kell to avoid sensitization to these antigens.[35] Patients with SCD should receive sickle cell–negative blood so that determinations of hemoglobin S are solely reflective of the patient and can be reliably used to guide management. Blood banks should be made aware of the patient's underlying disease, blood transfusion history, history of transfusion reactions or antibody formation, and any prior typing of minor antigens as these help guide them in choosing the best RBC units for the patient.

In patients with SCD, acute RBC transfusions are used to improve oxygen delivery to tissues during acute RBC aplasia or aplastic crisis, hemolytic crisis, or ACS. Chronic transfusions, often performed on a monthly basis, have been shown to decrease rates of primary and secondary strokes.[21,36] When performed chronically, the goals of transfusion are to improve baseline anemia as well as decrease percentage of circulating hemoglobin S through dilution and decreased RBC production. Often, the target is to decrease circulating hemoglobin S to less than 30%, which has been shown to be protective against complications of SCD. Chronic transfusion therapy has been shown to decrease the frequency of other SCD complications including VOC, ACS, and priapism. The role of chronic transfusion therapy to mitigate symptoms of renal disease, pulmonary hypertension, and retinopathy is less supported in the literature but often attempted given the severity of these complications.

Exchange transfusions, performed manually or with automated machines, may be used for acute transfusions during stroke, ACS, intrahepatic cholestasis/hepatic sequestration, or multiorgan failure.[37] This procedure is able to increase the hemoglobin in the patient while decreasing the hemoglobin S% in a short (<4 hours) period of time. It may be performed chronically on outpatients receiving chronic transfusion therapy to minimize iron overload, a universal complication of long-standing transfusion therapy. Exchange transfusions are generally well-tolerated but do require increased numbers of RBC units. Obtaining a sufficient number of appropriate units in patients with a history of alloimmunization may become challenging. Chelation therapies, which facilitate iron excretion, are available in IV, subcutaneous, and oral formulations, allowing for successful mitigation of transfusional iron overload in adherent patients. Patients receiving regular transfusions should be monitored closely for elevated ferritin levels, our closest noninvasive surrogate measure for assessing iron deposition in tissues. Other noninvasive measures, such as cardiac and liver magnetic resonance imaging (MRI) to measure iron load, are also helpful for optimizing chelation.[38]

To raise the hemoglobin 1 g/dL requires a 3–5 mL/kg transfusion of RBCs. For a child with hemoglobin in the range of 7–9 g/dL, a reasonable transfusion is 10–15 mL/kg. For patients with chronic anemia, such as SCD, symptomatic anemia may not occur until the hemoglobin falls 2 g/dL below their baseline as the body has multiple methods for compensating for chronic anemia. However, for SCD patients receiving chronic transfusion therapy, often their target post-transfusion hemoglobin is raised to 11–11.5 g/dL.[39] Prior to ordering a transfusion of blood, the volume to be transfused should be determined by the patient's condition, how quickly the anemia developed, the patient's pre-transfusion hemoglobin, and the post-transfusion goal hemoglobin. The volume of RBCs should be administered over 2–4 hours in most situations. Repeat transfusions may be required to adequately improve hemoglobin levels for patients with poor red cell production or ongoing red cell destruction. For more profound, chronic anemia, smaller aliquots of 5 mL/kg of RBCs each transfused over 4 hours may help prevent the development of congestive heart failure.

In addition to alloimmunization and iron overload, transfusions carry additional risks for reactions. The most common reactions are febrile reactions and allergic reactions. If a reaction is suspected, the first course of action is to stop the transfusion and evaluate the patient. Acute hemolytic reactions may have a fever as one of their earliest symptoms, so a temperature increase, defined as greater than 1°C and/or greater than 38.0°C, in any patient receiving RBCs warrants further evaluation by the blood bank.[40] Depending on the patient's underlying condition, further evaluation as to the source of the fever, empiric antibiotic administration, and admission to the hospital for observation may be necessary. Additional evaluation of the blood product may include a culture of the transfused unit depending on the likelihood of septic transfusion reaction. Prophylactic acetaminophen is often used to prevent febrile transfusion reactions; however, multiple studies have failed to demonstrate benefit.[41,42] Routine administration of acetaminophen prior to transfusion is not recommended unless the child has a personal history of transfusion reaction and there is no contraindication to using this medication.

Allergic reactions may vary from the appearance of a few hives to shortness of breath and bronchospasm to anaphylaxis. Mild reactions may resolve with diphenhydramine 0.5–1 mg/kg administered IV or orally, or hydroxyzine 0.5–1 mg/kg IV or 2 mg/kg orally. Severe reactions may require the additional administration of hydrocortisone or epinephrine, according to resuscitation protocols. Some institutions may premedicate patients with a history of allergic reaction with diphenhydramine prior to transfusion, if not contraindicated by patient condition, to try to prevent transfusion reactions. Washing, saline resuspension, or dilution of the product has been shown to prevent recurrent, severe allergic reactions; however, these manipulations may cause transfusion delays and loss of RBCs, thus decreasing transfusion efficacy.

Patients who are sensitive to fluid loading may require diuresis during or after transfusion to maintain fluid homeostasis Administration of furosemide 0.5–1 mg/kg immediately following a transfusion is frequently effective. Transfusion-related acute lung injury (TRALI) is a severe, rare complication of transfusion. Patients develop severe acute respiratory distress characterized by difficulty breathing and pulmonary infiltrates on chest x-ray. Patients experiencing TRALI may require intensive supportive care, such as intubation and ventilatory support.

Hemolytic transfusion reactions may be acute or delayed. They may start with fever accompanied by abdominal or flank pain. Patients may experience a general sense of feeling unwell or agitated. Routine blood counts may demonstrate hemolysis as evidenced by decreased hemoglobin and haptoglobin and increased lactate dehydrogenase (LDH) and unconjugated bilirubin. Urinalysis may demonstrate urine hemoglobin in the absence of RBCs. When these symptoms occur in a patient with SCD, it can be challenging to distinguish a transfusion reaction from underlying hemolysis; however, additional data such as trending laboratory values, repeating the type and screen and direct Coombs test, and calculating the hemoglobin A% and hemoglobin S% may help identify the root cause of the hemolysis.

Because of the potential for a variety of transfusion-associated reactions, patients receiving transfusion should receive blood products in a setting that can provide infusion services and respond in a timely manner to any transfusion reactions. This generally means an inpatient setting or outpatient infusion clinic.

BOX 34.1 FDA-APPROVED NOVEL THERAPIES

Endari (L-glutamine)[132]

- Oral medication that reduces oxidative stress in sickle cell erythrocytes
- Indicated to reduce the acute complications of SCD in adult and pediatric patients 5 years of age and older
- Can help to decrease the number of pain crises in patients with SCD

Adakveo (crizanlizumab)[133]

- Anti-P-selectin monoclonal antibody
- Lowers the rate of VOC in patients with SCD by 45% compared to placebo in the SUSTAIN trial
- 30-minute IV infusion given every 4 weeks
- For use in patients 16 years of age and older

Oxbryta (voxelotor, GBT440)[134]

- Oxygen-affinity modulator
- Inhibits Hb S polymerization
- Prevents red blood cells from becoming deformed
- Significantly increases hemoglobin concentration
- Once-daily, oral therapy in adults and children 12 years of age and older

ALTERNATIVES TO TRANSFUSION

HYDROXYUREA

HU has emerged as a useful, disease-modifying therapy in SCD. It was approved by the US Food and Drug Administration (FDA) in 1998 for adults, as a treatment option for patients with SCD,[43] and in 2017, it was approved for use in children. In sickle cell anemia, administration of HU switches on production of fetal hemoglobin, decreasing the percentage of hemoglobin S, reticulocyte, and neutrophil counts and altering expression of adhesion molecules.[44] It has been shown to reduce the frequency of acute painful episodes and ACS, reduce the need for hospitalization, and reduce the frequency of blood transfusions in patients with SCD.[45] HU has also been associated with increased life expectancy for patients with SCD.

NOVEL TREATMENTS

Three new medications have become FDA approved for SCD since 2017. These new medications have the potential to decrease pain and long-term complications in patients (Box 34.1).

ERYTHROPOIETIN

Erythropoietin is produced by the kidney in response to anemia. Hematopoietic stem cells differentiate along the erythroid lineage in response to erythropoietin. There are two erythropoietin formulations, epoetin-alpha, which is administered 2–3 times a week, and darbepoetin, which is longer acting. Unfortunately, recent studies have led to FDA warnings about increased thromboembolic events and increased risk for cardiovascular events in patients taking these medications.[46] Poor patient survival in some studies where epoetin was used has again raised questions about whether epoetin may be a growth factor for some types of cancer. The American Society of Hematology and the American Society of Clinical Oncology caution against the use of epoetins in patients with malignancy who are not receiving either chemotherapy or radiation therapy.[46]

There have been theoretic concerns about erythropoietin use in SCD, especially in the absence of use with HU. These concerns include increasing the Hb S concentration, the number of Hb S-containing reticulocytes, and the hematocrit, thereby increasing the risk of hypertension and hyperviscosity.[47]

However, epoetin-alpha may be useful for patients who object to blood transfusions on ethical or religious grounds, as do many of the Jehovah's Witness faith.[48] Indeed, patients of the Jehovah's Witness faith have taught us that severe anemia can be better tolerated than was initially supposed.[49,50] Additionally, they have helped drive the interest in development of blood conservation programs and blood alternatives. Blood alternatives, such as hemoglobin-based oxygen carriers, are acellular hemoglobin molecules and are in clinical trials in Africa and other countries. As yet, none is available for clinical use in the United States, but they may have a future role in treatment of anemia.

BLOOD AND MARROW TRANSPLANT AND GENE THERAPY

The goal of transplantation of hematopoietic stem cells in SCD is to provide a permanent source of red blood cells that do not sickle. Healthy red blood cells are produced by the hematopoietic stem cells on a continuous basis and, similar to transfusions, address SCD by stopping further injury. Following a successful transplant, the patient is protected from further chronic organ injury and acute sickling events. Transplantation may be more efficacious than red blood cell transfusion for some organs such as the brain[51] since the episodic nature of transfusions likely cannot match a constant delivery of healthy red blood cells as occurs following a transplant.

Donor hematopoietic stem cells sources include bone marrow, umbilical cord blood, and the peripheral blood of donors who have received a stem cell–mobilizing agent. The best blood and marrow transplant (BMT) donors are HLA-matched siblings. Transplants using these donors, especially in younger recipients, have excellent outcomes in SCD in the modern era with an approximate disease-free survival rate of 92%.[52,53] As such, the indications for BMT are being refined to be more inclusive and treat patients with a SCD genotype associated with a severe phenotype (HbSS and HbS/beta-zero thalassemia) early in the disease course.[54] Unfortunately, most patients do not have an HLA-matched sibling donor, and alternative donor options are being explored such as unrelated marrow donors, unrelated donor cord blood, and HLA half-matched or haploidentical donors (parents, siblings). These donor options are generally reserved for more severely affected patients to balance the risk-benefit ratio and are performed as part of a clinical trial.

The risks of BMT include acute complications that are primarily due to the chemotherapy or radiation used in the pre-transplant preparative regimen (e.g., mucositis, nausea, hair loss, cytopenias requiring blood and platelet transfusions, neutropenic infections). The main acute complication arising from the BMT graft is acute graft versus host disease (GVHD), which is an immune-mediated attack of the recipient's skin, gastrointestinal (GI) tract, or liver by the donor T cells in the graft. The risk of severe acute GVHD, manifested as widely disseminated erythematous maculopapular rash, severe vomiting and diarrhea, and/or liver dysfunction is lowest in recipients of HLA-matched donor grafts (15%)[53] and is managed with systemic immunosuppression. Acute complications of BMT are generally managed inpatient and include intravenously delivered antiemetics, nasogastric feeding tubes, total parenteral nutrition, and PCAs. Nonpharmacologic approaches for symptoms include aromatherapy for nausea, massage, acupressure, and acupuncture (in non-neutropenic patients with appropriate platelet counts). The most widely used approaches to BMT for SCD involve myeloablative chemotherapy, and the typical hospitalization period is 4–6 weeks. This period can be particularly stressful as the patient is restricted to the room for infection prevention. Thus, a concerted effort is made to include coping strategies facilitated by a variety of healthcare professionals such as child life specialists, art therapists, music therapists, and child psychologists.

In the long term, chemotherapy can also cause organ toxicity, and patients are monitored annually after BMT for organ dysfunction.[55] Due to the multiple organ systems that can be affected, a multidisciplinary team of specialists including pulmonologists, endocrinologists, neurologists, and cardiologists perform assessments of organ function. Most patients may not experience significant organ toxicity; however, gonadal function can be particularly affected and the majority of girls (>70%) need hormone supplementation.[56] Counseling about fertility preservation prior to BMT is thus of great importance, with sperm and oocyte collection being routinely offered pre-BMT. Testicular or ovarian tissue collection and cryopreservation may also be offered at select sites with the appropriate expertise. The main long-term complication from the graft is chronic GVHD. It is manifested as skin and connective tissue fibrosis, resembling rheumatologic diseases such as scleroderma. Fortunately, chronic GVHD requiring long-term immune suppression after matched sibling transplant is rare (3%),[52] but it is an important consideration since the manifestations are varied and can significantly impact quality of life. This complication may be more common with other donor types,[57] but rates of chronic GVHD remain to be determined given the ongoing optimization of non-sibling transplant approaches.

While the benefit of being cured of SCD is significant, further work is needed to limit the toxicity of BMT. Only 20–25% of the bone marrow needs to be replaced to achieve a cure since healthy red blood cells last longer than sickle red blood cells.[58,59] As a result, less intense BMT regimens are becoming more commonplace. The goal is to reduce the intensity of the preparative regimen while still maintaining good long-term engraftment, preferably without the need for prolonged immune suppression. There is growing experience with chemotherapy-free preparative regimens in adults and pediatrics,[60–63] with a multicenter trial in pediatrics under way (Clinicaltrials.gov, NCT03587272). In this trial, the health-related quality of life will be assessed with the expectation that, without chemotherapy, quality of life will be preserved and possibly improved.

To avoid acute and chronic GHVD, gene therapies using the patient's own cells are being developed for SCD. Gene-based therapies for SCD are still early in clinical trials and have primarily involved gene transfer or gene editing of patient hematopoietic stem cells.[64] The first requires addition of a globin gene that can restore normal hemoglobin function and, in some cases, impart an anti-sickling effect to the red cell. The other strategy is to reinduce expression of fetal hemoglobin by targeting the "off-switch" *BCL11A* that normally stops the high level of fetal hemoglobin expression after the first year of life. This approach is expected to be beneficial in some of the same ways that HU is helpful, as fetal hemoglobin is not affected by the sickle mutation and has an anti-sickling effect. Future approaches still being evaluated in preclinical testing include correction of the sickle mutation using gene editing such as inducing double strand breaks and repair with a donor template[65] and also making corrections by replacing single bases.[66] The current unknowns about gene therapy include how efficacious these modalities will be; the longevity of the effects, especially with gene addition where there may be silencing of the transferred gene over time; and the long-term safety of making changes to the genome, including unintended off-target effects. The FDA has mandated 15 years of follow-up for all patients receiving gene modification to better understand these aspects.

Currently, chemotherapy-based conditioning is still used for gene therapy, so acute and long-term concerns still exist. However, as with BMT, there is a push to evaluate non-chemotherapy, non-radiation–based approaches such as a monoclonal antibody-based preparative regimen. An antibody targeting the cell surface marker CD117 on hematopoietic stem cells has been encouraging in animal models as a way to prepare the body for BMT.[67] With an antibody-based preparative regimen, there is the hope that gene therapy will represent a low-toxicity, highly efficacious, potentially curative strategy that will be available to essentially all patients.

The decision to proceed with a potentially curative therapy is a complex one and may be the most challenging scenario patients and families face regarding care for SCD. On the one hand, BMT is elective, and families must weigh the potential risks of the many possible complications including debilitating and life-threatening ones against the chance of disease eradication. On the other hand, electing to not proceed with a BMT leaves the patient at risk of ongoing complications and early mortality from SCD. The decision is made even more complex when considering when to proceed with such a therapy. While the best outcomes with the fewest complications occur when patients receive BMT at a younger age, a major complication or death as a young child would be grave. Historically, medical providers have waited for patients to have significant sequelae from their SCD, such as a stroke, before recommending the family consider BMT. However, this approach is becoming less common given the significantly improved outcomes of potentially curative therapies over the past few decades. As a result, families are informed about these therapies much earlier in their course, leading to HLA typing within the first year of life to determine if a matched sibling donor is available. Many families also store sibling umbilical cord blood in the event the new sibling is HLA-matched to the patient, as cord blood can be used for transplantation. The decision to proceed with transplant remains based on how risk-averse a patient or family is. Interestingly, a majority of patients (~70%) may accept anywhere from 5–30% mortality risk to achieve long-term disease eradication, and this does not seem to be impacted by disease severity. In contrast, only approximately 40% of these patients would proceed with a transplant that would leave them infertile.[68] Factors that may influence how patients make the decision to proceed to a transplant include presence of a strong support system, the availability of a matched sibling donor, and the education received about transplant.[69]

CONSIDERATIONS FOR ADOLESCENTS AND YOUNG ADULTS

Although once a life-limiting disease, adolescents, and young adults (AYAs) with SCD now survive into adulthood.[8] As a result, one major health challenge is helping AYAs transition from pediatric to adult care. Studies show that AYAs leave pediatric care without adequate preparation or readiness to transition.[70] AYAs express fear that their new adult provider will not know them, understand their disease process, or adequately treat their pain. The time period shortly after transition to adult care has been identified as a time for increased morbidity and mortality as AYAs often do not attach to a new adult hematology provider and use the emergency room as their source of primary care.[71] Transition must be a coordinated, systematic process, and it is critical that healthcare providers develop transition plans to support comprehensive care. Plans should include disease education, assessing transition readiness for both patient and parent, developing self-care management skills and advocacy, finding a new hematology adult care team, and navigating insurance issues. Successful transition has been linked to improved health outcomes, resulting in significant reductions in morbidity and mortality with decreased healthcare cost.[72] Dedicated transition programs are necessary to ensure a successful transition, and longitudinal studies are needed to understand the impact of SCD across the lifespan.

Clinical Vignette

David is an 18-year-old man with sickle cell anemia (Hb SS), moderate-persistent asthma, silent infarcts, and avascular necrosis. He lives at home with his mother and eight siblings. At 10 years of age, he was hospitalized for ACS with respiratory failure. His respiratory status quickly decompensated, and he was placed on extracorporeal membrane oxygenation (ECMO) and given an exchange transfusion. He developed necrosis of his tongue and a tracheostomy was placed. Due to aspiration, he required nasogastric tube feeds. He was discharged to an inpatient rehabilitation facility and received physical therapy, occupational therapy, and speech therapy. He was given oral ibuprofen or oxycodone 30 minutes prior to physical therapy to help him to manage his pain. His ability to independently participate in his activities of daily living (ADLs) gradually improved, and, by discharge, he was able to walk comfortably with a walker. His physical medicine and rehabilitation physician made sure he had a wheelchair prior to discharge home to help with longer distances. His tracheostomy was eventually downsized, capped, and then removed. Speech therapy helped him to manage his secretions due to his enlarged tongue. He was gradually reintroduced to oral purees, and his nasogastric tube was removed. An occupational therapist helped him improve his fine motor skills, hand-eye coordination, and cognitive abilities.

After 3 months, David was discharged home with a visiting nurse 3 days per week for 1 month to monitor for complications and provide additional support and family education. He received monthly blood transfusions in hematology clinic to give his lungs time to heal. His hematologist discussed the possibility of a BMT given the severity of his disease. However, after several months of consideration, his mother opted to proceed with disease-modifying therapies and declined HLA typing. He continued to receive outpatient physical therapy, speech therapy, and occupational therapy. He was home-schooled for 3 months to allow him to have more time to complete his therapies and blood transfusions. He was eventually transitioned off chronic blood transfusions and onto oral HU therapy. When he returned to school full-time, an IEP was implemented to help him successfully achieve his academic goals.

The severity and prolonged nature of David's illness was a significant family stressor. His mother continued to work during his hospitalization, although eventually she lost her job due to frequent unanticipated absences related to his care. His family was at risk of being evicted due to their inability to pay for rent, and his sickle cell social worker helped his mother to obtain Social Security income. He required nightly bilevel positive airway pressure (BIPAP) and was at an increased risk for illness due to the crowded nature of his home, so his social worker helped his mother obtain subsidized housing with a private room for David. He developed frequent enuresis after his hospitalization, which was likely a result of severe stress and decreased ability to concentrate urine related to his SCD. He began seeing a psychologist, and his enuresis gradually resolved.

In 2016, he began having frequent hip and leg pain requiring increasing amounts of oral pain medication. An MRI was done of his hips which showed severe bilateral avascular necrosis. He was seen by orthopedics and scheduled for core decompression. His mother was anxious about the surgery due to his past history, and, on the morning of surgery, she asked for the procedure to be postponed. His mother began receiving counseling, and his surgery was completed a few months later without complication. After surgery he continued to receive physical therapy for pain management and no longer required frequent oral pain medication.

Today, David is a freshman in college and has straight A's; he is majoring in English. He continues to be hospitalized approximately twice per year, usually for ACS or pain crisis. At home, his pain crises are managed with as needed ibuprofen or oxycodone. In the hospital, severe pain is managed with IV morphine and ketorolac; on occasion he uses a PCA pump. He is followed by multiple specialists, including hematology, pulmonary, nephrology, cardiology, and ophthalmology. He takes eight daily medications and continues to receive physical therapy once per week. His pain is generally well-controlled, and he is learning to independently manage his disease on his own.

OTHER ANEMIAS

BACKGROUND

Other primary anemias result from either increased red cell destruction due to structural or enzymatic defects or from decreased production of red blood cells in the bone marrow (Box 34.2). The *beta-thalassemias* are a group of genetic disorders that occur due to decreased beta-globin production.[73] Red blood cells are subsequently unstable and reactive oxygen species are formed, which damages the red blood cell membrane. This leads to hemolysis and abnormal erythroid maturation. The phenotype of beta-thalassemia can range from asymptomatic to severe, transfusion-dependent anemia, depending on the degree of beta-globin production. Symptoms of beta-thalassemia occur due to a combination of anemia and ineffective erythropoiesis. Phenotypic presentation is classified as beta-thalassemia minor (mild microcytic anemia without symptoms), beta-thalassemia intermedia (moderate microcytic anemia, requiring intermittent transfusions especially during acute illness), and beta-thalassemia major (severe microcytic anemia requiring chronic monthly transfusions).

Bone marrow failure syndromes are a group of rare genetic disorders that are characterized by hematopoietic aplasia and cancer predisposition.[74] Inherited bone marrow failure syndromes are often due to progenitor/stem cell defects. The precise pathophysiology of bone marrow syndromes is unclear, although nearly all show accelerated hematopoietic cell apoptosis. Numerous genetic defects are linked to the various inherited bone marrow failure syndromes.

Primary anemias are no longer strictly childhood illnesses. The ability to treat children with transfusion therapy has revolutionized the care of these children, extending life expectancy well into the sixth decade or beyond. In addition, BMTs are potentially curative for many of these diseases, allowing many more children to survive into adulthood.

Children with other advanced chronic medical conditions may also develop secondary anemias (Box 34.2). An immobile child with neurologic deficits may become anemic because an absence of weight-bearing activity can weaken bones and lead to fatty replacement of bone marrow. These children may have nutritional deficiencies of iron, folic acid, or B_{12},

BOX 34.2 ANEMIAS

PRIMARY ANEMIAS

Increased red blood cell destruction

- SCD, hemoglobin SS, SC, S beta-thalassemia
- Thalassemia
- Pyruvate kinase deficiency
- Hereditary spherocytosis
- Hereditary elliptocytosis
- Glucose-6-dehydrogenase deficiency

Decreased production of red blood cells (bone marrow failure syndromes)

- Fanconi anemia
- Congenital aplastic anemia
- Diamond-Blackfan anemia
- Shwachman-Diamond syndrome

SECONDARY ANEMIAS

- Bone marrow failure due to previous and/or concurrent cytotoxic drugs and/or radiation therapy
- Lack of marrow due to immobility, non–weight bearing
- Nutritional deficiencies including iron, folic acid, vitamin B_{12}, protein
- Anemia of chronic disease, including suppressive cytokines
- Infectious myelosuppression, most characteristically parvovirus
- Erythropoietin deficiency due to renal failure
- Acute and/or chronic hemorrhage due to primary disease
- Acquired antibodies from transfused products
- Autoimmune antibodies
- Hepatorenal failure
- Hemophagocytosis
- Drug-induced

BOX 34.3 SYMPTOMS OF ANEMIA

- Pallor
- Difficulty feeding
- Decreased appetite
- Fussiness in infants and toddlers
- Irritability
- Increased number of hours spent sleeping
- Fatigue
- Tachycardia
- Headache
- Increased awareness of heartbeat
- Lightheadedness on sitting or standing quickly
- Orthostatic hypotension
- Hypotension
- Poor tissue oxygenation
- Cardiomegaly
- Decreased urine output
- Muscle weakness

which can also contribute to anemia. Kidney disease causes anemia due to decreased production of erythropoietin. In these situations, transfusion is rarely required. Appropriate steps should be taken to detect and correct the underlying cause of the anemia.

SYMPTOMS AND MANAGEMENT

For children, symptoms related to anemia can extend far beyond fatigue (Box 34.3). For infants and toddlers, symptomatic anemia may be expressed by a decreased ability to nurse, take a bottle, or eat. Many a mother has made the simple statement that their infant or toddler "probably needs to be transfused" because the child just is not eating as well as usual. Administration of a transfusion can be the difference between a child who is able to eat consistently and one who is not eating well. For other children, anemia may be recognized by longer nap times, changes in temperament, or limitations in ability to engage in activities or play. All of these are important contributors to quality of life for families of children with life-threatening illness all along the illness trajectory.

Teenagers are more likely to present with classic symptoms associated with anemia. While fatigue or need for increased hours of sleep may be a part of their symptoms, they may also experience headaches, fast heart rate, feeling like their heart is pounding, or lightheadedness when rising to sit or stand. For teens, symptoms related to anemia can be apparent when the hemoglobin drops below 9 gm/dL, a level where younger children are often relatively asymptomatic.

Children who are chronically anemic may tolerate a lower level of hemoglobin before exhibiting symptoms. Sequelae of uncorrected severe chronic anemia include cardiomegaly, progressive decrease in exercise endurance, congestive heart failure, growth abnormalities, and pulmonary hypertension. Patients with uncorrected beta-thalassemia major suffer bony deformities and massive hepatosplenomegaly from extramedullary hematopoiesis.

Treatment of symptomatic anemia includes supportive care and treatment of the underlying cause. The cardinal rule is to not to treat a number, but to consider if anemia is causing any uncomfortable symptoms or hemodynamic instability. Transfusion of RBCs can be used for severe symptomatic anemia; however, it should be used cautiously if the underlying etiology is unknown. For example, in the case of iron deficiency anemia, while transfusion can be used for severe symptoms and hemodynamic instability, the blood transfusion may delay the bone marrow's drive to make new reticulocytes. Therefore, treatment of iron deficiency should be focused on iron supplementation, and blood transfusion should be reserved for severe cases.[75]

Chronic, monthly transfusion therapy may be used for symptom management in certain primary anemias. Hemolytic anemias, where there is frequent RBC turnover, can lead to jaundice, icterus, and splenomegaly in addition to the typical signs and symptoms of anemia.[76,77] Patients with chronic hemolysis are also at risk of biliary sludging and gallstones and may require early cholecystectomy. In addition, splenectomy can help decrease hemolysis. However, the risk of infections, pulmonary hypertension, and thrombosis after splenectomy should be weighed against the potential benefits of decreased hemolysis and improved anemia.[78] Folic acid replacement should be considered for conditions with high red cell turnover. Autoimmune hemolytic anemia may lead to acute and severe drops in hemoglobin. Prompt treatment is often required and consists of corticosteroids, immunoglobulins, and/or immunosuppressants.

TRANSFUSION SUPPORT

Patients with beta-thalassemia major require chronic monthly RBC transfusions to decrease symptomatic anemia and avoid the complications of extramedullary hematopoiesis. These transfusions are life-long unless the patient receives BMT or gene therapy. Patients with beta-thalassemia intermedia may become significantly anemic in the setting of acute illness, requiring intermittent transfusion support. Abnormal RBC production, or dyserythropoiesis, in patients with beta-thalassemia increases iron absorption from the diet. These two mechanisms of increased iron loading underscore the critical need for appropriate chelation therapy in this population. Cardiac iron overload can lead to heart failure and arrhythmias. Iron overload can affect growth and cause pancreatic dysfunction, as well as lead to skin discoloration, which is why it historically was called "bronze diabetes." Hepatic iron overload may lead to cirrhosis and, ultimately, liver failure.

Unfortunately, the use of IV or subcutaneous chelation has been identified as a source of discomfort and decreased quality of life in several studies. Nearly 50% of patients identified iron chelator injections as the most disliked component of therapy.[79,80] However, novel oral chelation agents have improved tolerability, and these medications are approved for use in children as young as 2 years. Frequent absences from work or school to receive chronic transfusions also negatively impact quality of life, yet on measures of overall health, transfused patients report improved physical fitness and better performance on daily activities. Despite the complication of iron overload and the need for chelation, regular transfusions appear to improve the quality of life in some populations with primary anemia.

As with transfusions for patients with SCD, patients with other primary anemias should receive ABO and RhD group-appropriate, crossmatch compatible RBCs. Often, these are leukoreduced units. Extended matching at RhCE and Kell may be performed for patients receiving chronic transfusion therapy but may be less critical in this population compared to patients with SCD.

Even with leukoreduction, some lymphocytes may be passed from blood donor to recipient. These lymphocytes have the potential, in immunocompromised individuals, to cause transfusion-associated GVHD (TA-GVHD). To prevent TA-GVHD, RBCs and other cellular components (platelets or granulocytes) are irradiated with a minimum of 25 Gy.[34] Patients with intact immune systems may not be at risk of TA-GVHD when transfused from unrelated donors; however, some centers universally irradiate blood products to ensure all patients are protected.[81] Irradiation does shorten the shelf-life of RBCs to less than 28 days, which has impacts on inventory and availability of blood products.

Faced with their child's need for transfusions many families inquire about having blood directly donated to the patient by family donors or friends of the family. It is often useful to check the motivation behind the request. For some, it is a fear of unknown donors and potential transmission of infection. For others, it is a way for extended family to provide support during a crisis. It is often sufficient to educate them with regard to general issues, such as the need for blood types to match, the safety of the blood supply, and the need for complete testing even when blood donation is directed. Additionally, there are many situations where family members are not the ideal donors or may even increase the chance of complications for the child.

The ideal donation scenario for family members to fully meet the transfusion needs of the child would be where infrequent transfusions were required and the transfusion can be anticipated days or weeks ahead. When donated blood is directed to a specific recipient, the blood bank has increased administrative burden in tracking and storing the blood. A directed donation is still required to undergo testing and processing, which, in an urgent or emergent situation, may delay transfusion. In addition, irradiation of these units prior to transfusion to the child is critical as the risk of causing TA-GVHD is higher in related donors. For patients who are candidates for BMTs, transfusions from family members are strongly discouraged. Siblings and, in some cases, parents are potential BMT donors. Blood transfusions before BMT can sensitize the patient to minor histocompatibility antigens from that donor which increases the risk of future graft failure.

For patients with primary anemia, families are often not suitable donors. For example, in sickle cell anemia, other family members may also have SCD or sickle cell trait. This makes the parents, and most siblings, inappropriate candidates for directed donation. Similarly, the frequency of transfusions for children with primary anemias can be more often than an individual is allowed to make blood donations. Additionally, the physical demands of frequent blood donation may add additional burden on a family already under stress from caring for an ill child. Finally, due to the higher emotional incentives for family and friends to donate for a specific patient, there may be a higher risk of transfusion-related infections than from an altruistic donor. A safer product is likely to come from a donor who has donated multiple times and therefore has been frequently screened.[82]

Many friends and family want to donate blood in an effort to help. One recommendation is to encourage donation, but not designate the donation for a specific recipient. In this way, the precious resources are built up for the community and donors receive a sense of having helped someone in need. In fact, having a blood drive is an often-employed way for a community group to show support for a community member fighting illness.

ALTERNATIVES TO TRANSFUSION

Erythropoietin may be considered for some patients as an alternative to transfusion (see the section "Erythropoietin").

BLOOD AND MARROW TRANSPLANT AND GENE THERAPY (THALASSEMIAS, BONE MARROW FAILURE SYNDROMES)

As discussed with SCD, transplantation of hematopoietic stem cells from a healthy donor is an alternative option to transfusion in cases of primary anemias or bone marrow failure. In general, transfusion-dependent thalassemias are viewed as meeting criteria for BMT. Patients who need intermittent transfusions usually are not considered candidates as the benefits may not outweigh the risks. HLA-matched donor outcomes are best, and alternative donor options such as mismatched related or unrelated donors are still being evaluated.[83] BMT earlier in the disease course, prior to the development of the sequelae of iron overload, is associated with better outcomes. The same considerations regarding acute and chronic side effects of chemotherapy and radiation as discussed for SCD are applicable. An important consideration for thalassemia is that since the disease can be well managed in developed nations, the improvements in quality of life can be modest and make more risky transplants with alternative donors less appealing. Thus, gene therapy, which avoids the immune complications of graft rejection and GVHD, may become a more robust approach compared to alternative donor BMT. In general, the same gene therapy strategies that are being used for SCD are also applicable for thalassemia major. To date, gene addition strategies have been most effective in certain genotypes of beta-thalassemia, with some genotypes being more likely to become transfusion-independent following gene therapy.[84] Knowing a patient's genotype, as well as phenotype, may help in counseling the patient and their family about therapeutic options. In addition, gene editing trials are currently under way. Like SCD, efficacy and safety remain to be evaluated long term, and patients will be monitored for 15 years. Gene therapy is approved conditionally in Europe.[85]

Regarding bone marrow failure, while anemia may be addressed by RBC transfusion, there are other concerns such as other cytopenias and potential development of malignant hematological disease that make BMT more attractive. Given the potential benefit, both HLA-matched and alternative donor transplants are regularly pursued in patients with bone marrow failure. For patients with an inherited bone marrow failure syndrome, there may be a genetic predisposition not only for dysfunctional hematopoiesis, but also increased sensitivity and toxicity from chemotherapy in a preparative regimen. *Fanconi anemia* is particularly known for this, and attempts to improve mortality rates have led to greatly reduced chemotherapy-containing regimens prior to transplant.[86] To a lesser extent, the same is done for *dyskeratosis congenita* as the toxicity is not as severe as in Fanconi anemia.[87] In cases of idiopathic bone marrow failure, typically characterized as *aplastic anemia*, patients who meet the definition of severe aplastic anemia (absolute neutrophil count <500/mcL, reticulocyte count <20–40,000/mcL, platelets <20,000/mcL) are considered eligible for transplant. The preparative regimen is more immune targeted as opposed to myeloablative, so it is fairly well tolerated.

In the genetic-based diseases where the allogeneic donor transplant approaches continue to be challenging, gene therapy techniques are being developed. Fanconi anemia is characterized by a complex set of mutations in one of 16 different complementation groups and associated genes that ultimately lead to impaired DNA repair and genomic instability.[88] Thus, a universal gene-based strategy to cure the disease remains challenging, but there have been promising preclinical results that have recently led to early phase clinical trials.[89,90] The benefit of an autologous genetic therapy in combination with non-chemotherapy–based conditioning would be highly impactful and improve patient quality of life.

HEMOPHILIA/HEREDITARY BLEEDING DISORDERS

BACKGROUND

Primary plasma coagulation disorders are best represented by hemophilia. *Hemophilia* is an X-linked disorder that causes a deficiency of a plasma clotting factor. The most common type of hemophilia is hemophilia A, which is due to factor VIII deficiency. Hemophilia B is due to factor IX deficiency. Patients with severe hemophilia have less than 1% of normal factor VIII or IX in their blood. Patients with moderate hemophilia have 1–5% of normal factor levels. Patients with mild hemophilia have 6–49% of normal factor levels.[91]

In the past 70 years, hemophilia has transitioned from a potentially lethal disorder to a chronic illness, with a marked improvement in quality of life and normal life expectancy. In the 1960s, the average life expectancy of patients with hemophilia was less than 20 years. With the advent of plasma transfusion in 1950s, cryoprecipitate in the 1960s, and factor concentrate use in the early 1970s, the expected average life span increased to 68 years.[92]

Unfortunately, with the emergence of HIV/AIDS in the 1970s and 1980s, many patients with hemophilia were infected through plasma-derived factor infusions.[93] The safety of factor replacement products significantly improved after the introduction of widespread testing of blood donations for HIV-1 in 1985, hepatitis C in 1990, and HIV-2 in 1992.[94] The use of recombinant products, which are not derived from healthy blood donors, further improved the safety of these medications. However, adults with hemophilia may be living with the sequelae of these infections, requiring collaborative care between hematology providers and specialists in treating these infectious diseases.[95]

With improved life spans, people with hemophilia are becoming adults and need to cope with social pressures: employment, social adjustment, sexual function, and problems that come with aging, such as coronary artery disease, diabetes, and Alzheimer's. Hemophilia Treatment Centers (HTCs) now focus on quality of life due to advances in treatments for what was a lethal disorder 80 years ago.

Secondary failure of the plasma coagulation system, manifested by multiple factor deficiencies, is seen in severe liver disease, disseminated intravascular coagulation (DIC), or vitamin K deficiency. Testing specific factor levels, reviewing medication or ingestion history, as well as clinical history, may discriminate between these potential mechanisms of secondary coagulopathy.

SYMPTOMS AND MANAGEMENT

Patients with hemophilia may present with easy bruising and excessive bleeding even with mild injury. Spontaneous hemorrhage can also occur, which can present as large bruises and hematomas, severe pain and swelling of the joints, excessive nosebleeds, blood in the urine or stool, and irritability/neurologic changes. Bleeding in certain areas, such as the eyes, brain, throat, or GI tract, can be life-threatening.

Intra-articular hemorrhage is one of the most common clinical presentations in patients with hemophilia, especially those with severe factor deficiency. Typically, hemarthroses first present in infants and toddlers as they start to do weight-bearing activities. The affected joint is often painful, may have limited range of motion, and is inflamed, warm, and erythematous.[96] If hemarthrosis is suspected, the immediate treatment is factor replacement. In addition to bleeding control, pain management is crucial. Rest, ice, compression, and elevation (RICE) of the affected joint can relieve some pain. Splinting, temporary immobilization, and physical therapy may also provide some benefit. Cryo cuffs, which provide cooling and bracing to the involved joint, provide pain relief and decrease swelling and inflammation. In addition, acetaminophen and opioids can be used as needed for pain management. NSAIDs and aspirin should be avoided as these medications can further increase the risk of bleeding. Specific cyclooxygenase (COX)-2 inhibitors may be considered to treat inflammation.[97] Arthrocentesis may be considered for severe pain that does not respond to the aforementioned treatments, in cases of neurovascular compromise, or if there is concern for infection.

Target joints, which are joints with three recurrent episodes of intra-articular hemorrhage in 6 months or four episodes in 1 year may develop arthropathy. Arthropathy remains one of the most common morbidities in patients with hemophilia. Repeated joint bleeds lead to hemosiderin deposition within the joint, which in turn leads to chronic synovial inflammation. The iron deposition also leads to cartilage damage and degradation.[98] Arthropathy causes decreased range of motion and chronic joint pain and can severely impact ADLs and quality of life. Decreased mobility can lead to contractures, osteopenia, and muscular weakness. The best way to treat arthropathy is to prevent it altogether. Thus, prophylactic use of regular factor replacement is used to prevent recurrent joint bleeds and is generally used in patients with severe factor deficiency. Physical therapy and surgical intervention (i.e., synovectomy, total knee arthroplasty) may also be indicated.[96]

Acute muscle bleeds are treated in a fashion similar to that for acute intra-articular bleeds. Treatments include factor replacement, RICE, slow return to activity, physical therapy, and pain management. Particular attention should be given to iliopsoas hemorrhage because such bleeds can lead to large-volume blood loss into the muscle bed. Immediate factor replacement is often warranted for these bleeds. In addition, continuous infusion of factor and surgical intervention may be required.[96,97,99,100]

Intracranial hemorrhage (ICH) can contribute to significant morbidity and mortality.[101] The incidence of ICH in patients with severe hemophilia is approximately 4% in the neonatal period and 2–2.5% beyond the neonatal period. Symptoms of ICH include severe headaches, strokes, seizures, coma, or death. ICH is an emergency and should be treated promptly with factor replacement.[99,100] Of note, factor replacement should occur immediately if head trauma is suspected and should not be delayed for imaging to confirm the presence of ICH.[102] Neurosurgical consultation is required if imaging does show hemorrhage.

FACTOR REPLACEMENT THERAPY

Factor VIII and Factor IX replacement products include plasma-derived concentrates and recombinant products. Many patients with severe hemophilia self-infuse prophylactic factor three to four times per week. Novel factor products with longer half-lives are approved to treat hemophilia A and B. These products decrease the frequency of IV dosing which can significantly improve quality of life for patients with hemophilia.

Acute bleeds often require additional doses of factor. For minor bleeds, a single dose of factor may be sufficient to stop bleeding. Major hemorrhages require higher doses with subsequent infusions to maintain the patient at a sufficient trough factor level.

Some patients with hemophilia develop a neutralizing antibody, or inhibitor, to the treatment product.[103] Developing an inhibitor is one of the most serious complications of hemophilia because treatment of bleeds becomes more complicated. Patients with low titer inhibitors may be treated with higher amounts or increased frequency of factor. Bypassing agents can be used to treat bleeding episodes in patients with high titer inhibitors. Bypassing agents activate alternative coagulation factors, rather than replacing the missing factor. Some products are available that can mimic factor VIII without being affected by inhibitors. Immune tolerance induction therapy, which involves giving large amounts of daily factor, can be attempted to try to induce tolerance in the patient's immune system and decrease the levels of the inhibitor.

ALTERNATIVES TO FACTOR REPLACEMENT

Given the burden of frequent IV dosing and infusions, risk of inhibitor formation, and variable effect of bypassing agents in patients who have formed inhibitors, more effective and less burdensome medications have been developed. These new classes of agents enhance coagulation or inhibit anticoagulant pathways, circumventing the need for Factor VIII or Factor IX. In patients with and without inhibitors, treatment with these novel medications have resulted in significantly decreased bleeding episodes.[104] Emicizumab is a bispecific antibody that functions as a Factor VIIIa mimetic and brings together Factor IXa and Factor X to initiate coagulation. It is administered subcutaneously, at weekly, biweekly, or 4-week intervals.

Several additional medications are under development. Fitusiran is an RNA molecule that impairs expression of antithrombin, which is an innate anticoagulant. Tissue factor pathway inhibitor (TFPI) is an enzyme that controls clotting and slows clot initiation. Several agents have been developed to inhibit TFPI and are beginning to show clinical promise. Both of these mechanisms decrease the amount of endogenous anticoagulation and rebalance the hemostatic system, allowing for improved clot formation in patients with hemophilia.[104] These advances will hopefully decrease bleeding episodes, while also decreasing the therapeutic burden of treatment.

There are rare factor deficiencies that do not have recombinant or plasma-derived factor concentrates available. In these situations, or when a factor deficiency is suspected but has not yet been identified, replacement with plasma from healthy donors will replace any missing factors and resolve bleeding. Plasma is typically dosed at 10–15 mL/kg body weight infused over 2 hours. Cryoprecipitate, which is a concentrated blood product that contains high levels of Factor VIII, fibrinogen, and von Willebrand factor, may also be used to correct bleeding depending on the deficiency identified or suspected. One unit of cryoprecipitate per 5–10 kg of body weight is sufficient to raise the fibrinogen level. Prothrombin complex concentrates (PCCs) are enriched for several factors including Factor II, Factor VII, Factor IX, Factor X, protein C or protein S. These products are human-derived, but heat-treated and highly purified. They may be used to correct specific factor deficiencies and vitamin K–related deficiencies due to medications or diet or decrease bleeding in patients with hemophilia and inhibitors. Vitamin K administered IV or orally may also be indicated to promote hemostasis.[105]

Recombinant factor VIIa (rFVIIa) has also been successfully used to treat bleeding episodes in patients with bleeding disorders, including patients with hemophilia and inhibitors and platelet disorders. It has been studied in episodes of severe bleeding in patients who do not have an underlying coagulation defect, but clinical outcomes remain mixed.[106] rFVIIa and additional supportive measures to stop bleeding, such as local control, antifibrinolytics, and DDAVP, are further discussed later in this chapter.

GENE THERAPY

There have been great advances in the development of gene-based therapies for hemophilia in the past few decades.[107] Advances have been most notable in hemophilia B, owing to the smaller gene that would need to be transferred. The most common target organ for gene therapy in hemophilia has been the liver. The liver is a somatic organ with relatively low cell turnover, which allows for gene transfer that does not have to be permanently integrated into the cell. The benefit of keeping the gene expression in the cell, but not integrated into the genome, is that there is less risk for mutagenesis. However, given that the liver cannot be feasibly explanted for gene modification, the gene-transfer vectors are usually administered intravenously into a vessel that feeds the liver. The patient's immune system can limit the efficacy of this approach if either the viral vector for gene delivery or the actual factor protein to be produced leads to a neutralizing immune response. To date, these have been addressed by not performing gene therapy in patients with inhibitors, as well as treating recipients with a short course of systemic corticosteroids to mitigate the immune response.[108] Early-phase clinical trials have reported clinically relevant levels of factor which are expected to reduce the rate of severe bleeding episodes and need for infusion of factor.[107] However, there is still room for this approach to be optimized, such as restoring factor activity to a normal level with concomitant prevention of mild to moderate bleeding that can lead to morbidity. Long-term efficacy and safety data are still needed as development of neutralizing antibodies may occur later on, and there is also newer data suggesting that vector integration in the genome may occur.

Hemophilia A has been more challenging to treat despite being more common than hemophilia B due to the normal gene being too large to be delivered by vectors currently being explored. More recently, smaller genes have been tested in preclinical models and shown promise in hemophilia A.[109] This has led to ongoing clinical trials with encouraging results to date.[107]

CONSIDERATIONS FOR ADOLESCENTS AND YOUNG ADULTS

AYAs must learn to accept increasing responsibility for their condition, including self-injection, ordering supplies, and attending appointments. Adherence is often low during the transition period, and lack of adherence can lead to recurrent joint bleeds, decreased quality of life, and chronic pain.[110] Patients with hemophilia must consider restrictions when choosing employment opportunities, such as the inability to stand all day and the physical demands of a job. Approximately 80% of hemophilia patients reported that their condition had a negative impact on employment, and 22% believed they had lost a job because of it.[110] It is important to acknowledge these challenges and address them during the transition period. Transition programs should take an interdisciplinary approach and involve the entire family. Early planning and gradual transition help the patient begin to navigate the complexity of their disease and take full responsibility for their care.

BOX 34.4 THROMBOCYTOPENIA

PRIMARY THROMBOCYTOPENIA

- Amegakaryocytic thrombocytopenia
- Thrombocytopenia and absent radii syndrome
- Platelet dysfunction Glanzmann thrombasthenia
- Bernard-Soulier syndrome

SECONDARY THROMBOCYTOPENIA

- Aplastic anemia
- Autoimmune destruction
- Bone marrow failure due to previous and/or concurrent cytotoxic drugs and or radiation therapy
- Encroachment of marrow space with tumor
- Bone overgrowth, osteopetrosis
- Lack of marrow due to immobility and/or non–weight bearing
- Infectious myelosuppression
- Increased destruction associated with infection and fever

PLATELET DISORDERS

BACKGROUND

Platelet failure may be due to abnormal numbers or abnormal function (Box 34.4). Both of these may be primary, due to an intrinsic platelet disorder, or secondary due to underlying disease. Frequent platelet transfusions can lead to the development of alloimmunization against platelet antigens, which in turn can worsen thrombocytopenia due to increased platelet destruction.

PRIMARY THROMBOCYTOPENIA

Amegakaryocytic thrombocytopenia is a rare inherited failure of platelet production due to mutations in c-mpl, the thrombopoietin receptor, in about 50% of cases.[111] The disorder has a tendency for malignant transformation. Platelet transfusions are essential in the support of these patients as they await definitive therapy with BMT.

Thrombocytopenia and absent radii (TAR) syndrome is an inherited autosomal recessive disorder with characteristic radial abnormalities and thrombocytopenia. The disorder presents at birth, and, in most cases, the platelet count improves so that most patients achieve a platelet count sufficient to suppress hemorrhage by 1 year of age. Platelet transfusions to maintain platelet count greater than 20,000/mcL is both life-saving and greatly improves the quality of life of these children. The requirement for transfusion usually decreases during the first year of life.

PRIMARY PLATELET DYSFUNCTION

Primary platelet dysfunction, in general, causes mild bleeding problems. Only two disorders, *Glanzmann thrombasthenia* and *Bernard-Soulier syndrome*, could be classified as life-threatening.[112] Both are genetic defects affecting the critical platelet receptors for fibrin and von Willebrand factor, respectively. Infants with severe Glanzmann thrombasthenia present early in life. Severe hemorrhages are responsive to platelet transfusion, but sensitization to platelet antigens makes the long-term use of platelet transfusion therapy difficult. Bernard-Soulier syndrome is less severe, and patients have a reasonable quality of life when supported with the judicious use of platelets.[113]

SYMPTOMS AND MANAGEMENT

Thrombocytopenia first manifests with petechial rash on the skin and mucosal membranes which can coalesce into purpuric lesions. Bleeding gums and nosebleeds can result from thrombocytopenia and are primarily treated with supportive care. However, prolonged and severe bleeds may require a combination of platelet transfusion, otolaryngology consultation, and/or dedicated packing. Typically, the frequency and severity of bleeding improves after the platelet count improves.[114] Other bleeding manifestations can include hematuria, menorrhagia, scleral hemorrhage, and retinal hemorrhage. GI bleeding, when present, should be treated as an emergency, and patients with GI bleeding should be promptly evaluated by a medical provider. Administer platelet and RBC transfusions as required. Consider consulting gastroenterology for severe GI bleeds. Intracranial hemorrhage is the most significant and life-threatening form of bleeding (Box 34.5). Any head trauma in a patient with thrombocytopenia, especially in one whose level is lower than 30,000/mcL, should be evaluated promptly. Head imaging is required to rule out hemorrhage, and neurological status should be monitored closely. If hemorrhage is present, consult neurosurgery. Treat underlying causes of thrombocytopenia, and use platelet transfusions to maintain platelet counts above at least 100,000/mcL.[115] Of note, the platelet thresholds for transfusions may differ slightly in different institutions; therefore, refer to the institution's standard practice guidelines.

Causes of secondary platelet dysfunction, such as renal disease, medication administration, or autoimmune destruction, are far more common than primary platelet disorders though the symptoms often overlap. Hemorrhage secondary

BOX 34.5 SYMPTOMS OF THROMBOCYTOPENIA

- Petechiae
- Easy bruising
- Purpura
- Nosebleeds
- Gums bleeding
- Menorrhagia
- Hematuria
- Subconjunctival hemorrhage
- Retinal hemorrhage
- Intracranial hemorrhage

to platelet dysfunction is best exemplified by renal disease. As renal function decreases and blood urea nitrogen levels increases to higher than 50 mg/dL, platelet dysfunction becomes clinically significant.[116] Menorrhagia and nosebleeds are the most common clinical manifestation and the most disruptive to day-to-day living.

Bleeding, particularly visible bleeding, is a very distressing event for families, particularly for those involved in terminal care. However, home transfusion of platelets, though effective in resolving bleeding in thrombocytopenic patients, is not always available. In these circumstances, a few simple maneuvers can help minimize the distress of terminal bleeding should it occur. Most importantly, the caregivers should be warned of the possibility of terminal bleeding and plans discussed. They should be encouraged to remain calm and remain with the child rather than leave to seek help or supplies. Minor gum bleeding may be lessened by application of a dampened tea bag to the child's gums. Dark-colored towels and linens make the amount of blood lost less distressing for anyone present.

TRANSFUSION SUPPORT IN THROMBOCYTOPENIA

As needed, patients with thrombocytopenia or platelet dysfunction may benefit from platelet transfusions. Platelets may come as pools once separated from whole blood donations or from a single donor as an apheresis product. The goal of platelet transfusion is to decrease the incidence of spontaneous bleeding, which may be distressing to patients or families. Patients with platelet levels of less than 10,000/mcL are typically at highest risk of bleeding complications, but thresholds for transfusion may vary, especially if there is a need for invasive procedures or evidence of active bleeding. For high-risk bleeding, platelets may be maintained above a goal of 100,000/mcL. Single-donor apheresis platelets are preferred in many pediatric institutions to limit the number of donor exposures. Platelets are stored at room temperature in plasma and have a shelf life of 5–7 days. Newer storage solutions, called platelet additive solutions (PAS), dilute the amount of plasma in the platelet product, which has been shown to decrease rates of allergic reactions to platelets.[117,118] Platelet and plasma products which have undergone pathogen inactivation, which are additional steps to cause damage to potential infectious agents without harming the product, are becoming increasingly available worldwide. These represent an extra layer of protection for vulnerable patients, especially against emerging pathogens or pathogens to which no donor screening test is available.[119]

A dose of 5–10 mL/kg of platelets should result in a 50,000/mcL to 100,000/mcL increase in platelet count. Most patients weighing more than 50 kg can receive a single apheresis platelet and achieve an appropriate increase. Platelets can be transfused over 30–60 minutes. If platelets are being actively consumed due to the patient's condition, frequent transfusions may become necessary. Post-transfusion platelet counts can help identify the reason for the need for frequent platelet transfusions. Platelets from ABO, Rh, and HLA-matched donors may be used to improve platelet response by decreasing immune-mediated destruction. Platelets may be volume-reduced to avoid volume overload or excessive exposure to plasma.

ALTERNATIVES TO TRANSFUSION

In all patients with bleeding, first-line management is local control through the application of pressure, gauze, cauterization, sutures, topical thrombin, or fibrin sealants as appropriate. In patients with Glanzmann's thrombasthenia or Bernard-Soulier syndrome, platelet transfusions control bleeding; however, they may lead to sensitization to HLA antigens or to platelet specific antigens. This can compromise the efficacy of further platelet transfusions; therefore, other methods to control bleeding are essential. Recombinant Factor VIIa, which activates the extrinsic coagulation pathway, has been shown to successfully treat surgical and spontaneous bleeding in patients with platelet disorders.[120]

Antifibrinolytics, such as aminocaproic acid or tranexamic acid, prevent dissolution of clots. These medications are especially helpful with mucosal bleeding, such as epistaxis or oral bleeding, as well as prolonged menstrual bleeding in the setting of thrombocytopenia or functional platelet disorders. However, their potential role to limit surgical, postpartum, and traumatic bleeding is under active investigation.[121] Aminocaproic acid comes in tablets, liquid, and IV preparations. Typical dosing is 50–100 mg/kg every 6 hours; however, a loading dose of 200 mg/kg of body weight may be considered. Patients may experience nausea, vomiting, abdominal pain, and dizziness, especially at higher doses.

DDAVP (desmopressin) is available IV or subcutaneously and is administered at a dose of 0.03 mg/kg. It can also be delivered intranasally, one puff for children and two puffs for adults. It is a synthetic analogue of a pituitary hormone that controls renal water excretion, but it has been shown to increase Factor VIII levels in patients with hemophilia and von Willebrand disease. The mechanism of action in patients with platelet disorders is less well understood but may be through enhanced platelet/blood vessel interactions.[122] As DDAVP administration results in decreased water excretion, placing the patient on strict fluid restriction is important to avoid hyponatremia.

Hormonal contraception or intrauterine devices are also successful in limiting bleeding in patients with significant menorrhagia due to underlying platelet or bleeding disorders. Immune-mediated thrombocytopenia may be treated with expectant management in pediatric patients, or steroids or IV immunoglobulins in the setting of bleeding.

BLOOD AND MARROW TRANSPLANT

The use of BMT for thrombocytopenia outside of the context of bone marrow failure syndromes is limited to small case series in patients who have thrombocytopenia in the context of platelet dysfunction.[123] There are insufficient data to routinely consider BMT, and patients are generally considered if there are recurrent episodes of severe or life-threatening bleeds despite adequate medication use and transfusion therapy and/or the development of antiplatelet antibodies. In the latter case, there is risk of severe bleeding and graft failure with BMT. Additionally, BMT is likely to be reserved for the few patients who have a suitable HLA-matched sibling donor who is not affected by the same platelet disorder. Thus, BMT remains rarely used as it is not immediately clear that the benefits outweigh the risks for the majority of patients.

THROMBOSIS

BACKGROUND

Venous thromboembolism (VTE), including deep vein thrombosis (DVT) or pulmonary embolism (PE), are rare events in pediatric patients. However, rates in hospitalized children are 100–1,000 times greater than their peers. Inflammatory conditions such as inflammatory bowel disease or SCD, inherited thrombophilias, and anatomic variants such as May-Thurner anomaly, increase a patient's risk of VTE; however, up to 90% of pediatric VTEs are catheter-associated. Central lines are an essential component of the care of ill children. They can be accessed instead of placing IVs or drawing blood, limiting the number of sticks a patient must endure. However, these centrally placed, permanent or semi-permanent catheters disrupt the lining of blood vessels and impair flow through the vasculature, creating a perfect opportunity for a clot to form.[124]

SYMPTOMS AND MANAGEMENT

Acutely, patients may present with pain, swelling, or color change in the affected limb. The primary treatment for thromboses is anticoagulation, which is needed to hinder clot progression, embolization, and post-thrombotic syndrome (PTS).[125,126] Supportive care and clinical monitoring are used for symptomatic control. Pulmonary emboli can lead to chest pain, palpitations, and respiratory distress with hypoxia, shortness of breath, and increased work of breathing. Oxygen administration may alleviate some discomfort related to the respiratory distress, and pain medications can be helpful if there is any chest pain. As with DVTs, anticoagulation should be started as soon as possible.[125] Urgent evaluation is necessary if a clot is suspected.

Late effects of thromboses are influenced by the size, severity, and location of the VTE. PTS is a chronic condition that may develop weeks to months after a DVT. PTS is due to delayed venous return through the affected vein, in part due to valvular damage. Often occurring following a DVT in the leg, patients may experience chronic pain, swelling, skin changes, and ulceration. They may feel tingling, cramps, and heaviness in the limb, especially after long periods of standing. PTS is well described in adults, but underdiagnosed and poorly understood in children.[127] Recent studies have suggested that PTS occurs in about 26% of pediatric patients with DVTs and can lead to chronic pain even decades after the resolution of the DVT.[128] The symptoms of PTS have been shown to have a significant impact on quality of life. Mainstays of treatment for PTS include supportive management, examples being physical therapy and compression stockings. The use of pharmacologic treatments in PTS is debatable and currently does not show any significant benefits.[127,128]

Clots in other critical organs, such as the liver or kidney, may cause long-term damage that requires monitoring.

There is a long experience using anticoagulation in pediatric patients with acute VTEs; however, much of the data are extrapolated from adult studies. Initial therapy is often with unfractionated heparin, which potentiates endogenous anticoagulants to limit further clot formation and enhance clot resolution. Unfractionated heparin is administered as an IV infusion and frequent monitoring is necessary to adjust the dose. Patients may transition to low-molecular-weight heparins or fondaparinux, which are administered as subcutaneous injections, for outpatient management. Warfarin, a vitamin K antagonist, is an oral medication that has been used to treat acute VTEs in pediatric patients; however, levels are greatly affected by diet and concomitant medications. Close monitoring and dosing adjustments are required. At initiation of dosing, warfarin decreases levels of vitamin K-dependent anticoagulant factors in the blood faster than it decreases the procoagulant factors in the blood, which may result in an increased risk of thrombosis if a secondary anticoagulant (such as heparin) is not initially used.

Direct oral anticoagulants (DOACs), which work to directly inhibit thrombin (Factor IIa) or Factor Xa, require less routine monitoring or adjustment. Oral administration is desirable in a palliative setting so that injections can be avoided. In a pediatric study comparing rivaroxaban, an oral Factor Xa inhibitor, to standard anticoagulation in the treatment of VTE, there were similarly low VTE recurrence rates without evidence of increased bleeding.[129]

If the VTE is related to a catheter, but the catheter is no longer in use, it may be removed after initiation of anticoagulation. However, if the catheter is still functional and necessary, it may be possible to treat the patient with anticoagulation to resolve the symptoms without the need to replace the central line.[124] For catheter related VTEs, treatment for 3 months is generally recommended; however, duration of therapy may be varied depending on the presence of ongoing or additional risk factors, as well as response to therapy. Consultation with a specialist is recommended.

Early and aggressive anticoagulation with thrombolysis for acute VTE may decrease the likelihood of subsequent PTS; however, these treatments increase the risk of bleeding unless strict eligibility criteria are applied.[130] In a palliative setting, thrombolysis may not achieve the goals of care, so this therapy should be individualized. Patients suffering from PTS may derive some benefit from physical therapy, sequential compression devices, or graduated elastic compression stockings; however, response to therapies should be regularly assessed.[131]

PREVENTION

To prevent VTEs, patients being cared for in a hospital setting should engage in activities that encourage movement and early ambulation. Graduated compression stockings or mechanical compression devices may be used for those patients who are on bed rest, though skin care underneath should be optimized. In patients with a history of VTE, central venous line, or other risk factors, consideration should be given to the use of preventative low-dose anticoagulation while the patient is hospitalized or for the duration of the central venous line. Though studies are lacking, the DOACs may have a role in the prevention of VTEs in hospitalized patients.

CONCLUSION

Patients suffering from hematologic conditions require interdisciplinary care over the course of their lifetimes. The underlying disease guides clinicians in their therapeutic options. Symptom management needs to be individualized and tailored based on patient response. The psychological, emotional, and social needs of the patient need to be considered when developing a care plan as these all impact patient wellness and quality of life. AYA populations are particularly at risk for poor health outcomes, so patients in this critical period require developmentally appropriate support and care.

AUTHORS' NOTE

Authors JC, PP, LH, and JW have no relevant conflicts of interest to disclose. AA is a paid consultant with Sangamo Therapeutics. BSB is a paid speaker with Novartis Pharmaceuticals.

REFERENCES

1. Grant M, Elk R, Ferrell B, Morrison RS, von Gunten CF. Current status of palliative care: Clinical implementation, education, and research. *CA Cancer J Clin.* 2009;59(5):327–335.
2. Mohanti BK. Research focus in palliative care. *Indian J Palliat Care.* 2011;17(Suppl):S8–S11.
3. Muriel AC, Wolfe J, Block SD. Pediatric palliative care and child psychiatry: A model for enhancing practice and collaboration. *J Palliat Med.* 2016;19(10):1032–1038.
4. Gray NA, Horton JR, Dionne-Odom JN, Smith CB, Johnson KS. Update in hospice and palliative care. *J Palliat Med.* 2016;19(5):559–565.
5. World Health Organization (WHO). WHO Definition of Palliative Care. 2020. https://www.who.int/cancer/palliative/definition/en/
6. Ware RE, de Montalembert M, Tshilolo L, Abboud MR. Sickle cell disease. *Lancet.* 2017;390(10091):311–323.
7. Rees DC, Williams TN, Gladwin MT. Sickle-cell disease. *Lancet.* 2010;376(9757):2018–2031.
8. Shook LM, Farrell CB, Kalinyak KA, et al. Translating sickle cell guidelines into practice for primary care providers with Project ECHO. *Med Educ Online.* 2016;21:33616.
9. Centers for Disease Control and Prevention (CDC). Data & statistics on sickle cell disease. 2019. https://www.cdc.gov/ncbddd/sicklecell/data.html.
10. Fixler J, Styles L. Sickle cell disease. *Pediatr Clin North Am.* 2002;49(6):1193–1210, vi.
11. Benjamin L. Pain management in sickle cell disease: Palliative care begins at birth? *Hematology Am Soc Hematol Educ Program.* 2008:466–474.
12. Hargrave DR, Wade A, Evans JP, Hewes DK, Kirkham FJ. Nocturnal oxygen saturation and painful sickle cell crises in children. *Blood.* 2003;101(3):846–848.
13. Ballas SK, Darbari DS. Review/overview of pain in sickle cell disease. *Complement Ther Med.* 2020;49:102327.
14. Santos J, Jones S, Wakefield D, Grady J, Andemariam B. Patient controlled analgesia for adults with sickle cell disease awaiting admission from the emergency department. *Pain Res Manag.* 2016;2016:3218186.
15. Ballas SK, Kanter J, Agodoa I, et al. Opioid utilization patterns in United States individuals with sickle cell disease. *Am J Hematol.* 2018;93(10):E345–E347.
16. Masese RV, Bulgin D, Douglas C, Shah N, Tanabe P. Barriers and facilitators to care for individuals with sickle cell disease in central North Carolina: The emergency department providers' perspective. *PLoS One.* 2019;14(5):e0216414.
17. Wang WC. Minireview: Prognostic factors and the response to hydroxurea treatment in sickle cell disease. *Exp Biol Med (Maywood).* 2016;241(7):730–736.
18. Mahmood LA, Reece-Stremtan S, Idiokitas R, et al. Acupuncture for pain management in children with sickle cell disease. *Complement Ther Med.* 2020;49:102287.
19. Thompson WE, Eriator I. Pain control in sickle cell disease patients: Use of complementary and alternative medicine. *Pain Med.* 2014; 15(2):241–246.
20. Sil S, Lai K, Lee JL, et al. Preliminary evaluation of the clinical implementation of cognitive-behavioral therapy for chronic pain management in pediatric sickle cell disease. *Complement Ther Med.* 2020;49:102348.
21. Adams RJ, McKie VC, Hsu L, et al. Prevention of a first stroke by transfusions in children with sickle cell anemia and abnormal results on transcranial Doppler ultrasonography. *N Engl J Med.* 1998;339(1):5–11.
22. Ohene-Frempong K, Weiner SJ, Sleeper LA, et al. Cerebrovascular accidents in sickle cell disease: Rates and risk factors. *Blood.* 1998;91(1):288–294.
23. Lawrence C, Webb J. Sickle cell disease and stroke: Diagnosis and management. *Curr Neurol Neurosci Rep.* 2016;16(3):27.
24. Schatz J, Brown RT, Pascual JM, Hsu L, DeBaun MR. Poor school and cognitive functioning with silent cerebral infarcts and sickle cell disease. *Neurology.* 2001;56(8):1109–1111.
25. Switzer JA, Hess DC, Nichols FT, Adams RJ. Pathophysiology and treatment of stroke in sickle-cell disease: Present and future. *Lancet Neurol.* 2006;5(6):501–512.
26. Hogan AM, Pit-ten Cate IM, Vargha-Khadem F, Prengler M, Kirkham FJ. Physiological correlates of intellectual function in children with sickle cell disease: Hypoxaemia, hyperaemia and brain infarction. *Dev Sci.* 2006;9(4):379–387.
27. Cober MP, Phelps SJ. Penicillin prophylaxis in children with sickle cell disease. *J Pediatr Pharmacol Ther.* 2010;15(3):152–159.
28. Hord J, Byrd R, Stowe L, Windsor B, Smith-Whitley K. Streptococcus pneumoniae sepsis and meningitis during the penicillin prophylaxis era in children with sickle cell disease. *J Pediatr Hematol Oncol.* 2002;24(6):470–472.
29. Gladwin MT, Vichinsky E. Pulmonary complications of sickle cell disease. *N Engl J Med.* 2008;359(21):2254–2265.
30. Vichinsky EP, Neumayr LD, Earles AN, et al. Causes and outcomes of the acute chest syndrome in sickle cell disease. National Acute Chest Syndrome Study Group. *N Engl J Med.* 2000;342(25):1855–1865.
31. Madani BM, Al Raddadi R, Al Jaouni S, Omer M, Al Awa MI. Quality of life among caregivers of sickle cell disease patients: A cross sectional study. *Health Qual Life Outcomes.* 2018;16(1):176.
32. Crosby LE, Joffe NE, Irwin MK, et al. School performance and disease interference in adolescents with sickle cell disease. *Phys Disabil.* 2015;34(1):14–30.

33. Lebensburger JD, Grosse SD, Altice JL, Thierry JM, Ivankova NV. Understanding and improving health education among first-time parents of infants with sickle cell anemia in Alabama: A mixed methods approach. *J Pediatr Hematol Oncol.* 2015;37(1):35–42.
34. Wong E. *Pediatric Transfusion: A Physicians Handbook.* 4th ed. AABB; 2015.
35. The National Heart, Lung and Blood Institute (NHLBI). *Evidence-Based Management of Sickle Cell Disease: Expert Panel Report.* US Department of Health and Human Services; 2014.
36. Ware RE, Schultz WH, Yovetich N, et al. Stroke With Transfusions Changing to Hydroxyurea (SWiTCH): A phase III randomized clinical trial for treatment of children with sickle cell anemia, stroke, and iron overload. *Pediatr Blood Cancer.* 2011;57(6):1011–1017.
37. Padmanabhan A, Connelly-Smith L, Aqui N, et al. Guidelines on the use of therapeutic apheresis in clinical practice: Evidence-based approach from the Writing Committee of the American Society for Apheresis: The eighth special issue. *J Clin Apher.* 2019;34(3):171–354.
38. Stanley HM, Friedman DF, Webb J, Kwiatkowski JL. Transfusional iron overload in a cohort of children with sickle cell disease: Impact of magnetic resonance imaging, transfusion method, and chelation. *Pediatr Blood Cancer.* 2016;63(8):1414–1418.
39. Ware RE, Davis BR, Schultz WH, et al. Hydroxycarbamide versus chronic transfusion for maintenance of transcranial doppler flow velocities in children with sickle cell anaemia-TCD With Transfusions Changing to Hydroxyurea (TWiTCH): A multicentre, open-label, phase 3, non-inferiority trial. *Lancet.* 2016;387(10019):661–670.
40. Centers for Disease Control and Prevention (CDC). National Healthcare Safety Network Biovigilance Component Hemovigilance Module Surveillance Protocol v2.5.2. 2018. https://www.cdc.gov/nhsn/pdfs/biovigilance/bv-hv-protocol-current.pdf
41. Geiger TL, Howard SC. Acetaminophen and diphenhydramine premedication for allergic and febrile nonhemolytic transfusion reactions: Good prophylaxis or bad practice? *Transfus Med Rev.* 2007;21(1):1–12.
42. Sanders RP, Maddirala SD, Geiger TL, et al. Premedication with acetaminophen or diphenhydramine for transfusion with leucoreduced blood products in children. *Br J Haematol.* 2005;130(5):781–787.
43. Charache S, Terrin ML, Moore RD, et al. Effect of hydroxyurea on the frequency of painful crises in sickle cell anemia. Investigators of the Multicenter Study of Hydroxyurea in Sickle Cell Anemia. *N Engl J Med.* 1995;332(20):1317–1322.
44. McGann PT, Ware RE. Hydroxyurea for sickle cell anemia: What have we learned and what questions still remain? *Curr Opin Hematol.* 2011;18(3):158–165.
45. Wang WC, Ware RE, Miller ST, et al. Hydroxycarbamide in very young children with sickle-cell anaemia: A multicentre, randomised, controlled trial (BABY HUG). *Lancet.* 2011;377(9778):1663–1672.
46. Steinbrook R. Erythropoietin, the FDA, and oncology. *N Engl J Med.* 2007;356(24):2448–2451.
47. Telen MJ. Principles and problems of transfusion in sickle cell disease. *Semin Hematol.* 2001;38(4):315–323.
48. Michon J. Incidence of anemia in pediatric cancer patients in Europe: Results of a large, international survey. *Med Pediatr Oncol.* 2002;39(4):448–450.
49. Gannon CJ, Napolitano LM. Severe anemia after gastrointestinal hemorrhage in a Jehovah's Witness: New treatment strategies. *Crit Care Med.* 2002;30(8):1893–1895.
50. Knuti KA, Amrein PC, Chabner BA, Lynch TJ, Jr., Penson RT. Faith, identity, and leukemia: When blood products are not an option. *Oncologist.* 2002;7(4):371–380.
51. Whitehead MT, Smitthimedhin A, Webb J, et al. Cerebral blood flow and marrow diffusion alterations in children with sickle cell anemia after bone marrow transplantation and transfusion. *AJNR Am J Neuroradiol.* 2018;39(11):2132–2139.
52. Walters MC, De Castro LM, Sullivan KM, et al. Indications and results of HLA-identical sibling hematopoietic cell transplantation for sickle cell disease. *Biol Blood Marrow Transplant.* 2016;22(2):207–211.
53. Gluckman E, Cappelli B, Bernaudin F, et al. Sickle cell disease: An international survey of results of HLA-identical sibling hematopoietic stem cell transplantation. *Blood.* 2017;129(11):1548–1556.
54. Stenger EO, Shenoy S, Krishnamurti L. How I treat sickle cell disease with hematopoietic cell transplantation. *Blood.* 2019;134(25):2249–2260.
55. Shenoy S, Gaziev J, Angelucci E, et al. Late effects screening guidelines after hematopoietic cell transplantation (HCT) for hemoglobinopathy: Consensus statement from the Second Pediatric Blood and Marrow Transplant Consortium International Conference on Late Effects after Pediatric HCT. *Biol Blood Marrow Transplant.* 2018;24(7):1313–1321.
56. Bernaudin F, Dalle JH, Bories D, et al. Long-term event-free survival, chimerism and fertility outcomes in 234 patients with sickle-cell anemia younger than 30 years after myeloablative conditioning and matched-sibling transplantation in France. *Haematologica.* 2020;105(1):91–101.
57. Shenoy S, Eapen M, Panepinto JA, et al. A trial of unrelated donor marrow transplantation for children with severe sickle cell disease. *Blood.* 2016;128(21):2561–2567.
58. Abraham A, Hsieh M, Eapen M, et al. Relationship between mixed donor-recipient chimerism and disease recurrence after hematopoietic cell transplantation for sickle cell disease. *Biol Blood Marrow Transplant.* 2017;23(12):2178–2183.
59. Fitzhugh CD, Cordes S, Taylor T, et al. At least 20% donor myeloid chimerism is necessary to reverse the sickle phenotype after allogeneic HSCT. *Blood.* 2017;130(17):1946–1948.
60. Hsieh M, Kang E, Fitzhugh C, et al. Allogeneic hematopoietic stem-cell transplantation for sickle cell disease. *N Engl J Med.* 2009;361(24):2309–2317.
61. Hsieh MM, Fitzhugh CD, Weitzel RP, et al. Nonmyeloablative HLA-matched sibling allogeneic hematopoietic stem cell transplantation for severe sickle cell phenotype. *JAMA.* 2014;312(1):48–56.
62. Saraf SL, Oh AL, Patel PR, et al. Nonmyeloablative stem cell transplantation with alemtuzumab/low-dose irradiation to cure and improve the quality of life of adults with sickle cell disease. *Biol Blood Marrow Transplant.* 2016;22(3):441–448.
63. Guilcher GMT, Monagel DA, Nettel-Aguirre A, et al. Nonmyeloablative matched sibling donor hematopoietic cell transplantation in children and adolescents with sickle cell disease. *Biol Blood Marrow Transplant.* 2019;25(6):1179–1186.
64. Magrin E, Miccio A, Cavazzana M. Lentiviral and genome-editing strategies for the treatment of beta-hemoglobinopathies. *Blood.* 2019;134(15):1203–1213.
65. Hoban MD, Lumaquin D, Kuo CY, et al. CRISPR/Cas9-mediated correction of the sickle mutation in human CD34+ cells. *Mol Ther.* 2016;24(9):1561–1569.
66. Anzalone AV, Randolph PB, Davis JR, et al. Search-and-replace genome editing without double-strand breaks or donor DNA. *Nature.* 2019;576(7785):149–157.
67. Czechowicz A, Palchaudhuri R, Scheck A, et al. Selective hematopoietic stem cell ablation using CD117-antibody-drug-conjugates enables safe and effective transplantation with immunity preservation. *Nat Commun.* 2019;10(1):617.
68. Meier ER, Dioguardi JV, Kamani N. Current attitudes of parents and patients toward hematopoietic stem cell transplantation for sickle cell anemia. *Pediatr Blood Cancer.* 2015;62(7):1277–1284.
69. Khemani K, Ross D, Sinha C, Haight A, Bakshi N, Krishnamurti L. Experiences and decision making in hematopoietic stem cell transplant in sickle cell disease: Patients' and caregivers' perspectives. *Biol Blood Marrow Transplant.* 2018;24(5):1041–1048.
70. McPherson M, Thaniel L, Minniti CP. Transition of patients with sickle cell disease from pediatric to adult care: Assessing patient readiness. *Pediatr Blood Cancer.* 2009;52(7):838–841.
71. Brousseau DC, Owens PL, Mosso AL, Panepinto JA, Steiner CA. Acute care utilization and rehospitalizations for sickle cell disease. *JAMA.* 2010;303(13):1288–1294.

72. Telfair J, Alexander LR, Loosier PS, Alleman-Velez PL, Simmons J. Providers' perspectives and beliefs regarding transition to adult care for adolescents with sickle cell disease. *J Health Care Poor Underserved.* 2004;15(3):443–461.
73. Kwandros E, Kwiatkowski JL. Beta thalassemia: Monitoring and new treatment approaches. *Hematol Oncol Clin North Am.* 2019;33(3): 339–353.
74. Shimamura A, Alter BP. Pathophysiology and management of inherited bone marrow failure syndromes. *Blood Rev.* 2010;24(3):101–122.
75. Camaschella C. Iron deficiency: New insights into diagnosis and treatment. *Hematology Am Soc Hematol Educ Program.* 2015;2015:8–13.
76. Hill A, Hill QA. Autoimmune hemolytic anemia. *Hematology Am Soc Hematol Educ Program.* 2018;2018(1):382–389.
77. Hill QA, Hill A, Berentsen S. Defining autoimmune hemolytic anemia: A systematic review of the terminology used for diagnosis and treatment. *Blood Adv.* 2019;3(12):1897–1906.
78. Ho G, Brunson A, Keegan THM, Wun T. Splenectomy and the incidence of venous thromboembolism and sepsis in patients with autoimmune hemolytic anemia. *Blood Cells Mol Dis.* 2019;81:102388.
79. Pakbaz Z, Treadwell M, Yamashita R, et al. Quality of life in patients with thalassemia intermedia compared to thalassemia major. *Ann N Y Acad Sci.* 2005;1054:457–461.
80. Telfer P, Constantinidou G, Andreou P, Christou S, Modell B, Angastiniotis M. Quality of life in thalassemia. *Ann N Y Acad Sci.* 2005;1054:273–282.
81. Delaney M. How I reduce the risk of missed irradiation transfusion events in children. *Transfusion.* 2018;58(11):2517–2521.
82. Jacquot C, Seo A, Miller PM, et al. Parental versus non-parental-directed donation: An 11-year experience of infectious disease testing at a pediatric tertiary care blood donor center. *Transfusion.* 2017;57(11):2799–2803.
83. Li C, Mathews V, Kim S, et al. Related and unrelated donor transplantation for beta-thalassemia major: Results of an international survey. *Blood Adv.* 2019;3(17):2562–2570.
84. Thompson AA, Walters MC, Kwiatkowski J, et al. Gene therapy in patients with transfusion-dependent beta-thalassemia. *N Engl J Med.* 2018;378(16):1479–1493.
85. Harrison C. First gene therapy for beta-thalassemia approved. *Nat Biotechnol.* 37 2019:1102–1103.
86. Mehta PA, Davies SM, Leemhuis T, et al. Radiation-free, alternative-donor HCT for Fanconi anemia patients: Results from a prospective multi-institutional study. *Blood.* 2017;129(16):2308–2315.
87. Nelson AS, Marsh RA, Myers KC, et al. A reduced-intensity conditioning regimen for patients with dyskeratosis congenita undergoing hematopoietic stem cell transplantation. *Biol Blood Marrow Transplant.* 2016;22(5):884–888.
88. Longerich S, Li J, Xiong Y, Sung P, Kupfer GM. Stress and DNA repair biology of the Fanconi anemia pathway. *Blood.* 2014;124(18): 2812–2819.
89. Rio P, Navarro S, Guenechea G, et al. Engraftment and in vivo proliferation advantage of gene-corrected mobilized CD34(+) cells from Fanconi anemia patients. *Blood.* 2017;130(13):1535–1542.
90. Rio P, Navarro S, Wang W, et al. Successful engraftment of gene-corrected hematopoietic stem cells in non-conditioned patients with Fanconi anemia. *Nat Med.* 2019;25(9):1396–1401.
91. National Hemophilia Foundation for All Bleeding Disorders. Hemophilia A. 2020. https://www.hemophilia.org/Bleeding-Disorders/Types-of-Bleeding-Disorders/Hemophilia-A
92. National Hemophilia Foundation for All Bleeding Disorders. History of bleeding disorders. 2020. https://www.hemophilia.org/Bleeding-Disorders/History-of-Bleeding-Disorders
93. Gringeri A. Factor VIII safety: Plasma-derived versus recombinant products. *Blood Transfus.* 2011;9(4):366–370.
94. Perkins HA, Busch MP. Transfusion-associated infections: 50 years of relentless challenges and remarkable progress. *Transfusion.* 2010;50(10):2080–2099.
95. Shapiro S, Makris M. Haemophilia and ageing. *Br J Haematol.* 2019;184(5):712–720.
96. Srivastava A, Brewer AK, Mauser-Bunschoten EP, et al. Guidelines for the management of hemophilia. *Haemophilia.* 2013;19(1):e1–47.
97. Auerswald G, Dolan G, Duffy A, et al. Pain and pain management in haemophilia. *Blood Coagul Fibrinolysis.* 2016;27(8):845–854.
98. Goto M, Takedani H, Nitta O, Kawama K. Joint function and arthropathy severity in patients with hemophilia. *J Jpn Phys Ther Assoc.* 2015;18(1):15–22.
99. Kessler CM. New perspectives in hemophilia treatment. *Hematology Am Soc Hematol Educ Program.* 2005:429–435.
100. Manco-Johnson MJ. Advances in the care and treatment of children with hemophilia. *Adv Pediatr.* 2010;57(1):287–294.
101. Young G. New challenges in hemophilia: Long-term outcomes and complications. *Hematology Am Soc Hematol Educ Program.* 2012;2012:362–368.
102. Holme PA, Tjonnfjord GE, Batorova A. Continuous infusion of coagulation factor concentrates during intensive treatment. *Haemophilia.* 2018;24(1):24–32.
103. Centers for Disease Control and Prevention (CDC). Inhibitors and hemophilia. 2019. https://www.cdc.gov/ncbddd/hemophilia/inhibitors.html
104. Nogami K, Shima M. New therapies using nonfactor products for patients with hemophilia and inhibitors. *Blood.* 2019;133(5):399–406.
105. Menegatti M, Peyvandi F. Treatment of rare factor deficiencies other than hemophilia. *Blood.* 2019;133(5):415–424.
106. Goodnough LT, Levy JH. The judicious use of recombinant Factor VIIa. *Semin Thromb Hemost.* 2016;42(2):125–132.
107. Perrin GQ, Herzog RW, Markusic DM. Update on clinical gene therapy for hemophilia. *Blood.* 2019;133(5):407–414.
108. Miesbach W, Meijer K, Coppens M, et al. Gene therapy with adeno-associated virus vector 5-human factor IX in adults with hemophilia B. *Blood.* 2018;131(9):1022–1031.
109. Lisowski L, Dane AP, Chu K, et al. Selection and evaluation of clinically relevant AAV variants in a xenograft liver model. *Nature.* 2014;506(7488):382–386.
110. Brand B, Dunn S, Kulkarni R. Challenges in the management of haemophilia on transition from adolescence to adulthood. *Eur J Haematol.* 2015;95 Suppl 81:30–35.
111. Geddis AE. Congenital amegakaryocytic thrombocytopenia and thrombocytopenia with absent radii. *Hematol Oncol Clin North Am.* 2009;23(2):321–331.
112. Nurden AT. Glanzmann thrombasthenia. *Orphanet J Rare Dis.* 2006;1:10.
113. Simon D, Kunicki T, Nugent D. Platelet function defects. *Haemophilia.* 2008;14(6):1240–1249.
114. Beck R, Sorge M, Schneider A, Dietz A. Current approaches to epistaxis treatment in primary and secondary care. *Dtsch Arztebl Int.* 2018;115(1-02):12–22.
115. Silva F, Morais S, Sevivas T, Veiga R, Salvado R, Taborda A. Severe intracranial haemorrhage in neonatal alloimmune thrombocytopenia. *BMJ Case Rep.* 2011;2011:bcr0720114563.
116. Borawski J, Rydzewski A, Mazerska M, Kalinowski M, Pawlak K, Mysliwiec M. Inverse relationships between haemoglobin and ristocetin-induced platelet aggregation in haemodialysis patients under erythropoietin therapy. *Nephrol Dial Transplant.* 1996;11(12):2444–2448.
117. de Wildt-Eggen J, Nauta S, Schrijver JG, van Marwijk Kooy M, Bins M, van Prooijen HC. Reactions and platelet increments after transfusion of platelet concentrates in plasma or an additive solution: A prospective, randomized study. *Transfusion.* 2000;40(4):398–403.
118. Tobian AA, Fuller AK, Uglik K, et al. The impact of platelet additive solution apheresis platelets on allergic transfusion reactions and corrected count increment (CME). *Transfusion.* 2014;54(6): 1523–1529; quiz 1522.
119. Patel RM, Josephson C. Neonatal and pediatric platelet transfusions: Current concepts and controversies. *Curr Opin Hematol.* 2019;26(6): 466–472.
120. Zotz RB, Poon MC, Di Minno G, D'Oiron R. Glanzmann thrombasthenia registry I. The international prospective Glanzmann

thrombasthenia registry: Pediatric treatment and outcomes. *TH Open.* 2019;3(3):e286–e294.

121. Cai J, Ribkoff J, Olson S, et al. The many roles of tranexamic acid: An overview of the clinical indications for TXA in medical and surgical patients. *Eur J Haematol.* 2020;104(2):79–87.
122. Lee A, Poon MC. Inherited platelet functional disorders: General principles and practical aspects of management. *Transfus Apher Sci.* 2018;57(4):494–501.
123. Connor P, Khair K, Liesner R, et al. Stem cell transplantation for children with Glanzmann thrombasthenia. *Br J Haematol.* 2008;140(5):568–571.
124. Monagle P, Cuello CA, Augustine C, et al. American Society of Hematology 2018 Guidelines for management of venous thromboembolism: Treatment of pediatric venous thromboembolism. *Blood Adv.* 2018;2(22):3292–3316.
125. Bates SM, Greer IA, Middeldorp S, Veenstra DL, Prabulos AM, Vandvik PO. VTE, thrombophilia, antithrombotic therapy, and pregnancy: Antithrombotic Therapy and Prevention of Thrombosis, 9th ed: American College of Chest Physicians Evidence-Based Clinical Practice Guidelines. *Chest.* 2012;141(2 Suppl):e691S–e736S.
126. Bates SM, Jaeschke R, Stevens SM, et al. Diagnosis of DVT: Antithrombotic Therapy and Prevention of Thrombosis, 9th ed: American College of Chest Physicians Evidence-Based Clinical Practice Guidelines. *Chest.* 2012;141(2 Suppl):e351S–e418S.
127. Betensky M, Goldenberg NA. Post-thrombotic syndrome in children. *Thromb Res.* 2018;164:129–135.
128. Goldenberg NA, Donadini MP, Kahn SR, et al. Post-thrombotic syndrome in children: A systematic review of frequency of occurrence, validity of outcome measures, and prognostic factors. *Haematologica.* 2010;95(11):1952–1959.
129. Male C, Lensing AWA, Palumbo JS, et al. Rivaroxaban compared with standard anticoagulants for the treatment of acute venous thromboembolism in children: A randomised, controlled, phase 3 trial. *Lancet Haematol.* 2020;7(1):e18–e27.
130. Watson L, Broderick C, Armon MP. Thrombolysis for acute deep vein thrombosis. *Cochrane Database Syst Rev.* 2016;11:CD002783.
131. Azirar S, Appelen D, Prins MH, Neumann MH, de Feiter AN, Kolbach DN. Compression therapy for treating post-thrombotic syndrome. *Cochrane Database Syst Rev.* 2019;9:CD004177.
132. Niihara Y, Miller ST, Kanter J, et al. A Phase 3 trial of l-glutamine in sickle cell disease. *N Engl J Med.* 2018;379(3):226–235.
133. Kutlar A, Kanter J, Liles DK, et al. Effect of crizanlizumab on pain crises in subgroups of patients with sickle cell disease: A SUSTAIN study analysis. *Am J Hematol.* 2019;94(1):55–61.
134. Vichinsky E, Hoppe CC, Ataga KI, et al. A Phase 3 randomized trial of voxelotor in sickle cell disease. *N Engl J Med.* 2019;381(6):509–519.
135. Gordeuk VR, Castro OL, Machado RF. Pathophysiology and treatment of pulmonary hypertension in sickle cell disease. *Blood.* 2016;127(7):820–828.
136. Galie N, Hoeper MM, Humbert M, et al. Guidelines for the diagnosis and treatment of pulmonary hypertension: The Task Force for the Diagnosis and Treatment of Pulmonary Hypertension of the European Society of Cardiology (ESC) and the European Respiratory Society (ERS), endorsed by the International Society of Heart and Lung Transplantation (ISHLT). *Eur Heart J.* 2009;30(20):2493–2537.
137. McKie KT, Hanevold CD, Hernandez C, Waller JL, Ortiz L, McKie KM. Prevalence, prevention, and treatment of microalbuminuria and proteinuria in children with sickle cell disease. *J Pediatr Hematol Oncol.* 2007;29(3):140–144.
138. Alvarez O, Lopez-Mitnik G, Zilleruelo G. Short-term follow-up of patients with sickle cell disease and albuminuria. *Pediatr Blood Cancer.* 2008;50(6):1236–1239.

35 PRIMARY AND ACQUIRED IMMUNE DEFICIENCY DISORDERS

WEI LI ADELINE KOAY, NATELLA RAKHMANINA, MEGAN WILKINS, SARAH MATTHEWS, AND AMI DOSHI

My son has died from AIDS.

NELSON MANDELA

An AIDS-free generation would mean that virtually no child is born with HIV; that, as those children grow up, their risk of becoming infected is far lower than it is today; and that those who become infected can access treatment to help prevent them from developing AIDS and from passing the virus on to others.

ANTHONY S. FAUCI

INTRODUCTION

This chapter describes the role of palliative care in improving the quality of life (QOL) of the immunosuppressed child and their family. Immunodeficiencies result from a failure of the immune system to function appropriately. Primary immunodeficiencies (PIDs) generally have genetic causes that disrupt the immune system, while secondary immunodeficiencies are acquired as a result of medications, malnutrition, infections (e.g., HIV), or other external factors. The major focus of this chapter is on lessons learned about caring for families of children, adolescents, and youth living with HIV (YLHIV), which serves as a prototype to address the wide range of problems encountered by children experiencing other immunodeficiencies and provides the reader with insight and skills to address areas of palliative care.

Immunodeficiencies caused by inherent defects in immunity affect up to 1 in 2,000 individuals in the United States,[1] and the 10-year survival after a PID diagnosis is 93.5% in one population-based cohort study.[2] More than 300 PIDs have been identified and are categorized into nine groups by the International Union of Immunological Societies (IUIS) PID expert committee according to their clinical and immunologic phenotypes (Table 35.1).[3,4] Survival of people living with PIDs has improved over the years with the advancement of medical research and novel treatment modalities, resulting in a growing population of individuals who live with a chronic medical condition that requires daily, complicated medical management, many of whom may benefit from palliative and end-of-life care programs.

Secondary or acquired immunodeficiencies (Table 35.2) are more common than primary immunodeficiencies[4,5] and have a broad spectrum of clinical presentation depending on the underlying etiology and the host susceptibility. The most common secondary immunodeficiency, HIV, affected approximately 2.8 million children and adolescents globally in 2018, with 14.9 million children under the age of 18 years estimated to have lost one or both parents to acquired immune deficiency syndrome (AIDS)-related causes.[6] Of the estimated 770,000 people who died of AIDS-related illnesses in 2018, approximately 15% of them were under 20 years of age.[6] Vertically (or perinatally) acquired HIV is transmitted from the mother to the child during pregnancy, delivery, or breastfeeding, while horizontally acquired HIV is transmitted via blood transfusions (extremely rare in the United States), intravenous (IV) drug use, or through sexual contact. The latter is particularly important among adolescents, who constitute a significant proportion of horizontally acquired HIV in the United States.[7] The scale-up of national preventive strategies, including universal prenatal HIV screening for pregnant women and replacing breastfeeding with formula feeding has resulted in a significant decrease in the number of perinatally HIV infected infants in the United States from approximately 1,630 in 1993 to 44 infants in 2016.[7,8] With early diagnosis and increased availability and use of antiretroviral therapy (ART), the mortality rate among children living with perinatally acquired HIV has reduced by up to tenfold compared to the period before ART became available.[9]

Children with PIDs are usually diagnosed at a younger age compared to children with secondary immunodeficiencies,

TABLE 35.1 Characteristics of primary immunodeficiencies

CATEGORY	EXAMPLES OF DISORDERS	INHERITANCE	SELECTED CLINICAL FEATURES	TREATMENT
Immunodeficiencies affecting cellular and humoral immunity	Severe combined immunodeficiency	XL	Severe infections, failure to thrive, rash, alopecia	Enzyme replacement, gene therapy, HSCT, immunoglobulin replacement, prophylactic antimicrobials
	Adenosine deaminase deficiency	AR	Cartilage abnormalities, deafness, cognitive defects	
Combined immunodeficiencies with associated syndrome features	Wiskott Aldrich syndrome	XL	Recurrent bacterial and viral infections, diarrhea, eczema, lymphoma	Gene therapy, symptomatic management
	CHARGE syndrome	AD	Coloboma, heart defect, choanal atresia, intellectual disability, genital and ear anomalies, varying degrees of immune defects	Surgical intervention, hormonal replacement, thymic transplantation (clinical trial)
Predominantly antibody deficiencies	X-linked agammaglobulinemia	XL	Recurrent infections, chronic enteroviral meningoencephalitis	Prophylactic antimicrobials, immunoglobulin replacement, immunosuppressants
	Common variable immunodeficiency	AD, no defect specified	Presents after 2 years of age, recurrent infections, granulomatous disease	
Diseases of immune dysregulation	IPEX (immunodeficiency, polyendocrinopathy, enteropathy, X-linked)	XL	Autoimmunity, cytopenias, bacterial infections, eczema, diabetes	Immunosuppressants, biological agents, immunization, prophylactic antimicrobials
	Autoimmune Lymphoproliferative syndrome (ALPS)	AD, AR	Chronic adenopathy, splenomegaly, lymphomas	
Congenital phagocytic defects	Shwachman-Diamond syndrome	AR	Pancytopenia, exocrine pancreatic insufficiency, chondrodysplasia	Prophylactic antimicrobials, interferon gamma infusion, G-CSF, HSCT (CGD), gene therapy
	Chronic granulomatous disease (CGD)	XL, AR	Severe and recurrent infections	
Defects in intrinsic and innate immunity	Anhidrotic ectodermal dysplasia	XL, AR, AD	Predisposition to invasive bacterial, parasitic, fungal and viral infections	HSCT, prophylactic antimicrobials, immunizations, immunoglobulin replacement
Autoinflammatory disorders	Familial Mediterranean fever	AR, AD	Abdominal pain, arthritis, recurrent fevers, vasculitis	Corticosteroids, immunosuppressants, biological agents, supportive
	Neonatal-onset multisystem inflammatory disease	AD	Neonatal onset rash, chronic meningitis, arthropathy, deafness	
Complement deficiencies	C5, C6, C7, C8a, C8b, C9 deficiency	AR, AD	Neisserial infection, recurrent pyogenic infections	Immunizations, prophylactic antimicrobials
Phenocopies of primary immunodeficiencies	ALPS-sFAS	Somatic mutations, autoantibodies	Presents later in life, hepatosplenomegaly, lymphadenopathy, autoimmunity, lymphoma	Immunosuppressants, immunoglobulin replacement

AD, autosomal dominant; ALPS, autoimmune lymphoproliferative syndrome; AR, autosomal recessive; CHARGE, coloboma, heart defects, atresia choanae, growth retardation, genital abnormalities, ear abnormalities; G-CSF, granulocyte colony-stimulating factor; HSCT, hematopoietic stem cell transplant; XL, X-linked; CGD, chronic granulomatous disease; IPEX, immnuodeficiency, polyendocrinopathy, enteropathy, X-linked.

Adapted with permission from Bousfiha A, Jeddane L, Picard C, et al. The 2017 IUIS phenotypic classification for primary immunodeficiencies. *J Clin Immunol.* 2018;38(1):129–143; and Raje N, Dinakar C. Overview of immunodeficiency disorders. *Immunol Allergy Clin North Am.* 2015;35(4):599–623.

TABLE 35.2 Characteristics of secondary immunodeficiencies

RELATED CAUSES OF SECONDARY IMMUNODEFICIENCIES	EXAMPLES
Medications	Immunosuppressants, corticosteroids
Procedures	Splenectomy, hematopoietic stem cell transplantation
Infections	HIV infection, cytomegalovirus, Epstein Barr virus
Metabolic conditions	Diabetes mellitus, uremia
Nutrition conditions	Malnutrition, vitamin deficiency
Protein losing conditions	Nephrotic syndrome
Hereditary/genetic conditions	Sickle cell disease, Trisomy 21
Miscellaneous conditions	Burns, malignancies, systemic lupus erythematosus

Adapted with permission from Chinen et al., 2010 and Raje et al., 2015.

with the exception of infants with perinatal HIV infection who are diagnosed during infancy. Compared to children living with HIV who receive effective ART, children with PIDs tend to have earlier mortality, are at constant risk for opportunistic infections, and require more high-risk treatment interventions. As children with mild immunodeficiencies are less likely to require palliative care, this chapter focuses on palliative care for children living with severe immunodeficiencies. We specifically focus on YLHIV, acknowledging that physiological and psychological changes during adolescence are known to negatively impact HIV treatment outcomes and QOL.

Clinical Vignette

Daniel was the oldest of his mother's children and was diagnosed with HIV as an infant, which was also when his mother learned of her own HIV status. She vigilantly brought him to his appointments and gave him medications for many years, but his medication adherence waned over time. Daniel had attention deficit hyperactivity disorder (ADHD) and reading difficulties as a child. His teenage years brought health concerns for his mother and also a struggle for independence for him. During this time, Daniel admitted to depressive symptoms, which were also in his family history and likely compounded by community violence and other environmental stressors. He worried about his mother's declining health and watched her suffer through HIV-related renal failure and her complaints about dialysis. His mother eventually died when he was 12. Daniel showed increasing signs of depression over time, including social isolation, increased sleep, and irritability. When he was diagnosed with declining renal function himself, Daniel expressed concern about needing dialysis. He underwent a kidney transplant at age 16 and was fairly adherent to his post-transplant medications initially, but eventually showed signs of poor adherence and rejection. Once he turned 18, he expressed a desire to discontinue medications and dialysis. After graduating high school, Daniel made plans to reconcile and reconnect with his biological father, who lived in a nearby state. It was there that he chose not to take his medications any longer. Ethical concerns arose given his age, ADHD, and depression. An ethics consultation confirmed that Daniel was aware this decision might lead to his death, and he expressed the desire to see his mother again, in heaven, which he believed would happen should he die. Daniel also expressed that living with significant medical interventions, including the total number of medications taken daily and dialysis, was too much. Daniel was engaged with the palliative care team, who supported him and his family at the end of his life, primarily with pain management and facilitation of his end-of-life decisions and wishes. Daniel died at age 19 due to HIV-related renal failure, leaving behind his maternal grandmother, who cared for him after his mother's death, and a younger brother, who was uninfected.

PHYSICAL ASPECTS OF CARE

Most children living with primary or secondary immunodeficiencies require lifelong treatment unless they have received curative treatments not available for the majority of these morbidities. As with all children, children with immunodeficiencies should receive routine immunizations, except for live vaccines in those with PIDs or AIDS. For all children and their household members, maintaining good hygiene is vital. However, children with immunodeficiencies should not be isolated or "kept in a bubble."

With the advent and success of ART, most YLHIV on treatment are surviving into adolescence and adulthood. An estimated 50,900 youth had HIV in the United States in 2016,[7] all of whom were recommended to take daily ART, ranging from single to multiple pills or multiple suspensions for young children. Adhering to ART can be challenging for caregivers, who often share the burden of the disease within the family, and for YLHIV who may not understand why they need to take medication or see their medical team regularly or who struggle with treatment fatigue or HIV-related stigma in their community. The US Department of Health and Human Services guidelines for care of YLHIV summarize recommendations for assessment and intervention strategies to support medication adherence.[10] These guidelines and other meta-analyses of medication adherence in YLHIV suggest that medical providers assume a nonjudgmental approach to care, an example of which is the use of motivational interviewing strategies.[11] Routine assessment of medication adherence is recommended and, in addition to measurement of viral load, should also include one other type of measurement (e.g., self-report, pharmacy pill count, or pharmacy refill history assessment). Strategies to support adherence should be discussed at the initiation of therapy and at every medical visit thereafter. These strategies can take the form of regimen-specific changes (e.g., regimen simplification, reduction of pill burden) that could be offered, individual and family-level interventions (e.g., directly observed therapy, behavioral modification strategies, mobile phone applications), or healthcare provider–level interventions (e.g., providing multidisciplinary care, a youth-friendly environment and nonjudgmental approaches to discussion).[10]

Even though the life expectancy of YLHIV with effective ART in the United States has improved, with a 10-year survival rate of 94%,[12] living with HIV has long-term consequences on multiple organ systems including neurologic, cardiac, metabolic, and renal. YLHIV are not only at risk for bacterial infections, psychiatric diagnoses, and pain, but they also experience more subjective distress compared to their uninfected peers, including facing stigma, a sense of hopelessness, preoccupation with their illness, poor body image, and social withdrawal.[13] Some chronic pain experienced by YLHIV is related to the side effects and toxicities of ART, which can cause abdominal discomfort, nausea, diarrhea, headaches, and neuropathy.[14] With the introduction of new antiretroviral (ARV) drug classes, many older ARV drugs that were associated with more common toxicities are no longer in use. Side effects such as nausea and diarrhea typically resolve after the first few weeks of ART but may require antiemetics or antidiarrheal agents for symptom management. Insomnia and vivid dreams associated with certain regimens (e.g., efavirenz-based) can be abated by taking the ARV at bedtime and on an empty stomach. YLHIV with persistent symptoms for months or severe ART-related side effects can usually be managed by switching the presumed causative ARV for another agent, using ARVs with different side-effect and toxicity profiles when possible, or using dose reduction.[10] Management strategies of ART-related side effects must be individualized for each child and in consultation with the primary team.

AIDS is the outcome of chronic HIV infection and a depletion of CD4 cells to levels below 200 cells/mcL or the presence of any "AIDS-defining" condition regardless of the CD4 cell count. AIDS can occur at a young age in children who have not received effective ART, either due to poor adherence to medications or a late diagnosis of HIV. AIDS-defining conditions include opportunistic infections and malignancies that occur as a result of immunosuppression.[15] Clinical manifestations of poorly controlled HIV/AIDS in children include recurrent bacterial infections, neuro-psychiatric manifestations, malnutrition, respiratory problems, developmental delays, and pain (Box 35.1). Living with AIDS adds another layer of complexity to the management of YLHIV who require antimicrobial prophylaxis or treatment for opportunistic infections in addition to ART, which equates to requiring more daily medications and worse QOL.

Some YLHIV who initiate ART can develop an immune reconstitution inflammatory syndrome (IRIS), which manifests as a worsening of an opportunistic infection or new signs or symptoms and diagnosis of a previously occult opportunistic infection. The symptoms and opportunistic infections seen in people with IRIS are similar to those seen in people with AIDS. Although the data on IRIS in children are limited, a study in the United Kingdom showed that IRIS was relatively rare in children but was associated with a higher mortality rate compared to those who did not have IRIS.[16] Given the potential impact of symptoms associated with HIV and complicating infections, pain and side effects associated with ART, and the psychological stress of adherence to these complex regimens on QOL for YLHIV,[14] palliative care needs to be integrated with disease-directed care throughout the course of illness to improve QOL.

BOX 35.1 CLINICAL MANIFESTATIONS OF HIV AND AIDS IN CHILDREN

- Failure to thrive
- Developmental delay
- Encephalopathy
- Chronic pain
- Generalized lymphadenopathy
- Persistent candidiasis or *Candida* esophagitis
- Recurrent or protracted diarrhea
- Hepatosplenomegaly
- Parotitis
- Interstitial pneumonitis
- Recurrent bacterial infections (e.g., pneumonia, chronic otitis media)
- *Pneumocystis jirovecii* pneumonia
- Recurrent viral infections (e.g., herpetic stomatitis, varicella/herpes zoster, condyloma, molluscum contagiosum, disseminated cytomegalovirus infection)

STRUCTURE AND PROCESSES OF PALLIATIVE CARE IN HIV

In the past two decades, the trajectory of HIV in the setting of ART has shifted toward that of a chronic, incurable disease.[17] Longer survival brings with it challenges of non–HIV-related illness, psychosocial impact, problems with medication adherence, and need for decision-making that were not present early in the course of HIV. The physical symptoms and psychosocial factors impacting YLHIV can be expected to endure, persist, and evolve over the course of their lifetime. YLHIV in many ways now embody the "gravely ill but long surviving" patients described as the typical patient base for pediatric palliative care.[18] Despite recommendations to integrate palliative care into care of patients with HIV and evidence suggesting that palliative care improves psychosocial and physical outcomes,[19,20] the improved survival with ART has drawn some focus away from palliative care in HIV.

The preferred model for pediatric palliative care is a blended model in which palliative care is integrated into the care of the child starting at the time of diagnosis of serious illness and throughout the illness, alongside restorative or curative care. HIV carries an uncertain prognosis and can make end of life difficult to predict. Minor health problems can potentially evolve into life-threatening events, and it is not uncommon for YLHIV to experience frequent life-threatening episodes. HIV may be considered a "life-threatening condition" in that it requires intensive life-long treatment aimed at maintaining QOL, and thus it is appropriate for palliative care to be part of the standard of care.[21] HIV is a multigenerational disease where the child and parent(s) may witness each other's death. Thus, HIV may invoke application of the entire spectrum of palliative care, from the perinatal period through bereavement support.

Regular assessment of goals of care is necessary for YLHIV,[17] and older adolescents should be prepared to manage their own healthcare when approaching adulthood. Even when pediatric patients are successfully transitioned to an adult HIV clinic, there is a significant drop in retention over the first several years of adult care.[22] Providers should strive for a comprehensive hand-off process to an adult HIV care team to ensure that the patient and family feel supported through this transition and to enhance retention in adult care.

Decision-making, advance care planning (ACP), and documentation of the youth's and parent's wishes are important aspects of palliative care to integrate throughout the course of illness. The vast majority of YLHIV wish to discuss end-of-life decision-making early in the course of their illness and prefer their doctor to initiate these discussions. Yet their parents are often unaware of these preferences, suggesting a need for better integration of palliative care.[21] Facilitating communication between adolescents and their parents on these complex subjects represents a crucial area for intervention by the interdisciplinary care team. With HIV treatment teams representing a medical home for YLHIV and their families, patients and families may prefer early goals of care discussion to include or be initiated by the HIV care team or the primary palliative care team. Primary palliative care is palliative care provided by clinicians who are not palliative care specialists.[23] All clinicians caring for seriously ill patients, such as those with HIV, should have the skill set to perform some aspects of palliative care, such as basic symptom management, routine goals of care discussion, and referral to specialty-level palliative care or hospice.

YLHIV are typically supported by interdisciplinary teams. In pediatrics, the standard model is a family-centered model of an interdisciplinary HIV team which includes physicians, nurses, social workers, and mental health professionals, typically coordinated by an infectious disease specialist. Nutritionists, developmental specialists, and case managers are important members of the HIV team.[17,24] Members of the HIV team may also include outreach coordinators and peer advocates. The HIV team will likely represent the front-line team supporting the child and family and be the provider of primary palliative care. As the HIV team will be highly engaged as the medical home for the YLHIV, they will provide significant psychosocial support and primary medical management of HIV.

Due to the inherent complexity of HIV, the palliative care team (Box 35.2) may be consulted to provide specialty-level palliative care. The success of HIV treatment and the resulting lower morbidity and mortality may mean that HIV clinicians today have less first-hand experience or comfort in providing specialty-level palliative care compared to the era of poorer prognosis. Specialty palliative care may be required in more complicated situations requiring complex symptom management or difficult decision-making.[23] The multigenerational nature of HIV, complex family dynamics, and potential substance abuse or other psychosocial concerns in caregivers all influence goals of care, decision-making processes, and grief in YLHIV. This creates situations in which the additional expertise of specialty palliative care can be beneficial. The palliative care team can provide assessment of complex pain and other non-pain symptoms[23] that may be underrecognized and can result from HIV, HIV treatment, and associated comorbid conditions. Given the importance of and challenges with medication adherence, the palliative care team may facilitate decision-making regarding ART and other potentially burdensome treatments and document these discussions. Reassessment of pain, QOL, and goals of care will be important throughout the illness given its unpredictable and evolving nature. It is imperative that the palliative care team keep hospital staff informed of the family's understanding of illness and goals of care on an ongoing basis.

Care for YLHIV requires frequent medical appointments, developmental services, and in-home care, and it is often marked by frequent periods of acute illness

BOX 35.2 INTERDISCIPLINARY PALLIATIVE CARE TEAM

- *Physicians* focus on the illness trajectory, prognosis, and medical treatments, making patient visits or providing supervision in collaboration with advanced practice registered nurses or physician assistants.
- *Nurses* provide direct patient care, serving as patient advocate, care coordinator, and educator. Nurses are at the center of the immediate assessment and reassessment of patient needs.
- *Advanced practice providers* (physician assistants and advanced practice registered nurses) expand the capacity to deliver complex care and provide direct care.
- *Social workers* attend to family dynamics, assess and support coping mechanisms and social determinants of health, identify and facilitate access to resources, and mediate conflicts. In HIV, this may also include multigenerational impact, counseling regarding social stigma, addressing substance abuse.
- *Chaplains*, as the spiritual care specialists, assess and address spiritual and existential issues and help to facilitate continuity with the patient's faith community as requested. Chaplains facilitate meaning-making and provide pre-bereavement support.
- *Clinical pharmacists* optimize medication management through a thorough review of the patient's medications to identify therapies to further palliate symptoms, resolve or prevent potential drug-related toxicities, recommend dose adjustment, and de-prescribe where appropriate. In HIV, pharmacists are important in creating appropriate ART regimens.
- *Mental health professionals* assess and address depression, anxiety, substance use, and other mental health conditions and how they impact on medical care.
- *Child life specialists* address the child's and siblings' experience at developmentally appropriate level, providing assessment intervention and education. May facilitate meaning-making and memory-making; they provide coping mechanisms, especially for peer interaction and self-esteem in YLHIV.

Adapted with permission from Ferrell BR, Twaddle ML, Melnick A, Meier DE. National Consensus Project Clinical Practice Guidelines for Quality Palliative Care Guidelines, 4th edition. *J Palliat Med.* 2018; 21(12):1684–1689.[27]

and decompensation. An essential function of the palliative care team is to provide care coordination for a more seamless, family-centered experience. Children with immunodeficiency syndromes require complex care from a multitude of providers to manage the acute, chronic, and recurrent problems imposed by their underlying disorders. The presence of multiple existing clinical teams with competing priorities can create fragmentation and hamper effective communication. Improvement in the QOL for the child and family depends on the ability of interdisciplinary palliative care teams to collaborate with clinicians and subspecialists, schools, and community resources.

As with all palliative care, palliative care for YLHIV can be provided in all care settings: home, hospital, ambulatory, skilled nursing and assisted living facilities, and hospice. The goal is to provide palliative care in the setting that is preferred by and available to the child and family. Data in adults living with HIV suggest that embedding palliative care into the existing outpatient care of patients with HIV, via clinical training, teamwork, and availability of medications, favorably impacted on pain and symptom control and may represent a model for others to adopt.[25,26]

DEVELOPMENTAL CONSIDERATIONS

Children's experience with HIV, their understanding of their condition, and their sources of psychological and spiritual distress evolve as they grow older. Special attention needs to be paid to the developmental stage of YLHIV in providing palliative care and initiating discussions of understanding the illness, goals of care, and coping. The team should determine the child or adolescent's developmental status and parental preferences for communication with the child repeatedly throughout the trajectory of care, tailoring the assessment and intervention as developmentally appropriate.[27] Barriers to ART adherence change with age and developmental stage, ranging from palatability and tolerance of formulations in young children to social stigma and other concerns in adolescence. Understanding age-specific barriers is essential in creating strategies to promote adherence, which ultimately impacts QOL and mortality. Similarly, recommendations for disclosure of diagnosis also must account for the child's developmental stage, acknowledging that the need for and response to disclosure may differ significantly between young children and adolescents.[28]

CARE FOR THE MEDICAL TEAM

Clinicians caring for YLHIV are reported to experience difficulty caring for these patients and their families. Common healthcare provider challenges include inadequate palliative care training, inadequate resources for symptom management, difficulty watching suffering from symptoms, a need to share feelings of distress, feelings of helplessness, and suggestions of burnout, among other factors.[29,30] Similarly, surveys of palliative medicine practitioners also indicate significant risk of burnout, particularly of emotional exhaustion.[31,32] Assessment of burnout and compassion fatigue should be conducted in palliative care and other clinicians caring for YLHIV and children with other immunodeficiencies. Strategies to address distress or promote well-being in clinicians could include peer support groups, multidisciplinary team meetings, palliative care rounds, creation of sustainable models of care, systematic opportunities to debrief after crises, and staff training and education.[33]

PSYCHOLOGICAL AND PSYCHIATRIC ASPECTS OF CARE

The cognitive and behavioral functioning of YLHIV is heavily impacted by the environmental conditions in which youth develop. YLHIV in the United States are at high risk for living in poverty,[34] which is associated with experiencing marginalization, community violence, suboptimal educational experiences, family instability, and other stressful life events. The negative impact of poverty and stressful life events on cognitive and mental health functioning has been well-documented for youth in general and for YLHIV.[35,36] A host of other issues can affect the behavioral and cognitive functioning of YLHIV, including social stigma, which is a complex social phenomenon that can include devaluation and stereotyping of an individual and is related to lower social support, increased risk for mental health symptoms, and poorer physical health in people with HIV.[37–39] Given the number of risk factors often present for YLHIV, stigma can be intersectional, sourcing from the youth's primary medical diagnosis, their sexual or gender identity, race, or socioeconomic status, and it can contribute to increased risk for mental health diagnoses such as major depressive disorder and posttraumatic stress disorder (PTSD).

Historically, youth born with HIV were at risk for cognitive impairment due to viral impact on neurological functioning. This profound cognitive impairment observed was most often thought to be related to the presence of encephalopathy. More subtle impacts on cognitive functioning have been observed as advances in HIV treatment and detection have occurred, including executive functioning deficits, regardless of treatment patterns and medication adherence.[40,41] Specifically, a pattern of slower processing speed and working memory deficits has been reported.[42] On academic measures, YLHIV have not been found to perform lower than their uninfected counterparts on most measures, with the exception of youth with a history of encephalopathy and related profound cognitive impact, who perform significantly below the expected range for their age.[43] Among those with horizontally acquired HIV, cognitive impact has been reported, but treatment has not been shown to improve functioning over time.[41] Youth may be at risk for academic struggle and thus exhibit less educational and vocational success than their age peers. However, research on decisional capacity among YLHIV with documented cognitive deficits supports the idea that most YLHIV have the decisional capacity to participate meaningfully in their palliative care and healthcare, including at the end of life, despite possible deficits in intellectual and/or adaptive skills.[44]

YLHIV are at higher risk for psychiatric diagnoses, including anxiety disorders, mood disorders (e.g., depressive disorders), and ADHD.[45] When compared to youth exposed to but uninfected with HIV, rates of mental health disorders are similar,[46] suggesting environmental or other factors aside from HIV as contributing factors. While HIV status has not been strongly associated with mental health conditions,[46] the impact of mental health disorders on the treatment of HIV has been well-established. Depressive symptoms have been linked to poorer adherence and health outcomes.[47,48] Youth with mental health concerns may also be more likely to engage in risky sexual behaviors and less likely to disclose their illness status to partners.[49,50] Substance use, known to be more prevalent among youth with mental health conditions, may lead to decreased adherence to medication and HIV medical treatment. Compounded by increased risk for homelessness, trauma history, and marginalization due to sexuality, youth with horizontally acquired HIV have shown higher rates of substance use compared to their same-aged peers[49] and confer similar risks to their perinatally infected counterparts, including lower medication adherence rates and increased likelihood for engagement in risky sexual behaviors. Mental health disorders are underidentified and undertreated in this population, likely impacted by mental health stigma and the lower economic conditions already discussed. Providers need to be vigilant in screening for common mental health conditions, as well as for substance use and abuse, and refer appropriately to mental health providers for management when primary providers are unable to manage independently.

SOCIAL ASPECTS OF CARE

Stigma and discrimination are prevalent drivers of health outcomes for YLHIV and occur more frequently than in other health categories. Compared to people living with cancer, those living with HIV report more experiences of internalized shame, lower self-esteem, stigma including social rejection, social isolation, and financial insecurity associated with possible workplace discrimination.[51] YLHIV may experience stigma based on their HIV diagnosis, sexuality, mental health condition(s), race, or other personal characteristics. Youth experience of stigma is often chronic, additive, and far-reaching in nature. Stigma impacts social, romantic, familial, and vocational aspects of their lives. Stigma influences youth decision to disclose their diagnosis, a uniquely personal decision. Youth may fear the negative impact disclosure will have on relationships, possibly burdening these youth with secrecy and emotional distance in social relationships. Furthermore, nondisclosure also negatively impacts on youth's receipt of social support. Unintentional disclosure of diagnosis occurs when someone other than the youth themselves discloses their HIV diagnosis without their permission, thus impacting on the youth's trust in others significantly. Providers should explicitly assure that all those present in the treatment room have awareness of the diagnosis through personal and private conversation with the identified patient and should communicate clearly about youth and family disclosure status when referring to outside medical providers.

Another unique social feature for YLHIV is an increased risk for parental loss or serious parental illness. This risk is related to the route of infection and multigenerational impact of HIV in families and communities. The impact of parental loss on child functioning is well-documented and includes further risk of mental health diagnoses and other psychosocial difficulties,[52,53] as well as risk for increased viral load.[54] As a result of this illness and/or death, youth may have more experience with death and the end-of-life experience. Youth may view their own HIV differently following the loss of a parent who has died from the same disease—losing hope regarding their own prognosis or shifting motivation to improve medication adherence to avoid worsening symptoms themselves. YLHIV who have lost their parents may also be less likely to have social support during treatment, including near the end of life. Youth with horizontally acquired HIV are at risk for low social support (given the aforementioned low disclosure rates due to stigma) and higher rates of marginalization from family due to sexuality or gender identity.[55]

CULTURAL, SPIRITUAL, RELIGIOUS AND EXISTENTIAL ASPECTS OF CARE

CULTURAL, SPIRITUAL AND RELIGIOUS ASPECTS OF CARE

People living with primary and secondary immunodeficiencies come from diverse ethnic and cultural backgrounds, requiring the healthcare provider to take into account their patients' particular cultures. Learning about a patient's cultural beliefs and values allows the provider to be better equipped at helping the family and friends of their patients to adjust to end-of-life care and also improves the quality of medical care provided. For instance, it may be inappropriate and culturally insensitive in some cultures to discuss impending death, while some other cultures may express grief related to dying more openly. Culture, religion, and spirituality have a strong influence on decisions made by patients and their families and should be considered as part of the child's care. From a pain management standpoint, this can be particularly challenging as some cultures do not accept or encourage the use of opioids, which are commonly used for pain relief.[56]

Comprehensive palliative care for YLHIV requires attention to the spiritual domain through screening for spiritual or religious needs and identifying sources of support.[27] Indeed, YLHIV want their healthcare providers to inquire about their spirituality, especially in situations facing dying or chronic illness.[57] Literature suggests that spirituality in YLHIV, as in other chronic illnesses, may correlate with decreased depression and anxiety and improved QOL.[58] Positive spiritual coping appears to have a buffering effect against depression and poor coping strategies,[59] which may in turn impact adherence. No direct correlation between spirituality and adherence to ART has been shown,[60] although one study demonstrates that adolescents viewing HIV as a punishment demonstrated lower medication adherence.[61] Religiousness has also been associated with higher likelihood of a higher symptom burden, especially pain,[62] with the underlying reason being unclear. Meaning making is a key dimension of spirituality and fosters resilience. Throughout the course of the illness, YLHIV may carry a variety of beliefs surrounding their illness in an attempt to make meaning, including feeling "God's presence," feeling abandoned or punished by God, and being part of a larger force.[57,58] Clinicians should consider engaging a pastoral care provider for interested children and families to further explore and address their spiritual needs.

RESILIENCE IN END-OF-LIFE CARE

YLHIV demonstrate many patterns of resilience that are associated with better mental health and disease-specific outcomes. Coping mechanisms are an important factor in combatting HIV-related stressors and more generalized environmental stressors.[63] Coping self-efficacy, or the belief one has the ability to cope with a stressor, has been found to relate to resilience and decreased depressive symptoms.[64] Other factors that impact on youth resilience include self-esteem, perseverance, and positive parent–child relationships (e.g., active involvement and communication).[63,65] Similarly, social support from other adults in the life of youth reduces the risk of behavioral issues and increases coping efficacy.[66,67]

CARE OF REFUGEES, IMMIGRANTS, AND CHILDREN WHO ARE ADOPTED

A growing population of children living with HIV in the United States is comprised of immigrants, refugees, and internationally adopted children. According to the United States Department of Homeland Security, a refugee is a person who is unable to return to their home country due to "persecution or a well-founded fear of persecution on account of race, religion, nationality, membership in a particular social group, or political opinion."[68] In 2017, more than 53,000 refugees were resettled in the United States, with children making up 46% of that number.[69] International adoptions by American families totaled just over 4,000 in 2018.[70] Some of the refugees and adopted children entering the United States each year are YLHIV, although data are not available regarding the exact percentage. Modes of transmission other than perinatal (i.e., blood transfusions, sexual abuse, substance abuse, transactional sex) may be more common in YLHIV born in other countries.[71,72] Furthermore, international adoptees have been found to suffer from comorbidities that are relatively rare in the US pediatric population, including tuberculosis, hepatitis, and congenital syphilis.[73] One study of HIV-infected international adoptees and refugees in foster care in the United States identified unique healthcare needs of this population, with many of these children experiencing stunting, gastrointestinal disease including parasitic infections and diarrhea, and mental health or behavioral problems.[74] Another study of YLHIV found that refugee children are less likely to have virologic suppression than non-refugee children.[75] Overall, children born in other countries may be diagnosed less promptly and have less access to healthcare resources, resulting in more comorbidities, opportunistic infections, and drug resistance.

YLHIV born in other countries also face unique psychosocial and cultural aspects of their illness. Refugees have endured trauma which forced them to flee their home country, putting them at risk for PTSD and other trauma-related disorders. Immigrants from other countries may have unique cultural views of HIV and medical and spiritual care and face language barriers and culture shock from being immersed in an entirely new system.

The following reflection demonstrates the challenges faced by a family who immigrated to the United States and the psychosocial issues that the adolescent faced after learning of her diagnosis.

Clinical Vignette

Donisha and her mother immigrated to the United States when she was 4 years old. Donisha had recurrent ear infections, which led to the development of bacterial endocarditis requiring an artificial heart valve at 6 years of age. During this time, Donisha tested positive for HIV. Her mother had tested negative for HIV in her home country and later learned that she was positive and had most likely passed the virus to her daughter. No one else knew of their HIV diagnosis at the time, and both mother and daughter did well initially with ART. However, Donisha's mother passed away suddenly due to AIDS. Following her mother's death, Donisha's maternal grandmother brought her to clinic because of a clinic letter reminding her of a missed appointment. Until then, her grandmother did not know that Donisha and her mother had been living with HIV. The grandmother was overwhelmed and struggled with coping with the loss of her daughter and taking care of Donisha, so home nursing was arranged to assist her with Donisha's care. Donisha had difficulty tolerating her HIV medications; she developed several complications and required feedings through a gastric tube at night. She gradually became overweight and developed obesity, but her HIV was relatively well controlled over the years. Her grandmother died in a car accident when Donisha was 15 years old. Donisha then had her third caregiver—her 72-year-old grandfather. He was warm and caring, but also struggled to support her. Gradually, Donisha's obesity and depression became more prominent. She did not attend weight clinic or any fitness or diet programs recommended and arranged by her providers. She also refused to take any antidepressants or anticoagulants required for her artificial heart valve. At age 19 years, she had a boyfriend and kept her HIV a secret from him. She started smoking marijuana on a daily basis. Her immune status continued to worsen, and her lifestyle became increasingly sedentary. Through her HIV care team, she has begun to attend cooking classes where she met several young people living with HIV. During her meeting with her psychologist, she agreed to attend a peer support group, where transportation and food were provided. That experience has helped her to cope better with her HIV and comorbidities. She has an undetectable viral load for the first time in many years on treatment. What will happen to this young woman in the future? Will she find support in her partner? Will she be able to battle her substance use and depression? Or will she regress to being nonadherent to her medications? It is hard to know the future, but this young woman will continue to require support to stay on track. And that support must go well beyond the walls of the clinic into her community, home, and peer environment.

ETHICAL AND LEGAL ASPECTS OF CARE

Care of the YLHIV includes unique ethical and legal considerations. Many of these are intertwined with the particular social, cultural, and psychological aspects of this illness. Of specific note are confidentiality and privacy, disclosure of HIV status, the duty to warn controversy, transition to independent decision-making, and ethical issues regarding choosing to stop treatment. Legal confidentiality is complex for YLHIV. Generally speaking, parents and guardians have the right to give informed consent for medical care of their minor children. However, there are several exceptions to this rule which pertain to the healthcare of children. The first exception is emancipated minors, in which the parental right to the child has been renounced. The second is mature minors, who are deemed by the physician to have the maturity required to make independent decisions, typically in a situation where parental involvement is problematic. The third exception applies to certain categories of care, often including family planning, abortion, pregnancy, and delivery care, and care for sexually transmitted infections. Under these exceptions, many YLHIV have the right to their own health information and care decisions.[76]

The process of the disclosure of HIV status to a child is a controversial subject. Opinions regarding when to disclose HIV status often differ between healthcare providers and parents. Unlike disclosing a cancer or other life-threatening disease, disclosure of a child's HIV diagnosis often leads to disclosure of other family secrets, such as parent's HIV status, paternity, and parental sexual history or history of substance abuse.[77] Parents' decision to disclose is affected by their fears of the effect on their child's emotional state, but also fear of child anger toward a parent and social consequences for the child, including stigma and isolation.[77] There is a complex interplay between the ethical principles of autonomy, beneficence, nonmaleficence, and justice. For example, the principle of autonomy might argue that a child living with HIV has a right to know his or her diagnosis or that the parent has a right to decide. Beneficence might argue that the child deserves the positive effects of disclosure, such as empowerment, whereas nonmaleficence might argue that a child with HIV should be protected from negative effects of disclosure, such as psychological burden. The principle of justice might argue in favor of disclosure for public health reasons to protect potential partners.[78]

The American Academy of Pediatrics recommends that all adolescents need to know their HIV status and that disclosure should be considered for school-aged children as soon as it is developmentally appropriate.[79] However, there is limited guidance regarding when and how to disclose. For many parents, disclosure may be a fluid process that changes over time rather than a single divulgence. Some parents may opt for partial disclosure at a young age, telling their child something about their illness but not naming it and then progressing to full disclosure at an older age. Pressure to disclose builds as children approach adolescence, which carries unique risks of experimentation with sexual behavior and drug use, risk of transmission, and nonadherence that may result in drug resistance.[78] A conceptual framework of the disclosure process describes five steps:

1. *Information gathering and trust building*, characterized by the establishment and maintenance of a trust-based working relationship between the caregiver and the healthcare professional.
2. *Education*, beginning with initial assessments of caregivers and child knowledge and attitudes (including cultural and religious beliefs) and continuing through a gradual full disclosure to the child. This may take weeks to years.
3. *Determining when the time is right for disclosure*, a process that must include changes in the child's health status, parental health or relationships, and perhaps the initiation of experimental, risky, or more burdensome treatments.
4. *The actual disclosure event*, which may be accomplished by the caregiver in the presence of the healthcare professional.
5. *Monitoring post-disclosure coping* and disclosure-related bumps in the road, such as direct or indirect observations of behavior, school performance, and peer relationships and facilitating acceptance and adjustment with behavioral health professionals' consultation as needed.[28]

Many caregivers fear that disclosure will cause greater suffering for children living with HIV; however, evidence has not shown negative effects. In fact, some studies show that disclosure may help children cope with their illness. Furthermore, disclosure does not seem to decrease adherence as many caregivers fear. Benefits of disclosure include opportunity for open communication, patient involvement in care decisions, increased peer support, and increased trust in healthcare providers and caregivers.[80] Disclosure should be viewed as an ongoing process which takes the child's developmental stage and cultural needs into account. Trust and collaboration between healthcare providers, HIV-infected children, and their caregivers should be established to support adherence through the process of disclosure.[80]

Because HIV is a communicable and serious illness, this creates controversy regarding the "duty to warn" those who are at risk of being exposed. In 1969, Tatiana Tarasoff was murdered by a young man who had recently informed his psychologist of his plan to kill her. Neither Tarasoff nor her family received any warning of the threat. The court ultimately found that mental health providers were liable for failure to warn potential victims of their patients.[81] There is no consensus over whether this court ruling should be extrapolated to a Tarasoff-like "duty to warn" for healthcare providers of HIV-infected patients. Some states have laws where healthcare workers are permitted to warn sexual partners who are likely to have been exposed by a person living with HIV,[78] but it is controversial if they should do so. One approach is to work with YLHIV who exposed others by referring them to a partner notification program.

The decision to stop ART poses another ethical issue pertaining to care of YLHIV. Adolescents may take ART inconsistently due to perception of low life expectancy, treatment fatigue, fear of disclosure of their HIV status, mental health issues, and substance abuse.[82] Pediatric and adolescent HIV providers should provide a safe and nonjudgmental space for their patients to be candid about adherence. For some adolescents who are intentionally not taking ART consistently, shared decision-making regarding a planned temporary break in treatment may be an appropriate risk-reduction strategy to prevent drug resistance.

CARE OF THE PATIENT NEARING THE END OF LIFE

Issues specific to YLHIV at end of life include ACP, the transgenerational and psychosocial aspects of HIV manifesting at end of life, symptom management in final days, and complex grief and bereavement needs. In one study, 90% of YLHIV rate "being able to complete an advance directive to let loved ones know my wishes" as very important, however only 8% had completed an advance directive.[21] The vast majority of teenagers want their family to be involved in decisions about end-of-life care,[83] yet YLHIV have difficulty finding healthcare surrogates.[63] Adolescents are consistent in rating the importance of dying a natural death (77%) and being off machines that extend life, such as life support (71%).[21] Teenagers rate the following as somewhat to very important: being physically comfortable, being free from pain, being at peace spiritually, not being a burden to loved ones, knowing how to say goodbye, and having a sense of their own worth or value.[83] The use of trained staff to implement a structured interview discussion with YLHIV and their families using the Lyon Family Centered ACP survey, an adapted form of the Respecting Choices ACP interview and the Five Wishes advance directive document, was shown to increase congruence in end-of-life treatment preferences between adolescents and their surrogate decision-makers.[84] In addition to helping surrogate decision-makers honor their loved one's wishes, congruence in end-of-life treatment preference is also associated with fewer HIV-specific symptoms in YLHIV.[63]

Like other youth nearing end of life, YLHIV benefit from building a legacy and making memories. Care team members can assist caregivers with making key arrangements and deciding on location of death before the YLHIV is actively dying. Some adolescents may want to be involved in their own funeral arrangements. Pastoral care may provide valuable support to the child and family's spiritual welfare at end of life, if this is desired. Patients and their families should also have the opportunity to say goodbye in a way that is consistent with their cultural and spiritual practices. Most YLHIV think it is important to say everything they want to say to their family if they were dying and also to know how to say goodbye.[21]

The familial nature of HIV complicates a child's perspective on approaching end of life. Approaching one's own end of life may be triggering for a child who has memories of their family member dying in a similar manner. Similarly, YLHIV may have a support system in which friends or partners are also affected by the disease. Thus, they may witness loved ones in their community go through illness and end of life. Data are lacking on how these experiences affect YLHIV at end of life, but it is reasonable to suspect that these events complicate the child's grief and coping.

Despite the previous findings that most adolescents prefer a natural and pain-free death, only 3% of pediatric HIV patients die on hospice or have a do-not-resuscitate (DNR) order in place.[85] One study found that only 25% of the children who died of AIDS died at home, with the remainder dying in the hospital. The children who died in the intensive care unit underwent more invasive treatments over prolonged periods of time, were separated from their loved ones, and experienced more pain and suffering than those who died at home.[86] These trends show a need for both primary and specialty palliative care involvement in this population.

Comprehensive symptom management in the child's final days and hours is of paramount importance to effective palliative care. One study of YLHIV found that 71% feared dying painfully.[21] Worldwide, many children unfortunately die with uncontrolled symptoms. In one South African study, half of children with terminal AIDS received no analgesia, resulting in respiratory symptoms and painful skin conditions at the end of life.[87] The United States is fortunate to have greater access to opioids and other medications for comfort. A Malawian study of hospitalized children with HIV/AIDS found the most common presenting symptoms to be cough (30%), diarrhea (25%), pain (23%), mouth sores (22%), poor feeding (19%), fever (15%), and vomiting (15%). The most common site of pain was the abdomen. The most frequently appreciated clinical signs included wasting in 66%, oral candida in 38%, and skin rash in 30%.[88] Children with HIV/AIDS typically present with a larger variety of symptoms than those with cancer or other diagnoses, reflecting the effects of HIV/AIDS on multiple organ systems.[89]

During the child's final days and hours of life, the goal should be focused on providing a comfortable and pain-free death. Any interventions which cause discomfort should be discontinued. Pain should be frequently reassessed and vigorously managed. The World Health Organization provides a widely accepted pharmacologic approach to relieving pain in a stepwise ladder of treatment, escalating from mild analgesics up to gradually more potent opioids.[90] The pain caused by mouth sores may be addressed with various preparations of orally swished analgesics. Fever may be controlled with antipyretics. Diarrhea may be treated with antidiarrheals given that the child is near death and the benefits of increased comfort from reduced stool frequency and abdominal cramping likely outweigh the risks of antimotility. Soothing topical agents may be considered for relief of skin irritation. Decisions relating to the continuation of ART must balance the benefits against side effects and ultimate futility. It may be appropriate to stop ART in the final days to weeks of life if it is deemed that the regimen is contributing to toxicity and pill burden without providing further benefit. Most often it is appropriate to continue antibiotic prophylaxis against opportunistic infections as many of these infections carry significant morbidity.[91]

The unique challenges of HIV persist through the bereavement phase. Survivors may feel shame, rage, and fear and are more likely to be affected by stigmatization and multiple losses than with other illnesses. Survivors may also be affected by "disenfranchised grief," or grief that is not acknowledged by society.[92] Bereavement is complicated by the transgenerational nature of HIV as well as by the psychosocial issues discussed previously, such as resource limitations. In cases where parents with HIV have died and a child is in foster care, this separation from the family unit further complicates the grieving process. Bereavement support is a critical component of palliative care, both for the caregivers/family and for the care team.

PALLIATIVE CARE CONSIDERATIONS FOR SEVERE COMBINED IMMUNODEFICIENCY

Having a PID places children at risk for infections, autoimmune disorders, gastrointestinal disorders, malignancies, and hypersensitivities. They may face recurrent hospitalization, challenging symptoms, and difficult decision-making. Children with severe combined immunodeficiency (SCID) or other severe PIDs, especially those in which transplant is a consideration, should be referred to palliative care.[93] Children diagnosed with SCID require life-long immune globulin (IG) replacement and antimicrobial prophylaxis to prevent infections. The route of IG administration (i.e., subcutaneous vs. intravenous) has been found to play an important role in QOL of patients with PID. Compared to intravenous IG, children on subcutaneous IG miss fewer days of school,[94] spend fewer days in the hospital,[95] and have increased self-rated health.[96] Subcutaneous and home IG therapy should be made available for children with PIDs.

The only form of cure for SCID is hematopoietic stem cell transplantation (HSCT), which carries risks such as graft failure, secondary infections, and recurrent hospitalizations and is not guaranteed to be successful. Goals of care discussions can inform decision-making around HSCT and involving the palliative care team may help address parental hesitancies around HSCT. The palliative care team can also address symptoms associated with HSCT and its potential complications, particularly when not responding to first-line treatment. Involving an ethics committee may be necessary in cases where parents have declined a HSCT.[97] There has been minimal investigation of neuropsychological functioning in youth with PIDs. With the improving survival rate for those undergoing HSCT, it is important to monitor neurocognitive functioning post-HSCT, especially in those with other premorbid risk factors, such as youth from lower socioeconomic status and those with specific genetic defects (e.g., ADA deficiency[98]).

CONCLUSION

This chapter describes the complexities of palliative care when supporting a child living with primary or secondary immunodeficiencies. While the physical aspects of medical care are an important component of palliative care, they are part of a bigger picture which includes psychological, social, ethical, and cultural aspects of a patient's life. This chapter not only highlights the importance of family-centered care (see the Family Reflection), but also the need to educate healthcare providers across disciplines on how to manage the prognostic uncertainty of severe immunodeficiencies and the need to work as an interdisciplinary team when caring for children, adolescents, and families with life-threatening illnesses.

Family Reflection

A Parent's Perspective

My daughter was diagnosed with HIV at the age of 9 years. My daughter was always very small, but I was afraid to get tested myself and to test her. When they told me she had the virus, I did not want to believe it. Then they told me I must be positive as well, so I got tested. Then I knew that both of us had HIV. I did not want both of us to start taking medicines. I did not believe the doctors. When we tried to take the medicine, they only made us sick, so we skipped most of them and rarely went to the clinic. Then my daughter started getting sick. She first had chicken pox, but it ended badly and she became blind. Then she got some infection in her belly and needed to take many antibiotics, which made her deaf. Six months later she had a stroke and got paralyzed. Once I saw her laying in bed and they told me she will never walk, hear, or see, I got scared. I started taking my HIV medicines, as HIV and AIDS became a reality in our lives. I also did not want her to die. I refused palliative care again and again and again.

Two years passed, and she never went home. I finally agreed to let her go. She was the most beautiful girl, my daughter. I still see her in my dreams. She saved my life, but I did not save hers.

REFERENCES

1. Kobrynski L, Powell RW, Bowen S. Prevalence and morbidity of primary immunodeficiency diseases, United States 2001-2007. *J Clin Immunol.* 2014;34(8):954–961.
2. Joshi AY, Iyer VN, Hagan JB, St Sauver JL, Boyce TG. Incidence and temporal trends of primary immunodeficiency: A population-based cohort study. *Mayo Clin Proc.* 2009;84(1):16–22.
3. Bousfiha A, Jeddane L, Picard C, et al. The 2017 IUIS Phenotypic Classification for Primary Immunodeficiencies. *J Clin Immunol.* 2018;38(1):129–143.
4. Raje N, Dinakar C. Overview of immunodeficiency disorders. *Immunol Allergy Clin North Am.* 2015;35(4):599–623.
5. Chinen J, Shearer WT. Secondary immunodeficiencies, including HIV infection. *J Allergy Clin Immunol.* 2010;125(2 Suppl 2):S195–203.
6. UNICEF. Global and Regional Trends. 2019. https://data.unicef.org/topic/hivaids/global-regional-trends/
7. Centers for Disease Control and Prevention. Monitoring selected national HIV prevention and care objectives by using HIV surveillance data: United States and 6 dependent areas, 2017. *HIV Surveillance Supplemental Report.* 2018;29(3):1–74.
8. Davis SF, Byers RH, Jr., Lindegren ML, Caldwell MB, Karon JM, Gwinn M. Prevalence and incidence of vertically acquired HIV infection in the United States. *JAMA.* 1995;274(12):952–955.
9. Davies MA, Gibb D, Turkova A. Survival of HIV-1 vertically infected children. *Curr Opin HIV AIDS.* 2016;11(5):455–464.
10. Panel on Antiretroviral Therapy and Medical Management of Children Living with HIV. Guidelines for the use of antiretroviral agents in pediatric HIV infection. 2021. Updated April 7, 2021. https://clinicalinfo.hiv.gov/sites/default/files/guidelines/documents/PedARV_GL.pdf
11. Miller WR, Rollnick S. *Motivational Interviewing: Helping People Change.* Guilford; 2013.
12. Kapogiannis BG, Soe MM, Nesheim SR, et al. Mortality trends in the US Perinatal AIDS Collaborative Transmission Study (1986–2004). *Clin Infect Dis.* 2011;53(10):1024–1034.
13. Brown LK, Lourie KJ, Pao M. Children and adolescents living with HIV and AIDS: A review. *J Child Psychol Psychiatry.* 2000;41(1):81–96.
14. Barlow-Mosha L, Musiime V, Davies MA, et al. Universal antiretroviral therapy for HIV-infected children: A review of the benefits and risks to consider during implementation. *J Int AIDS Soc.* 2017;20(1):21552.
15. Centers for Disease Control and Prevention. Appendix A: AIDS-defining conditions. *MMRW Morb Mortal Wkly Rep.* 2008 Dec 5;57:RR10.
16. Gkentzi D, Tebruegge M, Tudor-Williams G, et al. Incidence, spectrum and outcome of immune reconstitution syndrome in HIV-infected children after initiation of antiretroviral therapy. *Pediatr Infect Dis J.* 2014;33(9):953–958.
17. Workgroup on Palliative and End-of-Life Care in HIV/AIDS. *Integrating Palliative Care into the Continuum of HIV Care: An Agenda for Change.* University of Montana; 2004.
18. Feudtner C, Kang TI, Hexem KR, et al. Pediatric palliative care patients: A prospective multicenter cohort study. *Pediatrics.* 2011;127(6):1094–1101.
19. Ahmed AA. *The Impact of Palliative Care on Health Status in HIV-Positive Children:* College of Health Sciences, Public Health Epidemiology, Walden University; 2017.
20. Carter BS, Oleske J, Friebert SE. Integrating Palliative Care into HIV Care and Treatment. In Carter BS, Levetown M, eds. *Palliative Care for Infants, Children and Adolescents: A Practical Handbook.* 2nd ed. Johns Hopkins University Press; 2011:465–487.
21. Lyon ME, Dallas RH, Garvie PA, et al. Paediatric advance care planning survey: A cross-sectional examination of congruence and discordance between adolescents with HIV/AIDS and their families. *BMJ Support Palliat Care.* 2019;9(1):e22.
22. Hussen SA, Chakraborty R, Knezevic A, et al. Transitioning young adults from paediatric to adult care and the HIV care continuum in Atlanta, Georgia, USA: A retrospective cohort study. *J Int AIDS Soc.* 2017;20(1):21848.
23. Quill TE, Abernethy AP. Generalist plus specialist palliative care--creating a more sustainable model. *N Engl J Med.* 2013;368(13):1173–1175.
24. Rivera DM, Frye RE. Pediatric HIV Infection. 2019. https://emedicine.medscape.com/article/965086-overview
25. Harding R, Simms V, Alexander C, et al. Can palliative care integrated within HIV outpatient settings improve pain and symptom control in a low-income country? A prospective, longitudinal, controlled intervention evaluation. *AIDS Care.* 2013;25(7):795–804.
26. Perry BA, Westfall AO, Molony E, et al. Characteristics of an ambulatory palliative care clinic for HIV-infected patients. *J Palliat Med.* 2013;16(8):934–937.
27. Ferrell BR, Twaddle ML, Melnick A, Meier DE. National Consensus Project Clinical Practice Guidelines for Quality Palliative Care Guidelines, 4th edition. *J Palliat Med.* 2018;21(12):1684–1689.
28. Gerson AC, Joyner M, Fosarelli P, et al. Disclosure of HIV diagnosis to children: When, where, why, and how. *J Pediatr Health Care.* 2001;15(4):161–167.
29. Amery JM, Rose CJ, Holmes J, Nguyen J, Byarugaba C. The beginnings of children's palliative care in Africa: Evaluation of a children's palliative care service in Africa. *J Palliat Med.* 2009;12(11):1015–1021.
30. Richter L, Chandan U, Rochat T. Improving hospital care for young children in the context of HIV/AIDS and poverty. *J Child Health Care.* 2009;13(3):198–211.
31. Back AL, Steinhauser KE, Kamal AH, Jackson VA. Building resilience for palliative care clinicians: An approach to burnout prevention based on individual skills and workplace factors. *J Pain Symptom Manage.* 2016;52(2):284–291.
32. Kamal AH, Bull JH, Wolf SP, et al. Prevalence and Predictors of Burnout among Hospice and Palliative Care Clinicians in the US. *J Pain Symptom Manage.* 2020;59(5):e6–e13.
33. Rushton CH, Reder E, Hall B, Comello K, Sellers DE, Hutton N. Interdisciplinary interventions to improve pediatric palliative care and reduce health care professional suffering. *J Palliat Med.* 2006;9(4):922–933.
34. UNAIDS. UNAIDS report on the global AIDS epidemic. 2012. http://www.unaids.org/en/media/unaids/contentassets/documents/epidemiology/2012/gr2012/20121120_UNAIDS_Global_Report_2012_en.pdf
35. Kang E, Mellins CA, Dolezal C, Elkington KS, Abrams EJ. Disadvantaged neighborhood influences on depression and anxiety in youth with perinatally acquired human immunodeficiency virus: How life stressors matter. *J Community Psychol.* 2011;39(8):956–971.
36. Mani A, Mullainathan S, Shafir E, Zhao J. Response to comment on "Poverty impedes cognitive function." *Science.* 2013;342(6163):1169.
37. Logie C, Gadalla TM. Meta-analysis of health and demographic correlates of stigma towards people living with HIV. *AIDS Care.* 2009;21(6):742–753.
38. Sherr L, Clucas C, Harding R, Sibley E, Catalan J. HIV and depression—a systematic review of interventions. *Psychol Health Med.* 2011;16(5):493–527.
39. Tanney MR, Naar-King S, MacDonnel K. Adolescent Trials Network for HIV/AIDS Interventions 004 Protocol Team. Depression and stigma in high-risk youth living with HIV: A multi-site study. *J Pediatr Health Care.* 2012;26(4):300–305.
40. Nichols SL, Bethel J, Garvie PA, et al. Neurocognitive functioning in antiretroviral therapy-naive youth with behaviorally acquired human immunodeficiency virus. *J Adolesc Health.* 2013;53(6):763–771.

41. Nichols SL, Bethel J, Kapogiannis BG, et al. Antiretroviral treatment initiation does not differentially alter neurocognitive functioning over time in youth with behaviorally acquired HIV. *J Neurovirol.* 2016;22(2):218–230.
42. Phillips N, Amos T, Kuo C, et al. HIV-Associated cognitive impairment in perinatally infected children: A meta-analysis. *Pediatrics.* 2016;138(5).
43. Garvie PA, Zeldow B, Malee K, et al. Discordance of cognitive and academic achievement outcomes in youth with perinatal HIV exposure. *Pediatr Infect Dis J.* 2014;33(9):e232–238.
44. Chenneville T, Sibille K, Lujan-Zilbermann J, Rodriguez C, Brown M, Emmanuel P. Medical decisional capacity among children with HIV. *AIDS Care.* 2010;22(11):1359–1366.
45. Mellins CA, Malee KM. Understanding the mental health of youth living with perinatal HIV infection: Lessons learned and current challenges. *J Int AIDS Soc.* 2013;16:18593.
46. Mellins CA, Elkington KS, Leu CS, et al. Prevalence and change in psychiatric disorders among perinatally HIV-infected and HIV-exposed youth. *AIDS Care.* 2012;24(8):953–962.
47. Carrico AW, Bangsberg DR, Weiser SD, Chartier M, Dilworth SE, Riley ED. Psychiatric correlates of HAART utilization and viral load among HIV-positive impoverished persons. *AIDS.* 2011;25(8):1113–1118.
48. Hosek SG, Harper GW, Domanico R. Predictors of medication adherence among HIV-infected youth. *Psychol Health Med.* 2005;10(2):166–179.
49. Gamarel KE, Brown L, Kahler CW, et al. Prevalence and correlates of substance use among youth living with HIV in clinical settings. *Drug Alcohol Depend.* 2016;169:11–18.
50. Lehrer JA, Shrier LA, Gortmaker S, Buka S. Depressive symptoms as a longitudinal predictor of sexual risk behaviors among US middle and high school students. *Pediatrics.* 2006;118(1):189–200.
51. Fife BL, Wright ER. The dimensionality of stigma: A comparison of its impact on the self of persons with HIV/AIDS and cancer. *J Health Soc Behav.* 2000;41(1):50–67.
52. Kranzler EM, Shaffer D, Wasserman G, Davies M. Early childhood bereavement *J Am Acad Child Adolesc Psychiatry.* 1990;29(4):513–520.
53. Rutter M. *Children of Sick Parents. An Environmental and Psychiatric Study.* Oxford University Press; 1966.
54. Elliott-DeSorbo DK, Martin S, Wolters PL. Stressful life events and their relationship to psychological and medical functioning in children and adolescents with HIV infection. *J Acquir Immune Defic Syndr.* 2009;52(3):364–370.
55. Lyon ME, Garvie PA, Briggs L, et al. Is it safe? Talking to teens with HIV/AIDS about death and dying: A 3-month evaluation of Family Centered Advance Care (FACE) planning—anxiety, depression, quality of life. *HIV AIDS (Auckl).* 2010;2:27–37.
56. Khosla N, Washington KT, Regunath H. Perspectives of health care providers on US South Asians' attitudes toward pain management at end of life. *Am J Hosp Palliat Care.* 2016;33(9):849–857.
57. Bernstein K, D'Angelo LJ, Lyon ME. An exploratory study of HIV+ adolescents' spirituality: Will you pray with me? *J Relig Health.* 2013;52(4):1253–1266.
58. Lyon ME, Garvie P, He J, Malow R, McCarter R, D'Angelo LJ. Spiritual well-being among HIV-infected adolescents and their families. *J Relig Health.* 2014;53(3):637–653.
59. Reynolds N, Mrug S, Hensler M, Guion K, Madan-Swain A. Spiritual coping and adjustment in adolescents with chronic illness: A 2-year prospective study. *J Pediatr Psychol.* 2014;39(5):542–551.
60. Gaines J, Cheng Y, Wang J, Lyon M. Does spirituality or religion hinder or help adherence to highly active antiretroviral therapy among adolescents living with HIV? *J Adolesc Health.* 2014;54:S59–S60.
61. Lyon ME, Garvie PA, Kao E, et al. Spirituality in HIV-infected adolescents and their families: FAmily CEntered (FACE) Advance Care Planning and medication adherence. *J Adolesc Health.* 2011;48(6):633–636.
62. Lyon ME, Garvie PA, D'Angelo LJ, et al. Advance care planning and HIV symptoms in adolescence. *Pediatrics.* 2018;142(5).
63. Betancourt TS, Meyers-Ohki SE, Charrow A, Hansen N. Annual Research Review: Mental health and resilience in HIV/AIDS-affected children: A review of the literature and recommendations for future research. *J Child Psychol Psychiatry.* 2013;54(4):423–444.
64. Murphy DA, Marelich WD. Resiliency in young children whose mothers are living with HIV/AIDS. *AIDS Care.* 2008;20(3):284–291.
65. Malee KM, Tassiopoulos K, Huo Y, et al. Mental health functioning among children and adolescents with perinatal HIV infection and perinatal HIV exposure. *AIDS Care.* 2011;23(12):1533–1544.
66. Battles HB, Wiener LS. From adolescence through young adulthood: Psychosocial adjustment associated with long-term survival of HIV. *J Adolesc Health.* 2002;30(3):161–168.
67. Orban LA, Stein R, Koenig LJ, et al. Coping strategies of adolescents living with HIV: Disease-specific stressors and responses. *AIDS Care.* 2010;22(4):420–430.
68. United States Department of Homeland Security. Refugees and Asylees. 2019. Updated November 2019. https://www.dhs.gov/immigration-statistics/refugees-asylees
69. United States Department of Homeland Security. Yearbook of Immigration Statistics 2017. 2019. Updated September 2019. https://www.dhs.gov/immigration-statistics/yearbook/2017
70. United States Department of State Bureau of Consular Affairs. Adoption statistics. 2019. Updated March 2019. https://travel.state.gov/content/travel/en/Intercountry-Adoption/adopt_ref/adoption-statistics1.html
71. Goldwater PN. Iatrogenic blood-borne viral infections in refugee children from war and transition zones. *Emerg Infect Dis.* 2013;19(6).
72. Martino SC, Tucker JS, Ryan G, Wenzel SL, Golinelli D, Munjas B. Increased substance use and risky sexual behavior among migratory homeless youth: Exploring the role of social network composition. *J Youth Adolesc.* 2011;40(12):1634–1648.
73. Staat MA. Infectious disease issues in internationally adopted children. *Pediatr Infect Dis J.* 2002;21(3):257–258.
74. Wolf ER, Beste S, Barr E, et al. Health outcomes of international HIV-infected adoptees in the US. *Pediatr Infect Dis J.* 2016;35(4):422–427.
75. Rogo T, DeLong AK, Chan P, Kantor R. Antiretroviral treatment failure, drug resistance, and subtype diversity in the only pediatric HIV clinic in Rhode Island. *Clin Infect Dis.* 2015;60(9):1426–1435.
76. Summers D, Alpert I, Rousseau-Pierre T, et al. An exploration of the ethical, legal and developmental issues in the care of an adolescent patient. *Mt Sinai J Med.* 2006;73(3):592–595.
77. Wiener L, Mellins CA, Marhefka S, Battles HB. Disclosure of an HIV diagnosis to children: History, current research, and future directions. *J Dev Behav Pediatr.* 2007;28(2):155–166.
78. Klitzman R, Marhefka S, Mellins C, Wiener L. Ethical issues concerning disclosures of HIV diagnoses to perinatally infected children and adolescents. *J Clin Ethics.* 2008;19(1):31–42.
79. American Academy of Pediatrics. Disclosure of illness status to children and adolescents with HIV infection. American Academy of Pediatrics Committee on Pediatrics AIDS. *Pediatrics.* 1999;103(1):164–166.
80. Nichols J, Steinmetz A, Paintsil E. Impact of HIV-status disclosure on adherence to antiretroviral therapy among HIV-infected children in resource-limited settings: A systematic review. *AIDS Behav.* 2017;21(1):59–69.
81. Tarasoff v. Regents of the University of California. 17 *Cal 3d* 425 [131 *Cal. Rptr.* 14, 551 *P.2d* 334].1976:429–464.
82. Yang E, Mphele S, Moshashane N, et al. Distinctive barriers to antiretroviral therapy adherence among non-adherent adolescents living with HIV in Botswana. *AIDS Care.* 2018;30(2):224–231.
83. Garvie PA, He J, Wang J, D'Angelo LJ, Lyon ME. An exploratory survey of end-of-life attitudes, beliefs, and experiences of adolescents with HIV/AIDS and their families. *J Pain Symptom Manage.* 2012;44(3):373–385 e329.
84. Lyon ME, D'Angelo LJ, Dallas RH, et al. A randomized clinical trial of adolescents with HIV/AIDS: Pediatric advance care planning. *AIDS Care.* 2017;29(10):1287–1296.

85. Lyon ME, Williams PL, Woods ER, et al. Do-not-resuscitate orders and/or hospice care, psychological health, and quality of life among children/adolescents with acquired immune deficiency syndrome. *J Palliat Med.* 2008;11(3):459–469.
86. Oleske JM, Czarniecki L. Continuum of palliative care: Lessons from caring for children infected with HIV-1. *Lancet.* 1999;354(9186):1287–1291.
87. Henley LD. End of life care in HIV-infected children who died in hospital. *Dev World Bioeth.* 2002;2(1):38–54.
88. Lavy V. Presenting symptoms and signs in children referred for palliative care in Malawi. *Palliat Med.* 2007;21(4):333–339.
89. Demmer C. Children and infectious diseases. In Balk D, Corr C, eds. *Children's Encounters with Death Bereavement and Coping.* Springer Publishing Company; 2010:131–146.
90. Michelson KN, Steinhorn DM. Pediatric end-of-life issues and palliative care. *Clin Pediatr Emerg Med.* 2007;8(3):212–219.
91. Carter BS, Oleske J, Czarniecki L, Grubman S. The child with HIV infection. In Carter BS, Levetown M, eds. *Palliative Care for Infants, Children and Adolescents: A Practical Handbook.* Johns Hopkins University Press; 2004:332–347.
92. Doka KJ. *Disenfranchised Grief: Recognizing Hidden Sorrow.* Lexington Books; 1989.
93. Friebert SE, Osenga K. Pediatric palliative care referral criteria. Center to Advance Palliative Care. 2019. Updated February 3, 2019. https://www.capc.org/toolkits/designing-a-pediatric-palliative-care-program/
94. Lingman-Framme J, Fasth A. Subcutaneous immunoglobulin for primary and secondary immunodeficiencies: An evidence-based review. *Drugs.* 2013;73(12):1307–1319.
95. Vultaggio A, Azzari C, Milito C, Finocchi A, Toppino C, Spadaro G, Trizzino A, Baldassarre M, Paganelli R, Moschese V, Soresina A, Matucci A. Subcutaneous immunoglobulin replacement therapy in patients with primary immunodeficiency in routine clinical practice: The VISPO Prospective Multicenter Study. *Clin Drug Investig.* 2015;35(3):179–185.
96. Gardulf A, Björvell H, Gustafson R, Hammarstrom L, Smith CI. The life situations of patients with primary antibody deficiency untreated or treated with subcutaneous gammaglobulin infusions. *Clin Exp Immunol.* 1993;92:200–204.
97. Nickels AS, Myers D, Johnson L, Joshi A, Sharp RR, Lantos JD. Can parents refuse a potentially lifesaving transplant for severe combined immunodeficiency? *Pediatrics.* 2016;138(1):e20160892.
98. Shah AJ, Kohn DB. Neurocognitive function of patients with severe combined immunodeficiency. *Immunol Allergy Clin North Am.* 2010;30(1):143–151.

INDEX

Note: Tables, figures, and boxes are indicated by *t*, *f*, and *b* following the page number. Italic page numbers indicate "Family Reflection," "Team Reflection," or "Clinical Vignette."

H

N

O

S

X

Y

Z